Microbial Control

of

Insects and Mites

Microbial Control
of
Insects and Mites

Edited by

H. D. BURGES
Pest Infestation Control Laboratory, Slough, Bucks, England

N. W. HUSSEY
Glasshouse Crops Research Institute, Agricultural Research Council, Littlehampton, Sussex, England

1971

ACADEMIC PRESS LONDON • NEW YORK

ACADEMIC PRESS INC. (LONDON) LTD
Berkeley Square House
Berkeley Square
London, W1X 6BA

U.S. Edition published by
ACADEMIC PRESS INC.
111 Fifth Avenue
New York, New York 10003

Library of Congress Catalog Card Number: 79-117132
Standard Book Number: 12-143350-1

Printed in Great Britain by
The Whitefriars Press Ltd., London and Tonbridge

to

Professor E. A. Steinhaus

in admiration of his illustrious services to

Invertebrate Pathology

Contributors

K. AIZAWA Institute of Biological Control, Faculty of Agriculture, Kyushu University, Fukuoka, Japan

T. A. ANGUS Insect Pathology Research Institute, Canada Department of Fisheries and Forestry, Sault Ste Marie, Ontario, Canada

L. BAILEY Rothamsted Experimental Station, Harpenden, Herts, England

G. BENZ Department of Entomology, Swiss Federal Institute of Technology, Zurich, Switzerland

R. P. M. BOND Shell Research Limited, Milstead Laboratory of Chemical Enzymology, Sittingbourne, Kent, England

C. B. C. BOYCE Shell Research Limited, Milstead Laboratory of Chemical Enzymology, Sittingbourne, Kent, England

J. D. BRIGGS Invertebrate Pathology Laboratory, Faculty of Entomology, The Ohio State University, Columbus, Ohio, U.S.A.

A. BURGERJON Station de Recherches de Lutte Biologique et de Biocoenotique, I.N.R.A., La Minière par Versailles, France

H. D. BURGES Pest Infestation Control Laboratory, Agricultural Research Council, Slough, Buckinghamshire, England

K. E. COOKSEY Division of Functional Biology, Rosenstiel School of Marine and Atmospheric Sciences, University of Miami, Virginia Key, Miami, Florida, U.S.A.

H. T. DULMAGE Entomology Research Division, Agricultural Research Service, U.S. Department of Agriculture, Brownsville, Texas, U.S.A.

L. A. FALCON Division of Entomology, University of California, Berkeley, California, U.S.A.

J. M. FRANZ Biologische Bundesanstalt für Land- und Forstwirtschaft, Institut für Biologische Schädlingsbekämpfung, Darmstadt, Germany

L. P. S. VAN DER GEEST Laboratory of Applied Entomology, University of Amsterdam, The Netherlands

P. GRISON Station de Recherches de Lutte Biologique et de Biocoenotique, I.N.R.A., La Minière par Versailles, France

M. GUSTAFSSON Värdsätravägen, Uppsala, Sweden

A. M. HEIMPEL United States Department of Agriculture, Agricultural Research Service, Entomology Research Division, Beltsville, Maryland, U.S.A.

T. J. HELMS Department of Entomology, University of Nebraska, Lincoln, Nebraska, U.S.A.

W. F. HINK Faculty of Entomology, Ohio State University, Columbus, Ohio, U.S.A.

N. W. HUSSEY Glasshouse Crops Research Institute, Littlehampton, Sussex, England

C. M. IGNOFFO International Minerals and Chemical Corporation, Libertyville, Illinois, U.S.A.

A. KRIEG Biologische Bundesanstalt für Land- und Forstwirtschaft, Institut für Biologische Schädlingsbekämpfung, Darmstadt, Germany

M. KUČERA Department of Insect Pathology, Institute of Entomology, Czechoslovak Academy of Sciences, Prague, Czechoslovakia

P. A. VAN DER LAAN Laboratory of Applied Entomology, University of Amsterdam, The Netherlands

M. LAIRD Memorial University of Newfoundland, St. John's, Newfoundland, Canada

J. J. LIPA Laboratory of Biological Control, Institute of Plant Protection, Poznań, Poland

A. E. LUND Texas Forest Products Laboratory, Lufkin, Texas, U.S.A.

P. LUTHY Canada Department of Fisheries and Forestry, Sault Ste. Marie, Ontario, Canada

O. LYSENKO Department of Insect Pathology, Institute of Entomology, Czechoslovak Academy of Sciences, Prague, Czechoslovakia

R. E. McLAUGHLIN Boll Weevil Research Laboratory, U.S. Department of Agriculture, Entomology Research Division, State College, Mississippi, U.S.A.

D. MARTOURET Station de Recherches de Lutte Biologique et de Biocoenotique, I.N.R.A., La Minière par Versailles, France

J. R. NORRIS Shell Research Ltd., Milstead Laboratory of Chemical Enzymology, Sittingbourne, Kent, England

G. O. POINAR, JR. Department of Entomology and Parasitology, University of California, Berkeley, California, U.S.A.

E. S. RAUN Department of Entomology, University of Nebraska, Lincoln, Nebraska, U.S.A.

R. A. RHODES U.S. Department of Agriculture, Northern Utilization Research and Development Division, Peoria, Illinois, U.S.A.

D. W. ROBERTS Boyce Thompson Institute for Plant Research, Yonkers, New York, U.S.A.

M. H. ROGOFF International Minerals and Chemical Corporation, Libertyville, Illinois, U.S.A.

T. R. SHIEH International Minerals and Chemical Corporation, Libertyville, Illinois, U.S.A.

G. R. STAIRS Faculty of Entomology, The Ohio State University, Columbus, Ohio, U.S.A.

E. A. STEINHAUS‡ Formerly at Centre for Pathobiology, University of California, Irvine, California, U.S.A.

E. M. THOMSON Pest Infestation Control Laboratory, Agricultural Research Council, Slough, Buckinghamshire, England

J. WEISER Laboratory of Insect Pathology, Institute of Entomology, Czechoslovak Academy of Sciences, Prague, Czechoslovakia

W. G. YENDOL Pennsylvania State University, University Park, Pennsylvania, U.S.A.

‡ Deceased.

Preface

Control of insects and mites faces on the one hand mounting concern about environmental pollution by poisons, and on the other, resistance of pests to pesticides. Consequently, alternatives to chemical control are being urgently sought. Among the most interesting are arthropod diseases. The study of these diseases has expanded rapidly in recent years, revealing their potential for control. This book is intended to assess the current knowledge, achievements and future prospects for this mode of control.

Attention is concentrated on the practical aspects of Insect Pathology, delving into fundamentals only when they are of potential practical significance. Two authors could hardly hope to treat authoritatively such a wide subject—embracing as it does most branches of microbiology, entomology, and acarology, with implications for the chemist, biochemist and ecologist. We have, therefore, brought together the expertise of many disciplines by eliciting the help of 41 authors, mostly practicing specialists, from 11 countries. We owe them thanks for their hard work and splendid co-operation.

We have attempted to cater for a wide audience, ranging from those concerned with practical insect control and general entomology to insect pathologists with detailed interests requiring a reference source. More general readers can obtain an insight into the subject from the introductory and concluding chapters. These cover not only present achievements and future prospects, but also suggestions for research and development, which we hope will not go unnoticed by those responsible for formulating and financing future work. For the more specialist readers the subject is divided into topics; some general, other narrower. The appendixes list sources of further information and training, and indicate centres willing to supply insects, micro-organisms and special materials—a list requested at an international meeting in Wageningen in 1966. Efforts have been made to cover unpublished research and to look to the future. It is hoped that the volume will become a handbook for the practical insect pathologist and so serve as a catalyst to the present momentum of the subject.

We wish to thank Misses S. D. Lole, E. M. Thomson, J. A. Hurst and S. A. Burges, Mr. R. Kelsall and M. J. Burges, and Mrs. S. M. Burges, who helped to check manuscripts and proofs; Misses I. K. Travis and S. F. Vahrman, who made the subject index; also editors' and contributors' families for patiently suffering preoccupation of their menfolk.

January, 1971

H. D. Burges
N. W. Hussey

Contents

8. Use of Nematodes for Microbial Control of Insects

9. Micro-organisms as Sources of New Insecticidal Chemicals: Toxins

10. The Protein Crystal Toxin of *Bacillus thuringiensis*: Biosynthesis and Physical Structure

CHAPTER 1

Introduction

H. D. BURGES and N. W. HUSSEY

Pest Infestation Control Laboratory, Slough, Buckinghamshire, England
and
Glasshouse Crops Research Institute, Littlehampton, Sussex, England

I. Development of Insect Pathology

From early times man has been aware that insects suffer from disease. This awareness has developed at an ever-accelerating rate into the science of insect pathology. Disease can be defined as a departure of the insect from a state of health and was first noticed among domesticated insects. In Europe, Aristotle was the first to mention that bees suffered disease and, in 1835, Agostino Bassi showed that animal disease could be caused by a micro-organism, when he found that the fungus *Beauveria bassiana* causes the muscardine disease of silkworms.

Early observations were largely concentrated on two domesticated insects, the honey-bee and the silkworm, in studies that became the foundation of fundamental work on the nature of insect disease and its role in the ecology of insects. Gradually these studies were extended to pest species too, and the concept of utilizing disease to control these insects was born. In 1879, the Russian, Metchnikoff, conducted the first significant experiments in the destruction of injurious insects with micro-organisms, by infecting larvae of the beetle *Anisoplia austriaca* with the fungus *Metarrhizium anisopliae* (Steinhaus, 1949). The first commercial product, Sporéine, containing *Bacillus thuringiensis*, was produced before 1938 (Jacobs, 1950). After the second world war, several commercial firms in the U.S.A. began to produce this bacterium. Today we can point to such achievements as the protection of over 50% of the cole-crops (brassicas) from the cabbage looper *Trichoplusia ni* in Southern California by *B. thuringiensis* in 1965 and 1966 (Angus, 1968), the commercial production of this bacterium, and the testing of 10 trial commercial products containing insect viruses (Ignoffo, 1967). Largely stimulated by these practical possibilities, many specialist insect pathology laboratories were created, beginning in 1945 with the establishment of a Laboratory of Insect Pathology by the University of California. The literature increased correspondingly (Rothman and Woodhead, 1968). Insect pathologists began to regard their subject as a distinct discipline and arranged their first International Conference in Prague in 1958. In 1959 a journal was produced specifically for insect pathology and in 1967 a society was formed in conjunction with students of other invertebrates. Insect pathologists increased in number from about 321 in 1948 (a total that included those who had died earlier) to about 551 working in 1967 or about 728 inclusive of all invertebrate pathologists. In 1966, Steinhaus envisaged that comparative pathology—the study of diseases of living organisms—could be regarded as a triad of vertebrate pathology, invertebrate pathology and plant pathology (Steinhaus, 1967), and more recently he has argued the case for the creation of centres combining the three disciplines as pathobiology (Steinhaus, 1968). He created the first centre at Irvine, California, in 1969. The microbial control of insects is a particularly active field of invertebrate pathology that profits from fundamental work in pathobiology.

The time is obviously ripe to assess (i) what part disease caused by micro-organisms can play in the control of insect pests, (ii) whether present attempts are correctly orientated, and (iii) future developments. Early work has been well documented by Steinhaus and others (see Appendix 1). It seems most useful, therefore, to concentrate on developments over the last 10 years, drawing on earlier work mainly to formulate principles and identify mistakes that should not be repeated.

II. Limitation of Insect Numbers

The reasons why some insects are regarded as pests, and the factors that confer this status, must be understood if pests are to be controlled intelligently. This applies to microbial no less than to other means of control. Accordingly the origins of pests and the use of non-microbial control methods will be analysed to establish general principles that should be considered in attempts to make the best use of microbial methods. For present purposes, a pest will be regarded as an insect or mite that either causes economic injury or nuisance to man, or endangers his health.

A. INSECT NUMBERS BEFORE THE ADVENT OF AGRICULTURAL MAN

From present knowledge it can be deduced that, before man's intervention, the numbers of an insect species depended on the balance between its capacity to breed and a combination of natural forces which, to greater or lesser degree, restrained its numbers. The natural forces comprised climate, weather, extent of the resources available for exploitation, competitors, natural enemies and pathogens.

Many prolific species fed on plants and themselves formed the animal bases of food chains. As such they were *naturally* numerous, some doubtlessly causing as much damage as certain present-day pests, such as those of virgin coniferous forests. Some increased so greatly as to temporarily destroy their own food supply as does the pine looper, *Bupalus piniarius,* occasionally in European pine forests today. Many fluctuated annually in response to the seasonal weather and food supply. Food chains were never static; some species experienced periodic abundance and scarcity over cycles of many years. There were, of course, even greater cycles over millions of years in response to major climatic shifts and evolution.

Many species were never abundant because of the interaction with a complex of natural enemies operating under the overriding influence of climate. All such interactions are complicated and influenced by many subsidiary factors including weather, habitat and faunal composition.

The forces limiting the numbers of an insect species were a complex of abiotic and biotic factors operating at widely different population levels. These forces collectively exerted natural control. Since, at the end of a round of seasons, numbers increase only if more than two of the descendants of a single female survive to breed, the overall increase or decrease of a species probably often depends on relatively small shifts of mortality. For instance, in the simple case of a univoltine species with a female laying 100 eggs, 98% of these offspring must die before breeding if the population is to remain steady. A deviation of only 0.5% in mortality could result in a 25% increase or decrease in numbers the next year.

B. IMPACT OF AGRICULTURAL MAN

Man used plants and animals for food and other purposes, but fell victim himself to a range of parasitic insects. These parasites and those insects that affect the quality and quantity of plant produce came to be regarded as pests. Since these insects could outstrip their natural controlling forces in numbers sufficient to cause annoyance, their numbers could be limited only by introducing new controlling factors into the environment: it would be useless to wait in the hope that natural forces would increase sufficiently of their own accord.

Man himself imposed a further series of complications. To facilitate harvesting and to take advantage of particular habitats for specialized crops he grew larger and larger areas of single crops. In addition to concentrating and extending the insect's food supply, this trend to monoculture reduced the floral and faunal complexity, and so increased the chance of imbalance in insect populations, caused by a failure of one controlling factor, being easily compensated by others. As his knowledge of varietal differences improved, he selected strains which gave improved and reliable yields. These modern high-yielding plant varieties tend to be less resistant to insect attack than their wild ancestors so that pests are able to multiply more rapidly on cultivated crops.

Until pesticides were developed the only possible controls available depended upon manipulation of the cultural techniques, e.g. early or late sowings. However, even lethal chemicals had limitations. Wide spectrum materials often produced undesirable side-effects by killing many useful species, so upsetting the natural restraints not only on the major pests species, which resurged in greater numbers, but also on the less important species, which themselves increased and became pests. The importance of tetranychid mites in the past 20 years stems from the widespread use of organochlorine pesticides. Pesticides have also brought other complications in the form of phytotoxicity to susceptible crop plants and hazards to man and wild-life through persistent toxic residues. These complications have restricted the choice of suitable pesticides, a choice further restricted by the appearance of resistant strains of insect which, in the case of protected crops for instance (in glasshouses, cloches, mushroom houses, etc.), has limited the useful economic life of many new chemicals to only two or three years.

Some of the most serious outbreaks of pests, however, have been caused by accidental geographical spread of insects without their full complex of natural enemies. This imbalance may be corrected by introductions from elsewhere, often with striking results as in the case of the European spruce sawfly, *Gilpinia (Diprion) hercyniae* in Canada (though the introduction of the virus was accidental).

C. CONTROL OF PESTS BY CHEMICALS

Extensive use of chemicals has revealed a number of principles that the insect pathologist should consider in applying microbial control. Disregard of these principles, listed briefly below, has already led to some failures.

1. The chemical must be active against the target species.
2. It should not be phytotoxic.
3. A lethal quantity must reach the pest in a suitable formulation.
4. Application should be made at a vulnerable stage of the pest, and so timed as to prevent economic damage to the crop.
5. Watch should be kept for the development of resistance by the pests.
6. Harm to natural enemies must be minimized.

7. Chemicals without undue hazard to operators and wild-life must be selected. Dangerous residues on the plants and in the soil must be avoided.
8. The chemical should be stable in storage prior to use.

The development of resistance to pesticides is largely responsible for the current interest in biological control. The increasing costs of developing new pesticides—caused in no small measure by the need for elaborate testing to ensure that any residues have no undesirable side-effects—demand that materials are suitable for use on large areas of important crops. These restrictions bear heavily on high intensity cropping systems and thus it is vital to prolong the economic life of existing chemicals.

Biological control is a promising alternative to chemicals but effective natural agents are available for only a few species within a pest complex. This restriction has opened the way for control systems which integrate all available methods to control the whole pest complex. One of the greatest difficulties in developing an integrated control programme is the scarcity of selective chemicals and the problem of using wide spectrum materials in a selective manner. The restricted host range of many pathogens holds promise that they could be conveniently used in integrated programmes.

D. BIOLOGICAL CONTROL

In this book the term "biological control" will be used in its commonest sense to mean the influence of predators, parasites and pathogens introduced or applied by man. Some authorities include the activities of naturally occurring biological agents in the term, but here these activities will be distinguished as "natural biological control". The classical approach to biological control has mainly encompassed predators and parasitic arthropods so that a new term "macrobial control" is proposed to distinguish these conveniently from "microbial control", i.e. the activities of micro-organisms. The qualification "natural" can also be applied to these terms.

A study of the macrobial control of pests reveals much information of potential use in microbial control, so much so that comparison of the two methods has been encouraged throughout this book. A successful macrobial control agent should have the following attributes:

1. Ability to spread among the pest population.
2. Ability to persist in the pest's environment.
3. Sufficient powers of search.
4. Ability to limit pest numbers below that causing economic damage to the plants when correctly introduced.
5. It must be possible to produce or collect sufficient numbers of healthy specimens of the agent.
6. The agent should not destroy other biological agents unless it is able to take their place adequately.
7. It should provide predictable control.

The degree of control actually obtained is usually difficult to determine, often impossible without information, or base-line data, about the situation before the introduction of the agent. Adequate base-line data should be obtained.

Accurate identification of the agent is vital, even at the level of strains and biotypes which may have different climatic requirements, behaviour patterns and reactions to type of prey or host. The agents themselves may fall prey to predators and parasitic arthropods or they may suffer from disease, so that agents must be examined before release to ensure that they are healthy.

III. Possibilities of Microbial Control

The considerations outlined above show that microbial agents need to be effective against naturally numerous pest insects and often to operate in highly artificial circumstances created by man. They must either become new lethal factors in the environment, or natural agents introduced to geographical areas freshly invaded by pests, or agents unaffected by chemical insecticides and thus invaluable in integrated control programmes.

Such agents can be used either as microbial insecticides, or as introductions leading to *enzootic establishment* and persistence of the pathogens in new environments. This distinction relates to the capabilities of the organisms. Those for introduction must spread from relatively small inocula and persist, so allowing nature to take its course. Those unable to spread and persist must be used as microbial insecticides both regularly and in larger quantities.

Experience from macrobial and chemical control, together with the known attributes of microbial agents, indicate several desirable attributes of those pathogens considered for use in control programmes (Table I). Unfortunately, no one organism has all these features. However, many have a combination of attributes making them suitable for an introduction, while others have alternative combinations befitting a microbial insecticide (Table I). Before the second world war, efforts were concentrated more on introductions, but subsequently the emphasis has shifted to microbial insecticides. This trend is perhaps not surprising. Microbial introduction is, perhaps, most akin to classical macrobial control, particularly when pathogens are taken to new geographical areas. Pathogens from different insect species, which may prove more virulent in foreign hosts, and existing pathogens improved by laboratory selection may also be used in this way. Recently, progress in protected cropping has demonstrated the value of introducing new lethal factors into environments. The value of microbial agents often depends to a great extent upon whether they are affected by chemical pesticides. With the advent of the chemical era, it is understandable that attention should turn to microbial insecticides, which have many features in

TABLE I

Desirable attributes of microbial control agents and nematodes

Attribute	Method of application of the agent
Rapid spread	
Power of search for host	
Persistence	Introductions
Safe and aesthetically acceptable	
Control to sub-economic levels	
Predictable control	
Virulence	Microbial insecticides
Easy production	
Low cost	
Good storage	
Easy application	

(The first bracket groups "Rapid spread" to "Predictable control" under Introductions; the second groups "Safe and aesthetically acceptable" to "Easy application" under Microbial insecticides.)

common with the chemical. We now wish to achieve a balance with due emphasis on both introduction and microbial insecticides.

Each major group of pathogens has a different potential for microbial control. Each will be assessed in the light of the attributes in Table I, adopting as far as possible comparative approaches. Thus a study of existing natural microbial control helps to predict what can be expected of *applied* microbial control. The introduction of pathogens can be compared with their use as microbial insecticides and finally the microbial insecticide can be compared with the chemical. The available micro-organisms include bacteria, viruses, fungi, protozoans and rickettsiae. Although not strictly micro-organisms, nematodes have often been included with pathogens particularly since some are associated with insect-pathogenic bacteria. In some ways, such as the ability of some species to search for hosts at some time in their life-cycles, they may be considered as intermediate between typical microbial and macrobial control agents.

While insects may be attacked by a variety of microbial agents, different ecological groups of insects are affected to different degrees by the different types of agent. For example, surface feeding phytophagous caterpillars, especially colonial species of moths and sawflies, are particularly vulnerable to bacterial and virus diseases which are ingested on contaminated leaf-material. They are, in general, less vulnerable to fungal diseases as their feeding habitat is less likely to provide the prolonged periods of high humidity essential for the germination of fungal spores. Bark-beetles, on the other hand, which are unlikely to consume bark superficially contaminated by bacteria or viruses, readily succumb to entomogenous fungi which thrive in the damp environment within their galleries. Ecological barriers to the artificial manipulation of epizootics occur widely and must be appreciated before man attempts to utilize microbial control in any particular situation. Special attention will be given to two groups of pests, plant sucking insects and termites, as examples of groups in which the biology of the insect might play a particularly important role in determining the feasibility of microbial control; to insects of medical importance because of recent research activity in this field; to mites because they commonly occur together with insect pests and show a marked tendency to become troublesome when broad spectrum insecticides are used.

More and more insect pathogens are being found to produce toxins, which have featured prominently in recent research. There is, of course, the possibility of synthesizing and using these toxins alone as specific insecticides. Microbial insecticides may eventually be divided into two groups, those containing the living organisms and those consisting only of toxins. Three chapters will be devoted specifically to toxins, which have many features in common with stomach poisons.

Variation is a special problem experienced in microbial control more severely than in most other forms of control. In addition to variations common to all methods of control, such as variation in the susceptibility of insects and the imperfect distribution of materials, other variations stem from the complexity of the host-pathogen relationship, the production of toxins and the fact that pathogens are living organisms and consequently variable. This variability makes the standardization of pathogenic preparations not only difficult, but also important, if predictable control is to be achieved.

Application of pathogens as microbial insecticides requires large quantities of the active agent, consequently production must be relatively easy and storage qualities must be good. When the pathogens are required for introduction smaller quantities are needed. Pathogen production depends on whether or not the organism will grow in artificial media, i.e. *in vitro.* If it will, it can often be produced easily using advances in modern fermentation technology developed for the manufacture of therapeutic antibiotics. Otherwise, the pathogen must be produced *in vivo,* in the living host or an alternative organism. This involves a very different technology and so will be considered separately. Such *in vivo* production has been made possible largely by modern methods for perennial breeding of disease-free insects, often on the artificial foods developed for larvae of Lepidoptera.

Whichever method of production is used, problems of formulation and the maintenance of strains are common to both. Methods and principles already developed for formulating chemical insecticides can largely be adopted for micro-organisms, although surprising mistakes have been made through ignoring some of these principles. In addition, pathogens present some special formulation problems, because they must be maintained alive and because they are harmed by factors which have no effect on most chemicals, such as ultra-violet light, and the temperature and pressure during the milling of powder formulations. Strain maintenance is of course vitally important, particularly among pathogens that tend to lose virulence during repeated culture *in vitro*. The variability, mutability and sometimes amenability to genetical manipulation of pathogens can provide an advantage over chemicals in that it may lead to improvement of the active ingredient. Furthermore, the life blood of microbial control is the continual discovery of new species and strains which must be preserved as a bank of material available to all. Luckily many new methods of preserving micro-organisms have recently been developed.

Man has always lived with insects and their diseases in varying degrees. Insects parasitic on man and warm-blooded animals, and those (like flies) associated with his dwellings are important vectors of human disease. Some of these disease organisms can multiply within the insect and so could also be regarded as pathogens of the insect. For present purposes, all disease organisms of warm-blooded animals normally transmitted by insects will be regarded as diseases of the larger host while organisms which cause diseases in insects, but not normally in higher animals, will be regarded as pathogens of the insect. A similar distinction can be made with plant diseases carried by insects. All aspects of the safety of microbial pest control to man and useful animals must be examined both for pathogenicity and toxicity. Among useful animals, domesticated insects and macrobial control agents are most likely to suffer harm and such possibilities should be carefully checked.

Microbial control may involve a number of interactions. More than one micro-organism may combine to produce a disease, particularly when a facultative pathogen, i.e. one without primary invasive powers, gains a foothold as a result of the activities of a primary pathogen. Pathogens may also interact with chemicals in a synergistic fashion. Another rather subtle form of microbial control which may become possible is that of eliminating essential symbiotic micro-organisms from insect pests by means of antibiotics.

In view of the frequent occurrence of acquired resistance to chemicals, the possibility that pests will also acquire resistance to microbial agents must not be ignored, particularly since "resistance to disease" is a phrase constantly used by pathologists and epidemiologists in all fields of pathology.

Ecology is as important to microbial control as it is to macrobial control, particularly in the establishment of base-line data, and more important than in chemical control. Disease influences most aspects of an insect's life at all stages of development, including its ability to utilize food, its productivity and its resistance to unfavourable climatic factors. Usually, insect control must be undertaken with either the environment or the crop requirements as the overriding consideration. On some crops a few surviving pests are important, whilst on others (or in forests) considerable populations can be tolerated. It may even be desirable for a proportion of the pests to survive, if introduced pathogens are to persist. This concept may be extended further in view of developments in the field of macrobial control which suggest that where pesticidal chemicals are to be restricted on intensively grown, protected crops of high value, it is most efficient to introduce the pest first so as to achieve an even distribution of macrobial agent. The subsequent pattern of population fluctuation is then predictable throughout the crop (Gould, Hussey and Parr, 1969). Despite some striking demonstrations of the power of this technique growers have been reluctant to adopt the practice in Britain. In some instances this technique might be applicable to micro-organisms and the problem of grower-acceptability would again arise.

However, whether or not a control technique comes into commercial use depends largely on economics, and no treatise on microbial control would be complete without an attempt to assess this difficult subject. The difficulties arise from the fact that, unlike pesticide chemicals, which are applicable to many pest species in many situations and so supply large markets, biological systems are usually applicable only to a few species or to localized pest problems. Among microbial insecticides, *Bacillus thuringiensis* has already attracted commercial interest in manufacture for profit. Its host spectrum is relatively large and the list of susceptible pest species in the Lepidoptera–and hence the commercial potential–has grown apace. Highly specific microbial insecticides may fail to provide a sufficiently large and continuous market to be attractive to invested capital and so give a reasonable return. Then microbial insecticides, together with micro-organisms used as introductions, depend on governmental or communal backing of one sort or another. Their development and use involves economics at the community level and therefore impinges on sociological problems. Development would benefit greatly from international co-operation especially at the research level.

Sound future planning is vital and throughout the text the various topics have been analysed with this in mind. Sources of training, knowledge (including the possibilities of searching literature by computer) and useful materials are summarized in the appendices, together with a bibliography of the recent literature in the active research field concerning medically important insects.

Whatever the future role of microbial control, it must be based on the accurate identification of pathogens which is as important as that of macrobial agents, perhaps more so, because pathogens may change when infecting different species of host as well as during culture *in vitro*. A large body of information on the identity of micro-organisms has accumulated, but has never been compiled. It is largely related to main divisions in the major groups of micro-organisms and scattered in specialist papers. Organisation into a whole is essential. This has been attempted to assist the non-specialist to ascertain the cause of disease observed in an insect, and to assist the specialist in one group of micro-organisms to tackle identification in another group–for few are specialist in more than a few groups–and so lead specialists to developments that may be of value in their own fields. Much diagnostic skill depends on personal know-how and an attempt has been made to include this wherever possible. Since logical treatment of pathogen identification involves the whole complex of organisms found in insects and mites, it forms the subject of the next chapter.

References

Angus, T. A. (1968). *Wldl. Rev. Pest Control* **7,** 11-26.
Gould, H. J., Hussey, N. W. and Parr, W. J. (1969). *Proc. 2nd Congr. Acarol.* 1967, 383-388.
Ignoffo, C. M. (1967). *In* "Insect Pathology and Microbial Control" (P. A. van der Laan, ed.), pp. 91-117. North-Holland Publ. Co., Amsterdam.
Jacobs, S. E. (1950). *Proc. Soc. appl. Bact.* **13,** 83-91.
Rothman, H. and Woodhead, M. (1968). *Nature, Lond.* **220,** 1053-1054.
Steinhaus, E. A. (1949). "Principles of Insect Pathology". McGraw-Hill, New York. Reprinted, 1967, Hafner Publ. Co. London.
Steinhaus, E. A. (1967). *J. Invertebrate Path.* **9,** i-v.
Steinhaus, E. A. (1968). *J. Invertebrate Path.* **11,** i-iv.

CHAPTER 2

Identification of Pathogens

JAROSLAV WEISER and JOHN D. BRIGGS

Laboratory of Insect Pathology, Institute of Entomology, Academy of Sciences, Prague, Czechoslovakia
and
Invertebrate Pathology Laboratory, Faculty of Entomology, The Ohio State University, Columbus, Ohio, U.S.A.

I. Introduction

Identification of a pathogen is an essential element in the diagnosis of an infectious disease. Where microbial control is the primary concern, the quantity and quality of knowledge about the agent affect its production, formulation and intelligent use. Identity is not only the key to important literature references, but also to ultimate success in the marketing of unique products based upon the organism causing the disease.

The recognition of infectious diseases in insects and determination of their causes depend upon correct identification of the pathogens. This requires a general knowledge of both the infectious pathogens and the non-infectious diseases affecting insects and mites. Detection of only one of several micro-organisms associated with a disease may prevent recognition of the primary agent or secondary infections responsible for the final effect on the host. Therefore, the preliminary requirements are three-fold:

1. A general knowledge of the morphology of the principal infectious pathogens in insects.
2. An awareness of the known pathogens in different insects before describing new pathogens.
3. Confirmation of the identification and, after initial study of the agent, a re-evaluation of its role in the host population.

After the isolation of an organism, it must be confirmed as the cause of the disease according to Koch's postulates: 1. The organism is always associated with the disease. 2. The organism can be isolated in a pure form in the laboratory. 3. The organism will produce the disease when inoculated into a susceptible animal. 4. It is possible to recover the same organism from the experimentally infected animals. In practice, positive results are definitive, but failure to produce the disease on inoculation must be regarded with caution, because an organism often requires a very specific set of conditions to achieve infection. These conditions include the route of inoculation, physical conditions, stage of development and the sort of food available to the insect. Steinhaus (1963) discusses the background for the diagnosis of insect diseases.

The important aspects of collecting and processing diseased insects for the identification of pathogens are described in this chapter. Also illustrated keys and descriptions are given to help a biologist, who is not necessarily an experienced insect pathologist, to make an identification in a logical fashion. However, identification is a skill developed with experience, the number of pathogens is great, and the causes of insect diseases complex. Depending largely on the experience of the investigator, the data presented will allow an identification to be made to a major group, to genus, or even to species. Wherever possible, additional information in the literature will be indicated. If there is any doubt about the identity of an infecting organism, a specialist for that group should always be consulted.

A distinction is made throughout these discussions between *signs* of a disease, which are the presence of the pathogen and changes in structure of the host; and *symptoms* of a disease, the response of the host to the effect of the pathogen involving aberration in behavior and function. A glossary of terms used in invertebrate pathology is given by Steinhaus and Martignoni (1967).

II. Processing of Material

The processing of material for diagnosis may differ according to whether the objective is to find the cause of an epizootic, or detect infrequent or irregular mortality; to select live infected animals in a population; to determine the frequency of diseases in a given population by regular monitoring, or to search for candidate organisms to use for control.

Epizootics are characterized by the high incidence of an infectious disease and host mortality. Occasionally the pathogen is not visible under the light microscope, as in some virus infections, and the cadavers resemble insects killed by poison, asphyxia, temperature extremes, or starvation.

Irregular mortality may be the result of the low incidence of a sporadic infection, or the beginning of an epizootic. Increasing incidence of a disease in a population is evidence for a developing epizootic.

The selection of infected specimens is possible where the infection is characterized by typical changes in appearance or behavior of the host, e.g. in color or morphology, unusual movement, or cessation of feeding. In aquatic insects the infected individuals may have opaque, or chalky white, cysts of protozoan spores, fungi or other organisms visible to the unaided eye in their transparent bodies. The entire host body may become milky white or appear iridescent, blackened, jaundiced, or pink to red. Infected lepidopterous larvae may move to the top of the host plants where they may die.

In determinations of the state of health of an insect population, it is essential to seek both apparent and inapparent infections. A suitable method of detection is the serial dissection and inspection of representative insect samples. If the situation in the field is to be determined accurately, the animals must be dissected immediately after collection. When held in the laboratory, samples of diseased insects may develop abnormally severe or atypical symptoms and infected individuals may transmit pathogens to healthy ones. In the field the development of infected individuals is generally retarded by the disease and unaffected larvae pupate, resulting in a predominance of infected late instar larvae. In cases where an infection appears to be rare, groups of 5, 10, 20 to 50 individual host specimens may be triturated together and samples examined for suspected pathogens. If spores or other stages of pathogens are detected, single hosts should be carefully dissected.

Candidate pathogens for microbial control of a given pest may be detected by another procedure: rearing hosts at high population densities. Groups collected from different localities, preferably having some mortality, may be united in one rearing unit (vessel or cage). All mortality should be recorded and dead animals examined. The rearing of specimens collected from widely separated areas may reveal inapparent or cryptic infections occurring in the field.

III. Collection of Diseased Insects and Mites

A. COLLECTION OF DEAD SPECIMENS

Dead insects may be found enclosed in webs, under bark, in plant stems or rolled leaves. They may be fixed to the surface of leaves by the pathogen involved; e.g. fungus infections; or by coagulated body fluids and feces. Most structures of the host and the pathogen are delicate and readily damaged when insects are separated from the substrate. Loss of essential symptoms and signs of infection may result. Dead insects should, therefore, be collected in vials as single specimens on, or with a part of, the substrate. To avoid excessive accumulation of moisture, the stopper of the collecting vial should be of cotton, perforated plastic, or other water permeable material. In many cases, gelatin capsules or pill vials are useful for collection. Aquatic insects are often very fragile when dead, and it is most effective to allow the dead specimens to dry on a cover-slip or to place them in a drop of 4% formalin in a small, stoppered vial. Specimens may be carefully placed upon absorbent paper (filter or bibulous paper) which can be folded to secure the specimen. The paper bearing the specimens is stored safely in a vial pending further processing. Dried specimens (not fixed with chemicals) are suitable for making smears for microscopic examination to determine the principal pathogens, and for experimental transmission of infectious diseases to healthy hosts.

Chemical fixation after death is useless because specimens in this condition cannot be used successfully for smears, or for experimental infections. Histology is difficult if animals are dead before fixation. Cadavers carrying the pathogen can be stored in aqueous solutions of antibiotics (penicillin, streptomycin, chloromycetin) thus retarding bacterial decomposition so that the specimen can be used for smears or for experimental infections. Treatment with antibiotics must be clearly indicated to assure accurate interpretation of the results of infection experiments. Alternatively, to avoid contamination, the dead host material should be dried rapidly to prevent saprophytic fungi becoming established, so altering the material and reducing the possibility of satisfactory isolation of pathogens. For example, they mask and obscure primary infections by the Entomophthoraceae or other entomophilic fungi. In the tropics, stored, dead specimens of insects are attractive to Diptera, which deposit eggs on decaying organic material and their larvae destroy the specimens. Dried, virus infected specimens, stored at 4° C, may remain for several years in a satisfactory state for electron microscopy. Many of the entomophilic fungi, protozoans, bacteria, or nematodes die a few days after death of the host. If the material is to be used for infection studies, the viability must be determined to avoid inaccurate bioassays. Resting stages of pathogens in the infected specimen store well (for example, thick-walled resting spores of fungi, spores or cysts of protozoans, spores of bacteria, and ensheathed infective forms of nematodes). Although low temperature may be used to extend the viability of pathogens in dead host specimens, further processing of collected hosts should be accomplished with dispatch.

B. COLLECTION OF LIVING INFECTED AND NON-INFECTED SPECIMENS

Where primary interest is in live infected animals, and their comparison with healthy specimens, diseased individuals should not be collected and held together with non-infected specimens. To avoid stress of high population density, specimens should never be crowded. The transportation of aquatic insects is facilitated by moist moss, water plants *(Montia, Sphagnum, Elodea, Chara)* or wet grass, in plastic bags. For transportation of torenticolous insects, the bags containing plants may be filled with snow or ice and maintained in a portable insulated cold box. In the laboratory, aquatic host specimens may be transferred to jars of water aerated by aquarium pumps. Animals from stagnant water may survive for long periods in aquarium jars without aeration. Storage of aquatic forms at 4° C for short periods provides an excellent means for retarding the development of the host and any associated pathogens.

Suitable containers for transportation of phytophagous animals are cylindrical cardboard boxes or other cellulose fiber containers (Ovaltine, dried milk, or salt boxes) provided with a tight-fitted cover. Minute perforations in covers to allow gas exchange while retaining the insects are essential. Host plants or other food for the specimens are added to the container in amounts necessary only for sustenance during shipment. Crowded animals or excess food which may decompose can deplete limited oxygen and cause asphyxia, so destroying the shipment or stressing the insects and stimulating bacterial infection by facultative pathogens. When animals are transported without food, the container must provide sufficient surface for their movement and rest, in addition to space for accumulation and desiccation of their feces. Adult insects, pupae, or late instar larvae can be successfully transported for short periods without food or water, provided that both items are available at their destination. Some animals, particularly species inhabiting soil or those which normally burrow in their substrate, will attack other individuals when in close confinement; e.g. armyworms, grubs, etc. Honeycomb-like constructions, similar to those used for chicken eggs or fishermen's hooks, may be used in transporting boxes so that each larva is retained in a separate compartment. For maintenance of boring larvae or other specimens with characteristic positive thigmotaxis, cardboard with a corrugated central layer is most suitable since it provides individual larvae with single galleries.

Moisture is essential for transportation of all animals, particularly small invertebrates. This may be provided by moistened sphagnum moss or vermiculite in layers around a smaller container of animals. Living plants, which are not a natural food for the insect, may provide a moisture source in a transporting container. It should be confirmed in advance that the plants, or other devices providing moisture, do not produce poisonous vapors. For insects of medical importance, the World Health Organization provides a collection and shipment kit for diseased vectors. This small, pocket-sized kit contains various useful small containers and an assortment of instruments and materials (forceps, brush, pipette, lancet, and chemicals for specimen preservation) and a document for recording observations. Cantwell and Laird (1966) describe the kit and its use.

All material should be transported without exposure to temperature extremes by the most direct and rapid means available. Where available, storage at 5° C, with adequate ventilation is a safe procedure during transport. Living material should not be distributed or transported without knowledge of the regulations for specimen transportation (particularly insects, snails, and acarines) and local quarantine requirements at the origin and destination. International shipments of living insects should be sent to designated quarantine laboratories.

Specimens should be numbered and labeled by their common or scientific names, date and locality of collection, name of collector, name of host plant or animal, collector's description of signs and symptoms of disease in individuals and incidence of disease in the host population and as much of the relevant history of the affected host population as possible. The diagnostician should acknowledge receipt of the specimen(s) and assign an accession number to which all subsequent studies, slides, isolates, etc. will be related.

IV. Preparation of Specimens for Diagnosis

The amount of infected material collected should be sufficient to allow specimens to be processed according to three procedures. First, gross assessment of the pathology and etiology, with a description of the host and apparent pathogen; second, histological sectioning for study of the pathogen, pathology and infected tissues; and third, use of etiological agents for infection of healthy susceptible hosts if available. The diagnosis itself may not require much material. A single caterpillar or larval mosquito can be divided into three parts for the three procedures, but more are desirable to permit adequate examination of the host population. If possible, field and diagnostic personnel should discuss sample size. A statement of the gross pathology should describe the disease in terms of the morphology, physiology and behavior of the host. For tissue examination, a host specimen is placed on a microscope slide, and with forceps and lancet, its posterior third is removed to a second slide. A portion of its adipose, gut, Malpighian and other tissues are squeezed beneath a cover-slip with a drop of water for microscopic examination. If a suspected pathogen is observed, the same material is used to prepare a series of smears on glass microscope slides or cover-slips, and dry-fixed or wet-fixed in a chemical fixative; e.g. Bouin's (Section VIII.A.5). The remains of the host specimen on the first slide are divided into two parts. One portion is placed immediately into a vial with a chemical fixative, the second is deposited in another vial without additional materials as a reference sample.

If there are many infected specimens with the same gross symptoms, each individual can be divided into three parts, or one-third of the entire collection may be used for each step. Dead host specimens should be used for preparation of smears and infectivity tests. Moribund individuals may be retained for a supply of infectious forms of the pathogen and some can be processed for histological examination.

V. General Examination of Whole Subject Specimens

The microscopic examination of whole specimens should be conducted under a dissecting microscope or other instruments providing magnification to about x80.

Key 1. Symptoms and Signs of Disease

1. Terrestrial, many aquatic, and aerial forms of host 2
   Aquatic hosts only 10

2. Dead 3
   Moribund 8

3. Fixed to a surface of a plant or other object 4
   Not fixed to the surface of a plant 5

4. Insects upright on legs, outgrowth of hyphal mycelium covering the cuticles, e.g. Fig. 3(c), (d) . . . . FUNGUS INFECTION
   Insects lying upon or hanging from a leaf or plant surface, no filamentous structures on cuticle . . . . .VIRUS INFECTION

5. Gray or white 6
   Brown, red, or black 7

6. Body soft and breakable, or body iridescent, or a dried scale in water yielding a milky mass . . .PROTOZOA, BACTERIA, OR VIRUS
   Body hard, cheese-like, not disintegrating in water . FUNGUS INFECTION

7. Insect brown, interior empty . . . . FUNGUS, *Tarichium, Entomophthora,* or ENTOMOPHAGOUS INSECTS
   Insect black, hollow, disintegrating to a black powder in water . . . . . FUNGUS, *Tarichium*

Insect brick red . . . .
FUNGUS, *Syngliocladium (Sorosporella)* (Fig. 4(a)) or *Tarichium*

8. Irregular movements, tremors, "knock-down" i.e. failure of co-ordination followed by recovery (when surface of insect washed in acetone and the wash evaporated and bioassayed, same symptoms result), not blackening . . . . INSECTICIDE POISONING
Insects with dark spots, without irregular movements 9

9. Many minute spots, black or brown . . . . . ACARINE WOUNDS
A few black areas spreading over body . . . .
EARLY INFECTION OF FUNGI, DEUTEROMYCETES

10. Dead 11
Moribund 13

11. Population appearing rose, pink, or white . . . . . .ASPHYXIATION
Iridescence of body . . . . VIRUS
Single dead larvae on bottom of container 12

12. White masses in the interior . . . . PROTOZOA OR FUNGUS
Without apparent masses in the interior . . . .
ENTOMOPHAGOUS INSECTS

13. Segmental or irregularly grouped cysts in place of the fat body . . . . .
PROTOZOA OR RICKETTSIAE
Spherical cyst-like sporangia within the body . . FUNGI, *Coelomycidium*
Hyphae or sculptured, thick-walled sporangia, mainly in posterior . . . .
FUNGI, *Coelomomyces*

Keys to individual groups of pathogens, illustrations and literature references are included later in this chapter.

VI. Examination of Specific Tissues from Host Specimens

In order to detect and accurately describe organisms present within the body of a host, a compound microscope providing x100 to x1000 magnification should be employed. In addition to examination of a drop of fluid from the hemocoel, the posterior part of the body is dissected with forceps and needles, separating the gut, Malpighian tubules, and fat body. Tissue fragments are separately compressed in a drop of water under a cover-slip on a microscope slide, but not sufficiently to rupture cells. All tissues should be specifically identified for examination. First detect and attempt to identify the non-pathogenic particles, commensals, and mutualists. For example, in the gut contents, which can be removed by dissecting the gut or extracting the peritrophic membrane, note the fragments of plant tissue, starch or passing algae, ciliate or flagellated protozoans, or gregarines (Figs 5(c), 9(f)). In the Malpighian tubes, note the size and shape of the urate crystals or granules, and in some cases also oval cysts of *Malpighamoeba*, microsporidia (Fig. 7(a)), or navicular cysts of schizogregarines (Fig. 5(d)), all protozoans. In the fat body, protein crystals or granules are conspicuous before pupation. These inclusions in the cytoplasm of the adipose cells are clearly differentiated from spherical fat droplets with Sudan III which stains fat (see Section VIII.C.8). The transparent silk glands become opaque and hypertrophied at points where a microsporidian infection (Protozoa) produces a cyst in the wall of the gland.

Continuing the examination of specific tissues by rupturing the cells in a wet-mount, note the nature of materials flowing from tissues. For example, from adipose and gut cells, in addition to fat droplets, urate crystals, and normal cellular inclusions, pathogens (signs of disease) may be present. Oval spores of protozoans, or streams of polyhedra (Fig. 1(a)) or granules (capsules)–virus inclusion bodies, motile nematodes (Fig. 7(c), (d)), and spores of fungi may be evident in tissue fluid.

Any generalization regarding the relative size of micro-organisms found associated with insects is subject to many specific exceptions. The following ranges of size, including all forms of the particular kind of organism, may help to provide the investigator with a perspective, while keeping in mind that a reference work treating a subject group should be consulted.

TABLE I

Approximate largest dimension of micro-organisms associated with insects

Virus inclusion bodies	1.0 μ-15 μ
Virus particles (rods or spheres)	0.01 μ-0.3 μ
Rickettsiae	0.3 μ-0.6 μ
Bacteria	0.5 μ-50 μ
Protozoa	2.0 μ-20 μ
Algae	1.0 μ-50 μ
Yeasts	5.0 μ-10 μ
Fungi	5.0 μ-several centimeters
Nematodes	1 mm-several centimeters

Within the abdomens of living and recently killed adult insects, ova or sperm can be observed frequently. Within inseminated females, individual or closely-packed groups of actively moving sperm may be released from the spermatheca, or a spermatophore with many sperm (often whirling *en masse*) will rupture upon dissection of an abdomen. Spermatozoa appear as long filamentous structures, thread-like and undifferentiated with light microscopy, except for a noticeable thickening at one end. Ova are not motile, and bear the chorionic surface sculpturing characteristic of the species.

Key 2 distinguishes the principal and most easily recognized infectious pathogens. Parasitic, commensal, and mutualistic organisms found in the lumen of the gut or Malpighian tubules have been excluded. Specific characteristics, literature references and a guide to methods for the groups of principal infectious pathogens are given in Sections VII and VIII.

Key 2. Principal Groups of Pathogens of Insects and Acarines

1. Body filled and/or covered with a film of hyphae 2
   Body not filled or covered with hyphae 6

2. Hyphae persist in water 3
   Hyphae disappear in water; oval spores with smooth or ridged wall, Fig. 2(c) *Coelomomyces*

3. Hyphae form on surface of insects or develop into long protrusions, possibly several times longer than the host, with fructifications, e.g. Fig. 2(d) 4
   Hyphae adjacent, fixing body to substrate. Fructifications on separate hyphae, on surface of insects, e.g. Figs 3(c), 8(b), (c), (d) 5
   Hyphae in the interior, but no other characteristic stages of fungus . . . *Mycelia sterilia*

4. Fructifications clublike, porous, most longer than the insect, e.g. Fig. 2(d) . FUNGI, *Cordyceps*
   Fructifications only simulated by sterile clubs of hyphae . . . . FUNGI, DEUTEROMYCETES

5. No resting spores or cysts, conidia form on conidiophores, not discharged around insect, Figs 3(c), (d), 8(b), (c), (d) . DEUTEROMYCETES
   Thick-walled resting spores, Figs 3(a), (b), conidia discharged around the insect from conidiophores, Fig. 3(b) . ENTOMOPHTHORACEAE

6. One or several worms in insects, Fig. 7(c), (d) 7
   No worms present .10

7. Long worms more than x100 longer than diameter, white or yellowish-brown; single or several, coiled in body 8
   Worms less than x100 longer than diameter, different stages together (adults, eggs, rhabditoid larvae) host dead 9

8. White, thin nemas or worms, smooth cuticula, Fig. 7(d) . MERMITHIDAE
   Brown, hard, coiled nemas, cuticula reticulated . . . . GORDIIDAE

9. Long, filarioid females and males, long thin larvae, Fig. 7(c) . . . . STEINERNEMATIDAE

Short, rhabditoid females and males, rhabditoid larvae . . . .
DIPLOGASTERIDAE

10. Host body soft; interior red, brown or black 11
Host body soft; interior white, yellow, pink or not colored 13

11. Interior of host body mass of red granules 12
Interior of host body black or brown, dispersing into spherical to lenticular resting spores in water . . . . *Tarichium megaspermum*

12. Red powder dispersing in water into prickly spherical cysts . . . .
Tarichium cleoni

Red powder dispersing in water to grape-like masses of minute spherical cells, Fig. 4(a) . . . . *Syngliocladium (Sorosporella) uvella*

13, White masses in host body visible at x25 magnification 14
No white masses in host body visible thus: sporangia of *Coelomomyces* and *Coelomycidium,* Fig. 2(b), (c), should not be confused with these masses 18

14. Masses formed of uniform stages, spores, Figs 7(a), 9(h) 15
Masses formed of tissue containing oval proteinaceous inclusions or milky mass 17

15. Spores oval, broad to elongate or crescent-shaped, single or in groups, Figs 6(c), (d), 7(a), 10 . . . . MICROSPORIDA (PROTOZOA)
Spores round or navicular 16

16. Spores round, vesicular, containing two sporozoites and a resting body. Spores in cysts to a total of 5-20, Fig. 9(h), (i) . . . .
COCCIDIA (PROTOZOA)

Spores navicular, single or in groups, in tissue or in the gut, Fig. 5(d) . . .
GREGARINIA (PROTOZOA)

17. Oval proteinaceous inclusions in some segmental lobes of fat body. Fine granules evident in inclusions after alkali treatment . . . .
INCLUSIONS OF POX-LIKE VIRUS

Milky mass in lobes of fat body, segmental distribution, Fig. 4(d) . . . .
Rickettsiella

18. Host body milky white 19
Host body or body fluid yellow or pink 22
No change in color of host body 24

19. Body fluid white 20
Body fluid not white. Body exhibiting bluish lavender iridescence . . . .
IRIDESCENT VIRUSES

20. Fluid containing oval to navicular bodies, refringent, thin-walled, regular; when stained polar vacuoles visible, Figs 6(c), (d), 7(a), 10 . . . . . MICROSPORIDA

Fluid containing thick-walled, navicular bodies, with a human shoeprint shape, 1-2 x 6 μ, Fig. 4(c) . . . . *Bacillus popilliae*

Fluid containing subspherical particles which do not stain on smears with Giemsa, shining in dark field 21

21. Particles sub-microscopic, in gray spherical vacuoles in fat body . . . . . GRANULOSIS VIRUSES

Particles 3-7 μ in diameter, subspherical to polyhedral, Fig. 1(a), (c), (d) . . POLYHEDROSIS VIRUSES

Particles not refringent in dark field and dissolve in water during processing of smears or of histological sections, yellow or green under polarized light (Smirnoff and Philogène, 1968) . . URIC ACID CRYSTALS

22. Spherical cystlike sporangia and free, uniflagellate round zoospores in blackflies, Fig. 2(b) . . . . *Coelomycidium*

Oval sporangia within host 23

23. Sporangia each with lateral tube or operculum, in ephemerids, 10 x 15-20 μ *Polycaryum ecdyonuris*

Sporangia without lateral tube, with surface ribs and ridges, about 25 x 40 μ, Fig. 2(c) . . . . COELOMOMYCETACEAE

24. Body filled with minute rods or spherules, mostly motile . . . . BACTERIAL SEPTICEMIA

Body filled with bacterial rods, 8-10 μ long, each with a spore and a diamond shaped body inside, Fig. 4(b), Lepidoptera only . . . . . *Bacillus thuringiensis*

Tissue without lesions and no free particles in hemolymph. Single cells in fat body or parts of fat body with bacteroid or yeast-like particles in dense masses . . . . SYMBIOTES IN MYCETOME

Local lesions in tissue or infiltration with stages of pathogens . . . 25

25. Oval refringent bodies, not shining in dark field, Figs 5(b), 7(a), 10 . . . MICROSPORIDA, *Malamoeba*

Other than oval bodies 26

26. Spherical cysts containing spherical spores, Figs 6(a), (b), 9(h) . . . . . COCCIDIA, *Chytridiopsis*

Spherical cysts without spores . . . . AMOEBAE

Spores navicular or tubular 27

27. Navicular spores, Fig. 5(d) . . . . GREGARINIA

Tubular spores, Fig. 10(a) . . . . *Monosporella, Mrazekidae*

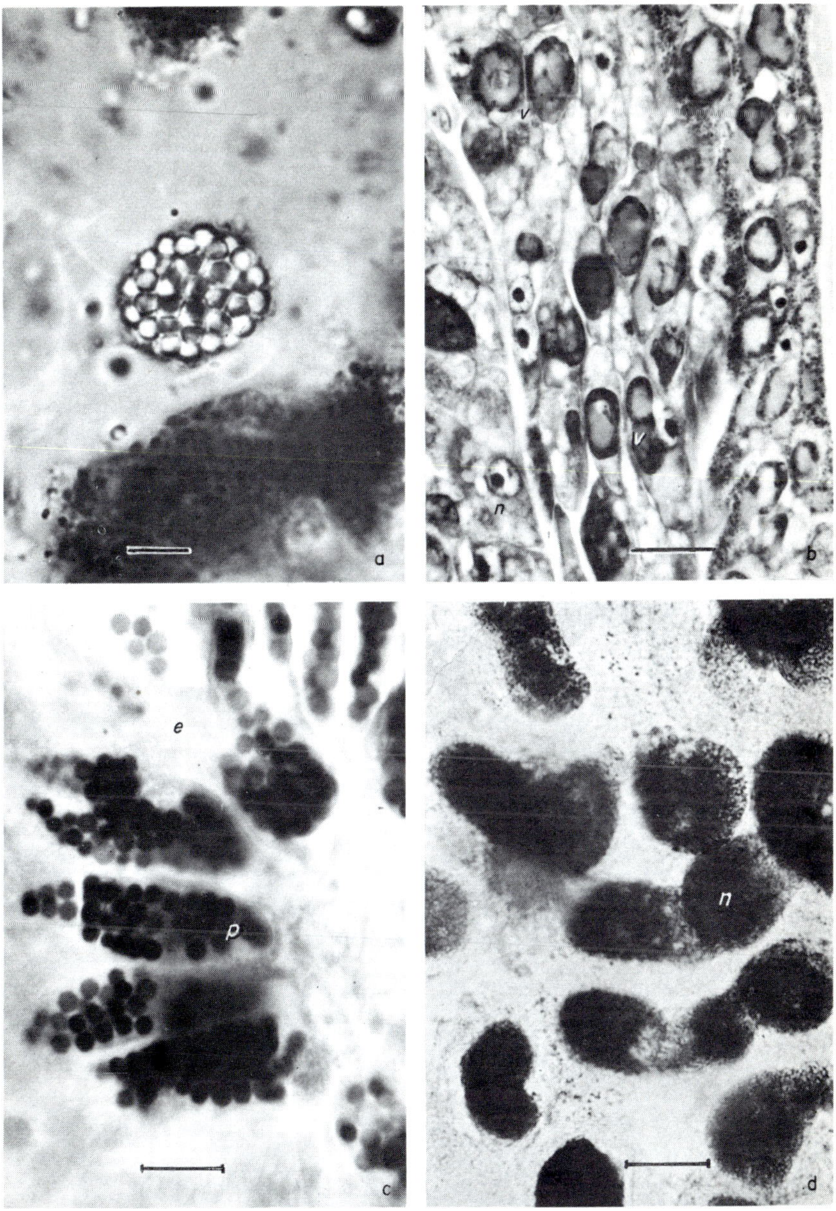

Fig. 1. (a): Nuclear polyhedrosis: one nucleus of fat body of *Stilpnotia salicis* filled with polyhedra. Line = 10 μ. (b): Mosquito iridescent virus in a section of fat body of *Aedes cantans*: dark virus stromata, *v*, in infected cells; nuclei, *n*, normal. Hematoxylin stain. Line = 10 μ. (c): Cross-section of midgut of *Tineola biselliella* larva with polyhedra, *p*, of a cytoplasmic polyhedrosis; empty spaces, *e*, are unstained nuclei. Line = 10 μ. Hematoxylin stain. (d): Smear of gut cells of sawfly with nuclear polyhedrosis: nuclei, *n*, are filled with minute polyhedra. Line = 10 μ. Watermount. Figs 1-10 from Weiser (1969, 1963) except as indicated on individual figures.

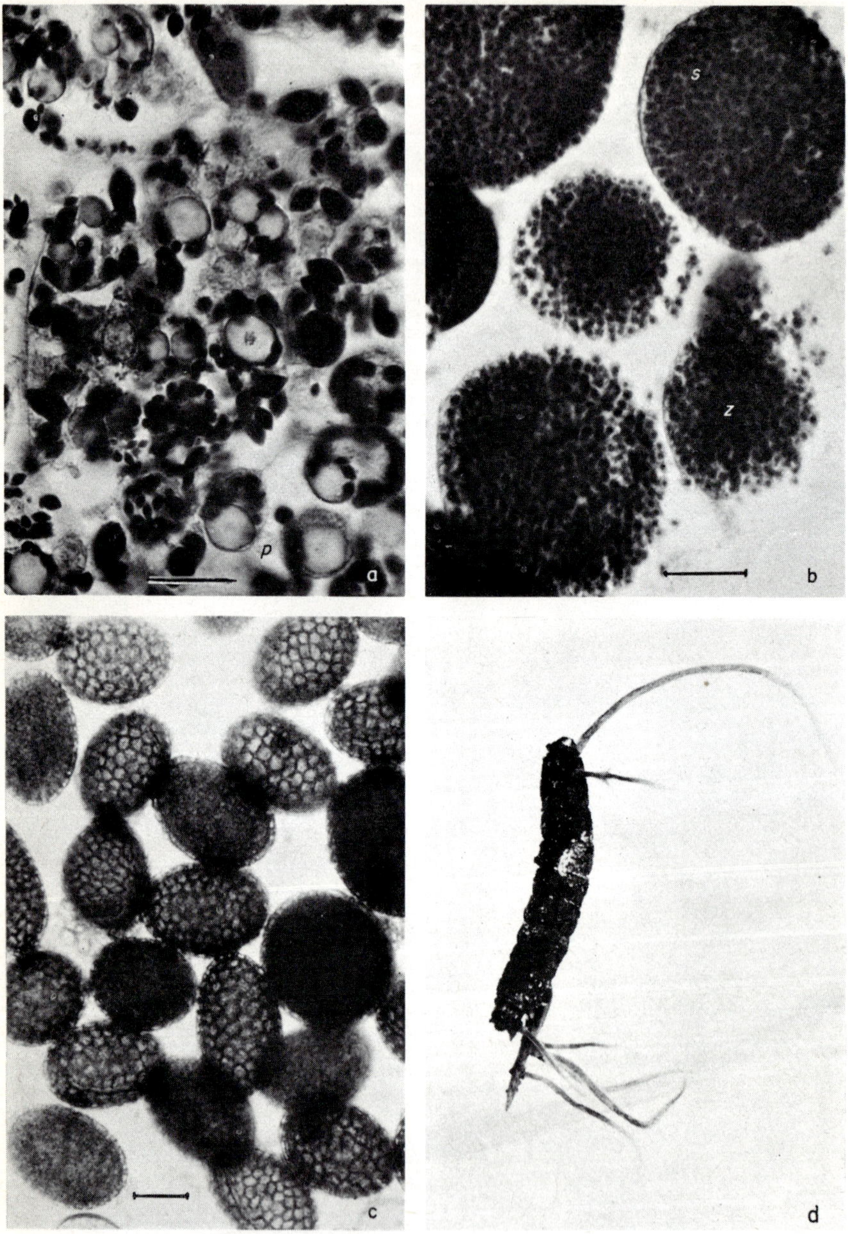

Fig. 2. (a): Spindle inclusion virus of *Melolontha melolontha*: young (dark) and mature (unstained) inclusions, *p*, in fat body. Line = 10 μ. Hematoxylin stain. (b): *Coelomycidium simulii*: sporangia, *s*, and zoospores, *z*, in infected blackfly larva. Line = 10 μ. Watermount. (c): *Coelomomyces chironomi*: oval sporangia with a reticulate surface wall. Line = 10 μ. Watermount. (d): Lepidopterous larva with stromata of *Cordyceps* sp. ×3. Fig. 2(d) by J. D. Briggs.

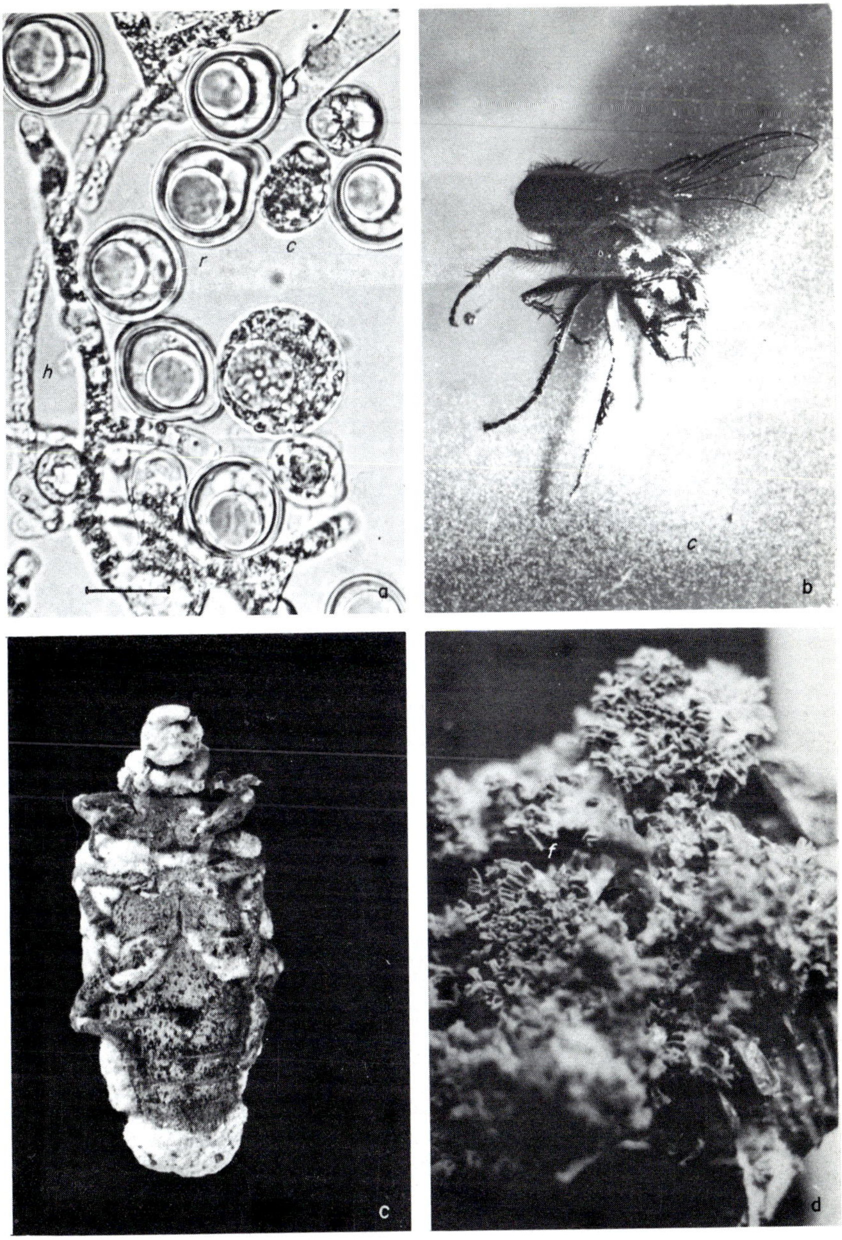

Fig. 3. (a): Resting spores, *r*, conidia, *c*, and hyphae, *h*, of *Entomophthora destruens* in cultures. Line = 10 μ. Watermount. (b): Blowfly fixed to substrate and infected with *Entomophthora muscae*: conidia, *c*, are distributed around the insect ×4. (c): *Bothynoderes punctiventris* with *Beauveria bassiana* ×3. (d): *Metarrhizium anisopliae* on adult *Melolontha melolontha*: spores deposed in long prismatic masses, *f*, ×4.

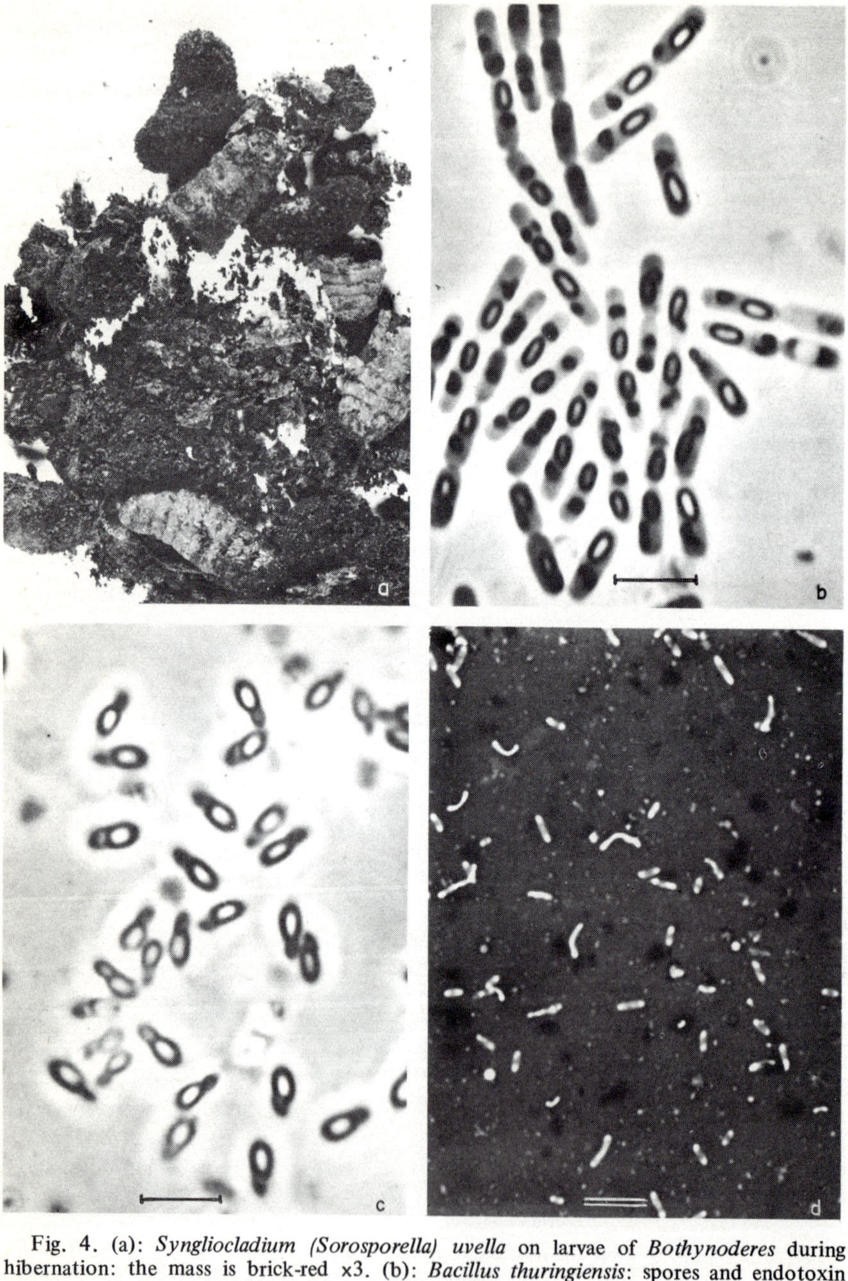

Fig. 4. (a): *Syngliocladium (Sorosporella) uvella* on larvae of *Bothynoderes* during hibernation: the mass is brick-red x3. (b): *Bacillus thuringiensis*: spores and endotoxin crystals inside sporulating rods. Line = 5 μ. Phase contrast. (c): *Bacillus popilliae*: sporangia with oval spores and polar parasporal bodies, producing the shoeprint pattern. Line = 5 μ. (d): *Rickettsia prowazekii*: cause of epidemic typhus in man, cells in India ink smear, showing the typical shape. Line = 1 μ.

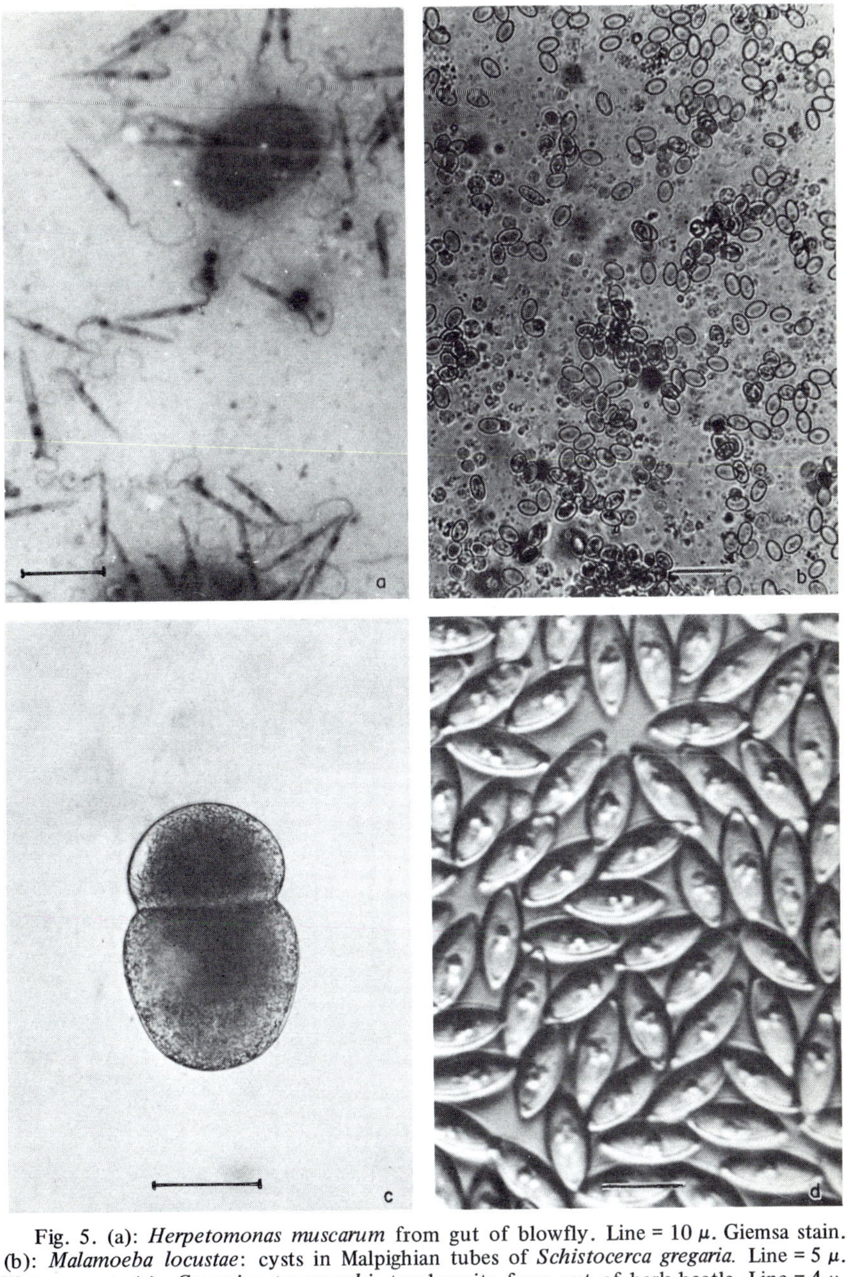

Fig. 5. (a): *Herpetomonas muscarum* from gut of blowfly. Line = 10 μ. Giemsa stain. (b): *Malamoeba locustae*: cysts in Malpighian tubes of *Schistocerca gregaria.* Line = 5 μ. Watermount. (c): *Gregarina typographi*: trophozoite from gut of bark beetle. Line = 4 μ. (d): Spores of gregarine, Phase contrast, *Monocystis* sp. in *Melolontha.* Line = 10 μ.

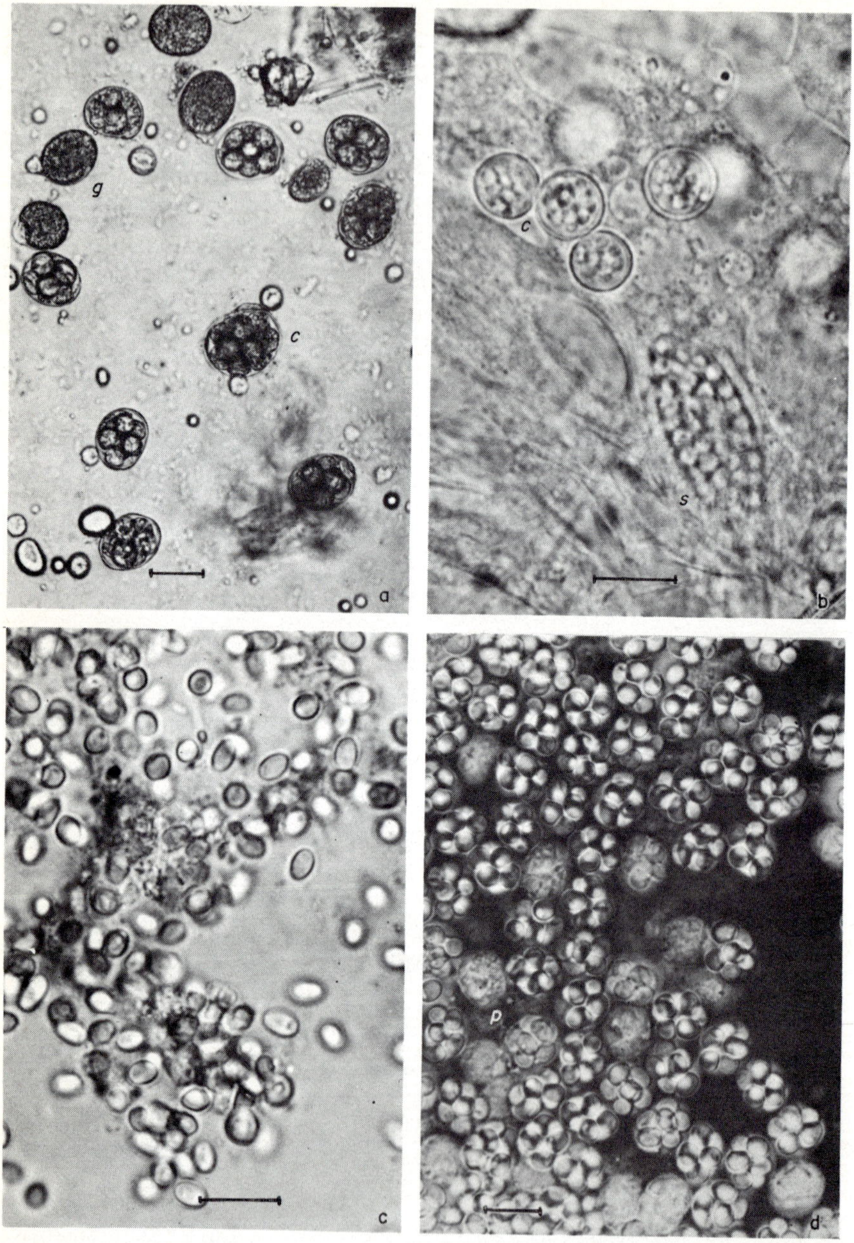

Fig. 6. (a): Cyst of *Adelina mesnili, c,* together with macrogametes, *g,* in the flour moth. Line = 10 μ. Watermount. (b): *Chytridiopsis*: cysts, *c,* and schizonts, *s,* in gut wall of *Ips typographus.* Line = 10 μ. Hematoxylin stain. (c): Spores of Microsporida: single spores of *Nosema* in watermount. Line = 10 μ. (d): *Thelohania lairdi,* an example of octosporous pansporoblasts and plasmodia, *p.* Line = 10 μ. India ink suspension.

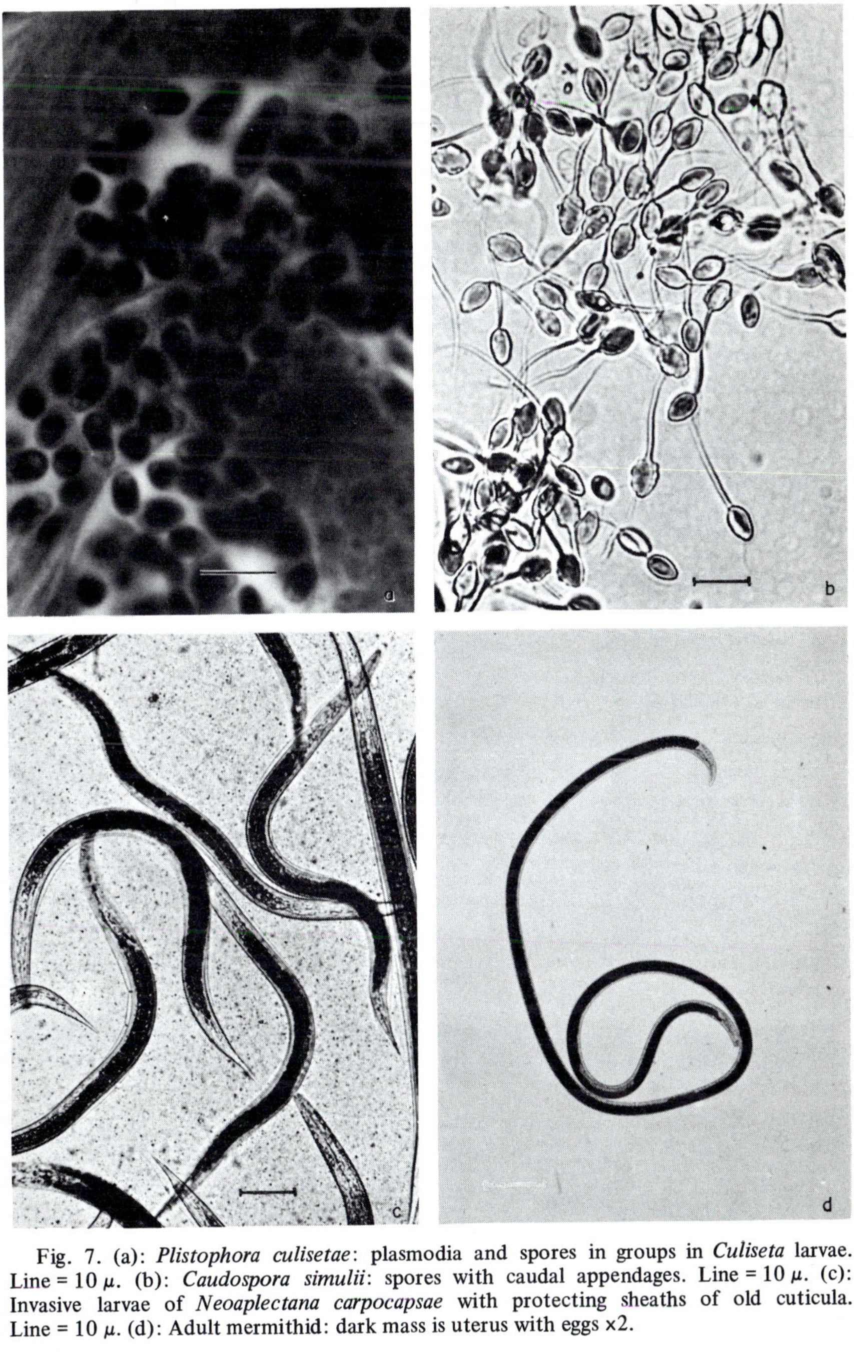

Fig. 7. (a): *Plistophora culisetae*: plasmodia and spores in groups in *Culiseta* larvae. Line = 10 μ. (b): *Caudospora simulii*: spores with caudal appendages. Line = 10 μ. (c): Invasive larvae of *Neoaplectana carpocapsae* with protecting sheaths of old cuticula. Line = 10 μ. (d): Adult mermithid: dark mass is uterus with eggs ×2.

VII. Description of the Principal Groups of Infectious Organisms

A. VIRUSES

The tissue of a host affected by a virus may be studied in watermounts for bright-, dark-field and phase contrast microscopy, or stained by Giemsa on smears either without or after previous treatment with 0.1% HCl or 0.1% NaOH. Samples of tissue in ultra-thin stained sections or stained centrifugation sediment after maceration of tissues and cells may be observed under the electron microscope on specimen grids.

Most viruses infecting invertebrates, particularly larvae of insects, are characterized by the occlusion of the virus particles (virions) within inclusion bodies; hence the terms "inclusion" viruses or "occluded" viruses. The inclusion bodies–polyhedra, granules or capsules, and spherule inclusions–are located in the nuclei or cytoplasm of the cells of adipose tissue, gut, hypodermis, muscles, and other tissues. Types of viruses with virions not occluded are referred to as "non-inclusion" or "non-occluded" viruses. The inclusion bodies are not stained with Sudan III solution. They are not stained by Giemsa if not pre-treated with 0.1% HCl or 0.1% NaOH for 2-5 min (see Section VIII for details of methods). After the pre-stain treatment, the inclusions are stained with Giemsa to a bluish color, with minute red areas in the interior. In wet mounts with dark-field microscopy, the inclusions are refringent and appear bright. Virus particles are visible within the inclusion bodies in thin sections under the electron microscope. The inclusions from moribund or dead and dry tissue, or a centrifugate, can be fixed in 2% osmic acid and embedded in resin; e.g. Epon, for sections for electron microscopy. Virus particles freed from inclusions, granules, polyhedra, or non-occluded viruses in tissue extracts or body fluids may be shown with an electron microscope on specimen grids when deposited in a dilute distilled water suspension. The water is absorbed from the grid after 5 min, and one drop of 2.0% uranyl acetate is added for 1 s and removed, or the grid is shadowed with a heavy metal; e.g. palladium. Using low magnification, about x8000, virus particles, granules or polyhedra are visible.

A similarly prepared specimen grid treated with 0.1% NaOH to dissolve the inclusion bodies and subsequently shadowed, will reveal remnants of inclusion bodies and the associated virus particles within or upon the inclusion body. Smith (1967) describes the insect viruses.

1. Nuclear Polyhedrosis, Borrelinavirus *Group, Occluded (Fig. 1(a))*

Description and Techniques: Tanada (1959). *Host:* Lepidoptera, larvae. *Symptoms:* Insects hanging from substrate, liquified body content, delicate, rupturing integument. *Tissue Site:* Fat body, hypodermis, tracheal matrix, hemocytes, other tissue in advanced infection. *Pathogen Morphology:* Subspherical polyhedra 3-7 μ in diameter, in groups in hypertrophic nuclei; virion rod 350 x 50 mμ. *Light Microscopy:* Polyhedra do not stain unless treated with 0.1% NaOH or hot 0.1% HCl, after which Giemsa stains polyhedra dark, other cellular inclusions or host structures light. *Electron Microscopy:* Bergold (1963). Virions rod-shaped in polyhedra dissolved on specimen grids, or in ultra-thin section. *Nucleic Acid:* DNA and RNA.

2. *Nuclear Polyhedrosis,* Birdiavirus *Group, Occluded (Fig. 1(d))*

Techniques and Illustrations: Bird and Whalen (1953). *Host:* Hymenoptera, Symphyta (sawfly) larvae. *Symptoms:* Infected insects stick to substrate by anus and legs, flaccid, some liquified and delicate. *Tissue Site:* Midgut epithelium, hypertrophic nuclei of cells. *Pathogen Morphology:* Minute subspherical polyhedra 0.5-1.2 μ in diameter, virion 250 x 50 mμ, frequent spherical particles. *Light Microscopy:* Treatment with 0.1% NaOH or hot 0.1% HCl facilitates inverse staining. *Electron Microscopy:* Polyhedra, dissolved or in sections, contain virus rods. *Nucleic Acid:* DNA.

3. *Granulosis (Capsule) Virus,* Bergoldiavirus *Group, Occluded*

Techniques and Illustrations: Steinhaus and Hughes (1953). *Host:* Lepidoptera, larvae. *Symptoms:* Infected insects white, milky hemolymph, often delicate integument and liquified body contents. *Tissue Site:* Fat body, hypodermis, and later other tissues. May be limited to single tissue. *Pathogen Morphology:* Granules (capsules) ovoidal 0.3-0.5 x 0.1-0.2 μ, can be cuboidal and a few may be 5.0 μ in largest dimension. Virion rods average 400 x 50 mμ. *Light Microscopy:* Huger (1963). Mass of particles at limit of resolution refringent in dark field; gray in normal microscopy; in hypertrophic nuclei and in spherical intracellular and extracellular vesicles. *Electron Microscopy:* Huger (1963). Solution in alkali reveals one virus rod in each granule. *Nucleic Acid:* DNA.

4. *Elastovirus,* Xerosia-virus *Group (Polyhedral Inclusion)*

Description, Illustration: Xeros (1954). *Phagocytosis, Techniques:* Xeros (1964). *Host:* Diptera, Tipulidae (leatherjacket) larvae. *Symptoms:* Host with hypertrophied lymphocytes, crescent-shaped inclusions on surface of nuclei, milky hemolymph, flaccid body. *Tissue Site:* Lymphocytes. *Pathogen Morphology:* Polyhedral inclusions free in hemolymph, 5-7 x 3-5 μ. When exposed to a drop of 4% NaOH, under a cover-slip, they change into sigmoid filaments up to 30 μ long. Neutralization restores the original shape. Virion 160 mμ long. *Electron Microscopy:* In ultra-thin sections, rod-like virus particles. *Nucleic Acid:* DNA.

5. *Cytoplasmic Polyhedrosis,* Smithiavirus *Group, Occluded (Fig. 1(c))*

Host: Lepidoptera (description and illustration, Bird, 1966), Diptera (Culicidae, *Culex tarsalis,* description and demonstration, Kellen *et al.,* 1966). *Symptoms:* Lepidoptera; host larvae active; gut hard, white, hypertrophied; feces chalky white, containing masses of polyhedra. Diptera; larvae sluggish, have difficulty in attaining surface attachment. *Tissue Site:* Midgut cells of Lepidoptera; hypodermal cells and imaginal discs of *C. tarsalis. Pathogen Morphology:* Polyhedral inclusions in same cell ranging from 1-7 μ. Virions spherical 50-70 mμ. *Light Microscopy:* Many polyhedral inclusions in gut wall cells, isolated in vacuoles. Inclusions stain with Giemsa after alkali treatment. *Electron Microscopy:* Polyhedra, with spherical depressions on surface easily seen in sections; dissolved show spherical virions in honeycomb-like polyhedral masses. *Nucleic Acid:* RNA.

6. Cytoplasmic Spindle-inclusion Virus, Vagoiavirus *Group, Occluded (Fig. 2(a))*

Description and Illustration: Weiser and Vago (1966). *Host:* Lepidoptera and Coleoptera. *Symptoms:* Host chalky white, hard, motionless on substrate. *Tissue Site:* Fat body. *Pathogen Morphology:* Early inclusion bodies needle to spindle-shaped. Final inclusion bodies oval, 0.7-13 x 0.7-6 μ; virions ovoidal, 400 x 250 mμ. *Light Microscopy:* Needle to spindle-shaped inclusions stain in the cytoplasm, final oval stages stain only after alkali treatment which reveals many granules refringent in dark-field illumination, nuclei not involved. *Electron Microscopy:* Virions ovoid with beaded surface in ultra-thin sections and in tissue sediment on EM grids. *Nucleic Acid:* Unknown.

7. Pox-like Viruses, Occluded

Techniques and Illustration: Roberts and Granados (1968). *Host:* Larval Diptera, Lepidoptera, and Coleoptera. *Symptoms:* Paralysis of abdominal region in Lepidoptera. *Tissue Site:* Adipose and hemocyte cytoplasm. *Pathogen Morphology:* Virions ovoidal 25 x 10 mμ, a beaded surface and an internal nucloid, oval inclusions, 4-10 μ. *Light Microscopy:* White, irregular cysts in fat body. Cytoplasm around the nuclei in cells packed with oval to cubic inclusions, refringent in dark-field, stain with Giemsa after alkali treatment. *Electron Microscopy:* In ultra-thin sections, virion cushion-shaped. *Nucleic Acid:* Unknown.

8. Grasshopper Inclusion-body Virus, Occluded

Pathology and Development: Henry *et al.* (1969). *Host:* Orthoptera, *Melanoplus sanguinipes, M. bivittatus, M. differentialis, Schistocerca americana. Symptoms:* High mortality, general torpor, delayed development, hypertrophied adipose tissue with distended abdomen in nymphs, hemolymph turbid in heavy infection. *Tissue Site:* Adipose, cytoplasm and nuclei; sublethal to terminal infections involve isolated portions to entire organ. *Pathogen Morphology:* Inclusion bodies irregular cuboidal crystalline, 2-10 μ in largest dimension. Virion rod 200-400 mμ. *Light Microscopy:* Inclusions insoluble in water, dissolve in 1.0% KOH. *Electron Microscopy:* Thin sections of inclusion body, virions continue development during occlusion, within enlarging polyhedra. *Nucleic Acid:* DNA.

9. Crystalline Array Virus, Occluded

Description and Techniques: Jutila *et al.* (1970). *Host:* Orthoptera, *Melanoplus bivittatus,* grasshoppers (Acrididae). *Symptoms:* Loss of appetite, vigor, and co-ordination. *Tissue Site:* Cytoplasm of tracheal matrix, muscle and pericardial cells. *Pathogen Morphology:* Elongate crystalline inclusions, 2-10 μ long; spherical virion, 13 mμ in diameter. *Light Microscopy:* Muscles atrophy, lose striated appearance, crystalline inclusions at ends of muscle fibers. *Electron Microscopy:* Thin sections of inclusions show crystalline-array in several planes. *Nucleic Acid:* RNA.

10. Densonucleosis and Morator-virus *Group, Non-occluded*

Description and Illustration: Vago *et al.* (1966). *Host: Galleria mellonella* (greater wax moth) larvae and other insects; e.g., honey-bee *(Apis mellifera)* larvae and adults. *Symptoms:* Dead larvae flaccid, brown to black; in sacbrood disease of honey-bees, living larvae float in watery liquid in the moulted skin, adult bees paralyzed. *Tissue Site:* Nuclei of fat body, and in adult bees, nerve ganglia are changed to dense uniform masses. *Pathogen Morphology:* Icosahedral, 20-30 mμ. *Light Microscopy:* Virions not visible; sections reveal the adipose tissue as dense, dark-stained uniform masses, nuclei appearing as homogeneous spheres. In bees, nerve tissues, ganglia, and some ventricular cells show similar changes. *Electron Microscopy:* Icosahedral virions free in body fluids, demonstrated after millipore filtration (0.45 μ). *Nucleic Acid:* DNA.

11. Iridescent Viruses, Pseudomorator-virus *Group, Non-occluded (Fig. 1(b))*

Host range and Development: Bird (1961). *Host:* Larvae of Diptera, Coleoptera, Lepidoptera. *Symptoms:* Host body with bluish-green, violet, or brown iridescence; infected tissues not hypertrophied, larvae sluggish and hidden. *Tissue Site:* Silk gland, fat body, tracheal epithelium, epidermis, muscle. *Pathogen Morphology:* Icosahedral virus, 130-180 mμ in diameter. *Light Microscopy:* Sections reveal virogenic stromata in tissues, staining black as porous masses in cytoplasm, 3-8 μ in diameter. Matta and Lowe (1969) review differential staining techniques, e.g. virus-infected mosquito tissue in sections can be stained dark purplish-brown under dark-field illumination. *Electron Microscopy:* Virus in cytoplasm of fat body, hypodermis, and some muscle cells. Hemolymph diluted with water contains masses of icosahedral virus particles. *Nucleic Acid:* DNA.

12. Viruses of Mites, Non-occluded

Host: Panonychus ulmi, the European red mite (description of virus, Steinhaus,

1959); *P. citri,* the citrus red mite (description of virus, Smith *et al.,* 1959). *Symptoms:* Paralysis of hosts; birefringent, irregular crystals, 3-7 μ to round bodies 50 μ in diameter, frequently observed in hemocoel of infected *P. citri* (Smith and Cressman, 1962). *Tissue Site:* Unknown. *Pathogen Morphology:* Spherical 30-60 mμ in diameter. *Electron Microscopy:* Filtrate of triturated mites dried and shadowed with palladium. *Nucleic Acid:* RNA (analysis, Estes and Faust, 1965).

B. RICKETTSIAE

Host: Diptera (midges, leatherjackets), larval Coleoptera and Lepidoptera (methods and description, Entwistle and Robertson, 1968). *Symptoms:* Cessation of feeding, diarrhoea, regurgitation, muscular spasms, and loss of tonus. *Tissue Site:* Cytoplasm of gut, fat body; rarely hypodermis. *Light Microscopy:* Submicroscopic particles with polar swellings in smears with India ink (Fig. 4(d)). In smears and sections bearing organisms of the genus *Rickettsiella,* numerous associated crystals in host cell stain red with neutral red or black with iron hematoxylin. Rickettsiae stain violet with Giemsa and Macchiavello's stains which differentiate them from granulosis inclusions of similar size; often occur in chains of up to 20 rickettsiae. Macchiavello's stain tends to be unreliable and that of Zdrodovski and Golinevich is better (Section VIII.C). Useful stains are reviewed by Krieg (1963). *Electron Microscopy:* Thin sections, all rickettsiae appear as oval bodies with an intracellular structure.

The different groups of rickettsiae are localized in different hosts and organs, and often exhibit pleomorphism. Rickettsial parasites of vertebrates (e.g. hemorrhagic and "spotted" fevers) may be detected in invertebrate vectors, in which they are localized in or upon the gut epithelial cells. The cells of the vector do not appear to be damaged. Certain rickettsiae infect Lepidoptera, in which thin sections for electron microscopy reveal the rickettsiae as oval to tubular, within granular host-cell cytoplasm of adipose or midgut cells. Rickettsiae occurring in adipose cells of midges (Diptera) are flat and bean-shaped with a sculptured surface.

The diagnostic features of rickettsiae can be summarized as failure to grow in bacteriological media, pathogenic species mainly intracellular, pleomorphism, averaging 300-500 mμ long and staining in Macchiavello's stain. For further literature see: Krieg (1963), Steinhaus (1946), Steinhaus (1949), Weiser (1966), and Weiser (1969).

C. BACTERIA

The bacteria regularly cause decomposition of dead insects. Those bacteria which are characteristic of the host environment are generally found within, and upon, dead specimens. Consequently, careful evaluation must follow the detection and isolation of bacteria from insects.

Except for a few species, bacteria do not infect and kill a host that ingests them. As a corollary, saprophytic aerobic species may cause mortal septicemia upon access to the hemocoel. Bacteria characterized as primary pathogens of insects are able to penetrate the gut or integument of the host, facilitated by the production of a toxin or enzyme which predisposes the host tissue to invasion by the proliferating bacteria.

Smears of infected, dying or dead insects should be stained with Giemsa or Gram's stain. Watermounts examined by phase contrast microscopy reveal the motility of vegetative bacteria, which appear dark, whereas spores appear bright and other cellular or sporangial inclusions (e.g. parasporal crystals of *Bacillus thuringiensis*) appear moderately bright (Fig. 4(b), Fig. 1 of Chapter 10). When the specimen is initially processed for diagnosis, nutrient agar and blood agar media should be inoculated with infected tissue to obtain isolated, *in vitro,* colonies of the bacteria. After 24-48 hr incubation at about 25°C, stained smears of *in vitro* colonies are compared with the bacteria in the primary smear of the host. A qualitative and quantitative evaluation or estimate is made of the micro-organisms present in the specimen and those which grow on artificial media. Quantitative relations between the morphological types of bacteria present both in host and on media are studied to detect types of bacteria which do, or do not, grow on nutrient media under aerobic conditions. The pure cultures are transferred to agar slants and stored at 5°C pending determination. A specialist for the bacterial group in question should be consulted for specific determination. Pathogenicity of the bacteria can be determined following Koch's postulates (Section I).

Key 3. The Principal Entomophilic Bacteria[1]

1. Bacteria grow on nutrient media 2
   Bacteria do not grow on nutrient broth and nutrient agar 5

2. Sporulating rods 3
   Non-sporulating rods 4

3. Oral infection in larval honey-bees, producing viscous cadavers, adhering to walls of cells; groups of undulated flagella evident when smears stained with Giemsa . . . . *Bacillus larvae*[2]
   Oral infection limited to larval Lepidoptera; elongate sporangia produce one terminal spore and one bipyramidal crystal, Fig. 4(b) . . . . *Bacillus thuringiensis*[3]

[1] These bacteria, and those omitted, are keyed and described by Breed *et al.* (1957).
[2] Description, also other bacterial pathogens of bees (Heimpel and Angus, 1963; Bailey, 1963; Bucher, 1963).
[3] Key to related species, key to strains (de Barjac and Bonnefoi, 1968; Heimpel, 1967; Krieg, 1968). Definition of strains by esterase pattern and flagellar antigens (Norris, 1964). Review, host range (Krieg, 1967).

4. Brick-red colonies at 72-120 hr on agar media . . . *Serratia marcescens*[4]
Bluish fluorescent colonies on nutrient agar at 72-120 hr . . . . *Pseudomonas aeruginosa*[4]
(Other colored or gray colonies are bacteria from the midgut growing in dead insects.)

5. In primary smears, navicular sporangia with oval spore and parasporal body, together appearing as a shoeprint shape. Infected hemolymph white. In terrestrial insects, scarabaeid grubs, Fig. 4(c) . . . . *Bacillus popilliae, B. fribourgensis*[5]
In primary smears, thick rods on food in gut in pin-cushion arrangement, restricted to the gut. Host body shortened, larvae of Lepidoptera . . . *Clostridium brevifaciens*[6]

D. FUNGI

Insects occupy virtually every ecological niche and a large proportion of the micro-organisms associated with them are characteristic of their immediate environment. Like bacteria, many fungi are opportunists; i.e. facultative parasites or saprophytes, and are not primary pathogens responsible for the disease condition. On the other hand, some primary fungal pathogens are responsible for restricting insect populations and sometimes cause impressive and conspicuous epizootics. Filaments of fungus mycelium, closely adhering to the host, and aerial hyphae with terminal conidia or spore-bearing structures above or within the mycelium are common (Figs 2(d), 3(c), (d)). Seeds and pollinia (stalked, pollen-bearing structures of plants such as orchids) attached to insects may be mistaken for fungal fructifications (illustrated in Steinhaus, 1949). They are easily recognized as they are readily detached—seeds without further treatment and pollinia after moistening the specimen with alcohol. A white dusting of pollen—soon recognized under the microscope—may also be mistaken for fungus.

The sexual and asexual reproductive elements, i.e. spores and conidia, have characteristic forms. Infectious or invasive motile spores each bearing a flagellum (zoospores, Fig. 2(b)) characterize species of Chytridiaceae and Blastocladiales, in aquatic insects, whose water habitat facilitates transmission of zoospores to susceptible hosts. Spores or conidia (Fig. 8) may be produced in asci (Ascomycetes), or on basal cells, phialides (Fig. 8(b), (f)), and conidiophores (Fig. 8(c)) characterizing the Fungi Imperfecti (Deuteromycetes) commonly isolated from moribund and dead insects.

[4] Review of species and related genera associated with insects and leads into taxonomic literature (Bucher, 1963).

[5] Descriptions, host range, culture (Steinhaus, 1949; Dutky, 1963).

[6] Review, description, host range, cultivation (Heimpel and Angus, 1963). Original descriptions, culture, pathology, etc. (Bucher, 1957, 1961). Serology (Hrubant and Rhodes, 1968). Non-pathogenic spp. (Stevenson, 1966).

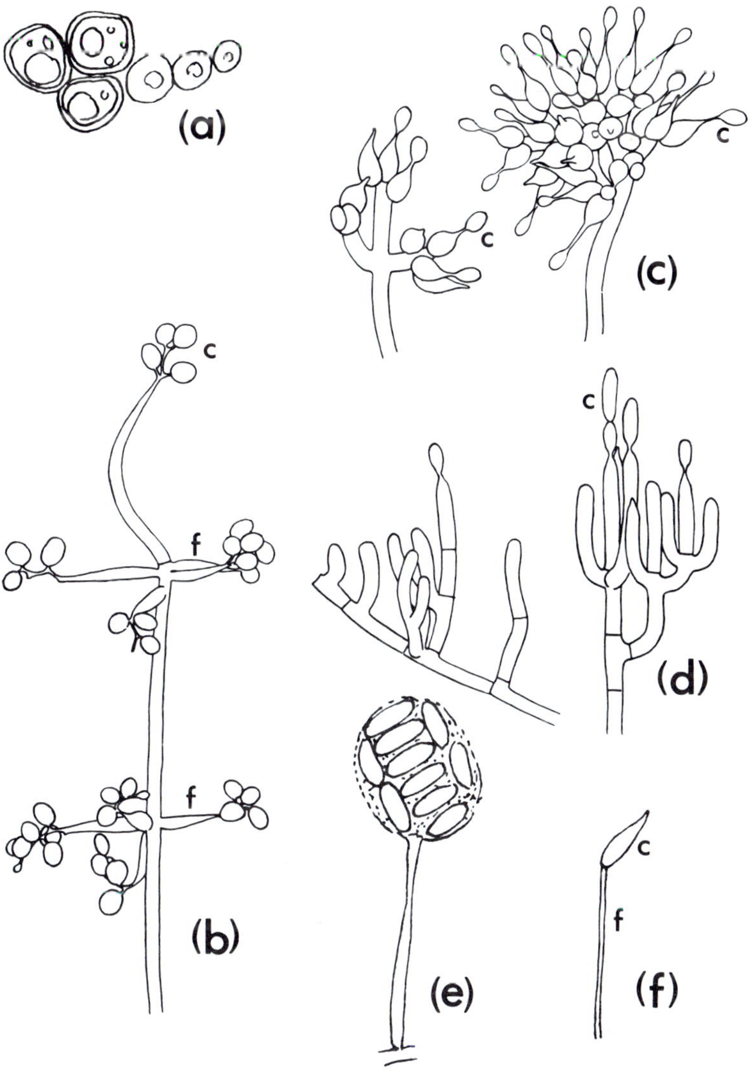

Fig. 8. (a): *Syngliocladium (Sorosporella)* hyphal bodies. (b): *Beauveria bassiana* from a slide culture on malt agar. (c): *Paecilomyces (Spicaria) farinosus* from coremia on naturally infected insects. (d): *Metarrhizium anisopliae* from a naturally infected froghopper. (e): *Cephalosporium* fruiting body within gelatinous sphere. (f): *Hirsutella* conidium. Phialides, f; conidia, c. Fig. 8(b), (c), (d) adapted from Madelin (1963).

Many of the fungi observed on moribund and dead hosts can be isolated and maintained on mycological media; e.g. maltose agar, potato-dextrose agar, or Sabouraud's medium.

Fungi of the genus *Entomophthora* (Zygomycetes, Entomophthorales), and their close relatives, regularly infect invertebrates. For cultivation, conidia of *Entomophthora* should be fresh. Infected insects are placed on small squares of agar stuck beneath the inside of the lid of a petri dish containing Sabouraud's agar or—better still—coagulated egg yolk. Conidia (Fig. 3(b)) fall to the surface of the medium in the sterile plate beneath and produce pure, uncontaminated cultures. Contamination of the isolation medium with other fungi will cause competition and loss of the culture (this also applies to many other entomogenous fungi). An *Entomophthora* colony has a characteristic "velvet-like" wavy surface growth. For identification of a fungus responsible for a mycosis, all developmental stages should be available. Whole mounts of infected small animals in cotton-blue lactophenol are important if resting spores, conidia, and hyphal bodies are present (Figs 3(a), 8). If the host specimen is fixed to the substrate, rhizoids or filaments attaching the insect body should be preserved. Often the conidia of the fungus are distributed in a ring around the host body (Fig. 3(b)). In many instances, when insects are not attached to the substrate, conidia may be distributed on the surface of the legs and wings. Resting spores (Fig. 3(a)) may be found in the interior of the host body, or also on its surface. It is important to detect the number of nuclei in the conidia and resting spores by fixing material and staining with Heidenhain's iron hematoxylin.

Another common genus, *Coelomomyces* (Chytridiomycetes, Blastocladiales), commonly infects invertebrates. Under a dissecting microscope, or low power of a compound microscope, the large, thick-walled, sculptured, 28-50 μ-long sporangia (Fig. 2(c)) may be seen, together with hyphal bodies, through the cuticle of aquatic insects. When an insect is dissected in water, the hyphal bodies, which do not possess a resistant surface membrane, appear to dissolve. To isolate the hyphal bodies, it is necessary to fix the insect in 7% formalin or alcohol before dissection. Sporangia may be isolated from dissected specimens or dried moribund hosts. Fixed, infected mosquito larvae can be mounted in Berlese's fluid or stained *in toto* with cottonblue-lactophenol, or borax-carmine, or other water-soluble stains, washed and passed through an alcohol series to xylol and mounted in balsam. *Coelomomyces* spp. are not cultivated *in vitro.*

Key 4. The Principal Entomophilic Fungi[1]

1. Host without external fungus growth 2
   Host with external hyphal growth, Fig. 3(c), (d) 11

[1] A number of genera containing some insect pathogens or facultative pathogens have been omitted (Table I in Chapter 5). These, and saprophytic fungi, can be identified to

2. Infected insect hard, dry or flaccid 3
   Infected insect soft, alive (aquatic insects) 9

3. Body intact 4
   Body with caverns, opening as holes or broken parts of cuticle . . . 8

4. Body color unchanged or white, with hyphal masses filling whole body . . IMMATURE FUNGUS INFECTION, FUNGI IMPERFECTI
   Body color changed 5

5. Body color yellow, in scale insects, with thick-walled spherical spores . . . *Myiophagus ucrainicus*[2]
   Body color brown or red 6

6. Body color brown to black, interior empty, layer of dark resting spores beneath cuticle . . . . *Tarichium*[3]
   Body color red 7

7. Interior of body filled with red, dust-like prickly spores . . . . *Tarichium cleoni*[3]
   Interior of body filled with red yeast-like cells, Figs 4(a), 8(a) . . . . . *Syngliocladium (Sorosporella)*[4]

8. Body opens in one or two spherical caverns . . . . *Strongwellsea*[5]
   Abdomen broken ventrally, brown dust of spores . . . . *Massospora*[6]

9. Many spherical pink sporangia filling body cavity, mature sporangia contain multinucleated masses or uniflagellate zoospores, in blackflies, Fig. 2(b) *Coelomycidium simulii*
   Body containing a yellow cheesy mass 10

10. Dense yellow mass of smooth oval cysts with a lateral tube and operculum, Ephemerids . . . . *Polycaryum ecdyonuris*

---

genera and often to species using keys and descriptions by Ainsworth (1967); Bessey (1952) incorporates a good guide to identification literature; Clements and Shear (1931); Barron (1968, Fungi Imperfecti, difficult to use); Barnett (1960, Fungi Imperfecti, easy to use); Raper and Fennell (1965, monograph on *Aspergillus*); Raper and Thom (1949) and Kulik (1968) on *Penicillium*; Booth (1966, *Fusarium*). See also chalkbrood (*Ascosphaera apis*) and stonebrood (*Aspergillus flavus*) diseases of honey-bee (Bailey, 1963); monograph of *Sporotrichum* (Müller, 1964-65), key to species (Fassatiová, 1967); taxonomy of *Tilachlidium* and *Synnematium* (Mains, 1951).

[2] Description of species (Karling, 1948).

[3] Forms only resting spores in the host. Recent record (Müller-Kögler, 1962).

[4] Morphology, pathology (Speare, 1920).

[5] Description, comparison with related genera (Batko and Weiser, 1965).

[6] Description of species (Soper, 1963). Review, morphology, pathology, hosts etc. (Macleod, 1963).

Long delicate hyphal branches and oval, irregular, sculptured sporangia, in mosquitoes and midges, Fig. 2(c) . . . . *Coelomomyces*[7]

11. Long, horn-like protrusions from host body, no mycelium over body . 12
Body covered by cotton-like mycelium, with hyphae and conidia . . 13

12. Few wire-like protrusions with thickened ends, Fig. 2(d) . . *Cordyceps*[8]
Brush-like groups of protrusions, tapering, without hyphae inside insect, on living insects . . . . LABOULBENIACEAE

13. Conidia discharged around host body, Fig 3(b) . . . *Entomophthora*[9]
Conidia fixed to hyphae 14

14. Blue-green conidial masses in columns, Fig. 3(d) *Metarrhizium anisopliae*[10]
White or pink conidial masses 15

15. Hard fungus cushion on surface of scale insects, conidia fusoid, septate . . *Aschersonia*[11]
Powdery conidial masses 16

16. Conidia not in chains 17
Conidia in chains on ends of phialides, Fig. 8(c) . *Paecilomyces (Spicaria)*[12]

17. Conidia single on end of solitary phialides, Fig. 8(f) . . . . *Hirsutella*[13]
Conidia in groups on phialides, Fig. 8(b), (e) 18

18. Conidia in gelatinous spheres on ends of phialides, Fig. 8(e) . . . . . *Cephalosporium*[14]

[7] Aquatic fungi only. Morphology, cytology (Umphlett, 1962, 1964; Lum, 1963). Comprehensive review, lists of species and hosts, morphology, biology, etc. (Couch and Umphlett, 1963). Review of more recent information (Madelin, 1966). New Zealand species (Pillai and Smith, 1968). Key to species (Laird, 1959).

[8] Review of taxonomy, morphology, pathogenesis, culture, species and hosts (McEwen, 1963). Taxonomy, generic characters, species and host lists (Kobayasi, 1941; Mains, 1958). Good account of a single species (Mathieson, 1949) and species found on the cicada (Kobayasi and Shimizu, 1963).

[9] Key to order Entomophthorales, family Entomophthoraceae, review of genus *Entomophthora,* species list, morphology etc. (MacLeod, 1963). Key to Entomophthoraceae, recognizing many new genera, mostly not distinguished in the present book (Weiser, 1966). Key to 39 species of *Entomophthora,* distribution map, host list, cultivation (Hutchison, 1963). Key, descriptions of species on aphids (Gustafsson, 1965). Generic characters, culture (Srinivasan *et al.,* 1964).

[10] Review of taxonomy, morphology, sporulation, host etc. (Madelin, 1963). Good description (Radha *et al.,* 1956). Selective isolation medium (Veen and Ferron, 1966). Monospore culture and determination of nucleus numbers (Veen, 1967).

[11] Description of N. American species on Aleyrodidae (white flies) (Mains, 1959).

[12] Review of taxonomy, morphology, sporulation, host etc. (Madelin, 1963). Taxonomy of species and genus, key (Brown and Smith, 1957); extension of Brown and Smith's key (Leatherdale, 1965).

[13] Review of taxonomy (Mains, 1951).

[14] Comprehensive accounts of *C. lecanii* (Ganhaõ, 1956).

Conidia not in gelatinous masses 19

19. Conidia in whorl on end of conidiophore . . . . *Isaria*[15]
Conidia on elongated phialide, alternately attached on either side, Fig. 8(b) . *Beauveria*[16]

E. PROTOZOANS

The diversity in form (Figs 5, 6, 7, 9, 10) among the protozoans associated with insects and their functional association as host or vector is unparalleled in documented biology. Three groups predominate among the parasitic forms associated with invertebrates, particularly insects: Sarcomastigophora (amoebae, flagellates), Sporozoa (gregarines, coccidia), and Cnidospora (microsporida). These are broadly distinguished in Key 2. The obligate parasites and entomophilic groups in each of these major categories are characterized by a resistant sporulated or encysted stage, and frequently intracellular reproductive forms. During the cyclic development of the parasite, resistant forms (Figs 5, 6, 7) may be detected within the gut lumen and hemocoel of the host, and reproductive forms within host cells (Figs 9, 10).

For diagnosis, insects are dissected and tissues are mounted in water under a cover-slip. When protozoan specimens appear to be present, a portion of the infected host tissue is used for smears and another portion fixed for histology. The organ and tissue site of the parasite should be identified; e.g. the lumen of the gut, gut cells, Malpighian tubules, the fat body, or hemocytes. The obligate parasitic protozoans develop in tissues, and only the spores or encysted forms are shed from the host tissues and are moved with feces or urate crystals in the gut or the Malpighian tubes, or are free in the hemolymph. Many commensal and mutualistic flagellates (Fig. 5(a)), amoebae, and eugregarines (Figs 5(c), 9(f)) occur only in the lumen of the gut. The Eugregarinida are commensals, oval to elongate, flat, the body divided into two sections with a nucleus in the larger portion (Figs 5(c), 9(f)). The small section may bear a small protuberance, the epimerite (Fig. 9(f)), attaching the eugregarine to the host gut wall at certain periods in its development. Thus the investigator is obliged to distinguish a great variety of commensals from the parasitic forms. Since they are not described here, the researcher is referred to introductory literature and reference volumes such as Kudo (1966), and Grassé (1952-53). Other works include Théodoridès (1955), Watson (1916, 1922), Lipa (1967) and Berberet and Helms (1969), who describe two *Eugregarina*.

Extensive taxonomic descriptions of representatives of the whole phylum are

[15] Taxonomic study (Brown and Smith, 1957).

[16] Thorough taxonomic study (MacLeod, 1954). Review of mycelial form, spore formation, perithecia etc. (Madelin, 1966). Review of signs and symptoms, host range, strains, life-cycle, cultivation etc. (Madelin, 1963). Selective medium for *B. tenella* (Veen and Ferron, 1966). Media, good biological study (Schaerffenberg, 1964).

given by Kudo (1966), Grassé (1952-53) and Jahn and Jahn (1949); those found in insects are described by Steinhaus (1946, 1949) and Weiser (1966, 1969).

1. Ciliates

Ciliata are rarely parasites of insects. They are commonly encountered in dead animals (e.g. the genus *Colpoda*). The free-living forms develop from cysts that are eaten with the food. Sessile ciliates, often with contractile stalks (e.g. *Vorticella* and the colonial *Carchesium*), are epibionts on the surface of aquatic insects. As infectious agents (Lipa, 1963), ciliates must be described and evaluated from the living host (e.g. *Tetrahymena chironomi* in chironomids, Corliss, 1960). Watermounts of hosts bearing ciliates, or isolated ciliate specimens, should be examined by phase contrast microscopy to detect fine structure. The rapid movements of the protozoan ciliation or contractions may be retarded by adding a drop of an aqueous methyl-cellulose solution to the watermount. India ink, mixed in approximately equal parts with the fluid containing the protozoans, spread on a slide, allowed to dry, then sealed with a cover glass and mounting medium provides "relief staining" where the parts of the protozoans are visible against a dark background.

2. Amoebae

Parasitic amoebae in insects occur in the Malpighian tubules or the gut. Amoeboid forms adhere to the surface or pass into the tubule cells. Terminal cyst forms (Fig. 5(b)) of the parasite leave with the excretory products of the Malpighian tubes and mix with feces. Two important, frequently detected, amoebae infections occur in some Orthoptera and Hymenoptera.

Key 5. Amoebae Diseases of Orthoptera and Hymenoptera

Malpighian tubes of Orthoptera; oval, regular cysts, Fig. 5(b) refringent uninucleate 7-10 μ long; trophozoites (motile forms) with broad round pseudopodia . . . . *Malamoeba locustae*

Malpighian tubes of honey-bee; broadly oval to spherical, thin-walled spores (cysts); trophozoites with finger-like pseudopodia and a motile flagellum . *Malpighamoeba mellificae*

Lipa (1963) reviews insect-parasitic amoebae. Henry (1968) illustrates *M. locustae* and describes its incidence and control. Giordani (1959) and Bailey (1963) illustrate *M. mellificae*, its biology and control.

3. Sporozoans

Parasitic sporozoans in insects occur in three groups, Haemosporina, Neogregarinida and Coccidia. The stages in their development are schizogonic

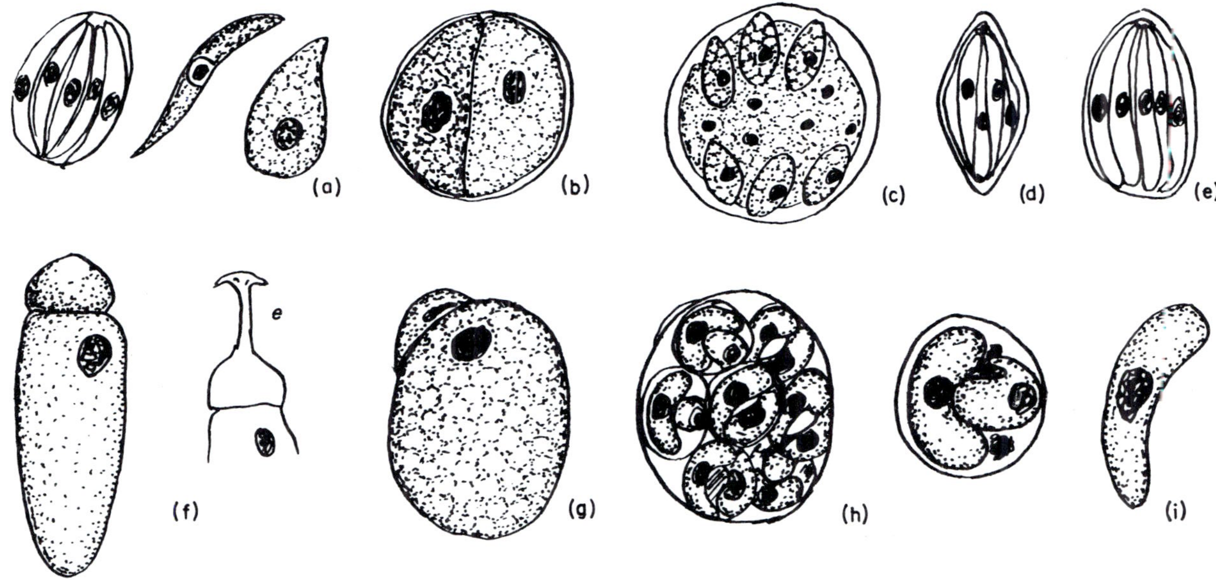

Fig. 9. (a)-(e): Neogregarinida ((a) schizogony; (b) zygote; (c) cyst with developing spores; (d) navicular; and (e) sac-like spore with sporozoites). (f): Trophozoite of an eugregarine; *e*, another with epimerite. (g)-(i): Coccidia zygote and spore formation in *Adelina*. Schematic, different magnifications.

(Fig. 9(a)), which divide vegetatively by fission and rapidly increase the number of parasites in the host, and sporogonic (Figs 9(b), (c), (d), (e)), involving gametes and the production of spores. The most important forms for initial detection of sporozoan infections are the resting or resistant forms, the cysts and spores. The detection and identification of additional stages in the life-cycle of a particular parasite serves to support a diagnosis.

Key 6. Principal Sporozoan Pathogens of the Class Telosporea Infecting Insects

Parasites within cysts on gut wall, multinucleate ookinetes (motile worm-shaped zygotes) within body cavity and elongate sporozoites (infective stage) in salivary glands of blood-sucking insects; no spores formed and no schizogony in insects . . . . .SUB-ORDER HAEMOSPORINA

Parasites in wall of gut, wall of Malpighian tubes or in fat body; oval to navicular spores; eight sporozoites in interior of spores; isogametes, Figs 5(d), 9(a)-(e) . . ORDER NEOGREGARINIDA (SCHIZOGREGARINIDA)

Parasites in fat body, occasionally in wall of gut, spores spherical to sub-oval, with resting body; microgametes and macrogametes, Figs 6(a), 9(g)-(i) . . SUB-CLASS COCCIDIA

Haemosporina, which are primarily parasites of vertebrates, occur in their insect vectors and may be pathogenic insofar as they invade the tissues of the vector in the process of transmission; e.g. a malaria parasite in mosquitoes. The determination of forms of a parasite in a vector is possible only if its cycle and localization in the insect are known or proven by experiment.

Neogregarinida (Schizogregarina) are parasites of the fat body, Malpighian tubes or gut of insects. Weiser (1955d) revised the order. Large numbers of schizogonic forms (Fig. 9(a)) are produced and schizogony continues as long as susceptible tissue is available. Nuclei of different sizes may occur in schizogonic trophozoites. Eventually the offspring of schizogony join in pairs and encyst. Gametes, of equal size and shape, are formed, giving rise to zygotes within the cyst (Fig. 9(b)). Each zygote becomes a multinucleate plasmodium which divides and forms spores (Fig. 9(c)). As soon as the spores have access to oxygen outside the host body, the sporoplasm differentiates and each produces up to 128 sporozoites (Fig. 9(d), (e)). When ingested by a new host, spores burst at one or both poles. For light microscopy, the parasite may be detected in smears or watermounts, fixed in Bouin's and stained with Heidenhain's hematoxylin, or identified in histological sections of host tissue.

Key 7. Neogregarinida

1. Two distinct schizogonic cycles (macro- and micronuclear), family Ophryocystidae 2

One distinct schizogonic cycle (macronuclear), family Schizocystidae . 3

2. Gametes mononucleate at initiation of syzygy (end-wise association) . 4
Gametes multinucleate at initiation of syzygy 5

3. Spores vesicular, thin-walled 8
Spores navicular, thick-walled 9

4. Trophozoites and schizonts attached to host cells by rhizopodia multinuclear, cysts monosporous . . . . *Ophryocystis*[1]
Trophozoites without rhizopodia, intracellular 6

5. Worm-like trophozoites with longitudinal myonemes, four spores in cyst . . *Machadoella*[2]
Spherical trophozoites without myonemes, eight spores in cyst . . . . . *Farinocystis*[3]

6. Trophozoites with pseudomerite, 1-2 spores in cyst . . . . *Mattesia*[4]
Trophozoites without pseudomerite, more than two spores in cyst . . 7

7. Up to 40 spores in cyst . . . . *Menzbieria*[5]
More than 10, less than 20 spores in cyst . . . . *Lipocystis*[6]

8. Cyst with one spore only . . . . *Tipulocystis*[7]
Cyst with eight spores . . . . *Caulleryella*[8]

9. Trophozoites spherical to subspherical cysts elongated with 32 spores . . . *Schizocystis*[9]
Trophozoites worm-like, bud into pyriform merozoites 10

10. Spores with polar spines . . . . *Syncystis*[10]
Spores without spines . . . . *Lipotropha*[11]

Coccidia infect cells of the fat body and gut wall of insects. Schizogony is similar to that of the Neogregarinida. The final stages are the micro- and macrogamete. The final microgamete is a minute crescent-shaped body which adheres to the oval macrogamete (Figs 6(a), 9(g)) where its remnant can be

[1] Description of genus, Leger (1907).
[2] Description of genus, biology, and techniques, Reichenow (1935).
[3] Illustration of single species in *Tribolium* sp., Dissanaike (1955).
[4] Pathology of infection, Finlayson (1950).
[5] Illustration and methods, Weiser (1955a).
[6] Description of single species, Grell (1938).
[7] Description, illustration, and parasitology, Kramář (1950).
[8] Description of single species, Bresslau and Buschkiel (1919).
[9] Description and methods for study in larval Diptera, Keilin (1923a).
[10] Description of single species, Weiser (1955b).
[11] Biology and methods for study, Keilin (1923b).

observed on the surface of the zygote until sporulation. Spores are contained within the oocyst (Figs 6(a), 9(h)) which is formed within the wall of the zygote. Each spore (Fig. 9(i)) bears two or more sporozoites and a resting body which functions by enlargement, as a bursting organ, releasing the sporozoites (Fig. 9(i)), when the spore is ingested by the host. The stages of the coccidia have the staining properties characteristic of the Neogregarinida.

Key 8. Coccidia

1. Gametocytes similar, microgametocytes with several hundred nuclei; one sporozoite in a bivalve spore in gut wall . . . . *Barrouxia*[1]
   Gametocytes dissimilar, microgametocytes with five nuclei; spores not bivalve, containing 2-6 sporozoites, Figs 6(a), 9(g)-(i) 2
2. Spores in cysts 3
   Spore wall not formed, sporozoites within oocyst wall . . . *Legerella*[2]
3. Cyst with three spores, each with 4-6 sporozoites . . . . *Chagasella*[3]
   Cyst with four spores . . . . *Ithania*[4]
   Cyst with 10 or more spores, each with two sporozoites, Figs 6(a), 9(g)-(i) . *Adelina*[5]

4. Cnidospora

The subphylum Cnidospora includes the Order Microsporida (Class Microsporidea), which is most commonly adapted and widely distributed in invertebrates, particularly insects. Transmission of the parasite from host to host may be oral or transovarial.

The microsporida are characterized by a brief schizogony (Fig. 10(k), left) resulting in stages that have closely adjacent, paired nuclei, the diplokaryon. The stage is considered by some authorities to be the autogametes (Fig. 10(k), centre). The nuclei separate, produce chromosomes, and divide. Meiotic figures have been observed by some authorities in thin sections by electron microscopy, the resulting stage being considered to be the gametes. Initiation of the sporogony by gamete fusion produces a sporont (Fig. 10(l), (n), (o), left) from which a series of plasmodia (Fig. 10(q), centre) or uninucleate stages (Fig. 10(k), fourth right) are formed prior to spore formation. The plasmodia divide into elongated uninucleate elements, the sporoblasts (Fig. 10(o), second left), around

[1] Biology, parasitology, and techniques, Reyer (1937).
[2] Illustration and identification, Vincent (1927).
[3] Life-cycle and biology, Machado (1913).
[4] Biology and techniques for several tipulid protozoa, Ludwig (1947).
[5] Biology and identification, Yarwood (1937).

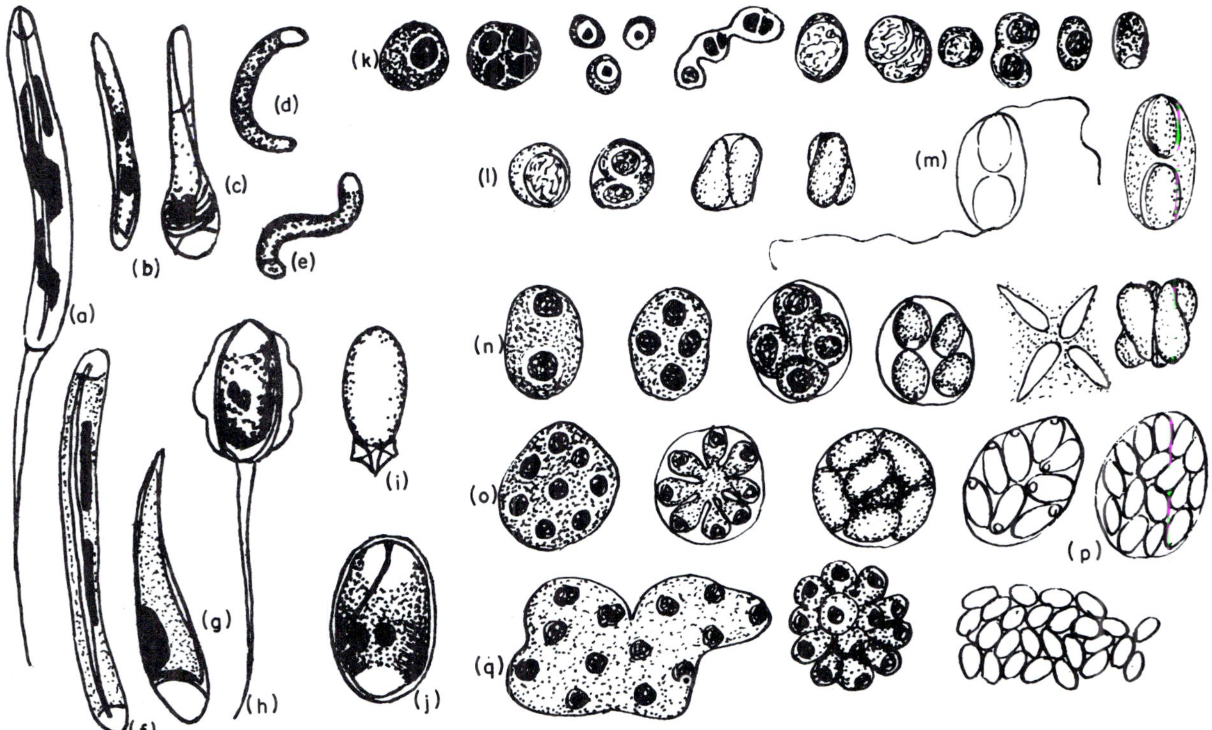

Fig. 10. Microsporida. (a): *Mrázekia.* (b): *Octosporea.* (c): *Cougourdella.* (d): *Toxoglugea.* (e): *Spiroglugea.* (f): *Bacillidium.* (g): *Pyrotheca.* (h): *Caudospora.* (i): *Weiseria.* (j): *Nosema.* (k): Development of *Nosema.* (l): *Perezia.* (m): *Telomyxa.* (n): *Gurleya.* (o): *Thelohania.* (p): *Duboscquia.* (q): *Plistophora.* Schematic drawings.

each of which a resistant spore wall is formed (Fig. 10(j)). Within the spore it is possible to detect the end of a polar filament, crossing an anterior polar vacuole (Fig. 10(c)) the posterior vacuole and the sporoplasm (Fig. 10(j)). In fixed and stained smears where spores have not released the polar filaments, the spores are characterized by two unstained regions at the poles and the stained sporoplasm is distributed in a central cone (Fig. 10(j)). A nucleus, or the nuclei, are stained with Giemsa after hydrolysis with *N*-HCl for 8 min at 61-62° C. The extrusion of the polar filament (Fig. 10(m)) from the spore is necessary to confirm that spores are those of a microsporidan. The filament may be forced from the spore when pressure, which may need to be very great, is applied on the cover-slip of a watermount preparation, or by drying a watermount and rewetting after about 30 min, or after exposure of the spores to hydrogen peroxide, Lugol's solution, or the saliva of insects. All stages of microsporidan parasites stain well with Giemsa on dry smears. For moribund host specimens, smears can be fixed in Bouin's fluid and stained with iron hematoxylin on a microscope slide and mounted under a cover-glass. Paraffin-embedded tissue, sectioned and stained with iron hematoxylin, provides excellent definition of the parasite life stages *in situ.* The taxonomy of microsporida is based upon the number and morphology of spores within each pansporoblast (Fig. 10(k)-(q), right). Detailed taxonomic studies were made by Kudo (1924) and Weiser (1961), and Thomson (1960) reviewed the host range of species, with short descriptions.

Key 9. Genera of the Order Microsporida

1. Spores oval to spherical, not more than twice longer than broad; range 0.5 μ-6.0 μ long 2
   Spores more than twice longer than broad 12

2. Spores with lateral or polar crests and appendages, Fig. 10(h), (i) . . 3
   Spores without appendage or crest 4

3. Spores each with a long caudal appendage and lateral gelatinous crests, Figs 7(b), 10(h) . . . . *Caudospora*[1]
   Spores without appendages, each with a membranous polar crest, Fig. 10(i) . *Weiseria*[2]

4. Spores single, Figs 6(c), 10(k), or in pansporoblasts, Figs 7(a), 10(q), with more than 16 spores, number of spores varying widely (64-128) . 5
   Two, four, eight, Fig. 6(d), 16 or rarely 32 spores in each pansporoblast . 6

5. Spores mature singly, sporonts only mono- or binucleate, Figs 6(c), 10(j), (k) . . . . *Nosema*[3]

[1] Illustration of species in a new genus, Weiser (1947).
[2] Biology and techniques, Doby and Saguez (1964).
[3] Life-cycle and techniques, Kramer (1959a).

Spores in groups or pansporoblasts with irregular numbers of spores, plasmodia with irregular number of nuclei, Figs 7(a), 10(q) . . . . . *Plistophora*[4]

6. Pansporoblasts with four and eight, or eight and 16 spores present at once . *Stempellia*[5]
Only one type of pansporoblast present 7

7. Pansporoblasts with two spores 8
Pansporoblasts with more than two spores 9

8. Spores part under pressure, not in a common capsule, Fig. 10(1) . . . . *Perezia*[6], *Glugea*[6]
Spores end to end in a resistant common capsule, Fig. 10(m) . *Telomyxa*[7]

9. Pansporoblasts with four spores, Fig. 10(n) . . . . . . *Gurleya*[8]
Pansporoblasts all with eight or all with 16 spores 10

10. Pansporoblasts with eight spores, Figs 6(d), 10(o) . . . . *Thelohania*[9]
Pansporoblasts with 16 spores 11

11. Pansporoblasts with four long needles in walls . . . *Trichoduboscquia*[10]
Pansporoblasts without appendage, Fig. 10(p) . . . . . *Duboscquia*[11]

12. Spores tubular each with a needle-like structure (manubrium) inside; 2-20 μ in length, Fig. 10(a), (f) 13
Spores rod-shaped, Fig. 10(b), (c), (g), arched, Fig. 10(d), or sigmoidal, Fig. 10(e), without manubrium 14

13. Spores with caudal appendage, Fig. 10(a) . . . . *Mrázekia*[12]
Spores tubular without caudal appendage 4-7 μ, Fig. 10(f) . *Bacillidium*[13]

14. Spores rod-shaped, Fig. 10(b), (c), (g) 15
Spores sigmoidal, or deeply arched, Fig. 10(d), (e) 17

15. Spores rod-shaped, both ends similar, Fig. 10(b) . . . . *Octosporea*[14]

[4] Description of single species, Canning (1957).
[5] Description and illustration of original genus determination, Paillot (1941).
[6] Life history and morphology, Kramer (1959b), McLaughlin (1969), Canning (1968).
[7] Biology and description, Codrenau (1961).
[8] Description and techniques for demonstration, Gibbs (1953).
[9] Description of single species in *Culex tarsalis,* Kellen and Lipa (1960).
[10] Occurrence and description, Leger (1926).
[11] Life history and techniques, Kudo (1941).
[12] Biology and morphology, Leger and Hesse (1916).
[13] Biology and life history, Jirovec (1936).
[14] Illustration and identity, Thomson (1935).

One end of spore broadened 16

16. Spores with clublike broadening at base, Fig. 10(c) . . *Cougourdella*[15]
Spores wedge-like, fore-end tapering, Fig. 10(g) . . . . *Pyrotheca*[16]

17. Spores deeply arched, eight in pansporoblast, Fig. 10(d) . *Toxoglugea*[17]
Spores sigmoidal, Fig. 10(e) . . . . *Spiroglugea*[18]

5. *Haplosporea (Class)*

A few insect pathogens have developmental stages very similar to microsporida but their spores have no polar filament and so are placed in the subphylum Sporozoa. They are on the borderline between primitive protozoans and fungi. They produce similar pansporoblasts to microsporida, with almost spherical spores. Their schizogony is similar to microsporida. *Haplosporidium bayeri,* with spherical multisporal pansporoblasts, is found in the fat body of ephemerid nymphs; *Haplosporidium typographi,* with spherical cysts of 20-40 spores occurs in the gut wall of bark beetles; and *Haplosporidium tipulae* (described and illustrated by Huger, 1961) occurs in the leatherjacket *(Tipula paludosa).* Weiser (1963) describes the group.

F. NEMATODES

Insects may be vectors of nematode parasites of vertebrates, associated phoretically with nematodes, hosts of entomophilic forms, or subject to combinations of these relationships. Five super-families of the phylum Nematoda may be intimately associated with insects, in addition to the groups identified primarily as parasites of vertebrates, yet found in insects. The latter are not considered here, and the interested investigator is referred to Chandler and Read (1961).

Nematodes of the super-family Oxyuroidea develop and reproduce within the gut of the host, the eggs passing with feces. Lesions of the gut may be detected in histological sections, although the nematodes are not documented as pathogenic. Orthoptera, Coleoptera, and rarely Lepidoptera are hosts. Members of the Aphelenchoidea, principally the gravid females, invade the hemocoel of bark beetles through the gut and enter the gonads where oocytes are sites of oviposition by the nematode.

Parasitic Tylenchoid nematodes invade the insects through a gravid female which produces eggs and miniature or juvenile forms in the hemocoel. Gonad tissue is a frequent site for juvenile development resulting in host reproductive

[15] Biology and description, Hesse (1935).
[16] Biology and description, Hesse (1935).
[17] Description of single species, Poisson (1940).
[18] Biology and description, Fantham and Porter (1958).

sterility. The juveniles leave the host and mature. Larval or juvenile forms often are found encapsulated in a connective tissue sheath or cyst within the host. Hosts occur among the Coleoptera (frequently bark beetles), Hymenoptera, Diptera, and Lepidoptera.

The families Diplogasteridae and Steinernematidae (super-family Rhabditoidea), and the Mermithidae (super-family Mermithoidea) are the specimens frequently detected in diagnosis.

Diplogasteridae and Steinernematidae (Fig. 7(c)) characteristically introduce bacteria into the host insect, initiating a fatal septicemia which kills the host in several hours, providing the substrate for nematode development and reproduction. Their infecting and invading forms (Fig. 7(c)) can be "trapped" for collection and isolation when larvae of the greater wax moth *(Galleria mellonella)* are placed in an environment infested with the nematodes. The invasive forms of the nematode, generally ensheathed larval forms (juveniles) enter the wax moth larvae, mature and reproduce for continued rearing in the laboratory. If the host body is not dried entirely and is placed on a moistened filter paper, the nematode larvae emerge on the paper from which they can be collected, washed in water and used to infect more moth larvae in fresh dishes. Inside the larvae, a "giant" generation of long nematode females (10-15 mm) develops, followed by subsequent generations, small by comparison, yet overwhelming the host with ensheathed (infective stage) larvae, in 24-40 hr. The pathogenic members of the Mermithidae (Fig. 7(d)) enter and develop in the insect body, and mortally wound the host on emerging.

Nematodes are isolated from insects during dissection of the host. If the host is dead, dissection in glycerine or lactophenol is useful. Upon detection of a nematode specimen, carefully remove it to a microscope slide beneath a glass cover-slip. Identify its internal organization and determine if it is a mature form with ovaries or testes (the male possessing spicules on the bent end of the body), or an undifferentiated juvenile form. Immature forms may be short (rhabditoid) or long (filaroid). The important diagnostic characters of nematodes are concentrated on the anterior and caudal portions of their bodies (Fig. 11). The stoma is protected with lip papillae and a musculature envelops the esophagus, divided morphologically into a procorpus, metacorpus and the posterior bulb. Between the procorpus and metacorpus there may be a slight constriction. The isthmus is the region between the metacorpus and bulb. The nerve ring or brain encloses the isthmus. A distinct valve functions between the bulb and the intestine. Ventral and dorsal esophageal ducts are important taxonomic characters, as in the presence or absence of a stylet and its position within the stoma. Males bear a row of anal papillae and a filamentous tail, the morphology of both characters is important taxonomically. Further literature is to be found in the following good comprehensive texts: Chitwood and Chitwood (1950), good for the higher taxonomic categories; Filipjev and Schuurmanns Stekhoven

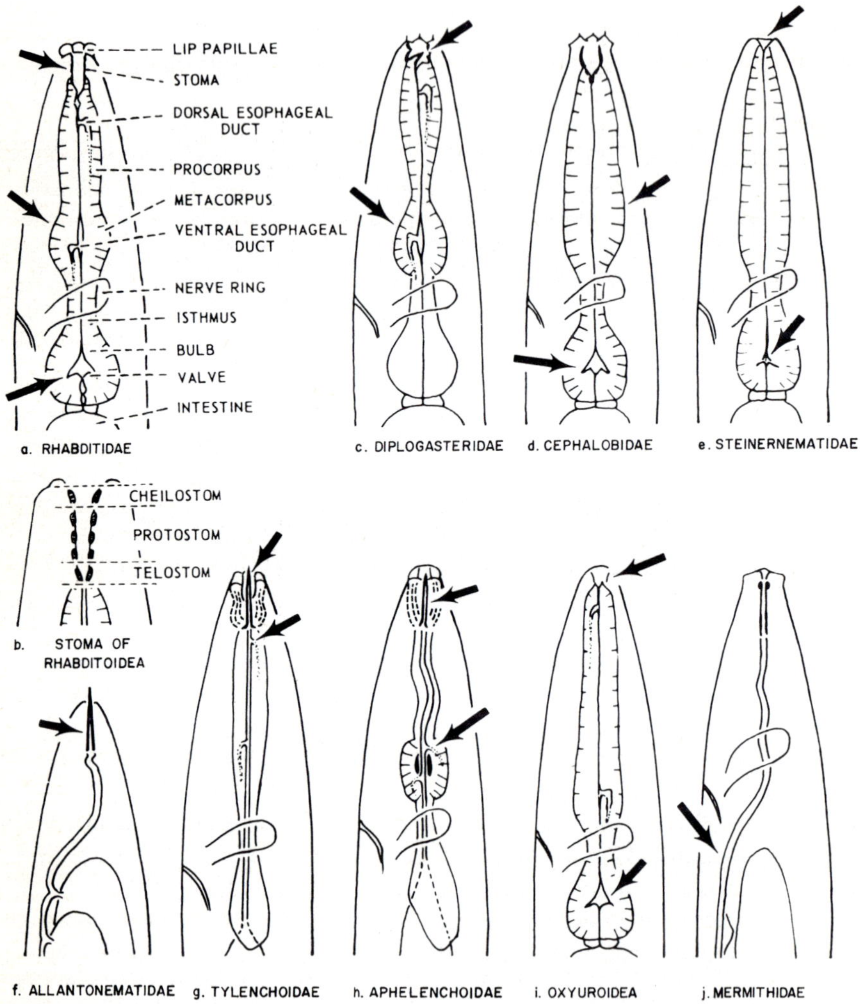

Fig. 11. Schematic representation of the heads of representatives of nine super-families and families of nematodes. The arrows indicate diagnostic characters. (Adapted from Welch, 1963.)

(1941); Goodey (1957) and Thorne (1961), good for preservation and mounting techniques and treatment of some major divisions; Ruhm (1956) gives a useful key to larvae; Skryabin *et al.* (1954); Weiser (1966, 1969), Welch (1963, 1965) treat insect-pathogenic forms. Nickle (1967) revised the classification of the Sphaerulariidae.

Key 10. Principal Groups of Adult Entomophilic Nematodes

1. Long, thread-like nemas, more than x100 longer than thick, coiled in insect body, Fig. 7(d) 2
   Nemas less than x100 longer than thick, both ends tapering. In insect or on its surface; mature nemas and larvae found 3

2. Hard, chord-like nemas with regular surface pattern, usually brown, sexual stages in insect . . . . GORDIOIDEA[1]
   Thin, white nemas with smooth, soft surface, musculature degenerated in whole esophagus, only a thin esophageal duct; larval stages in insect, Figs 7(d), 11(j) . . . . MERMITHIDAE[2]

3. Oral opening with three lips, short stoma, no stylet, esophagus with corpus, isthmus, and bulb well-musculatured, Fig. 11(a), (b), (c), (d), (e), (i) 4
   Stoma with stylet fixed near base of esophageal duct, Fig. 11(g), (h) . 8

4. Short, tubular stoma; esophageal bulb with valve; nemas in anal ampule and gut content of insect, non-parasitic, Fig. 11(i) . . OXYUROIDEA[3]
   Stoma variable; six, three, or two lips, esophageal bulb with or without valve, in hemocoel or on surface of insect 5

5. Stoma deep 6
   Stoma shallow; metacorpus not swollen, bulb with reduced valve, giant females in first generation; bacteria kill host (neoaplectanoid nematodes with specific bacteria transmitted by larvae), Fig. 11(e) . . . . . . STEINERNEMATIDAE[4]

6. Smooth lips, deep stoma, sclerotized; metacorpus thickened, esophageal bulb with valve; in gut and Malpighian tubes of insect, non-parasitic, Fig. 11(a), (b). . . . . RHABDITIDAE[5]
   Lips with minute spines 7

7. Deep stoma with tooth-like valve, constriction between procorpus and

[1] Systematics, illustration (Sacchitano, 1958).
[2] Biology, techniques (Polozhentsev and Artyukhovskii, 1963).
[3] Biology, systematics, techniques (Basir, 1956; Leibersperger, 1960).
[4] Systematics, biology (Veremchuk, 1962); comparison of six species of *Neoaplectana* (Weiser, 1955c).
[5] Systematics, descriptions (Osche, 1952); cultivation, biology (Dougherty, 1960).

metacorpus, no valve in bulb, Fig. 11(c) . . . DIPLOGASTERIDAE[6]
(*Pristionchus l'heritieri* is a bacteria-transmitting pathogen in wood-boring and soil insects)

Deep stoma without valve, no constriction after procorpus, bulb with valve, non-parasitic, Fig. 11(d) . . . . CEPHALOBIDAE[7]

8. Dorsal esophageal duct opens in procorpus, at base of stylet, Fig. 11(a) (TYLENCHOIDEA) 9

Dorsal esophageal duct opens in musculatured metacorpus (APHELENCHOIDEA), Fig. 11(h). 10

9. Well-formed tubular esophagus; larvae in gut, adults in frass of beetles, Fig. 11(g) . . . . TYLENCHIDAE[8]

Esophagus reduced to only a thin tube; organs except gonads reduced and absorbed; parasitic, Fig. 11(f) . . . . . .ALLANTONEMATIDAE[9]
(*Bradynema, Allantonema, Howardula* have a free sexual generation and free fertile females deposit eggs in insects. *Sphaerulariopsis* has hypertrophic evaginate uterus)

10. Esophageal bulbus absent, fused with intestine (many genera of nematodes living in hemocoel of insect), Fig. 11(h) . APHELENCHOIDIDAE[10]

Esophageal bulbs soft, fusing with gut; gonads hypertrophic and uterus evaginated, the nema itself being a small appendage of it . . . . . SPHAERULARIIDAE[11]

VIII. Methods

In this section a selection of methods of particular use with insect pathogens is described. The practical use of some of them is detailed by Martignoni and Steinhaus (1961). General reference works recommended for further information on histological techniques are Humanson (1967), Lillie (1965) and Reimer (1966).

A. FIXATIVES

The object of fixation is to preserve the physical structure of the living system, and to prepare it for chemical treatment that should aid the detection of

[6] Parasitic associations, biology (Bovien, 1937); systematics, description of species (Weingartner, 1955).
[7] Biology of the genus *Panagroliamus* Fuchs (Lazarevskaya, 1960).
[8] Biology, techniques for the super-family (Thorne, 1961).
[9] Biology, systematics (Wachek, 1955).
[10] Classification of species (Allen, 1960).
[11] Hosts of *Sphaerularia bombi* (Stein, 1956); biology of *S. bombi* (Pouvreau, 1962). Revision of classification transferring the Sphaerulariidae from the Aphelenchoidea to the Tylenchoidea (Nickle, 1967).

structures using light or electron microscopy. In addition, the nature and location of chemical entities characterizing life processes may be preserved by fixation. The nature of the organisms and structures of interest will influence the selection of materials and methods.

Material should be fixed rapidly and immediately to avoid deterioration of structures. Fixation should start in all parts of the organism simultaneously. To achieve the best definition of structure, maximal specimen surface area must be exposed to the fixative, and enzyme activity in host cells minimized by low temperature. For example, resolution of subcellular structure requires that individual cells be exposed by finely chopping tissue in cold chemical fixative, with further processing in an ice bath. In contrast, the setae on the surface of a mosquito larva may be easily distinguished on a specimen killed and fixed with any preservative.

Formalin is a universally available fixative, simple to prepare. Whole insects or tissues, fixed and held in formalin, do not degenerate in storage and may be transported easily because the tissues are hard. Exposure to high tropical temperatures or saprophytic organisms does not threaten the quality of the specimens. However, distortion of structure and shrinkage of tissue may characterize a formalin-fixed specimen. The definition of tissue structure and the quality and variety of staining for tissues fixed with formalin are inferior to tissues fixed with either Bouin's or Zenker's solutions. The latter should be used for small specimens, 3-4 mm in the largest dimension, and processed for histology immediately. Bouin's solutions (alcoholic and aqueous) provide for fixation and short-term storage, with indefinite storage of specimens in 70% alcohol. Alcoholic Bouin's penetrates better than the aqueous preparation, which minimizes distortion and shrinking of tissues. The glutaraldehyde-osmium tetroxide fixation procedure is best for maximum resolution using electron microscopy. The availability of reagents and the prevailing conditions may determine the choice of fixative: experience with a particular technique may outweigh all other considerations for selection of a method.

1. Heat

Air-dried smears of bacteria may be fixed by passing the slide rapidly, five or six times through the flame of a bunsen burner. Smears should be stained immediately; e.g., Gram's stain.

2. Methyl Alcohol

Flood air-dried smear with a thin film and allow to air dry before staining with Giemsa stain.

3. Formalin

Histological sections: 4% aqueous solution for 12 hours (hr) or more. Whole mount (e.g. mosquito larvae): 7% aqueous solution for 24 hr or more. A neutral solution (pH 7.0) is a useful emergency fixative for preparing tissue for electron microscopy when other preferred chemical fixatives are not available.

4. Zenker's

To 100 ml H_2O add: potassium bichromate 2.5 g, sodium sulfate 1.0 g, mercuric chloride 5.0 g. Before use add: 80% acetic acid 5 ml. Fix pieces of tissue not thicker than 3-4 mm for 12-24 hr, and wash tissue in running water for 2 hr before further processing. To eliminate precipitates, sections may be washed in Lugol's solution for several minutes.

5. Bouin's, Aqueous

Saturated aqueous picric acid solution 75 ml, formalin (40% solution) 25 ml, glacial acetic acid 5 ml. Fix for 12-24 hr or store the material in fixative. Before further processing, wash in H_2O for 4-6 hr to elute fixative.

6. Bouin's, Alcoholic (Bouin-Duboscq)

Ethyl alcohol (80%) 150 ml, formalin (40% solution) 60 ml, glacial acetic acid 15 ml, picric acid crystals 1 g. Fix for 1-3 days. Specimens may be removed directly to 95% EtOH for further processing or stored indefinitely by removing from the fixative to 70% EtOH.

7. Glutaraldehyde-Osmium Tetroxide

Fixation and embedding for electron microscopy are described below together for the sake of continuity. A source of the chemicals is Polysciences, Inc., Rydal, Pennsylvania, 19046, U.S.A.

i. Cut tissue, covered with glutaraldehyde fixative, into pieces not more than 1 mm in the largest dimension.

ii. Fix for 2-4 hr in 5% buffered glutaraldehyde (19 ml 0.2 *M*-monobasic sodium phosphate, 81 ml 0.2 *M*-dibasic sodium phosphate, 60 ml distilled H_2O, 40 ml glutaraldehyde 25% solution).

iii. Wash tissue for 1 hr in buffer (19 ml 0.2 *M*-monobasic sodium phosphate, 81 ml 0.2 *M*-dibasic sodium phosphate, 100 ml distilled H_2O).

iv. Fix for 6-8 hr in 1% buffered OsO_4. (The following aqueous solutions should be mixed immediately before use: 37.3 ml of 2.26% $NaH_2PO_4 \cdot H_2O$, 7.7 ml of 2.52% NaOH, 5.0 ml of 5.4% glucose, 0.5 g OsO_4 crystal.)

v. Wash tissue in distilled H_2O for 5 min, with subsequent immersion for 5 min in each of the following methyl alcohols, 35, 50, 70, 80, 95%; then absolute 10 min; finally propylene oxide 30 min.

vi. Embed tissue in resin (Vestopal, Araldite) for sectioning as follows: Epoxy Resin : propylene oxide, 1 : 2, 1 hr. Epoxy Resin : propylene oxide, 1 : 1, 1 hr. Epoxy Resin : propylene oxide, 2 : 1, 1 hr. Overnight in pure resin. Next day, put freshly mixed resin in gelatin capsules and drop single pieces of tissue into each capsule. The resin consists of 20 ml Epon 812, 20 ml Araldite (Epoxy Resin 506), 60 ml dodecenylsuccinic anhydride (freshly mixed) with 2.0 ml DMP 30 added to accelerate just before use.

vii. Place capsules at 74° C for 3 days. Remove and cool for 1 hr. Drop hardened capsules into warm water to dissolve gelatin capsules. Trim resin with embedded tissues and section on ultramicrotome for electron microscopy.

B. EMBEDDING

An experienced histologist with good facilities will provide maximum return upon the effort of collecting and protecting specimens for analysis. The selection of embedding procedures depends upon whether priority is given to specificity of pathogen location in the host, within an organ, tissue, or cell; morphology of the pathogen and the need for measurements and photographic record; dispatch with which the information is required; and also the nature of the specimen. General procedure: EtOH 70% 12 hr, EtOH 96% 6 hr, EtOH : ButOH 1 : 1 12 hr, ButOH 6 hr, ButOH : paraffin 1 : 1 12 hr, paraffin 6 hr under vacuum.

1. Paraffin

Paraffin wax is universally available and handled with most hydrocarbon solvents. Routine techniques are treated in all histology reference works. Intact sections less than 6 μ thickness cannot be expected, therefore precise definition of the morphology of a microbial pathogen or its location within specific cells should not be pursued by paraffin embedding.

2. Paraplast

A paraffin base medium compounded with plastic polymers (m.p. 56°-57° C), Paraplast, may be substituted for paraffin in a procedure for the latter. Sections to 6 μ thick may be expected if the tissue is of nearly equal hardness throughout. For example, the exoskeleton on the abdomen of a specimen should be removed before embedding in Paraplast to avoid excessive compression where thin sections are desired. Intact sections can be rapidly produced if the thickness of sections is acceptable.

3. Ester Wax

Ester wax, 1960, is a diethylene glycoldisterate base medium, harder than paraffin and with melting point slightly lower, from The British Drug Houses, Ltd., BDH Laboratory Chemicals Division, Poole, Dorset, Great Britain. It is used to obtain sections to 4 μ thickness from a specimen characterized by tissues of different hardness; e.g. a head capsule. The identity of soft tissue is maintained without compression of thin sections. Good resolution of intracellular parasites is routinely obtained; e.g. to determine morphology and size of protozoan spores or proliferate forms. However, sections are produced more slowly than with Paraplast or paraffin. Details may be obtained from Steedman (1960).

4. *Electron Microscopy*

Embedding procedures for electron microscopy are included with the appropriate techniques for fixation (Section VIII.A.7).

C. STAINS

1. *Giemsa*

Dry smears fixed with methyl alcohol are stained for 30-60 min with a fresh solution of 1-2 drops of stock stain to 1 ml of distilled water. Wash with running water and dry. Permanent preparations may be mounted with a cover glass and a neutral medium (Caedax, Euparal). Immersion oil, used with light microscopy, must be washed from the surface of stained smears with chloroform. Smears pre-treated with *N*-HCl for 8 min at 61-62°C and stained with Giemsa will show nuclei in the spores of protozoans. Smears of polyhedra, treated with 1% HCl (80-100°C) or cold 1% NaOH, and stained with Giemsa will reveal the virions in the interior of polyhedra.

2. *Hematoxylin (iron)*

The mordant is 4% aqueous ferric ammonium sulfate. Stock stain is made by dissolving 10 g hematoxylin (basic) in 100 c.c. 95% EtOH and adding 900 c.c. H_2O. Smears or sections are soaked in mordant for 6-12 hr, washed in water, stained for 4-6 hr and rewashed in water. Differentiate with mordant to obtain a dark-gray color in sections and wash again in running water for 5 min. Repeat if necessary. For staining proteinaceous virus inclusions, pre-treat sections with 1% HCl (80-100°C) or cold 1% NaOH and stain as above.

3. *Cotton Blue Solution*

0.1-1% in water or lactophenol, for staining fungi and nematodes.

4. *India Ink Negative Staining*

One small drop of India ink is mixed with a drop of water containing tissues with microsporida or schizogregarines and a cover glass is applied. The preparation reveals any gelatinous capsules around spores, pansporoblasts and vegetative stages. After inspection, the cover-slip can be removed and the material dried as a smear, which may be fixed to provide the same staining properties as a normal smear.

5. Gram Stain

Air dry and heat fix a smear, then flood with 1% aqueous crystal violet on a staining rack for 1 min, wash in water 5 seconds (s), rinse in Lugol's iodine 1 min, differentiate 2 min in *n*-propyl alcohol bath, rinse in 2% aqueous safranin 1 min and rinse in tap water for 5 s. Gram positive bodies stain dark violet; gram negative red. When the gram reaction is used as a diagnostic character for bacteria, the portion of colonies from which smears are made must be actively growing because the gram reaction often alters with the age of cells. Colonies of unknown age should be subcultured and the age of the sampled colony and conditions of growth recorded with the Gram stain reaction.

6. Neutral Red

0.5-1% solution in absolute EtOH for 10-15 min stains the NR-bodies in rickettsial infections.

7. Zdrodovski and Golinevich (1960) Stain

Stock carbol fuchsin is 1 g basic fuchsin, 5 g phenol, 10 ml EtOH and 100 ml distilled water. For use, dilute stock by 10-15 drops to 10 ml double glass distilled water or phosphate buffer, pH 7.4. Air dry a smear, heat fix, stain 5 min, wash quickly in water, differentiate 1-3 s in weak acid (e.g. 0.5% citric or 0.15% acetic), wash well in water, counterstain 10 s in aqueous methyl blue, wash, blot dry, allow to air dry, wash in euparal essence and mount in euparal.

8. Sudan III

Saturated aqueous solutions for 10-15 min, stain fat droplets red.

D. SPECIMEN MOUNTING

1. Canada Balsam or Synthetic Resins (Caedex, Euparal, Piclolyte)

For preparation of permanent mounts of smears or sections, material must be dehydrated and brought to xylol before transfer to the mounting media. Specimens from water; e.g. mosquito larvae with spores of *Coelomomyces* fungi can be brought to Canada balsam containing 1% crystalline phenol without dehydration. This avoids the formation of water droplets and functions well for all kinds of moist materials.

2. Amann's Lactophenol

Amann's lactophenol is a mixture of 20 g crystalline phenol, 20 ml lactic acid, 10 c.c. glycerin and 20 ml water. Useful for fungi and nematodes, it is commonly used with 0.1% cottonblue for fixation of fungi prior to permanent mounting. After desiccation of the medium beneath the cover-glass, the edge of the cover-glass should be sealed with lacquer.

3. Berlese's (Hoyer's) Medium

Used for permanent whole mounts of small invertebrates, this medium has the excellent characteristic of clearing pigmented and sclerotized integument, thus revealing the internal structure of the specimen or the presence of certain parasites and pathogens. Specimens fixed in formalin can be removed directly to Berlese's medium. The ingredients should be mixed in the following sequence, adding the chloral hydrate after all the gum arabic is dissolved: gum arabic (flakes) 8 g, H_2O 8 ml, glycerin 5 ml, chloral hydrate 70 g, glacial acetic acid 3 ml. Filter with lint-free material. Berlese's medium can be thinned with water. Mounts on glass slides may be reclaimed by soaking slides in water.

E. COMPLEX MEDIA *IN VITRO*

Nutrient media for bacteria are given in special lists of commercial suppliers (e.g. Oxoid, 1965; Difco, 1953). A large array of special media for isolation and maintenance of bacteria and fungi are supplied as dry powders. The most common medium for isolation of fungi is coagulated egg yolk used in slant tube preparations. Egg yolk is separated from fresh surface sterilized eggs, shaken with glass beads in sterile flasks and dispensed into pre-sterilized vials. The substance is coagulated as slants in 20-40 min at 80° C, depending upon the quality of the eggs. Müller-Kögler (1965) reviews media for fungi and Goodey (1957) and Welch (1963) those for nematodes. Special media for *in vitro* cell or tissue cultivation may be used for survival of isolated organs of insects. Glycerin or 1% agar without other ingredients are useful for keeping infected cadavers in the refrigerator for further use. In some cases addition of 0.1-1.0% Streptomycin, chloramphenicol or Nipagin for suppression of secondary growth of bacteria or molds is necessary.

F. MISCELLANEOUS MATERIALS

1. Methyl Cellulose

Methyl cellulose is used for immobilizing protozoans and other microorganisms. 10 g Methocel (15 centipoises viscosity rating) is mixed in 45 ml boiling water, and the mixture allowed to cool 20-30 min; then an equal amount of cold water is added and the mixture stirred until smooth. A ring of the solution, a little smaller than a cover-glass, is made on a slide and a drop of water with the organisms is placed inside the ring, then the cover-glass is added. Slowing down occurs progressively as the methyl cellulose diffuses inward.

2. Lugol Solution

To 100 ml water add 6 g of potassium iodide and 4 g of iodine.

References

Ainsworth, G. C. (1967). "Dictionary of the Fungi", 5th Edn. Commonwealth Mycological Institute, Kew.

Allen, M. W. (1960). *In* "Nematology" (J. N. Sasser and W. R. Jenkins, eds), pp. 220-211. University North Carolina Press, Chapel Hill, North Carolina.

Bailey, L. (1963). "Infectious Diseases of the Honey Bee". Land Books, London.

Barjac, H. de and Bonnefoi, A. (1968). *J. Invertebrate Path.* **11**, 335-347.

Barnett, H. L. (1960). "Illustrated Genera of Imperfect Fungi". Burgess Publ. Co., Minneapolis.

Barron, G. L. (1968). "The Genera of Hyphomycetes for Soil". Williams and Wilkins, Baltimore.

Basir, M. A. (1956). *Zoologica* **38**, 1-79.

Batko, A. and Weiser, J. (1965). *J. Invertebrate Path.* **7**, 455-463.

Berberet, R. C. and Helms, T. J. (1969). *J. Invertebrate Path.* **14**, 395-401.

Bergold, G. H. (1963). *In* "Insect Pathology. An Advanced Treatise" (E. A. Steinhaus, ed.), Vol. I, pp. 413-456. Academic Press, New York.

Bessey, E. A. (1952). "Morphology and Taxonomy of Fungi". Blakiston Co., Philadelphia.

Bird, F. T. (1961). *Can. J. Microbiol.* **7**, 827-830.

Bird, F. T. (1966). *Can. J. Microbiol.* **12**, 337-345.

Bird, F. T. and Whalen, M. M. (1953). *Can. Ent.* **85**, 433-437.

Booth, C. (1966). "Provisional Key to Fusaria". Commonwealth Mycological Institute, Kew.

Bovien, P. (1937). *Vidensk. Meddr dansk naturh. Foren.* **101**, 1-114.

Breed, H. S., Murray, E. G. D. and Smith, N. R. (1957). "Bergey's Manual of Determinative Bacteriology", 7th Edn. Williams & Wilkins, Baltimore.

Bresslau, M. and Buschkiel, M. (1919). *Biol. Zbl.* **39**, 325-336.

Brown, A. H. S. and Smith, G. (1957). *Trans. Brit. mycol. Soc.* **40**, 17-89.

Bucher, G. E. (1957). *Can. J. Microbiol.* **75**, 499-509.

Bucher, G. E. (1961). *Can. J. Microbiol.* **7**, 641-655.

Bucher, G. E. (1963). *In* "Insect Pathology. An Advanced Treatise" (E. A. Steinhaus, ed.), Vol. 2, pp. 117-147. Academic Press, New York.

Canning, E. U. (1957). *Riv. Malar.* **XXXVI 1-3**, 39-50.

Canning, E. U. (1968). *Parasitology* 58, 341-347.

Cantwell, G. E. and Laird, M. (1966). *J. Invertebrate Path.* **8**, 442-451.

Chandler, A. C. and Read, C. P. (1961). "Introduction to Parasitology", 10th Edn. John Wiley, New York.

Chitwood, B. G. and Chitwood, M. B. (1950). "An Introduction to Nematology". Monumental Printing Co., Baltimore.

Clements, F. E. and Shear, C. L. (1931). "The Genera of Fungi". Wilson Co., New York.

Codrenau, R. (1961). *C.r. hebd. Séanc. Acad. Sci. Paris* **253**, 1613-1615.

Corliss, J. O. (1960). *Parasitology* **50**, 111-153.

Couch, J. N. and Umphlett, C. J. (1963). *In* "Insect Pathology. An Advanced Treatise" (E. A. Steinhaus, ed.), Vol. 2, pp. 149-188. Academic Press, New York.

Difco Laboratories (1953). Difco Manual of Dehydrated Culture Media and Reagents for Microbial and Clinical Laboratory Procedures, 9th Edn. Difco Laboratories, Detroit, Michigan.

Dissanaike, A. S. (1955). *J. Protozool.* **2**, 150-156.

Doby, J. M. and Saguez, F. (1964). *C.r. hebd. Séanc. Acad. Sci. Paris* **259**, 3614-3617.

Dougherty, E. C. (1960). *In* "Nematology" (J. N. Sasser and W. R. Jenkins, eds), pp. 297-318. University North Carolina Press, Chapel Hill, North Carolina.

Dutky, S. R. (1963). *In* "Insect Pathology. An Advanced Treatise" (E. A. Steinhaus, ed.), Vol. 2, pp. 75-116. Academic Press, New York.

Entwistle, P. F. and Robertson, J. S. (1968). *J. Invertebrate Path.* **10**, 345-354.

Estes, Z. E. and Faust, R. M. (1965). *J. Invertebrate Path.* **7**, 259-260.

Fantham, H. B. and Porter, A. (1958). *Proc. Zool. Soc. Lond.* **130**, 153-168.

Fassatiová, O. (1967). *J. Invertebrate Path.* **9,** 563-566.
Filipjev, J. N. and Schuurmans Stekhoven, P. H. (1941). "A Manual of Agricultural Helminthology". Brill, Leiden.
Finlayson, L. H. (1950). *Parasitology* **40,** 261-264.
Ganhaõ, J. F. P. (1956). *Broteria* **25,** 71-135.
Gibbs, A. J. (1953). *Parasitology* **43,** 143-147.
Giordani, G. (1959). *J. Insect Path.* **1,** 245-269.
Goodey, J. B. (1957). "Laboratory Methods for Work with Plant and Soil Nematodes". H.M. Stationery Office, London.
Grassé, P. P. (1952-53). "Traité de Zoologie, I. Protozoaires, 1,2", pp. 1071-1158. Masson, Paris.
Grell, K. G. (1938). *Arch. Protistenk.* **91,** 526-545.
Gustafsson, M. (1965). *LantbrHögsk. Annlr* **31,** 102-212.
Heimpel, A. M. (1967). *J. Invertebrate Path.* **9,** 364-375.
Heimpel, A. M. and Angus, T. A. (1963). *In* "Insect Pathology. An Advanced Treatise" (E. A. Steinhaus, ed.), Vol. 2, pp. 21-73. Academic Press, New York.
Henry, J. E. (1968). *J. Invertebrate Path.* **11,** 224-233.
Henry, J. E., Nelson, B. P. and Jutila, J. W. (1969). *J. Virology* **3,** 605-610.
Hesse, E. (1935). *Archs Zool. exp. gén.* **75,** 651-661.
Hrubant, G. R. and Rhodes, R. A. (1968). *J. Invertebrate Path.* **11,** 371-376.
Huger, A. (1961). *Proc. 1st Int. Conf. Protozool.* 506-509.
Huger, A. (1963). *In* "Insect Pathology. An Advanced Treatise" (E. A. Steinhaus, ed.), Vol. 1, pp. 531-575. Academic Press, New York.
Humanson, G. H. (1967). "Animal Tissue Techniques", 2nd Edn. Freeman Co., San Francisco.
Hutchison, J. A. (1963). *Trans. Kans. Acad. Sci.* **66,** 237-254.
Jahn, T. L. and Jahn, F. F. (1949). "How to Know Protozoa". C. Brown Co., Dubuque.
Jirovec, O. (1936). *Věst. čsl. zool. Spol.* **4,** 1-75.
Jutila, J. W., Henry, J. E., Anacker, R. L. and Brown, W. R. (1970). *J. Invertebrate Path.* **15,** 225-231.
Karling, J. S. (1948). *Am. J. Botany* **35,** 246-254.
Keilin, D. (1923a). *Parasitology* **15,** 103-116.
Keilin, D. (1923b). *Proc. Camb. phil. Soc. biol. Sci.* **1,** 18-29.
Kellen, W. R., Clark, T. B., Lindegren, J. E. and Sanders, R. D. (1966). *J. Invertebrate Path.* **8,** 390-394.
Kellen, W. R. and Lipa, J. J. (1960). *J. Insect Path.* **2,** 1-12.
Kobayasi, Y. (1941). Sci. Repts. Tokyo Bunrika Daigaku Sect. B5, 53-260.
Kobayasi, Y. and Shimizu, D. (1963). *Bull. natn. Sci. Mus., Tokyo* **6,** 286-314.
Kramář, J. (1950). *Věst. čsl. zool. Spol.* **16,** 55-75.
Kramer, J. P. (1959a). *J. Insect Path.* **1,** 297-303.
Kramer, J. P. (1959b). *Trans. Am. Microsc. Soc.* **78,** 336-343.
Krieg, A. (1961). "Grundlagen der Insektenpathologie". Steinkopf, Darmstadt.
Krieg, A. (1963). *In* "Insect Pathology. An Advanced Treatise" (E. A. Steinhaus, ed.), Vol. 1, pp. 577-617. Academic Press, New York.
Krieg, A. (1967). "Neues über *Bacillus thuringiensis* und seine Anwendung". Mitt. Biol. Bundesanstalt f. Land- u. Forstwirtschaft 7-86.
Krieg, A. (1968). *J. Invertebrate Path.* **12,** 366-378.
Kudo, R. R. (1924). "A Biologic and Taxonomic Study of the Microsporidia", 9, 268 pp. Illinois Biol. Monographs.
Kudo, R. R. (1941). *J. Parasitol.* **27,** 32.
Kudo, R. R. (1966). "Protozoology", 5th Edn. Thomas, Springfield.
Kulik, M. M. (1968). Agric. Handbk U.S. Dep. Agric., Agric. Res. Service, No. 351, 80 pp.
Laird, M. (1959). *Can. J. Zool.* **37,** 781-791.
Lazarevskaya, S. L. (1960). *Helminthologia* **2,** 169-176.
Leatherdale, D. (1965). *J. Invertebrate Path.* **7,** 325-328.
Leger, L. (1907). *Arch. Protistenk.* **8,** 159-202.

Leger, L. (1926). *Trav. Lab. Hydrobiol. Piscic. Univ. Grenoble* **21,** 210.

Leger, L. and Hesse, E. (1916). *C.r. Séanc. Soc. Biol.* **79,** 345-348.

Leibersperger, E. (1960). *Parasit. SchrReihe* **11,** 1-150.

Lillie, R. D. (1965). "Histopathologic Technic and Practical Histochemistry" McGraw-Hill, New York.

Lipa, J. (1963). *In* "Insect Pathology. An Advanced Treatise" (E. A. Steinhaus, ed.), Vol. 2, pp. 335-361. Academic Press, New York.

Lipa, J. J. (1967). *Acta Protozoologica* **5,** 97-179.

Ludwig, F. W. (1947). *Trans. Am. Microsc. Soc.* **45,** 22-33.

Lum, P. T. M. (1963). *J. Insect Path.* **5,** 157-166.

McEwen, F. L. (1963). *In* "Insect Pathology. An Advanced Treatise" (E. A. Steinhaus, ed.), Vol. 1, pp. 273-290. Academic Press, New York.

Machado, A. (1913). *Mems Inst. Oswaldo Cruz* **5,** 32-44.

McLaughlin, R. E. (1969). *J. Protozool.* **16,** 84-92.

MacLeod, D. M. (1954). *Can. J. Bot.* **32,** 818-890.

MacLeod, D. M. (1963). *In* "Insect Pathology. An Advanced Treatise" (E. A. Steinhaus, ed.), Vol. 2, pp. 189-231. Academic Press, New York.

Madelin, M. F. (1963). *In* "Insect Pathology. An Advanced Treatise" (E. A. Steinhaus, ed.), Vol. 2, pp. 233-271. Academic Press, New York.

Madelin, M. F. (1966). *Ann. Rev. Ent.* **11,** 423-448.

Mains, E. B. (1951). *Mycologia* **43,** 691-718.

Mains, E. B. (1958). *Mycologia* **50,** 169-222.

Mains, E. B. (1959). *J. Insect Path.* **1,** 43-47.

Martignoni, M. E. and Steinhaus, E. A. (1961). "Laboratory Exercises in Insect Microbiology and Insect Pathology". Burgess Publ. Co., Minneapolis.

Mathieson, J. (1949). *Trans. Brit. mycol. Soc.* **32,** 113-136.

Matta, J. F. and Lowe, R. E. (1969). *J. Invertebrate Path.* **13,** 457-458.

Müller, G. (1964-65). *Math.-Naturw. Reihe* **13,** 611-638; **13,** 843-860; **14,** 753-798.

Müller-Kögler, E. (1962). *Gesunde Pfl.* **14,** 198.

Müller-Kögler, E. (1965). "Pilzkrankheiten bei Insekten". Parey, Hamburg.

Nickle, W. R. (1967). *Proc. helminth. Soc. Wash.* **34,** 72-94.

Norris, J. R. (1964). *J. Appl. Bact.* **27,** 439-447.

Osche, G. (1952). *Zool. Jber. Abt.* **1, 81,** 190-280.

Oxoid Ltd. (1965). "The Oxoid Manual". Oxoid Ltd., London.

Paillot, A. (1941). *C.r. Séanc. Soc. Biol.* **135,** 1041-1043.

Pillai, J. S. and Smith, J. M. B. (1968). *J. Invertebrate Path.* **11,** 316-320.

Poisson, R. (1940). *Archs Zool. Exp. gén.* **82,** 30-35.

Polozhentsev, P. A. and Artyukhovskii, A. K. (1963). *In* "Metody Issledovaniya Nematod Rastenii, Pochvy i Nasekomykh", 70-90 (Izdatel'stvo Akad. Nauk S.S.S.R., Moskva).

Pouvreau, A. (1962). *Annls Abeille* **5,** 181-199.

Radha, K., Nirula, K. K. and Menon, K. P. V. (1956). *Indian Cocon. J.* **9,** 83-89.

Raper, K. B. and Fennell, D. I. (1965). "The Genus *Aspergillus*". Williams & Wilkins, Baltimore.

Raper, K. B. and Thom, C. (1949). "Manual of the *Penicillia*". Williams & Wilkins, Baltimore.

Reichenow, E. (1935). *Arch. Protistenk.* **84,** 431-445.

Reimer, L. (1966). "Elektronenmikroskopische Untersuchungs- und Präparationsmethoden". Springer Verl., Berlin.

Reyer, W. (1937). *Z. ParasitKde* **9,** 478-522.

Roberts, D. W. and Granados, R. R. (1968). *J. Invertebrate Path.* **12,** 141-143.

Ruhm, W. (1956). "Die Nematoden der Ipiden". G. Fischer, Jena.

Sacchitano, I. (1958). *Annls Mus. r. Congo Belge Sér. 8vo Sci. zool.* **67,** 1-111.

Schaerffenberg, B. (1964). *J. Insect Path.* **6,** 8-20.

Skryabin, K. I., Shichobalova, N. P., Sobolev, A. A., Paramonov, A. A. and Sudarikov, V. E. (1954). "Opredelitel parasiticheskich nematod", Vol. IV. Izd. Akad. Nauk, Moskva.

Smirnoff, W. A. and Philogène, B. J. R. (1968). *Can. Ent.* **100,** 69-74.

Smith, K. M. (1967). "Insect Virology". Academic Press, New York.
Smith, K. M. and Cressman, A. W. (1962). *J. Insect Path.* **4**, 299-236.
Smith, K. M., Hills, G. J., Munger, F. and Gilmore, J. E. (1959). *Nature, Lond.* **184**, 70.
Soper, R. S. (1963). *Can. J. Bot.* **41**, 875-878.
Speare, A. T. (1920). *J. agric. Res.* **18**, 399-440.
Srinivasan, M. C., Narasimhan, M. J. and Thirumalachar, M. J. (1964). *Mycologia* **56**, 683-691.
Steedman, H. F. (1960). "Section Cutting Microscopy". Blackwell, Oxford.
Stein, G. (1956). *Z. ParasitKde* 17, 383-393.
Steinhaus, E. A. (1946). "Insect Microbiology". Comstock Publ. Co., Ithaca, New York.
Steinhaus, E. A. (1949). "Principles of Insect Pathology". McGraw-Hill, New York.
Steinhaus, E. A. (1959). *J. Insect Path.* **1**, 435-437.
Steinhaus, E. A. (1963). *In* "Insect Pathology. An Advanced Treatise" (E. A. Steinhaus, ed.), Vol. 2, pp. 549-588. Academic Press, New York.
Steinhaus, E. A. and Hughes, K. M. (1953). *J. econ. Ent.* **45**, 744.
Steinhaus, E. A. and Martignoni, M. E. (1967). "An Abridged Glossary of Terms used in Invertebrate Pathology". Pacific N.W. Forest Range Expt. Stn, U.S.D.A.
Stevenson, J. P. (1966). *J. Invertebrate Path.* **8**, 205-211.
Tanada, Y. (1959). *J. Insect Path.* **1**, 197-214.
Théodoridès, J. (1955). *Vie et Milieu* Suppl. **4**, 1-310.
Thomson, J. G. (1935). *Trans. R. Soc. trop. Med. Hyg. Lond.* **29**, 6.
Thomson, H. M. (1960). *J. Invertebrate Path.* **2**, 346-385.
Thorne, G. (1961). "Principles of Nematology". McGraw-Hill, New York.
Umphlett, C. J. (1962). *Mycologia* **54**, 540-554.
Umphlett, C. J. (1964). *Mycologia* **56**, 488, 497.
Vago, C., Duthoit, J. L. and Delahaye, F. (1966). *Archiv für die Gesamte Virusforschung* **18**, 344-349.
Veen, K. H. (1967). *J. Invertebrate Path.* **9**, 276-278.
Veen, K. H. and Ferron, P. (1966). *J. Invertebrate Path.* **8**, 268-269.
Veremchuk, G. V. (1962). *Tezisy Dokladov, Nauchn. Konf. Vsesoyuznogo Obshchestva Gel'mintologov Akad. Nauk S.S.S.R., Chast I,* 24-25.
Vincent, M. (1927). *Parasitology* **19**, 394-400.
Wachek, F. (1955). *Parasit. SchrReihe* **3**, 1-119.
Watson, M. (1916). *Illinois Biol. Monographs* **2**, 215-468.
Watson-Kamm, M. (1922). *Illinois Biol. Monographs* **7**, 1-105.
Weingartner, I. (1955). *Zool. Jber. Abt.* **1**, **83**, 248-317.
Weiser, J. (1947). *Ann. Parasitol.* **22**, 11-15.
Weiser, J. (1955a). *Věst. čsl. zool. Spol.* **19**, 374-380.
Weiser, J. (1955b). *Czech. parasitol.* **2**, 181-184.
Weiser, J. (1955c). *Věst. čsl. zool. Spol.* **19**, 44-52.
Weiser, J. (1955d). *J. Protozool.* **2**, 6-12.
Weiser, J. (1961). "Mikrosporidien als Parasiten der Insekten". Parey, Hamburg.
Weiser, J. (1963). *In* "Insect Pathology. An Advanced Treatise" (E. A. Steinhaus, ed.), Vol. 2, pp. 291-234. Academic Press, New York.
Weiser, J. (1966). "Nemoci hmyzu" (Diseases of Insects). Academia, Praha (in Czech).
Weiser, J. (1969). "An Atlas of Insect Diseases". Academia, Praha.
Weiser, J. and Vago, C. (1966). *J. Invertebrate Path.* **8**, 314-318.
Welch, H. E. (1963). *In* "Insect Pathology. An Advanced Treatise" (E. A. Steinhaus, ed.), Vol. 2, pp. 363-392. Academic Press, New York.
Welch, H. E. (1965). *Ann. Rev. Ent.* **10**, 275-302.
Xeros, N. (1954). *Nature, Lond.* **174**, 562.
Xeros, N. (1964). *J. Insect Path.* **6**, 225-236.
Yarwood, E. E. (1937). *Parasitology* **29**, 370-390.
Zdrodovski, P. F. and Golinevich, H. M. (1960). "The Rickettsial Diseases" (Translation from Russian by B. Haigh). Pergamon Press.

CHAPTER 3

Use of Bacteria for Microbial Control

L. A. FALCON

Division of Entomology, University of California, Berkeley, California, U.S.A.

I. Introduction

Our knowledge of bacteria causing diseases in insects began in the late nineteenth century with Pasteur's (1870) study of flacherie of the silkworm, and with Cheshire and Cheyne's (1885) description of *Bacillus alvei* and its role in European foulbrood disease of the honey-bee. Since then over 90 species and varieties of pathogenic bacteria have been described from insects (Anonymous,

1969). Of these, *Bacillus popilliae* and *B. lentimorbus,* the causative agents of Types A and B milky disease in the Japanese beetle, *Popillia japonica,* and certain varieties of the crystal forming bacterium, *Bacillus thuringiensis,* which infect a wide range of Lepidoptera, have been developed for commercial pest control. Currently the major research effort in the use of bacteria for microbial control continues to be concentrated on these bacteria. For the milky spore disease bacteria, emphasis is on the development of efficient mass production techniques and for *B. thuringiensis* to further development of its use as a "broad spectrum" bacterial insecticide. Today, the subject of *B. thuringiensis* is extensive and so much knowledge has accumulated in recent years that three papers in this book have been devoted exclusively to it. In comparison, little research has been done with other bacterial pathogens as regards their practical use. Consequently, a discussion on the use of bacteria for microbial control will be dominated by the *B. thuringiensis* complex and somewhat less by the milky spore disease bacteria.

In "Insect Pathology. An Advanced Treatise", edited by the late E. A. Steinhaus (1963), several chapters were devoted in whole or part to entomogenous bacteria, i.e. taxonomy, certain spore-forming bacteria, milky diseases, non-sporulating bacterial pathogens, epizootiology, microbial control and commercial production. Since then several reviews have appeared. Some cover the use of entomogenous bacteria for microbial control (Afrikan, 1963; Burges, 1964b; Jaques, 1964; Heimpel, 1964; Angus, 1965a; Krieg, 1965); others are concerned specifically with *B. thuringiensis* (Heimpel, 1963, 1967; Martouret and Milaire, 1963; Doane, 1964; Fedorinchik, 1964; Vankova, 1964; Herfs, 1965a, 1967; Norris, 1965; Kreig, 1967; Martouret, 1967; Angus, 1968). Many review the general aspects of microbial control with considerable reference to bacteria (Cameron, 1963, 1967, 1969; Hall, 1964, 1967; Franz, 1964, 1966; Prokhorov, 1964; Heimpel, 1965; Hurpin, 1966; Grison, 1967; Rivers, 1967; Tanada, 1967; Anonymous, 1969).

II. Characteristics of Bacterial Pathogens of Insects

A. CLASSIFICATION

Entomogenous bacteria are generally classified as either sporeformers or non-sporeformers and are further differentiated as obligate or facultative pathogens. In a classification proposed by Bucher (1960), the pathogenic bacteria of insects were grouped by properties or requirements of pathogenic significance, such as infective dose, site of infection, host specificity and specific mode of action. He proposed four categories of bacterial pathogens: (1) obligate pathogens; (2) crystalliferous sporeformers; (3) facultative pathogens; and (4) potential pathogens. In Table I, representative bacteria of the various groups proposed by Bucher are arranged in accordance with their spore-forming

TABLE I

Classification of some bacterial pathogens of insects

Sporeformers			Non-sporeformers	
Obligate	Facultative			
	Crystalliferous	Non-crystalliferous	Potential	Facultative
Bacillus euloomarahae	*B. thuringiensis*	*B. cereus*	*Pseudomonas aeruginosa*	*Serratia marcescens*
B. fribourgensis	var. *aizawai*		*P. chlororaphis*	
B. lentimorbus	var. *amuscatoxicus*		*P. fluorescens*	
B. lentimorbus var. *australis*	var. *anagastae*		*P. reptilivora*	
	var. *dendrolimus*		*P. septica*	
B. popilliae	var. *entomocidus*		*P. putida*	
Clostridium brevifaciens	var. *galleriae*		*Aerobacter* spp.	
	var. *pacificus*		*Cloaca* spp.	
C. malacosomae	var. *sotto*		*Proteus vulgaris*	
	var. *subtoxicus*		*P. mirabilis*	
	var. *thuringiensis*		*P. rettgeri*	

characteristics. The crystalliferous bacteria are grouped as varieties of *B. thuringiensis* according to Heimpel (1967).

B. MODE OF ACTION

All spore-forming bacteria produce endospores which allow them to persist in a dormant or quiescent state outside the intended host. Upon ingestion by a susceptible host the spores germinate in the gut. In obligate pathogens in the genus *Bacillus,* the vegetative cells produced by the germinating spores enter the hemocoel where they multiply rapidly, destroy certain tissues, and soon fill much of the cavity. This stage of the infection is termed "septicemia". Prior to death of the host, thick-walled refractile spores are formed which appear white through the integument, thus the name "milky disease". Following death, the host disintegrates and the spores are released into the soil. The mode of action of obligate pathogens of the genus *Clostridia* differs in that these bacteria multiply only in the gut and do not invade the hemocoel. After death, the cadaver becomes shrunken, dry and mummified. As a group, the spore-forming obligate pathogens are highly virulent for specific insect hosts and kill apparently without producing highly poisonous toxins that aid in infection or cause death.

The crystalliferous sporeformers, in addition to forming endospores, produce a proteinaceous parasporal crystal in the sporangium at the time of sporulation. The crystal contains an endotoxin capable of paralyzing the gut of most lepidopterous larvae. This material has been labeled as δ-endotoxin (Heimpel,

1967). During the process of infection, susceptible insects are either killed by the toxic crystals or so weakened that the bacteria can readily invade the hemocoel from the gut and produce a lethal septicemia (Heimpel and Angus, 1963). In addition to the crystal, at least three other substances toxic to insects may be produced by crystalliferous bacteria. Following the nomenclature proposed by Heimpel (1967) these are: α-exotoxin, an enzyme of the growing bacterium, phospholipase C, that breaks down essential phospholipids in insect tissue; β-exotoxin, a small, water-soluble, heat stable, dialyzable molecule that is secreted outside the bacterial cell into the surrounding medium, and kills larvae and pupae of Diptera and some Lepidoptera; and γ-exotoxin, an unidentified phospholipase that affects phospholipids, probably releasing fatty acids from the molecule.

B. cereus, a spore-forming facultative pathogen, also produces phospholipase C in quantities sufficient to damage gut cells of susceptible species thus aiding entry of the bacterium into the hemocoel (Heimpel 1955b; Heimpel and Angus, 1963).

The non-spore-forming bacteria are a heterogeneous group that usually infect insects only under extraordinary circumstances. Although they occur in the gut of the host, they do not multiply readily there and probably do not produce enzymes or toxins in sufficient quantities to cause damage or to aid invasion of the hemocoel. They do, however, multiply in the hemocoel of the insect once they have invaded it (Bucher, 1963a).

C. METHODS OF PROPAGATION

The obligate pathogens, among species of *Bacillus* and *Clostridium,* are fastidious organisms that can be propagated in artificial media only with extreme difficulty. The commercial preparations of *B. popilliae* produced in the U.S.A. are made by injecting or feeding bacteria to grubs of the Japanese beetle. The bacteria multiply to great numbers in the grubs and are recovered by grinding up the host.

Most other bacterial pathogens are much less fastidious and can be readily propagated on simple bacteriological media. This is one reason why the facultative bacterial pathogens are likely candidates for microbial control (Ignoffo, 1967).

D. HOST RANGE

Obligate pathogens of the genus *Bacillus* have a narrow host range and infect only certain closely related beetles of the family Scarabaeidae. Dutky (1963) provides an extensive list showing the susceptibility of different species to these bacteria. Clostridial pathogens were originally isolated from *Malacosoma californicum (pluviale)* (Bucher, 1957). Other than experimental infections in other tent caterpillars and the possible presence of these bacteria in *Thymelicus lineola* (Heimpel and Angus, 1963) little is known about their host range. *B. thuringiensis* and its varieties have been tested successfully against more than 137 insect species from the orders Lepidoptera, Hymenoptera, Diptera, and Coleoptera (Heimpel, 1967). Most of these pathogenicity tests have been conducted in the laboratory. The most susceptible insects are those lepidopterous larvae having alkaline gut contents (pH 9.0-10.5) and enzymes which dissolve the crystals and release the toxin (Angus, 1956; Angus and Heimpel, 1959; Heimpel and Angus, 1959).

B. cereus is a common, widely distributed soil saprophyte with an extensive host range including insect species from the orders Coleoptera, Hymenoptera and Lepidoptera (Heimpel and Angus, 1963). Its host range is also limited by the pH of the gut as a highly alkaline gut content can inactivate the toxic exoenzyme, phospholipase C (Heimpel, 1955a).

The non-spore-forming bacteria attack a wide range of hosts from the Acarina, and the insect orders Coleoptera, Diptera, Hymenoptera, Isoptera, Lepidoptera, and Orthoptera (Bucher, 1963a).

E. SAFETY

The milky spore disease bacteria are registered for use in the U.S.A. on crops not used for human food and *B. thuringiensis* is exempt from tolerance limits on a number of food crops. The latter registration is based on evidence, developed by the manufacturers, that *B. thuringiensis* is both effective and safe to use. Safety to man, other vertebrates and plants has yet to be established for all other entomogenous bacteria.

III. Current Status

A. MILKY DISEASES

The discovery and practical application of the milky disease bacteria for control of grubs of the Japanese beetle in the U.S.A. (White and Dutky, 1940) provided the first real encouragement for the use of bacteria as a reliable means of insect control. Furthermore, the success of this program has become one of the classic examples of microbial control by the colonization of a microorganism (Dutky, 1963; Beard, 1964). In the period 1939-1953, 109 tons of spore powder were distributed to over 90,000 sites in 13 eastern states and the District of Columbia as part of a Government program (Anonymous, 1952). In Maryland, for example, the disease was applied in 1940 to the fairway of a golf course. At the time of application there were 20-60 grubs/sq ft of turf. The infestation was reduced to 1-3 grubs/sq ft of turf and remained at this level for at least nine years after application (Cory and Langford, 1955). In Connecticut, the milky disease was first applied 29 years ago. Subsequently the beetle decreased markedly in importance. The numbers of beetles are now greatly reduced and there are few new major infestations. However, cultivated grass is still damaged to some extent, possibly by larvae hatching from eggs laid by beetles that bred in neighboring untreated cultivated or rough ground. Although most of these larvae are slowly killed by the disease, control is too protracted to prevent a certain amount of damage to the grass. Thus the disease has been very successful from the point of view of the state as a whole, but less so from that of individual lawn or grass owners (Beard, 1964).

For many years, spore dusts containing no less than 10^8 viable spores of either or both *B. popilliae* and *B. lentimorbus* per gram have been produced by Fairfax Biological Laboratories in the U.S.A. and marketed under the name of Doom®.

The milky disease bacteria in general are a promising group of bacterial pathogens, their potential use extending far beyond control of the Japanese beetle. The host range for *B. popilliae* is wide (Dutky, 1963) and, in addition, several other similar bacteria have been isolated from scarab larvae in several parts of the world. These include *B. euloomarahae* from *Heteronychus sanctae-helenae* and *B. lentimorbus* var. *australis* from *Sericesthis geminata (pruinosa)* (Australia); New Zealand milky disease from *Odontria zealandica* (New Zealand) and *B. fribourgensis* from *Melolontha melolontha* (Switzerland) (Steinkraus and Tashiro, 1967).

Goodwin (personal communication) conducted a three-year initial investigation of diseases of scarab populations in Australian pastures. The studies concentrated on milky disease bacteria because of their prolonged survival in the soil and potential for artificial cultivation. He concluded that the soil environment is the most promising habitat for microbial insect control. The major obstacle to further development of the work in Australia, as elsewhere, remains the development of artificial culture techniques for milky disease bacteria (Steinkraus and Tashiro, 1967; Rhodes, 1968).

B. *BACILLUS THURINGIENSIS*

Early commercial development of *B. thuringiensis* was well reviewed by Hall (1963). In recent years commercial preparations containing *B. thuringiensis* have been produced by at least 12 manufacturers in five countries (Appendix 6 IV). In the U.S.A., hundreds of tons are manufactured each year with production rising annually. One firm, for example, increased production more than 200-fold over the past eight years. Commercial preparations of *B. thuringiensis* are currently registered in the U.S.A. for use on more than 20 agricultural crops in addition to shade trees, ornamentals and forests for the control of at least 23 insect species (Table II). It is significant that the registration of a product in the U.S.A. requires that the U.S.D.A. registration authority is satisfied not only that the product is safe, but also that field testing has shown that it gives effective control of the registered pest species. The estimated cost for material to the user

TABLE II

Some registered uses for B. thuringiensis *products in the U.S.A.*[a]

Pest		Crop
	VEGETABLE AND FIELD CROPS	
Alfalfa caterpillar	*Colias eurytheme*	alfalfa
Artichoke plume moth	*Platyptilia carduidactyla*	artichokes
Bollworm	*Heliothis zea*	cotton
Cabbage looper	*Trichoplusia ni*	beans, broccoli, cabbage, cauliflower, celery, collards, cotton, cucumbers, kale, lettuce, melons, potatoes, spinach, tobacco
Diamondback moth	*Plutella maculipennis*	cabbage
European corn borer	*Ostrinia nubilalis*	sweet corn
Imported cabbageworm	*Pieris rapae*	broccoli, cabbage, cauliflower, collards, kale
Tobacco budworm	*Heliothis virescens*	tobacco
Tobacco hornworm	*Manduca sexta*	tobacco
Tomato hornworm	*Manduca quinquemaculata*	tomatoes
	FRUIT CROPS	
Fruit-tree leaf roller	*Archips argyrospilus*	oranges
Orange dog	*Papilio cresphontes*	oranges
Grape leaf folder	*Desmia funeralis*	grapes
	FORESTS, SHADE TREES, ORNAMENTALS	
California oakworm	*Phryganidia californica*	
Fall webworm	*Hyphantria cunea*	
Fall cankerworm	*Alsophila pometaria*	
Great Basin tent caterpillar	*Malacosoma fragile*	
Gypsy moth	*Lymantria (Porthetria) dispar*	
Linden looper	*Erannis tiliaria*	
Salt Marsh caterpillar	*Estigmene acrea*	
Spring cankerworm	*Paleacrita vernata*	
Winter moth	*Operophtera brumata*	

[a] From information supplied, in part, through the kindness of International Minerals and Chemical Corp., Libertyville, Illinois and Nutrilite Products Inc., Buena Park, California, U.S.A.

lies between \$1.75 and \$7.50 per acre, which in many situations is competitive with chemical insecticides.

C. OTHER SPORE-FORMING BACTERIA

The obligate spore-forming clostridial pathogens are also potentially useful bacteria as shown by Bucher (1961) who obtained excellent control of the eastern tent caterpillar, *Malacosoma americanum,* in the field. He concluded that artificial distribution of the disease was not economically practical so long as the bacterial spores cannot be produced cheaply in mass culture.

Despite the fact that the facultative sporeformer *B. cereus* is a widely distributed, commonly occurring bacterium which has frequently been isolated from diseased insects, little effort has been made to develop its potential in microbial control. *B. cereus* can be readily propagated on standard bacteriological media and has a wide host range.

D. NON-SPOREFORMERS

These bacteria are common in the digestive tracts of insects but seldom cause pathogenic infection because they lack the invasive power to penetrate through the midgut wall. However, when the insect is stressed by such factors as starvation, ingestion of contaminated food, infection with other pathogens, and mechanical rupturing of the gut, these bacteria may enter the hemocoel and cause septicemia.

Raun and Brooks (1963) isolated bacteria of several genera including *Aerobacter, Streptococcus, Achromobacter, Pseudomonas* and *Serratia* from dead larvae of *Ostrinia nubilalis, Agrotis ipsilon* and *Heliothis zea* collected on corn in Iowa. Infectivity tests indicated that these bacteria probably aided in the natural reduction of these insects in the field. Bucher (1967) reported that the bacteria *S. marcescens, P. fluorescens, P. aeruginosa* and *Enterobacter aerogenes* were the predominant pathogens in the majority of samples of hornworm larvae *(Manduca sexta* and *M. quinquemaculata)* from tobacco growing areas near Ontario, Canada. The bacteria caused little harm unless the insects were also exposed to certain stress factors.

These examples suggest that under certain conditions non-spore-forming bacteria can be important mortality factors. Little is known about the factors influencing these bacterial pathogens and few investigations have been made to develop their use in microbial control.

IV. Factors Which Influence Effectiveness

Several factors influence the effectiveness of entomogenous bacteria employed for microbial insect control. The manner in which these factors influence bacteria and other pathogens is discussed in several chapters of this book. In this chapter it will suffice to review some of the recent contributions as regards the bacteria.

A. SELECTION OF BACTERIA

The efficiency of a bacterium in insect control is influenced by many factors related to the characteristics of the species or variety selected, the method of propagation, and the manner of formulation. Great variation exists between the activities of current commercial preparations of *B. thuringiensis* against any one host species as demonstrated by Morris (1969a) who investigated the susceptibility of several species of forest insects to five commercial preparations of

B. thuringiensis. In some comparisons a preparation poor against one host was good against another. Standardization of commercial preparations of *B. thuringiensis* is a major problem. For this reason, two international study groups have met to discuss the subject (Vago and Burges, 1964; Burges, 1967). At the 1966 meeting several resolutions were adopted, but whether they can or will be implemented remains to be seen.

B. thuringiensis consists of a number of closely related varieties (Heimpel and Angus, 1958; Norris, 1964; de Barjac and Bonnefoi, 1967; Angus and Norris, 1968). Insect susceptibility differs not only to varieties (Herfs, 1963; Vaňková, 1964; Burgerjon and Biache, 1967), but may also differ within a single variety (Angus and Norris, 1968). Rogoff *et al.* (1969) reported major differences in insecticidal activity for 31 isolates of *Bacillus* tested against several important pests. Evaluation of *B. thuringiensis* varieties for specific insecticidal activity may prove to be of great value to the future of microbial control. From this approach arises the possibility that several specific varieties will be made available as commercial products–more than now on the market–each for control of a single or several closely related pest species.

B. SUNLIGHT AND TEMPERATURE

In the application of a bacterium, a suspension of minute particles is deposited on plant foliage. From the time the bacterium leaves the application equipment until it is consumed by the target species, it is exposed to all the physical elements of the environment. The period of exposure will vary depending on the feeding habits and activities of the insect host. During this period, sunlight appears to be a major deleterious environmental factor. For *B. thuringiensis,* Cantwell and Franklin (1966) found that spores on membrane filters or glass slides were rapidly inactivated by exposure to ultraviolet irradiation in the laboratory (1 min–12%; 2 min–50%; 10 min–99.9%), but less quickly when exposed to natural sunlight (30 min–50%; 60 min–80%). Raun *et al.* (1966) reported drastic effects on spores and paraspores of *B. thuringiensis* exposed to a 15-W germicidal lamp. Irradiation for 24 and 48 hr progressively reduced pathogenicity, while exposure for 72 hr eliminated measurable pathogenic effects. Crystals of *B. thuringiensis* var. *sotto* exposed to a germicidal ultraviolet lamp for up to 120 min lost no toxicity to the silkworm (Cantwell, 1967).

Temperature is another limiting factor which acts not only on the spore, but also on the insect and its development. Using the commercial preparations Agritrol and Thuricide, Ignoffo (1964) tested the physical effects of temperature and water on the viability and virulence of *B. thuringiensis* at a decimal dilution of 1 g of the spore preparations per 9 ml of water. Spores in dry Agritrol exposed to 10° or 30° C for 200 days showed no loss in viability. Suspended in water at 10° C, the Agritrol showed an initial reduction in viability of spores after 30 days exposure, whereas the Thuricide suspension lost no viability after 500 days exposure. At 30° C spore viability of Thuricide was reduced and, at 50° C, completely destroyed. The Thuricide spore suspension exposed from 1 to 500 days at 10° C produced 100% mortality of pink bollworm larvae, *Pectinophora gossypiella*, over the entire period.

Ignoffo (1962) reported 40.1° C as the optimum temperature for larval mortality caused by spores of *B. thuringiensis* injected into pink bollworm. No septicemia was detected at 51.2° and 8.6° C. Exposure of spore-injected larvae to different relative humidities (100, 69, 24, 7%) had no effect on the progression of mortality. Raun *et al.* (1966) reported that *B. thuringiensis* spores mixed into food were more effective, and resulted in more rapid mortality of fourth instar larvae of the fall armyworm, *Spodoptera frugiperda*, at 32° than at 21° C. Similarly, greater mortality for *O. nubilalis* larvae occurred at 34° than at 27° or 20° C. Thus pathogenicity of *B. thuringiensis* was greatest at temperatures where growth of the bacterium and metabolic rate of the insects are most rapid. Herfs (1965a) stated that, in the field, temperatures of 18°-20° C were most favorable for application of *B. thuringiensis.*

Under field conditions, the effects of ultraviolet irradiation and temperature interact on the spore. Raun *et al.* (1966) stated, "Low temperatures in the field would allow more exposure of the bacterium to solar radiation, rainfall, etc. and would reduce the effectiveness of the bacterium. Higher temperatures would allow the bacterium to kill the insect before solar radiation could have its effect." In 1969, Pinnock and Milstead (in press) compared three commercial preparations (Biotrol dust, wettable powder: Thuricide 90TS) for control of California oakworm *(Phryganidia californica)* on oak in three areas of differing climate in northern California. The climatic areas were: area 1–coastal with frequent sea mists and mean daily temperatures of about 20° C; area 2–further inland, dry with mean daily temperatures of about 24° C; and area 3–in a sunny interior valley where daily temperatures averaged about 37° C. There was no rainfall in any of the study areas. Control was similar in all areas and the preparations were about equally effective, but differed in persistence. Viable spores of the wettable powder could not be detected on treated foliage one week after application. The flowable preparation, which contained a protective compound against ultraviolet light, persisted up to three weeks, although with a steadily declining viable spore count. The dust preparation persisted significantly longer than the flowable formulation. Consequently, the differences in persistence appeared to be due more to formulation and less to climatic factors.

C. PHYTOCIDES

Kushner and Harvey (1960, 1962) tested foliage extracts obtained from ten species of conifers and eight species of deciduous trees on the development of

B. cereus and *B. thuringiensis*. They demonstrated that phytocides (anti-bacterial substances) were present in the plants and within the insects feeding on these plants. These phytocides protect insects against bacterial disease. Smirnoff and Hutchison (1965) and Smirnoff (1965a, 1967, 1968) showed that phytocides are plant products with a wide range of properties which can inhibit *B. thuringiensis* and other bacteria. Morris (1969a) concluded that the high acidity of certain foliage extracts may lower the normally high alkalinity of the midgut of Lepidoptera so that toxic crystals cannot be dissolved. Even if the crystals do dissolve, bacterial growth in the gut may be inhibited, allowing survival of the insect.

D. FIELD APPLICATION TECHNIQUES

Application of bacterial pathogens is one of the most important, yet frequently neglected, aspects in field use. In addition to the bacterial preparation, one must consider habits and susceptibility of the target insect, host crop and environment, use of adjuvants, type of application equipment and methods for evaluation of the effectiveness of the bacterium.

The milky disease bacteria were introduced for the long-term control of a soil inhabiting beetle larva by seeding a powder, containing spores from diseased larvae, at intervals over permanent turf. One treatment was sufficient because the spores survive a long time and spread in the soil: larvae succumbing to the disease increase the bacterial inoculum, giving a slow, long-lasting control. Once established, the disease spreads naturally to neighboring areas.

In contrast, microbial insecticides for short-term control neither persist from year to year nor spread, and so must be applied very efficiently to give thorough coverage of the crop. This is particularly so with bacteria since they take effect only when eaten. The previous discussion has shown that great differences can exist between bacterial preparations of *B. thuringiensis*. Recent research has demonstrated that the effectiveness and persistence of such preparations can also be affected by the addition of adjuvants such as spreaders, stickers, wetting agents, etc. (Chapter 28). The performance of *B. thuringiensis* was enhanced by several of these agents, including cornmeal baits (Creighton *et al.*, 1961), Lovo® (amine stearate) spray additives (Geering and Lloyd, 1962), Plyac®, Triton B-1956, polybutenes L-100 and H-35 (Begg, 1964), corn oil (Creighton *et al.*, 1964), Triton B-1956 and Cellosize QP 4400 (Meyer, 1964), boric acid (Doane and Wallis, 1964), surfactant oils (Wolfenbarger, 1965); and Pinolene® (Lewis, 1966). Morris (1969a) tested several sticker-spreaders with various commercial preparations of *B. thuringiensis* and found that most not only mixed poorly, but had some adverse effects on the physiological characteristics of the bacteria. Falcon (unpublished) improved the effectiveness and persistence of a Biotrol wettable powder against *H. zea* on cotton by the addition of 5% crude molasses to the finished spray. However, the molasses also seemed to attract more egg-laying females to the treated plots as compared to the untreated controls.

Bacterial preparations are commonly applied with the same equipment used for application of chemical insecticides. Little attention has been given to the characteristics of such equipment which may influence spray droplet or dust particle size, deposit, coverage, drift, etc. Several methods for assessing spray coverage have been tried with varying degrees of success. These include: direct count or culture of spore deposits removed from treated foliage; use of culture plates in the field to collect spores at the time of application (Connola *et al.*, 1966); employment of adhesive transparent tape to trap spores for counting under the microscope (Pinnock, unpublished); and use of fluorescent materials to detect spray coverage (Lewis and Connola, 1966; Bullock and Dulmage, 1969). The latter two methods appear to be the most practical as they provide a rapid means for assessing coverage immediately after application.

Employing a fluorescent particle technique (Himel *et al.*, 1965), Fisher (personal communication) assessed deposits of Thuricide 2.5 B tagged dust applied (50 lb/acre) to broccoli. He estimated that 540-1330 spores/mm^2 should have been deposited on the upper surface of the leaves and 40-60 on the under surface. More than twice the amount of dust was deposited on the downwind swath than the upwind swath in a 2.5-m.p.h. crosswind. A rainfall of 0.14 in on the third day after application almost completely removed the top deposit, but had little effect on the underleaf deposit. The deposits were fairly wind resistant requiring about a 30-m.p.h. wind to remove 49-80% of the deposit. Drift was also measured and several fluorescent particles per plant were found 630 ft downwind.

Proper evaluation of the effect of the bacterial pathogens used in microbial control is of utmost importance. For most lepidopterous pests, the larval stage is the only target for assessment. However, some recent studies have shown that mortality does not always occur during the larval stage, but may be delayed until after pupation and even eclosion. This has been demonstrated with several lepidopterous species including the Siberian silkworm, *Dendrolimus sibiricus* (Tyumentsev, 1963); the eye-spotted budmoth, *Spilonota ocellana* (Legner and Oatman, 1962; Oatman and Legner, 1964); *Malacosoma disstria, Sarrothripus (Nycteola) cinereana, Nymphalis antiopa* (Angus, 1965b), *Choristoneura fumiferana* (Klein and Lewis, 1966), and *Vanessa cardui* (Morris, 1969b). Studies by Hitchings (1967) indicated that a water-soluble toxin found in Bakthane, when applied to the surface of soil, inhibited the reproductive potential of southern armyworm, *Prodenia eridania,* pupating in the soil. The activity of the toxin was undiminished after four months in the soil.

V. Practical Application

In the classical sense of biological control, bacterial pathogens can be introduced and so colonized for long-term regulation and suppression of pest species. Conversely, bacterial pathogens can be used in a manner similar to chemical insecticides for short-term or temporary suppression of insect pests. They can be applied as sprays, dusts or baits, alone, or in conjunction with parasites, predators or other pathogens. Bacterial pathogens can be used compatibly and possibly synergistically with many chemical insecticides as well as with most other control procedures such as radiation-induced sterilization, chemosterilants, pheromones, etc. Stressors may enhance their pathogenicity or activate chronic infections (Tanada, 1967). As with most other insect pathogens, bacteria have many features which make them useful tools in integrated control and pest management systems (Hurpin, 1966).

A. COMBINATIONS AND INTERACTIONS

1. Interaction with Macrobial Agents

Entomogenous bacteria interact with parasites and predators and can be (1) harmful; (2) have no effect; or (3) beneficial to the abundance and density of these macrobial agents. A harmful or deleterious effect is seldom direct destruction as with broad-spectrum chemical insecticides. Instead, it is due to competition where, for example, a bacterial infection may make the host nutritionally or physiologically unsuitable for parasite development or consumption by predators. In addition, the bacterium may cause premature death of the host and so indirectly cause death of parasitic larvae or so lower the abundance of the host that the predators are starved out.

There is much documented evidence that entomogenous bacteria do not directly destroy parasites and predators, *B. popilliae* (White, 1943); *B. thuringiensis* (Biliotti, 1956; Ankersmit *et al.*, 1962; Lappa, 1963; Kurstak, 1964a; Falcon *et al.*, 1965, 1968; Jaques, 1965; Isakova and Moisejeva, 1966; Wiackowski and Wiackowska, 1966); *S. faecalis* (Bucher and Williams, 1967). Conversely, a few reports suggest that the use of commercial preparations of *B. thuringiensis* may be detrimental to macrobial agents, but these have not been substantiated (Shorey and Hall, 1963; Jaques, 1965).

This high degree of specificity permits the use of bacteria in combination with macrobial agents in several ways, most of which have been demonstrated with commercial preparations of *B. thuringiensis.* They may be applied (1) for control of a specific pest so as not to interfere with control of other pests by macrobial agents, as in British glasshouses where control of whole pest complexes by biological means is being developed (Gould *et al.*, 1969); (2) to augment control by parasites and predators (Kurstak, 1964a; Isakova and Moisejeva, 1966, 1967; Falcon *et al.*, 1968); (3) in conjunction with artificial releases of parasites and predators (Shchepetilnikova and Fedorinchik, 1963). Parasites may disperse a bacterium (White, 1943; Bucher, 1963b; Isakova, 1965), a bacterium may weaken insect immunity to bacterial infection (Isakova and Moisejeva, 1967), or both weakening of the host and transmission of spores may occur simultaneously (Shchepetilnikova and Fedorinchik, 1963).

2. Combination with Other Microbial Agents

Under natural conditions, mixed infections in which several causative agents are present simultaneously are not uncommon. This has led to investigations on the use of combined microbiological preparations for insect control. *B. thuringiensis* combined with a nuclear polyhedrosis virus enhanced control of the alfalfa caterpillar (Steinhaus, 1951). A combination of *B. thuringiensis* and nuclear polyhedrosis virus was effective for control of *Malacosoma fragile* (Stelzer 1965, 1967). Kalyuga (1968) found a combination of *B. thuringiensis* and the fungus, *Beauveria bassiana,* provided more effective control of *P. brassicae* than either agent alone.

Applications of *B. thuringiensis* have also activated latent infections as with granulosis virus in *Hyphantria cunea* (Kreig and Schmidt, 1962). Conversely, one pathogen may adversely affect the development of another as reported by Sicker *et al.* (1965) who suspected *B. thuringiensis* of retarding the development of nuclear polyhedrosis virus in *Malacosoma neustria.*

3. Use with Chemicals

B. thuringiensis is compatible with a wide range of chemical pesticides and supplements (Chapter 28). In a review by Herfs (1965c), 36 pesticide agents comprising fungicides, insecticides, herbicides and acaricides were listed. Of these, 26 were considered to be compatible with *B. thuringiensis.* Of 40 supplements listed, including wetting agents, emulsifiers and adhesives, 35 were compatible. As a consequence, *B. thuringiensis* preparations can be used in combination with many pesticides and supplements, a factor of great importance for use in integrated control programs.

In addition to being compatible with chemical pesticides the combining of pathogen and chemical may increase the effectiveness of one or both over either alone (Chapter 14). Furthermore, this may be accomplished by using lower dosages of each with a resultant synergistic effect. However, this area is controversial as pointed out in the fine review by Pristavko (1967). Additional reviews on this subject include Vaňková (1964) and Herfs (1965c).

4. Use with Other Control Procedures

Bacteria may also be combined with the sterile male technique although apparently little research has been conducted in this area. By their selective nature, bacteria can be used to control other pests in a sterile male program without interfering with the program. The sterility technique for control of codling moth is being intensively investigated in the U.S.A. and Canada and may possibly be practical soon. Yet there are many other pests in the orchard ecosystem at present suppressed by broad spectrum chemicals used against the codling moth. With the sterile male approach, use of these chemicals must be reduced or eliminated, resulting in the upsurge of other insect pests. The fruit tree leaf roller, *Archips argyrospilus,* appears to be such a pest (Madsen and Downing, 1968) and *B. thuringiensis* may prove to be a useful adjunct to the codling moth-sterile male program for the control of this and other species.

Jafri (1964) reported increased susceptibility of irradiated insects to *B. thuringiensis* and suggested integration of biological and radiation control of stored grain pests.

B. LONG-TERM CONTROL

No recent work rivals that classical example of long-term insect control, the supression of the Japanese beetle in the U.S.A. by the milky disease bacteria. Recently, several Russian papers have reported permanent control of the Siberian silkworm, *Dendrolimus sibiricus,* following the introduction of *B. thuringiensis* var. *dendrolimus* (Talalaev, 1958, 1959; Gukasyan, 1961; Talalayev, 1966). After application to forests, the bacterium persisted in the soil in the remains of dead caterpillars and pupae (Talalayeva, 1966).

Reports of natural bacterial epizootics suggests a potential for further research in this field. Kurstak (1964b) discovered a natural bacterial epizootic disease in populations of the Mediterranean flour moth, *Ephestia (Anagasta) kuehniella,* caused by *B. thuringiensis.* In Russia, Talalayeva (1967) reported an epizootic of *B. thuringiensis* in field populations of the lepidopteran forest pest, *Selenephera lunigera.* On cabbage, an epizootic in *Mamestra (Barathra) brassicae* resulted in 80-100% mortality of caterpillars and was caused by several species of bacteria, *Streptococcus subtilissimus, S. liquifaciens, Pseudomonas aeruginosa,* and *Bacillus laterosporus* (Sirko *et al.*, 1966).

C. SHORT-TERM CONTROL

Research and development of bacteria for temporary suppression of economic pests has been made almost exclusively with commercial preparations of *B. thuringiensis.* Investigations have been made in many countries on a wide variety of pests of vegetable, field, fruit, forest and ornamental plants, as well as pests of stored products and insects of medical importance. Hall (1963, 1964) reviewed the research undertaken during the 1950's. Much has been learnt from early failures in the field with *B. thuringiensis* preparations and with this as background information, recent rapid developments will be explored in the next few pages.

1. Vegetable and Field Crops

In crucifers, tests with spray and dust formulations of *B. thuringiensis* have provided generally good to excellent control of the cabbageworm, *Pieris brassicae* (Vaňková, 1962; Herfs and Krieg, 1963), *P. rapae* (Creighton *et al.*, 1964; Cass, 1965; Frye and Scholz, 1965), and *Plutella maculipennis* (Cass, 1962, 1965). Results with *Trichoplusia ni* have been less consistent, ranging from poor control reported by Rolston and Mayes (1965), erratic control by Chalfant and Brett (1965), some suppression, but at excessive cost (Cass, 1965), sprays of *B. thuringiensis*-surfactant combinations warranted further study (Wolfenbarger, 1965), to effective control (Greene *et al.*, 1969). Creighton *et al.* (1964) reported that *B. thuringiensis* decreased feeding by *T. ni* and was usually more effective in preventing damage than in reducing populations. In a laboratory study, Ignoffo *et al.* (1968) determined the relationship between laboratory and field doses of Thuricide® 90TS to control *T. ni* on cabbage. They demonstrated that proper application of 1-2 quarts (qt) per acre should kill 98% of larvae younger than 24 hr; 3-4 qt/acre should kill in excess of 90% of four-day-old larvae with a minimum of 50% of the population dying within two days following application. Their data indicated that frequent applications (three-day intervals) at low doses (1-2 qt/acre) possibly provided more effective seasonal control than emergency applications at high doses of 3-4 qt/acre.

In recent years products containing *B. thuringiensis* have been used rather extensively for the control of foliage-chewing species of Lepidoptera, especially cabbage looper, on lettuce and cole crops in the U.S.A. (Angus, 1968; personal communications from representatives for International Minerals and Chemical Corp., and Nutrilite Products, Inc.). This is especially so in areas where *T. ni* is resistant to once effective insecticides, or where legal restrictions limit the use of persistent insecticides. In these areas a common practice is to combine *B. thuringiensis* with a chemical insecticide and presumably by "synergistic action", obtain better control than if either agent is used alone. Hall (1968) questions this approach and feels that improved control probably results from a summation of the marginal reduction provided by each control agent. In his opinion, a more practical approach is being taken in an integrated program under development in southern California. In this program, chemical insecticides are employed until the plants reach a certain stage of maturity (approximately 30 days from harvest), and from this period until harvest, *B. thuringiensis* is applied as needed.

Use of *B. thuringiensis* for the control of corn pests has received considerable attention. Tanada and Reiner (1962) reported control of the corn earworm, *Heliothis zea,* in sweet corn by heavy dosages of *B. thuringiensis.* They concluded that earlier workers had failed because of (1) insufficient dosage and (2) differences in potency of the preparations used. Subsequent reports continued to show poor control of *H. zea* in corn (Anderson *et al.*, 1963; Staples *et al.*, 1968; Janes and Greene, 1969). Extensive studies employing *B. thuringiensis* for the control of the European corn borer, *Ostrina nubilalis,* have recently been made. McConnell and Cutkomp (1954) reported that concentrations of *B. thuringiensis* which produced heavy larval mortality in the laboratory could not be relied upon to produce significant control in the field. This was due to the behavior of the small larvae which go deep into the whorl of the plant and thus avoid exposure to the spores. Subsequently, inconsistent, but generally poor results were reported with *B. thuringiensis* for the control of this insect (Hudon, 1962, 1963; Raun, 1963). Success was later achieved with an encapsulated formulation, as well as standard clay granular and emulsifiable formulations (Raun and Jackson, 1966).

For tobacco insect control, commercial preparations of *B. thuringiensis* are as effective as chemical insecticides for control of the tobacco hornworm, *Manduca sexta* (Guthrie *et al.*, 1959; Creighton *et al.*, 1961; Begg, 1964; Rabb and Guthrie, 1964) and for tobacco budworm, *Heliothis virescens* (Creighton *et al.*, 1961). In recent years, commercial preparations have been used extensively for control of these pests in tobacco in the U.S.A., especially in the production of chemical insecticide-free tobacco. *B. thuringiensis* is also an important tool in integrated control programs being developed for tobacco (Gentry *et al.*, 1969).

During the past decade, commercial preparations of *B. thuringiensis* have been tested extensively for control of several cotton pests. Good suppression of the cotton leafworm, *Alabama argillacea,* was reported (Cowan *et al.*, 1960; Ignoffo *et al.*, 1964; Aragon, 1964). Leaf damage by *T. ni* was reduced significantly in a large-scale field test (Falcon *et al.*, 1968). Significant reductions in larval populations of the cotton leaf perforator, *Bucculatrix thurberiella,* were obtained (Aragon, 1964). Ignoffo and Graham (1967) showed marked reductions in overwintering populations of the pink bollworm, *Pectinophora gossypiella,* with high dosages of *B. thuringiensis* applied to the soil. Subsequently, Bullock and Dulmage (1969) obtained good control of pink bollworm on cotton in field cages with foliar applications of 1 and 2 qt/acre. They suggested that early season application of *B. thuringiensis* may be useful in reducing numbers sufficiently, so that other techniques, such as sterile-male releases, may then be used to further reduce populations.

Numerous tests with *B. thuringiensis* have been conducted to develop its use as a selective control of the bollworm, *H. zea,* on cotton (Falcon *et al.*, 1965, 1966, 1968). In early tests, Thuricide at high doses (4 gal/acre) gave encouraging results, but the cost was excessive. Consequently, a major effort was devoted to reducing cost by testing lower dosages, improving timing of application through the use of light traps (Falcon *et al.*, 1967), and developing better sampling techniques to assess bollworm populations (González *et al.*, 1967). In addition, the manufacturers of *B. thuringiensis* improved formulations by selecting strains more pathogenic to *H. zea* and improving the chemical and physical properties of their formulations. In 1968, low dosages (1 qt or 1 lb/acre) of improved formulations of Thuricide and Biotrol applied at 4-6 day intervals significantly reduced worm populations. In 1969, a low dosage (1.5 lb/acre) of Biotrol wettable powder combined with crude molasses (to filter ultraviolet light) suppressed worms in four out of five fields in which it was tested (Falcon, unpublished). A formulation of *B. thuringiensis* produced by a new isolate of

B. thuringiensis var. *alesti,* termed HD-1 (Dulmage, 1970) looked particularly promising for control of *Heliothis* species on cotton (McGarr *et al.,* 1970; Dulmage *et al.,* in press). Thuricide is registered in the U.S.A. for use against the bollworm but has not been employed extensively. It is anticipated that, with additional research, *B. thuringiensis* will be developed as an effective, efficient and economical tool for the control of *H. zea* in cotton.

In two years of field testing, Middlekauff *et al.* (1963) compared *B. thuringiensis* with chemical insecticides for the control of several tomato pests and obtained good control of the western yellow-striped armyworm, *Prodenia praefica,* poor control of *M. sexta* and little or no control of *T. ni, H. zea,* the tomato pinworm, *Kieferia lycopersella,* and the beet armyworm, *Spodoptera exigua.* In this season-long evaluation, *B. thuringiensis* was applied twice in the first year but only once in the second year. Conversely, Shorey and Hall (1963) made weekly applications using high rates of Biotrol dust and wettable powder. They reported good control of *T. ni* and *S. exigua* and fair to good control of *H. zea.* Spray applications were inferior to dust but still provided adequate control.

In other field crops, commercial preparations of *B. thuringiensis* have shown some promise for control of the sugarcane borer, *Diatraea saccharalis,* in the U.S.A. (Long *et al.,* 1961) and for several pests of sugar in India (Kalra and Kumar, 1963) and Taiwan (Yen, 1962). Follow-up research appears to be lacking. The European skipper, *Thymelicus lineola,* a recently introduced pest of timothy in Canada, was effectively controlled with commercial preparations of *B. thuringiensis* (Arthur and Angus, 1965). However, further research showed that the present cost of *B. thuringiensis* preparations makes their use uneconomical on this low cash value crop (Arthur, 1968).

In field studies for the control of insect pests of castor bean, applications of *B. thuringiensis* reduced populations of the leptidopteran, *Euproctis lunata* (Venkatraman *et al.,* 1963), and provided better control of the castor semi-looper, *Achaea janata,* than the insecticide benzene hexachloride (BHC) (Kulshreshtha *et al.,* 1965). In preliminary studies on the integrated control of the pest complex of cowpea (Taylor, 1969), three applications of *B. thuringiensis* followed by three applications of BHC resulted in 60% mortality of the lepidopteran, *Maruca testulis,* compared to 30% reduction where six applications of BHC alone were used.

2. Fruit Crops

Since the late 1950's, *B. thuringiensis* has been tested for control of over 20 species of lepidopterous pests on more than 10 kinds of fruit crops. The codling moth, *Cydia (Laspeyresia) pomonella,* because of its great economic importance, has received considerable attention. In most tests, worm damage to apples was reduced considerably, but insufficiently, by western world standards, to justify its use (McEwen *et al.*, 1960; Jaques, 1961, 1965; Meyer, 1964; Oatman, 1965). The susceptibility of codling larvae to *B. thuringiensis* is similar to that of the cabbage looper. Larval behavior in the field is quite different because codling larvae feed only slightly on the surface before tunneling into an apple, 2-24 hr after eclosion. On walnuts, the pattern of behavior is somewhat different. Newly-hatched larvae may take 2-7 days to enter a nut once the shell has differentiated (Boyce, 1935). Larval entry is usually restricted to the natural openings of the shell at the stem end of the nut, forcing larvae to feed on, and tunnel about, the outer husk seeking a point of entry. Thus, they are more exposed and more likely to ingest spores deposited on the surface of the nut. Falcon (in press) obtained good control of codling moth using three to four applications per season during a three-year study with commercial preparations of *B. thuringiensis.* This provided a selective control agent around which to begin to develop integrated control programs for walnuts in California.

Apple is one of the few crops in which commercial preparations of *B. thuringiensis* have been tested in continuous season-long programs. Jaques (1965) applied Thuricide five to seven times during a growing season for each of four years. Compared to the untreated controls, this had a considerable effect on several species: (1) species reduced for two or more years were the tent caterpillar, *M. americanum,* fall webworm, eye-spotted budmoth, winter moth, codling moth, tentiform leaf miner, *Lithocolletis blancardella,* and the apple rust mite, *Vasates schlechtendali*; (2) no apparent differences were found in the abundance of the European red mite, *Panonychus ulmi,* the brown mite, *Bryobia arborea,* and *Typhlodromus* mite; and (3) population increases were observed for a predaceous mite, *Anystis agilis,* and the mirid, *Philophorous perplexus.* Oatman (1965) reported similarly but with certain exceptions: populations of the European red mite were consistently higher and those of predatory mites (Phytoseiidae) were consistently lower in the *B. thuringiensis* treated areas. In addition, *B. thuringiensis* retarded development of summer larvae and pupae of *Spilonota ocellana,* which greatly reduced moth emergence the following year (Legner and Oatman, 1962; Oatman and Legner, 1964). In still another similar study Cleveland (1966) reported moderate to good control of the red-banded leaf roller, *Argyrotaenia velutinana,* eastern tent caterpillar, and fall webworm.

In Europe, several apple pests have been successfully controlled in field tests with *B. thuringiensis,* including a budmoth, *Argyroplace variegana, S. ocellana, Operophtera brumata,* a small ermine moth, *Hyponomeuta malinellus,* a web moth, *H. padellus,* and *H. cunea* (Herfs, 1964a, b, 1965b). For most species, the commercial preparations of *B. thuringiensis* were about as effective as chemical insecticides.

In peaches, Caltagirone and Falcon (unpublished) did not control the oriental fruit moth, *Grapholitha molesta,* even with several concentrations of Thuricide and Biotrol used alone and in combination with Ryanicide® or Guthion®.

Unexpectedly, populations of the phytophagous mite, *Tetranychus telarius,* were significantly reduced in the *B. thuringiensis*-treated plots compared to the untreated control. Possibly this was due to the exotoxin present in the *B. thuringiensis* preparations as discussed by Krieg (1968). In the same study an important lepidopteran pest of peaches, the peach twig borer, *Anarsia lineatella,* was susceptible to *B. thuringiensis.* Subsequent testing of *B. thuringiensis* against this pest on almond was promising.

On other fruit crops, work by Stafford *et al.* (1960) and Jensen (1966, 1969) led to the use of *B. thuringiensis* to control the grape leaf folder on grapes in California. Both dust and wettable formulations of Thuricide and Biotrol are as effective against this pest as the chemicals carbaryl and lead arsenate. The bacterium is now an important part of the integrated pest control program for grapes. Yamvrias (1967) conducted extensive research with "Bactospéine bonillie", a wettable powder formulation of *B. thuringiensis,* to control the olive moth, *Prays oleae,* in Greece. He reported 80% reductions in the larval population with two treatments applied 4-6 days apart during the flowering period. For control of the citrus-flower moth, *Prays citri,* on citrus in Italy, Giammanco *et al.* (1965, 1966) reported 91% and 72% larval kill with *B. thuringiensis.* In Malaysia, Conway (1969) obtained suppression of larvae of the bagworm complex (Psychidae) on cocoa with Thuricide.

3. Forest, Shade and Ornamental Plants

The gypsy moth, *Lymantria (Porthetria) dispar,* is an important pest of fruit, shade, and forest trees, including conifers, in Europe and north-eastern North America. In the U.S.A., it was effectively controlled by area-wide programs employing DDT. Due to the unfavorable public reaction plus the undesirable side-effects of DDT, researchers were forced to seek more selective methods of control and so commercial formulations of *B. thuringiensis* have been tested extensively. Inconsistent results were obtained with early wettable powders, primarily because of their poor spray characteristics (Cantwell *et al.*, 1961; Lewis *et al.*, 1961). These problems were reduced when a flowable preparation, Thuricide 90T, became available (Doane and Hitchcock, 1964; Lewis, 1964). During three years of field work, Lewis and Connola (1966) and Connola *et al.* (1966), concluded that for control with *B. thuringiensis* (a) protection of foliage was more important than larval kill, (b) timing of application was critical, (c) retreatment was necessary to prevent reinfestation, and (d) the presence of polyhedrosis virus in field populations of the gypsy moth did not enhance control by *B. thuringiensis.* In addition, they employed a fluorescent dye-tracer technique to assess spray coverage and found that certain stabilizers and adjuvants improved effectiveness and persistence of spray deposits. During this period commercial preparations were further improved and good control of gypsy moth was reported in field tests with Thuricide 90TS (Doane, 1966).

In eastern North America the spruce budworm, *Choristoneura fumiferana,* is a serious pest of balsam fir and red fir. In laboratory tests, *C. fumiferana* proved to be susceptible to *B. thuringiensis* (Angus *et al.*, 1961) and *B. cereus* (Smirnoff, 1963, 1965b). Smirnoff also reported that temperature and precipitation, as well as possible bacteriostatic effects from the foliage, were probably the most important factors limiting the control of this pest in the forest. Efforts to develop the use of *B. thuringiensis* to control this species have met with mixed success. Mott *et al.* (1961) reported that aerial applications of Thuricide in water killed some larvae. The addition of oil assisted passage through the spray apparatus, better coverage, deposition and a slightly higher kill. Control was not sufficient, however, to consider its use in place of DDT. Klein and Lewis (1966) found water mixtures to be superior in control compared to oil formulations. Even though neither method provided adequate control they found that *B. thuringiensis* spores would carry-over from field-treated larvae to pupae. A recent personal communication (Cameron) suggests that repeated applications of *B. thuringiensis* may yet provide adequate control of this species.

The black-headed budworm, *Acleris variana,* a pest of hemlock *(Tsuga heterophylla)* is highly susceptible to *B. thuringiensis* (Morris, 1961, 1962; Schmiege and Hard, 1966). In British Columbia, Kinghorn *et al.* (1961) demonstrated that aerial applications of an oil formulation of Thuricide wettable powder left a lethal deposit of the bacterium on the foliage, but the clumping tendency of the formulation and the short residual life of the deposits were detrimental to control efficiency. Morris (1969a) found that foliage extracts from *T. heterophylla* inhibited spore and crystal formation of *B. thuringiensis.* Morris (1969b) field tested Thuricide in conjunction with various sticker-spreaders. The materials were sprayed on three occasions to each of two test plots during early summer. Spray coverage was good. Effectiveness was assessed in several ways: (1) prespray and postspray egg and larval samples from the treated trees, (2) assay of treated foliage with healthy larvae, (3) larvae were transferred from sprayed trees to unsprayed foliage, and (4) healthy larvae were moved to sprayed trees. Morris attempted to separate larval mortality due to natural causes from mortality caused by *B. thuringiensis* in the natural population. That due to the bacterium ranged from 66% to 95% and additional mortality could be expected in the pupal and adult stages. Persistence studies indicated that the spore deposits on the foliage killed some larvae 38 days after application. Morris concluded that Thuricide was a highly promising control agent for *A. variana.*

On broadleaf trees, commercial *B. thuringiensis* has been field tested for control of several insect species, most with positive results. Duda (1962) claimed 100% control of the linden looper, *Erannis tiliaria,* on American elm, nine days after treatment with Bakthane. Thuricide and Biotrol used alone and in combination with field-collected nuclear polyhedrosis virus in small-scale experiments on the Great Basin tent caterpillar, *Malacosoma fragile incurva,* produced encouraging control (Stelzer, 1965). This was followed by a large-scale forest test with a combination of Thuricide and polyhedrosis virus in a corn syrup-water mixture plus a wetting agent (Triton B-1956) (Stelzer, 1967). One year later, populations were 95% lower in the sprayed portion compared to the untreated area. Morris (1969b) tested *B. thuringiensis* (Thuricide 90TS) against the western tent caterpillar, *M. pluviale,* and also found greatly reduced populations one year following treatment. Natural mortality from parasites was low, but mortality caused by unknown factors was high. There was no mention of virus in the population. In California, *B. thuringiensis* proved highly effective against the California oakmoth, *Phryganidia californica,* on coast live oak (Pinnock and Milstead, in press). One application of either Thuricide 90TS flowable, Biotrol BTB wettable powder or dust, timed to coincide with the early third instar larva, provided complete control. The cost for application of these materials is competitive with that for currently used chemicals.

In Europe and the U.S.S.R., *B. thuringiensis* has been widely tested for control of several forest insect pests. Franz and Krieg (1967) discussed the success of large-scale efforts against the Siberian silkworm, *Dendrolimus sibiricus* (U.S.S.R.), the oak tortricid, *Tortrix viridana* (U.S.S.R. and Europe) and the grey larch tortricid, *Eucosma diniana* (Europe). In addition, they discuss the testing of *B. thuringiensis* against several other insect species including *Cacoecia murinana, Thaumetopoea pityocampa, T. wilkinsoni, Lymantria dispar, L. monacha, Panolis flammea* and *Archips crataegana.*

4. Stored Products

B. thuringiensis has been tested for control of several insect pests of stored products and has suppressed populations of the Mediterranean flour moth, *Ephestia (Anagasta) kuehniella* (Burges, 1964a; van der Laan and Wassink, 1964; Gibson and Wolf, 1964); the tobacco moth, *Ephestia elutella* (Burges, 1964a; van der Laan and Wassink, 1964); the almond moth, *Ephestia (Cadra) cautella* (Godavaribai *et al.,* 1962; Loaiza-Mercado, 1962; Burges, 1964a; van der Laan and Wassink, 1964); the Indian meal moth, *Plodia interpunctella* (Kantack, 1959; Burges, 1964a; van der Laan and Wassink, 1964); the Angoumois grain moth, *Sitotroga cerealella* (Zagatto *et al.,* 1963); the greater wax moth, *Galleria mellonella* (Burges, 1964a; van der Laan and Wassink, 1964; Burges and Bailey, 1968); and the lesser wax moth, *Achroia grisella* (van der Laan and Wassink, 1964; Burges and Bailey, 1968). Use of this bacterium for control of these pests has been only on an experimental scale, because it is too expensive and possibly too selective. Burges (1964a) stated, "Specificity of this bacterium almost entirely to Lepidoptera is a great disadvantage in food stores where Coleoptera are common and where there are no predatory insects worth preserving." In addition he states, "Bacteria are probably more suitable for the prevention of infestation by insects than for the treatment of food already containing well-established infestations, which are often best eradicated by fumigation."

5. Insects of Medical Importance

Considerable testing of *B. thuringiensis* in recent years has shown that the thermostable exotoxin kills several dipterous pests in animal droppings. As a feed additive, the bacterium does not affect steers (Dunn, 1960; Gingrich, 1965; Gingrich and Eschle, 1966), poultry (Sherman and Ross, 1961; Millar, 1965), and Japanese quail (Borgatti and Guyer, 1963). Sufficient exotoxin appeared in animal droppings to kill larvae of the common housefly, *Musca domestica* (Millar, 1965; Gingrich, 1965), face fly, *Musca autumnalis* (Yendol and Miller, 1967; Hower and Cheng, 1968) and hornfly, *Siphona (Haematobia) irritans* (Gingrich, 1965; Gingrich and Eschle, 1966).

Species in several other insect groups are affected by the exotoxin (Heimpel, 1967). Some of the symptoms described include inhibition of development, death following moulting and prevention of pupation. The exotoxin is not present in all commercial preparations of *B. thuringiensis* and its safety for vertebrates has not been fully established. If it is found to be harmful it may be removed by washing at harvest of the bacteria (Angus, 1968).

Another area in which *B. thuringiensis* has shown promise is for control of chicken body, shaft and wing lice (Mallophaga). Hoffman and Gingrich (1968) found that one or more dustings of 3.5 g of Bakthane per bird controlled lice effectively. The component in Bakthane causing death was not determined, but other tests had demonstrated that inert diluents similar to those in the Bakthane preparation did not affect lice when applied as dusts to poultry.

VI. Appraisal

About 100 years have passed since man first learnt that bacteria cause diseases in insects. Even though efforts to use them for insect control were made from 1910, there was no real encouragement until the discovery and practical use of the milky disease bacteria against the Japanese beetle in 1940. This accomplishment helped to establish insect pathology as an important discipline on an international scale. Then came the major effort by the late E. A. Steinhaus, and others in the 1950's, which led to the development of *B. thuringiensis* as a useful microbial control agent. In the last decade much of the research effort in microbial control has been concerned with this bacterium.

The early commercial preparations of *B. thuringiensis,* first made available in 1958, were not uniform, tended to settle quickly in spray containers and varied in potency. Research with spreaders, stickers, anti-weathering agents, emulsifiers and stabilizing agents, as well as the selection of more potent strains, and improved production methods, resulted in better and more reliable commercial products. In the field, information on how and when to use them for effective insect control was and is being developed. These efforts, plus the need to replace certain dangerous chemical insecticides, have led to increased usage of *B. thuringiensis* both in research and in commercial pest control in recent years.

With the current interest in preventing environmental contamination and the need to develop integrated control and pest management programs, *B. thuringiensis* is one of the few available "broad spectrum", yet selective and ecologically safe, insect control agents. As a result, its use should accelerate during the 1970's. Furthermore, its successful development has given researchers and industry experience and confidence to develop other microbial agents.

On the negative side, it may be said that interest in *B. thuringiensis* has not only detracted significantly from the development of other bacteria but also from many other aspects of microbial control as well. Most other entomogenous bacteria have not shown the same potential as the crystalliferous bacteria and their use certainly presents difficult problems. Given the same intensive research effort as devoted to the development of *B. thuringiensis,* many other bacteria would find a place in the pest control arsenal.

Research problems facing the further development of bacteria for use in microbial control are many. For the highly promising obligate bacteria, efficient artificial mass culture techniques must be found. As concerns the non-sporeformers, methods must be sought to improve their virulence and persistence under field conditions. Also, more information is needed on their host range and safety. Little is known about the importance of bacteria as natural control agents and how to initiate infection or enhance their effectiveness. Most recent research has concentrated on short-term control: sorely neglected, is the selection, importation and colonization of bacteria for long-term control of exotic insect pests. In the short-term, additional exploration is needed on methods of application, the use of bacteria in combination with chemical, macrobial and other microbial agents for improved pest control. The potential of bacteria in integrated control and pest management programs is great and should be fully exploited, as should the development of bacterial toxins as "natural insecticides".

The past quarter century has seen entomogenous bacteria play an increasing role in insect control and make significant contributions to microbial control and insect pathology. In the dawning era of ecological-pest control, their future looks even brighter.

References

Afrikan, E. K. (1963). *Arm. Akad. Nauk S.S.S.R. Izv. Biol. Inst.* **16,** 23-38.
Anderson, L. D., Nakakihara, H. and Hall, I. M. (1963). *J. econ. Ent.* **56,** 40-42.
Angus, T. A. (1956). *Can. Ent.* **88,** 280-283.
Angus, T. A. (1965a). *Bacteriol. Rev.* **29,** 364-372.
Angus, T. A. (1965b). *Proc. ent. Soc. Ontario* **95,** 133-134.
Angus, T. A. (1968). *World Rev. Pest Control* **7,** 11-26.
Angus, T. A. and Heimpel, A. M. (1959). *Can. Ent.* **91,** 352-358.
Angus, T. A. and Norris, J. R. (1968). *J. Invertebrate Path.* **11,** 289-295.

Angus, T. A., Heimpel, A. M. and Fisher, R. A. (1961). *Can. Dep. Forest. Bi-monthly Progr. Rep.* **17**, 1-2.
Ankersmit, G. W., Locher, J. T., Velthuis, H. H. W. and Zwart, K. W. R. (1962). *Entomophaga* **7**, 251-255.
Anonymous. (1952). *Farmer's Bulletin* No. 2004. U.S.D.A. 14 pp.
Anonymous. (1969). *In* "Principles of Plant and Animal Pest Control", Vol. 3, pp. 165-195. National Academy of Sciences, Washington, D.C.
Aragon, J. H. (1964). *Acta agron. Palmira* **14**, 103-224.
Arthur, A. P. (1968). *J. Invertebrate Path.* **10**, 146-150.
Arthur, A. P. and Angus, T. A. (1965). *J. Invertebrate Path.* **7**, 180-183.
Barjac, H. de and Bonnefoi, A. (1967). *C.r. hebd. Séanc. Acad. Sci., Paris* **264**, 1811-1813.
Beard, R. L. (1964). *Mém. hors Sér. Entomophaga* No. 2, pp. 47-49.
Begg, J. A. (1964). *J. econ. Ent.* **57**, 646-649.
Biliotti, E. (1956). *Entomophaga* **1**, 45-53.
Borgatti, A. L. and Guyer, G. E. (1963). *J. Insect Path.* **5**, 377-384.
Boyce, A. M. (1935). *J. econ. Ent.* **28**, 864-873.
Bucher, G. E. (1957). *Can. J. Microbiol.* **3**, 695-709.
Bucher, G. E. (1960). *J. Insect Path.* **2**, 172-195.
Bucher, G. E. (1961). *J. Insect Path.* **3**, 439-445.
Bucher, G. E. (1963a). *In* "Insect Pathology. An Advanced Treatise" (E. A. Steinhaus, ed.), Vol. 2, pp. 117-147. Academic Press, New York.
Bucher, G. E. (1963b). *J. Insect Path.* **5**, 277-283.
Bucher, G. E. (1967). *J. Invertebrate Path.* **9**, 82-89.
Bucher, G. E. and Williams, R. (1967). *J. Invertebrate Path.* **9**, 467-473.
Bullock, H. R. and Dulmage, H. T. (1969). *J. econ. Ent.* **62**, 994-995.
Burgerjon, A. and Biache, G. (1967). *In* "Insect Pathology and Microbial Control" (P. A. van der Laan, ed.), pp. 294-296. North-Holland Publ. Co., Amsterdam.
Burges, H. D. (1964a). *Mém. hors Sér. Entomophaga* No. 2, pp. 323-327.
Burges, H. D. (1964b). *World Crops* **16**, 70-76.
Burges, H. D. (1967). *In* "Insect Pathology and Microbial Control" (P. A. van der Laan, ed.), pp. 306-314. North-Holland Publ. Co., Amsterdam.
Burges, H. D. and Bailey, L. (1968). *J. Invertebrate Path.* **11**, 184-195.
Cameron, J. W. M. (1963). *Ann. Rev. Ent.* **8**, 265-286.
Cameron, J. W. M. (1967). *In* "Insect Pathology and Microbial Control" (P. A. van der Laan, ed.), pp. 182-196. North-Holland Publ. Co., Amsterdam.
Cameron, J. W. M. (1969). *Proc. ent. Soc. Ontario* **95**, 73-79.
Cantwell, G. E. (1967). *J. Invertebrate Path.* **9**, 138-140.
Cantwell, G. E. and Franklin, B. A. (1966). *J. Invertebrate Path.* **8**, 256-258.
Cantwell, G. E., Dutky, S. R., Keller, J. C. and Thompson, C. G. (1961). *J. Insect Path.* **3**, 143-147.
Cass, L. M. (1962). *Proc. ent. Soc. Ontario* **93**, 85-87.
Cass, L. M. (1965). *Phytoprotection* **46**, 1-4.
Chalfant, R. B. and Brett, C. H. (1965). *J. econ. Ent.* **58**, 28-33.
Cheshire, F. R. and Cheyne, W. W. (1885). *J. R. Microscop. Soc.* **5**, 581-601.
Cleveland, M. L. (1966). United States Dep. Agric., Agric. Res. Service, Ent. Res. Div., Fruit and Vegetable Insects Res. Branch, Vincennes, Indiana (mimeo), 37 pp.
Connola, D. P., Lewis, F. B. and McDonough, J. L. (1966). *J. econ. Ent.* **59**, 284-287.
Conway, G. R. (1969). *Natur. Hist.* **78**, 46-51.
Cory, E. N. and Langford, G. S. (1955). *Univ. of Maryland Extension Bull.* **156**, 20 pp.
Cowan, C. B., Jr., Davis, J. W. and Parencia, C. R., Jr. (1960). *J. econ. Ent.* **53**, 747-749.
Creighton, C. S., Cuthbert, F. P., Jr. and Reid, W., Jr. (1964). *J. Insect Path.* **6**, 102-110.
Creighton, C. S., Kinard, W. S. and Allen, N. (1961). *J. econ. Ent.* **54**, 1112-1114.
Doane, C. C. (1964). *Frontiers Plant Sci.* **16**, 6-7.
Doane, C. C. (1966). *J. econ. Ent.* **59**, 618-620.
Doane, C. C. and Hitchcock, S. W. (1964). *Conn. Agric. Exp. Stn Bull.* **665**, 20 pp.
Doane, C. C. and Wallis, R. C. (1964). *J. Insect Path.* **6**, 423-429.

Duda, E. J. (1962). *Scient. Tree Top.* (Stamford, Conn.) **2,** 14.
Dulmage, H. T. (1970). *J. Invertebrate Path.* **15,** 232-239.
Dulmage, H. T., Lukefahr, M. J., Graham, H. M. and Hernandez, N. S. (1970). *J. econ. Ent.* (In press.)
Dunn, P. H. (1960). *J. Insect Path.* **2,** 13-16.
Dutky, S. R. (1963). *In* "Insect Pathology. An Advanced Treatise" (E. A. Steinhaus, ed.), Vol. 2, pp. 75-115. Academic Press, New York.
Falcon, L. A. (1970). *J. econ. Ent.* (In press.)
Falcon, L. A., Leigh, T. F., van den Bosch, R., Black, J. H. and Burton, V. E. (1965). *Calif. Agric.* **19,** 12-14.
Falcon, L. A., van den Bosch, R., Etzel, L. K., Ferris, C. A. and Stromberg, L. K. (1967). *Calif. Agric.* **21,** 12-14.
Falcon, L. A., van den Bosch, R., Ferris, C. A., Stromberg, L. K., Etzel, L. K., Stinner, R. E. and Leigh, T. F. (1968). *J. econ. Ent.* **61,** 633-642.
Falcon, L. A., van den Bosch, R., Leigh, T. F., Etzel, L. K. and Stinner, R. E. (1966). *In* "Cotton Insect Control—A Progress Report on Research", pp. 17-22. Div. Agric. Sci. Univ. Calif.
Fedorinchik, N. S. (1964). U.S.S.R. Min. Agric. "Kolos" publications, Moscow. pp. 1-6.
Franz, J. M. (1964). *In* "Global Impacts of Applied Microbiology" (M. P. Starr, ed.), pp. 256-266. John Wiley and Sons, New York.
Franz, J. M. (1966). *Rijksfaculteit Landbouwwetenschappen. Mededelingen.* (Ghent) **31,** 512-525.
Franz, J. M. and Krieg, A. (1967). *Gesunde Pfl.* **19,** 175-182.
Frye, R. D. and Scholz, E. W. (1965). *North Dakota Farm Res.* **23,** 21.
Geering, Q. A. and Lloyd, J. H. (1962). *J. econ. Ent.* **55,** 786-790.
Gentry, C. W., Thomas, W. W. and Stanley, J. M. (1969). *J. econ. Ent.* **62,** 1274-1277.
Giammanco, G., Militello, M. and Mineo, G. (1965). *Boll. Dell'Istituto Ent. Agr. Dell'Osservatorio Fitopathologia Palermo* **6,** 17-28.
Giammanco, G., Militello, M. and Mineo, G. (1966). *Entomophaga* **11,** 211-212.
Gibson, N. H. E. and Wolf, J. (1964). *Mém. hors Sér. Entomophaga* No. 2, 329-336.
Gingrich, R. E. (1965). *J. econ. Ent.* **58,** 363-364.
Gingrich, R. E. and Eschle, J. L. (1966). *J. Invertebrate Path.* **8,** 285-287.
Godavaribai, S., Krishnamurthy, K. and Majumder, S. K. (1962). *Pest Technol.* **4,** 155-158.
González, R., van den Bosch, R., Orphanides, G. M., Dawson, L. and White, C. (1967). *Calif. Agric.* **21,** 12-14.
Gould, H. J., Hussey, N. W. and Parr, W. J. (1969). *Proc. 2nd Congr. Acarol.* **1967,** 383-388.
Greene, G. L., Genung, W. G., Workman, R. B. and Kelsheimer, E. G. (1969). *J. econ. Ent.* **62,** 798-800.
Grison, P. (1967). *Phytiat.-Phytopharm.* **16,** 63-74.
Gukasyan, A. B. (1961). *Akad. Nauk S.S.S.R. Vestnik* **31,** 58-59.
Guthrie, F. E., Rabb, R. L. and Bowery, T. G. (1959). *J. econ. Ent.* **52,** 798-804.
Hall, I. M. (1963). *In* "Insect Pathology. An Advanced Treatise" (E. A. Steinhaus, ed.), Vol. 2, pp. 477-518. Academic Press, New York.
Hall, I. M. (1964). *In* "Biological Control of Insect Pests and Weeds" (P. DeBach, ed.), pp. 610-628. Chapman and Hall, London.
Hall, I. M. (1967). *Mushi* (Suppl.) **39,** 75-84.
Hall, I. M. (1968). Proc. Joint U.S.-Japan Semin. Microbial Control Insect Pests. U.S.-Japan Committee Sci. Cooperation. Panel 8, Fukuoka, 165-167.
Heimpel, A. M. (1955a). *Can. J. Zool.* **33,** 99-106.
Heimpel, A. M. (1955b). *Can. J. Zool.* **33,** 311-326.
Heimpel, A. M. (1963). *In* "New Approaches to Pest Control and Eradication". *Bull. Am. chem. Soc.* **41,** 64-74.
Heimpel, A. M. (1964). *Mém. hors Sér. Entomophaga* No. 2, 23-33.
Heimpel, A. M. (1965). *Wld Rev. Pest Control* **4,** 150-161.
Heimpel, A. M. (1967). *Ann. Rev. Ent.* **12,** 287-322.
Heimpel, A. M. and Angus, T. A. (1958). *Can. J. Microbiol.* **4,** 531-541.

Heimpel, A. M. and Angus, T. A. (1959). *J. Insect Path.* **1,** 152-170.
Heimpel, A. M. and Angus, T. A. (1963). *In* "Insect Pathology. An Advanced Treatise" (E. A. Steinhaus, ed.), Vol. 2, pp. 21-73. Academic Press, New York.
Herfs, W. (1963). *Entomophaga* **8,** 163-181.
Herfs, W. (1964a). *NachrBl. dt. PflSchutzdienst. Braunschw.* **16,** 147-149.
Herfs, W. (1964b). *Z. PflKrankh.* **71,** 332-344.
Herfs, W. (1965a). *Mitt. Biol. Bundesanstalt Land- Forstwirtsch. Berlin-Dahlem* **115,** 60-70.
Herfs, W. (1965b). *Z. PflKrankh.* **72,** 65-77.
Herfs, W. (1965c). *Z. PflKrankh.* **72,** 584-599.
Herfs, W. (1967). *Mém. hors Sér. Entomophaga* No. 3, pp. 113-117.
Herfs, W. and Krieg, A. (1963). *NachrBl. dt. PflSchutzdienst. Braunschw.* **15,** 49-54.
Himel, M., Vaughn, L., Miskus, R. P. and Moore, A. D. (1965). U.S.D.A. Forest Serv. Pacific Southwest Forest Range Exp. Stn. Res. Note PSW-87, 10 pp.
Hitchings, D. L. (1967). *J. econ. Ent.* **60,** 596-597.
Hoffman, R. A. and Gingrich, R. E. (1968). *J. econ. Ent.* **61,** 85-88.
Hower, A. A., Jr. and Cheng, Tien-Hsi. (1968). *J. econ. Ent.* **61,** 26-31.
Hudon, M. (1962). *J. econ. Ent.* **55,** 115-117.
Hudon, M. (1963). *J. econ. Ent.* **56,** 804-808.
Hurpin, B. (1966). *Proc. FAO Symp. Integrated Pest Control (1965).* Part 2, pp. 149-165.
Ignoffo, C. M. (1962). *J. Insect Path.* **4,** 63-71.
Ignoffo, C. M. (1964). *Mém. hors Sér. Entomophaga* No. 2, 293-298.
Ignoffo, C. M. (1967). *In* "Insect Pathology and Microbial Control" (P. A. van der Laan, ed.), pp. 91-117. North-Holland Publ. Co., Amsterdam.
Ignoffo, C. M. and Graham, H. M. (1967). *J. Invertebrate Path.* **9,** 390-394.
Ignoffo, C. M., Garcia, C. and Gasparotto, V. A. (1968). *J. Invertebrate Path.* **11,** 97-103.
Ignoffo, C. M., McGarr, R. L. and Martin, D. F. (1964). *J. Insect Path.* **6,** 411-416.
Isakova, N. P. (1965). *Zashch. Rast. Vredit. Bolez.* **3,** 51.
Isakova, N. P. and Moisejeva, T. S. (1966). *9th Int. Congr. Microbiol. Moscow 1966, Abstr.,* pp. 321-322.
Isakova, N. P. and Moisejeva, T. S. (1967). *In* "Insect Pathology and Microbial Control" (P. A. van der Laan, ed.), pp. 281-282. North-Holland Publ. Co., Amsterdam.
Jafri, R. H. (1964). *Mém. hors Sér. Entomophaga* No. 2, 351-354.
Janes, M. J. and Greene, G. L. (1969). *J. econ. Ent.* **62,** 1031-1033.
Jaques, R. P. (1961). *J. Insect Path.* **3,** 167-182.
Jaques, R. P. (1964). *Ann. ent. Soc. Quebec* **9,** 17-29.
Jaques, R. P. (1965). *Can. Ent.* 97, 795-802.
Jensen, F. L. (1966). *Calif. Agric.* **20,** 2-3.
Jensen, F. L. (1969). *Calif. Agric.* **23,** 5-6.
Kalra, A. N. and Kumar, S. (1963). *Indian J. Sugarcane Res.* **8,** 75.
Kalyuga, M. V. (1968). *Ent. Rev.* **47,** 274-276.
Kantack, B. H. (1959). *J. econ. Ent.* **52,** 1226-1227.
Kinghorn, J. M., Fisher, R. A., Angus, T. A. and Heimpel, A. M. (1961). *Can. Dep. Forest. Bi-monthly Progr. Rep.* **17**(3), 3-4.
Klein, W. H. and Lewis, F. B. (1966). *J. Forestry* **64,** 458-462.
Krieg, A. (1965). *Dtsch. Bienenwirtsch.* **16,** 27-30.
Krieg, A. (1967). *Mitt. biol. BundAnst. Ld- u. Forstw. B.* **125,** 1-106.
Krieg, A. (1968). *J. Invertebrate Path.* **12,** 478.
Krieg, A. and Schmidt, L. (1962). *NachrBl. dt. PflSchutzdienst. Braunschw.* **14,** 177-182.
Kulshreshtha, J. P., Sanghi, P. K. and Ravindranath, V. (1965). *Indian J. Ent.* **27,** 353-354.
Kurstak, E. S. (1964a). *C.r. hebd. Séanc. Acad. Sci. Paris* **259,** 211-212.
Kurstak, E. S. (1964b). *Mém. hors Sér. Entomophaga* No. 2, 245-247.
Kushner, D. J. and Harvey, G. T. (1960). *Can. Dep. Agr. Bi-monthly Progr. Rep.* **16**(5), 2-3.
Kushner, D. J. and Harvey, G. T. (1962). *J. Insect Path.* **4,** 155-184.
Laan, P. A. van der and Wassink, H. J. M. (1964). *Mém. hors Sér. Entomophaga* No. 2, 315-322.
Lappa, N. V. (1963). *Zoologicheskii Zhurnal* **52,** 1064-1070.

Legner, E. F. and Oatman, E. R. (1962). *J. econ. Ent.* **55**, 677-678.
Lewis, F. B. (1964). Northeastern Forest Exp. Stn. (New Haven, Conn.), 3 pp.
Lewis, F. B. (1966). Northeastern Forest Exp. Stn. 4500-FS-NE-2202.23, 10 pp.
Lewis, F. B. and Connola, D. P. (1966). U.S. Forest Service Res. Paper NE-50, 38 pp.
Lewis, F. B., Connola, D. P. and Swett, R. C. (1961). Northeastern Forest Exp. Stn. (New Haven, Conn.) Special Report, 19 pp.
Loaiza-Mercado, V. M. (1962). *Fitofilo* **15**(34), 30-48; (35), 5-29.
Long, W. H., Hensley, S. D., Concienne, E. J. and McCormick, W. J. (1961). *J. econ. Ent.* **54**, 1155-1156.
McConnell, E. and Cutkomp, L. K. (1954). *J. econ. Ent.* **47**, 1074-1081.
McEwen, F. L., Glass, E. H., Davis, A. C. and Splittstoesser, C. M. (1960). *J. Insect Path.* **2**, 152-164.
McGarr, R. L., Dulmage, H. T. and Wolfenbarger, D. A. (1970). *J. econ. Ent.* **63**, 1357-1358.
Madsen, H. F. and Downing, R. S. (1968). *J. ent. Soc. Brit. Columbia* **65**, 19-21.
Martouret, D. (1967). *Académie d'Agriculture de France. C.r. hebd. Séanc.* **53**, 154-159.
Martouret, D. and Milaire, H. (1963). *Phytiat. Phytopharm.* **12**, 71-80.
Meyer, R. H. (1964). *Diss. Abstr.* **24**, 3896-3897.
Middlekauff, W. W., Gonzales, C. Q. and King, R. C. (1963). *J. econ. Ent.* **56**, 155-158.
Millar, E. S. (1965). *New Zealand J. Agric. Res.* **8**, 721-722.
Norris, O. N. (1961). *Can. Dep. Forest. Bi-monthly Progr. Rep.* **17**(3), 2-3.
Morris, O. N. (1962). *Can. Ent.* **94**, 686-690.
Morris, O. N. (1969a). *J. Invertebrate Path.* **13**, 134-146.
Morris, O. N. (1969b). *J. Invertebrate Path.* **13**, 285-295.
Mott, D. G., Angus, T. A., Heimpel, A. M. and Fisher, R. A. (1961). *Can. Dep. Forest. Bi-monthly Progr. Rep.* **17**(3), 2.
Norris, J. R. (1964). *J. appl. Bacteriol.* **27**, 439-447.
Norris, J. R. (1965). *Ann. appl. Biol.* **56**, 335.
Oatman, E. R. (1965). *J. econ. Ent.* **58**, 1144-1147.
Oatman, E. R. and Legner, E. F. (1964). *J. econ. Ent.* **57**, 294.
Pasteur, L. (1870). "Etudes sur la maladie des vers à soie". Tome I, 322 pp. Tome II, 327 pp. Gauthier-Villars, Paris.
Pinnock, D. E. and Milstead, J. E. *J. econ. Ent.* (In press.)
Pristavko, V. P. (1967). *Ent. Rev.* **46**, 443-446.
Prokhorov, M. I., ed. (1964). ["The Use of Micro-organisms to Control Agricultural Pests"] "Kolos" publications, Leningrad, 86 pp.
Rabb, R. L. and Guthrie, F. E. (1964). *J. econ. Ent.* **57**, 995-996.
Raun, E. S. (1963). *Iowa State J. Sci.* **38**, 141-150.
Raun, E. S. and Brooks, D. L. (1963). *J. Insect Path.* **5**, 66-71.
Raun, E. S. and Jackson, R. D. (1966). *J. econ. Ent.* **59**, 620-622.
Raun, E. S., Sutter, G. R. and Revelo, M. A. (1966). *J. Invertebrate Path.* **8**, 365-375.
Rhodes, R. A. (1968). *In* "Proc. Joint U.S.-Japan Semin. Microbial Control Insect Pests". U.S.-Japan Committee Sci. Cooperation. Panel 8. Fukuoka, 85-92.
Rivers, C. F. (1967). *In* "Insect Pathology and Microbial Control" (P. A. van der Laan, ed.), pp. 252-263. North-Holland Publ. Co., Amsterdam.
Rogoff, M. H., Ignoffo, C. M., Singer, S., Gard, I. and Prieto, A. P. (1969). *J. Invertebrate Path.* **14**, 122-129.
Rolston, L. H. and Mayes, R. (1965). *Farm Res.* **14**(3), 7.
Schmiege, D. C. and Hard, J. S. (1966). U.S. Dep. Agric. Forest Serv., Northern Forest Exp. Stn. Res. Note NOR-17, 4 pp.
Shchepetilnikova, V. A. and Fedorinchik, N. S. (1963). Thèses 5e. Conf. Soc. Ent. Union, pp. 132-134.
Sherman, M. and Ross, E. (1961). *J. econ. Ent.* **54**, 573-578.
Shorey, H. H. and Hall, I. M. (1963). *J. econ. Ent.* **56**, 813-817.
Sicker, W., Magnoler, A. and Huger, A. (1965). *Z. PflKrankh.* **71**, 332-344.
Sirko, L. A., Poltev, V. I. and Sheukunova, V. S. (1966). *9th Int. Congr. Microbiol. Moscow 1966, Abstr.*, p. 317.

Smirnoff, W. A. (1963). *Can. Ent.* **95**, 127-133.
Smirnoff, W. A. (1965a). *J. Invertebrate Path.* **7**, 71-74.
Smirnoff, W. A. (1965b). *J. Invertebrate Path.* **7**, 266-269.
Smirnoff, W. A. (1967). *In* "Insect Pathology and Microbial Control" (P. A. van der Laan, ed.), pp. 179-180. North-Holland Publ. Co., Amsterdam.
Smirnoff, W. A. (1968). *J. Invertebrate Path.* **11**, 513-515.
Smirnoff, W. A. and Hutchison, P. M. (1965). *J. Invertebrate Path.* **7**, 273-280.
Stafford, E. M., Jensen, F. L. and Kido, H. (1960). *J. econ. Ent.* **53**, 531-534.
Staples, R., Kindler, S. D. and Kantack, B. H. (1968). *J. econ. Ent.* **61**, 774-776.
Steinhaus, E. A. (1951). *Hilgardia* **20**, 359-381.
Steinhaus, E. A. (ed.) (1963). "Insect Pathology. An Advanced Treatise", Vol. 1, 2. Academic Press, New York.
Steinkraus, K. H. and Tashiro, H. (1967). *Appl. Microbiol.* **15**, 325-333.
Stelzer, M. J. (1965). *J. Invertebrate Path.* **7**, 122-125.
Stelzer, M. J. (1967). *J. econ. Ent.* **60**, 38-41.
Talalaev, E. V. (1958). *Ent. Obozr.* **37**, 641-652.
Talalaev, E. V. (1959). *Trans. 1st Int. Conf. Insect Path. and Biol. Control Praha 1958*, pp. 51-57.
Talalayev, E. (1966). *Int. Congr. Microbiol. Moscow 1966, Abstr.*, pp. 324-325.
Talalayeva, G. B. (1966). *9th Int. Congr. Microbiol. Moscow 1966, Abstr.*, p. 317.
Talalayeva, G. B. (1967). *Ent. Rev.* **46**, 191-192.
Tanada, Y. (1967). *In* "Pest Control" (W. W. Kilgore and R. L. Doutt, eds), pp. 31-88. Academic Press, New York.
Tanada, Y. and Reiner, C. (1962). *J. Insect Path.* **4**, 139-154.
Taylor, T. A. (1969). *J. econ. Ent.* **62**, 900-902.
Tyumentsev, S. N. (1963). *Mikrobiologiya* **32**, 879-884.
Vago, C. and Burges, H. D. (1964). *Entomophaga* **9**, 305-308.
Vaňková, J. (1962). *Ústav Vĕdeckotechnických Informaci Ministerstva Zemĕdĕlstvi, Rostlinná Výroba* **8**, 571-576.
Vaňková, J. (1964). *Mém. hors Sér. Entomophaga* No. 2, 271-291.
Venkatraman, T. V., Mathur, V. K. and Chander, R. (1963). *Indian J. Ent.* **24**, 274-277.
White, R. T. (1943). *J. New York Ent. Soc.* **51**, 213-218.
White, R. T. and Dutky, S. R. (1940). *J. econ. Ent.* **33**, 306-309.
Wiackowski, S. K. and Wiackowska, I. (1966). *Entomophaga* **11**, 261-267.
Wolfenbarger, D. A. (1965). *J. Invertebrate Path.* **7**, 33-38.
Yamvrias, C. (1967). *In* "Insect Pathology and Microbial Control" (P. A. van der Laan, ed.), pp. 284-285. North-Holland Publ. Co., Amsterdam.
Yen, D. F.-Y. (1962). *Q. J. Taiwan Mus.* **15**, 117-122.
Yendol, W. G. and Miller, E. M. (1967). *J. econ. Ent.* **60**, 860-864.
Zagatto, A. G., Orlando, A. and Coutinho, J. M. (1963). *Biológico*, Sao Paulo **29**, 234-236.

CHAPTER 4

Use of Viruses for Microbial Control of Insects

GORDON R. STAIRS

Faculty of Entomology, The Ohio State University, Columbus, Ohio, U.S.A.

I. Introduction

The occurrence of viruses in insect populations is well documented and new viruses are being discovered as pest species are studied more intensively. Much information has been obtained on the natural distribution and dispersal of a few viruses but very little for the great majority. The nuclear-polyhedrosis viruses (NPV) have been studied most and enough basic information is available for some to permit their intelligent manipulation to control pests. Studies of the granulosis (GV) and cytoplasmic-polyhedrosis viruses (CPV) indicate that they also can be used. Always, a sufficient body of knowledge must be built by a quantitative, scientific approach to ensure that we take full advantage of viruses.

In this chapter emphasis will be placed on basic host-virus relationships, the use of viruses in both long-term and short-term pest control. Specific pest species and their respective viruses will be discussed in detail as models to further our understanding of other virus-host systems and of the best application for population regulation.

Laboratory experiments and field trials with insect viruses all have some aspects in common. The virus is propagated in living larvae, the dead and dying larvae being triturated in water, often followed by a purification procedure like that described on page 99, or the insects may be dried and the virus formulated as a dust. Polyhedra are counted in standard counting chambers, but the granulosis capsules are too small to be counted in this way, dosage being expressed as the number of larval bodies. In the following descriptions of studies of different viruses, any deviations will be specifically mentioned.

II. Tenthredinoidea (Sawflies)

A few species of these plant-feeding Hymenoptera are susceptible to nuclear-polyhedrosis viruses (NPV), which cause destructive disease of the larval midgut epithelium (Balch and Bird, 1944; Bird, 1949, 1953; Dowden, 1940; Smirnoff, 1961). These viruses often cause high mortality and may play an important role in the natural regulation of host populations (Bird and Elgee, 1957; Bird and Burk, 1961; Neilson and Morris, 1964). Many more species of sawflies are probably infected by these viruses, which await discovery. A few species of the families Tenthredinidae and Diprionidae are susceptible (Bird, 1949; Smirnoff, 1962) and most species of the family Neodiprionidae (Bird, 1950, 1952; Escherich, 1913; Forrslund, 1945; Smirnoff, 1961; Hughes, 1957). Some of the viruses have been used against pest species (Bird, 1953, 1961, 1964; Smirnoff *et al.*, 1962; Bird and Burk, 1961; Rivers, 1962).

A. *GILPINIA (DIPRION) HERCYNIAE*, EUROPEAN SPRUCE SAWFLY

Studies on the NPV of this species have provided a fine model for investigation of diseases of other sawflies. When this sawfly threatened to destroy the spruce forests of north-eastern North America following its accidental ingress during the early part of the twentieth century, entomologists sought its natural parasites in Europe. The virus accompanied the introduction of these parasites. It spread rapidly to cause a spectacular disease epizootic that reduced the sawfly populations and saved many valuable acres of spruce forests (Balch and Bird, 1944). Populations of the sawfly, its parasites, and the virus have been monitored continuously since 1939 (Bird and Elgee, 1957; Neilson and Morris, 1964). The virus has persisted and it is considered to be a major control factor.

G. hercyniae is parthenogenetic, males occurring very infrequently–less than 1%. The eggs are laid singly in the needles of spruces and the larvae feed almost exclusively on the one- and two-year-old foliage. Full-grown larvae drop to the ground, form pupal cells in the duff layer and mature to the adult or enter diapause. Larvae that contract virus just before maturity often develop to adults. Many of their eggs are contaminated by virus so causing infection and mortality among the hatched larvae (Bird, 1953; Neilson and Elgee, 1968a, b). This is the chief mode of transmission of the virus from one host generation to the next (Bird, 1961). The virus seems to be on the surface of the eggs only (Neilson and Elgee, 1968a).

This sawfly species can be artificially reared using aseptic techniques and large quantities of virus obtained by feeding contaminated spruce foliage to last instar larvae. After one week, dead and dying larvae can be harvested daily and allowed to putrify in water at room temperature. The polyhedra rapidly sink as a whitish sediment. The supernatant can be carefully poured off leaving most of the sediment which may be further purified by slow-speed, differential centrifugation. All the supernatants should be kept and allowed to stand because more virus will usually settle out.

For a particularly high yield of relatively pure virus, the mid-gut tissues may be removed from heavily diseased, but living, larvae. This is easily accomplished by cutting off the head and the posterior prolegs and pulling the alimentary tract through either end. Virus obtained in this way often requires little or no further purification.

Quantitative field and laboratory tests have shown this NPV to be highly infectious for larvae of all ages and it has been successfully introduced into virus-free populations (Bird and Burk, 1961). In 1950, three infested spruce trees were sprayed with virus and one year later (three generations) heavy mortality from virus disease occurred on all trees within 500 ft of those sprayed. Diseased larvae were found 2000 ft from the treated area. The virus has persisted and exerted a regulating force ever since (Bird and Burk, 1961). There is no doubt that this virus is an important factor in regulating populations of the European spruce sawfly and that, if necessary, it can be artificially disseminated to suppress excessively high populations.

B. *NEODIPRION SERTIFER*, EUROPEAN PINE SAWFLY

This sawfly was introduced into North America during the early part of the century and was causing serious damage to pines in New Jersey, Ohio and Michigan by 1943. By 1949 it had spread throughout most of south-western Ontario (Bird, 1953). All these populations appeared to be free from virus disease. Since virus was known to cause high mortality in certain European populations (Escherich, 1913; Forrslund, 1945), it was introduced into North America. In 1949, a few diseased larvae were shipped from Sweden to Ontario and laboratory studies showed the virus to be very virulent for the populations there. The oral LD_{50} was between 100 and 500 polyhedra/larva (Bird and Whalen, 1954). This virus was mass-produced as described on page 99 for *G. hercyniae.* Since the polyhedra are large enough to be seen under the light microscope, the concentrations of suspensions were measured in a bacteria-counting chamber.

In trials the virus was disseminated from either a pressure sprayer, mist blower, or aircraft. Results in all tests were favorable and the virus effectively suppressed sawfly populations (Bird, 1953). Several important results regarding fundamental aspects of the virus-host association were obtained. These trials produced dosage-mortality data; 10^6 polyhedra/ml caused rapid and high mortality among newly-hatched larvae and 10^4 caused high mortality but less rapidly. The latter was adopted as the most economical dosage.

This virus is now routinely applied by hand sprayers and portable mist blowers for effective short-term control and it persists like that of *G. hercyniae* (Bird, 1961). Trees less than 3 ft high do not produce enough foliage to support high sawfly populations and virus introduced into these young plantations will not persist. The host population must be above a certain density threshold before the virus is able to survive from one generation to the next; hence, young trees may require repeated treatment for complete protection.

Aircraft have been used to disseminate virus over Scots pine plantations, achieving good control of sawflies (Bird, 1953). The most effective procedure for short-term control is the application of at least 10^6 polyhedra/ml at 0.5 gal/acre by aircraft flying strips no wider than 300 ft (Bird, 1961). For initiation of long-term epizootics much lower concentrations of virus will suffice, since a few infected individuals provide foci from which the virus spreads naturally (Bird, 1961).

The virus of *N. sertifer* is a very effective control agent and several private organizations and individuals are marketing it for use by plantation owners.

C. *NEODIPRION SWAINEI,* SWAINE'S JACK PINE SAWFLY

This species is a serious defoliator of jack pine particularly in the north-eastern part of its range. An NPV was isolated from dead larvae collected from a population at Lac Gagnon in 1956, and mass produced as described on page 99 (Smirnoff, 1962).

In a large-scale experiment, virus was sprayed from aircraft over relatively large stands of infested jack pines. An attempt was made to control or measure as many factors as possible that could affect the mechanical dissemination of virus over the foliage (Smirnoff *et al.,* 1962). Two formulations of 2×10^6 polyhedra/ml were used: (1) water-based, with latex (Geon 652, B. F. Goodrich Chemical Co.) and dried beef blood (Soluble Dried Blood, Canada Packers Ltd., Toronto); and (2) an invert emulsion with an aqueous magma of bentonite clay, emulsified with Span 80 (Atlas Powder Co., Wilmington, Delaware) in 80% No. 2

fuel oil at pH 6.7. Both preparations were applied at equivalent rates, and droplet number and size were monitored in the treated stands by special dye cards so that the actual amount of material reaching the foliage could be estimated.

Generally, the water suspension was good at high deposit levels but the oil-bentonite suspension was better at lower levels. A dosage-mortality relationship could not be determined because all applications caused high mortality, and the results suggested that both suspensions could have been more effective as finer sprays at lower rates per acre. For example, the oil-based suspension applied at the rate of 0.001 gal/acre (about 10^7 polyhedra/acre) may have given adequate control. If this is so, a given amount of virus could be used to treat a much larger area.

Sawfly populations were assessed continuously after treatment and no cocoons were found. In the next generation, diseased larvae were found two miles from the points of introduction indicating that the virus had persisted and spread in the host populations.

These field tests certainly indicate that the virus of *N. swainei* can be utilized successfully for large-scale control. This is particularly interesting because this sawfly is a native species in contrast to the others that were introduced, deficient in natural controlling enemies. This species has probably evolved a relatively homeostatic association in the ecosystem with a full complement of parasites, predators and diseases, one that should not be disturbed by the use of chemical insecticides.

D. *NEODIPRION PRATTI PRATTI,* VIRGINIA PINE SAWFLY

This sawfly attacks Virginia pine, pitch pine, and short-leaf pine, in the eastern U.S.A. It has caused extensive damage to pine stands over 14 million acres of North Carolina and Virginia. NPV-diseased larvae were found in Montgomery County, Maryland, in 1955 and 1956. These were used to mass-produce the virus. Small-scale field tests showed 77% larval mortality from virus 11 days after 5×10^8 polyhedra/tree had been applied. Then stands of 25-50 acres of the Beltsville Experimental Forest were sprayed by helicopter at 1 gal/acre to give 20, 10, 5, all $\times 10^9$ polyhedra/acre, when larvae were hatching and beginning to feed (McIntyre and Dutky, 1961). In all treated areas at all dosages, disease mortality began in 8-10 days and was nearly 100% in 16 days, very few cocoons being found afterwards.

These tests leave little doubt that the Virginia pine sawfly can be controlled by dissemination of the NPV into outbreak populations. Concentrations of less than 10^9 polyhedra/acre will probably be effective if good coverage of the foliage is obtained.

E. *NEODIPRION PRATTI BANKSIANA,* JACK PINE SAWFLY

An NPV of this other pest of jack pine was found near Sault Ste. Marie,

Ontario. Although it did not appear to be highly pathogenic in the laboratory, a large quantity was propagated and disseminated into an outbreak of sawflies. On trees drenched with suspensions of virus of concentrations in excess of 3×10^6 polyhedra/ml, less than 70% of the sawfly larvae were killed. The use of this virus as a control measure, therefore, is not practical. The virus was not even transmitted from one generation to the next (Bird, 1955) indicating that it has not evolved a very close relationship with this species of sawfly. Since several sawfly species occur on jack pine and since they are often difficult to distinguish from one another, it is possible that the original virus was not isolated from *N. p. banksiana* but from another species. Also, the sawfly infestation into which the virus was introduced may have contained larvae of more than one species. This problem should be investigated before the virus is labeled useless.

F. *NEODIPRION LECONTEI*, RED-HEADED PINE SAWFLY

This sawfly is particularly injurious to young plantations of red pine. Trees may be completely defoliated and destroyed within a single season. It probably also occurs in stands of larger trees without causing noticeable damage. An NPV was isolated from this species, multiplied in the laboratory, and sprayed into heavy host populations. It was highly pathogenic, causing high larval mortality, and a natural epizootic developed the next year causing even higher larval mortality. In another test, mortality was very high in the year of spraying and there was no residual population (Cameron, 1962). The concentrations of virus were similar or lower than those used for *N. sertifer.* The immediate results were similar, but the epizootics that followed were even more devastating, practically eradicating the sawfly from the treated plantations. Well-adapted parasites and predators occurred in these sawfly populations and they undoubtedly played an important role in the spread of virus. There is no doubt that this virus can be used with great success for control of *N. lecontei.*

III. Lepidoptera (Butterflies and Moths)

A. *LYMANTRIIDAE* (TUSSOCK MOTHS)

1. Lymantria (Porthetria) dispar, *Gypsy Moth*

This species is indigenous to Europe and damages many different kinds of trees. It appeared in the New England states at the beginning of this century and has extensively damaged oak, maple and beech stands. *L. dispar* is considered a serious pest in both Europe and North America and many attempts have been made to control outbreak populations on both continents. A nuclear-polyhedrosis virus (NPV) producing wilt symptoms often causes high mortality (Chapman and Glaser, 1915) and recent studies indicate that this virus reaches epizootic levels in high host populations (Campbell, 1963). Epizootics are often spectacular causing many larvae to die with typical "wilt" symptoms. In the laboratory larval instar I is about 10 times more susceptible than II and III (Doane, 1966). The virus was sprayed into a mixed-oak stand in the White Memorial Forest, Litchfield, Connecticut, infested with instars II and III during the spring of 1963 (Rollinson *et al.*, 1965). Large quantities of virus were obtained and counted as described for sawflies on page 99.

Using food treated in the laboratory, a median lethal concentration (LC_{50}) of 2.3×10^7 polyhedra/ml was obtained for instar II larvae and an LC_{95} of 1.0×10^{10}.

This virus was disseminated by a truck-mounted mist blower at the rate of 4 U.S. gal/acre and a concentration of 2.7×10^8 polyhedra/ml, with 4 fl. oz of Lovo 192 (an amine stearate) as sticker. Excessive defoliation was prevented. The first virus-killed larvae were observed 15 days after spraying and deaths continued for 34 days. The highest rate of mortality occurred after 19 days. Residual populations, as measured by the number of egg masses per acre, were reduced 80% (treated plot, 40 egg masses/acre; control plot, 200; Rollinson *et al.*, 1965).

Tests in Europe were similarly effective. Tests in heavily infested stands of cork oak were conducted in Sardinia during 1965 and 1966. Concentrations of 10^8-10^9 polyhedra/ml caused a 90-100% mortality, provided the foliage was well covered with the spray while most of the larvae were in instar II (Magnoler, 1967). Excessive defoliation by this species in either Europe or North America can be prevented by aqueous suspensions of 10^9-10^{10} polyhedra/ml at the rate of 4 gal/acre. Fresh suspensions of virus may be more effective than those treated by centrifugation or stored (Magnoler, 1968). Epizootics can probably be initiated with much lower concentrations (Stairs, 1965).

2. Lymantria fumida

This species, a major pest of Japanese fir, is susceptible to a nuclear (NPV) and a cytoplasmic (CPV) polyhedrosis virus (Koyama and Katagiri, 1967). The NPV often reaches epizootic proportions two or three years after host populations reach high levels, and usually reduces them to very low levels (Koyama and Katigiri, 1959; Katigiri and Koyama, 1959). The CPV has recently been discovered and very little is known of its etiology.

During the summer of 1966, the mixed viruses were sprayed in the second year of an outbreak. Mass-production of the virus mixture was by feeding laboratory-bred instar V larvae on contaminated fir foliage and storing the diseased larvae at 0°C until needed to make an aqueous suspension of 5×10^5 polyhedra/ml. Just before spraying 0.05% of a neutralized sticker solution was added. A helicopter sprayed 6.2 gal/acre over 135 acres when host larvae were young.

Mortality by the disease began in about one week and had reached a maximum in two or three weeks. Larval mortality by NPV averaged 59% and by CPV 24%, totalling 83%. Many pupae were killed by the NPV but only a few by the CPV. Data on transmission of the viruses to the next generation were not obtained but, as a result of the treatment, the pest population collapsed and excessive damage was prevented (Koyama and Katagiri, 1968). These viruses may be useful in the control and management of *L. fumida* populations.

3. Hemerocampa (Orgyia) pseudotsugata, *Douglas-fir Tussock Moth*

This insect often causes serious defoliation and damage to valuable fir stands in western North America. Its larvae are susceptible to an NPV, which kills many insects under natural conditions. Attempts to disseminate it into pest populations were not considered successful because an epizootic was already under way (Morris, 1963). Enough information was obtained, however, to indicate that epizootics could be initiated in incipient outbreak populations.

B. NOTODONTIDAE (PROMINENTS)

1. Thaumetopoea pityocampa, *Pine Processionary Caterpillar*

A specific cytoplasmic-polyhedrosis virus (CPV) attacks larval populations of this pest of pines in Europe (Grison *et al.*, 1959; Biliotti, 1959). Large quantities of virus were propagated in larvae on contaminated pine foliage in the laboratory and formulated with bentonite dusts. These dusts were applied by helicopter over 1250 acres of infested pine plantation at Mont-Ventoux, France, at about 4.8×10^8 polyhedra/acre.

Within three weeks of treatment, larval mortality by virus reached high levels, and after 2-4 months the living larvae were found to be heavily infected. This virus controlled the pest without harming its natural parasitic insects and predators (Biliotti, 1959). Virus production, assay and storage in the cold is easy. This virus can now be used routinely for the control of *T. pityocampa* (Grison, 1960).

C. TORTRICIDAE

1. Argyrotaenia velutinana, *Red-banded Leaf-roller*

This species is often a pest of apples, particularly since broad spectrum insecticides have been used for the control of other apple pests. A granulosis virus (GV) isolated by Sibold (1950) was prevalent in most leaf-roller populations in Virginia and southern Indiana during 1949, 1950, 1951 and may have exerted a regulating influence in these areas (Schoene and Sibold, 1952), but not in New York state (Glass, 1958).

In laboratory tests in New York, foliage treated with one diseased mature larva per 20 ml of water caused 60% mortality of newly-hatched larvae within a week, and 24% pupated but no adults emerged. On the other hand, one cadaver in 135 U.S. gal of water caused heavy infection and mortality but more slowly

(Glass, 1958). Also most fungicides had no effect on the pathogenicity of the virus, although one (glyodin) appeared to inactivate virus.

Based on these data, suspensions of virus were sprayed with conventional equipment into the crowns of apple trees, at 5, 10 and 100 cadavers/100 U.S. gal of water when the larvae were young. All these suspensions killed many larvae, but not before the fruit had been damaged. Mortality was very high at the highest concentrations, but a few insects survived to the adult stage at the lowest concentration. Data on the persistence of the virus from one generation to the next were not obtained.

These suspensions were too dilute to cause rapid and high mortality among young larvae. The laboratory tests showed that higher concentrations caused the most rapid mortality and so, if all damage to apples is to be prevented, very high concentrations must be used. Also, the suspensions may be more efficiently disseminated by mist blowers than by conventional spray machines. Until these points are studied further, we should not conclude that this virus will be useless in short-term control. Based on the short-term results, the virus certainly has potential in the long-term control of leaf-roller populations.

2. Choristoneura fumiferana, *The Spruce Budworm*

This is the most serious defoliator of the spruce-fir forests of North America (Elliott, 1960; Blais, 1968). It is susceptible to three diseases, a nuclear-polyhedrosis–NPV–(Bergold, 1951), a granulosis–GV–(Bergold, 1950; Bird, 1959b) and a cytoplasmic-polyhedrosis–CPV–(Bird and Whalen, 1954).

In 1960, following laboratory tests and small-scale field trials, the NPV and GV were sprayed into natural host populations on balsam fir in north-western Ontario when larvae were in instars III and IV and the current year's foliage was beginning to elongate. The viruses were applied singly or mixed at 0.08 U.S. gal/30-ft tree using a hand sprayer or a small, portable mist blower, and several trees were treated with each preparation. The concentrations were determined by protein analyses and the viruses were applied singly at 0.76 g protein/U.S. gal of water or in mixtures of about 0.38 g each (0.76 g protein = approximately 10^{10} polyhedra). Weekly samples of branch tips were taken from the mid-crown of each tree and all living and dead larvae were examined using phase contrast optics.

Infected living larvae were found on all sprayed trees 14-20 days after treatment. GV caused the highest rate of infection (40-60%) but the NPV killed more rapidly and the virus spread to other larvae on the trees but not to other trees. These results are encouraging considering the late stage of larval development when the virus was disseminated, but discouraging considering that an equivalent of about 10^9 polyhedra were sprayed on to each tree. Better results may be obtained if larvae are treated in instar II when they are beginning to mine needles and buds. The practical use of these viruses will depend on (i) the development of efficient virus propagation, (ii) knowledge of the best concentrations to apply to young larvae and (iii) whether the viruses persist from year to year (Stairs and Bird, 1962).

Large numbers of larvae can now be reared the year around on artificial food (McMorran, 1965), and used for virus propagation. An efficient technique for infecting larvae, however, must be developed because much virus must be fed to mature larvae to obtain a high percentage of diseased individuals (Bergold, 1951). Possibly, free virus particles could be injected directly into the body cavity of mature larvae to cause high and uniform mortality as with tent caterpillars (Stairs, 1964).

At present, the use of viruses to control *C. fumiferana* does not appear promising but intensive quantitative laboratory and field studies should be made before a definite conclusion is reached. For example, the NPV from *C. fumiferana* will infect the jack pine budworm, *Choristoneura pinus* (Stairs, 1960) and field tests may be more successful against this species.

D. OLETHREUTIDAE

1. Cydia (Carpocapsa) pomonella, *Codling Moth*

This is a very important, world-wide pest of apples, walnuts and other deciduous fruits. Recently a granulosis virus appeared in populations in Central and North America (Falcon *et al.*, 1968), but nowhere else in the world. Larvae of all ages are highly susceptible and the virus has been tried in the control of field populations (Falcon *et al.*, 1968).

Larvae were reared in the laboratory on artificial food (modified from Ignoffo, 1965a) and infected by contaminating the food with virus. The average yield was 4×10^9 capsules per mature larva and suspensions were stored in the dark at 6°C. Virus was sprayed into an apple orchard near Placerville, California by the handgun of a standard orchard sprayer at 150 p.s.i., with 0.03% Triton X-100 (Rohm and Haas Co.) as wetting agent.

In 1966, five virus applications were made; the first on May 2 when trees were in 90% petal fall, the second on May 16 when the first larval feeding was observed, the third, fourth and fifth coincided with high peaks of adult populations on June 22, July 20 and August 17. Fruit was harvested on August 24. This treatment reduced the codling moth population and prevented excessive damage to the apples. In the untreated control, approximately 50% of the crop was damaged by larval feeding, compared with only 10% on treated trees, although about 50% showed signs of early feeding (strings) by very young larvae (Table I). Apparently, the young larvae became infected and died before causing excessive damage.

In 1967 and 1968, successive increases in the number of applications at reduced concentrations greatly improved the result, while the total amount of virus used was decreased (Table I). Thus the key factor was more applications at reduced dosage, the final level being equal to eight mature cadavers/gal.

TABLE I

Effects of frequency of treatment with granulosis virus on populations of Cydia pomonella *and damage to apples (Falcon* et al., *1968)*

Year	1966	1967	1968
Concentration (capsules/gal)	3.4×10^{11}	1.2×10^{11}	9.5×10^{9}
Dosage (gal/tree)	5	5	5
Number of applications	5	7	12
Total virus capsules used	8.5×10^{12}	4.2×10^{12}	5.7×10^{11}
Relative virus capsules used	17	8	1
Apples damaged at harvest	10%	5%	2.3%

It is important to note that many other pests, such as phytophagous mites, aphids, cutworms, fruit worms and leaf-rollers were present in the orchards and none caused excessive damage. The virus was the only control measure applied so these species must have been curbed by their natural parasites and predators (Falcon *et al.*, 1968). Although this virus should be tested in populations of *C. pomonella* in other parts of the world the Californian studies certainly indicate its potential in the short-term management of apple orchards. The virus persists in overwintering populations but whether long-term epizootics can be artificially initiated remains to be seen.

E. LASIOCAMPIDAE

1. Malacosoma fragile, *Great Basin Tent Caterpillar*

This moth is an important pest of the valuable, range-browse bitterbrush. Larvae are susceptible to a nuclear-polyhedrosis virus (NPV), which has been tested near Truckee, Nevada County, California (Clark and Thompson, 1954; Clark and Reiner, 1956).

A supply of virus was obtained by spraying a suspension of polyhedra into an abandoned orchard infested with *Malacosoma californicum.* One week later larvae were brought into the laboratory, reared in wooden boxes, and processed in the usual way (p. 99).

Virus sprayed among populations of *M. fragile* in 1952 killed about 80% of the larvae. Further tests in 1953 and 1954 caused heavy larval and pupal mortality, but in 1955 no virus mortality was observed, demonstrating that little, if any, virus reached the plant surfaces upon which larvae were feeding (Table II). This was because a much lower dosage and concentration was used and the aircraft flew at 150-200 ft instead of 10-15 ft as in 1954.

These studies demonstrated that virus concentrations above 10^{11} polyhedra/acre sprayed among young larvae cause 80-90% mortality, provided the virus reaches the surface of the plant. Since the authors made no mention of damage, it is presumed that considerable damage was caused by feeding larvae during the

TABLE II

Results of dissemination of a NPV into populations of Malacosoma fragile *on bitterbrush*

	1953 Ground	1954 Airplane	1955 Airplane
Concentration (polyhedra/gal)	2×10^{10}	2×10^{10}	2×10^{9}
Dosage (gal/acre)	10	5	2
Total (polyhedra/acre)	2×10^{11}	1×10^{11}	4×10^{9}
Control (larvae/test) survived	80	70	No deaths by virus
Treated (larvae/test) survived	15	21	No deaths by virus
Reduction of population	80%	70%	0%
Pupae/test survived: control	–	0.11	–
Pupae/test survived: treated	–	0.01	–
Reduction of pupae	–	90%	–

period of virus mortality. Subsequent studies showed that the virus could be introduced into pest populations to start long-term epizootics (Clark, 1956, 1958). The relatively high concentrations of virus required to cause short-term reductions in population levels and the difficulty of obtaining large quantities indicate that this virus may not be used effectively in the short-term over large range areas.

2. Malacosoma disstria, *Forest Tent Caterpillar*

Widely distributed in North America, high populations of this moth develop in the aspen forests of Canada and northern U.S.A. After 4-6 years of high insect population an NPV often reaches epizootic proportions and within two or three years reduces the numbers to very low levels (Chapman and Glaser, 1915; Bergold, 1951; Sippell, 1952). Since the natural occurrence of virus epizootics is frequent and regular, attempts have been made to start epizootics in incipient caterpillar populations and thus reduce them before they cause excessive damage (Stairs, 1964, 1965). Studies were also made on short-term control.

The virus, obtained in 1962 from diseased larvae in the Peace River area of Alberta, was mass-produced in the laboratory during February to April of 1963. Eggs were collected in the fall and stored at 0° C until February. Larvae, emerged after incubation for one week at 22° C, were fed fresh strips of agar-base diet every two or three days (McMorran, 1965).

Virus particles were injected into the body cavity of last instar larvae with a fine glass or 28-gauge steel needle. The virus particles were released by dissolving polyhedra in 0.004 *M* sodium carbonate and 0.05 *M* sodium chloride. Bacteria were removed by filtration through an HA Millipore filter (0.45 μ pore size). Dead larvae were processed in the usual way (p. 99).

More virus was obtained with minimal effort by injecting virus into several thousand full-grown larvae from the field. They were not fed, but were kept in 20-lb size paper bags (about 100 larvae/bag). Dead and dying larvae were removed daily beginning four days after injection and processed. This procedure eliminated the work of feeding the larvae, one man collected about 1000 larvae/hr and one technician injected 50-100 larvae/hr. Surplus healthy larvae were stored at 4° C for several weeks without undue mortality. Enough virus to treat an acre could thus be obtained for less than 10 cents, enabling relatively large infestations to be treated at a cost competitive with those of chemical insecticides.

In field tests, 10^5, 10^6 and 10^7 polyhedra/ml were tried against instar I larvae and 5 x 10^6 polyhedra/ml against instars III and IV, all at 150 ml/aspen tree (bole diameter 3.5 in). In each plot, 20-40 trees were sprayed with a small pack-sack-type mist blower (Micro Hart) in the early morning or late evening when air movement was minimal. Plots were at least ¼ mile apart, in the Graham and Bigwood townships, of the Sudbury district of Ontario.

The highest concentration (10^7 polyhedra/ml) rapidly killed instar I larvae (92% in 17 days), before they reached instar IV and before they could cause excessive damage (Stairs, 1964). The 10-times weaker spray (10^6 polyhedra/ml) killed only 28% of the larvae and considerable damage was done by the survivors. Virus disseminated during instars III and IV killed few larvae (0.6%).

These studies showed that this NPV can be used to reduce pest populations at 10^{11} polyhedra/acre, or more, and it is essential to spray as soon as larvae hatch and begin to feed. Small isolated infestations around tourist resorts and on individual trees can be sprayed with a conventional pressure sprayer. Mist blowers may also be used and large infestations may be treated by aircraft. Small incipient outbreaks of *M. disstria* (a few square miles) could probably be reduced by introducing the virus at a high concentration (10^7 polyhedra/ml) and 5-10 gal/acre.

Although the lower concentrations of virus did not cause rapid mortality, they did initiate epizootics. In one area, the virus spread more than 20 miles from the point of introduction and epizootics developed in succeeding generations (Stairs, 1965).

3. Dendrolimus spectabilis, *Pine Caterpillar*

Severe infestations often completely defoliate and kill pines in Japan (Koyama and Katagiri, 1967). In 1956, some overwintering larvae from several pine forests in the Kanto District were found infected with a cytoplasmic-polyhedrosis virus (Koyama, 1961). Further investigations showed that nearly all the larvae were infected at a low level and that only those containing large quantities of virus died from the disease. No natural epizootiological patterns were observed.

In many attempts to utilize the virus, 5 x 10^{10} polyhedra/acre generally reduced survival rates when disseminated while larvae were in instar VII (Koyama and Katagiri, 1967). The virus was applied with conventional equipment or by helicopter either in aqueous suspension with a neutralized sticker, as a wettable powder or as a dust.

Large quantities of the virus were obtained from instar VII larvae in the laboratory. The larvae were reared on pine foliage or on a synthetic diet. When 10^6 polyhedra/ml were applied to the foliage or diet surface, most larvae became heavily infected. After 20 days, all larvae were processed, yielding about 5×10^8 polyhedra/larva. Thus 100 larvae yielded enough virus to treat one acre.

The virus was applied at various times during the life cycle and the best effects were obtained when 5×10^{10} polyhedra/acre were disseminated in June, when larvae were in instars VII and VIII.

F. PIERIDAE

1. Colias philodice eurytheme, *Alfalfa Caterpillar*

A wilt disease of this serious pest of alfalfa has been known for over 60 years and identification of the agent as an NPV in 1948 was soon followed by field trials (Steinhaus and Thompson, 1949).

A large amount of virus was obtained by collecting larvae from naturally infested fields and rearing them in laboratory traps where they were crowded together with previously infected individuals. The virus was processed (p. 99) and stored at 4° C.

Four plots of alfalfa in the north-west part of the San Joaquin Valley, California, ranging in size from 0.2 to 6.2 acres, were treated by back-pack hand sprayer during the summer of 1948 at 4-5 U.S. gal/acre and $1.9\text{-}3.6 \times 10^{11}$ polyhedra/gal. The results from these tests reveal that nearly all larvae were infected four days after spraying, deaths began after 6-8 days, mortality was high between 8-15 days, resulting in 75-93% reduction of population. The virus treatment kept populations below economic levels. Cadavers were collected for use next year (Thompson and Steinhaus, 1950) and stored in water at +2°, −30° or −70° C without inactivating the virus.

One test in 1949 tried lower concentrations, 190, 90, 19, 3.8 all $\times 10^9$ polyhedra/gal at 5 gal/acre on one-acre plots. Larval populations were effectively reduced on all plots.

Other tests were made by airplane. On August 17, 40 acres were sprayed at 1.9×10^{10} polyhedra/gal (boom type sprayer, 5 gal/acre, height 6 ft, swath width 45 ft, wind 5 m.p.h.). Populations were greatly reduced, but because most of the larvae had entered instar II at spraying some damage was done to the crop, indicating that the virus should have been sprayed a day or two earlier. An epizootic developed, however, and larval populations were reduced to very low levels seven days after treatment (Thompson and Steinhaus, 1950).

These tests showed that this NPV can be used to control pest populations of the alfalfa caterpillar. Applied by ground sprayers, 3.8 x 10^9 polyhedra/gal of water at 5 gal/acre will reduce populations before they cause economic damage provided that larvae are sprayed when most are in instars I and II. On a larger scale, aircraft may be used, but more virus is required (1.9 x 10^{10} polyhedra/gal, 5 gal/acre).

The NPV of *C. p. eurytheme* may be used against other Pierids since it infects the South American species, *Colias lesbia* (Steinhaus, 1952), the imported cabbage worm, *Pieris rapae* (Tanada, 1954) and possibly other Pierids too.

2. Pieris rapae, *Imported Cabbage Worm or Small White Butterfly*

This cosmopolitan species, a pest of cruciferous crops everywhere, suffers from a wilt disease caused by a granulosis virus (GV) (Thompson, 1951; Tanada, 1953).

In 1953 and 1954 field tests were made on the island of Oahu, Hawaii (Tanada, 1956). Infested broccoli plants were thoroughly wetted with virus suspensions prepared from recently dead, large larvae at 2, 4 and 8 cadavers/ U.S. gal and an unmeasured rate. After about six days, the virus killed many larvae, the numbers per plant being reduced by 50-80%, with no differences between the different concentrations.

In another study at Geneva, New York, the virus was applied with a tractor-mounted, low-volume sprayer (Tee-jet nozzles, No. 8002 tips, 85 p.s.i., McEwen and Hervey, 1959). A suspension of 0.13 diseased, large larvae/gal of water was sprayed at 38 gal/acre over broccoli and cauliflower plants 18-24 in high. Larval populations were reduced 50-70% by a single application and two applications (two weeks apart) were little better than one. Survivors caused excessive damage indicating that higher concentrations of virus are necessary to control pest populations, at least, in New York state.

In 1957, this GV was found at Canberra, Australia. In trials epizootics were induced on infested cabbage and the virus persisted for 3-7 weeks. Populations were markedly reduced and relatively few larvae pupated. The protection afforded by the virus was as good as that by DDT (Wilson, 1960).

Also in 1957, small-scale field experiments were made in New Zealand (Kelsey, 1958). Two GV's were used; one isolated from *P. rapae* in New Zealand (Kelsey, 1957) and the other from *Pieris brassicae* in England (Smith and Rivers, 1956). Both viruses were virulent in the laboratory. An 0.035-acre plot of rape was sprayed with 2 gal of the New Zealand virus at 50 large, diseased larvae/gal of water with a wetting agent. After 11 days the virus had killed all the 3881 larvae. In an adjacent control area, virus killed many larvae (2047) but there were 311 survivors, all of which appeared healthy. Observations on the natural occurrence of the virus in New Zealand indicate that severe virus epizootics commonly develop greatly reducing larval populations (Kelsey, 1958).

Recent studies in Canada have shown that the virus is a major mortality factor in the long-term regulation of *P. rapae* populations on cabbage (Harcourt, 1966). Comprehensive analyses of data collected over several generations show that the incidence of virus disease among larvae increases with larval density. High host populations are consistently reduced by natural epizootics of the virus.

These studies indicate that the GV of *P. rapae* may be used in the control and regulation of pest populations and that the virus may be more useful in certain parts of the world than others, although this impression may be the result of the different concentrations used.

3. Pieris brassicae, *Large White Butterfly*

Larvae of this butterfly occasionally infest brassica (Cruciferous) crops in Britain and in other European countries. They may cause severe damage particularly to gardens. A granulosis virus causing mortality of larvae was discovered by Paillot (1926) and it has recently been studied in some detail. The virus is not easily washed off leaves or leached out of the upper layer of the soil (David, 1965; David and Gardiner, 1966, 1967a). It is stable in the soil from one season to the next and capable of withstanding winter and summer temperatures (David and Gardiner, 1967b). On the other hand, the virus is rapidly inactivated by ultra-violet light. Purified virus suspension applied to the upper surface of leaves had lost most of its activity after 3-6 hr exposure to direct sunlight (David *et al.*, 1968).

Laboratory populations constantly exposed to the virus became resistant to the disease (David and Gardiner, 1960, 1965) but it is not known how rapidly this would occur under field conditions. Wild strains from Oxford, England and the Canary Islands were about 100 times more susceptible than the laboratory strain at Cambridge (David and Gardiner, 1965). This indicates that much more virus would be required to cause infection and mortality if any wild populations proved to be as resistant as the Cambridge laboratory stock. If this virus is to be used for control purposes, qualitative tests should be made to ensure that adequate dosage levels are used.

G. NOCTUIDAE (PHALAENIDAE)

This family of moths comprises many species of diverse life habit. Some are serious pests, e.g. the cabbage "looper", armyworm and cotton bollworm. Many are susceptible to viruses of both the NPV and GV groups (Hughes, 1957; Steinhaus and Marsh, 1962, 1967). Several of these viruses have been tried for long- and short-term control of pest populations (Coaker, 1958; Hafez, 1958; Abul-Nasr, 1959; Hall, 1957; Chamberlin and Dutky, 1958; Graham, 1961).

1. Trichoplusia ni, *Cabbage Looper*

This species is susceptible to NPV (Chapman and Glaser, 1915) and a GV

(Hamm and Pashke, 1963). The NPV has been observed to decimate looper populations on cole (brassica) crops throughout North America and it has been used successfully to suppress pest populations (Hall, 1957; Hofmaster and Ditman, 1961; Elmore, 1961; Getzin, 1962).

The first field tests with the NPV were made in 1953 and 1954 at Meloland, California. In a small test young lettuce plants were sprayed by hand sprayer at 18, 12 and 3 all x 10^8 polyhedra/U.S. gal of water and 150 gal/acre, causing high larval mortality in 6-9 days. The average temperature was 22° C, but a similar test during November at 16° C showed that the virus acted more slowly at the lower temperature.

Larger tests in 1954 involved higher concentrations (30, 15 and 3 all x10^9 polyhedra/gal at 12 gal/acre) applying one or two treatments spaced two weeks apart. Larval populations were reduced by all treatments; two applications were more effective than one; the higher virus concentrations were more effective than the lower ones. It was concluded the virus would have killed more larvae if the undersides of the plant leaves had received more thorough coverage.

For tests in eastern U.S.A., larvae were mass-reared on broccoli plants and when nearly full-grown they were transferred to plants that had been dipped in a virus suspension (5 large cadavers/100 gal of water). Within a week the larvae were ready for processing (p. 99) and storage at 0° F. About 150 acres of broccoli, kale and collards were sprayed (e.g., Table III; 1 large cadaver/10 gal water = about 10^8 polyhedra/gal; 75-100 gal/acre; high pressure–300 p.s.i.– boom-type sprayer). In both the treated areas the looper populations were reduced to low levels within three weeks of the first application of virus

TABLE III

Effect of weekly applications of NPV on larval populations of Trichoplusia ni *on cole crops at three places in Virginia at 10^8 polyhedra/gal (1 mature cadaver/10 gal of water and 75-100 gal/acre)*

Sampling date (1960)	No. of larvae per 100 plants		
	Treated		Untreated
	Keller	Cape Charles	Painter
August 16	437 (date treated)	–	–
August 24	1	1612 (date treated)	1361
September 8	1	20	453
September 13	0	1	30
September 20	0	0	212
September 28	1	0	1165
October 5	0	1	1022
October 11	1	1	563
October 19	0	0	118
October 26	0	0	20

(Table III). A decrease of more than 98% was observed in the Cape Charles area. The virus was also applied with chemical insecticides, without adverse effects on the activity of the virus (Hofmaster and Ditman, 1961).

Further studies in California demonstrated that the NPV could be used successfully at any time of the year to reduce populations on cabbage, cauliflower and lettuce (Elmore, 1961). A wetting agent, Colloidal X-77, was added at 4 oz/100 gal, and virus suspension was sprayed at 50-85 gal/acre, with vertical and horizontal nozzles to obtain good coverage of the whole plant surface, immediately following plant thinning. At 5, 25 and 50, all x 10^9, the higher concentrations were more effective in reducing larval populations when a single application was made, but when three applications were spaced 9-12 days apart, all concentrations were equally effective in reducing long-term population levels. In all tests, 60-98% of the larvae were killed and leaf injury was correspondingly reduced.

In the lower Rio Grande Valley of Texas, *T. ni* is the major pest of cruciferous crops. Large populations of larvae often occur and chemical control is unsatisfactory during the spring and fall, hence the NPV was tested (Getzin, 1962). Water suspensions containing 0.01% Triton X-100 as a wetting agent were sprayed on to the plants from the top and the sides with a carbon dioxide-pressured sprayer at 30 p.s.i., weekly and bi-weekly throughout the growing season at 30 gal/acre, 3, 30 and 300, all x 10^8, polyhedra/gal. In some tests the chemical insecticides, parathion and toxaphene, were combined with the virus. All treatments reduced larval populations, but the highest virus concentrations were more effective than the lowest. Weekly applications were slightly better than bi-weekly and the virus-chemical combinations were only slightly better than virus alone. An interesting and peculiar observation indicated that young larvae are less susceptible than are the older ones. The populations fell by 55-70% after treatment, but this is inadequate for successful commercial production of cabbage. The results are, however, encouraging, particularly in view of other studies with this virus. Higher virus concentrations, at more frequent intervals and higher rates, may be more effective.

Studies on the epizootiology of this virus have shown that it will persist on plants up to one month without losing all its activity (Jaques, 1964, 1967b). It will also survive at least five years in soil which, of course, provides a readily available source of virus for the initiation of epizootics (Jaques, 1967a). Further ecological studies on this virus-host complex should be encouraged, because they should reveal basic information essential to the understanding of other virus-host systems.

2. Heliothis *and* Helicoverpa *spp., Cotton Bollworm, Corn Earworm, Tobacco Budworm, Tomato worm*

Six species of *Heliothis* and *Helicoverpa* are susceptible to NPV (Allen, 1968).

Species from various parts of the world are susceptible to each other's virus strains suggesting that one virus is capable of causing disease in all *Heliothis* and *Helicoverpa* spp. These two genera are distinguished here, following Hardwick (1965) because the degree of difference between the species may explain some of the results obtained with the virus. Elsewhere in this book all six species are regarded as *Heliothis*.

The virus caused disease in *Helicoverpa armigera* on cotton in Uganda in 1955 and was used in small-scale tests (Coaker, 1958). Cotton plants were sprayed by low-volume hand sprayer at 20 ml/plant and 1, 2, 5, 10, 20 and 40, all $\times 10^5$ polyhedra/plant when larvae were in instars III and IV. The ED_{50} was approximately 10^6 polyhedra/plant and the ED_{80} about 10^7. Similar experiments in field populations gave discouraging results, presumably because the bollworm populations were very light.

In 1963, studies were begun to determine whether another strain of this virus could control the cotton bollworm, *Helicoverpa zea,* and the tobacco budworm, *Heliothis virescens,* on cotton in southern U.S.A. (Ignoffo, 1965a, b; Ignoffo *et al.,* 1965). Techniques for rearing both species on semi-synthetic diets and for the propagation of large quantities of virus were developed.

Large quantities of the virus were propagated in larvae of *H. zea.* Larvae were reared on the food in 2-oz plastic cups with flexible plastic lids (Ignoffo, 1965a). At instar IV the food was contaminated with 3.6×10^6 polyhedra. Each infected larva, usually last instar, contained about 10^{10} polyhedra at death, thus a 3000-fold multiplication of virus was realized. Diseased larvae were processed in the usual way (p. 99), stored at 8° C, and used within a week of processing. A wetting agent, Triton X-100, was added. Grain sorghum was sprayed once, corn every two or three days and cotton every 4-5 days using a tractor-type sprayer or a compressed-air hand sprayer.

In two tests on cotton the virus was combined with methyl parathion and in a third test it was used alone. Results were evaluated by estimating injury to cotton squares and bolls and by measuring the amount of cotton seed produced. The cotton was infested with *H. zea* and *H. virescens.*

Using 10^{11} polyhedra plus 0.04 lb of methyl parathion/U.S. gal at 6 gal/acre on June 7, 11, 20, 26 and July 6, 10, 15 and 19, damage was reduced and seed yields were nearly as high (1775 lb/acre) as those obtained with insecticides alone (1950 lb/acre). In a second similar experiment (sprays on June 21, 27, July 5, 9, 13, 17, 22, 26 and 31), while seed yields were as good as those following standard insecticide treatment, damage to bolls and squares was higher.

In the third test the cotton had not received sufficient spring moisture but following June and July rains it began to grow and produce a good crop. Because boll weevils were not abundant, virus alone was used at 10^{11} and 10^{12} polyhedra plus 0.7 ml Triton X-100/gal, 6 and 12 gal/acre, on July 3, 6, 11, 16, 20 and 25.

Population levels and damage were reduced by all treatments. Applications totalling 3.6×10^{13} polyhedra/acre were more effective in preventing damage to bolls and squares and higher yields were obtained, than at 3.6×10^{12}. It is possible that more frequent applications at the lower concentrations would have provided adequate protection, and this aspect should be investigated to determine how best to use a given amount of virus.

Although the higher doses of virus (3.6×10^{13} polyhedra/acre) were more effective than the lower doses, further tests have shown that seed-cotton yields were not substantially increased by applying them (Ignoffo, 1966). Some tests were made in the High Plains Area of Texas using lower doses of virus applied nine times during the season at intervals of four or five days (Chapman and Bell, 1967). Yields of cotton seed were significantly increased (50%) by a total of only 5.4×10^{11} polyhedra = 90 larval equivalents/acre. Yields were almost doubled (86%) by 10 times this amount of virus (900 larval equivalents). These increased yields were similar to those obtained by standard insecticide treatment. Allen *et al.* (1966) also reported control by virus that compared favorably with insecticide treatment.

There is no doubt that this virus could be useful in the management of *H. zea* and *H. virescens* on cotton. Under most conditions, concentrations of virus ranging from 10^{10} to 10^{11} polyhedra (1.7-17 larval equivalents/gal) applied eight or nine times at 6 or 7 gal/acre will ensure adequate yields of cotton seed.

On grain sorghum in 1963, *H. zea* populations were reduced 86-88% 13 days after treatment and a continuing epizootic was initiated (parallel tests to those on cotton, page 115, late May near Brownsville, Texas, 0.4 ml Triton X-100 and 9.96×10^{10} polyhedra = 16.6 cadavers/gal, at the rate of 10 gal/acre).

Tanada and Reiner (1962) tried another strain of the virus against the corn earworm, *Helicoverpa zea,* in California from 1957 to 1960, on sweet corn, variety Golden Cross Burtam, in field plots at Albany and Davis. Suspensions with a wetting agent, Colloidal X-77, were applied by paint-gun sprayer or force oil-can applicator directly to the silks or silk channels. Dust formulations were applied to the silks with a stiff shaving brush. At 3.6×10^6 to 14.3×10^6 polyhedra/ml and 1.2 ml/ear, six and nine applications reduced crop damage significantly. In 1958, higher concentrations were used (2.5×10^7, 1×10^8 and 2×10^8 polyhedra/ml) at 1 ml/ear. Three applications applied topically, or one inoculation of 1 ml/silk channel, reduced crop damage and further tests showed that two to four applications were most effective. In 1959, the corn ears were thoroughly covered with a dust formulation of 2×10^8 polyhedra/g. Five to six applications of the dust were as effective as the water suspensions in preventing damage. In 1960, six applications were made with a knap-sack powder duster at 60 lb/acre (4.48×10^{12} polyhedra/acre/application totalling 2.7×10^{13} polyhedra/acre). The first application was made when tassels were just visible. This treatment also reduced damage significantly and appeared to be as good as the previous procedures. None of the tests, however, reduced damage as much as did 5% DDT dust.

In 1963, three tests were made on corn in parallel with tests on cotton (p. 115) using 2.5-3 ml Triton X-100 in 16 gal spray/acre as follows:

Test	Ears silked	Applications First	Applications No.	Polyhedra/gal	Reduction in: Population	Reduction in: Damage
1	28	27 April	5	3.7×10^{10}	64%	54%
2	0	1 May	8	1.9×10^{10}	68%	48%
3	?	1 May	8	3.7×10^{10}	86%	83%

In all tests, larval populations were reduced substantially. Eight applications appeared to be more effective than five but this improvement was lost at the lower concentration. Apparently, 4×10^{10} polyhedra/gal at 16 gal/acre will effectively control *H. zea* on corn. Higher application rates at this concentration may produce better results. However, it is clear that this virus can be used for short-term control of the corn earworm though it should be established whether effective epizootics can be initiated to reduce *H. zea* populations over wide corn-growing areas.

Thus a series of applications is required on cotton and corn, but only one on sorghum, all three crops requiring similar concentrations, but different rates of application.

Despite all the testing of this virus, little is known about its natural ecology. It is inactivated very rapidly by exposure to sunlight (Allen, 1968; Bullock, 1967), therefore, dissemination during the late afternoon and evening may be more effective than routine daily application. Certainly, the possibility of initiating epizootics among these host species over wide areas should also be explored.

3. Pseudaletia unipuncta, *Cosmopolitan Armyworm*

The viruses of this armyworm have been studied primarily in Hawaii (Tanada, 1956, 1959a, b, 1961, 1968). Natural epizootics have been followed and the data suggest that viruses could be used to control this species effectively. Outbreaks of virus diseases of the typical "wilt" type have been frequently reported from various parts of North America (Chapman and Glaser, 1915; Steinhaus, 1951). NPV, GV and CPV have been isolated and sometimes the three viruses occur in the same larva. Interactions of these viruses have been studied in the laboratory and all the viruses are often prevalent in field populations (Tanada, 1966). Usually, the NPV seemed to be more prevalent than the GV. Both high and low host populations were regulated by the combined action of viruses and parasitic insects, and the reduction of high armyworm populations was rapid.

4. Prodenia litura, *Cotton Leafworm*

This serious pest of cotton in Egypt is susceptible to a polyhedrosis virus, which has been used to control larvae on cotton, sweet potatoes, clover and corn (Abul-Nasr, 1956, 1959). The virus was obtained from large numbers of larvae collected from a severely diseased field population, diluted 1 : 500 in water, and sprayed on the plants. Although polyhedra were not counted nor the rate of application measured, it is probable that about 10^7 polyhedra/ml were sprayed at 30-50 liters/acre.

On cotton a single spray on 7 July 1958, when larvae were in instars II and III, reduced the larval population by about 70% and prevented excessive damage to the crop for the rest of the season. A single application on sweet potato plants was made on 8 August 1958. Larvae were in instars II and III. Mortality by virus began a week later and continued at high levels for the rest of the season, reducing larval populations by about 80%. The virus was relatively ineffective against full-grown larvae in mid-August 1958, on corn. It may be useful in the management of *P. litura* populations.

5. Spodoptera exempta, *African Armyworm*

Outbreaks of armyworm occur about every two years in Kenya (Graham, 1961). Damage is usually confined to pastures and cereal crops. In 1961, a severe outbreak damaged agricultural land so much that many cattle were lost. An NPV killed larvae early in the outbreak and infectious spray was prepared from the cadavers at 10/Imp. gal. This was applied from aircraft and from the ground; 7-10 days later there was widespread mortality by virus among the young larvae. Once established, the virus appeared to reach epizootic proportions and to spread rapidly. Tachinid parasites were very active and may have contributed to the spread of the virus. In later studies, Brown and Swaine (1965) concluded that there was insufficient evidence to show whether the virus could be used for control and Brown (1966) reported unsatisfactory results in one field trial. However, owing to the migratory habit of *S. exempta* and the need to find and treat infestations soon after the larvae have hatched, it remains uncertain to what extent it will be practicable to exploit this virus for control (Brown, 1970).

H. PSYCHIDAE

1. Kotochalia junodi, *Wattle Bagworm*

Plantations of black wattle, *Acacia mollisima,* in southern Africa are often heavily infested (Ossowski, 1957). Outbreaks occur at intervals of 6-8 years and are often terminated by a combination of factors including overcrowding, unfavorable climate, parasites, predators and diseases. An NPV causes natural epizootics and attempts have been made to use it to control bagworm populations (Ossowski, 1957, 1960).

Large quantities of virus were propagated by feeding contaminated foliage to mature larvae, and prepared and counted in a typical way (p. 99) (Ossowski, 1957). In a small field test, about 25 x 10^9 polyhedra in 100 ml of aqueous suspension were sprayed on a 10-ft tree with a hand atomizer having a jet nozzle. Fifty larvae were placed on the tree and their feeding activity was monitored by counts of frass pellets.

After five days the number of pellets began to decrease and by 10 days had reached low levels. After 20 days 44 out of 50 larvae died by virus disease on the sprayed tree and only four on an unsprayed tree, demonstrating that the virus was highly effective.

Subsequent tests showed that both newly-hatched and 14-day-old larvae were highly susceptible to 10^9 polyhedra/10-12-ft tree (10^7 polyhedra/ml at 100 ml/tree) or higher.

Large-scale field tests were made in 1957. The plantations were either 3-5 or 7-8 years old and contained either 550-600 or 450 trees/acre, respectively. The average size of the plots was about 25 acres. All the virus suspensions contained 0.5% methyl cellulose and were applied at 5 gal/acre against bagworms in instar I and 10 gal/acre where they were in instars II and III, using a 150-h.p. aircraft equipped with 46 spray nozzles with D8 orifices. One series of concentrations gave 0.475, 0.95, 1.9 and 19; another gave 0.95, 1.9, 3.8 all x 10^{11} polyhedra/acre. Applications were made at six places in Natal, South Africa. All sprays on larvae in instar I caused high mortality and prevented damage. The lowest concentration, 4.75 x 10^9 polyhedra/acre, was less satisfactory than 10^{10}/acre and higher. At 3.8 x 10^{11}/acre on instars II and II, only a slight increase in mortality by virus disease was observed, indicating that the susceptibility of larvae to virus infection decreases with age.

Heavy rainfall did not wash the virus off the foliage even where suspensions were applied without skim milk powder as a sticker. In fact, the milk powder was a nuisance because it clogged the sprayer nozzles. Comparisons of the virulence of viruses against instar I larvae from different sources did not demonstrate appreciable differences; all were highly virulent and caused high mortality.

There is no doubt that the NPV of the wattle bagworm can be used to suppress damaging populations provided the virus is applied early in the larval cycle at rates of 10^{10} polyhedra/acre and higher.

IV. Acarina: Tetranychidae: *Panonychus citri*, Citrus Red Mite

A spherical type non-inclusion virus attacks this major pest of citrus and is discussed in detail in Chapter 15. It is of interest here because it is a non-inclusion type and consequently relatively unstable. It rapidly loses activity both in sunlight and in slightly alkaline suspensions (pH 8), although infectivity lasts several days in slightly acid ones (pH 6). This instability probably explains why the release of infected mites was more effective in spreading the disease than spraying of virus suspensions. The virus is transmitted more rapidly in dense host populations than in sparse ones, probably because transmission is not transovarial. The release of infected mites neither increases the feeding damage, nor adds to the biotic potential of wild mite populations, nor affects the activity of three predatory phytoseiid mites. This virus could be a valuable control agent, although the actual reduction in numbers of mites achieved is not clear.

V. Synopsis, Conclusions and Suggestions for Research

This review covers only instances where viruses have been used, successfully or unsuccessfully, for regulation of pest species. Most have been used only on an experimental scale and not over extensive commercial areas. The sawfly viruses are an exception. They have been employed extensively in Canada. Officially, viruses cannot be used in the United States without registration and approval of health authorities. None have been approved, so their use is still on an experimental basis. Several nuclear-polyhedrosis viruses are being mass-produced in the United States on a relatively large scale, e.g. cotton bollworm, corn earworm, tobacco budworm, cabbage looper and Douglas fir tussock moth, but their registration for unlimited use has not been approved. Safety data and acceptable protocols are being gathered and most of the viruses mentioned above should be registered in the near future. The great value of the insect viruses lies in their being part of the natural environment of pest species, and their artificial introduction will provide control of the pest without causing massive (often detrimental) changes in the ecosystem. For this reason, their development and use should be vigorously pursued.

Although each pest species and its relation to a virus must be considered as a specific case, certain general trends and similarities are evident. Most of the nuclear-polyhedrosis viruses liquefy host larvae, releasing the polyhedra to spread over the host plant. This seems to be a characteristic mode of action that might be essential to the survival and spread of the viruses. The pathophysiological reactions may be similar in the different species, even among sawflies and Lepidoptera. The polyhedra resist normal putrefaction processes and can contain and protect infectious virions for a long time, in some cases for several years. The upper layers of the soil, therefore, are probably impregnated with large amounts of infectious polyhedra, which may initiate epizootics. Similarly, granulosis virus survive in the uppermost layers of the soil.

In all instances, it is important to determine the numerical relationships between virus particles and host susceptibility, because the successful utilization of a virus often depends on accurate knowledge of this relationship. Some viruses may be suspended in oil emulsions, etc.—a topic requiring more research—and prepared in dust formulations to facilitate even dissemination over the host plants, thereby increasing availability of the virus. Aqueous suspensions, however, are adequate provided that large dosage rates (5-15 U.S. gal/acre) are used. For short-term control, it may be necessary to apply viruses frequently, particularly if the host insect has a number of overlapping generations or larval emergence occurs over a long period. Also, virus on foliage is rapidly inactivated by sunlight so that inoculum must be replenished to maintain it over extended periods. Research on protectants against sunlight should be rewarding. Virus preparations may be applied by conventional pressure sprayers, mist blowers, or by aircraft. All methods have advantages and disadvantages. However the development of specialized equipment to treat the undersurfaces of leaves and force the virus into cracks and crevices should be investigated, because this is where many species feed most when young and where the virus is most protected from sunlight.

Generally recently propagated virus gives best results, because virus may lose virulence during storage. If necessary, however, storage in the dark and cold (4° C) will minimize loss of infectivity. Production of large quantities of virus is often difficult and each virus-host system is different. For example, large quantities of *Heliothis* virus may be obtained by feeding larvae contaminated food, upon which most of the larvae die by disease (Ignoffo, 1965b). On the other hand, when half grown larvae of *Malacosoma disstria* are fed heavily contaminated food (10^9 + polyhedra), only a few become diseased (Stairs, 1965). Most mature larvae, however, die by disease within 10 days of injection with small quantities of virus (particles from 10^5 polyhedra). Large quantities of virus are thus obtained very efficiently. Different systems will require different approaches to ensure that the most efficient technique is applied.

Many insect viruses are highly host-specific and usually do not affect more than one insect in a pest complex. This is advantageous on the one hand and disadvantageous on the other. When a virus is artificially introduced, a pest species may be controlled with a minimum of disruption of the ecosystem, but other pest species in the complex may not be influenced. This disadvantage could be overcome by combining the virus with other control agents. The high degree of host-specificity is important when the hazard of broad spectrum insecticides to other organisms in the ecosystem is considered. A virus pathogen of an insect can be used with great safety and precision. This fact far outweighs any disadvantage.

Much more attention should be paid to the long-term effects of virus. Long-term studies on the viruses of the sawflies are splendid examples of what might be attained. As well as studies during the current season of a test, search should be made in subsequent crops and seasons. Also, we need to know the long-term effects of successive applications of virus over large areas of agricultural crops with minimum use of chemicals against other pests. Will the virus build up in the area and keep populations below economic levels? Will build-up allow dosage rates to be progressively decreased? Will the reduced use of chemicals cause less harm to natural enemies, allowing them to play a greater role in controlling pest populations?

Ideally, the more that is known about an ecosystem, the better it can be manipulated to our advantage. This is probably true for the utilization of many insect viruses. The bio-ecology of the host species should be known as fully as possible. The presence of other pathogens, parasites, predators, and scavengers may be important to the success of a virus introduction. Simple presence or absence data are important, but precise quantitative data will be more useful. Should we not be embarking on comprehensive, long-term quantitative research on the bio-ecology of insect viruses, particularly the nuclear-polyhedrosis and granulosis types?

References

Abul-Nasr, S. (1956). *Bull. Soc. Fouad I. Ent.* **40,** 321-332.
Abul-Nasr, S. (1959). *J. Insect Path.* **1,** 112-120.
Allen, G. E. (1968). Proc. Joint U.S.-Japan Semin. Microbial Control Insect Pests. U.S.-Japan Committee Sci. Cooperation. Panel 8. Fukuoka, 37-41.
Allen, G. E., Gregory, B. G. and Brazzel, J. R. (1966). *J. econ. Ent.* **59,** 1333-1336.
Balch, R. E. and Bird, F. T. (1944). *Sci. Agric.* **25,** 65-80.
Bergold, G. H. (1950). *Can. J. Res. E* **28,** 5-11.
Bergold, G. H. (1951). *Can. J. Zool.* **29,** 17-23.
Biliotti, E. (1959). *Revue Path. vég. Ent. agric.* **38,** 149-155.
Bird, F. T. (1949). Ph.D. Thesis McGill University.
Bird, F. T. (1950). Bi-Monthly Progress Report, Canadian Department of Agriculture, Division of Forest Biology, Vol. 6, No. 5.
Bird, F. T. (1952). Bi-Monthly Progress Report, Canadian Department of Agriculture, Division of Forest Biology, Vol. 8, No. 3.
Bird, F. T. (1953). *Can. Ent.* **85,** 437-446.
Bird, F. T. (1955). *Can. Ent.* 87, 124-127.
Bird, F. T. (1959a). *Can. J. Microbiol.* **4,** 267-272.
Bird, F. T. (1959b). *J. Insect Path.* **1,** 406-430.
Bird, F. T. (1961). *J. Insect Path.* **3,** 352-380.
Bird, F. T. (1964). *Mém. hors Sér. Entomophaga* No. 2, 465-473.
Bird, F. T. and Burk, J. M. (1961). *Can. Ent.* **93,** 228-238.
Bird, F. T. and Elgee, D. E. (1957). *Can. Ent.* **89,** 371-378.
Bird, F. T. and Whalen, M. M. (1954). *Can. J. Microbiol.* **1,** 170-174.
Blais, J. R. (1968). *For. Chron.* **44,** 1-7.
Brown, E. S. (1966). Rept. XIIth Specialist Entomological and Insecticides Committee, Mombasa, Sept. 1966, Appendix 16.
Brown, E. S. (1970). *E. Afr. agic. for. J.* **35,** 237-245.
Brown, E. S. and Swaine, G. (1965). *Bull. ent. Res.* **56,** 95-116.
Bullock, H. R. (1967). *J. Invertebrate Path.* **9,** 434-436.
Cameron, J. W. M. (1962). Proc. Int. Congr. Ent. 11th Vienna **2,** 769-776.
Campbell, R. W. (1963). *Can. Ent.* **95,** 426-434.
Chamberlin, F. S. and Dutky, S. R. (1958). *J. econ. Ent.* **51,** 560.

Chapman, A. J. and Bell, R. A. (1967). *J. econ. Ent.* **60**, 655-656.
Chapman, J. W. and Glaser, R. W. (1915). *J. econ. Ent.* 8, 140-150.
Clark, E. C. (1956). *Ecology*, **37**, 728-732.
Clark, E. C. (1958). *Ecology*, **39**, 132-139.
Clark, E. C. and Reiner, C. E. (1956). *J. econ. Ent.* **49**, 653-659.
Clark, E. C. and Thompson, C. G. (1954). *J. econ. Ent.* **8**, 140-149.
Coaker, T. H. (1958). *Ann. appl. Biol.* **46**, 536-541.
David, W. A. L. (1965). *Ann. appl. Biol.* **56**, 331-334.
David, W. A. L. and Gardiner, B. O. C. (1960). *J. Insect Path.* **2**, 106-114.
David, W. A. L. and Gardiner, B. O. C. (1965). *J. Invertebrate Path.* **7**, 285-290.
David, W. A. L. and Gardiner, B. O. C. (1966). *J. Invertebrate Path.* 8, 180-183.
David, W. A. L. and Gardiner, B. O. C. (1967a). *J. Invertebrate Path.* **9**, 342-347.
David, W. A. L. and Gardiner, B. O. C. (1967b). *J. Invertebrate Path.* **9**, 555-562.
David, W. A. L., Gardiner, B. O. C. and Woolner, M. (1968). *J. Invertebrate Path.* **11**, 496-501.
Doane, C. C. (1966). *In* "Insect Pathology and Microbial Control" (P. A. van der Laan, ed.), pp. 200-203. North-Holland Publ. Co., Amsterdam.
Dowden, P. B. (1940). *J. For.* **38**, 971-972.
Elliott, K. R. (1960). *For. Chron.* **36**, 61-82.
Elmore, J. C. (1961). *J. econ. Ent.* **54**, 47-50.
Escherich, K. (1913). *Naturw. Z. Forst- u. Landwirtsch.* **11**, 86.
Falcon, L. A., Kane, W. R. and Bethell, R. S. (1968). *J. econ. Ent.* **61**, 1208-1213.
Forrslund, K. H. (1945). *Medd. skogs-forsoksanst.* **34**, 365.
Getzin, L. W. (1962). *J. econ. Ent.* **55**, 442-445.
Glass, E. H. (1958). *J. econ. Ent.* **51**, 454-457.
Graham, J. F. (1961). *Pl. Prot. Bull. F.A.O.* **9**, 182-184.
Grison, P. (1960). *Z. angew. Ent.* **47**, 24-31.
Grison, P., Maury, R. and Vago, C. (1959). *Revue for. Fr.* **5**, 353-370.
Hafez, M. (1958). *Bull. Soc. ent. Égypte* **42**, 357-370.
Hall, I. M. (1957). *J. econ. Ent.* **50**, 551-553.
Hamm, J. J. and Pashke, J. D. (1963). *J. Insect Path.* **5**, 187-197.
Harcourt, D. G. (1966). *Can. Ent.* **98**, 653-662.
Hardwick, D. F. (1965). *Mem. ent. Soc. Canada* No. 40, p. 247.
Hofmaster, R. N. and Ditman, L. D. (1961). *J. econ. Ent.* **54**, 921-923.
Hughes, K. M. (1957). *Hilgardia* **26**, 597-629.
Ignoffo, C. M. (1965a). *J. Invertebrate Path.* **7**, 315-319.
Ignoffo, C. M. (1965b). *J. Invertebrate Path.* **7**, 209-216.
Ignoffo, C. M. (1966). *J. Invertebrate Path.* **8**, 531-536.
Ignoffo, C. M., Chapman, A. J. and Martin, D. F. (1965). *J. Invertebrate Path.* **7**, 227-235.
Jaques, R. P. (1964). *J. Insect Path.* **6**, 251-254.
Jaques, R. P. (1967a). *Can. Ent.* **99**, 785-794.
Jaques, R. P. (1967b). *Can. Ent.* **99**, 820-829.
Kelsey, J. M. (1957). *N.Z. Jl Sci. Technol.* 38, 644-646.
Kelsey, J. M. (1958). *N.Z. Jl Agric. Res.* **1**, 778-782.
Katagiri, K. and Koyama, R. (1959). *J. Jap. For. Soc.* **41**, 17-18.
Koyama, R. (1961). *J. Jap. Forest Soc.* **43**, 91-96.
Koyama, R. and Katagiri, K. (1959). *J. Jap. For. Soc.* **41**, 1-17.
Koyama, R. and Katagiri, K. (1967). Bull. Govt. Forest Expt Stn No. 207, Tokyo.
Koyama, R. and Katagiri, K. (1968). Proc. U.S.-Japan Semin. Microbial Control Insect Pests. U.S.-Japan Committee Sci. Cooperation. Panel 8. Fukuoka, 63-69.
Magnoler, A. (1967). *Entomophaga* **12**, 199-207.
Magnoler, A. (1968). *J. Invertebrate Path.* **11**, 326-328.
McEwen, F. L. and Hervey, G. E. R. (1959). *J. econ. Ent.* **51**, 626-631.
McIntyre, T. and Dutky, S. R. (1961). *J. econ. Ent.* **54**, 809-810.
McMorran, A. R. (1965). *Can. Ent.* **97**, 58-62.
Morris, O. N. (1963). *J. Insect Path.* **5**, 401-414.

Neilson, M. M. and Elgee, D. E. (1968a). *J. Invertebrate Path.* **10,** 70-75.
Neilson, M. M. and Elgee, D. E. (1968b). *J. Invertebrate Path.* **12,** 132-139.
Neilson, M. M. and Morris, R. F. (1964). *Can. Ent.* **96,** 773-784.
Ossowski, L. L. J. (1957). *Ann. appl. Biol.* **45,** 81-89.
Ossowski, L. L. J. (1960). *Ann. appl. Biol.* **48,** 299-313.
Paillot, A. (1926). *C.r. hebd. Séanc. Acad. Sci. Paris,* **182,** 180-182.
Rivers, C. F. (1962). *Mém. hors Sér. Entomophaga* No. 2, 476-480.
Rollinson, W. D., Lewis, F. B. and Waters, W. E. (1965). *J. Invertebrate Path.* **7,** 515-517.
Schoene, W. J. and Sibold, N. J. (1952). *J. econ. Ent.* **45,** 1081.
Sibold, N. J. (1950). *Va J. Sci.* **1,** 226.
Sippell, W. L. (1952). *Bi-monthly Prog. Rep. Forest Biol. Div., Canada Dep. Agric.* **8,** 1-2.
Smirnoff, W. A. (1961). *J. Insect Path.* **3,** 29-46.
Smirnoff, W. A. (1962). *J. Insect Path.* **4,** 192-200.
Smirnoff, W. A., Fettes, J. J. and Haliburton, W. (1962). *Can. Ent.* **94,** 477-486.
Smith, K. M. and Rivers, C. F. (1956). *Parasitology* **46,** 235-242.
Stairs, G. R. (1960). *Can. Ent.* **92,** 906-908.
Stairs, G. R. (1964). *Can. Ent.* **96,** 1017-1020.
Stairs, G. R. (1965). *Can. Ent.* **97,** 1059-1062.
Stairs, G. R. and Bird, F. T. (1962). *Can. Ent.* **94,** 966-969.
Steinhaus, E. A. (1951). *Hilgardia* **20,** 629-678.
Steinhaus, E. A. (1952). *J. econ. Ent.* **45,** 897-899.
Steinhaus, E. A. and Marsh, G. A. (1962). *Hilgardia* **33,** 349-490.
Steinhaus, E. A. and Marsh, G. A. (1967). *J. Invertebrate Path.* **9,** 436-437.
Steinhaus, E. A. and Thompson, C. G. (1949). *J. econ. Ent.* **42,** 301-305.
Tanada, Y. (1953). *Proc. Harv. ent. Soc.* **15,** 235-260.
Tanada, Y. (1954). *Ann. ent. Soc. Am.* **47,** 553-574.
Tanada, Y. (1956). *J. econ. Ent.* **49,** 52-57.
Tanada, Y. (1959a). *J. Insect Path.* **1,** 197-214.
Tanada, Y. (1959b). *J. Insect Path.* **1,** 215-231.
Tanada, Y. (1961). *J. Insect Path.* **3,** 310-323.
Tanada, Y. (1966). *Proc. Hawiian ent. Soc.* **19,** 302-308.
Tanada, Y. (1968). Proc. Joint U.S.-Japan Semin. Microbial Control Insect Pests. U.S.-Japan Committee Sci. Cooperation. Panel 8. Fukuoka, 25-31.
Tanada, Y. and Reiner, C. (1962). *J. Insect Path.* **4,** 139-154.
Thompson, C. G. (1951). *J. econ. Ent.* **44,** 255.
Thompson, C. G. and Steinhaus, E. A. (1950). *Hilgardia* **19,** 411-445.
Wilson, F. (1960). *Aust. J. agric. Res.* **11,** 485-497.

CHAPTER 5

Use of Fungi for Microbial Control of Insects

DONALD W. ROBERTS AND WILLIAM G. YENDOL

Boyce Thompson Institute for Plant Research, Yonkers, N.Y., U.S.A., and Pennsylvania State University, University Park, Pennsylvania, U.S.A.

I. Introduction

Recently Whittaker (1969), in a departure from the traditional division of the entire living world into plant and animal kingdoms, proposed a five-kingdom system. Significantly, he considered the fungi sufficiently unique to warrant placing them in a separate kingdom. Their uniqueness is also apparent when entomogenous fungi are compared with other entomogenous micro-organisms. The most significant difference is the mode of host invasion, which, in most cases, is directly through the cuticle. This, in turn, imposes rather rigid tolerances in the environmental conditions which permit disease induction because spores must germinate outside their hosts. These environmental tolerances are more strict than with other entomogenous micro-organisms or viruses which usually invade via the alimentary tract. Attempts to use fungi for microbial control, as will be discussed later, must take account of these requirements.

Although, at first glance, the consideration of entomogenous fungi might appear a very restricted topic, there is a very large body of literature extant on the subject. The most thorough review to date (Müller-Kögler, 1965) cited approximately 1200 publications, and this excluded the Laboulbeniales, nonpathogenic fungus-insect interrelationships, and microbial control studies reported before 1937 or after 1963. Some areas, such as unquantified field observations of catastrophic population reductions of insects, are widely represented in the literature, while areas which are ripe for the application of modern technology, such as cuticle penetration, toxins, and genetics, are but scantily studied. The most recent reviews are those of Madelin (1966, 1968) and Ferron (1967a).

Entomogenous fungi have played a uniquely important role in the history of microbial control of insects (Steinhaus, 1956; Chapter 1).

One field trial of considerable historical importance was a project conducted by the state of Kansas about 1890 in which *Beauveria bassiana* was provided to many farmers for use against the chinch bug *(Blissus leucopterus).* The significance of this event lies in its failure. The results of the first two years (1891 and 1892) were considered promising, but the outlook changed in succeeding years. The dramatic reductions in chinch bug populations which had been induced by the fungus in the same locality a few years earlier without the aid of man could not be reproduced. This apparently led to two conclusions, one an extension of the other. First, the mere presence of a microbial control agent is not adequate to insure death of exposed insects, i.e. the environment is a factor of paramount importance in disease induction. And second, since man has no control over the environment, there is little hope for microbes, particularly fungi, as dependable microbial control agents. The recognition of the importance of microclimates and the possibility of increasing the virulence of the fungus have, to some extent, modified this negative feeling. Nevertheless almost 80 years later, these points are still very much in evidence when microbial control with fungi is discussed (e.g. Bucher, 1964).

II. Fungal Disease

A. ENTOMOGENOUS FUNGI

The majority of publications on insect mycoses discuss *Entomophthora, Beauveria, Metarrhizium,* or *Aspergillus.* These are the genera most commonly encountered in nature. All four major taxonomic groups of true fungi (slime molds excluded) contain entomopathogenic species (Table I). The fungal genera most frequently associated with insect disease are printed boldly in Table I, and some species used in microbial control attempts are shown in Table II. Several of

TABLE I

List of the major taxa which contain insect-parasitizing species. (The main genera are shown in **bold** *type.)*

PHYCOMYCETES	*Podonectria*	*Cephalosporium*
Coelomomyces	*Sphaerostilbe*	*Gibellula*
Myiophagus	*Torrubiella*	**Hirsutella**
Entomophthora[a]	Laboulbeniales[b]	*Hymenostilbe*
Massospora		**Isaria**
	BASIDIOMYCETES	**Metarrhizium**
ASCOMYCETES	**Septobasidium**	*Microcera*
Ascosphaera (Pericystis)	*Uredinella*	**Paecilomyces**
Calonectria	FUNGI IMPERFECTI[c]	*Penicillium*
Cordyceps	*Acrostalagmus*	**Spicaria**
Hypocrella	*Aegerita*	*Synglíocladium (Sorosporella)*
Myriangium	*Aschersonia*	*Synnematium*
Nectria	**Aspergillus**	*Tetracrium*
Ophiocordyceps	**Beauveria**	*Verticillium*

Table slightly modified from Madelin, 1968.
[a]Divided into more than one genus by some authors (see text for literature).
[b]Approximately 125 genera.
[c]Many species in the genera listed are asexual states of ascomycetous insect-parasites.

these genera are principally or exclusively associated with scales and mealybugs, and will be treated in Chapter 16. The host ranges of some species of *Coelomomyces, Entomophthora, Massospora, Hirsutella,* and *Septobasidium* are limited to a single family, genus, or a few species of insects. Wide host ranges, however, are the rule with the most commonly isolated pathogenic fungi, e.g. the host range of *M. anisopliae* exceeds 200 species of insects (Veen, 1968). There are many strains among the various species and some vary considerably in their host ranges. This is particularly well illustrated by the recent report of

TABLE II

Entomogenous fungi most commonly used for microbial control, excluding those used primarily for scale and whitefly control

Species	Remarks
Beauveria bassiana	Most widely used fungus
Beauveria tenella	Mostly used against *Melolontha* in soil
Metarrhizium anisopliae	Second most widely used fungus
Paecilomyces farinosus	
Spicaria rileyi	
Entomophthora spp.	Conidia generally too short-lived for use as microbial insecticides; colonization has been attempted
Coelomomyces stegomyiae and *C. indiana*	Insufficient inoculum available for use as microbial insecticide; colonization has been attempted

Ferron and Diomandé (1969), in which a strain of *M. anisopliae* isolated from *Oryctes* beetles was the only strain of several tried which infected *Oryctes* in the laboratory (see also Aoki, 1968; Latch, 1965).

The Laboulbeniales is a very specialized order of Ascomycetes which produce small determinant thalli on the cuticle of insects and send haustoria into the underlying tissue for nourishment. They are generally considered rather innocuous to their hosts, and this assumption has been verified for *Stigmatomyces ceratophorus* on adults of the muscid fly, *Fannia canicularis* (Whisler, 1968). Nevertheless, field populations of a coccinellid beetle reportedly were reduced considerably by lethal infections of *Hesperomyces virescens* (Kamburov *et al.*, 1967). This report is unique in the literature of the group, and efforts to verify it in closely related fungi would appear to be worth while.

The taxonomy of the entomogenous fungi is not static. The most important proposed revisions of recent years involve *Spicaria* and *Entomophthora.* Many of the species formerly placed in *Isaria* and *Spicaria* are now called *Paecilomyces* (Brown and Smith, 1957); however, the rather common insect pathogen *S. rilyei* is still unassigned (Behnke and Paschke, 1966). Two different approaches have been taken with *Entomophthora,* (1) division into several genera (Batko, 1964a, b, c, d; Batko and Weiser, 1965) and (2) moving some species to the pre-existing genus *Conidiobolus* (Srinivasan *et al.,* 1964; Srinivasan and Thirumalachar, 1967). Recent publications on experimental studies with *Entomophthora* have not employed either of these proposals and they will not be adopted in this book, though they may find acceptance in the future. As noted in Table I, the generic name of the chalk-brood fungus of bees has been changed from *Pericystis* to *Ascosphaera,* and *Sorosporella,* the causative agent of red muscardine, is actually the resting spore stage of *Synggliocladium.*

B. INSECT HOSTS

Incidence of fungal disease varies considerably in different groups of insects. In some cases, such as the seldom observed Strepsiptera (twisted-wing flies or stylopids), absence of reports of fungal disease probably is merely an indication that the insects are seldom observed. On the other hand, most medically important insects have been observed closely by many workers, and yet mycoses have seldom or never been reported for Mallophaga (lice), Siphonaptera (fleas), Tabanidae (horse flies), and *Glossina* (tsetse flies) (Jenkins, 1964). The warm, moist habitat of house-dwelling cockroaches should be optimal for fungal disease initiation, but these insects are relatively disease-free. The very dry habitats of Thysanura (fire brats and silver fish) and larval Siphonaptera probably account for their lack of fungal disease. On the other hand, mycoses are common with certain taxonomic groups, e.g. Lepidoptera (moths and butterflies, particularly larvae), Homoptera (particularly aphids, cicadas, and scale insects), Hymenoptera (bees), Coleoptera (beetles), and Diptera (flies, such as *Hylemya* and mosquitoes).

C. DISEASE DEVELOPMENT

1. General Description

In general disease is induced by the entomogenous fungi as follows. The infective unit in most fungi is a spore, usually a conidium. Invasion through the respiratory or alimentary tract has been reported (Müller-Kögler, 1965; Veen, 1966; Yendol and Paschke, 1965), but these are relatively rare invasion sites. Conidia usually germinate on the cuticle or form appressoria (see p. 130) and then penetrate. Enzymes and mechanical forces are involved. In most cases, but not all, yeast-like fragments of mycelium called hyphal bodies are produced which usually float free and apparently multiply in the hemocoel (Prasertphon and Tanada, 1968). Some strains produce sufficient toxins in this stage to cause death, though no major organs have been invaded. When organ invasion does occur, the fat body almost invariably is the preferred site. After death, or even before, in those strains which are weak toxin producers, normal thread-like mycelium ramifies throughout the internal organs. This continues until the insect is virtually filled with fungus and quite firm to the touch. Conidiophores are then produced which erupt through the cuticle and produce spores on the outside of the insect. With the Fungi Imperfecti, conidiophores and conidia are not produced unless the dead insect is in a moist environment. The genus *Coelomomyces* differs from the above description in that infection is probably induced by free swimming zoospores from sporangia rather than by conidia. These sporangia, like most resting spores of *Entomophthora*, are formed within the host rather than on the outside.

2. Spore Germination

The influence of environmental conditions on germination will be discussed on page 136. The outermost (epicuticular) layer of the cuticle is of special significance in disease induction since it is here that, in most cases, the fungal spore must germinate before it can reach the underlying hemocoel and vital organs. This layer contains various lipids, mostly still uncharacterized (David, 1968; Locke, 1964; Noble-Nesbitt, 1968); and alteration of this layer by light abrasion or washing with nonpolar solvents reduces the resistance of certain insects to entomogenous fungi (Evlakhova and Chekhourina, 1964; Müller-Kögler and Huger, 1960; Sussman, 1951; Koidsumi, 1957). In exuviae, Koidsumi (1957) found antifungal, medium-chain saturated fatty acids, presumably caprylic or capric acid, and he attributed reduction of resistance to loss of these materials. Excised cuticle of *Tenebrio* larvae was not invaded more readily after wiping with solvents (Robinson, 1966), but invasion took place without wiping and these results can probably be explained by damage incurred by the epicuticular layer during excision and mounting. Technology in lipid research has advanced significantly in recent years, and insect cuticle warrants close scrutiny with these techniques (e.g. Bursell and Clements, 1967). David (1968) has suggested that abrasions may expose openings of pore canals and open dermal glands, thereby facilitating entrance of fungi. Penetration via the pores of sense organs has been demonstrated, but was considered to be rare (McCauley *et al.,* 1968). Non-lipid compounds which might be inhibitory to fungi are also found in the cuticle, e.g. phenols and 3,4-dihydroxybenzoic acid. These materials, however, are probably present in the endocuticle only and therefore would not be expected to affect spore germination.

In addition to inhibition, the cuticle of insects ought to enhance germination of at least some entomogenous fungi. This aspect has not been studied carefully, but the lipoid layer of *Cossus cossus* reportedly stimulated germination of *M. anisopliae* spores (Notini and Mathlein, 1944). Spores from this fungus can also germinate on glass slides covered with ether-soluble compounds from the cuticle of locusts, and of particular interest is the significantly better germination of one strain on the lipids if the spores were produced on an inorganic nitrogen medium instead of on an organic nitrogen medium (Veen, 1968).

Fungal spores are very active metabolically just before germination. Typically spores swell, and *M. anisopliae* reportedly has some effect upon the cuticle of its host at this stage, as evidenced by lightening of the cuticle color (Wallengren and Johansson, 1929). With some nonentomogenous fungi, enzyme activity at this time is high enough for commercial fermentations to be carried out, even in conditions not permitting germ tube production by the spores (Johnson *et al.,* 1968). It is conceivable that physiological activities such as the enzyme or toxin production of spores from insect-parasitizing fungi are very important to disease induction (Roberts, 1967). At germination one or more germ tubes (short hyphae) are produced from each spore.

3. Penetration of Cuticle

Germ tubes may grow on the surface of the insect for short distances or may begin to penetrate the cuticle immediately. Appressoria have been found recently in some entomogenous fungi (Robinson, 1966; Madelin *et al.*, 1967). These are swellings produced at the end of short germ tubes which attach to the cuticle and send "infection pegs" into the host (Fig. 1). They are considered to provide the firm attachment that the fungus needs to physically force its way into the host. Appressoria are not always formed even in those species which can produce them. The invading mycelium is frequently more narrow within the cuticle than in the hemocoel and it sometimes penetrates between lamellae of the cuticle rather than proceeding directly to the hemocoel. These two traits indicate that physical forces are involved in penetration. A further indication is given by experiments in which depth of penetration of paraffin by *Paecilomyces farinosus* was directly related to its hardness (Robinson, 1966; Madelin *et al.*, 1967).

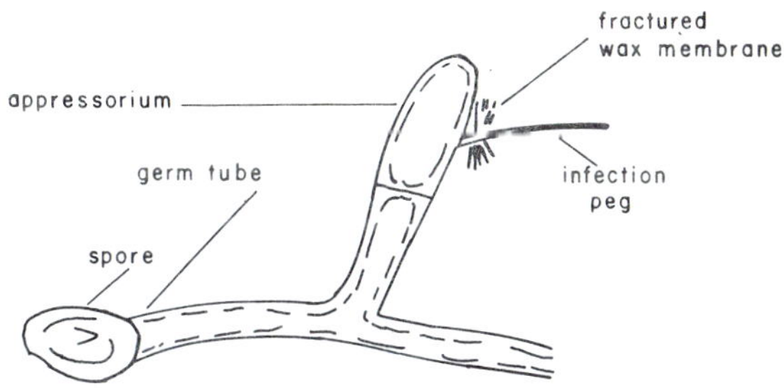

Fig. 1. Appressorium of a *Paecilomyces farinosus* spore on a wax membrane (redrawn from Robinson, 1966).

Enzyme studies are still in the exploratory stage, but several classes of compounds present in the insect cuticle are attacked *in vitro* by all entomogenous fungi tested to date. These include chitin, protein, and lipids for several species of *Entomophthora, Cordyceps militaris, B. bassiana, M. anisopliae,* and *A. flavus* (Ali *et al.,* 1965; Claus, 1961; Huber, 1958; Gabriel, 1968a). Species examined by Gabriel (*Entomophthora* spp., *B. bassiana,* and *M. anisopliae*) did not produce chitinase in the presence of protein; the lipase and protease activity, however, was constitutive. The enzymes involved have neither been isolated nor tested against specific constituents of insect cuticle, except chitin. Nevertheless, histological and histochemical evidence points to enzyme activity in cuticle penetration (Gabriel, 1968b; David, 1968). Robinson (1966) suggested that with several Fungi Imperfecti the epicuticle was attacked by mechanical forces alone, while penetration of the lower layers was facilitated by enzymes. Recently reported histochemical tests with cuticle infected by *E. coronata* indicated that lipase was produced at the point of penetration (Gabriel, 1968b). In accordance with the *in vitro* studies, chitin was not extensively dissolved in the cuticle, presumably because of the proteins present (Gabriel, 1968b). Hydrolysis of protein was restricted to the area surrounding the invading fungus, and Gabriel (1968b) suggested that only certain kinds of protein were digested, thereby loosening exo- and endocuticular lamellae to permit penetration by mechanical means.

A major difference between fungi which can infect insects and those which cannot appears to be whether or not they can penetrate the exoskeleton of the host. It has been suggested that it is the exocuticular layer which serves as the main line of defense (Robinson, 1966). Some normally nonpathogenic fungi can penetrate wounds (Müller-Kögler and Huger, 1960; Heitor, 1962), and this may prove a significant problem in mass rearing of insects.

4. Toxins

Insect pathogenic fungi produce toxins in two overlapping categories, those toxic *per os* and those toxic on injection. The former may have potential as insecticides while the latter are useful in elucidating the modes of action of pathogens.

One of the first workers to study toxins active *per os* was Burnside (1930), who established that honey-bees were susceptible to an ether-soluble compound produced *in vitro* by a strain of *Aspergillus flavus.* The characteristics of his material indicate that he was working with aflatoxins, compounds discovered from strains of *A. flavus* about a decade ago (Chapter 9). These compounds are not specific, being toxic for insects, birds, mammals, micro-organisms, and plants. In addition, certain nonentomopathogenic fungi also produce materials toxic *per os* for insects, e.g. Damodar *et al.* (1964), Kishaba *et al.* (1962), Beard (1968), Chapter 9 (p. 223), but the toxicity of these materials to other life forms is unknown. There are many fully characterized materials from fungal cultures which have not been, but should be, tested for toxicity for insects, including metabolites from genera containing insect pathogenic species, e.g. isarins and isarolides from *Isaria.* To date we know of no insect-specific fungal toxins, active *per os,* that could be used alone as insecticides or in combination with pathogenic organisms, but a search should be made. Such compounds will be particularly useful if they prove less persistent in the environment than DDT and its relatives. Many antibiotics proved lethal to phytophagous mites and, since no symbiotes are known in these mites, the antibiotics may have the indirect effect of disturbing the gut microflora or a direct toxic effect on the mites (Chapter 31).

The observation that death sometimes occurs while infection is confined to the hemolymph and hypodermis led some authors to conclude many years ago that toxins are important. In these cases, the normal site for toxin production is the hemolymph. Nevertheless, in all the toxin work before that of Kodaira (1961), culture filtrates were fed to test insects rather than injected directly into the hemocoel. This simple oversight retarded the development of the field for a number of years. Toxins harmless by contact or *per os* but toxic on injection have no use for direct application to crops, but explain in part the modes of action of certain fungi and may enable more effective pathogens to be produced by selection for high toxin production.

Materials toxic on injection are produced *in vitro* by several insect pathogens and are discussed in Chapter 9. Four such materials of known chemical composition from entomogenous fungi are destruxins A and B from *M. anisopliae* (Tamura and Takahashi, 1970; Roberts, 1969), beauvericin from *B. bassiana* (Hamill *et al.,* 1969; Dorschner and Lardy, 1969), and cordycepin from *C. militaris* (Hanessian *et al.,* 1966; Roberts, unpublished). The destruxins and beauvericin are toxic to mosquito larvae on addition to their culture water, and are probably active *per os* (Roberts, 1967, 1970; Hamill *et al.,* 1969). Destruxin-contaminated leaves were not readily eaten by *Epilachna* (beetle) larvae (Kodaira, 1961) or young stick insects *(Carausius)* (Roberts, unpublished), but the insects died, probably from toxins obtained by ingestion. *Metarrhizium* and *Beauveria* produce additional compounds which are toxic to *G. mellonella* by injection only (West and Briggs, 1968; Roberts, 1969). Cordycepin has not been tested *per os*. It is slightly toxic to *G. mellonella* by injection and with sublethal doses the ensuing pupae have badly deformed appendages (Roberts, unpublished). Unlike the toxins listed above, those from *Entomophthora* are proteinaceous (Prasertphon, 1967b; Prasertphon and Tanada, 1969; Yendol *et al.*, 1968). They cause color changes in their hosts and may be enzymes. The classification of toxins by some authors expressly excludes enzymes (e.g. Bonventre *et al.*, 1967), but in at least one case, the proteases of *Beauveria*, they have been referred to as toxins (Kučera and Samšiňáková, 1968; Chapter 9). Numerous entomogenous fungal species have yet to be examined for toxins. Variations in culture morphology and pigments indicate that some fungal genera are metabolically diverse, e.g. *Beauveria* (MacLeod, 1954; El Basyouni *et al.*, 1968). Accordingly, future isolation of more toxins can be expected.

D. EPIZOOTIOLOGY

Entomogenous fungi may occur in insect populations at consistent but rather low levels (enzootics) or may flare up into outbreaks which involve large proportions of the population (epizootics). Although very time consuming, the level of disease incidence and particularly the impact on host numbers is best determined by the construction of life tables.

An understanding of why and how natural epizootics occur will suggest how a fungus can be used most efficiently in microbial control. The study of epizootiology, however, can be very complicated because, in the field, the various aspects of the three main agents—pathogen, host, and environment—interact and change at the same time. Comparatively few comprehensive field studies have been made, although a very interesting example is currently under way on *Coelomomyces punctatus* infecting *Anopheles quadrimaculatus* larvae in North Carolina, U.S.A. (Umphlett, 1968, personal communication). The study is facilitated by regular outbreaks of disease occurring in one area of a lake, but not in another area of the same lake, where larvae are virtually disease-free. Of the various physical factors observed, high level of dissolved oxygen, temperatures in the 30's and possibly shading appear to be associated with scarcity of disease. These clues suggest hypotheses which now can be tested in the laboratory. Also, host susceptibility will be checked to determine if resistance to the fungus has occurred (Couch, personal communication).

Most field studies do not go beyond the recording of temperature and sometimes humidity. It must be emphasized, however, that even though these are two of the most important factors in the microclimate, there are many more which influence development of epizootics (MacLeod and Soper, 1965; MacLeod *et al.*, 1966). These include light, air currents, host population density, stress, host activity, antagonism or synergism of other pathogens, and genetic make-up of host and pathogen. Specific studies on these topics in relation to epizootics will provide important new information about entomogenous fungi. Available information on some of these topics is summarized below and in more detail by MacLeod *et al.* (1966), Müller-Kögler (1965), and Tanada (1963).

1. Pathogen

a. Dispersal. Spores of many, if not most fungi, are widely disseminated by wind (e.g. Hirst *et al.*, 1967) and this is considered important with entomogenous fungi as well. Environmental conditions, particularly sunlight and humidity, may kill spores during transport. Splashing of rain also accounts for some spreading. In addition, there are active means such as spore discharge (Entomophthorales), climbing of hosts to high places before death (some *Entomophthora* infections), and sporulation while the host is still mobile *(Massospora).*

b. Viability. Viable inoculum is maintained in the environment by the production of conidia, ascospores, sclerotia, chlamydospores, or resting spores in or on the host. The first of these are relatively short-lived (a few hours to several months) spores. The others survive long storage and adverse conditions. The resting spores of certain *Entomophthora* are of particular interest since they obviously incite infections in the field, but most are extremely difficult to germinate in the laboratory (Krejzová, 1968).

Under controlled environmental conditions longevity of the muscardine conidia has been clearly related to temperature and humidity (Kawakami, 1960b; Kawakami and Mikuni, 1965; Thontadarya, 1966). Clerk and Madelin (1965) found that the viability of conidia of *Beauveria bassiana, Paecilomyces farinosus* and *Metarrhizium anisopliae* decreased as the storage temperature increased from 8° to 25° C. After conidia of *M. anisopliae* were exposed to light fewer germinated, and this effect was more pronounced with *B. bassiana.* Conidia of *B. bassiana* and *P. farinosus* lived longer at a relative humidity of 0% or 34%, than at 75%. On the other hand, conidia of *M. anisopliae* survived longest at extreme high and low humidities and least at humidities near 45%. These species store best at about 4° C, in the dark and at very low humidity. Drying of thin-walled blastospores of *B. bassiana* (defined on p. 140) reduces their effectiveness, and Müller-Kögler (1967a) suggests storage at a high humidity and low temperature. The value of applying *Entomophthora* conidia in the conventional manner as a microbial insecticide is still questionable, since even brief storage at humidities below 80% reduces their germination greatly (Sawyer, 1931; Yendol, 1968). However, on artificial media, *E. virulenta* produces resting spores which germinate without a period of dormancy, and these may prove more useful for microbial control than conidia (Gustafsson, 1965).

c. Inoculum size. As with other pathogens, a minimum number of infective units (spores) must contact a host before disease is induced, and exposure to lower numbers will permit its escape. Counts from environments where epizootics occurred have not been reported, but microbial control experiments indicate that these numbers may be higher than normally expected. Ferron (1967c) and Jaques *et al.* (1968) used about 10^{10} spores/m^2 or ft^2 of soil surface. LD_{50} values in the laboratory also tend to be rather high, but since they usually include spores which do not actually contact the test insect, they probably offer little clue as to the precise number needed to incite disease in a single animal. The method of Veen (1968) obviates this problem to some extent, and he estimated an LD_{50} of about 150,000 *M. anisopliae* spores per *Schistocerca gregaria* in instar II.

d. Virulence. Within single fungal species, strains exist which differ in virulence for a given insect species (e.g. Rockwood, 1950; Aoki, 1962; Paschke, 1965; Ferron, 1967b; Ferron and Diomandé, 1969; Latch, 1965; Veen, 1968). Factors which may account for this phenomenon include heterokaryosis and/or somatic recombination from the anastomosis of hyphae of differing genotypes, and the amount of saprobic growth the fungus has undergone in the environment prior to encountering insects. The latter is known to cause reduced virulence in certain fungi (e.g. Kawakami, 1960a; Latch, 1965).

2. Host

a. Population density. Entomogenous fungi are only imperfectly density-dependent. Infected larvae occur in scattered areas even with low populations of the host. This is particularly true of *Beauveria* where the inoculum apparently is widespread in certain environments (e.g. Hurpin, 1967; Jaques and MacLellan, 1965). However, the density of aphids infected with *Entomophthora* affects the rate of mortality (MacLeod *et al.*, 1966).

b. Susceptibility to fungi. Insecticide resistance studies have demonstrated conclusively that not all populations of an insect species are identical Also the composition of the insect's cuticle varies somewhat with nutrition and crowding, as evidenced by the "phases" of insects such as armyworms and locusts, and these changes may alter the susceptibility of the insect. Closely related insects or insects with similar behavior (e.g. pupation in soil) may demonstrate different degrees of susceptibility to a given fungus (e.g. Jaques *et al.*, 1968; Zacharuk and Tinline, 1968; McCauley *et al.*, 1968; Latch, 1965). Survivors of epizootics of fungi theoretically should be more resistant to the disease than the pre-epizootic population as has been proposed for viruses (Martignoni and Schmid, 1961), but no information is available on this point.

Susceptibility to infection only at the time of ecdysis has been reported (e.g. Rockwood, 1950; Clark *et al.*, 1968), but generally infection occurs during intermolt periods as well (e.g. Roberts, 1970). Lepidopterous larvae tend to be more susceptible than eggs, pupae, or adults, whereas with elaterid beetles pupae and adults were most susceptible (Zacharuk and Tinline, 1968). Young cockchafer beetles *(Melolontha)* were more resistant than older ones (Ferron, 1967b; Hurpin, 1968).

Inapparent infections, which manifest themselves after insects are brought into the laboratory, often occur (Crow *et al.*, 1968; Surany, 1960). It would be of great interest to verify these observations histologically or with procedures to prevent cross-contamination, such as rearing insects individually and sterilizing tools and external surfaces of the insects.

3. Environment

It must be emphasized that the microclimate around the fungus is the critical environment. The best illustration of this is the fungal epizootics affecting aphids in humid, irrigated alfalfa fields situated in desert areas (Hall and Dunn, 1958).

a. Temperature. Much information is available on the effects of temperature on germination and/or growth of entomogenous fungi *in vitro* (Müller-Kögler, 1965). In general, the limits for growth range between 5° and 35°C and the optima fall between 20° and 30°C. *B. bassiana,* however, kills overwintering insects in environments where temperatures average well below the optimum. Interestingly, the optimum for growth of strains of this species is reduced from south to north in the U.S.S.R. (Yevlakhova and Shvetsova, 1965). This may account for the bark-beetle mortality noted with a Finnish isolate at temperatures below 14°C and averaging considerably less than 10°C (Nuorteva and Salonen, 1968). Large numbers of mosquito adults overwintering in caves were also killed at low temperatures by *Entomophthora* (= *Entomophaga* of Batko) (Novak, 1967; Weiser and Batko, 1966; Teernstra-Eeken and Engel, 1967). Temperatures which support only moderate growth of the fungus are adequate for disease initiation and development. The rate of mortality is affected by temperature, being seriously lowered at low temperatures (e.g. Zacharuk and Tinline, 1968; Stimmann, 1968; Ferron, 1965, 1967b; Roberts, 1970). Total mortality may or may not be affected, and this may depend upon whether or not the optima of the host and parasite coincide.

Optimum temperatures for spore germination are less well documented than for mycelium development. With three species of *Entomophthora,* the germination ranges (Yendol, 1968) were found to be slightly more restricted than those for growth (Hall and Bell, 1961). Also, the surface had a marked influence. Agar afforded much higher germination in most cases when compared to glass slides. Since both types of surface were held over water, it is assumed that humidity was not the limiting factor.

b. Humidity. Humidity can be limiting at two periods in an epizootic. First, high humidity is needed by most fungi to germinate and cause disease. Second, the new spores needed to spread and heighten the epizootic usually are produced on cadavers only at very high humidities. It has been claimed, but not fully documented, that these limitations can be obviated in microbial control by introducing large quantities of spores into the environment (microbial insecticide) (Dunn and Mechalas, 1963; Schaerffenberg, 1966). As pointed out in the literature surveys of Müller-Kögler (1965) and Baird (1958a), epizootics are usually associated with periods of high humidity, particularly rainy periods, and microbial control is usually "successful" where the application took place shortly before wet weather.

As mentioned on page 134, humidity affects longevity of spores. Germination is also seriously affected, since most fungi germinate only at very high relative humidity—usually 90% or higher. It is likely that some of the published figures for entomogenous fungi are too low, since, as pointed out by Veen (1968), a reduction of 1°C in a test chamber at very high humidity will permit condensation, and therefore only data obtained at carefully controlled temperatures are valid. Germination of *M. anisopliae* on insect cuticle and on ether extracts of cuticle could be obtained only when free water was present (Veen, 1968), and certain other pathogens may have the same requirements, as indicated by recent studies with *E. apiculata* and *E. virulenta* (Yendol, 1968). The requirement for high humidity is not as restrictive as it would appear at first glance, since the humidity is needed for less than 48 hr for infection to begin (Getzin, 1961; Kawakami and Mikuni, 1965), after which fungal development can proceed on the moisture within the insect. In some cases a heavy dew is adequate, in others rain is needed.

c. Light. Light appears to affect both longevity of spores and sporulation on the host after its death. The latter has been documented with *P. farinosus* and *Cordyceps militaris* recently by Cohen (1967) and Basith and Madelin (1968) who found light essential to spore production, and the former by Clerk and Madelin (1965) (p. 134). Sunlight (presumably the ultra-violet component) is known to kill spores (Müller-Kögler, 1965), and neglect of this fact may be responsible for some of the microbial control failures recorded with fungi. Proper formulation and/or application in the evening should alleviate this problem.

III. Microbial Control

A. CONCEPTUAL APPROACHES TO MICROBIAL CONTROL

Many attempts have been made to use entomogenous fungi to control economically important insects, e.g. Baird (1956, 1958a, b) lists 41 successful attempts to control 28 species or groups of insects with fungi. Nevertheless, few of the fungi listed as successful are utilized in control programs today. Most of the successful trials used *Beauveria bassiana, Metarrhizium anisopliae* or one of a few species of *Entomophthora.* As with other biological control agents, entomogenous fungi can be used in three different ways for insect control. The method of choice will be determined by the characteristics of the fungus and insect involved. (1) Colonization: the fungus is introduced into an insect population where it becomes permanently established. Pest insects, therefore, are killed year after year from one or a few introductions. (2) Microbial Insecticide: as with chemical insecticides, applications are made repeatedly as required to control pest populations. And (3) Integrated Control: control techniques are selected which have minimal adverse effects on natural mortality factors such as parasites, predators, and pathogens. The entomogenous fungus can play a role as a desirable applied control agent or as a naturally occurring mortality factor which warrants protection.

1. Colonization

The introduction of natural insect enemies to control arthropod pests is well established with state and federal organizations. Nevertheless, few biological control projects in the past have seriously considered foreign exploration for beneficial micro-organisms. Most introductions and colonizations have been restricted to the redistribution of indigenous groups or to those fungi that were accidentally introduced along with the insect host. The primary objective in introducing new fungal pathogens into disease-free areas is their permanent establishment, which allows them to spread naturally and also to serve as a source for further artificial distribution. The use of this concept is best exemplified by the transfer of *Coelomomyces* into mosquito populations free of this parasite (Laird, 1967; Muspratt, 1963). Unfortunately, the effect of the fungus on the numbers of adult mosquitoes was inconclusive (Chapter 18, p. 394), but the fungus became established in the *Aedes polynesiensis* population of the Tokelau island where colonization was attempted.

2. Microbial Insecticide

Colonization, being cheap and not laborious, is the preferred method of microbial control, but it is not always feasible. It has been well established with nuclear polyhedrosis viruses and *Bacillus thuringiensis* that repeated applications of insect pathogens can be effective in insect control. This is in agreement with the observation of Baird (1956) that applications of indigenous entomogenous fungi may be useful in initiating epizootics before they would normally occur or in increasing the amount of fungus in areas where insufficient inoculum is present to start epizootics. Many of the "successful" microbial control attempts cited by Baird (1958a, b) and Müller-Kögler (1965) resulted in short-term reductions of pest populations, and, although not always mentioned, repeated treatment apparently would be needed to maintain the lower pest levels.

In considering instances of successful pest control with *Beauveria* spores,

Dunn and Mechalas (1963) suggested that there was a massive field inoculation employed in each case. They have proposed that many of the failures with *Beauveria* occurred because applications were made utilizing only the colonization concept and secondly, where crops were treated with fungal materials, too little inoculum was applied. These workers have proposed two principles for the practical application of this pathogen. First, reduction of the population to a point below the economic threshold is, in many instances, a direct function of dosage and time of observation. And second, the larger the dosage applied the wider the spectrum of pests that can be expected to be controlled. Moisture is generally regarded as limiting with fungal microbial-insecticide applications in that relative humidity must be very high, at least in the microclimate (MacLeod *et al.*, 1966). A dissenting viewpoint (Dunn and Mechalas, 1963; Schaerffenberg, 1964), however, suggests that infection can occur with low humidity if large numbers of spores are used. Laboratory and field tests to evaluate the validity and significance of these statements with *Beauveria* and other fungi are needed.

Combined applications of entomogenous fungi and low doses of chemical insecticides may result in synergism between the two, an approach considered promising in Eastern Europe, but little studied in the West (Chapter 14).

3. Integrated Control

When considering chemicals for pest control, it should be remembered that fungicides used to control plant-attacking fungi have often been considered limiting factors in the development of fungal epizootics in insect pest populations. For example, fungicide sprays on citrus trees in Florida reduced infection of the scale insects by entomogenous fungi (Holloway and Young, 1943; Fisher and Griffiths, 1950). Some fungicides appear to have less effect on naturally occurring epizootics than others, and Jaques and Patterson (1962) have shown that infection by *E. sphaerosperma* killed more apple suckers when orchards were treated with glyodin than with captan or ferbam. Also, in potato fields treated weekly with the fungicides zineb, nabam and zinc sulfate, Shands *et al.* (1962) were still able to find more than 11% of the potato aphids infected with several species of *Entomophthora.*

Laboratory experiments have repeatedly demonstrated the inhibition of entomogenous fungi by commercial insecticides and fungicides. The insecticides commonly used against the spotted alfalfa aphid definitely inhibited many of the entomophthoraceous fungi isolated from this aphid (Hall and Dunn, 1959). The vegetative growth of these fungi was restricted in varying degrees by the fungicides wettable sulfur, Dithan Z-78, ferbam, Bordeaux 5-5-50 and captane. The dominant pathogen of the spotted alfalfa aphid, *E. exitialis* was particularly susceptible. Both the chlorinated hydrocarbon and organic phosphate insecticides retarded the germination of *E. virulenta* resting spores, but eventually good vegetative growth resulted. Conidial germination of *E. coronata* is inhibited by the insecticide malathion, and in general the germination of entomophthoraceous conidia was significantly reduced by fungicides (Yendol, 1968). The development of the muscardine fungi *Beauveria* and *Metarrhizium* is also restricted by certain insecticides (Ten, 1961; Urs *et al.*, 1967).

Susceptibility of parasites and predators to fungi scheduled for microbial control should be considered in the final choice of fungal species. Strains of even broad spectrum fungi are known which are much more virulent with one insect as compared to others (e.g. Ferron and Diomandé, 1969; Veen, 1968; Latch, 1965; Aoki, 1968).

B. PRODUCTION OF INFECTIOUS MATERIAL

1. Culture

An important consideration in the mass culture of a fungus for microbial control is the selection of strains that maintain a high degree of virulence *in vitro* and produce good growth with abundant sporulation. The spore yield is often determined by the type of medium used to culture the fungus (e.g. Dresner, 1949; Schaerffenberg, 1964; Gustafsson, 1965).

Methods for mass-producing spores of *Beauveria* and *Metarrhizium* have been successfully developed (Martignoni, 1964). The basic culture substrates were usually wheat, corn or potato products. Müller-Kögler (1967a) suggests that loose (bran or corn grains) rather than solid substrates like agar yield more spores, since spores/unit weight of medium is related to the surface area of the medium. Three main methods of mass-producing *B. bassiana* are currently used (Pristavko and Goral, 1967). (1) Reproduction on solid nutrient media in sterile conditions with natural aeration, a method acceptable only for small-scale laboratory production. (2) Growth under semi-sterile conditions on liquid, pasty and solid nutrient media in flat vessels of various sizes. This method can be satisfactorily used to produce enough material for laboratory and field tests. (3) Production in liquid media on a shaking machine or in industrial type fermentation tanks with artificial aeration. Spreading in shallow vessels for spore production after growth in submerged cultures has been suggested (Pristavko and Goral, 1967).

Some entomogenous fungi are dimorphic and, when grown in submerged cultures that are shaken and aerated, produce yeast-like cells instead of mycelium. These yeast-like cells are called blastospores and can be mass-produced relatively quickly. The disadvantage for microbial control is that dried blastospores are shorter lived than conidia (Müller-Kögler, 1967a). Mass culture of blastospores has been accomplished with *B. bassiana* (Samšináková, 1966; Kawakami, 1962), *B. tenella* (Cordon and Schwartz, 1962), *M. anisopliae* (Adamek, 1965), *Spicaria prasina* (Kawakami, 1962), and *Paecilomyces (Spicaria) farinosus* (Kerner, 1959).

2. Maintaining and Increasing Virulence

Virulence may be reduced or lost by repeatedly culturing certain entomogenous fungi on artificial media, e.g. several muscardines (Kawakami, 1960a; Latch, 1965). This is best documented with *B. bassiana* where reduction in virulence began after 16 transfers (Schaerffenberg, 1964) and toxin production was reduced after repeated culturing (West and Briggs, 1968). On the other hand, brown strains of *M. anisopliae* remained virulent after 7 and 30 years (unknown number of transfers) of artificial culture (Rockwood, 1950; Latch, 1965). *Entomophthora* spp. with broad host spectra, e.g. *E. coronata,* appear to maintain their virulence over long periods (e.g. Prasertphon, 1963).

In most cases virulence is reduced rather than totally destroyed and can be restored to the original high level by passage through insect hosts. The mechanism of the loss and reacquisition is unknown, but its occurrence with single spored cultures (Kawakami, 1960a) indicates it is not accomplished by selection of specific genotypes such as could occur with mixed cultures. Since virulence can be reduced on artificial media, spores obtained shortly after isolation from infected insects should be maintained as seed for further spore productions. This can be accomplished by low temperature and/or drying techniques or reduction of oxygen (e.g. Perkins, 1962; Mizrahi and Miller, 1968; Ellis and Roberson, 1968; Lange and Boyd, 1968; Hwang, 1968; Goos *et al.*, 1967; Prasertphon, 1967a; review by Müller-Kögler, 1967a).

Incorporation of lard (animal fats) into or on the nutrient substrate has been proposed to maintain virulence (Schaerffenberg, 1964). Also addition of various chemicals such as insecticides or chitin, as well as more standard treatments such as irradiation of spores, has apparently induced stable mutants with increased virulence (Evlakhova, 1966; Evlakhova and Chvetzova, 1964; Yevlakhova and Shvetsova, 1965). Genetic recombination with various strains of entomogenous fungi to alter virulence has not been attempted. Since the perfect stage is absent, mitotic recombination may prove useful for this type of study with Fungi Imperfecti (Roper, 1966; Roberts, 1968) (see also Chapter 30).

Enhancement of virulence is a particularly neglected area of research with the entomogenous fungi. Naturally occurring strains of fungi are currently used almost exclusively, whereas tailor-made strains would obviously be better suited for microbial control in certain conditions.

3. Storage

Tests of viability of stored spores are frequently not quantitative. A simple dead or alive designation, however, can be very misleading since strong cultures will appear on normally streaked test plates even though less than 10% of the inoculated spores are viable. The use of material with low viability for microbial control, of course, is wasted effort, and percentage viability should be determined for spore preparations prior to use. As mentioned on p. 134 spore longevity is related to temperature, humidity, gaseous atmosphere, and probably light during storage. Unless expensive methods of storage such as extreme cold or lyophilization are employed to assure high viability, spores should be used within a few weeks or months of their production. Also, when possible, spores should be held at 4°C after harvesting until use. If spores are frozen they should be thawed quickly (Goos *et al.,* 1967). Dead spores from improper storage probably account for some of the failures reported in microbial control attempts using fungi.

4. Formulation

In general, spores can be applied in dusts, sprays or granules. The best formulation depends primarily upon the fungal species. Dusts offer a slight advantage, in that they can be stored in a formulated condition, and their swirling in air jets tends to adhere them to lower as well as upper surfaces of foliage. Caution should be used in selecting a diluent since some materials inhibit spore germination (Dresner, 1949). Talc, flour, and milk powder have served as suitable diluents for dusts (Kerner, 1959; Bartlett and Lefebvre, 1934; Dresner, 1949; York, 1958; Chapter 28).

Aqueous sprays of *B. bassiana* spores are generally unsuitable unless a wetting agent is included, although it is advisable to test its effect on spore viability first. Hall (1954) suggested that the failure of *B. bassiana* spores to infect *Crambus* larvae was due to the wetting agent. Some compounds which have proved satisfactory include Triton X-100, DuPont Spreader-sticker with *Spicaria rileyi* (Getzin, 1961). Triton X-155 and the household detergent "Trend" at 1% in water had no detectable adverse effect on the spores of *B. bassiana* (York, 1958).

York (1958) found granules (corn meal or attapulgite) to be more effective than sprays or dusts when treating corn with *B. bassiana* for corn borer control.

Compounds which shield spores from ultra-violet rays of the sun, increase moisture in the microclimate of the spore, and reduce the allergenicity hazard from spores should be given special consideration by formulators of entomogenous fungi. Encapsulation (Raun and Jackson, 1966), which conceivably could satisfy some of these requirements, has not been reported for fungi.

C. APPLICATION

Colonization is usually attempted with relatively small inocula in the form of diseased insects or cultured material (e.g. Hall and Dunn, 1958; Laird, 1960, 1966, 1967). For the microbial insecticide approach, large amounts of material are needed, which can be applied satisfactorily with equipment designed for application of chemical insecticides. The observations of Dunn and Mechalas (1963), Ferron (1967c, d), and Jaques *et al.* (1968) indicate that large doses are advisable, but the precise amount has been established for few situations and, in the present dearth of guidelines, the worker will be well advised to devise recommendations to meet his specific conditions. Timing of applications must, of course, coincide with the presence of susceptible stages of the host; but timing should also be related to the environment. For example, immediately after rain or irrigation would be better than in dry periods. Also, treatment in the evening will take advantage of the absence of sunlight (for those fungi most susceptible to it) and of the moisture afforded by dew. For soil insects which remain underground, the mere application of spores to the soil surface may be unsatisfactory since certain fungal spores move downwards very little (Burges, 1950).

D. ISOLATION AND LABORATORY EVALUATIONS

Identification of entomogenous fungi is described in Chapter 2. Success in infecting insects with an entomogenous fungus depends largely on (1) obtaining a pure culture of a fungal isolate which is pathogenic for a given insect host, (2) positioning the infective stage on or within the host and (3) duplicating the environmental conditions which are conducive to infection. As in any pathogenic relationships, Koch's postulates should be satisfied whenever possible.

Experimental techniques used to infect insects with fungi have varied greatly among investigators. A commonly used method is exposure of insects for a standard time on a sporulating fungal culture of specific age (Prasertphon, 1963; Yendol and Paschke, 1965). This method is especially suitable for evaluating species of *Entomophthora,* where the fragility of spores makes their transfer difficult; but for exact quantitative studies it is poor. Where spore material is easily harvested and formulated into a dust, as with *Metarrhizium* and *Beauveria,* a vacuum duster as suggested by Dunn and Mechalas (1963) can be used. However, it is not known to what extent the release of vacuum draws spores into the trachea. Suspensions of spores can be applied directly to the cuticle by spraying, or in a drop of liquid of known volume, or, as is more common, by "painting" the insect with a small brush. Except for "painting", these methods have the advantage that a known number of spores is used for each dosage. With insects living in stored food or soil the spore material can be mixed quantitatively into these substrates. Injection of spores into the hemocoel also affords known doses, but circumvents the normal portal of entry—the cuticle. A number of methods for inoculating insects with fungi have been used, but few have been critically evaluated. It is evident that more research is needed for the development of satisfactory bioassay techniques (Müller-Kögler, 1967a; Chapter 27).

E. EFFECTS ON MAN AND HIGHER ANIMALS

Although most insect pathogenic fungi are considered to be harmless to man, allergenic reactions have been reported after the harvesting of *B. bassiana* spores (Hall, 1954; York, 1958). Hall suggested that this reaction resulted from inhaling spores, but Dresner (1949) indicated no harmful effects when spores were inhaled and York (1958) found that long sleeves and gloves halted the response, whereas the use of a respirator alone did not. Proper attire and careful formulation should reduce the hazard to operators from this fungus (Schaerffenberg, 1968). *B. bassiana* blastospores are apparently non-allergenic (Müller-Kögler, 1967b).

Some species of *Aspergillus* and one species of *Entomophthora, E. coronata,* are known to infect vertebrates (Chapter 22).

Aspergillus spp. and *E. coronata* obviously should not be used for microbial control. In addition, before strains of other fungi are used in large-scale microbial control programs they should be tested for ability to infect and cause side-effects to vertebrates. Such tests have been particularly suggested for fungi able to grow at temperatures approaching that of man (Müller-Kögler, 1967b). Past experience indicates that the results of such tests will be negative except for the allergenicity of certain people to *B. bassiana* spores, which can be alleviated or avoided as mentioned above. Obviously all fungi should not be discarded as potential microbial control agents because of the vertebrate pathogenicity of *Aspergillus* spp. and *E. coronata,* neither of which, for different reasons, is likely to be used for massive field applications, and both of which are already cosmopolitan in distribution. To discard all fungi on these grounds would be as unwise as it would be to rule out viruses because arboviruses multiply in both man and arthropods.

F. CURRENT RESEARCH NEEDS

Nine areas of research are in need of study before the promising potential for microbial control with entomogenous fungi is likely to be consistently attained: (1) elucidation of aspects of disease induction, including chemical constituents of the insect cuticle which inhibit or enhance spore germination, penetration of the cuticle by germ tubes, and production and mode of action of toxins; (2) use of genetic manipulation (including mitotic recombination) to produce fungal strains well suited to microbial control; (3) methods for maintaining virulence in mass cultures; (4) standardization of microbial control products; (5) study of the effects of environment on viability and disease induction; (6) discovery of additives which preserve viability, enhance virulence, and reduce the allergenic hazard of spores to man; (7) examination of the effects of massive amounts of spores on pest-insect mortality and on ecosystems; (8) determination of the effects on insect mortality of combinations of fungal species, fungi with other pathogens, and fungi with sublethal doses of insecticides; and (9) systematic examination of the effects of entomogenous fungi on vertebrates to document the failure of the majority to invade living vertebrate tissue, and to critically assess their allergenic characteristics (Roberts, 1968).

Because the pathogens' requirements for high humidity are usually adequately met in the soil and in water, these habitats should merit more emphasis in microbial control studies than they have received in the past. Some recent reports of work in these habitats have been encouraging (Couch, 1968; Umphlett, 1968; Ferron, 1967b; Jaques *et al.*, 1968; Anderson and Ringo, 1969; Roberts, 1970).

The pathogens chosen will still be those species used in the past, but current knowledge as to the variations on virulence between strains of the same species indicates that a strain highly virulent for the specific target insect should be selected or induced before embarking upon large-scale field trials.

One group, the genus *Coelomomyces*, has long been of interest because of its activity against mosquito larvae. Reproducible laboratory infections were unattainable until recently (Couch, 1968), as the information basic to understanding natural epizootics and the proper methods for microbial control were not available. The combined field and laboratory studies of Umphlett (1968) and Couch (1968) will probably strengthen worldwide interest in the group and provide the guidelines needed to capitalize on the microbial control potential of these fungi.

IV. Conclusions

One of the most important concepts to be gleaned from work in the past decade is the realization that a single fungal species can contain strains which are widely divergent in physiology and virulence. Accordingly, success or failure in microbial control, or the requirements for germination, etc. of a given strain are not necessarily applicable to other strains of that species. It is obvious that strains should be specified in publications and single-spore or single-nucleus isolates used for experiments. Also, these isolates should be stored by methods which require only infrequent transfer to reduce the chance of spontaneous mutation.

Virtually every experienced field entomologist has witnessed "spontaneous" epizootics of fungal diseases which dramatically decimated large insect populations. The apparently effortless success of the fungi in these instances has been very tantalizing to those interested in controlling insect pests. This has resulted in field trials without adequate basic knowledge of how the fungus performs the task it is asked to do, viz. kill insects. It should come as no surprise, nor should it cause pessimism as to the potential of fungi in microbial control, that many of these field trials yielded negative results. For example, in most instances death occurs only after penetration by the fungus, so that fungal spores must be alive at the time of contact with their prospective host. Nevertheless, past field trials have been made without quantifying the viability of the spores prior to application, nor were the effects on viability of environmental stresses, such as sunlight, evaluated. In our view, the modes of disease induction constitute a study which will be essential to the rational use of fungi in microbial control.

References

Adamek, L. (1965). *Folia microbiol. Praha,* **10,** 255-257.

Ali, B. S., Heitefuss, R. and Fuchs, W. H. (1965). *Z. PflKrankh. PflSchutz,* **72,** 201-207.

Anderson, J. F. and Ringo, S. L. (1969). *J. Invertebrate Path.* **13,** 386-393.

Aoki, J. (1962). *J. seric. Sci., Tokyo* **31,** 221-227.

Aoki, K. (1968). Proc. Joint U.S.-Japan Semin. Microbial Control Insect Pests. U.S.-Japan Committee Sci. Cooperation. Panel 8, pp. 115-118. Fukuoka, Japan.

Baird, R. B. (1956). "A List of Attempts to Control Insects by Means of Entomogenous Fungi. A Supplement to Use of Fungus Diseases in Biological Control of Insects." *Int. Congr. Ent.,* 10th, Montreal, 1956. Mimeo.

Baird, R. B. (1958a). "The Artificial Control of Insects by Means of Entomogenous Fungi: a Compilation of References with Abstracts." Entomology Laboratory, Belleville, Ontario.

Baird, R. B. (1958b). *Proc. Int. Congr. Ent.,* 10th, Montreal, 1956, **4,** 689-692.

Bartlett, K. A. and Lefebvre, C. L. (1934). *J. econ. Ent.* **27,** 1147-1157.

Basith, M. and Madelin, M. F. (1968). *Can. J. Bot.* **46,** 473-480.

Batko, A. (1964a). *Bull. Acad. pol. Sci. Cl. II Ser. Sci. biol.* **12,** 319-321.

Batko, A. (1964b). *Bull. Acad. pol. Sci. Cl. II Ser. Sci. biol.* **12,** 323-326.

Batko, A. (1964c). *Bull. Acad. pol. Sci. Cl. II Ser. Sci. biol.* **12,** 399-402.

Batko, A. (1964d). *Bull. Acad. pol. Sci. Cl. II Ser. Sci. biol.* **12,** 403-406.

Batko, A. and Weiser, J. (1965). *J. Invertebrate Path.* **7,** 455-463.

Beard, R. L. (1968). *J. Invertebrate Path.* **10,** 438-439.

Behnke, C. N. and Paschke, J. D. (1966). *J. Invertebrate Path.* **8,** 103-108.

Bonventre, P. F., Lincoln, R. E. and Lamanna, C. (1967). *Bacteriol. Rev.* **31,** 95-109.

Brown, A. H. S. and Smith, G. (1957). *Trans. Br. mycol. Soc.* **40,** 17-89.

Bucher, G. E. (1964). *Ann. ent. Soc. Quebec* **9,** 30-42.

Burges, A. (1950). *Trans. Br. mycol. Soc.* **33,** 142-147.

Burnside, C. E. (1930). U.S. Dept. Agr. Tech. Bull. No. 149, 1-42.

Bursell, E. and Clements, A. N. (1967). *J. Insect Physiol.* **13,** 1671-1678.

Clark, T. B., Kellen, W. R., Fukuda, T. and Lindegren, J. E. (1968). *J. Invertebrate Path.* **11,** 1-7.

Claus, L. (1961). *Arch. Mikrobiol.* **40,** 17-46.

Clerk, G. C. and Madelin, M. F. (1965). *Trans. Br. mycol. Soc.* **48,** 193-209.

Cohen, J. (1967). *Ann. Bot.* **31,** 455-468.

Cordon, T. C. and Schwartz, J. H. (1962). *Science, N.Y.* **138,** 1265-1266.

Couch, J. N. (1968). Proc. Joint U.S.-Japan Semin. Microbial Control Insect Pests. U.S. Committee Sci. Cooperation. Panel 8. pp. 93-105. Fukuoka, Japan.

Crow, W. R., Puttler, B. and Daugherty, D. M. (1968). *J. econ. Ent.* **61,** 576-577.

Damodar, P., Perti, S. L. and Agarwal, P. N. (1964). *Indian J. Ent.* **26,** 110-112.

David, W. A. L. (1968). *In* "Insects and Physiology" (J. W. L. Beament and J. E. Treherne, eds), pp. 17-35. American Elsevier, New York.

Dorschner, E. and Lardy, H. (1969). Eighth Interscience Conference on Antimicrobial Agents and Chemotherapy, New York, 1968, p. 19.

Dresner, E. (1949). Contr. Boyce Thompson Inst. *Pfl. Res.* **15,** 319-335.

Dunn, P. H. and Mechalas, B. J. (1963). *J. Insect Path.* **5,** 451-459.

El Basyouni, S. H., Brewer, D. and Vining, L. C. (1968). *Can. J. Bot.* **46,** 441-448.

Ellis, J. J. and Roberson, J. A. (1968). *Mycologia* **60,** 399-405.

Evlakhova, A. A. (1966). *Trudý mosk. Obshch. ispýt. Prir.* **22,** 257-262. [Abstr. in *Biol. Abstr.* **50,** 16795. 1969.]

Evlakhova, A. A. and Chekhourina, T. A. (1964). *Mém. hors Sér. Entomophaga.* No. 2, 137-141.

Evlakhova, A. A. and Chvetzova, O. I. (1964). *Mém. hors Sér. Entomophaga.* No. 2, 521-529.

Ferron, P. (1965). *Ann. Soc. Ent. Fr. (N.S.)* **1,** 619-625.

Ferron, P. (1967a). *Ann. Épiphyt.* 18, 361-382.

Ferron, P. (1967b). *Entomophaga* **12,** 257-293.
Ferron, P. (1967c). *In* "Insect Pathology and Microbial Control" (P. A. van der Laan, ed.), pp. 204-209. North-Holland Publ. Co., Amsterdam.
Ferron, P. (1967d). *Phytiat.-Phytopharm.* **16,** 115-123.
Ferron, P. and Diomandé, T. (1969). *C.r. Sér. D.* **268,** 331-332.
Fisher, F. E. and Griffiths, J. T., Jr. (1950). *J. econ. Ent.* **43,** 712-718.
Gabriel, B. P. (1968a). *J. Invertebrate Path.* **11,** 70-81.
Gabriel, B. P. (1968b). *J. Invertebrate Path.* **11,** 82-89.
Getzin, L. W. (1961). *J. Insect Path.* **3,** 2-10.
Goos, R. D., Davis, E. E. and Butterfield, W. (1967). *Mycologia* **59,** 58-66.
Gustafsson, M. (1965). *LantbruksHögsk. Annlr* **31,** 405-457.
Hall, I. M. (1954). *Hilgardia* **22,** 535-565.
Hall, I. M. and Bell, J. V. (1961). *J. Insect Path.* **3,** 289-296.
Hall, I. M. and Dunn, P. H. (1958). *J. econ. Ent.* **51,** 341-344.
Hall, I. M. and Dunn, P. H. (1959). *J. econ. Ent.* **52,** 28-29.
Hamill, R. L., Higgens, C. E. and Gorman, M. (1969). Eighth Interscience Conference on Antimicrobial Agents and Chemotherapy, New York, 1968, pp. 18-19.
Hanessian, S., DeJongh, D. C. and McCloskey, J. A. (1966). *Biochim. biophys. Acta* **117,** 480-482.
Heitor, F. (1962). *Ann. Épiphyt.* 13, 179-203.
Hirst, J. M., Stedman, O. J. and Hurst, G. W. (1967). *J. gen. Microbiol.* **48,** 357-377.
Holloway, J. K. and Young, T. R., Jr. (1943). *J. econ. Ent.* **36,** 453-457.
Huber, J. (1958). *Arch. Mikrobial.* **29,** 257-276.
Hurpin, B. (1967). *Ann. Épiphyt.* 18, 127-173.
Hurpin, B. (1968). *J. Invertebrate Path.* **10,** 252-262.
Hwang, S-w. (1968). *Mycologia* **60,** 613-621.
Jaques, R. P. and Patterson, N. A. (1962). *Can. Ent.* **94,** 818-825.
Jaques, R. P. and MacLellan, C. R. (1965). *J. Invertebrate Path.* **7,** 291-296.
Jaques, R. P., Stultz, H. T. and Huston, F. (1968). *Can. Ent.* **100,** 813-818.
Jenkins, D. W. (1964). *Bull. Wld Hlth Org.* 30 (Suppl.), 1-150.
Johnson, D. E., Nelson, G. E. N. and Ciegler, A. (1968). *Appl. Microbiol.* **16,** 1678-1683.
Kamburov, S. S., Nadel, D. J. and Kenneth, R. (1967). *Israel J. Agric. Res.* **17,** 131-134.
Kawakami, K. (1960a). *Bull. seric. Exp. Stn Japan* **16,** 83-99.
Kawakami, K. (1960b). *Sanshi-Kenkyu* **33-12,** 43-47.
Kawakami, K. (1962). *Bull. seric. Exp. Stn Japan* **18,** 147-156.
Kawakami, K. and Mikuni, T. (1965). *Sanshi-Kenkyu* **56,** 42-46.
Kerner, G. (1959). *Trans. Int. Conf. Insect Path. Biol. Control,* 1st, Prague, 1958, pp. 169-176.
Kishaba, A. N., Shankland, D. L., Curtis, R. W. and Wilson, M. C. (1962). *J. econ. Ent.* **55,** 211-214.
Kodaira, Y. (1961). *J. Fac. Textile Sci. Technol., Shinshu Univ.,* No. 29, Ser. E. (5), 1-68.
Koidsumi, K. (1957). *J. Insect Physiol.* **1,** 40-51.
Krejzová, R. (1968). *J. Invertebrate Path.* **12,** 460.
Kučera, M. and Samšiňáková, A. (1968). *J. Invertebrate Path.* **12,** 316-320.
Laird, M. (1960). Conference on Biological Control of Insects of Medical Importance, Washington, D.C., 1960. Tech. Rep., pp. 84-92.
Laird, M. (1966). "Integrated Control and *Aëdes polynesiensis*: an Outline of the Tokelau Islands Project, and its Results." W.H.O./EBL/66: 69, pp. 1-9.
Laird, M. (1967). *Int. Pest Control.* **9,** 21, 23, 25, 27. [Reprinted from *W.H.O. Chronicle* **21,** 18-26. 1967.]
Lange, B. J. and Boyd, W. J. R. (1968). *Phytopathology* **58,** 1711-1712.
Latch, G. C. M. (1965). *N.Z. Jl agric. Res.* **8,** 384-396.
Locke, M. (1964). *In* "The Physiology of Insecta" (M. Rockstein, ed.), Vol. 3, pp. 379-470. Academic Press, New York.
MacLeod, D. M. (1954). *Ann. N.Y. Acad. Sci.* **60,** 58-70.
MacLeod, D. M. and Soper, R. S. (1965). *Proc. Int. Congr. Ent.,* 12th, London, 1964, pp. 724-726.

MacLoed, D. M., Cameron, J. W. and Soper, R. S. (1966). *Rev. Roumaine Biol., Sér. Botan.* **11,** 125-134.

Madelin, M. F. (1966). *Ann. Rev. Ent.* **11,** 423-448.

Madelin, M. F. (1968). *In* "The Fungi" (G. C. Ainsworth and A. S. Sussman, eds), Vol. 3, pp. 227-238. Academic Press, New York.

Madelin, M. F., Robinson, R. K. and Williams, R. J. (1967). *J. Invertebrate Path.* **9,** 404-412.

Martignoni, M. E. (1964). *In* "Biological Control of Insect Pests and Weeds" (P. De Bach, ed.), pp. 579-609. Reinhold, New York.

Martignoni, M. E. and Schmid, P. (1961). *J. Insect Path.* **3,** 62-74.

McCauley, V. J. E., Zacharuk, R. Y. and Tinline, R. D. (1968). *J. Invertebrate Path.* **12,** 444-459.

Mizrahi, A. and Miller, G. (1968). *Appl. Microbiol.* **16,** 1100-1101.

Müller-Kögler, E. (1965). "Pilzkrankheiten bei Insekten. Anwendung zur biologischen Schädlingsbekämpfung und Grundlagen der Insektenmykologie." Paul Parey, Berlin.

Müller-Kögler, E. (1967a). *In* "Insect Pathology and Microbial Control" (P. A. van der Laan, ed.), pp. 339-353. North-Holland Publ. Co., Amsterdam.

Müller-Kögler, E. (1967b). *Entomophaga* **12,** 429-441.

Müller-Kögler, E. and Huger, A. (1960). *Z. angew. Ent.* **45,** 421-429.

Muspratt, J. (1963). *Bull. Wld Hlth Org.* **29,** 81-86.

Noble-Nesbitt, J. (1968). *In* "Insects and Physiology" (J. W. L. Beament and J. E. Treherne, eds), pp. 3-16. American Elsevier, New York.

Notini, G. and Mathlein, R. (1944). *Statens Växtskyddsanstalt, Medd.* **43,** 1-58.

Novák, D. (1967). *Z. Tropenmed. Parasitol.* **18,** 488-491.

Nuorteva, M. and Salonen, M. (1968). *Ann. ent. fennici* **34,** 49-55.

Paschke, J. D. (1965). *J. Invertebrate Path.* **7,** 101-102.

Perkins, D. D. (1962). *Can. J. Microbiol.* **8,** 591-594.

Prasertphon, S. (1963). *J. Insect Path.* **5,** 174-181.

Prasertphon, S. (1967a). *J. Invertebrate Path.* **9,** 140-142.

Prasertphon, S. (1967b). *J. Invertebrate Path.* **9,** 281-282.

Prasertphon, S. and Tanada, Y. (1968). *J. Invertebrate Path.* **11,** 260-280.

Prasertphon, S. and Tanada, Y. (1969). *Hilgardia* **39,** 581-600.

Pristavko, W. P. and Goral, V. M. (1967). *In* "Insect Pathology and Microbial Control" (P. A. van der Laan, ed.), pp. 118-119. North-Holland Publ. Co., Amsterdam.

Raun, E. S. and Jackson, R. D. (1966). *J. econ. Ent.* **59,** 620-622.

Roberts, D. W. (1967). *In* "Insect Pathology and Microbial Control" (P. A. van der Laan, ed.), pp. 243-246. North-Holland Publ. Co., Amsterdam.

Roberts, D. W. (1968). Proc. Joint U.S.-Japan Semin. Microbial Control Insect Pests. U.S. Committee Sci. Cooperation. Panel 8, pp. 129-134. Fukuoka, Japan.

Roberts, D. W. (1969). *J. Invertebrate Path.* **14,** 82-88.

Roberts, D. W. (1970). Conference on Anopheline Biology and Malaria Eradication, Walter Reed Army Institute of Research, Washington, D.C. Misc. Publ. Ent. Soc. Am. 7, 140-155.

Robinson, R. K. (1966). *Pest Articles and News Summaries, Sect. B.* **12,** 131-142.

Rockwood, L. P. (1950). *Ann. ent. Soc. Am.* **43,** 495-498.

Roper, J. A. (1966). *In* "The Fungi: An Advanced Treatise" (G. C. Ainsworth and A. S. Sussman, eds), Vol. 2, pp. 589-617. Academic Press, New York.

Samšiňáková, A. (1966). *J. Invertebrate Path.* **8,** 395-400.

Sawyer, W. H., Jr. (1931). *Mycologia* **23,** 411-432.

Schaerffenberg, B. (1964). *J. Insect Path.* **6,** 8-20.

Schaerffenberg, B. (1966). *Z. angew. Ent.* **58,** 362-372.

Schaerffenberg, B. (1968). *Entomophaga* **13,** 175-182.

Shands, W. A., Hall, I. M. and Simpson, G. W. (1962). *J. econ. Ent.* **55,** 174-179.

Srinivasan, M. C. and Thirumalachar, M. J. (1967). *Mycologia* **59,** 698-713.

Srinivasan, M. C., Narasimhan, M. J. and Thirumalachar, M. J. (1964). *Mycologia* **56,** 683-691.

Steinhaus, E. A. (1956). *Hilgardia* **26**, 107-160.
Stimmann, M. W. (1968). *J. econ. Ent.* **61**, 1558-1560.
Surany, P. (1960). South Pacific Commission, Noumea, New Caledonia, Techn. Paper No. 128, 1-62.
Sussman, A. S. (1951). *Mycologia* **43**, 338-350.
Tamura, S. and Takahashi, N. (1970). *In* "Naturally-occurring Insecticides" (M. Jacobson and D. G. Crosby, eds), pp. 499-539. Marcel Dekker Inc., New York.
Tanada, Y. (1963). *In* "Insect Pathology: An Advanced Treatise" (E. A. Steinhaus, ed.), Vol. 2, pp. 423-475. Academic Press, New York.
Teernstra-Eeken, M. H. and Engel, A. (1967). *J. Invertebrate Path.* **9**, 431-432.
Ten, G. J. (1961). *Bull. Plant Protect. Ass.* **3**, 53-55.
Thontadarya, T. S. (1966). *Dissertation Abstr.* **27**, 849-B.
Umphlett, C. J. (1968). *J. Elisha Mitchell Sci. Soc.* **84**, 108-114.
Urs, N. V. R., Govindu, H. C. and Shastry, K. S. S. (1967). *J. Invertebrate Path.* **9**, 398-403.
Veen, K. H. (1966). *J. Invertebrate Path.* **8**, 254-256.
Veen, K. H. (1968). *Mededel. Landbouwhogeschool Wageningen* **68-5**, 1-77.
Wallengren, H. and Johansson, R. (1929). *Sor. Int. Corn Borer Invest. Sci. Rept.* **2**, 131-145.
Weiser, J. and Batko, A. (1966). *Folia Parasitol. Praha* **13**, 144-149.
West, E. J. and Briggs, J. D. (1968). *J. econ. Ent.* **61**, 684-687.
Whisler, H. C. (1968). *Mycologia* **60**, 65-75.
Whittaker, R. H. (1969). *Science, N.Y.* **163**, 150-160.
Yendol, W. G. (1968). *J. Invertebrate Path.* **10**, 116-121.
Yendol, W. G., Miller, E. M. and Behnke, C. N. (1968). *J. Invertebrate Path.* **10**, 313-319.
Yendol, W. G. and Paschke, J. D. (1965). *J. Invertebrate Path.* **7**, 414-422.
Yevlakhova, A. A. and Shvetsova, O. I. (1965). *Ent. Rev. (U.S.S.R.)* (Eng. Transl.) **44**, 423-426.
York, G. T. (1958). *Iowa State Coll. J. Sci.* **33**, 123-129.
Zacharuk, R. Y. and Tinline, R. D. (1968). *J. Invertebrate Path.* **12**, 294-309.

CHAPTER 6

Use of Protozoans for Microbial Control of Insects

ROY E. McLAUGHLIN

Boll Weevil Research Laboratory, U.S. Department of Agriculture, Entomology Research Division, State College, Mississippi, U.S.A.

I. Introduction

The protozoans associated with insects are diverse both in type and relationship. Our interest lies in pathogenic types, but even when the protozoan horizon is thus restricted, a myriad of forms and relationships confront us. Here, the major insect pathogenic protozoans and their potential use as control agents will be discussed, with an analysis of specific successes and failures. Areas where further research would be most valuable are emphasized.

Excellent reviews of protozoans as insect pathogens and of their status and potential as control agents have been written by Tanada (1959), Hall (1963), Weiser (1963a), Lipa (1963) and Tanada (1963).

II. General Characteristics of Protozoan Pathogens and Control Systems

As described in Chapter 1, when a pathogen cannot maintain itself in the insect population it must be repeatedly applied. Alternatively when it can maintain itself naturally it can be used as an introduction as in a long-term population control system.

The characteristics of protozoan pathogens suggest that they cannot be used as short-term, quick acting microbial insecticides. With few exceptions, they can be produced only *in vivo* and such large quantities are relatively difficult to produce (Chapter 25). Few act with sufficient speed to prevent severe damage to crops, unless applied when pest populations are low, or to developmental stages that cause no damage. *Immediate* damage control cannot be the prime object with introductions. Damage must be circumvented by introducing pathogens in the season or developmental stage prior to an expected outbreak of the pest. Protozoans are, therefore, likely to be most useful as introductions.

Protozoans depend upon their insect hosts for energy, although they may exist outside them for a time, usually relatively inactive. The total biomass of the pathogen in any ecosystem depends not only upon successful infection and the number of hosts present but also upon dispersal within the host population. The basic problem, then, in any control attempt is one of dispersal.

The primary route of infection by a protozoan is the alimentary tract–to reach the proper environment most protozoans must be eaten. In some cases, congenital or trans-ovum transmission may be the primary method of dispersion though transmission by parasites and predators also occurs. Protozoans, once thought to be highly host and tissue specific, are now known to cross-infect not only genera, but even orders of insects. From a control standpoint, the larger and more variable the host substrate the greater should be the resilience and persistence of the pathogen in nature.

In contrast to the rapid action of viruses or *Bacillus thuringiensis,* protozoans act rather slowly on their hosts. Few are highly virulent, some have a post-infection time to death of a week (i.e. virulent) or more commonly much longer (i.e. avirulent pathogens). Seldom are vital functions of the host disrupted quickly, rather a slow debilitation occurs. Vitality is sapped, fecundity reduced, the life span shortened, movement decreased and responses to stimuli gradually impaired.

These characteristics may be advantageous if properly exploited. Dispersal of the pathogen and infection of new hosts may be greatest in a persistent disease, which continues to provide a source of inoculum–rather than rapid death of the host–which tends to eliminate the pathogen. Ultimately, mortality is desired, but only after optimum dispersal of the pathogen has been achieved. Protection of the insect to ensure foci of infection is not beyond credibility. Stability becomes the keyword. Man must manage the system to preserve the balance of host and pathogen, which may require additional introductions of the pathogen, and possibly also the addition of some host material. Limited release of insects might be cheaper than widespread reintroduction of the pathogen. Protection of the pathogen would be vital and might involve protection of the free-living stages that may be susceptible to the physical environment.

III. Principal Types of Protozoan Pathogens

Readers interested in taxonomy and morphology are referred to the general scheme of Honigberg *et al.* (1964) and for families and lower groupings to Pearse (1936), Jahn and Jahn (1949), Hall (1953), and Kudo (1954).

A. FLAGELLATES LIMITED TO INSECTS

Most insect-pathogenic forms belong to the order Kinetoplastida, mostly in the suborder Trypanosomatina. Further studies may reveal pathogens in the other eight orders and they should not be ignored. Lipa (1963) reviewed other flagellates. Wallace (1966) revised the trypanosomatid parasites of insects and arachnids. Kramer (1963) reviewed the pathologies of the insect vectors. The genera include *Leptomonas, Herpetomonas, Crithidia, Blastocrithidia* and *Rhynchoidomonas,* and a few of uncertain position.

1. Pathogenesis and Epizootiology

Little is known about pathogenesis. The symptoms are mild or undetectable; there may be some diarrhoea or loss of activity. The primary tissue involved is usually the gut, sometimes the hemocoel, salivary glands, Malpighian tubules and ovaries. Death of the host is infrequent, not necessarily caused directly by the pathogen, and no epizootics have been recorded. The insect-limited trypanosomatids are widespread geographically, primarily in Hemiptera and Diptera. Wallace (1966) accounts for 85% of the records from these two orders, recognizing 123 species and varieties from over 270 insect species. *B. raabei* (Lipa, 1966) and *B. vagoi* (Tuzet and Laporte, 1965) can also be added.

2. Control Considerations

Flagellates may be useful as introductions, since they are slowly debilitative and spread in infected fecal pellets of pests. Also, from cross-infection experiments, Wallace concluded that flagellates have very little specificity within a family of insects, and even between families and between orders there was some interchange of hosts. In feeding tests, *Herpetomonas muscarum* infected nine species (mostly flies) and *C. fasciculata* infected mosquito adults of a number of species. *L. pyrrhocoris* was cross-infectious among several hemipterans, and also infected many insect species on injection, lethally so in larvae of the wax moth, *Galleria mellonella* (Zotta, 1921).

The culture of flagellates on artificial media improves their usefulness in microbial control (Guttman and Wallace, 1964; Wallace and Clark, 1959). Moreover, Wallace and Johnson (1961) found that *C. fasciculata* remained infectious after 2·44 years on artificial media. A suitable environment, preferably frequented by the host, might be found or created in which a ready reservoir of infection could be maintained.

B. INSECT PATHOGENIC CILIATES

Most reports of ciliates parasitizing insects concern the genus *Tetrahymena* (order Hymenostomatida; family Tetrahymenidae). Corliss (1960) reviewed the systematics and parasitism in the genus. The hosts are mainly mosquitoes and midges. Lichtenstein (1921) reported *Ophryoglena collini* destroying tissues, including the gonads, of larval *Baetis* sp. (Ephemeridae). Mercier and Poisson (1923) found *Colpoda* sp. in the hemipteran *Nepa cinerea.*

1. Pathogenesis and Epizootiology

Some tetrahymenid ciliates are free-living, but may also parasitize tissues and may have limited invasive ability, as distinct from other species histophagous in moribund, wounded or dead insects.

T. stegomyiae is the only species that invades through the mosquito cuticle. Muspratt (1945, 1947) found invasion of the host (tree-hole breeding culicine mosquitoes) by direct penetration of the cuticle from the cyst. Mosquito larvae became infected when placed in containers with the ciliates. The other species all enter by wounds, or possibly weak areas in the intersegmental membranes following molting as suggested by Corliss (1960) in the midge, *Chironomus plumosus,* fatally attacked by *T. chironomi.*

Once inside the host the ciliates multiply rapidly for two days or so, then reach a rather constant level, much like the standard growth curve in a culture medium. The host larvae live for some time, but few become pupae or adults. The ciliates are present in the hemocoel, visible as generally distributed "white spots", or aggregated in certain locations, e.g. the anal papillae (Corliss, 1961; Kellen *et al.*, 1961; Muspratt, 1945; Keilin, 1921; listed by Corliss, 1960).

Few ciliate infections have been found among samples collected from nature. Kellen *et al.* (1961) reported one of several hundred *Aedes sierrensis* larvae infected with a tetrahymenid. Corliss (1960) found *T. pyriformis* and *T. chironomi* in 0.0-11.8% of larvae in eight samples of the midge, *C. plumosus.* The incidence was greatest in larger larvae—43.2% of early instar III in one sample. *T. pyriformis* was never found alone but *T. chironomi* did occur alone in about half the larvae. The true incidence was probably greater than in the samples, since Corliss collected only the larger, healthiest larvae in the early samples. No epizootics have been reported as controlling a population.

2. Control Considerations

Ciliates have very similar characteristics as well as the small control potential of the flagellates, but with the additional attractions of usually killing the hosts and almost certainly of living free in natural aquatic habitats. Once seeded into a niche they may multiply by using available nutrients and Corliss (1961) suggested attempts to control certain tropical mosquitoes, which well deserve investigation.

Special mention should be made of *T. chironomi.* It undergoes a lethal conjugation in the host, and all exconjugants die. Corliss (1960) noted that when all the ciliates in an individual midge larva were *T. chironomi,* they all underwent conjugation with high mortality. Infection by a single ciliate, or lack of equal numbers of proper complementary mating types of normal conjugation, could cause the selfing effect. Selection of proper strains of the ciliate might prevent this.

C. INSECT PATHOGENIC AMEBAE

The best-known entomopathogenic ameba is perhaps *Malpighamoeba mellificae,* the honey-bee ameba. Also widely known is *Malamoeba locustae,* the grasshopper ameba. Other genera containing entomophilic amebae are *Malpighiella, Dobellina, Hartmanella, Amoeba, Entamoeba, Endamoeba,* and *Endolimax. Dobellina mesnili* attacks the winter gnat, *Trichocera hiemalis,* and in one instance 92% of gnats collected in January were infected whereas the disease had disappeared in May (Bishop and Tate, 1939; Keilin, 1917). *Naegleria* sp. was found in boll weevils, *Anthonomus grandis,* from winter hibernation sites in Louisiana (McLaughlin, unpublished) but no distinct pathology was confirmed. The most important ameba at present seems to be *M. locustae,* a serious pathogen of grasshoppers.

1. Pathogenesis and Epizootiology

After cysts of *M. locustae* are eaten, the cells of the Malpighian tubules and the gut become heavily infected. In severe cases, the cells may rupture, liberating the amebae into the hemocoel, where they may produce tumorous masses in fat body and muscles. The disease is generally debilitative and in *Locustana pardalina,* the brown locust, it limits sexual maturity. Infected *L. pardalina* failed to copulate or produce many eggs (Venter, 1966), and the proportion of diapausing eggs decreased (Prinsloo, 1961).

A natural epizootic of *M. locustae* in the brown locust was accredited with stopping a potential outbreak (Venter, 1966). Lea (1958), studying the causes of brown locust outbreaks, pointed out that low rainfall in the early summer favored locust build-ups, and that population fluctuations were most closely associated with weather conditions during the previous season; dry conditions were considered to be more harmful to natural enemies such as birds, predators and disease organisms than to locusts. Taylor and King (1937) increased the incidence of ameba disease in field populations of grasshoppers by distributing cysts in a bran and molasses bait. Henry (1968) reported *M. locustae* in several laboratory colonies of *Melanoplus* sp. and in *Schistocerca vaga vaga* from the wild in California and Montana. (See also King and Taylor, 1936; Taylor and King, 1937; Steinhaus and Marsh, 1962; Prinsloo, 1960; these involved some 40 species of grasshoppers.)

2. Control Considerations

M. locustae apparently infects *per os* quite easily. Many cysts are produced in each host, and spread by cannibalism or by eating food contaminated by feces. The effect on the host is severe though slow. Reductions in fecundity, numbers of diapausing eggs and possible prevention of aggregation and swarming are important.

Production of cysts may seem a problem, but they should lend themselves to culture *in vitro*. It may be practical to use cysts in baits and to release severely infected hoppers at strategic points during the optimum period for survival and dissemination of the pathogen.

D. INSECT PATHOGENIC COCCIDIA

The Sporozoa contain by far the largest number of entomophilic protozoans, as well as the most potentially useful. Coccidians in insects mostly belong to the family Adeleidae. The genus *Adelina* is known from a wide range of insects, with about 11 species, some in more than one host. *A. tribolii* infects *Tribolium castaneum, T. confusum* and possibly also *Tenebrio molitor* and *Trogoderma* sp. *A. sericesthis,* from a scarabaeid grub *Sericesthis geminata (pruinosa),* was also infective to *Aphodius howetti* and *Melolontha hippocastani* (Weiser and Beard, 1959; Weiser, 1963a). Very few studies have been made on host specificity.

1. Pathogenesis, Epizootiology and Control Possibilities

In storage insects, *Adelina* spp. attack the fat body and other coccidians the Malpighian tubes (*Legerella* spp.) or gut epithelium (*Chagasella* and *Ithania*). Infection occurs *per os* in all cases reported. Larvae tolerate infection and are often able to form fecund adults. The effect is that of devitalization and reduction of fecundity. The epizootic effects of *A. tribolii* in *T. confusum* can be striking–a cyclical heavy kill and gradual increase of the insect. Weiser (1959, 1963a) reported a high incidence of *A. sericesthis* among grubs in lawns in Canberra, Australia, and in over 30% of *M. hippocastani* grubs in Prague.

E. HAPLOSPORIDA AS INSECT PATHOGENS

Haplosporida are primarily known from freshwater invertebrates. Sprague (1963) revised the genus. Beaudoin and Wills (1968) reported *Haplosporidium simulii* from the blackfly, *Simulium venustum,* and Huger (1963) *H. tipulae* from the crane fly, *Tipula paludosa. H. typographi* from the bark beetle, *Ips typographus,* may have control potential. Weiser (1954a) studied its epizootiology and reported transmission by ingestion of contaminated feces, used by the female to plug the egg gallery. Hatching from contaminated eggs also infected larvae. Old bark beetle infestations may be heavily infected, but not new ones. Artificial dissemination of spores would seem the best approach to control. Again, this aims to circumvent the slow natural spread of the disease. Other methods will be discussed later, but the current interest in bark beetle pheromones suggests that the beetles might become infected at a bait station.

F. NEOGREGARINES AS INSECT PATHOGENS

In the subclass Gregarinia only the Neogregarinida have considerable pathogenicity and potential for control. Weiser (1955a, b) and Grassé (1953) reviewed infections in insects among 10 genera; Ashford (1965) has since reported *Lymphotropha tribolii* n.g., n. sp. from *Tribolium castaneum.* Other species include *Mattesia trogodermae* (Canning, 1964), from the khapra beetle, *Trogoderma granarium*; *M. grandis* (McLaughlin, 1965) from the boll weevil, *Anthonomus grandis*; unidentified neogregarines from the grasshoppers *Melanoplus bivittatus* and *M. bilituratus* (Bucher, 1966), and from the southern potato wireworm, *Conoderus falli* (Bell *et al.*, 1967); a new species of *Ophryocystis* from the monarch and Florida queen butterflies *(Danaus plexippus* and *D. gillipus berenice)* (McLaughlin and Myers, 1970); and a new species of *Mattesia* from the corn earworm, *Heliothis zea* (McLaughlin, Phillips and Yearian, unpublished). Neogregarines are undoubtedly widespread.

1. Pathology and Epizootiology

The neogregarines infect various host tissues. Infection usually occurs by eating spores. Loss of function of target tissues and organs as a result of schizogonic multiplication is the major cause of host illness. The protozoan life-cycle is usually rather long, requiring up to several weeks for sporulation. Some species act rapidly, killing larvae and reducing the life-span and fecundity of adults, in contrast to others that utilize less vital organs. For instance, the neogregarines in the monarch and Florida queen butterflies, and in *H. zea,* infect only the larval hypodermal tissue. Some larvae are killed, but adults, once emerged, are no longer harmed because all the spores are on the external hairs and scales.

The most damaging species can greatly reduce both laboratory colonies and field populations. In the laboratory, epizootics proceed slowly, reaching a peak and decimating the population. A few insects survive and the population remains at a low level, e.g. *M. dispora* in the Mediterranean flour moth, *Ephestia kuehniella* (Weiser, 1954b). Many species occur in cultures of stored-grain insects, and some in natural infestations. In experiments, *F. arinocystis tribolii* soon superseded *L. tribolii,* but all larvae died. Weiser (1963a) claimed that *Tribolium castaneum* is a less common flour beetle than *T. destructor* and *T. confusum* because *T. castaneum* is highly susceptible to *F. tribolii* while others are not. *M. dispora* attacks several hosts besides the original. *T. molitor,* including *Plodia interpunctella.* Most neogregarines infect several hosts, though the host list is not extensive. In laboratory tests *M. grandis* infected several lepidoptera (Ignoffo and Garcia, 1965) and a Hymenopteran (McLaughlin and Adams, 1966).

Infections in natural populations range from low incidences to epizootics. Bucher (1966) found a neogregarine in 10% of *M. bivittatus* and 15% of *M. bilituratus,* from a total of 427 hoppers collected in 1960. This high disease incidence was rare, and had not been observed since. Steinhaus and Marsh (1962) and Henry (unpublished) reported other infections. *Mattesia povolnyi* was found in the sunflower moth, *Homeosoma nebulellum,* by Weiser (1953a). He successfully established this disease over a wide area infested by one larva per 50 sunflower plants by release of infected moths, because moths surface-contaminated their eggs during oviposition. In another case, nearly all adult bollworms, *H. zea,* carried spores in a population that had failed to develop as it had previously every year for 15 years (Phillips and Yearian, unpublished).

2. Control Considerations

The neogregarines cause a slow, devitalizing disease requiring 1-6 or more weeks for full expression. Spread of intestinal infections usually depends upon local or general crowding. The sunflower moth readily spreads the disease by fecal contamination of eggs (Weiser, 1953a); the monarch and Florida queen butterflies, as well as the bollworm, do so by contaminated scales. Storage insects are good subjects for control attempts (p. 164).

G. MICROSPORIDA AS INSECT CONTROL AGENTS

Spores of the order Microsporida are unicellular in origin, and have a polar filament and sporoplasm. Infection occurs by emergence of the sporoplasm through the everted polar filament after the spore is taken into the gut of the host. Microsporida are very common in insects, and have the greatest reported range of host and tissue relationships among protozoans. This diversity will not be described in detail, but some specific cases will be considered to illustrate the opportunities, inadequacies and potentials for control.

The spore stage is of paramount interest in control. Spore life-span and resistance to environmental factors vary among species. Some, particularly those associated with mosquitoes, require special conditions for infection not provided by the host, such as preconditioning in preparation for germination in a host.

Kudo (1954) and Hall (1953) give excellent details of microsporidan taxonomy and host relationships. A monograph on Microsporida in insects

(Weiser, 1961), and a comprehensive listing (Thomson, 1960a), provide specific host-pathogen information, as do Weiser (1963a) and Tanada (1963).

1. Pathogenicity and Epizootiology

In their pathogenicity, the Microsporida are much like other protozoan pathogens but they outnumber them in species and so involve a wider range of host-pathogen relationships. They kill the host in a few days to many months after infection; all host stages may be infected, or only eggs and larvae may be killed with a few survivors maturing to adults and so transmitting the disease to further generations. Cases are known where only one sex is killed (p. 163). For convenience the target tissues may be classified into several groups. Some Microsporida infect the alimentary tract and Malpighian tubules; other adipose tissue, hemocytes or muscles; some germinal tissues; while some eventually infect all tissues in sequence. Death usually ensues, though preceded by other important effects—loss of vigor, different behavior, less mating and fewer eggs. Microsporida are transmitted to progeny more often than other protozoans, an important characteristic for control purposes. Other effects include reduced host-resistance to weather, insecticides, predation and parasitism.

2. Control Considerations

Specific systems in natural populations and attempts at control will be discussed in the next section. Some Microsporida are extremely host specific, others have a rather broad host spectrum. Unfortunately each species has only some of the desirable attributes listed above; some readily infect upon ingestion while others will not infect in the laboratory; some are transmitted only *per os* while others are passed on congenitally to nearly all progeny; the spores of some species have remained viable for three years, while the spores of others have died in a few weeks. Kramer is preparing a review of the longevity of microsporidan spores. Nevertheless, some species control insects without assistance by man. The Microsporida offer the greatest potential for control among protozoans because of the large number of species, the well-known instances of control, and the excellent attributes of several species.

IV. Assessment of Protozoans as Control Agents

Analysis of natural infections and attempts at control should permit analysis of the reasons for success or failure. We may then better understand how to employ protozoa, or at least to identify those areas of research most likely to prove fruitful.

A. NATURALLY-OCCURRING SYSTEMS

1. Glugea pyraustae *in the European Corn Borer,* Ostrinia nubilalis

This microsporidan was found in the European corn borer in the U.S.A. in the early 1950's. It is a protozoan causing consistent suppression of a crop pest without dramatic epizootics. Decker (1960) postulated that this disease was the most important factor maintaining corn borer populations at a level facilitating economic control by other means.

Decker (1960), Kramer (1959), Raun (unpublished), Van Denburgh and Burbutis (1962), York (1961), Zimmack *et al.* (1954) and Zimmack and Brindley (1957) provided the following information. Larvae and adults can become infected by ingestion of spores. Infection of early instars or ingestion of massive doses of spores by later instars prevents formation of adults. Infected larvae develop slower and are less able to infest the plant. Infection reduces infestation under stress conditions; hybrid corn lines resistant to borers were less attacked by diseased than by healthy larvae (Raun, unpublished). Diseased adults died sooner, mated less often and laid fewer eggs than did healthy ones on the resistant corn. Zimmack found, in two separate tests, that infected borers laid 47-48% fewer eggs and that over half of the egg masses carried infection. Kramer confirmed these results and found that infection was transmitted to progeny by contaminated egg surfaces as well as by schizonts within. Both Raun and Van Denburgh showed that frass from infected larvae contaminated others near by. Extensive surveys of corn borer populations in the midwestern states have shown a remarkable persistence of the disease. In the early 1950's, Decker successfully established the disease in all counties of Illinois by distribution of infected female moths. The records of Raun, Van Denburgh and Zimmack revealed the disease in almost all sampled areas and a definite decline of the number of borers–sometimes to very low levels. Surveys in all Illinois counties show great fluctuation in disease incidence (Illinois State Natural History Survey staff, unpublished), though the disease persists.

The host-pathogen relationships that bear on epidemiology are primarily: (1) effective transmission and spread of the pathogen trans-ovum, congenitally, and from larva to larva; (2) reduction of the number of larvae able to infest plants or to become adults; and (3) reduced vitality and fecundity of the adults. On the other hand, infection of parasites may have been an adverse factor. Although analysis of these factors suggests that the disease should decrease in a population (because parents infect only half of the progeny, and diseased larvae succumb to stress conditions at a greater rate than healthy larvae), in practice, the disease increases to 85% or more of the population in some cases. Cross-contamination of larvae feeding near infected larvae, close deposition of egg masses, and other density-related factors no doubt assist this increase.

The effect of *G. pyraustae* might be increased in several ways. First, Decker's success in establishing the disease in a corn borer population suggests that further increase of disease is possible. Raun placed spores in the leaf axils and so infected instar 1, which almost completely prevented infestation. Control might be improved by assisting the pathogen during certain critical periods. Adequate surveys showing little disease in a rather high borer population would suggest that further introduction of disease would be valuable. Application of spores to leaf axils to coincide with the hatch of the first new generation, release of infected female moths, and use of borer resistant corn lines might be valuable.

2. Glugea fumiferanae *in the Spruce Budworm,* Choristoneura fumiferana

This is another excellent example of a protozoan persisting in, and controlling, a host population. Thomson (1958, 1960b) and Morris (1963) documented the natural occurrence of the disease in Ontario, Canada. This microsporidan is perhaps even more closely associated with the habits of its host than is that of the European corn borer.

Larvae become infected from their parents or by eating spores. Those infected via their parents do not mature, but their frass and broken cadavers are rich inocula in the feeding galleries of active late IV and early V instar larvae. These produce infected adults. All infected females and some males transmit the pathogen to their progeny. Adults may also become infected by eating spores. Increase of disease in the population is normally by ingestion of spores but congenital transmission perpetuates the disease. The spring environment of instar II larvae emerging from the hibernaculum is almost devoid of spores, but infected larvae begin to spread the spores in frass. The young larvae are usually isolated, but older ones move to new feeding sites almost daily and so have a better chance to acquire spores from frass and cadavers. The disease in studied populations increased in incidence from 1955 to 1958, i.e. 36.5%, 43.6%, 56.1% to nearly 80%. The ultimate collapse of the population was attributed to the depressing effect of the protozoan.

Again, as with the corn borer, the protozoan readily persisted and spread. The studies on spruce budworm populations are excellent examples of the type of information needed to understand a biologically controllable system. Methods could perhaps be devised to optimize the spread of the pathogen to produce the desired effect—a spruce budworm population stabilized at an acceptably low level, with restraining factors curbing infestations above a selected level. Dissemination of infected instar II larvae early in the spring, release of infected moths late in the year into areas deficient in disease, spraying spores in a suitable formulation, or even release of infected males so as to outnumber healthy males and thus induce disease might be considered.

3. Microsporida in Other Lepidotera

Several other Lepidoptera are controlled, to some extent, by protozoans. Epizootiological data are sparse, thus precluding meaningful analysis. Certainly, the protozoans do exert a suppressant effect and the need for detailed study becomes increasingly acute. *G. mesnili* infected the European cabbage worm, *Pieris brassicae,* in scattered locations (Paillot, 1918) and was widespread in the imported cabbage worm, *P. rapae,* in Hawaii (Tanada, 1955). At two locations 58.6% of the larvae were infected by *G. mesnili,* and an additional 22.1% by both *G. mesnili* and a braconid parasite.

Two virus diseases, a microsporidan and combined infections were diagnosed in an epizootic in the armyworm, *Pseudaletia unipuncta,* in Hawaii (Tanada and Chang, 1962). The incidence of microsporidan infections alone was 25.5% and of a virus and microsporidan 29.1%, so that 54.6% of the individuals were infected with the microsporidan. The protozoan had not been observed in the previous four years. Later (1964) Tanada found 23% with the protozoan alone, 2.4% with both and less than 1% with only virus in field populations in Hawaii. Kramer (1965a) described two microsporida, *Nosema necatrix* and *Thelohania diazoma,* from this insect and reported that infected larvae ate normally for 3-4 days, ceased feeding in the next 1-2 and died by the 5th-7th. Maddox (1966) reported these diseases in Illinois. In an outbreak of armyworm in August 1964, 64% of 346 larvae had the disease, but in a sparse population only 1% of 51 in June 1965. Both outbreaks of armyworm studied by Maddox and Tanada were unseasonal.

4. Nosema melolonthae *in the Common Cockchafer,* Melolontha melolontha

An epizootic of this disease was observed by Hurpin and Vago (1958) and Hurpin (1965). A different ecological system is involved because the grubs live in meadow soil. A five-year study of the grub population in a meadow revealed that the disease rose in three years from 2.5% to an average of 20%, with 50-60% occurring in some samples. The infection spread in "oil-stain" fashion from a few inoculated plots (4 x 4 m) until nearly the entire 12.5 acres contained infected grubs. The *Nosema* persisted for 10 months, from September 1961 when most of the grubs had died, until July 1962 when a new series of eggs hatched. Hurpin concluded that spores persisted in the soil and that trans-ovum transmission did not account for the persistence of infection.

The microsporidan epizootic in a soil insect is an excellent example of the potential control value of a protozoan in an environment that could be highly protective to the spore, and in which larger numbers of the pest may be tolerated than is usual in a food crop. The success of the milky disease organism, *Bacillus popilliae,* against Japanese beetle grubs, *Popillia japonica,* should stimulate hope for such a control method. Release of infected adults or grubs might be acceptable method of spore dissemination, since the adults would be more likely than man to find grub populations and the ability of the disease to spread obviates the need for even distribution.

5. Octosporea muscaedomesticae *in Muscoid Flies*

Kramer's excellent investigations reveal that this microsporidan may be an important limiting biotic factor for a number of hosts. Kramer (1964) listed at least five species of muscoid flies infected in nature: *Phormia regina*, *Cochliomyia macellaria*, *Pollinia rudis*, *Musca domestica* and *Phaenicia sericata*. Spores from wild individuals of each species infected all the other species as well as *Drosophila melanogaster*. In detailed studies on *P. regina* Kramer found the following key features: the spore-to-spore development time may be as short as three days (1965b); the activity of adult flies is normal up to two weeks after infection but then declines (1965c); the fly dies after the proximal gut epithelium has been reduced to a shapeless pathogen-filled mass (1966); longevity of flies is halved by disease; fall-infected flies probably carry the pathogen through the winter and viable spores were found in fecal spots 120 days after deposition (1967), overwintering of the disease is thus assured; the flies are very mobile disseminators of spores. Most impressively a female adult that ingests spores in her first post-eclosion meal does not lay eggs! The disease affects larvae severely, since those infected in instars I or II never become adults. The variety of hosts and their varied bionomics lend stability to the system and host populations normally need not be drastically reduced in a short time. Kramer (1968) surveyed Illinois field populations of *P. regina* in 1963 and 1964 and found up to 13% infection, which included mainly flies infected less than two weeks because older, infected flies are less mobile and might not find the trap.

6. Microsporidan Pathogens of Mosquitoes and Other Aquatic Diptera

The aquatic habitat, biology of host mosquitoes and their Microsporida are quite different from the types discussed so far. These are unique host relationships and induction of experimental infections is extremely difficult. Species of floodwater mosquitoes pose the problem of protozoan persistence during periods of drought (often quite prolonged) when the mosquito eggs provide the only protected survival niche. Multi- and univoltine mosquitoes each present different situations for persistence, dissemination, infection and multiplication of the pathogen. Despite the difficulties of studying fluctuating host populations, unstable communities and the intricate associations between the protozoan and host, some investigations have revealed potentially useful pathogens.

Kellen *et al.* (1965) categorized the relationships between mosquitoes and Microsporida of the genus *Thelohania* into four types. Transovarial infections were found in each type, though not universally. In type I, males died and sporogony occurred, but females transmitted the pathogen transovarially without sporogony; II, sporogony in both sexes but progressive infections occurred mostly among males; III, disease usually fatal with sporogony in both sexes and some females surviving to pass on the disease; and IV, sporogony in both sexes but disease usually benign. In nature up to 80% of larvae of *Culiseta incidens* were infected with *Thelohania* (Kellen, 1963). Kellen *et al.* (1966)

concluded that type III relationships result in death of transovarially infected larvae before pupation. The disease could therefore be expected to die out in one generation as it requires reinfection of larvae. Type I is potentially useful because infected males die, while females transmit the disease, so that management to increase the disease among larvae might create a sexual imbalance to the detriment of the host. The need for detailed study of the host-pathogen bionomics is again sharply apparent.

Infections via spore ingestion have been difficult to produce, indicating a period of "conditioning" of the spore for infection. Often, attempts at laboratory infections have failed or have been difficult to reproduce. Kellen *et al.* (1965) concluded (1) that spores play a minor role in the overwintering of *Thelohania* in certain univoltine mosquito species, infected females being most important, (2) transovarial infection of larvae is lethal, infection of adults by spore ingestion must occur if disease is to be maintained in the population; and (3) those *Thelohania* which are primarily dependent upon peroral transmission have the best chance for a continuous host-parasite association in multivoltine hosts.

Microsporida no doubt play an important role in the regulation of aquatic insect populations. In addition to the mosquitoes, Chironomidae (midges), Simuliidae (black flies) and Chaoboridae (gnats) are infected by Microsporida. Weiser (1961) reported 16 microsporidan species from midges. An example of the potential value of such infections is the annihilation of midges in three semi-permanent ponds three weeks after initial detection of diseased larvae (Hunter, 1968). Sikorowski and Madison (1968) reported on the seasonal occurrence of *T. corethrae* in the Clear Lake gnat, *Chaoborus astictopus.* The incidence was highest in early spring among overwintered larvae, reaching 9.9% in one sample and declining to less than 1% in the summer generations. Hilsenhoff and Lovett (1966) reported *Thelohania* sp. in a Chironomid in Lake Winnebago, Wisconsin. Disease was commonest in the fall but declined during the spring and summer when the insect was breeding. Incidence ranged from 0.9% to 9.5%. Mortality was greatest in instar IV, and no viable adults matured from infected larvae, confirming the report of Weiser (1963b). Early instars were readily infected in laboratory tests, and transovarian transmission was a negligible factor in disease spread. Thus, in these relationships, the management of disease must depend upon maintaining contaminated larval habitats when each generation of young larvae is present.

7. Protozoan Pathogens of Stored Products Insects

Stored products provide a unique habitat. The insect's food is evenly distributed within definite boundaries, usually those of the storage container. The insects often populate small foci which gradually expand. The pathogen's substrate is thus initially localized but dense. Consequently, in undisturbed materials, the natural course of disease eventually produces an epizootic, but only after extensive insect damage to the product. Initially, only a few insects are affected and so the pathogen is absent from most foci. If the host does not move between foci the pathogen will not spread. Thus, stored products present a prime opportunity to use protozoans—as a pre-infestation prophylactic—by distributing infective quantities of the pathogen. It may be too great a task to treat successive loads of materials in storage, but national food reserves in long-term storage might offer opportunities. Many of the obstacles to pathogen distribution in other biotopes are absent or minimal. Thorough studies of carefully selected combinations of pathogens are needed to establish parameters by proper records of physical conditions and insect populations. Reduction of primary invaders from residual populations would not only lessen the chances of their causing bulk food to heat and so create a better environment for themselves, but would also lessen the attack of secondary pests normally unable to breed rapidly in sound grain. Protozoans are promising in this field of control.

Natural infections are usually sparse but occasionally may become epizootics. Laboratory colonies have been destroyed or greatly reduced. Storage insects have an impressive variety of protozoan pathogens, including coccidia, neogregarines and microsporida, as follows. The Indian meal moth, *Plodia interpunctella,* is attacked by *Adelina mesnili* (Steinhaus, 1947), *Mattesia dispora* (Musgrave and Mackinnon, 1938), *M. grandis* (McLaughlin, 1965), *Glugea* sp. and *Nosema plodiae* (Kellen and Lindegren, 1968), and *Nosema* sp. (Steinhaus and Marsh, 1962); the Mediterranean flour moth, *Ephestia kuehniella,* by *M. dispora* (Naville, 1930), *A. mesnili* (Steinhaus, 1947), *Thelohania ephestiae* (Mattes, 1928), and *M. grandis* (McLaughlin, 1965); the mealworm, *Tenebrio molitor* by *A. tribolii* (Bhatia, 1937), *Ophryocystis mesnili* (Leger, 1907), *Farinocystis tribolii* (Huger, 1967), *Sporomyxa tenebrionis* (Rietschel, 1935) and the same or a similar organism (Huger, 1967); the flour beetle, *Tribolium castaneum* by *A. tribolii* (Bhatia, 1937), *F. tribolii* (Weiser, 1953b), *Lymphotropha tribolii* (Ashford, 1965), *Nosema* sp. (Thomson, 1960a) and *Nosema oryzaephili* (Burges, 1971). Other flour beetles may be infected by some of the same pathogens: *T. confusum* by *A. tribolii, F. tribolii* and a *Nosema* (Thomson, 1960a); *T. destructor* and *T. madens* by *F. tribolii* (Weiser, 1953b; Tyler, 1962). The khapra beetle, *Trogoderma granarium* is attacked by *M. trogodermae* (Canning, 1964) and *Ophryocystis* sp. (Steinhaus and Marsh, 1962). The latter report also included this protozoan in *T. inclusum, simplex* and *parabile. M. dispora* (or possibly *M. trogodermae*) occurred in *T. glabrum* and *inclusum* (Burkholder and Dicke, 1964), and *A. tribolii* in *Trogoderma* sp. (Bhatia, 1937). Seven species of storage beetle, and three of moth, are infected by *Nosema oryzaephili* (Burges *et al.,* 1971).

Pathogens infective in several species differ in pathogenicity and virulence from host to host (p. 158). A dual infection in a single host may result in eventual dominance of one pathogen. Some hosts yield greater numbers of spores, while the pathogens have varying effects on longevity of hosts.

B. ATTEMPTS TO USE PROTOZOANS AS CONTROL AGENTS

1. Control of Lepidopteran Pests of Fruit Trees by Spore Application

Attempts to manipulate the protozoan-host system or to use protozoans as "microbial insecticides" are few. Weiser and his coworkers have conducted experiments on lepidopteran pests in the crowns of fruit trees in Europe. This biotope contains a group of insects that feed on numerous host trees and in turn are susceptible to several microsporida. Weiser (1957) described the cross-infectivity of microsporida to several pest insects. Weiser and Veber (1957) summarized their previous work and described attempts at control by spraying spore suspensions. These accounts are assessed as follows.

The fall webworm, *Hyphantria cunea,* was a new introduction into a region already inhabited by a number of other lepidopteran pests of fruit trees. It acquired *Thelohania hyphantriae* probably from the moth *Nygmia phaeorrhoea, Malacosoma neustria,* or *Hyponomeuta malinellus.* This microsporidan did not infect *Lymantria dispar, Aporia crataegi, Bombyx mori, Eriogaster lanestris* or *Leucoma (Stilpnotia) salicis.* A series of treatments in which small infestations of *H. cunea* were sprayed with spores controlled damage and caused very high mortality. In further tests in a region very highly populated with *H. cunea,* a relatively small number of the nests were sprayed. Infections spread slowly and, although the sprayed nests suffered from the disease, the total pest population was neither infected nor controlled.

The host-pathogen relationships in this complex biotope explain these successes and failures. Infection occurs only *per os* but spores are not shed in feces. *H. cunea* larvae die rapidly in five days, mostly from septicemia, but a few pupate or, rarely, form adults. The other hosts are similarly affected but after five days do not feed and live for a month or so. The later in larval life the infection occurs, the further the host develops. Host biology plays a major role in the system. *H. cunea* and *M. neustria* overwinter as pupae. Normal winter mortality is high and as survival of infected pupae is negligible, the disease is removed from the biotope. However, *M. neustria,* when also infected by a nuclear polyhedrosis in summer, distributes spores effectively by its wet, disintegrating cadavers. *N. phaeorrhoea* carries the disease through the winter. It overwinters in instar I, and when infected by spraying egg masses, the disease was maintained until spring. Unfortunately, the infected larvae were selectively preyed upon and birds removed the microsporidan from the environment. This contrasts with the spruce budworm controlled by *Glugea fumiferanae.* Weiser and Veber concluded that direct spraying of the larval nests of the three species was an effective control measure but the slow spread and disappearance of the disease prevented long-term control. Repeated applications, or thorough coverage of all nests, are required.

In further work along these lines, Weiser (personal communication) reported negative results using *Plistophora schubergi* against *Euproctis chrysorrhoea* and fair results using *Nosema serbica* against instar I of *L. dispar* and *P. schubergi* against instar I of *L. dispar* before hibernation. Failures were due to removal of the pathogen by rain and inactivation by sunlight. Generally, infections disappear after hosts die and fall to the ground so that transmission in eggs is a more consistent method of maintaining the disease in a population.

2. Use of Protozoans in Feeding-baits to Control the Boll Weevil, Anthonomus grandis

Effective spread of the pathogen throughout the entire host substrate is a vital requirement for pest control by a protozoan. A suitable method has been developed in *A. grandis.* McLaughlin (1966) first demonstrated the effective use of a bait containing a feeding stimulant and the protozoan. Subsequently, better feeding stimulants and formulations improved the effectiveness, progressing from cages to season-long open field tests (Daum *et al.*, 1967; McLaughlin, 1967; McLaughlin *et al.*, 1968; McLaughlin *et al.*, 1969). The adult feeds within the cotton plant fruit, so even complete spray coverage could not induce infection. In contrast, use of the feeding stimulant in large, viscous drops of bait was extremely effective in the spring against overwintered adults and again in the fall against weevils entering diapause in preparation for overwintering. At these times 50-70% infection was frequently attained, and sometimes 80-98% in the fall in open field tests. Weevil populations were suppressed during the spring and late fall and, in one test, disease in the overwintering population reduced the surviving population next spring. Average winter mortality for the area was 84% but in the treated area it was 96%. Mid-season failure may be due to a difference in behavior of the weevils or inadequate bait strength, and improvement of the bait may help. The initial weevil populations in these tests were very large, providing extensive data but precluding control.

The important factor I wish to emphasize here is the principle of using response–eliciting baits to induce infection in a population. Present emphasis on insect pheromone research is providing materials which may open the door to the use of many insect pathogens previously regarded as laboratory curiosities because they could not be introduced into a target insect population. Now the habits of the host itself may be harnessed to infect, carry and spread disease throughout the entire population. Small quantities of a pathogen may be sufficient if concentrated and protected at a few bait stations visited by the insects which spread the disease. Various responses may be used besides that of feeding, e.g. copulatory to contaminate egg masses, or mere contact with the pathogen to spread it to natural feeding surfaces. The possibilities are great, and research on each specific host-pathogen system may reveal different methods of using the same principle.

V. Research Needed for Use of Protozoans as Control Agents

Perhaps the hardest practical problem requiring solution is that of infecting a sufficient proportion of the population. *Thorough studies are needed on distribution by contamination of food, parasites and predators, parent to progeny, use of attractive materials, and release of carrier insects.* A selection of systems that appear most promising for control is given in Table I.

TABLE I

A list of protozoans considered to be the most promising research candidates for use in control of their insect hosts

Protozoan	Insect host(s)
Adelina tribolii, Farinocystis tribolii and others selected for pests in the total complex	Stored product pest complex
Malamoeba locustae	Suitable grasshopper species
Thelohania hyphantriae	*Hyphantria cunea* and associated susceptible species
Nosema melolonthae	*Melolontha melolontha*
Glugea pyraustae	*Ostrinia nubilalis*
Glugea gasti	*Anthonomus grandis*
Mattesia povolnyi	*Homeosoma nebulellum*
Haplosporidium typographi	*Ips typographus*
Octosporea muscaedomesticae	Muscoid flies
Tetrahymena pyriformis, and *T. stegomyiae,* possibly also *T. chironomi*	Aquatic insects, probably mosquitoes, Chironomids

Another major problem is persistence of the protozoan in the environment, mostly involving protection of infective quantities of spores in the proper sites. Suitable formulations should be available among the vast array of protectants against drying, wetting, ultra-violet light, washing, etc. available to the chemical industry today. Just as chemical insecticides are carefully formulated to foster their activity for specific usages, equal attention, if not more, should be given to a living organism if it is to survive.

More critical assessment procedures must be established, because infections characteristically tend to be underestimated. Observations on the incidence and course of disease are difficult. Diseased insects are often not caught in samples designed to obtain healthy insects; dead and moribund insects may be quickly scavenged from the niche; diagnosis may be difficult because saprophytic bacteria or fungi often obscure the picture; another pathogen (such as a virus) may be present and the microsporidan remain undetected because few spores are produced. Disease incidence and epizootics may, therefore, exceed their apparent significance.

Research is needed to determine what levels of infection are required to cause a desired suppression. For instance, Smirnoff (1966) reported a decrease in numbers of the larch sawfly, *Pristiphora erichsonii,* when the incidence of infection increased to 25% from less than 5% over three years. Distribution of the pathogen throughout the host population may not be required. There are more subtle effects than death—the avirulent organism may be more useful than the highly virulent one (p. 152) because it lowers biotic potential (Veber and Jasic, 1961). This is probably the major reason for the slow decline in insect numbers as disease incidence increases.

The role of protozoans in integrated control must be studied. Control need not depend on a protozoan alone, rather the whole arsenal of controlling factors should be used. The insect may be weakened by protozoans, then thwarted by resistance of the plant to insect attack, or killed by low insecticide doses or even by another disease lethal to the infected pest but harmless to the beneficial parasites or predators. Protozoan infections often occur with viral, fungal and bacterial infections, some in synergism, a pathogen being able to infect only a host weakened by another disease.

Research is needed on the host range of candidate protozoans: all possible agents should be screened for effectiveness against the target insect. I know of no program to screen protozoans against a series of insect species comparable to that used by insecticide companies for chemicals. Surely such effort would discover protozoans pathogenic to unrecognized hosts, and identify some with potential as control agents. Already a number of microsporida, neogregarines and coccidia are known to infect several hosts, which could lead to a stable disease complex (p. 152). Screening programs should be supplemented by research on selection and mutation of protozoan pathogens.

VI. Conclusions

Protozoans are most likely to be useful in insect control as introductions of low virulence, mostly unspectacular, some exerting major control and others reducing populations to levels that permit economic control by other means. A measurable degree of microbial control by protozoans, both natural and at the hand of man, has been described in seven insect species. In some of these, and in others where host mortality appears low, control could be greater than that revealed by usual sampling techniques, because these methods tend to miss diseased insects. An analysis of examples showed that by far the most important factors in successful control were transmission of disease (directly from parent to offspring in some cases, and persistence of spores in others), resulting in infection of a sufficient proportion of the population for decimation by disease to counteract the host's ability to increase. The relatively slow action of the disease was beneficial, for, besides death of the host, the disease has other important effects, such as reduction in fecundity. The use of attractive spore baits is extremely promising. Protozoans offer a wide range of species that await trial.

Biology today is a dynamic field, and the use of protozoans for control of insects should be boldly approached, learning from past failures and advancing to further successes.

References

Ashford, R. W. (1965). *J. Protozool.* **12,** 609-615.

Beaudoin, R. L. and Wills, W. (1968). *J. Invertebrate Path.* **10,** 374-378.

Bell, J. V., Day, A. and Hamalle, R. J. (1967). *J. Invertebrate Path.* **9,** 567.

Bhatia, M. L. (1937). *Parasitol.* **29,** 239-246.

Bishop, A. and Tate, P. (1939). *Parasitol.* **31,** 501-510.

Bucher, G. E. (1966). *J. Invertebrate Path.* **8,** 127-129.

Burges, H. D., Canning, E. U. and Hurst, J. A. (1971). *J. Invertebrate Path.* (In press).

Burkholder, W. E. and Dicke, R. J. (1964). *J. econ. Ent.* **57,** 818-819.

Canning, E. U. (1964). *J. Insect Path.* **6,** 305-317.

Corliss, J. O. (1960). *Parasitol.* **50,** 111-153.

Corliss, J. O. (1961). *Trans. R. Soc. trop. Med. Hyg. Lond.* **55,** 149-152.

Daum, R. J., McLaughlin, R. E. and Hardee, D. D. (1967). *J. econ. Ent.* **60,** 321-325.

Decker, G. C. (1960). *Agric. Chemicals* **30-33,** 93.

Grassé, P. P. (ed.) (1953). "Traité de Zoologie, Anatomie, Systématique Biologie". 1,(fasc. 1,2). Masson et Cie, Paris.

Guttman, H. N. and Wallace, F. G. (1964). *In* "Biochemistry and Physiology of the Protozoa" (S. Hutner, ed.), Vol. 3, pp. 459-474. Academic Press, New York.

Hall, I. M. (1963). *In* "Insect Pathology–An Advanced Treatise" (E. A. Steinhaus, ed.), Vol. 2, pp. 477-517. Academic Press, New York.

Hall, R. P. (1953). "Protozoology". Prentice-Hall, New York.

Henry, J. E. (1968). *J. Invertebrate Path.* **11,** 224-233.

Hilsenhoff, W. and Lovett, O. L. (1966). *J. Invertebrate Path.* **8,** 512-519.

Honigberg, B. M., Balamuth, W., Bovee, E. C., Corliss, J. O., Gojdics, M., Hall, R. P., Kudo, R. R., Levine, N. D., Loeblich, A. R., Jr., Weiser, J. and Wenrich, D. H. (1964). *J. Protozool.* **11,** 7-20.

Huger, A. M. (1963). *In* "Progress in Protozoology". Proc. 1st Int. Congr. Protozool., Prague, 1961, pp. 506-509. Academic Press, New York.

Huger, A. M. (1967). *J. Invertebrate Path.* **9,** 572-574.

Hunter, D. K. (1968). *J. Invertebrate Path.* **10,** 387-389.

Hurpin, B. (1965). *J. Invertebrate Path.* **7,** 39-44.

Hurpin, B. and Vago, C. (1958). *Entomophaga* **3,** 285-330.

Ignoffo, C. M. and Garcia, C. (1965). *J. Invertebrate Path.* **7,** 260-262.

Jahn, T. L. and Jahn, F. F. (1949). "How to Know the Protozoa". Brown, Dubuque, Iowa.

Keilin, D. (1917). *C.r. Séanc. Soc. Biol.* **80,** 133-136.

Keilin, D. (1921). *Parasitol.* **13,** 216-224.

Kellen, W. R. (1963). *Proc. and Papers, 31. Ann. Conf. Calif. Mosquito Control Ass.,* pp. 23-25.

Kellen, W. R., Chapman, H. C., Clark, T. B. and Lindegren, J. E. (1965). *J. Invertebrate Path.* **7,** 161-166.

Kellen, W. R., Chapman, H. C., Clark, T. B. and Lindegren, J. E. (1966). *J. Invertebrate Path.* **8**, 355-359.
Kellen, W. R. and Lindegren, J. E. (1968). *J. Invertebrate Path.* **11**, 104-111.
Kellen, W. R., Wills, W. and Lindegren, J. E. (1961). *J. Insect Path.* **3**, 335-338.
King, R. L. and Taylor, A. B. (1936). *Trans. Am. microsc. Soc.* **55**, 6-10.
Kramer, J. P. (1959). *J. Insect Path.* **1**, 25-33.
Kramer, J. P. (1963). *In* "Insect Pathology–An Advanced Treatise" (E. A. Steinhaus, ed.), Vol. 1, pp. 251-272. Academic Press, New York.
Kramer, J. P. (1964). *J. Insect Path.* **6**, 331-342.
Kramer, J. P. (1965a). *J. Invertebrate Path.* **7**, 117-121.
Kramer, J. P. (1965b). *Z. f. Parasitenk.* **25**, 309-313.
Kramer, J. P. (1965c). *Entomophaga* **10**, 339-342.
Kramer, J. P. (1966). *Am. Midland Naturalist* **75**, 214-220.
Kramer, J. P. (1967). U.S.-Jap. Commit. Sci. Coop., Panel 8, Res. Pesticides, Fukuoka, p. 48.
Kramer, J. P. (1968). *Z. f. Parasitenk.* **30**, 33-39.
Kudo, R. R. (1954). "Protozoology". 4th ed. Thomas, Springfield, Illinois.
Lea, A. (1958). *J. ent. Soc. S. Africa* **21**, 162-213.
Leger, L. (1907). *Arch. Protistenk.* **8**, 159-202.
Lichtenstein, J. L. (1921). *C.r. Séanc. Soc. Biol.* **85**, 794-796.
Lipa, J. J. (1963). *In* "Insect Pathology–An Advanced Treatise" (E. A. Steinhaus, ed.), Vol. 2, pp. 335-361. Academic Press, New York.
Lipa, J. J. (1966). *Acta Protozool.. Warszawa* **4**, 19-23.
Maddox, J. V., Jr. (1966). Ph.D. Thesis, Dep. Ent., Univ. Illinois, Urbana, Illinois.
Mattes, O. (1928). *Zeit. wiss. Zool.* **132**, 526-582.
McLaughlin, R. E. (1965). *J. Protozool.* **12**, 405-413.
McLaughlin, R. E. (1966). *J. econ. Ent.* **59**, 909-910.
McLaughlin, R. E. (1967). *J. Invertebrate Path.* **9**, 70-77.
McLaughlin, R. E. and Adams, C. H. (1966). *Ann. ent. Soc. Am.* **59**, 800-802.
McLaughlin, R. E., Cleveland, T. C., Daum, R. J. and Bell, M. R. (1969). *J. Invertebrate Path.* **13**, 429-441.
McLaughlin, R. E., Daum, R. J. and Bell, M. R. (1968). *J. Invertebrate Path.* **12**, 168-174.
McLaughlin, R. E. and Myers, J. (1970). *J. Protozool.* **17**, 300-305.
Mercier, L. and Poisson, R. (1923). *C.r. hebd. Séanc. Acad. Sci. Paris* **176**, 1838-1841.
Morris, R. F. (ed.) (1963). "The Dynamics of Epidemic Spruce Budworm Populations". *Mem. ent. Soc. Can.* No. 31, 332 pp.
Musgrave, A. J. and Mackinnon, D. L. (1938). *Proc. R. ent. Soc., Lond.* (A). **13**, 89-90.
Muspratt, J. (1945). *J. ent. Soc. S. Africa* **8**, 13-20.
Muspratt, J. (1947). *Parasitol.* **38**, 107-110.
Naville, A. (1930). *Z. Zellforsch. mikrosk. Anat.* **11**, 375-396.
Paillot, A. (1918). *C.r. Séanc. Soc. Biol.* **81**, 66-68.
Pearse, A. S. (ed.) (1936). "Zoological Names. A List of Phyla, Classes and Orders". Duke University Press. Durham, N.C.
Prinsloo, H. E. (1960). *Suid-Afrik. Tydskr. Landbouwetensk.* **3**, 551-560.
Prinsloo, H. E. (1961). *Suid-Afrik. Tydskr. Landbouwetensk.* **4**, 225-230.
Rietschel, P. (1935). *Arch. Protistenk.* **86**, 349-358.
Sikorowski, P. and Madison, C. H. (1968). *J. Invertebrate Path.* **11**, 390-397.
Smirnoff, W. A. (1966). *J. Invertebrate Path.* **8**, 360-364.
Sprague, V. (1963). *J. Protozool.* **10**, 263-266.
Steinhaus, E. A. (1947). *J. Parasitol.* **33**, 29-32.
Steinhaus, E. A. and Marsh, G. A. (1962). *Hilgardia* **33**, 349-490.
Tanada, Y. (1955). *Proc. Hawaiian ent. Soc.* **15**, 609-616.
Tanada, Y. (1959). *Ann. Rev. Ent.* **4**, 277-302.
Tanada, Y. (1963). *In* "Insect Pathology–An Advanced Treatise" (E. A. Steinhaus, ed.), Vol. 2, pp. 423-475. Academic Press, New York.
Tanada, Y. (1964). *Proc. Hawaiian ent. Soc.* **18**, 435-436.
Tanada, Y. and Chang, G. Y. (1962). *J. Insect Path.* **4**, 129-131.

Taylor, A. B. and King, R. L. (1937). *Trans. Am. microsc. Soc.* **56**, 172-176.
Thomson, H. M. (1958). *Can. J. Zool.* **36**, 309-316.
Thomson, H. M. (1960a). *J. Insect Path.* **2**, 346-385.
Thompson, H. M. (1960b). Bi-monthly Prog. Rep. Can. Dep. Agric., Res. Branch, Forest Biol. Div. 16, No. 1.
Tuzet, O. and Laporte, M. (1965). *Arch. Zool. exp. gén. Paris* **105**, 77-81.
Tyler, P. S. (1962). *J. Insect Path.* **4**, 270-272.
Van Denburgh, R. A. and Burbutis, P. O. (1962). *J. econ. Ent.* **55**, 65-67.
Veber, J. and Jasic, J. (1961). *J. Insect Path.* **3**, 103-111.
Venter, I. G. (1966). *South African J. Agric. Sci.* **9**, 429-433.
Wallace, F. G. (1966). *Exp. Parasitol.* **18**, 124-193.
Wallace, F. G. and Clark, T. B. (1959). *J. Protozool.* **6**, 40-42.
Wallace, F. G. and Johnson, A. (1961). *J. Insect Path.* **3**, 75-80.
Weiser, J. (1953a). *Zool. ent. Listy* **1**, 252-264.
Weiser, J. (1953b). *Věst. čsl. zool. Spol.* **17**, 199-211.
Weiser, J. (1954a). *Acta Soc. zool. čechoslov.* **18**, 217-224.
Weiser, J. (1954b). *Arch. Protistenk.* **100**, 127-142.
Weiser, J. (1955a). *J. Protozool.* **2**, 6-12.
Weiser, J. (1955b). *J. Protozool.* **2**, 88.
Weiser, J. (1957). *Z. angew. Ent.* **40**, 509-521.
Weiser, J. (1961). "Die Mikrosporidien als Parasiten der Insekten". *Monograph. Angew. Ent.* **17**, 149 pp.
Weiser, J. (1963a). *In* "Insect Pathology–An Advanced Treatise" (E. A. Steinhaus, ed.), Vol. 2, pp. 291-334. Academic Press, New York.
Weiser, J. (1963b). *Zool. Anz.* **170**, 226-230.
Weiser, J. and Beard, R. L. (1959). *J. Insect Path.* **1**, 99-106.
Weiser, J. and Veber, J. (1957). *Z. angew. Ent.* **40**, 55-70.
York, G. T. (1961). *J. Insect Path.* **3**, 101-102.
Zimmack, H. L., Arbuthnot, K. D. and Brindley, T. A. (1954). *J. econ. Ent.* **47**, 641-645.
Zimmack, H. L. and Brindley, T. A. (1957). *J. econ. Ent.* **50**, 637-640.
Zotta, G. (1921). *C.r. Séanc. Soc. Biol.* **85**, 135-137.

CHAPTER 7

Possible Use of Rickettsiae for Microbial Control of Insects[1]

ALOYSIUS KRIEG

Biologische Bundesanstalt für Land- und Forstwirtschaft,
Institut für biologische Schädlingsbekämpfung, Darmstadt, Germany

I. Advances in the Microbiology of Rickettsiae

Rickettsiae represent a group of micro-organisms which, like viruses, are known to be obligate pathogens, though they also have many features characteristic of bacteria. Rickettsiae have cellular structure, contain both types of nucleic acids (DNA and RNA), and are bound by a typical cell wall containing muramic acid. Moreover, they possess an active metabolism (including respiration) and are, therefore, sensitive to antimetabolic inhibitors including special antibiotics. But their metabolism is so heterotrophic that cultivation on simple artificial media is not usually possible. However, *Rochalimaea quintana,* which induces trench fever in man, has been propagated on a cell-free blood medium (Ito and Vinson, 1965). This rickettsia, which is non-pathogenic to its arthropod host, also grows extracellularly within the gut of the louse. Nearly all other rickettsiae, however, show intracellular development. For example, *Rickettsia typhi,* which induces typhus fever in man, usually grows within the cytoplasm of

[1] A more detailed account of earlier work is given by Krieg, 1963.

gut epithelium cells of the louse. According to recent investigations of Weyer (1968), however, special forms of *R. typhi,* which are able to grow extracellularly, may dissociate. But these forms (which may also multiply on a cell-free blood medium) are unable to grow further intracellularly or to induce pathological effects.

Rickettsiae of the standard type are very small (mostly 0.2 μ in diameter) spherical to rod-shaped micro-organisms, single or arranged in chains. Recently, Huger and Krieg (1967) demonstrated that rickettsiae multiplied not only by binary fission, but also in a more complex way. This life-cycle implies development of a rickettsiogenic stroma from "initial bodies" (pleomorphic forms derived from typical rickettsiae after invasion of the host cell). This stroma is subsequently transformed into discrete, typical rickettsiae or into pleomorphic "large-bodies". The latter may undergo binary or multiple fission so producing pleomorphic or typical rickettsiae. In some species of rickettsiae (genus *Rickettsiella*) the formation of proteinic crystals within the "large-bodies" has been reported.

II. Propagation of Entomopathogenic Rickettsiae

Rickettsiae can be propagated in susceptible hosts *in vivo* or in tissue cultures *in vitro.* Haemolymph, or ultrafiltered tissue-homogenates of diseased insects, are useful as inocula. Separation and purification of rickettsiae from diluted haemolymph or tissue homogenates is possible by stepwise ultrafiltration, by differential centrifugation or by density gradient centrifugation.

A simpler technique to obtain infectious material, especially for oral application, is homogenizing whole insects affected by rickettsiosis and using the supernatant after low-speed centrifugation. After ultrafiltration, or incubation with antibiotics, such supernatants are also useful for parenteral inoculation.

III. Stability and Resistance of Entomopathogenic Rickettsiae

In contrast to most of the other rickettsiae (Krieg, 1963) some species of the genus *Rickettsiella* are extremely stable despite environmental changes. Hurpin (1965a) observed the effects of different factors such as pH, desiccation, temperature, irradiation, antibiotics, disinfectants, etc., on *Rickettsiella melolonthae.* He stated that soil contaminated by homogenized infected larvae retained its infectivity for over a year under natural conditions. This has been confirmed by Niklas and Brammanis (1969) who demonstrated viability of *R. melolonthae* in contaminated soil over a period of more than three years. Hurpin (1965a) reported that an aqueous dilution of contaminated haemolymph (pH 5.0-8.5) retained its infectivity over a period of two weeks at room temperature. Contaminated haemolymph dried on slides was still infective after storage at +2° C for about 12 months, or at 20° C for about six months. Under more favourable storage conditions *R. melolonthae* may retain its activity for as long as four years at +2° C. Thermoresistance is also very high; *R. melolonthae* may survive 1 hr at 85° C. Ultra-violet irradiation could not effectively kill *R. melolonthae,* dried on slides, even after one week's exposure (germicidal lamp; 30 cm distance) at 20° C.

In addition, *R. melolonthae* shows high chemoresistance. It is not only very resistant to ethanol treatment (30 min at 45° C), but also may survive 4% formaldehyde solution for 30 min (Hurpin, 1965a). Of all antibiotics tested, only dihydrostreptomycin at a dose of 2500 γ/larva will inactivate *R. melolonthae.* Penicillin 10,000 U/larva, streptomycin 1000 γ/larva, oxytetracycline 1000 γ/larva, and chlorotetracycline 2000 γ/larva have had little influence on the effectivity of *R. melolonthae* (Hurpin, 1965b).

IV. Insect Pathology of Rickettsiae

The taxonomy of rickettsiae is closely related to their pathogenic properties (for details see Krieg, 1963). The species of the tribes Rickettsieae and Ehrlichieae, which mostly show host alternation, are predominantly pathogenic to vertebrates including man, but only in some cases (e.g. *Rickettsia prowazekii*) are they also harmful to their arthropod vector. In the tribe Wolbachieae, however, no host alternation between vertebrates and arthropods is known. Some genera in this tribe *(Rickettsoides* and *Wolbachia)* are more commensals than pathogens of their arthropod hosts. But others, *Enterella* and *Rickettsiella,* to which we must pay attention here, are highly pathogenic for their arthropod hosts.

Species of *Enterella* grow intracellularly in the epithelial cells of the gut of susceptible insects, causing variable pathogenic effects. A rickettsia of this type, *Enterella (Rickettsiella) stethorae,* was isolated from Coleoptera by Hall and Badgley (1957).

Species of *Rickettsiella* mostly grow intracellularly in the fat body cells of insects, though not in the gut epithelium cells. Associated crystals are frequently produced. *Rickettsiella* spp. usually have a deleterious effect on their hosts. Species of this type have been isolated from Coleoptera, e.g. *R. popilliae* by Dutky and Gooden (1952), *R. melolonthae* by Wille and Martignoni (1952), *R. tenebrionis* by Krieg (1965); from Diptera, e.g. *R. chironomi by* Weiser (1949), *R. tipulae* by Müller-Kögler (1958); and from Orthoptera, e.g. *R. grylli* by Vago and Martoja (1963), *R. blattae* by Huger (1964), *R. schistocercae* by Vago and Meynadier (1965).

One of the best-known insect pathogenic rickettsiae is *R. melolonthae* which induces the "Lorsch disease" in white grubs of *Melolontha melolontha, Melolontha hippocastani,* and other species of lamellicorn beetles (*Amphimallon solstitiale, Amphimallon majalis, Anomala dubia, Phyllopertha horticola, Serica brunnea* etc.) (Hurpin, 1962; Niklas, 1963). Orally infected larvae of *Melolontha* spp. show first symptoms of disease after 2-3 months and about 85% die at 20°C after 4-6 months. The temperature optimum of the disease is about 14°-20°C; over 24°C the host withstands infection better than at lower temperatures (Hurpin and Robert, 1967). Older grubs are more resistant to infection than younger ones, but pupae and adults are also susceptible (especially after injection). If rickettsiae are injected into the haemocoele, the disease develops in a relatively short time and induces almost 100% mortality. According to Hurpin (1962), successive passages by the parenteral route may enhance the virulence of rickettsiae: after the seventh passage through grubs, manifestation of the disease could be reduced from three months to three weeks. A morphological variation, chains of spherical forms superseding bacillary forms, accompanied this increase in virility.

A striking sign of diseased larvae is the opalescent discoloration of the larvae due to masses of free rickettsiae in the haemolymph. They are released from infected cells in which rickettsiae have multiplied. Propagation of rickettsiae in insects occurs only in the cytoplasm of the cells, where rickettsia-filled vacuoles may occur, and not within nuclei. In ticks, however, rickettsiae may also multiply in cell nuclei. During their life-cycle, beside standard type rickettsiae ($0.2 \times 0.6\,\mu$ in size) smaller spherical forms ("minute forms") and larger pleomorphic forms ("large-bodies") have also been observed. In the latter, bipyramidal crystals of protein, mostly 1-2 μ in size, may originate (Huger and Krieg, 1967). With the exception of the gut epithelium, nearly all the tissues (including ganglia cells) of all the developmental stages of susceptible hosts may be invaded. Heavily infected grubs often die before they are able to undergo another larval moult. Others die as pupae or as young malformed adults.

A very interesting symptom of diseased larvae is a change in behaviour (Niklas, 1964): whereas low temperatures cause healthy grubs to move deeper into the ground, diseased larvae come up to the surface. Generally, the mobility of grubs and adults suffering from rickettsiosis is progressively reduced. These changes may be due to development of rickettsiosis in the nervous system (see above).

V. Epizootiology of Entomopathogenic Rickettsiae

Studies in this field are largely limited to *R. melolonthae.* Because this pathogen multiplies (like viruses) only in its host (species of Lamellicornia), it could be assumed that the effect of epizootics (caused by *horizontally* transmitted rickettsiae between contemporaries) depends largely on the density of the host population. In his epizootiological studies in the forest region of Lorsch (Western Germany), however, Niklas (1960) could not verify density-dependence by annual estimates of population density and mortality of the host. A lower degree of density-dependence of obligate pathogens could be easily explained if *vertical* transmission occurred from one generation to the next.

Krieg (1966) found that, in adults of *Melolontha* spp. and *Amphimallon* spp. suffering from rickettsiosis, the reproductive organs and their products (ovarioles, and cyst cells of testes, respectively) may also be infected. If such infection does not induce sterility, *vertical* transmission of rickettsiae from diseased males, via the spermatophores, to the eggs of a healthy female *post coitum* is as possible as transmission by the eggs of a diseased female infected *in situ*. The degree of contamination governs the further development of fertilized, infected eggs. The viability of heavily infected beetles is greatly reduced, but it is not known whether they are still able to mate and to lay eggs.

In spite of these difficulties, by carefully selecting dose and time of application Niklas (1969) was able to rear heavily infected larvae of *Amphimallon solstitiale* of which 62% developed to rickettsia-infected adults. Only three of 74 pairs laid eggs. Most of the young grubs (45) died, largely between instars I and II. Of the remaining seven larvae, six pupated and three matured, although suffering from rickettsiosis. As suggested by previous epizootiological and ultrahistological investigations, these laboratory studies demonstrated vertical transmission to offspring from parents infected as larvae. Infected adults may not only play an important role in vertical transmission, but also by spreading *R. melolonthae* from place to place, and eventually by infection of the soil when their cadavers break up.

VI. Aspects of the Microbial Control of Insects by Rickettsiae

From laboratory infection experiments (in which the effectiveness of *R. melolonthae* was compared with that of other pathogens such as bacteria, fungi, protozoans, and viruses) Hurpin and Robert (1967) calculated that *R. melolonthae* was more effective than *Bacillus popilliae* var. *fribourgensis*, but less effective than *Beauveria tenella* for the control of *Melolontha melolontha* larvae. In their experiments one rickettsia-diseased larva was homogenized and mixed into 1000 ml of substrate (peat); 160 ml of the substrate were placed in each container with a single healthy larva. As food pieces of carrot were used. The LT_{50} of third instar larvae was about 15 weeks at 20°C and the total mortality (after correction by Abbott's formula) about 85%. At 17° and 25°C *R. melolonthae* induced 92% and 45% mortality, respectively. From this study on the epizootiology of "Lorsch disease" it can be assumed that the artificial application of *R. melolonthae* to soil should establish the disease as an enzootic one in areas bearing permanently high populations of subterraneous lamellicorn larvae.

Pilot field trials with *R. melolonthae* on populations of *M. melolontha* were started in Southern Sweden in 1966. At a population density level of 85-95 larvae (instar III) per m^2 the dosage used was three rickettsiae-dead grubs (instar III) per m^2. One year later, when the first infected grubs had been found, this project was unavoidably discontinued (Niklas and Brammanis, 1969).

VII. Medical and Veterinary Problems Associated with the Application of Entomopathogenic Rickettsiae

A handicap of all microbial control experiments with *Rickettsiella*-species is their pathogenicity for vertebrates, especially warm-blooded animals. It is well known that the host specificity of rickettsiae is relatively low and not limited to arthropods. Many rickettsiae *(Rickettsia prowazekii, Rochalimaea quintana)* show host alternation between vertebrates and arthropods. But *R. melolonthae* and *R. grylli* (other species have not been tested so far) are also able to infect mammals lethally: details are given on page 485, Chapter 22. Although in regions where *R. melolonthae* occurs at enzootic or epizootic levels, for example in the forests near Lorsch (Western Germany), no significant death of small rodents was evoked, it is my opinion that application of rickettsiae for microbial control is not without danger because their pathogenicity for vertebrates is directly related to their low host specificity. Further research should be undertaken to decide whether animals really would be harmed following *Rickettsiella* application under field conditions. Serological techniques may be useful for checking the infection of small mammals living in areas infested by *Rickettsiella.*

References

Dutky, S. R. and Gooden, E. L. (1952). *J. Bacteriol.* **63,** 743-750.
Hall, I. M. and Badgley, M. E. (1957). *J. Bacteriol.* **74,** 452-455.
Huger, A. M. (1964). *Naturwissenschaften* **51,** 22.
Huger, A. M. and Krieg, A. (1967). *J. Invertebrate Path.* **9,** 442-445.
Hurpin, B. (1962). *Verhandlg. 11. Int. Kongr. Ent., Wien 1960,* **2,** 875-880.
Hurpin, B. (1965a). *Proc. 12. Int. Congr. Ent., London 1964,* p. 727.
Hurpin, B. (1965b). *Entomophaga* **10,** 311-315.
Hurpin, B. and Robert, P. H. (1967). *Phytiat.-Phytopharm.* **16,** 105-113.
Ito, S. and Vinson, J. W. (1965). *J. Bacteriol.* **89,** 481-495.
Krieg, A. (1963). *In* "Insect Pathology. An Advanced Treatise" (E. A. Steinhaus, ed.), Vol. 1, pp. 577-617. Academic Press, New York.
Krieg, A. (1965). *Naturwissenschaften* **52,** 144-145.
Krieg, A. (1966). *Naturwissenschaften* **53,** 484-485.
Müller-Kögler, E. (1958). *Naturwissenschaften* **45,** 248.
Niklas, O. F. (1960). "Standorteinflüsse und natürliche Feinde als Begrenzungsfaktoren von *Melolontha* Population etc.". *Mitt. biol. BundAnst. Ld-u. Forstw.* **101,** 66 pp.
Niklas, O. F. (1963). *Beitr. Ent.* **13,** 395-401.
Niklas, O. F. (1964). *Anz. Schädlingsk.* **37,** 22-24.
Niklas, O. F. (1969). *Entomophaga* **14,** 225-228.

Niklas, O. F. and Brammanis, L. (1969). *NachrBl. dt. PflSchutzd.* **21**, 11-12.
Vago, C. and Martoja, R. (1963). *C.r. hebd. Séanc. Acad. Sci. Paris* **256**, 1045-1047.
Vago, C. and Meynadier, G. (1965). *Entomophaga* **10**, 307-310.
Weiser, J. (1949). *Ann. Parasitol.* **24**, 259-264.
Weyer, E. (1968). *Acta virol. (Bratislava)* **12**, 44-48.
Wille, H. and Martignoni, M. E. (1952). *Schweiz. Z. Path. Bakt.* **15**, 470-474.

CHAPTER 8

Use of Nematodes for Microbial Control of Insects

GEORGE O. POINAR, JR.

Department of Entomology and Parasitology, University of California, Berkeley, California, U.S.A.

I. Introduction

The subjects of this chapter are those representatives of the class Nematodea which are parasites of insects, the effect they exert on insect populations, how they have been used to control insect pests in the past and prospects for the future.

The potential use of nematodes as natural regulators of insect populations was discussed years ago by Glaser and Wilcox (1918) who, with regard to a mermithid infection of grasshoppers, stated "...we firmly believe that the nematodes accomplished an immense reduction in the number of grasshoppers ... this worm might offer possibilities for introduction into regions where it does not occur and where grasshoppers are a pest".

Although our knowledge of the life-history and ecological factors affecting entomophilic nematodes leaves much to be desired, we have accumulated considerable evidence illustrating the role some nematodes play in the natural control of insect populations and are now at the threshold of deciding if these agents can be used for directed control against specific insect pests.

Thus far, there is no evidence of any entomogenous nematode causing damage to plants or vertebrates. Animals preying on insects parasitized by the nematode groups discussed here will not become secondarily infected.

II. Range of Nematode-Insect Associations

Nematodes have been found associated with representatives of most of the insect orders as well as with mites. However, our knowledge of the nematode parasites of mites is so limited that discussion on this topic will be withheld at this time. An early list of nematode-insect associations was presented by van Zwaluwenburg (1928) and later continued by La Rivers (1949). There is no up-to-date host list and present-day reports are widely scattered in the literature.

The widespread occurrence of nematodes with certain insect groups can be readily illustrated. The nematode associates of bark beetles have attracted much attention, with Théoridoridès (1950) citing over 100 species and sub-species of nematodes associated with these insects in France, and Rühm (1956) listing a similar number associated with scolytids in Germany. In a recent examination of 35 insect species in Egypt, Mohamed Ali (1968) found 17 of them associated with nematodes. The above reports include nematodes found externally on the insect or in the insect environment and since these usually cause no detrimental effect to the host, such associations will not be discussed further here. Also, those nematodes which utilize insects as intermediate hosts and later continue their development in vertebrates will not be covered here, although in rare instances a massive invasion of the insect may cause damage.

Nematodes may occur in low numbers in insect populations. An average of 12% of 3332 grasshoppers collected in certain regions of Virginia contained nematodes (Cobb *et al.*, 1923), and higher rates of grasshopper parasitism have been reported in Japan (Sugiyama, 1956). About 20% of the cucumber beetle population in eastern Canada and throughout most of the U.S.A. was reported attacked by nematodes (Cobb, 1921). Nematode parasitism of alfalfa weevil larvae reached 33% in one locality in New York and the parasite was also found in other eastern states (Poinar and Gyrisco, 1962). A survey of grasshopper parasites in three Quebec localities showed nematodes to be widely distributed and occurring much more frequently than other parasites (Briand and Rivard, 1964).

Besides terrestrial pests, aquatic insects of medical importance are also attacked by nematodes. Jenkins and West (1954) reported a nematode infection of three species of mosquitoes in Canada and listed a number of earlier records. More recently Artyukhovsky and Kolcheva (1965) found a nematode parasite of *Aedes communis* in the U.S.S.R. and Petersen *et al.* (1968) recorded 13 species of mosquitoes serving as natural hosts to nematodes in southern U.S.A. Nematode parasites of chironomids from a number of lakes in the central U.S.A. have been studied by Johnson (1955) and recently Poinar (1968) described a new nematode parasitizing chironomid larvae from percolation ponds in California. Simuliids are also subject to attack by parasitic nematodes, and Phelps and DeFoliart (1964) recently completed a detailed study on the bionomics of the nematode parasites of simuliids in Wisconsin, while Rubtsov (1966, 1967) described many nematodes from Russian blackfly populations.

The few examples cited above show how widespread insect-nematode associations are and the following sections will be devoted to a more detailed discussion of some of these relationships.

III. Biology of Entomogenous Nematodes and Their Regulatory Role in Nature

A. MERMITHIDAE

Representatives of this family are parasites of invertebrates (mainly insects) during part of the nematodes' development. The infective juvenile generally enters directly through the host cuticle and after an active period of growth, leaves the host and enters the soil (Fig. 1). The final molt to the adult stage, mating and oviposition occur outside the host. Since the host invariably dies when the parasite emerges, mermithids have considerable potential as biological control agents. Nearly 300 records of mermithid parasitism of medically important insects (mainly Culicidae, Simuliidae, and Chironomidae) occur in the world literature (Welch and Poinar, 1965). Mermithids are distributed among only a few of the available culicid populations, but an infected population is usually severely attacked.

The incidence of infection of arctic mosquito larvae attacked by mermithids reached 100% in one pool and after reviewing previous reports of mermithid infections in mosquitoes, the authors concluded that these parasites would offer an effective means of natural control if they could be mass-reared for artificial introductions (Jenkins and West, 1954). Welch (1960) remarked that a mermithid parasite of *Aedes communis* in Manitoba occurred in no more than half of the pools sampled, thus artificial introductions would have to be undertaken to achieve a significant degree of control. In studying African tree hole mosquitoes, Muspratt (1945) found that in infected holes parasitism of most mosquito larvae reached as high as 70-80%, although the number of sampled tree holes infected with mermithids was only 10%. Later, Muspratt (1965) described a technique that could be used for mass-rearing mermithids attacking *Culex pipiens*, so allowing introductions to be attempted. The sparse

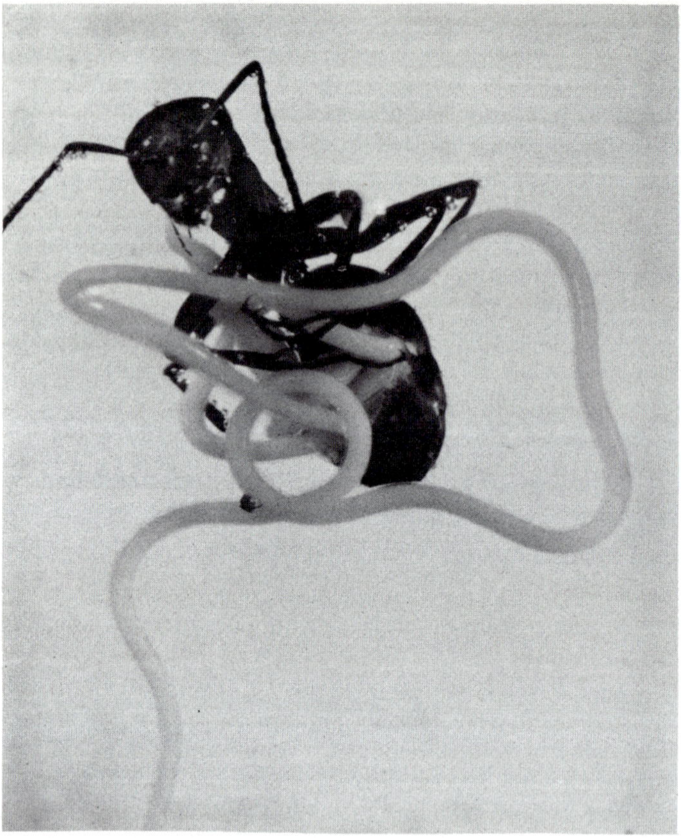

Fig. 1. A juvenile mermithid emerging from the abdomen of an ant. (Photo by H. Lyons.)

distribution of mermithids was again emphasized in a recent study by Petersen *et al.* (1968). Although hundreds of locations were examined, infected larvae were found in only five ponds. The incidence of infection varied considerably, depending on environmental factors, but reached as high as 93% in a single population of the culicids *Psorophora confinnis* and *Uranotaenia sapphirina.* Recently, Hagen and Hoopingarner (in press) found a mermithid parasite of *Aedes stimulans* in the north-eastern United States. All eight ponds examined contained parasitized mosquitoes and the average infection in these ponds was slightly over 25%.

Investigations of the mermithid parasites of chironomids have also been conducted. Natural mermithid infections at certain times of the year have been reported as high as 100% in populations of *Tanytarsus* larvae in Germany (Wülker, 1961). Johnson (1955) studied the monthly infection rate of

Hydromermis contorta in the midge, *Chironomus plumosus,* and found a range of 0-24.8% parasitism throughout the year. Wülker (1963) considered the possibility of liberating a palearctic mermithid into the tropics for biological control, but stressed the need for more preliminary studies. Recently, investigations were made on mermithids in chironomid populations in percolation ponds in California. These ponds were essentially isolated from direct stream action and were fairly uniform throughout the year. The incidence of larval infection reached 45% (n = 150) in one spring month and it was concluded that the parasites controlled the midge population about two years after the ponds were first flooded (Poinar, 1968; Chapman and Ecke, 1969).

Similar high levels of mermithid infection have also been reported for blackflies (Simuliidae). At least 153 records of mermithid parasites of blackflies exist in the world literature, with hosts mainly in the genera *Simulium, Prosimulium, Eusimulium* and *Cnephia* (Welch, 1963). After reviewing the rates of parasitism reported by earlier authors, Welch concluded that mermithids could be a significant factor in the natural regulation of certain species of blackflies. Rubtsov (1964) found that the incidence of infection for a particular host fluctuated markedly, depending on the local stream environment. However, when infection levels reached peaks of 80-90% blackfly populations often vanished from a given biotope for two or three years. In four Wisconsin streams, Phelps and DeFoliart (1964) recorded 37-63% adult blackflies parasitized by mermithids, while larval mortality from nematodes was estimated at 50%. With such high infection rates, virtual elimination of blackfly larvae occurred on two occasions.

Mermithids have been reported as exerting control on agricultural pests as well. A list of insects parasitized by mermithids in India was presented by Mathur (1959) who considered these parasites of considerable economic importance.

In 1917, a natural mermithid epizootic was observed among grasshopper populations in north-eastern U.S.A. (Glaser and Wilcox, 1918). The incidence of parasitism rose to 76% in some areas and the authors concluded that the nematodes greatly reduced the number of grasshoppers in that locality.

Christie (1937) stated that "there is little doubt that both *Mermis subnigrescens* and *Agamermis decaudata* are important factors in grasshopper control throughout the regions where these parasites occur".

In Japan, Kaburaki and Imamura (1932) found 285 out of a total of 372 rice borers, *Chilo suppressalis (simplex)* (76.61%) parasitized by a mermithid nematode and felt that the nematodes were important in controlling this moth. Cutworm (noctuid) larvae also may be heavily attacked by mermithids. Infection rates reaching 92.8% held cutworm larvae in check during pest outbreaks in India (Khan and Hussain, 1964), and similar infection rates were reported by Chatterjee and Singh (1965). From 587 cutworm larvae collected during two summers in Mexico, an average of 39% was parasitized (Gómez and Villa, 1965), while heavy mermithid parasitism of *Feltia subgothica* in southern U.S.A. may be the main reason why this cutworm is not a major economic pest in that region (Puttler, personal correspondence).

A study made of mermithid parasitism of the alfalfa weevil in one locality showed that on the average 21.7% of 584 fourth instar larvae collected were infected (Poinar, 1962). Recently, a new mermithid was found parasitizing larvae of the banded cucumber beetle, *Diabrotica balteata,* in southern U.S.A. and Cuthbert (1969) felt that, under certain conditions, the parasite was capable of exerting a profound influence on populations of this insect.

B. RHABDITIDA

Nematodes belonging to the order Rhabditida are commonly found associated with insects, but most of these associations are strictly phoretic and are innocuous to the insect. The following section discusses the biology and natural control of those rhabditids responsible for insect mortality.

In 1941, larvae of the white fringed beetle, *Pantomorus peregrinus,* from southern U.S.A. were found containing nematodes. These nematodes, which were undetermined rhabditids, were cultured in the laboratory and killed the host in a manner similar to *Neoaplectana* infections. These nematodes were recovered from six insect species in six south-eastern states and could kill larvae of *P. peregrinus* and the vegetable weevil, *Listroderes obliquus* (Littig and Swain, 1943).

Perhaps the most interesting group of entomogenous nematodes in the Rhabditida, from the evolutionary and economic standpoint, are those of the genus *Neoaplectana.* The first representative was found in 1929 in dead larvae of the Japanese beetle *(Popillia japonica),* and Glaser soon succeeded in cultivating the new nematode, *N. glaseri,* on artificial media. Preliminary field experiments indicated that the nematodes could be established in a previously non-infected area and were capable of producing high insect mortality (Glaser, 1932).

Since the distribution of *N. glaseri* was decidedly limited, very little data were given on natural field infections. The successful achievements of this nematode therefore fell heavily on the efforts of Glaser and his coworkers who established it in new areas from cultures reared on veal medium (Glaser *et al.,* 1940). This work will be covered in the section on the uses of nematodes for insect control.

Various species of *Neoaplectana* have been found throughout the northern hemisphere, yet little is known of their effect on insect populations. Swain (1943) reported a complex of *Neoaplectana* in the gulf coastal region of the U.S.A. but found less than 1% parasitism after examining more than 60,000 larvae of the white fringed beetle. However, in such surveys, the rapid deterioration of diseased insects may account for their low recovery rate. The incidence of natural infection of *Neoaplectana* reached 33% in pronymphs of the sawfly, *Acantholyda nemoralis* in Poland (Weiser and Koehler, 1955) and 25%

(n = 104) in larvae of the tussock moth, *Crambus simplex,* in New Zealand (Hoy, 1954).

In the U.S.S.R., Kirjanova and Puchkova (1955) found, on the average, from 13-67% of beet weevil larvae infected with *N. bothynoderi* and at certain times recovered up to 19 infected larvae in a square meter of soil in a beet field. In Poland, Stanuszek (1967) collected 126 cutworm caterpillars from a sugar beet plantation and found 55% parasitized by *Neoaplectana feltiae.*

Rhabditids of the family Diplogasteridae possess a characteristic muscular metacorpus and a glandular basal bulb. Like other saprobic forms, they commonly occur in soil or decomposing plant or animal matter, where they feed on bacteria and other micro-organisms. Some authors attribute insect mortality to the actions of these nematodes, although many reports were never substantiated and remain questionable. Davis (1919) found a nematode disease of *Phyllophaga* (scarabaeid) grubs that killed 90% of the insects in one field and suggested that the infection was caused by the diplogasterid, *Mikoletzkya aerivora.* Juveniles of the same nematode were also found in the head of active, normal-looking termites, *Reticulitermes flavipes,* while adult nematodes occurred in sick and dead insects (Banks and Snyder, 1920). *Diplogasteritus labiatus* entered the gut of adult long horned beetles, *Saperda tridentata* and caused a high rate of insect mortality in 120 beetles when the developing nematodes ruptured the host intestine and entered the hemocoel (Merrill and Ford, 1916). These authors also found *M. aerivora* in the head of the termite, *Leucotermes lucifugus* and observed that the insects died when nematode numbers were high.

Recently, Sander and Stanuszek (1967a, b) found a diplogasterid nematode killing hibernating adults of the Colorado potato beetle, *Leptinotarsa decemlineata* and found 90% of the adults attacked in some regions. Niklas (1960) considered *Diplogasteroides berwigi* as playing an important role in the biological control of chafers of the genus *Melolontha,* yet the exact nature of the association remains unclear. Further information on the relationship of diplogasterid nematodes to insect disease has been summarized by Poinar (1969b).

Other rhabditids parasitic in insects have been recovered from natural host populations and additional information on their distribution and effect on host would be interesting (Körner, 1954; Stammer and Wachek, 1952).

C. TYLENCHIDA

Although members of the Tylenchida have not hitherto been considered as biological control agents, there is growing evidence that they are important in the regulation of insect populations. Due to their host specificity and difficulties involved in culturing these nematodes, their artificial spread by man has not yet been undertaken.

Goodey (1930) remarked that the great majority of frit-flies, *Oscinella frit,* parasitized by the nematode, *Howardula oscinellae,* were sterile, with the incidence of infection ranging from 5.18 ($n = 3477$) to 14.7% ($n = 966$). Hussey (1965) referred to the potential of an undescribed *Bradynema* sp. for the control of the mushroom-infesting phorid *Megaselia halterata.* This eelworm sterilizes female phorids and may affect as many as 90% of the population on mushroom farms in the autumn.

Also in England, Oldham (1930) examined *Scolytus scolytus (destructor)* ($n = 385$) and *Scolytus multistriatus* ($n = 180$) and found that 40% of both species were sterilized by nematodes. He considered the parasite as having an appreciable controlling effect upon these bark beetles. Schvester (1957) noted that the nematode, *Parasitylenchus dispar rugulosi,* totally sterilized adult bark beetles in France and more recently, Massey (1966) recorded several instances where nematode parasites considerably reduced the reproductive potential of bark beetles by rendering them sterile and in one instance, by killing the host. In the latter instance the nematode, *Parasitylenchus elongatus,* was thought to be responsible for the decline of the scolytid, *Scolytus ventralis,* in southern New Mexico. The nematode, *Howardula aptini,* was capable of rendering its host, *Aptinothrips rufus,* sterile with the incidence of infection ranging from 21.4% ($n = 377$) in the spring to 32% ($n = 415$) in the summer (Sharga, 1932).

Recently, attention has been focused on two species of *Heterotylenchus.* One of these is a new species that was described from the face fly, *Musca autumnalis* in eastern U.S.A. Surveys showed that from over 3000 flies collected, an average of 23% were parasitized by the nematode (Stoffolano and Nickle, 1966; Nickle, 1967). The nematode appears to occur in fly populations throughout the U.S.A. (Stoffolano, 1968), and in Missouri, the average infection of *M. autumnalis* by this nematode throughout the year was approximately 40% (Puttler, personal communication). The parasite is capable of partial sterilization of female flies and the ease of rearing the host insect may lend itself to the favorable propagation of the nematode under laboratory conditions. A similar species of *Heterotylenchus* has recently been found parasitizing the Australian bushfly, *Musca velustissima,* over wide areas of Australia (Hughes and Nicholas, 1969). Since all of these muscoids are serious pests, attempts at controlling them by artificially applying nematodes to the breeding sites of the fly will be a challenging goal for the future.

The second nematode which offers potential as a biological control agent is a parasite of wood wasps of the genus *Sirex.* While dissecting *Sirex noctilio* females in New Zealand, Zondag (1962) found nematodes in the hemocoel and reported that parasitism resulted in castration of the adult insect. High rates of parasitism resulted in investigations on the possibility of utilizing the nematode as a biological control agent. Bedding (1967) then discovered that nematode juveniles removed from adult hosts could be cultured on the symbiotic fungus carried by the sawfly. These nematodes (*Deladenus* sp.) continued to reproduce on the fungus, *Amylostereum,* until environmental conditions promoted the formation of an infective stage female capable of entering a new insect host. Such a condition would be beneficial from the standpoint of biological control since the nematodes could remain in the environment in the absence of hosts. The only unfortunate circumstance in this case was the wide host range of the nematodes which enables them to attack the hymenopterous parasites of the wood wasps (Hocking, 1967).

The employment of a tylenchid nematode for insect control on a limited scale was initiated by Poinar (1965) when he introduced a nematode parasite of sciarid flies infesting beet seedlings in a glasshouse at Rothamsted Experimental Station, England. Shortly after releasing the nematode, *Tripius sciarae,* the fly populations began to decrease and after four weeks, the weekly insecticide spraying program against these insects could be discontinued. The nematode killed most of the host larvae before they reached the pupal stage, while the few infected adult flies that survived were invariably sterile (Fig. 2).

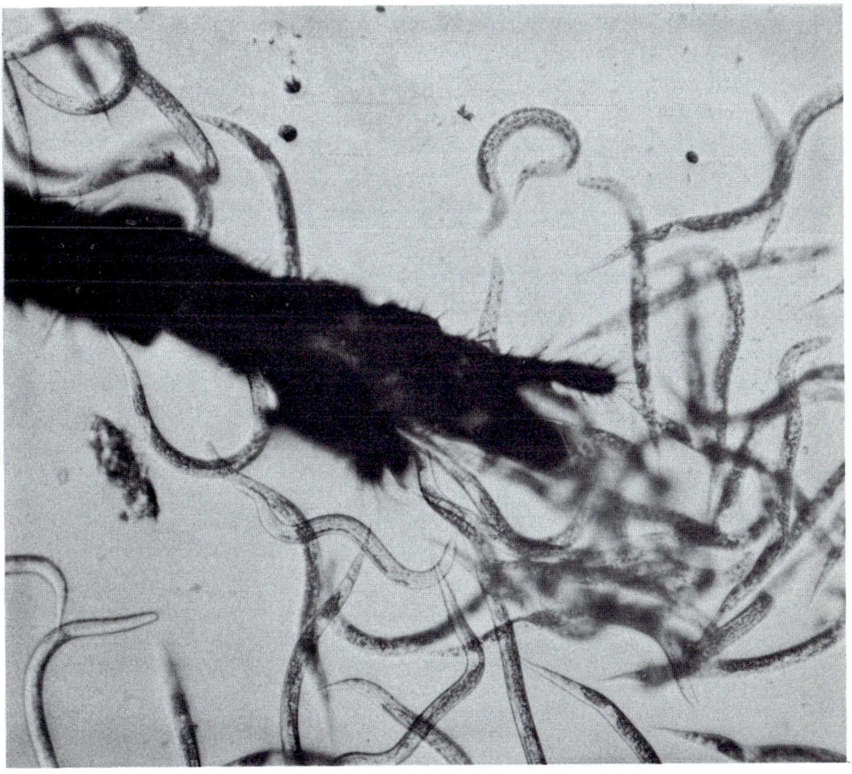

Fig. 2. Juveniles of the sphaerulariid, *Tripius sciarae,* being expelled through the ovipositor of an infected sciarid fly, *Bradysia paupera.* (Photo by C. C. Doncaster.)

It is obvious that entomogenous Tylenchida are important in insect control and have great potential for use against selected insect pests.

IV. Entomogenous Nematodes as Vectors of Micro-organisms

Entomogenous nematodes invariably have a free-living soil stage which picks up bacteria and other micro-organisms on its cuticle. This might seem to be a problem with the infective stages of mermithids and sphaerulariids, which must enter the host without bringing about secondary infections. However, those nematodes which kill the host first and then develop in or on the cadaver may even require bacteria for their nutrition. A specialized condition has developed with some of the neoaplectanid nematodes which have become symbiotically bound to specific bacteria.

Such a condition has recently been described for a strain of *Neoaplectana carpocapsae* (Poinar, 1967a) (Fig. 3). This strain was originally known as the DD-136 nematode, and its relationship with an associated bacterium was first reported by Dutky (1959) while the bacterium was later described by Poinar and Thomas (1965). Cells of *Achromobacter nematophilus* are carried in the ventricular portion of the intestinal lumen of the infective stage nematodes and

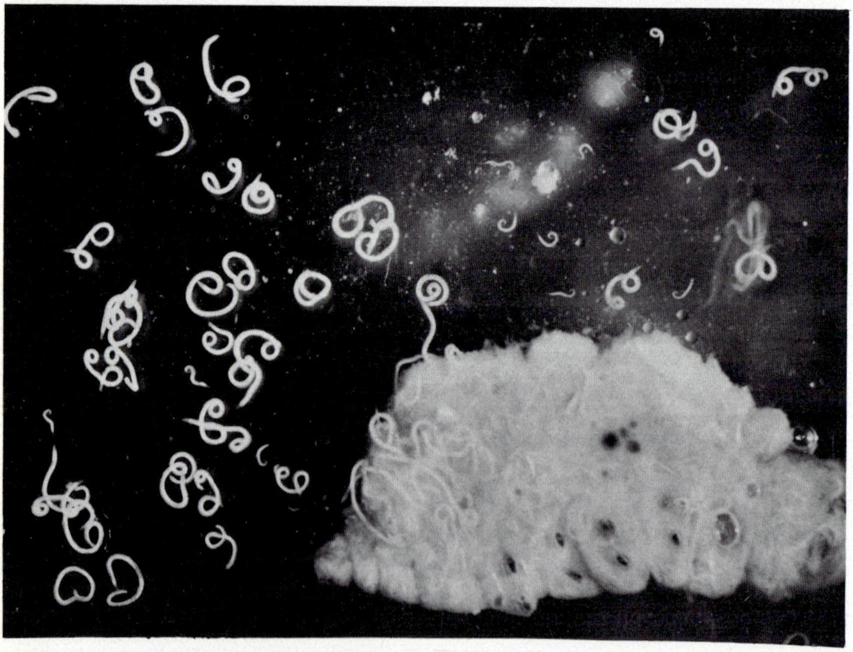

Fig. 3. Adults of *Neoaplectana carpocapsae* removed from the body cavity of a last instar *Galleria mellonella* larva. (Photo by A. Blaker.)

are released through the anus when the nematode enters the body cavity of a host (Poinar, 1966). It was shown that the relationship between nematode and bacterium is a case of mutualism, since the bacterium is protected in nature by the nematode, which then releases it into the hemolymph of an insect host. In turn, the bacterium provides the necessary environment for nematode reproduction (Poinar and Thomas, 1966). An almost identical bacterium was found in another neoaplectanid recently collected in Mexico (Poinar, 1967b). The bacterium imparts a characteristic light tan color to the insect cadaver. This particular color and lack of putrefaction after death are typical of an infection with *A. nematophilus* and may indicate parasitism by certain neoaplectanid nematodes (Poinar and Thomas, 1967).

Dutky (1937) recovered diseased Japanese beetle grubs attacked by an undescribed neoaplectanid and noticed a characteristic bacterium in the dead insects. He postulated that the nematode might serve as a means of introduction into the body cavity of the insect. In the same year, Bovien (1937) described two species of *Neoaplectana* and remarked that the infective juveniles of one species contained bacteria-like bodies in the anterior portion of the intestine. He suggested the possibility of a symbiotic relationship but did not investigate the situation further. These two observations can now be better understood in the light of the recent findings with the DD-136 strain of *N. carpocapsae.*

Although bacteria were never mentioned, their presence was suggested in *N. bothynoderi* when Kirjanova and Puchkova (1955) reported that the body of infected weevil larvae became soft and pulpy, pinkish yellow. Weiser (1966) recovered a number of bacteria from the invasive juveniles of the Czechoslovakian strain of *N. carpocapsae* and felt that these were carried into the body cavity of *Galleria mellonella* larvae. Swain (1945) thought that an insect-infecting *Diplogaster* was associated with bacteria responsible for insect mortality, yet such a relationship was never confirmed.

However, contrary to general opinion, not all described species of *Neoaplectana* are known to be associated with specific bacteria. The relationship of *N. glaseri* with bacteria will remain unclear until fresh material is found from naturally infected insects.

The ability of entomogenous nematodes to transmit fungal, viral and protozoan pathogens into insects remains to be discovered by future workers.

V. Trials of Nematodes for Insect Control

Although mermithid and sphaerulariid nematodes are promising agents for the biological control of insect pests, the difficulty of producing mass numbers for distribution severely limits their usefulness. Since growth on artificial media has been unsuccessful, large numbers for field work must be obtained from living hosts, requiring considerable time and effort.

TABLE I

Trials of entomogenous nematodes for control of field populations of insects

Host	Substrate	Dosage and site	Culture method	Results	References
		NEOAPLECTANA GLASERI			
Larva of the Japanese beetle, *Popillia japonica*	Pasture turf; 2 test, 2 control plots, each 6 ft^2	Approx. 27,000 nemas/ft^2; soil surface	Dextrose veal infusion agar seeded with yeast	Nemas established, high mortality	Glaser, 1932
Larva of *Popillia japonica*	Pasture turf; 2 test, 1 control plot, 110 x 20 ft each	3-4 inches in the soil	Dextrose veal infusion agar seeded with yeast	Significantly reduced grub populations by about 40%	Glaser and Farrell, 1935
Larva of white fringed beetles, *Pantomorus* spp.	Soil; 31 plots, 1000 ft^2 each	25,000/ft^2; soil surface	Veal infusion agar seeded with yeast or ovarian substance	Nemas established in 29 plots	Swain, 1944, unpublished
Grass grub, *Costelytra zealandica*	Grass plot; 2500 ft^2	80,000 nemas/ft^2; soil surface	Veal infusion agar seeded with yeast or ovarian substance and veal pulp	Infected grubs found, but no reduction over controls	Hoy, 1955
		DD-136 Strain of *NEOAPLECTANA CARPOCAPSAE*			
Codling moth larva, *Cydia pomonella*	Trunks and branches of apple trees	Sprayed on trunk	Wax moth larvae, *Galleria mellonella*	60% and higher mortalities	Dutky, 1959; Anon., 1956
Potato beetle larva, *Leptinotarsa decemlineata*	500 potato plants	20,000 nemas/plant; sprayed on plants	Wax moth larvae	Infection obtained; at least 14% reduction over control plot	Welch, 1958
Potato beetle larva, *Leptinotarsa decemlineata*	640 potato plants	5×10^4, 10×10^4, 20×10^4, 40×10^4 nemas/plant; sprayed on plants	Wax moth larvae	Small reductions, not significantly different from control	Welch and Briand, 1961a

Tobacco budworm, *Heliothis viescens*	Tobacco leaves	5 x 10^6 nemas/100 plants; water suspensions by hand sprayers to leaf	Wax moth larvae	Gave 80-85% reduction under very moist conditions only	Chamberlin and Dutky, 1958
Cabbage root maggot, *Hylemya brassicae*	Cabbages, radishes, rutabagas; soil	1.0 x 10^5 to 5.1 x 10^5 nemas/plant; water application and cadaver burial	Wax moth larvae	Reduction in plant damage over control	Welch and Briand, 1961b
European corn borer, *Ostrinia nubilalis*	Leaf sheath of corn plants	Water application; 10,000 nemas/leaf sheath	Wax moth larvae	Reduction of cob-damage in treated plants	Welch and Briand, 1961b
Imported cabbage-worm, *Pieris rapae*	Cabbage head	3.4 x 10^5 to 1.5 x 10^5 nemas/plant	Wax moth larvae	No significant reduction of larvae over controls	Welch and Briand, 1961b
Root collar weevil larva, *Hylobius radicis*	Base of pine trees; 10 trees	10,000 infective nemas/tree	Wax moth larvae	Infection obtained but experiment limited	Schmiege, 1962
Pruinose scarab, *Sericesthis geminata (pruinosa)*	Turf plot 150 x 300 ft^2	35 x 10^3, 70 x 10^3 nemas/ft^2	Wax moth larvae	No nema-infected larvae found	Reed and Carne, 1967
Banded cucumber beetle, *Diabrotica balteata*	Sweet potato field; 8 field plots, each 12 x 25 ft	1.09 and 0.54 x 10^9 nemas/acre; hand sprinkler	Wax moth larvae	Reduction of damage but protection inadequate	Creighton *et al.*, 1968
Imported cabbage-worm, *Pieris rapae*	Cabbage heads	1840-3120 nemas/ml; air-hand sprayer	Wax moth larvae	Significant reduction of larvae over controls	Fox and Jaques, 1966
Winter moth, *Operophtera brumata*	Apple trees (each tree 10 ft tall)	11.25 x 10^6 nemas/tree	Wax moth larvae	No significant reduction on treated over untreated leaves	Jaques, 1967
Artichoke plume moth, *Platyptilia carduidactyla*	Head of 202 artichoke plants	2000 and 4000 nemas/plant; pipetted on plants	Wax moth larvae	No significant reduction over control	Tanada and Reiner, 1960
Corn earworm, *Heliothis zea*	Corn silk; 4-7 rows of plants (each row 30-40 ft)	2000-6000 nemas/ear	Wax moth larvae	Mortality high, damage to corn ears not prevented	Tanada and Reiner, 1962

However, the neoaplectanids are fairly easy to grow on artificial media and this aspect, along with their wide host range (for an up-to-date host list, see Niklas, 1967) has promoted interest in their introduction into new localities. Attempts to use neoaplectanid nematodes to control field populations of insects are summarized in Table I.

Initial field studies were carried out by Glaser with the nematode, *N. glaseri*. This species was first applied to experimental plots against Japanese beetle in pasture turf on two farms in New Jersey. Although the actual percentage mortality could not be determined due to insect losses from birds, over half of the grubs from the treated plots were killed by the nematodes (Glaser, 1932). In a more extensive field trial, the authors again found that the grub population had been significantly reduced in nematode treated plots by about 40% (Glaser and Farrell, 1935). After these preliminary trials, 73 different experimental plots in various soil types were treated with *N. glaseri* at different seasons and parasitized beetle grubs were recovered from 72 of these experiments (Glaser *et al.*, 1940). Soil surface applications proved more successful than sub-surface ones, provided that fresh water followed the nematode suspension. Natural distribution could also occur since it was discovered that the nematodes could be transported by the adult beetles to new localities. A program releasing the nematodes at 2.5-mile intervals over the state of New Jersey was then conducted in an attempt to widely distribute the parasites (Glaser *et al.*, 1940). With all this effort, it is unfortunate that at present there are no known field sites where *N. glaseri* can be found. Through the courtesy of W. Metterhouse, F. Soraci and H. B. Girth of the New Jersey Department of Agriculture, the author visited several fields in 1967 where *N. glaseri* had been previously released, but beetle infestations were difficult to find. Insect infestations still remained at the Tavistock golf course, the original "home" of the nematode, but nematode-infected grubs were not found. The last time *N. glaseri* was recovered from beetle larvae appears to be in 1953 (Girth, 1954).

N. glaseri was tried elsewhere against grubs in soil. It was applied to field plots in Alabama, Florida, Louisiana, Mississippi, and North Carolina for control of larvae of the white fringed beetles, *Pantomorus* spp. Although the nematodes were established in 29 plots, as determined by soil extraction methods, Swain *et al.*, (1944) felt that the widespread application of *N. glaseri* as an eradication measure was not feasible, although crop protection could be obtained in limited areas. Later, cultures of *N. glaseri* were sent to New Zealand where they were liberated in 1952 for control against the grass grub, *Costelytra zealandica* (Table I). Although nematode infected grubs were recovered from field plots, there was no over-all reduction in population when compared with controls.

At this time, another species of Neoaplectanid was gaining popularity. Initially termed the DD-136 nematode-bacterium complex (Dutky, 1959), it was later shown to be a strain of *N. carpocapsae* Weiser (Poinar, 1967a) and initial trials with agricultural pests above, as well as below ground, gave promising results, e.g. against larvae of the codling moth, *Cydia (Carpocapsa) pomonella* (Table I).

In some trials humidity was believed to be important. In 1958, Welch reported initial success with the DD-136 strain against larvae of the Colorado potato beetle. However, further tests failed, apparently due to environmental factors, particularly atmospheric moisture at the time of application (Welch and Briand, 1961a). After applying it to leaves of tobacco plants, Chamberlin and Dutky (1958) observed an 80-85% reduction in larvae of the tobacco budworm under conditions of high humidity but remarked that little or no control was obtained when the leaves were dry.

However in a number of experiments, environmental moisture was not considered a limiting factor. Trials of DD-136 against the cabbage root maggot, *Hylemya brassicae,* resulted in a decrease in plant damage as compared to treated controls and applications into the leaf sheaths of corn plants to combat the European corn borer, *Ostrinia (Pyrausta) nubilalis* resulted in a significant reduction of cob damage between nematode-treated and untreated plants. However, field trials against the imported cabbageworm resulted in no significant reduction of larvae on cabbage heads over the control (Welch and Briand, 1961b).

At soil level, DD-136 was successful in some trials (Table I). The susceptibility of a number of forest pests was tested and the nematodes could locate and kill larvae of the root weevil, *Hylobius radicis,* when applied to the base of pine trees. Reed and Carne (1967) added DD-136 to turf containing larvae of the scarabeid, *Sericesthis geminata,* but never recovered nematode-infected insects and concluded that it was adapted for attacking insects on the surface, rather than soil-ingesting species. Its application to field plots of sweetpotatoes reduced insect damage to the root, but Creighton *et al.* (1968) considered that the protection provided was not adequate.

Above ground success was also variable. DD-136 significantly reduced numbers of the imported cabbageworm in Nova Scotia (Fox and Jaques, 1966). However, when it was sprayed on leaves of apple trees to combat larvae of the winter moth no significant reductions in insect larvae were observed. Against larvae of the artichoke plume moth it gave no significant control in the field and the authors concluded that the nematodes were relatively ineffective against this insect. It caused high mortality of corn ear worms, but did not prevent insect damage to corn ears.

It is surprising that rhabditoid nematodes have not been more widely utilized for biological control of medically important insects, since the aquatic habitat would solve the problem of desiccation so frequently encountered on land.

Preliminary studies with DD-136 against woodland mosquitoes have been made and Briand and Welch (1963) observed that both larval populations and adult emergence were reduced in field trials with this nematode.

VI. Factors Influencing the Effectiveness of Entomogenous Nematodes

A. PHYSICAL CONDITIONS

The major factors governing the natural distribution of entomogenous nematodes and limiting their usefulness as biological control agents are physical, with moisture probably being the most important.

Natural infestations of entomogenous neamatodes are often localized in a given area. Painter (1929) noticed that nematode-infected plant bugs came from a very poorly drained waste area that was more or less wet throughout the season. Vandel (1930) emphasized the local distribution of mermithid parasites which appeared to be limited to a particular soil type. By knowing the geological nature of the underlying rock, Vandel could predict where mermithid parasites might be found. Smith (1965) remarked that significantly higher numbers of grasshopper hosts were infected by mermithids in two areas where the vegetation was heavier, and conditions were presumably damper, than elsewhere in the field. Christie (1936) noticed that *Agamermis decaudata* was confined to localities usually saturated with water throughout the winter. Théodoridès (1952) presented some data from previous workers who related the presence of mermithid nematodes to the occurrence of underlying limestone in, or near, an infested locality and suggested a possible cause and effect relationship.

After conducting a survey on the natural distribution of *Neoaplectana,* it was found that insect parasitism was greatest at high soil temperatures with abundant soil moisture. The heaviest nematode populations occurred in areas where the water table was within a few feet of the soil surface during much of the year (Swain *et al.,* 1944). Welch and Briand (1961a) reported that because of desiccation, the infective stage neoaplectanids probably did not survive more than 1 hr when sprayed on the leaves of potato plants for control of the Colorado potato beetle. Ideal conditions would require relative humidities in excess of 80%, little air movement and a temperature range of 70°-80°F. These authors concluded that the use of nematodes on exposed plant surfaces would, in general, be impractical.

Tolerances of temperature and physical stress have been determined for some entomogenous nematodes. Schmiege (1962) found that the activity of infective stage neoaplectanids began to decrease above 32°C, and exposure of 16 hr at 37°C caused 100% mortality. The juveniles survived six months in sterile soil under conditions of high humidity and could overwinter at the latitude of Minnesota. After making tests with the Czechoslovakian strain of

N. carpocapsae, Weiser (1966) found that the survival of infective stages was less than 1 hr at 38° C and, although freezing temperatures killed them in water, they were able to survive temperatures below 10° C if protected in the dead insect. The infective juveniles are much more resistant to chemicals than the normal stages and will tolerate a 2% formaldehyde solution for 3 hr. The DD-136 strain has also been found resistant to the physical stress of application to substrates with conventional high pressure spray equipment and to many commonly used insecticides and fungicides (Dutky, 1959).

It is now evident that, aside from simple infectivity tests, we must know the environment of the insect we are attempting to control and the effect of that environment on any nematodes we may attempt to introduce. The microclimate of the plant leaf and the first few inches of soil is extremely important to nematode survival.

The importance of knowing the biology of the parasite was emphasized by Reed and Carne (1967), when they discovered that infective stages of the DD-136 strain tended to migrate to the soil surface after being introduced into the ground. The authors felt that this behavior was the cause of poor success with soil inhabiting scarabeid beetle larvae and this habit eliminated the possibility of their use in controlling soil-ingesting insects.

Although migratory movements and temperature are important, there is general agreement that moisture is still the greatest single factor to be considered in making field trials with nematodes (Welch, 1962; Jaques, 1967).

The possibility of retarding the rate of evaporation from exposed surfaces and thus increasing the longevity of the infective stage nematodes was mentioned by Welch and Briand (1961b). However, initial trials were halted because of problems involving nematode and plant toxicity. After testing various substances for their suitability as additives to suspensions of infective stage neoaplectanids, Webster and Bronskill (1968) selected Gelgard M Polymer as the most suitable compound. When used at a rate of 1.3 g of Gelgard/liter of tap water, optimum viscosity was obtained for spraying on plant surfaces. A compound for retarding the rate of evaporation and a surfactant were added to the Gelgard, thus allowing the spray mixture to maintain a water film on the foliage for a longer period. It was then possible to extend the survival period of the nematode and increase insect mortality.

B. INSECT DEFENSE REACTIONS

Insect immunity to nematodes may be an important factor limiting the usefulness of nematodes as biological control agents. Such defense reactions as encapsulation and melanization occur against all major groups of entomogenous nematodes by a wide range of insect hosts (Poinar, 1969a). When Welch and Bronskill (1962) infected mosquito larvae with the DD-136 strain of *N. carpocapsae,* a number of the nematodes were melanized and killed soon after entering the host. Although many of the insects still died, some infected mosquitoes remained unharmed, indicating that they had successfully defended themselves against the parasite.

There are also reports of host reactions directed against mermithids, and there is no doubt that these reactions are important in limiting the host range of these and other entomogenous nematodes.

C. DISEASES OF NEMATODES

Nematodes are attacked by a number of parasitic animals and plants. However, just how important diseases are in limiting nematode populations is unknown. Many of the earlier observations have been discussed by Dollfus (1946) and recently, Esser and Sobers (1964) presented recent findings on this subject.

The free-living stages of mermithid nematodes are frequently attacked by fungi or parasitic protozoans and this sometimes presents a serious problem in rearing these worms under laboratory conditions. Fungi of the Saprolegniales and Chytridiales have been found attacking mermithids and Steiner (1926) also reports some of the Actinomyxida (Protozoa) attacking species of *Agamermis* and *Pseudomermis.* Crowding may bring about conditions which favor disease and at room temperatures it may be necessary to add copper sulfate to storage water containing neoaplectanid nematodes to inhibit fungi (Swain *et al.*, 1944). A possible bacterial disease that deformed neoaplectanid nematodes under storage conditions has also been reported. When these nematodes were later placed on artificial culture media, they did poorly and eventually died (Swain *et al.*, 1944). Veremtchuk and Issi (1968) produced a microsporidan infection in a neoaplectanid by feeding caterpillars microsporidan spores, then infecting them with nematodes.

VII. Practical Considerations for the Use of Entomogenous Nematodes

One of the prerequisites for the use of entomogenous nematodes as biotic insecticides is the necessity to produce large numbers at relatively little cost. The main reason why members of the Mermithidae and Tylenchida have not been used in field trials is the difficulty involved in mass production, since methods for breeding these parasites on artificial media are still unknown. Mass production of an entomogenous nematode was initiated by Glaser (1931) who successfully cultivated *N. glaseri* on standard meat infusion agar plates containing 1% dextrose and a water suspension of actively growing yeast. Swain *et al.* (1944) used essentially this method for propagating a strain of *N. glaseri* collected from the white fringed beetle, *P. perigrinus,* and remarked that the cost of production was approximately one dollar/million nematodes. However, because of increased production demands and the necessity for finding a cheaper and continuous means of culturing *N. glaseri,* McCoy and Glaser (1936) developed a potato technique, consisting of a yeast-fermented mixture of ground, raw Irish and sweet potatoes. The production averaged about 2000 nematodes/cm^2 of culture surface.

Later, a third medium consisting of chopped, infused raw veal with preservatives provided from 9000 to 12,000 nematodes/cm^2 of culture area, and had the added advantages of being inexpensive and of providing uniform cultures (McCoy and Girth, 1938). Shortly afterwards, Glaser (1940) achieved bacteria-free culture of *N. glaseri* on pieces of sterile raw meat and axenic development was continued by Stoll (1953) who successfully cultivated *N. glaseri* in liquid media. However, the added cost involved with axenic development did not compensate for the more uniform development.

The DD-136 strain of *N. carpocapsae* was initially propagated in wax moth larvae, *G. mellonella,* which yielded up to 160,000 infective stage nematodes per insect (1,500,000/g). These yields were about five times higher than those obtained on sterile media inoculated with the associated bacterium (Dutky, 1959). Recently, House *et al.* (1965) described a method for rearing *N. carpocapsae* on a dog food medium and this method also proved successful with another brand of dog food when only pure cultures of *Achromobacter nematophilus* accompanied the nematodes (Poinar and Leutenegger, 1968). Nutrilite Products, Inc., Lakeview, California, have established a mass breeding program of the DD-136 strain of *N. carpocapsae* using this latter method. Since 1967, more than 100 million infective stage juveniles have been sent to various agencies throughout the U.S.A. for laboratory and field tests against a number of insect pests. One technician can adequately handle 200 petri dishes of dog food medium per day and collect 100 million nematodes each week. The cost of production (mainly labor) is about one dollar for 1 million nematodes. Research is now under way to develop cheaper culture methods involving semi-solid media and mammalian pathogenicity tests with these nematodes are also in progress (Chauthani, personal correspondence).

The Miller Chemical and Fertilizer Corporation in Hanover, Pennsylvania did some culture work with the DD-136 strain of *N. carpocapsae* in 1958 in an attempt to commercially produce the nematodes. However, the work has since been abandoned (McGrew, personal correspondence).

The infective stages of many neoaplectanid nematodes can be stored under refrigeration for several years without a significant decrease in infectivity. Swain *et al.* (1944) stored the infective stages of *N. glaseri* in 1- or 5-gallon jugs of aerated water. Up to 3500 nematodes/ml were safely stored at room temperature for 4-6 weeks, but high summer room temperatures resulted in almost complete mortality within a few months. With the DD-136 strain of *N. carpocapsae,* Dutky *et al.* (1964) adjusted the suspension to 50,000 nemas/ml in oxygenated water with formaldehyde and, after storage at 7.1°C (45°F), found viable nematodes after five years. Our results indicate that if the suspension is fairly clean and not too thick, the nematodes can survive without oxygenation or formaldehyde.

VIII. Conclusions

The above examples illustrate that insect-nematode associations are widespread and that, in many instances, nematodes play no small role in controlling natural populations of insects. Although I have discussed the effect of nematodes alone, on insect populations, under certain conditions these agents would be excellent candidates in integrated control programs. Difficulties in obtaining large numbers of inocula for field releases have limited the practical use of entomogenous nematodes to members of the genus *Neoaplectana.* Although initial successes have been reported, we now realize the importance of

TABLE II

Promising nematodes as candidates for insect control

Nematode group or species	Host group or species	Special points for consideration
Aquatic Mermithidae (*Hydromermis* spp., *Isomermis* spp.)	Culicidae, Simuliidae and Chironomidae	Mass-rearing of parasites for more widespread distribution. Effect of various aquatic environments on the nematodes.
Terrestrial Mermithidae (*Filipjevimermis, Hexamermis, Agamermis*)	Insects which live in or near the soil	Same as above, with addition of soil moisture.
Neoaplectanidae (*Neoaplectana carpocapsae*)	Insects with chewing mouthparts living on the soil surface or on leaf surface under humid conditions.	Longevity of infective stage in the soil under various conditions. Additions of substances with nematode inocula to retard evaporation.
Heterotylenchus spp.	Muscoid flies	Mass-rearing of parasites. Distribution of nematodes and factors affecting survival in insect environment.
Deladenus spp.	*Sirex* woodwasps	Host range of parasites. Factors affecting formation of entomogenous females.
Tripius sciarae	Fungus gnats (Sciaridae)	Longevity of infective stage in greenhouse flats. Host range of parasites.

environmental factors in determining the fulfilment of these efforts. Not only is the impact of the host environment on the nematode important, but nematode behavior as well as host specificity need also be investigated. The future use of entomogenous nematodes for insect control will depend on our ingenuity, imagination and efforts to surmount these present difficulties. Some of the host-parasite relationships which appear promising from the standpoint of biological control are cited in Table II. Also listed are special points which need consideration and further investigation before we can accurately utilize these parasites for insect control.

References

Anonymous. (1956). *Agric. Res.* **4,** 3-4.
Artyukhovsky, A. K. and Kolcheva, R. V. (1965). *Zool. Ž.* **44,** 454-455. [In Russian.]
Banks, N. and Snyder, T. E. (1920). *Bull. U.S. natn. Mus.* **108,** 228 pp.
Bedding, R. A. (1967). *Nature, Lond.* **214,** 174-175.
Bovien, P. (1937). *Vidensk. Meddr dansk naturh. Foren.* **101,** 114 pp.
Briand, L. J. and Rivard, I. (1964). *Phytoprotection* **45,** 73-76.
Briand, L. J. and Welch, H. E. (1963). *Phytoprotection* **44,** 37-41.
Chamberlin, F. S. and Dutky, S. R. (1958). *J. econ. Ent.* **51,** 560.
Chapman, J. and Ecke, D. H. (1969). *Calif. Vector Views* **16,** 83-88, 92.
Chatterjee, P. N. and Singh, P. (1965). *Indian Forestry* **91,** 714-721.
Christie, J. R. (1936). *J. Agric. Res.* **52,** 161-198.
Christie, J. R. (1937). *J. Agric. Res.* **55,** 353-364.
Cobb, N. A. (1921). *Contr. Sci. Nematol.* No. 10, 345-352.
Cobb, N. A., Steiner, G. and Christie, J. R. (1923). *J. Agric. Res.* **23,** 921-926.
Creighton, C. S., Cuthbert, F. P., Jr. and Reid, W. J. (1968). *J. Invertebrate Path.* **10,** 368-373.
Cuthbert, F. P., Jr. (1969). *J. Invertebrate Path.* **12,** 283-287.
Davis, J. J. (1919). *Ill. Nat. Hist. Surv.* **13,** 53-138.
Dollfus, R. P. (1946). "Encyclopedia Biologique" (P. Lechevalier, ed.), Vol. 27, 480 pp.
Dutky, S. R. (1937). Ph.D. Thesis. Rutgers Univ. 113 pp.
Dutky, S. R. (1959). *Adv. appl. Microbiol.* **1,** 175-200.
Dutky, S. R., Thompson, J. V. and Cantwell, G. E. (1964). *J. Insect Path.* **6,** 417-422.
Esser, R. P. and Sobers, E. K. (1964). *Soil Crops Sci. Soc. Florida* **24,** 326-353.
Fox, C. J. S. and Jaques, R. P. (1966). *Can. J. Plant Sci.* **46,** 497-499.
Girth, H. B. (1954). *Ent. News* **65,** 97.
Glaser, R. W. (1931). *Science* **73,** 614-615.
Glaser, R. W. (1932). *New Jersey Dept. Agric. Bureau Plant Industry, Cricular* **211,** 3-34.
Glaser, R. W. (1940). *Proc. Soc. exp. Biol. Med.* **43,** 512-514.
Glaser, R. W. and Farrell, C. C. (1935). *J. New York ent. Soc.* **43,** 345-371.
Glaser, R. W. and Wilcox, A. M. (1918). *Psyche* **25,** 12-15.
Glaser, R. W., McCoy, E. E. and Girth, H. B. (1940). *J. Parasitol.* **26,** 479-495.
Gómez, L. A. and Villa, M. M. (1965). *Fitofilo* **48,** 5-20.
Goodey, T. (1930). *Philo. Trans. R. Soc. Lond.* **218,** 315-343.
Hagen, N. and Hoopingarner, R. (In press.) *Ann. ent. Soc. Am.*
Hocking, H. (1967). *J. Aust. ent. Soc.* **6,** 52-56.
House, H. L., Welch, H. E. and Cleugh, T. R. (1965). *Nature, Lond.* **206,** 847.
Hoy, J. M. (1954). *Parasitology* **44,** 392-399.
Hoy, J. M. (1955). *N.Z. Sci. Rev.* **13,** 56-58.
Hughes, R. D. and Nicholas, W. L. (1969). *J. econ. Ent.* **62,** 520-521.

Hussey, N.W. (1965). Proc. XII Int. Congr. Ent. Lond.1964, p. 752.
Jaques, R. P. (1967). *J. econ. Ent.* **60,** 741-743.
Jenkins, D. W. and West, A. S. (1954). *Mosquito News* **14,** 138-143.
Johnson, A. A. (1955). Ph.D. Thesis. Univ. Illinois, 92 pp.
Kaburaki, T. and Imamura, S. (1932). *Proc. Imp. Acad. Japan* **8,** 109-112.
Khan, M. Q. and Hussain, M. (1964). *Indian J. Ent.* **26,** 124-125.
Kirjanova, E. S. and Puchkova, L. B. (1955). *Trudi Zool. Inst. Akad. Nauk S.S.S.R.* **18,** 53-62. [In Russian.]
Körner, H. (1954). *Zool. Jb. (Syst.)* **82,** 245-353.
La Rivers, I. (1949). *Wasmann Collector* **7,** 177-206.
Litig, K. S. and Swain, R. B. (1943). Unpubl. Rep. U.S. Dep. Agric. Gulfport, Mississippi, 17 pp.
Mathur, R. N. (1959). *Curr. Sci. Bangalore* **28,** 255-256.
Massey, C. L. (1966). *Bull. ent. Soc. Am.* **12,** 384-386.
McCoy, E. E. and Girth, H. B. (1938). New Jersey Dep. of Agric., Circular **285,** 3-12.
McCoy, E. E. and Glaser, R. W. (1936). New Jersey Dep. of Agric. Bureau of Plant Industry. Circular **265,** 1-10.
Merrill, J. H. and Ford, A. L. (1916). *J. Agric. Res.* **61,** 115-127.
Mohamed Ali, M. A. (1968). M.S. Thesis. Al-Azhar Univ. Egypt. 228 pp.
Muspratt, J. (1945). *J. ent. Soc. S. Africa* **8,** 13-20.
Muspratt, J. (1965). *Bull. Wld Hlth Org.* **33,** 140-144.
Niklas, O. F. (1960). *Mitt. biol. BundAnst. Ld- u. Forstw.* **101,** 60 pp.
Niklas, O. F. (1967). *Mitt. biol. BundAnst. Ld- u. Forstw.* **124,** 40 pp.
Nickle, W. R. (1967). *J. Parasitol.* **53,** 398-401.
Oldham, J. N. (1930). *J. Helm.* **8,** 239-248.
Painter, R. H. (1929). *Ann. Rept. Quebec Soc. Protect. Plants* **21,** 53-55.
Petersen, J. J., Chapman, H. C. and Woodard, D. B. (1968). *Mosquito News* **28,** 346-352.
Phelps, R. J. and DeFoliart, G. R. (1964). *Univ. Wis. Res. Bull.* **245,** 78 pp.
Poinar, G. O., Jr. (1962). Ph.D. Thesis. Cornell Univ. 82 pp.
Poinar, G. O., Jr. (1965). *Parasitology* **55,** 559-569.
Poinar, G. O., Jr. (1966). *Nematologica* **12,** 105-108.
Poinar, G. O., Jr. (1967a). *Proc. helminth. Soc. Wash.* **34,** 199-209.
Poinar, G. O., Jr. (1967b). *In* "Insect Pathology and Microbial Control" (P. A. van der Laan, ed.), pp. 197-199. North-Holland Publ. Co., Amsterdam.
Poinar, G. O., Jr. (1968). *Ann. ent. Soc. Am.* **61,** 593-598.
Poinar, G. O., Jr. (1969a). *In* "Immunity to Parasitic Animals" (G. J. Jackson and R. Herman, eds), Vol. 1 Appleton-Century-Crofts. pp. 173-210.
Poinar, G. O., Jr. (1969b). *J. Invertebrate Path.* **13,** 447-454.
Poinar, G. O., Jr. and Gyrisco, G. G. (1962). *J. Insect Path.* **4,** 469-483.
Poinar, G. O., Jr. and Leutenegger, R. (1968). *J. Parasitol.* **54,** 340-350.
Poinar, G. O., Jr. and Thomas, G. M. (1965). *Int. Bull. Bact. Nomen. Taxon.* **15,** 249-252.
Poinar, G. O., Jr. and Thomas, G. M. (1966). *Parasitology* **56,** 385-390.
Poinar, G. O., Jr. and Thomas, G. M. (1967). *J. Invertebrate Path.* **9,** 510-514.
Reed, E. M. and Carne, P. B. (1967). *J. Invertebrate Path.* **9,** 196-204.
Rubtsov, I. A. (1964). WHO mimeogr. docum., WHO/EBL/19: 6 pp.
Rubtsov, I. A. (1966). *In* "New Species of the Fauna of Siberia and Adjoining Regions" (A. I. Cerepanov, ed.), pp. 109-147. Izd. Nauka Sib. Otd. Novosibirsk. [In Russian.]
Rubtsov, I. A. (1967). *Tran. Zool. Inst.* **43,** 59-92. [In Russian.]
Rühm, W. (1956). *Par. Schriftenreihe* **6,** 437 pp.
Sandner, H. and Stanuszek, S. (1967a). *In* "Insect Pathology and Microbial Control" (P. A. van der Laan, ed.), pp. 210-212. North-Holland Publ. Co., Amsterdam.
Sandner, H. and Stanuszek, S. (1967b). Proc. IXth Int. Nematol. Symp. Warsaw 1967, p. 34.
Schmiege, D. C. (1962). Ph.D. Thesis, Univ. Minnesota, 97 pp.
Schmiege, D. C. (1963). *J. econ. Ent.* **56,** 427-431.
Schvester, D. (1957). *Ann. Epiph.* 8th année, 162 pp.

Sharga, U. S. (1932). *Parasitology* **24,** 268-279.
Smith, R. W. (1965). *Can. J. Zool.* **43,** 179-201.
Stammer, H. J. and Wachek, F. (1952). *Zool. Anz.* **148,** 185-193.
Stanuszek, S. (1967). Abst. IXth Int. Nematol. Symp. Warsaw 1967, p. 40.
Steiner, G. (1926). *J. Parasitol.* **12,** 181.
Stoffolano, J. G., Jr. (1968). *J. econ. Ent.* **61,** 861-863.
Stoffolano, J. G., Jr. and Nickle, W. R. (1966). *J. econ. Ent.* **59,** 221-222.
Stoll, N. R. (1953). *J. Parasitol.* **39,** 422-444.
Sugiyama, K. (1956). *Dobuts. Zasshi, Tokyo* **65,** 386-391.
Swain, R. B. (1943). Unpubl. Rep. U.S. Dep. Agric. Gulfport, Mississippi, 6 pp.
Swain, R. B. (1944). Unpubl. Rep. U.S. Dep. Agric. Gulfport, Mississippi, 8 pp.
Swain, R. B. (1945). *J. econ. Ent.* **38,** 488-490.
Swain, R. B., Littig, K. S., Bartlett, F. J. and Gordon, M. F. (1944). Unpubl. Rep. U.S. Dep. Agric. Gulfport, Mississippi, 33 pp.
Tanada, Y. and Reiner, C. (1960). *J. Insect Path.* **2,** 230-246.
Tanada, Y. and Reiner, C. (1962). *J. Insect Path.* **4,** 139-154.
Théodoridès, J. (1950). *Vie et Milieu* **1,** 53-68.
Théodoridès, J. (1952). *Vie et Milieu* **3,** 288-291.
Vandel, A. (1930). *Bull. Soc. Zool. France* **55,** 244-252.
Veremtchuk, G. V. and Issi, I. V. (1968). Abst. 13th Int. Congr. Ent. Moscow, 1968, 287-288.
Webster, J. M. and Bronskill, J. F. (1968). *J. econ. Ent.* **61,** 1370-1373.
Weiser, J. (1966). *Nemoci Hmyzu.* Academia, Prague, 554 pp.
Weiser, J. and Koehler, W. (1955). *Roczniki Nauk Lesnych* **11,** 93-110.
Welch, H. E. (1958). *Ann. Rep. ent. Soc. Ontario* 88, 53-54.
Welch, H. E. (1960). *Can. J. Zool.* **38,** 465-474.
Welch, H. E. (1962). *Proc. ent. Soc. Ontario* **92,** 11-19.
Welch, H. E. (1963). WHO mimeogr. docum., WHO/EBL/16 pp.
Welch, H. E. and Briand, L. J. (1961a). *Can. Ent.* **93,** 759-763.
Welch, H. E. and Briand, L. J. (1961b). *Proc. ent. Soc. Ontario* **91,** 197-202.
Welch, H. E. and Bronskill, J. F. (1962). *Can. J. Zool.* **40,** 1263-1268.
Welch, H. E. and Poinar, G. O., Jr. (1965). Proc. XII Int. Congr. Ent. Lond. 1964, p. 732.
Wülker, W. (1961). *Arch. Hydrobiol. Suppl.* **25,** 127-181.
Wülker, W. (1963). WHO mimeogr. docum., WHO/EBL/11 pp.
Zondag, R. (1962). New Zealand Forest Service Interim Research Release, pp. 1-6.
Zwaluwenburg, R. H. van (1928). *Bull. exp. Sta. Hawaiian Sugar Planters Ass.* **20,** 68 pp.

CHAPTER 9

Micro-organisms as Sources of New Insecticidal Chemicals: Toxins

O. LYSENKO and M. KUČERA

Department of Insect Pathology, Institute of Entomology, Czechoslovak Academy of Sciences, Prague, Czechoslovakia

I. Introduction

Toxins are sometimes supposed to be chemical weapons either for defence of the micro-organism or attack of the host. This opinion is a rough anthropomorphism exemplifying our lack of knowledge. Even though these compounds are harmful to higher organisms in many respects and in different intensities, it is uncertain whether their original purpose is to damage a host. Many are produced as more or less usual microbial metabolites, even in normal nutrient media. Their toxicity can be considered a secondary effect of their occurrence in a susceptible host. Thus *Clostridium tetani*, which produces highly lethal toxins, is a natural inhabitant of soil and it would be rather foolish to consider its presence there merely as waiting to infect man. The same may be said about *C. botulinum*, which produces one of the most active biological compounds known and finds tinned meat a more favourable medium than living animals. It is, therefore, more justifiable to regard toxins as normal bacterial products harmful to sensitive hosts, without adjudging them any other ecological role *a priori*. Anthropomorphic explanations of their functions are an unimportant philosophic aspect of our topic, but their application to ecology may lead to misleading statements. Sometimes, however, it is impossible to distinguish with certainty between cause and effect.

Since toxins are one of the possible mechanisms of pathogenicity, all attributes of pathogenicity must be considered when thinking about toxicity. Pathogenicity itself is not an exclusive feature of a micro-organism, but the result of a relationship between the micro- and macro-organism, therefore the susceptibility of a host to a toxin must automatically be taken into account. From this viewpoint the terms "toxicity" and "susceptibility" are valid only for the system in question and all statements are largely dependent on the methods used. Therefore criteria like "highly toxic" or "atoxic" are variable in meaning and precise quantitative data are necessary for comparisons to be made. This criterion is often neglected by insect pathologists, who often publish mortality diagrams from which it is impossible to establish an LD_{50} unit.

Different hosts vary in susceptibility to the same toxin. Equally some toxins have a broad, others a narrow, spectrum of susceptible hosts and even in phylogenetically closely-related animals some toxins cause different mortality.

To explain such diversity it is necessary, however, to know the mechanisms of the mode of action of toxins. The solution of this problem depends more on progress in biochemistry and physiology, than on the number of people involved. It is, therefore, a typical interdisciplinary project. If this is true of our knowledge of toxins affecting man, the more it concerns insect pathology.

We shall refer only to papers about toxins harmful to insects, and in discussing more general questions, only to comprehensive papers containing references to more detailed literature.

II. Classification of Bacterial Toxins

The word "toxin" was derived from the Greek *toxikon* which meant a poison. In Ehrlichian times, all substances were called toxins if produced by bacteria and causing similar symptoms on injection to those caused by injection of living microbes. Here, as often in biology, the less is known the clearer the term appears to be. With increasing knowledge, this term underwent its "Babylonian stage" and now its usage is completely confused. It acquired different meanings in pharmacology, bacteriology, chemistry, mycology, etc. As we are dealing only with bacteria here, we will try to use this word in the bacteriological sense.

Most of our terminology is derived from a brilliant, up-to-date and exhaustive discussion by Bonventre *et al.* (1967). Toxins are usually regarded either by common parlance as any poisonous or harmful materials obtained from a living organism, or in a scientific sense (especially in bacteriology) as a specific class of antigenic poisons of cellular origin, with high molecular weight. Poisons are defined as "any substances, either organic or inorganic in nature, which when ingested, inhaled, adsorbed through the skin, or injected parenterally produce damage to tissues or disruption of normal physiological functions" (Bonventre *et al.*, 1967). Animal poisons inflicted either by sting or bite are called venoms. These are mixtures of distinct, chemically unrelated entities, which may include one or more toxins in the scientific sense.

As knowledge of true bacterial toxins damaging insects is poor and as our purpose is to deal with all insecticidal substances produced by micro-organisms, we shall also review here substances, mixtures of compounds and even particles of microbial origin, which cannot scientifically be classified as toxins. Although we shall cover the toxins of common parlance, we shall try to distinguish in terminology between toxins valid in the scientific sense and those which can be included only by common usage, although some are described insufficiently to permit even this distinction. A classification of toxins based primarily on that used in medical microbiology seems most apt for present purposes and toxins important to insects will be dealt with after describing this classification.

Considered either as in common parlance or scientifically, toxins are variously classified according to different criteria. Each classification is made from a different viewpoint, each taking into account only one of these possible criteria. Consequently the same compound may be listed in different classes according to which criterion is used in the classification. Three main criteria are in vogue: (i) anatomical location–where toxins are produced by the cell; (ii) mode or site of action in the sensitive host; and (iii) structure of the toxin molecule.

A. CLASSIFICATION BY ANATOMICAL LOCATION

Two main groups of toxins are distinguished according to where they occur or where they are produced in the bacterial cell: (a) endotoxins are bound to the bacterial cell, from which they may be extracted; while (b) exotoxins are soluble compounds excreted outside the bacterial cell during its active growth in a medium.

1. Endotoxins

In medical microbiology endotoxins are regarded as a distinct group of toxins. The prefix "endo" denotes that they ought to be produced within the cell. Really, the endotoxins are a part of the bacterial cell wall from which they may be extracted by means of trichloracetic acid or phenol-water. The toxic macromolecular complex has a molecular weight of up to 10^6 and 10^7, and usually consists of three fractions, a protein, a lipid and a polysaccharide, respectively. The fractions may be separated though loss of the lipid results in a loss of the toxic activity. The polysaccharide fraction determines the antigenic characteristic by which the immunological specificity of the endotoxin is explained. Injection of an endotoxin into a sensitive host produces typical syndromes like fever, leucopenia, skin reaction, shock and death.

The mechanisms of endotoxin activity have been studied extensively, but results are not yet explicit. It is supposed that the toxic effect is expressed only by antigenicity, to which a sensitive host responds by reactions generally resembling an allergic or anaphylactic reaction. Mice kept without normal intestinal pathogens are insensitive to endotoxins in the usual way, so that their reactivity is dependent on the presence of the normal gut microflora. As the problems of endotoxins are very complicated and exceed our theme, the reader should consult more specialized literature, e.g. Landy and Braun (1964).

The term "endotoxin", in its medical sense, meets problems with the toxins of insect pathogens. In medical microbiology the term is reserved for a very special group of toxins, i.e. those whose mode of action is based on a distinct reaction of a sensitive host–a humoral response–rather than on a direct pharmacological activity of the endotoxin. Therefore, if in insect pathology we follow this established terminology, as we should, we ought to know whether insects have protective mechanisms similar to those in mammals, because it will be shown later that the prefixes "endo" and "exo" lose much of their original meaning as descriptions of the place where the toxin is formed–now the nomenclature is based mainly on other criteria. In reality endotoxins are a part of the cell surface and the prefix "endo" only explains that the toxin is bound to the bacterial cell in contrast to exotoxins which are excreted into the medium.

2. Exotoxins

Classical exotoxins are secreted into the medium by the bacterial cell during its active growth phase. At present exotoxins may be defined by several properties: (i) they are separate antigens, i.e. immunochemically they are chemical entities; (ii) they pass into the culture filtrate, i.e. they are not bound to the bacterial cell; (iii) they are proteins of high molecular weight; and (iv) in low doses they are able to damage the sensitive host in a specific way.

It is now known that the excretion of exotoxins outside the cell is not immediate, because they are proteins formed inside the cell on ribosomes. For instance, the toxin yield from young cells of *Clostridium botulinum* (type A) is as much as nine times that from the filtrate. This fact is used in a routine method for obtaining large amounts of botulinum toxin.

Another problem, not yet solved, is the mechanism by which a toxin is excreted from the cell into the medium. Realizing that some toxins are big molecules (the molecular weight reaches 10^6) it is difficult to imagine that the toxin can pass by simple diffusion through the cytoplasmic membrane and the cell wall. In the light of present knowledge we should expect a permease mechanism or some mechanical "holes" in the cell wall or both. But neither have been demonstrated and much more evidence is needed.

B. CLASSIFICATION BY THE SITE OR MODE OF ACTION

According to the site or mode of action, toxins may primarily damage a structure (i.e. a morphological entity) or a function (i.e. a metabolic pathway). Often the damage to a structure may be only another site of the damage of a function or vice versa. In practice, this theoretically correct criterion has all the shortcomings of distinguishing between cause and effect. In practice, however, it is still useful, especially when based on a site of action, because it is much easier to find morphological symptoms of the toxic effect than metabolic ones.

1. Classification by Site of Action

This is one of the oldest criteria for differentiating toxins, as it refers to the target tissues and its veracity is based on clinical and pharmacological evidence. Thus toxins affecting the nervous system are neurotoxins (tetanotoxin, botulotoxin), those affecting the gastro-intestinal tract are enterotoxins, those causing lysis of erythrocytes are haemolysins, those with necrotic effect are necrotoxins and so on.

This nomenclature, taking advantage of the tissue affinity of toxins, seems very simple and useful but it may be very misleading. Some toxins produce several morphological or clinical symptoms. A toxin may be a haemolysin with a necrotic effect, another may be both necrotoxic and neurotoxic and so on. This is due to the nature of the classification–it describes only the morphological symptoms and nothing about the *real* cause of the change. It does not differentiate primary and secondary effects as was mentioned earlier. For example, the staphylococcal enterotoxin affects intestinal tissues, but these tissues are also sensitive to nervous-system stimuli. Therefore precise experiments investigating all possibilities are necessary to localize the correct site of action of this toxin.

The site of action of a toxin can be defined not only at the tissue level but also within the cell organization. For example haemolysins damage the erythrocyte cell wall. Chemically, haemolysins are lecithinases and by splitting lecithin, which is a component of the cell wall, they damage the cell.

2. Classification by the Mode of Action

This criterion is biochemical and seems to augur the most correct for the future. Biochemically toxins are, according to their chemical activity, either enzymes or enzymic inhibitors. Presumably, if the substrate or metabolic mechanism upset by each toxin could be found, all the basic problems of primary modes of action could be described in biochemical or biophysical terms. But this is still a goal, in most cases far from fulfillment.

If some toxins are enzymes it is necessary to find a boundary line between an enzyme and a toxin. Obviously an enzymic toxin must have all the attributes of an enzyme as well as of a toxin. In this context it is worth mentioning the term "auxiliary virulence factor", which refers to those enzymes of pathogenic bacteria that do not exert a direct, specific toxic effect upon the sensitive host in small doses, and thus do not contribute to the pathogenesis of the infection (Miles, 1955). In particular cases, therefore, it is better to speak of "toxic enzymes" until we know the mechanism of their action and whether they may be classified as true toxins. On the other hand, it would be unwise to limit the term "toxin" only to the few commonly accepted toxins (botulotoxins, tetanotoxins, enterotoxins, leucocidin, plague murine toxin, anthrax toxin etc.), because knowledge about their mechanisms of activity is also limited.

The enzymic activities of toxins are defined by the substrates attacked in the host cells. But for an enzyme to be a toxin, it should also be toxic, which means that small doses must damage the host in a specific way. For example, lecithinases split lecithin in four different ways. For the enzyme to evince a toxic activity, its substrate must occur in the sensitive host and this substrate must be physiologically important to the host. Thus different lecithinases may have different potencies for different erythrocytes and their potencies depend not only on the presence of the substrate, but also on the way in which the substrate is built into the cell.

We should also mention that the activities of particular toxins may combine to give a final toxic effect.

C. CLASSIFICATION BY THE STRUCTURE OF THE TOXIN MOLECULE

This is a recent and most complicated criterion, developed by Bonventre *et al.* (1967). It is based on the molecular structure of the toxin and on the part played by this structure in the toxic effect. We shall describe only the main principle: the original paper gives details and examples (Bonventre *et al.*, 1967). Three main types of toxin molecules, simple toxins, complex toxins, and toxic mixtures are recognized (Fig. 1).

1. Simple Toxins

These comprise one sort of toxic molecule synthesized in a biologically active form, sometimes aggregated in dimers or polymers, all active. This sort of molecule completely poisons a sensitive host, as probably with tetanus toxin.

The toxin molecule may exist in an atoxic precursor form—protoxin. This is activated by some mechanism which either unmasks toxotrophic chemical groups, or changes the configuration of the polypeptide chain, or splits the molecule into smaller toxic fragments. The resulting effect is always an activation. Some proteases were described as activators for toxins of *Clostridium perfringens* or botulotoxin.

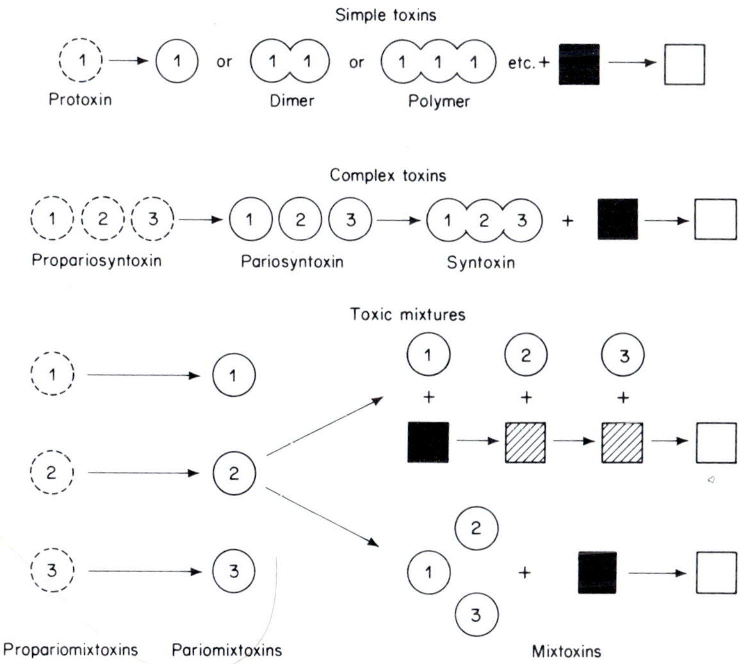

Fig. 1. Schematic classification of bacterial toxins by the structure of the toxin molecule (after Bonventre *et al.*, 1967). A susceptible host is represented by ■, an altered but not fully poisoned host by ▨, and a fully poisoned host by □. For details, see text, p. 210 *et seq.* Reprinted by courtesy of Bonventre *et al.* (1967).

2. *Complex Toxins*

These toxins exist as several atoxic components, which must unite to exhibit a biological activity.

3. *Toxic Mixtures*

These are most complicated toxic systems. In contrast to the complex toxins, the individual components of toxic mixtures retain their molecular identity and do not undergo a chemical union. They may act in two ways on the sensitive host: (i) the toxic effect depends on the sequence in which the individual components act on the susceptible host, and they produce the final effect by subsequent alterations of the host; (ii) individual components can act independently in the host but they cannot exhibit the symptoms elicited by the whole mixture; if one of the components loses its activity, so does the whole mixture, e.g. anthrax toxin and staphylococcal leucocidin.

III. The Problem of Toxins in Insect Pathology

Toxins have been extensively studied for several generations in medical and veterinary microbiology and recent progress in biochemistry, immunochemistry and other boundary disciplines not only brings new methods but also opens new questions and perspectives. Therefore it is not surprising that much less is known about insecticidal toxins.

In insect pathology only a few microbes have been studied as toxin producers. Results often vary in quality which hampers any comparison. The mode of action as well as the nature of the substances are usually only roughly determined so that it is sometimes difficult to classify them definitely as toxins. Some are isolated only as crude preparations of uncertain chemical nature and physiological function. The problem is also complicated by the patchy knowledge of the physiology and pathophysiology of insects.

As in medical microbiology, we may assume that toxins or toxic substances may take part in different ways in the pathogenesis of insect disease. Smith (1968) distinguishes four different categories. Even when he defines a toxin as in common parlance, his division is primarily justifiable from the viewpoint of methodology. His first category comprises toxins of overriding importance in disease, the second those that are significant but not the only factors responsible for the disease. The first category resembles exotoxins, the second endotoxins as defined above. In his third category are toxins produced *in vitro*, but of unknown importance in disease. Most of the toxins of insect pathology may perhaps be put in this group. The fourth is the opposite of the third, namely "toxic effects *in vivo* of bacteria which appear to produce no relevant toxin *in vitro*" (Smith, 1968, p. 171). Theoretically the third and fourth categories may be doubtful, as these compounds are either not toxins at all, or toxins that cannot be produced in nutrient media. But experimentally they are valuable, as they show all the possible combinations in the study of a pathogenicity. This statement results in a practical conclusion that "for dealing with unsolved problems of pathogenicity, the behaviour of bacteria *in vivo* should be examined for virulence attributes which might then be reproduced *in vitro* for closer investigation" (Smith, 1968, p. 172). The same is true for the determination of toxic activity. Therefore, before a compound isolated *in vitro* is called a toxin, we should be sure that it plays a role in the pathogenesis of the disease *in vivo*.

IV. Bacterial Toxins Harmful to Insects

This section reviews toxins, or even toxic enzymes, of bacteria that have been described as harmful to insects. At the beginning it must be emphasized that most of these substances cannot be scientifically defined as toxins. This is due to inadequate knowledge of their chemical nature as well as of their mode of biological action in the pathogenesis of the disease in question. Therefore we shall deal with all the toxic substances described, including those which cannot be scientifically defined.

A. TOXINS OF *BACILLUS THURINGIENSIS*

This classical bacterium has been studied most intensively during the last two decades because of its promising application in biological control. Its literature has been regularly and extensively reviewed (Heimpel, 1963, 1967; Krieg, 1961, 1967). As two separate chapters of this book are devoted to these toxins we shall consider only their more important aspects in order to orientate them in the above scheme.

Taxonomically *B. thuringiensis* can be defined as a *B. cereus* producing an "endotoxin", a crystalline parasporal body. As the taxonomy is a compromise of accepted conventions and theoretical statements gleaned from present knowledge, the toxin formation became a fundamental criterion for the definitions of species within the "*B. cereus* group". In some schemes (e.g. Heimpel, 1967) the species *B. thuringiensis* is characterized as having parasporal bodies in contrast to other species of the "*B. cereus* group". The parasporal body is called an endotoxin. Together with a few biochemical characteristics, sub-specific division of *B. thuringiensis* is based on H serotypes, esterase types and production of "toxins" other than the crystal. Some 11 different varieties have been described to date and it may be expected that other new ones are certain to be created. This taxonomic conception is an ideal organ for that brand of taxonomist dubbed a "splitter" to create new varieties with new combinations of characters, including new "toxins". This resembles in many ways the taxonomic situation in the salmonellas; every good town has its own salmonella species! It is of doubtful value to regard serotypes and toxotypes as new varieties. These are better labelled by letters or numbers, which are more explanatory.

In *B. thuringiensis* strains, five different toxins have been described: lecithinase C (Toumanoff, 1953), a "thermostable exotoxin" (McConnell and Richards, 1959), an endotoxin (Hannay, 1953), an unidentified enzyme which may not be toxic (Heimpel, 1965) and a "labile exotoxin" (Smirnoff and Berlinguet, 1966).

1. Lecithinase C

As this enzyme is not exclusive to *B. thuringiensis*, it will be discussed later (p. 215).

2. "Thermostable Exotoxin"

This is the subject of Chapter 12. It is almost certainly a family of chemically very closely-related compounds[1], some details about the identity of which have still to be determined. These compounds include the nucleotide of de Barjac and Dedonder (1965), that of Benz (1966), the compound of Cantwell *et al.* (1964) and the phosphorylated allaric acid bound to adenosylglucose isolated by the Czechs, Šebesta *et al.* (1969) and chemically determined by their colleagues, Farkaš *et al.* (1969). It is certainly not a protein, as it is thermostable and of low molecular weight. It is formed only by some strains of *B. thuringiensis.* As this species is defined within the *B. cereus* group only on crystal production, the exotoxin may appear in strains of *B. cereus* and most probably also in other species. By the scientific definition (p. 208) it is not a toxin, only a toxic metabolite. Also, its role in the pathogenesis of *B. thuringiensis* infections is unknown. Speculations about its interference with insect hormones are not confirmed. As it is perhaps a nucleotide-like compound, it probably damages the ATP metabolism of susceptible hosts. Also, it should be verified whether it plays a part in the pathogenesis of *B. thuringiensis in vivo.* If it proves to be harmless for vertebrates in acceptable doses, it might be applied as an insecticide.

3. The Crystal

The parasporal body of *B. thuringiensis* is called an "endotoxin", because it is formed inside the bacterial cell during sporulation. This is, however, not an exclusive property of this species. Other bacilli may form parasporal bodies too, e.g. *B. subtilis, B. laterosporus, B. popilliae, Clostridium cochlearium* (Pope *et al.*, 1968) etc. That of *B. thuringiensis* is toxic for susceptible hosts, but its mode of action is not fully explained (Chapter 11). It is antigenic and more than one antigen can be distinguished. As far as the criteria of toxin classification are concerned the crystal may be regarded as a toxin, but it would be wiser not to use the term endotoxin for the reasons noted above (p. 208). The crystal is of course formed within the cell, but the toxin is not bound over the whole cell, nor is it likely to show toxicity inside the cell, for to be toxic it must not only be liberated from the cell, but also activated (is this an analogy to a protoxin–Fig. 1?). Thus it more closely resembles the exotoxins. Formed inside the cell, in a way perhaps not bound to the sporulation mechanism, the crystal seems to be a waste product of cell metabolism. For these reasons it would be better not to classify it until much more is known about its formation and mode of action. Introduction of even a tentative nomenclature may mislead those unfamiliar with this toxin; those who know it well need no classification. A typical example of premature nomenclature is the gamma toxin of *B. thuringiensis* (Heimpel, 1967, p. 294), which is "the unidentified enzyme(s)

[1] Editor's note: see contrasting view in Chapter 12, p. 278.

responsible for clearing egg yolk agar . . . Since there is no proof of toxicity, it is debatable whether this substance should be recognized".

4. "Labile Exotoxin"

Smirnoff and Berlinguet (1966) found a toxic compound in two unrepeatable lots of Thuricide powder, a commercial preparation of *B. thuringiensis.* It was extracted in water and was toxic for sawfly larvae fed on treated foliage. The first three larval instars were the most susceptible. The compound was sensitive to air, sunlight, oxygen, 40° C for 144-264 hr, and temperatures above 60° C for 10-15 min. Rough chemical analysis revealed free amino acids and one or more peptides of low molecular weight (200-2000). In an acid hydrolysate 17 amino acids were detected. It is not clear whether the toxic entity is the whole mixture or only one particular peptide. Its mode of action is not yet explained, neither do we know whether it is really formed by *B. thuringiensis* or is an artefact of the fermentation. It may be concluded that this "labile exotoxin" cannot be classified as an exotoxin. It may be of use in biological control but much more data are naturally required.

B. LECITHINASES

In medical microbiology lecithinases are known as toxins exhibiting a variety of activitics, e.g. as haemolysins. Erythrocytes of different vertebrates vary in susceptibility to the same haemolysin. The sites of action in the erythrocyte are not the same for different lecithinases, which means that each haemolysin may have its own receptor in the cell, but two different haemolysins show the same enzymic activity on lecithin as a substrate *in vitro.* Consequently: (i) toxicity is determined not only by the enzymic specificity, but also by the manner in which the substrate is built into the sensitive structure; and (ii) the sensitive structure plays the basic role in the total pathological effect.

Lecithinase production as a biochemical property has been demonstrated in many bacterial species *in vitro.* In insect pathology this enzyme has been studied only in connection with the pathogenicity of *B. thuringiensis* and *B. cereus.* Toumanoff (1953) was the first to point out the analogy between the production of lecithinase by *B. thuringiensis (cereus)* var. *alesti* and the alpha toxin of *Clostridium perfringens* in man. Later, Heimpel (1954, 1955) demonstrated the coincidence between the pH optimum for lecithinase and the pH inside the gut of sawfly larvae. Sawfly species, whose gut pH was higher than the optimum for the enzyme, were not susceptible to *B. cereus.* The LD_{50} for instar V of susceptible larvae was 21 times higher than that for the mouse (both per mg of body weight). Also, histological examination of insect gut revealed enzymic destruction. The mechanism of lecithinase formation by bacterial cells was studied by Kushner (1960, 1962) and Kushner and Heimpel (1957). As well as other enzymes lecithinase was found to be primarily cell-bound, and released from the cell and activated by a low-molecular weight activator, which was thermolabile and most probably a lipid. This suggests that the activity of this bacillus is determined not only by the pH in the insect gut, but also by other mechanisms.

Slein and Logan (1963) described two lecithinases in *B. cereus,* one with a phosphatasaemia activity in mammals, and the other inhibiting this activity *in vitro*. The activity of the phospholipase C of *Pseudomonas aeruginosa* may be increased by a haemolysin, also produced by the bacterium. Since other bacteria produce lecithinase, it may be expected that this enzyme may take part in the bacterial pathogenicity for insects in a more complex manner than now postulated.

C. PROTEASES

Proteases, i.e. hydrolases of peptide bonds, are produced by many bacterial species in many genera. Also other micro-organisms, especially fungi, are significant producers of these enzymes, a property used in industrial microbiology. *Pseudomonas aeruginosa, Proteus vulgaris, Serratia marcescens,* some bacilli, enterococci, clostridia, etc. are examples of outstanding producers of extracellular proteases. Many of them produce elastases and collagenases, which from the biochemical point of view may be regarded as proteases.

In 1960, Bucher pointed out that the protease of *B. thuringiensis* may be involved in pathogenesis, because when bacteria invade the haemocoel the enzyme may destroy phagocytes. This suggestion was based more on speculation than on evidence. He also thought that bacterial species with prominent proteolytic activity, established by a microbiological technique on gelatin, are more virulent than others when injected into the body cavity. But all such statements suffered from lack of precise experimental evidence.

When the mechanism of pathogenicity of *P. aeruginosa* was studied, this bacterium sometimes proved to be pathogenic in different insect larvae and also, in field experiments, it was claimed to be an important facultative pathogen. It produced, extracellularly, a compound toxic by injection into the haemocoel of *Galleria mellonella.* This compound was believed to be a protein which, together with its antigenic characteristics and influence on the oxygen consumption of larvae, suggested that it was an extracellular toxic antigen with all the attributes of an exotoxin (Lysenko, 1963a, b, c, d). Later, after isolation, it was found to be a protease, more toxic than that of *Bacillus subtilis* (Lysenko, 1965). Even when the proteolytic activity of these two proteases was the same on the reference substrate *in vitro,* the toxic activities *in vivo* were different, indicating that the protease of *P. aeruginosa* had a specific affinity to proteins of *G. mellonella* larvae. This led to a study of this model system in detail.

The conditions under which the enzyme was produced and its properties were described (Lysenko, 1967). From the culture filtrate of the strain in use, five different proteolytic fractions were isolated by DEAE cellulose chromatography, gel filtration, and disc electrophoresis. Molecular weights and pH optima suggested that four of these are most probably a monomer and corresponding oligomers of the same enzyme (Kučera and Lysenko, 1968). On the other hand, the toxicities of these fractions to *G. mellonella* larvae were unequal. The fraction with a molecular weight of 26,000 was the most toxic. Enzymic inhibition led to a proportional decrease of toxicity and thus a fair correlation between proteolytic activity and toxicity could be established (Lysenko and Kučera, 1968).

As, theoretically, toxins may interfere with a function or attack a structure, further research was focused on changes in the haemolymph, after treatment with the enzymes. Examining the enzymic kinetics of the enzyme, with haemolymph as a substrate, aroused a suspicion that the enzyme did not attack all the proteins of the haemolymph. Disc electrophoresis showed that the enzyme attacked only two of a total of 18 protein bands. This was substantiated by electrophoresis of haemolymph of larvae treated with enzymes *in vivo*. Further examination of terminal amino acids in proteins of larval haemolymph digested by the enzyme showed that the enzyme split the same peptidic bonds in some haemolymph proteins *in vitro* as it did in the synthetic peptides (Kučera and Lysenko, unpublished).

Even though this research is unfinished some conclusions may be drawn. The protease of *P. aeruginosa* is toxic for *G. mellonella* larvae by injection; in this respect it resembles the kappa and lambda toxins of *Clostridium welchii*. Different proteases of different organisms (bacteria, fungi, plants, animals) show different toxicity for *G. mellonella* larvae (Fig. 2). These experiments suggest that the modes of action of these toxic enzymes concern insect haemolymph, but the nature of the mechanism is still uncertain. Two possible explanations may be considered: that death is caused either (i) by the resulting lack of proteins sensitive to the enzyme; or (ii) by the breakdown products liberated from these proteins. Whether the cause of death is direct or indirect, is difficult to say. On the other hand, it cannot be excluded that the primary or a parallel effect is on the function of lymphocytes or on another sensitive structure. However, the toxicity in *G. mellonella* larvae may differ from that in other insect species. For instance, the instar V larvae of *Mamestra brassicae* are as much as x100 more sensitive than those of *G. mellonella* (Lysenko and Kučera, unpublished).

D. OTHER ENZYMES

As bacteria produce many extracellular enzymes which may find a fairly well matching substrate in the insect body, it may be anticipated that some of them may be toxic. Among other enzymes, hyaluronidase, phosphatase and other

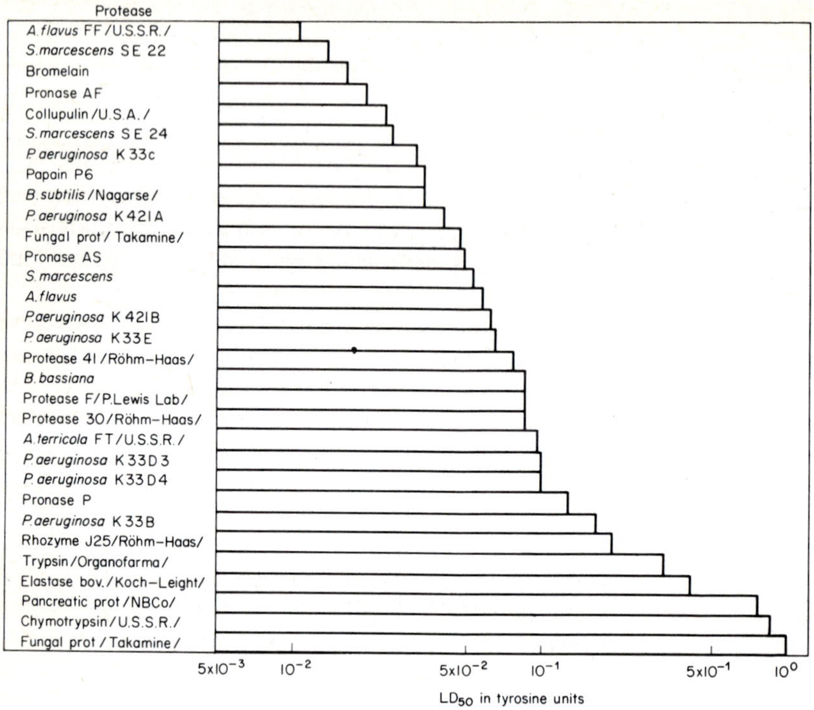

Fig. 2. Toxicity of different proteases for larval instar VII of *Galleria mellonella* by injection into the haemocoele. The origin of each protease is given by the organism from which it was isolated, or for commercial preparations, by the firm. The LD_{50} is expressed in proteolytic activity as tyrosine units (t.u.). 1 t.u. = 10^{-4} mmoles of tyrosine liberated from 2% casein in 0.2 molar phosphate buffer, pH 7.4, at 30° C/min. (Lysenko and Kučera, unpublished.)

esterases may be considered. But whether they will be toxins or only auxiliary factors is unknown; for a correct appreciation of their role in pathogenesis, all the criteria mentioned earlier should be considered.

V. Fungal Toxins

In fungi, classical toxins like those in bacteria have not been described and so the nomenclature is also different. We shall follow common practice and call any toxic compound produced by a fungus a toxin, as it is not our purpose to attempt to unify the nomenclature.

In fungal, as in bacterial, diseases of insects the production of metabolites exhibiting a distinct toxic effect on the insect host is an important factor in pathogenicity. Since Wallengren and Johansson (1929), Toumanoff (1931), and Burnside (1930) attributed pathogenicity of some fungi *(Metarrhizium anisopliae* and *Aspergillus flavus)* to toxins, a series of papers have appeared, but much less has been done in this field than with bacterial diseases of insects. An exhaustive review up to 1965 appears in the book by Müller-Kögler (1965). Etiological aspects of fungal toxins and their importance in insect control are also discussed in Chapter 5. Even though many papers deal with insect pathogenic fungi, only a few describe a distinct metabolic product toxic to the insect host when used as a pure preparation.

Since some fungi produce several toxic compounds, which may act simultaneously to cause various toxic effects, it is necessary to study the components of the toxic complex step by step. For this reason, the use of modern biochemical methods for isolation and characterization of these compounds is vital as in the key papers of Kodaira (1961, 1962). The more a toxin can be purified and defined the more precisely the mechanism of its action may be judged without interference from other biologically active compounds that contribute to the complete toxic effect. This is important because some toxic breakdown products, from nitrogen or carbon sources of high molecular weight, may be present when a medium in which a fungus has been cultivated is examined for toxicity (Kodaira, 1961). On the other hand, such toxic products can be formed in the insect body and the toxic action of several hydrolytic enzymes may be explained in this way.

A. CHEMICALLY DEFINED TOXINS OF LOW MOLECULAR WEIGHT

Long before the discovery of the highly toxic aflatoxins, some moulds (especially the *Aspergillus flavus* group) were known to produce a series of substances toxic *per os.* Both their ubiquity and presence as contaminants in foods attracted serious world-wide attention. As the history of aflatoxins appears to be classical, and as aflatoxins appear to be toxic even for insects, it will be useful to briefly review these important toxins of low molecular weight.

1. Aflatoxins

Research on aflatoxins has been active since the outbreak of "turkey X" disease in 1960 (Sargeant *et al.,* 1961). The generic name "aflatoxins" was subsequently applied to the group of toxic compounds produced by some aspergilli and penicillia (Kulik and Holaday, 1966); recently aflatoxin was demonstrated only from *A. flavus* and *A. parasiticus* (Wilson *et al.,* 1968). A series of papers dealt with the production of aflatoxins on natural solid substrates such as ground peanuts, crushed wheat and rice, with optimal yields up to 200 mg aflatoxin/kg substrate. Yeast extract and corn-steep liquor play an important role in semi-synthetic media, influencing both yield and the ratio of the aflatoxin components. A submerged culture yielded up to 212 mg/litre

(Hayes *et al.*, 1966). The original aflatoxin was soon shown to be a complex of closely-related toxic compounds, aflatoxins B_1, B_2, G_1 and G_2. The production ratio of these components depends on the strain, medium and other conditions of growth. B_1 and B_2 emit blue visible light, and G_2 fluoresces yellow-green. The complex is usually richest in B_1 and poor in B_2 and G_2. Chemical structures have been proposed for B_1 and G_1 (Fig. 3); B_2 and G_2 are the dihydro derivatives of the parent compounds (Asao *et al.*, 1965).

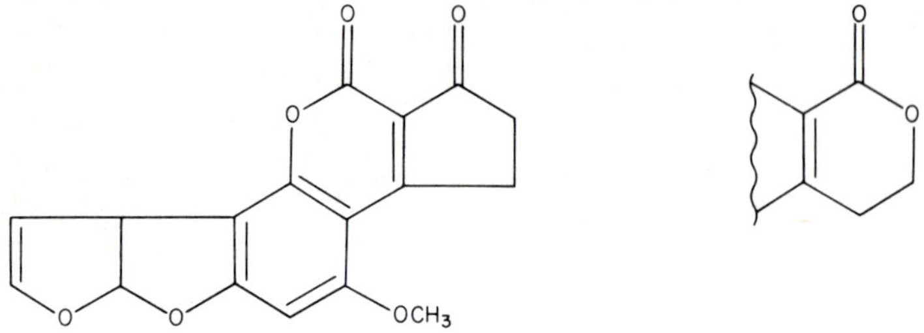

B_1 G_1

Fig. 3. Chemical structures of aflatoxin B_1 and G_1.

Aflatoxins are hepatotoxins, lethal *per os* to most animal species in large doses and causing histological changes in small doses. The toxicity is relatively high: the LD_{50} of B_1 *per os* for ducklings is 0.36 mg, B_2 1.69 mg, G_1 0.78 mg, and G_2 3.45 mg/kg body wt (Carnaghan *et al.*, 1963). Toxicity to a series of laboratory animals has been examined and many symptoms described. Of great general interest is the suppression of DNA synthesis and mitosis, an abnormal production of giant cells and an induction of bacteriophage in lysogenic bacteria (Legator, 1966). Also, they decrease the activity of certain mitochondrial enzymes (Brown, 1965), inhibit the incorporation of leucine-^{14}C into protein (Smith, 1963), inhibit a RNA polymerase (Sporn *et al.*, 1966), and cause precancerous lesions (Richir *et al.*, 1964). Detailed information about aflatoxins is reviewed by Carnaghan (1964), Abrams (1965) and Wogan (1966).

As mentioned above, aflatoxins cause serious changes in metabolic activity of vertebrates and they may also be important in insects. Pure B_1 and a mixture of aflatoxins are potent toxins for *Heliothis virescens* (Gudauskas *et al.*, 1967). The most sensitive stage is the newly-hatched larva and the toxic effect decreases with larval age. A chemosterilizing activity in insects was recently reported by Matsumura and Knight (1967). As the aflatoxin complex exhibits no specific activity on distinct groups of animals–it is toxic and carcinogenic in vertebrates–it is unlikely to be used in microbial control, but its activity in mammals is so interesting that it poses many questions which may be solved in insect pathology.

2. Destruxins

Destruxin B is another insecticidal metabolite of fungi with a defined molecule. Beginning in 1954, Kodaira wrote a comprehensive series of papers about fungal toxins (reviewed in Müller-Kögler, 1965). He isolated two toxic substances, destruxin A and destruxin B, from the culture filtrate and mycelium of *M. anisopliae* (Kodaira, 1961, 1962). Tamura *et al.* (1965) and Tamura and Takahashi (1969) also isolated them from *M. anisopliae (Oospora destructor)* on Czapek-Dox medium containing 0.5% peptone. The culture filtrate was treated with charcoal, the toxin eluted with *n*-butanol, extracted with benzene and purified on a neutral alumina column. Yields of 13-15 mg/litre culture broth were obtained. Both the toxins, when applied intraperitoneally, killed mice at 1.8 and 17.0 mg/kg body wt, a level very similar to that of aflatoxin. When injected into silkworm larvae in instar V these toxins caused immediate paralysis and death at the lowest dose of 0.3 μ/g body wt; orally or by contact they were atoxic. With *G. mellonella,* destruxin A is approximately twice as toxic as destruxin B (D. W. Roberts, personal communication).

Suzuki *et al.* (1966) have elucidated the structure of destruxin A. Chemically, destruxin B is a cyclic depsipeptide (Tamura *et al.*, 1965). In Fig. 4, parallels can

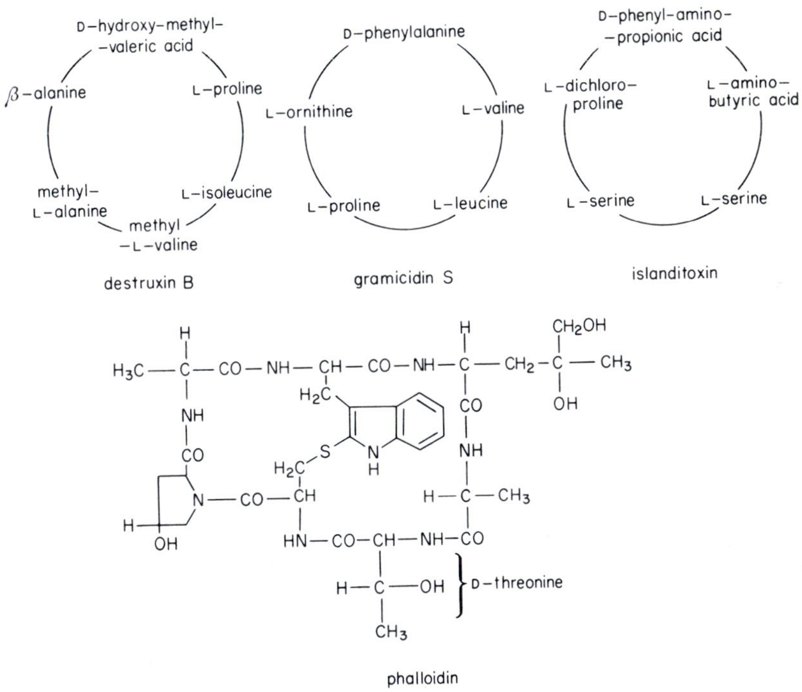

Fig. 4. Chemical structures of some toxic compounds from fungi and bacteria.

be drawn between the structures of destruxin B and other polypeptidic toxic substances, such as Gramicidin S, a cyclopentapeptide antibiotic from *Bacillus brevis*; phalloidin from the agaric fungus *Amanita phalloides* (Wieland, 1963); or islanditoxin, a chlorine-containing cyclopeptide from *Penicillium islandicum* (Kobayashi *et al.*, 1958). All these peptides are highly toxic *per os* for mammals, all contain one D-amino acid, but only one, destruxin B, was studied in insect pathology and adjudged entomotoxic; the toxicity of the others to insects is still doubtful. (See also Suzuki *et al.*, 1966; Tamura and Takahashi, 1970.)

Another toxic depsipeptide "beauvericin" has just been described by Hamill *et al.* (1969). It was removed from the mycelium of *Beauveria bassiana* with methanol, extracted into ethyl acetate and purified by chromatography on basic alumina. The compound contains three units each consisting of (L)-*N*-methyl phenylalanine and (D)-α-hydroxy isovaleric acid in a macrocyclic ring. It possesses weak activity against gram-positive micro-organisms, is toxic to the brine shrimp *(Artemia salina)* and slightly toxic to mosquito larvae.

3. Other Substances

In the literature many substances of low molecular weight toxic to vertebrates are described, but they have not been studied in insects. For example sporidesmin from potato-carrot cultures of *Pithomyces chartarum* resembled another fungal toxin, gliotoxin (Bell *et al.*, 1958). In their molecules, both toxins have disulphide bridges, the destruction of which detoxifies the molecule. Miyake *et al.* (1940) and Tsunoda (1951) isolated several toxigenic strains from mouldy "yellowed" rice, namely *Penicillium islandicum, P. rugulosum, P. toxicarium, P. citreoviride* and *P. citrinum,* and their toxins were named islanditoxin (Fig. 4) and luteoskyrin. In 1964-65 other fungal toxins were discovered such as those from *Aspergillus amstelodami* (Rabie *et al.*, 1964), *A. wentii,* and ochratoxin A from *A. ochraceus.* The toxicity of the latter when fed to ducklings is of the same order as that of aflatoxin B_1 (van der Merwe *et al.*, 1965). *A. flavus* is a potent source of other mycotoxins of low molecular weight. For example: oxalic acid, aspergillic acid, tremorgenic substance, kojic acid (gamma pyrone) and neurological toxin have been found in various foods contaminated with this fungus. All toxins of *A. flavus,* other than aflatoxins, were reviewed by Wilson (1966), some other fungal toxins by Wright (1968).

B. UNDEFINED TOXINS

A toxin acting on *Musca domestica, Gastrophysa cyanea* and *Gnorimoschema operculella* was thought to be present in germinating spores of *Beauveria bassiana* by Dresner (1950). It seemed to be stable and acted both as a stomach and a contact poison. However, Steinhaus and Bell (1953) were unable to confirm these results. Schaerffenberg (1957) extracted an acetone-soluble toxin from cockchafers, *Melolontha* sp., infected with *B. bassiana.* It was given orally to larvae of the Colorado beetle *Leptinotarsa decemlineata,* which died with typical symptoms of toxic action. A toxin produced *in vitro* by isolates of *B. bassiana* was bioassayed by injection into *Galleria mellonella* larvae by West and Briggs (1968). They found that isolates from infected insect hosts were better toxin producers than were isolates repeatedly subcultured on media and that the toxin titre varied with aging of the culture. Roberts (1966a, b, 1969) described a toxin produced by *M. anisopliae* which was more abundant in submerged than in surface cultures in a medium with either an inorganic or an organic nitrogen source. On injection into larvae of *G. mellonella* the culture filtrates induced paralysis similar to that occurring in infected larvae. By injection, Yendol *et al.* (1968) found freeze-dried filtrates from cultures of *Entomophthora apiculata* toxic to both *G. mellonella* larvae and the face fly *Musca autumnalis,* whereas similar preparations from *E. virulenta* were toxic only to adult face flies; the filtrates caused blackening and death after two days. Beard and Walton (1965) described the effect of the mycotoxin from *A. flavus* var. *columnaris* in cultures of the house fly. In these affected cultures eggs hatched, but the maggots soon died. The same result was obtained when eggs were added to fly medium on which the fungus had been allowed to grow to an advanced stage. In a new paper on the milkweed bug, *Oncopeltus fasciatus,* Beard (1968) stated that the toxic metabolite affecting milkweed bugs was unlikely to be the same as that toxic for fly maggots, because the medium on which the fungus is grown affects the metabolic end-products. However, he found that the toxin formed in modified Diener's medium, that from milkweed seed and that from the fly medium (dog meal and yeast) acted similarly, although none of them is similar in their physical properties to aflatoxins. Identification of these toxins is in progress. All these results are interesting and some may serve as the starting points of further investigations, which may reveal a series of biochemical problems.

C. THE TOXINS OF HIGH MOLECULAR WEIGHT: ENZYMES

Various fungal enzymes can be of considerable interest in insect pathology. They are often secreted in significant quantities into the culture media and into the host body, from both of which they can be isolated by reliable methods of protein chemistry. Therefore they can be deemed a potent means of penetration into the insect body and of digesting tissues or haemolymph. Thus one might anticipate many hydrolytic enzymes in the culture filtrates of entomopathogenous fungi (Burnside, 1930; Sawyer, 1933; Turian, 1952 and others). Huber (1958) found a pronounced lipolytic enzyme (splitting soya oil) from *M. anisopliae* and *A. flavus*; a glycogenase from *M. anisopliae*; a proteolytic enzyme acting on gelatine from *A. flavus*; a proteolytic enzyme acting on milk and an urease activity from *Cordyceps militaris, B. bassiana* and *A. flavus*; a considerable amount of amylase from *B. bassiana* and *A. flavus*; and a low asparaginase activity from all four fungi. In submerged and stationary cultures of *B. bassiana,* excretion of chitinase depended on the age of the culture (Samšiňáková, unpublished 1968). Liberation of *N*-acetylglucosamine from pure chitin and from integument of *G. mellonella* larvae was estimated by titration and chromatography.

Jönsson (1968) studied proteolytic enzymes of 10 insect-pathogenic species of *Entomophthora,* of which *E. coronata* gave the highest yield: the best medium was liver extract medium. The increase of pH during cultivation and the optimal temperature were established, including scaled-up fermentation. Prasertphon (1967) and Yendol *et al.* (1968) also reported proteinous toxins *in vitro* from the Entomophthorales. Culture filtrates of *E. coronata* and *E. apiculata* were toxic to *G. mellonella* by injection, but *E. virulenta* and *E. thaxteriana* filtrates were not. Adult face flies, *Musca autumnalis,* were susceptible to both *E. coronata* and *E. virulenta* filtrates.

Kučera and Samšiňáková (1968) separated proteases of *B. bassiana* from compounds of low molecular weight in culture broth by gel filtration. They showed that the proteolytic complex toxic to *G. mellonella* could be separated on Sephadex G-75 into two components, which differed in their molecular weight and in the inhibition by ethylenediaminetetraacetate (Kučera, unpublished). The LD_{50} of the toxic protease preparation when injected was 90×10^{-3} tyrosine units of proteolytic activity per larva, which places it among the proteases of moderate toxicity (Fig. 2). Obviously proteases may be one type of active toxic component in the enzymic complex and they damage very quickly and specifically some principal physiological functions by attacking biologically active proteins. Investigation of their properties would be useful and may solve some questions about the mechanisms of pathogenicity of fungi.

VI. Practical Possibilities and Perspectives

Knowledge of toxins or toxic metabolites can be exploited in biological control in two different ways: either directly to produce commercial microbial insecticides, or indirectly for deeper understanding of the mode of pathogenicity of a toxin producer.

As far as commercial preparations of toxins are concerned, the only practical achievements have been the use of microbial insecticides based on *B. thuringiensis* (Chapter 3). The crystalline toxin, which is extremely potent and *specific* to a wide range of Lepidoptera, could be applied safely even to processed foodstuffs. At present it plays a key role in the pathogenesis of microbial insecticides. The "heat stable exotoxin" might be of practical use in insect control, if it proves to have a very low toxicity to mammals. The cardinal criterion for judging the practical possibilities of application is economic and depends in many respects not only on the biological effectiveness of the preparation in question, but also on the trade situation and local public health regulations. In many respects the latter may be a limiting factor, although such limitations are sometimes a result of the novelty of the method, rather than practical experience.

Even though the use of partially purified toxins or toxic metabolites in biological control may appear expensive financially, it may be profitable under certain circumstances. For instance, it may be undesirable to use the live micro-organisms or their whole toxin complex if they form, as well as the desirable toxin, other toxins dangerous to mammals or other insects. The commercial production of toxins and toxic metabolites is the exclusive realm of fermentation technology or chemical synthesis. It should be discussed and considered by experts qualified in these fields, because the laboratory techniques so often used by insect pathologists are frequently too remote from industrial requirements.

At present, indirect employment of recent knowledge of toxins is much more rewarding, as it can contribute to many branches of insect pathology. Knowledge of the nature of particular toxins helps to explain their modes of action, to develop the optimal conditions for their production, and enables a tendentious selection of productive strains. Study of toxic metabolites may lead to discoveries of biologically active compounds, which may be fully or partly synthesized by the chemical industry as purely chemical products. Since the "antibiotics" include compounds very potent against some micro-organisms, while being of very low toxicity to mammals, some entomotoxic compounds—atoxic to mammals—might also occur in the repertoire of micro-organisms in general, not only insect pathogens. Furthermore, study of the modes of action of such relatively insect-specific compounds might reveal valuable new pathways for control, unique to the insect's physiology.

Also, studies of toxins as model systems, with insects as experimental animals, may contribute to some general biological discoveries. Insects are still not fully appreciated as experimental animals—they might play a similar role in general biology to that of bacteria and evince another broader goal to insect pathology. For these manifold reasons a closer tie with modern biochemistry, microbiology and physiology is sorely needed.

VII. Conclusions

Our purpose has been to review recent knowledge of bacterial and fungal toxins harmful to insects. Since concrete results in this field are limited compared with, for instance, medical microbiology, we have focused our main attention on the more general and basic problems. Our main task has been to bring a brief but comprehensible treatise to this scientific field, which would enable an insect pathologist to get a broader orientation of the problem. It is our wish that the reader should find this review useful for his further work. If his interest is stimulated in this promising field, this chapter will have fulfilled its purpose.

References

Abrams, L. (1965). S.Afr. Dep. Agric. Tech. Servs Tech. Commun. No. 35, pp. 1-8. Pretoria.

Asao Toyonobu, Büchi, G., Abdel-Kader, M. M. and Wogan, G. N. (1965). *J. Am. chem. Soc.* **87,** 882-886.

Barjac, H. de and Dedonder, R. (1965). *C.r. hebd. Séanc. Acad. Sci. Paris* **260,** 7050-7053.

Beard, R. L. (1968). *J. Invertebrate Path.* **10,** 438-439.

Beard, R. L. and Walton, G. S. (1965). *J. Invertebrate Path.* **7,** 522-523.

Bell, M. R., Johnson, J. R., Wyldi, B. S. and Woodward, R. B. (1958). *J. Am. chem. Soc.* **80,** 1001.

Benz, G. (1966). *Experientia* **22,** 81-82.

Bonventre, P. E., Lincoln, R. E. and Lamana, C. (1967). *Bact. Rev.* **31,** 95-109.

Brown, J. M. M. (1965). S.Afr. Dep. Agric. Tech. Servs Tech. Commun. No. 35, pp. 33-46. Pretoria.

Burnside, C. E. (1930). *U.S. Dep. Agric. Tech. Bull.* **149,** 1-42.

Cantwell, G. E., Heimpel, A. M. and Thompson, M. J. (1964). *J. Insect Path.* **6,** 466-480.

Carnaghan, R. B. A. (1964). *Proc. R. Soc. Med.* **57,** 414-416.

Carnaghan, A., Hartley, R. D. and O'Kelly, J. (1963). *Nature, Lond.* **200,** 1101.

Dresner, E. (1950). *J. New York ent. Soc.* **58,** 269-278.

Farkaš, J., Šebesta, K., Horská, K., Samek, Z., Dolejš, L. and Šorm, F. (1969). *Colln. Czech. chem. Commun. Engl. Edn.* **34,** 1118-1119.

Gudauskas, R. T., Davis, N. D. and Diener, U. L. (1967). *J. Invertebrate Path.* **9,** 132-133.

Hamill, R. L., Higgens, C. E., Boaz, H. E. and Gorman, M. (1969). *Tetrahedron Lett.* No. 49, 4255-4258.

Hannay, C. L. (1953). *Nature, Lond.* **172,** 1004.

Hayes, A. W., Davis, N. D. and Diener, U. L. (1966). *Appl. Microbiol.* **14,** 1019-1021.

Heimpel, A. M. (1954). Ph.D. Thesis, Queen's Univ., Kingston, Canada, 155 pp.

Heimpel, A. M. (1955). *Can. J. Zool.* **33,** 311-326.

Heimpel, A. M. (1963). *Bull. Am. chem. Soc.* **41,** 64-74.

Heimpel, A. M. (1965). *Proc. 12th Int. Congr. Ent.,* 1964, p. 736. London.

Heimpel, A. M. (1967). *Ann. Rev. Ent.* **12,** 287-332.

Huber, J. (1958). *Arch. Microbiol.* **29,** 257-276.

Jönsson, A. G. (1968). *Appl. Microbiol.* **16,** 450-457.

Kobayashi, Y., Uraguchi, K., Tatsuno, T., Sakai, F., Tsukioka, M., Sakai, Y., Yonemitsu, O., Sato, T., Miyaka, M., Saito, M., Enomoto, M., Shikata, T. and Ishiko, T. (1958). *Proc. Japan Acad.* **34,** 736-741.

Kodaira, Y. (1961). *J. facult. Text. Sci. Technol. Shiushu Univ.,* Ser. E. Agric., Sericult. **5,** 1-68.

Kodaira, Y. (1962). *Agric. Biol. Chem. (Tokyo)* **26,** 36-42.

Krieg, A. (1961). *Mitt. biol. BundAnst. Ld- u. Forstw.,* Berlin-Dahlem **103,** 1-79.

Krieg, A. (1967). *Mitt. biol. BundAnst. Ld- u. Forstw.,* Berlin-Dahlem **125,** 1-106.

Kučera, M. and Lysenko, O. (1968). *Folia microbiol.* **13,** 288-294.

Kučera, M. and Samšiňáková, A. (1968). *J. Invertebrate Path.* **12,** 316-320.

Kulík, M. M. and Holaday, C. E. (1966). *Mycopathol. Mycol. appl.* **30,** 137-140.

Kushner, D. J. (1960). *Biochem. J.* **75,** 386-395.

Kushner, D. J. (1962). *Can. J. Microbiol.* **8,** 674-688.

Kushner, D. J. and Heimpel, A. M. (1957). *Can. J. Microbiol.* **3,** 547-551.

Landy, M. and Braun, W. (eds) (1964). "Bacterial Endotoxins". Rutgers State Univ., New Brunswick, N.J.

Legator, M. (1966). *Bact. Rev.* **30,** 471-477.

Lysenko, O. (1963a). *J. Insect Path.* **5**, 78-82.
Lysenko, O. (1963b). *J. Insect Path.* **5**, 83-8.
Lysenko, O. (1963c). *J. Insect Path.* **5**, 89-93.
Lysenko, O. (1963d). *J. Insect Path.* **5**, 94-97.
Lysenko, O. (1965). *Proc. 12th Int. Congr. Ent.*, 1964, p. 717. London.
Lysenko, O. (1967). *In* "Insect Pathology and Microbial Control" (P. A. van der Laan, ed.), pp. 219-237. North-Holland Publ. Co., Amsterdam.
Lysenko, O. and Kučera, M. (1968). *Folia microbial.* **13**, 295-299.
Matsumura, F. and Knight, S. G. (1967). *J. econ. Ent.* **60**, 871.
McConnell, E. and Richards, A. G. (1959). *Can. J. Microbiol.* **5**, 161-168.
van der Merwe, K. J., Steyn, P. S. and Fourie, L. (1965). *Nature, Lond.* **205**, 1112-1113.
Miles, A. A. (1955). *In* "Mechanisms of Microbial Pathogenicity" (J. W. Howie and A. J. O'Hea, eds), pp. 1-16. Cambridge Univ. Press, London.
Miyake, I., Naits, H. and Tsunoda, H. (1940). *Beikoku Riyo Kenkyuto Hokoku,* **1**, 1.
Müller-Kögler, E. (1965). "Pilzkrankheiten bei Insekten". Paul Parey, Berlin and Hamburg.
Pope, L., Yolton, D. P. and Rode, L. J. (1968). *J. Bacteriol.* **96**, 1859-1862.
Prasertphon, S. (1967). *J. Invertebrate Path.* **9**, 281-282.
Rabie, C. J., Deklerk, W. A. and Terblanche, M. (1964). *S. Afr. J. agric. Sci.* **7**, 341-346.
Richir, C., Martineaud, M., Toury, J. and Dupin, H. (1964). *C.r. Séanc. Soc. Biol.* **158**, 1375-1379.
Roberts, D. W. (1966a). *J. Invertebrate Path.* **8**, 212-221.
Roberts, D. W. (1966b). *J. Invertebrate Path.* **8**, 222-227.
Roberts, D. W. (1969). *J. Invertebrate Path.* **14**, 82-88.
Sargeant, K., O'Kelly, J., Carnaghan, R. B. A. and Allcroft, R. (1961). *Vet. Rec.* **73**, 1219-1223.
Sawyer, W. H. Jr. (1933). *Ann. Bot., Lond.* **47**, 799-809.
Schaerffenberg, B. (1957). *Z. angew. Ent.* **41**, 395-402.
Šebesta, K., Horská, K. and Vaňková, J. (1969). *Colln. Czech. chem. Commun.* **34**, 1118.
Slein, M. W. and Logan, G. F., Jr. (1963). *J. Bacteriol.* **85**, 369-381.
Smirnoff, W. A. and Berlinguet, L. (1966). *J. Invertebrate Path.* **8**, 376-381.
Smith, R. H. (1963). *Biochem. J.* **88**, 50P-51P.
Smith, H. (1968). *Bact. Rev.* **32**, 164-184.
Sporn, M. B., Dingman, C. W., Phalps, H. L. and Wogan, G. N. (1966). *Science* **151**, 1539.
Steinhaus, E. A. and Bell, C. R. (1953). *J. econ. Ent.* **46**, 582-598.
Suzuki, A., Kuyama. S., Kodaira, Y. and Tamura, S. (1966). *Agric. Biol. Chem. (Tokyo)* **30**, 517-518.
Tamura, S., Kuyama, S., Kodaira, Y. and Higashikawa, S. (1965). *Proc. 12th Int. Congr. Ent.*, 1964, pp. 749-750. London.
Tamura, S. and Takahashi, N. (1970). *In* "Naturally-occurring Insecticides" (M. Jacobson, and D. G. Crosby, eds). pp. 499-539. Marcel Dekker, Inc. New York.
Toumanoff, C. (1931). *Ann. Parasitol.* **9**, 462-482.
Toumanoff, C. (1953). *Ann. Inst. Pasteur* **85**, 90-99.
Tsunoda, H. (1951). *Jap. J. Nutr.* **8**, 186-199.
Turian, G. (1952). *Mitt. schweiz. ent. Ges.* **25**, 44-46.
Wallengren, H. and Johansson, R. (1929). *Int. Corn Borer Invest.; Sci. Rep.* **2**, 131-145.
West, E. J. and Briggs, J. D. (1968). *J. econ. Ent.* **61**, 684-687.
Wieland, T. (1963). *Pure appl. Chem.* **6**, 339-349.
Wilson, B. J. (1966). *Bact. Rev.* **30**, 478-484.
Wilson, B. J., Campbell, T. C., Hayes, A. W. and Hanlin, R. T. (1968). *Appl. Microbiol.* **16**, 819-821.
Wogan, G. N. (1966). *Bact. Rev.* **30**, 460-470.
Wright, D. E. (1968). *Ann. Rev. Microbiol.* **22**, 269-282.
Yendol, W. G., Miller, E. M. and Behnke, C. N. (1968). *J. Invertebrate Path.* **10**, 313-319.

CHAPTER 10

The Protein Crystal Toxin of *Bacillus thuringiensis:* Biosynthesis and Physical Structure

J. R. NORRIS[1]

Shell Research Ltd., Milstead Laboratory of Chemical Enzymology, Sittingbourne, Kent, England

I. Introduction

The existence of a parasporal body or "Restkörper" in sporulated cells of *Bacillus thuringiensis* was noted by Berliner (1915) and Mattés (1927) at an early stage in the development of our knowledge of this insect pathogen, but the observation attracted little attention. It was not until 1953, when Hannay (1953) re-discovered the extra-sporal inclusion body, that it was really characterized and attention was paid to its nature and significance. With the realization that the parasporal body was a toxic, proteinaceous crystal, it became the centre of considerable attention. Subsequent work concerning the toxic characteristics of the crystal, and of its digestion products, is described by Cooksey in Chapter 11.

[1] I am indebted to Dr. H. J. Somerville and Dr. A. McKay for valuable discussions concerning the subject matter of this chapter.

The crystal itself proved difficult to study and it is only in the last few years that much progress has been made in determining its nature and the details of its biosynthesis.

II. Growth of *Bacillus thuringiensis*

B. thuringiensis grows only slowly and sporulates poorly on completely defined media containing glucose and salts (Singer *et al.*, 1966). Growth is improved by the addition of amino acids or casein hydrolysate but unless care is taken to balance the nitrogen content of the medium with an appropriate source of carbon and energy such as glucose, sporulation remains poor. Some studies have concerned the effects of varying amino acid composition of media on growth. Thus the presence of leucine or isoleucine produces growth inhibition which is counteracted by valine. Either threonine or serine added alone are inhibitory, but a mixture of the two is not, and serine inhibition can be overcome by methionine (Singer and Rogoff, 1964, 1968). These effects have not been explained and the observations seem to be at variance with what might be expected from known growth control mechanisms.

Most of the metabolic studies with *B. thuringiensis* have been carried out on various forms of simple semi-defined media. A particularly useful medium for this work contains 0.1% glucose, 0.2% yeast extract, 0.2% ammonium sulphate, 0.05% di-potassium hydrogen phosphate and mineral salts. During the exponential phase of growth in a medium of this kind, glucose is utilized and acetic and pyruvic acids accumulate, lowering the pH to a value of approximately 5.0 (Yousten *et al.*, 1969). The acetic acid is later metabolized and the pH again rises to reach neutrality after some 2 or 3 hr. Agents which interfere with the metabolism of acetate prevent sporulation of *B. thuringiensis* and such agents also inhibit crystal synthesis. An example is fluoroacetate, which may prevent acetate metabolism by inhibiting aconitate hydratase and is an effective inhibitor of both spore and crystal formation. In the presence of this inhibitor acetate continues to accumulate during the exponential growth phase and pH fails to rise. Another inhibitor of spore and crystal formation in *B. thuringiensis* is α-picolinic acid (Yousten *et al.*, 1969).

Erythromycin, at concentrations too low to inhibit growth of the bacterium, prevents the development of mature spores but allows crystal formation to proceed normally. Sporangia do not lyse in the presence of the antibiotic and the crystals remain inside remnant cell walls (Arescaldino, 1969).

Synthesis of an exocellular proteolytic enzyme is one of the early events associated with the onset of sporulation and the appearance of this enzyme is obligatory for the successful completion of the process. Mutants failing to produce the protease neither sporulate nor produce crystals. There is ample evidence of an extensive turnover of vegetative cell protein contributing towards the synthesis of both spores and crystals. Monro (1961) first showed that proteins, related antigenically to the crystal proteins, are not present in extracts of vegetative cells and do not appear until crystals are detected in the electron microscope. He also demonstrated that labelled amino acids, added during sporulation, are incorporated into crystal proteins. When labelled glutamate is added during vegetative growth or later during crystal formation, the label appears in the same peptides in the crystal protein irrespective of the time at which the amino acid was added to the medium. For details of the chemical structure of the crystal the reader is referred to Chapter 11.

Although defined and semi-defined media play an important part in investigations of the metabolism of growing cultures of *B. thuringiensis,* commercial production of spores and crystals for use as insecticides calls for the use of cheaper media in industrial-scale submerged fermentations, which are readily applicable to the production of *B. thuringiensis.* Media based on such cheap substrates as molasses, corn steep liquor, fishmeal and soybean have all been successful in promoting extensive growth and sporulation of the organism. The size of crystals forming in the individual cells varies somewhat from medium to medium. One successful medium for submerged fermentation contains 2% fishmeal, 1% starch, 0.1% calcium carbonate, 0.001% niacin and a salts mixture (Pendleton, 1969). Such media are usually used in fermentation tanks whose capacity may be measured in thousands of gallons. The optimum growth temperature for *B. thuringiensis* is about 30° C and good aeration is necessary at all stages of the culture if a high sporulation rate is to be achieved. Lowering the growth temperature to below 15° C can lead to an inhibition of spore formation although crystals may still be produced (Smirnoff, 1963).

III. Methods of Studying the Crystal

A. LIGHT MICROSCOPY

The mature crystal differs somewhat in shape in the various varieties of *Bacillus thuringiensis.* In many varieties it is a regular bi-pyramid and obviously crystal-shaped as seen in the light microscope. In other cases, however, particularly in some isolates of var. *thuringiensis* (serotype I), the crystal is much more irregular and it may be difficult to identify as seen in the light microscope. The mature crystal often exceeds one micron in length and half a micron in width and may account for some 30% of the total dry weight of the sporulated cell. It is therefore easily visible in the light microscope and the experienced microscopist has no difficulty in detecting the crystal, either within the sporulating cell, or freely lying after breakdown of the cell wall has released it from the sporangium.

In smears prepared from laboratory cultures the distinction between spore and crystal is relatively easy. Heat fixed smears stained with strong carbol fuchsin, naphthalene black, giemsa, crystal violet or victoria blue show the crystals deeply stained with the oval unstained spores clearly outlined by their coloured margins. The crystals do not stain well with the relatively mild reagents used, for instance, as the counter stain in a Gram stain. For observation within the sporangium, phase contrast microscopy of wet mounted preparations is the method of choice (Fig. 1) and indeed most workers today prefer it for all observations on the crystal. Hannay (1953) used nigrosin as a negative stain to

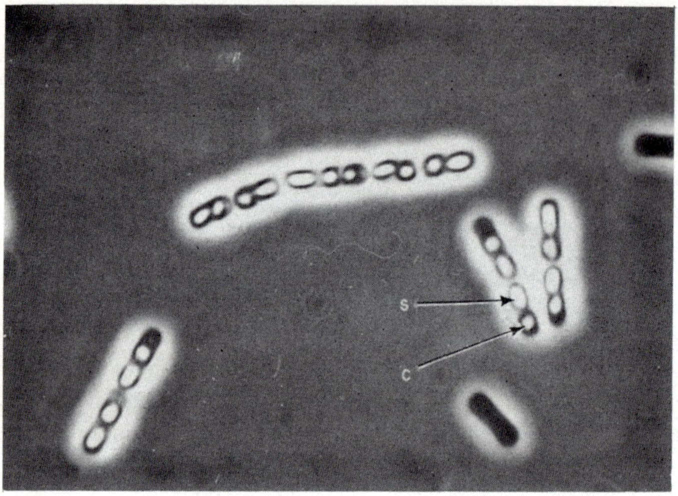

Fig. 1. Phase contrast photomicrograph of *Bacillus thuringiensis* sporangia (x3500). s = spore; c = protein crystal.

facilitate observation of the crystal within the sporangium. A method which I have found useful, particularly for observing crystals in commercial formulations containing a great deal of extraneous organic material, is to stain a heat fixed smear with strong carbol fuchsin and observe it with phase contrast optics. Then the crystals develop a characteristic refractility which makes them easy to distinguish from the amorphous background material. Using this technique it is possible to make accurate spore and crystal counts from material which is extremely difficult to analyse by other methods, although powder formulations still present problems.

B. ELECTRON MICROSCOPY

The first electron micrographs of the *B. thuringiensis* crystal were published by Hannay and Fitz-James (1955) who showed that the parasporal body was a regular bi-pyramidal crystal with surface structure in the form of rather coarse striations parallel to the base plane of the crystal. They used the relatively harsh technique of metal shadowing, the resolution of which is not great by modern standards and damage to the crystals was undoubtedly responsible for some artefacts. Labaw (1964) used the more sensitive carbon replica technique to study the surface structure of intact crystals and revealed more detail, which he interpreted as meaning that the basic protein unit of the crystal was a sphere with a diameter of approximately 8.7 nm.

Thin sections of sporulating cells containing crystals in various stages of development were studied by Norris and Watson (1960). These showed that the crystals of *B. thuringiensis* var. *alesti* (serotype III) were produced outside the exosporium of the developing sporangium and illustrated the maturation and release of the spores and crystals during the later stages of growth of the organisms. No details of the internal structure of the crystals were seen in these sections and indeed considerable effort was required before any details of internal structure of crystals were seen in thin sections (Norris, 1969). The technique used for fixation and embedding of crystal material is apparently critical. The best pictures of internal structure, either of free lying crystals or of crystals within sporangia, have been obtained using gluteraldehyde/osmium fixation and embedding in araldite by the method of Luft (1961). Sections were stained with lead citrate and uranyl acetate. Interpretation of thin sections of this kind has been considerably aided by a photo-optical system fully described by Norris (1969). Features seen in electron micrographs are of two types; real features representing structures actually present in the material being observed and non-systematic artefacts resulting from the processes of fixation, embedding and sectioning. If multiple copies of electron micrograph negatives showing crystal lattice structure are prepared and superimposed in such a way that the sub-units are out of phase by multiples of the lattice spacings, the real features superimpose and emphasize one another while the non-systematic artefacts tend to cancel one another out, and the real structure emerges more clearly (cf. Figs 2(a) and (b), and Fig. 3). Using these techniques Norris (1969) examined crystals of *B. thuringiensis* var. *Tolworthi* (serotype IX) and found ample evidence of regular arrangement of sub-units within the crystal.

IV. Biosynthesis of the Protein Crystal

The ability to produce one or more protein crystals per cell is the main character which separates members of the *Bacillus thuringiensis* group from the closely similar, but non-entomopathogenic, *Bacillus cereus*. Growth and sporulation of *B. thuringiensis* follows the course which is well described for *B. cereus* (Fitz-James and Young, 1969). The first detailed study of the changes which occur during spore and crystal formation was that by Young and Fitz-James (1959) using phase contrast microscopy, differential staining and electron microscopy. Chromatin material forms into an axial filament which becomes

(a)

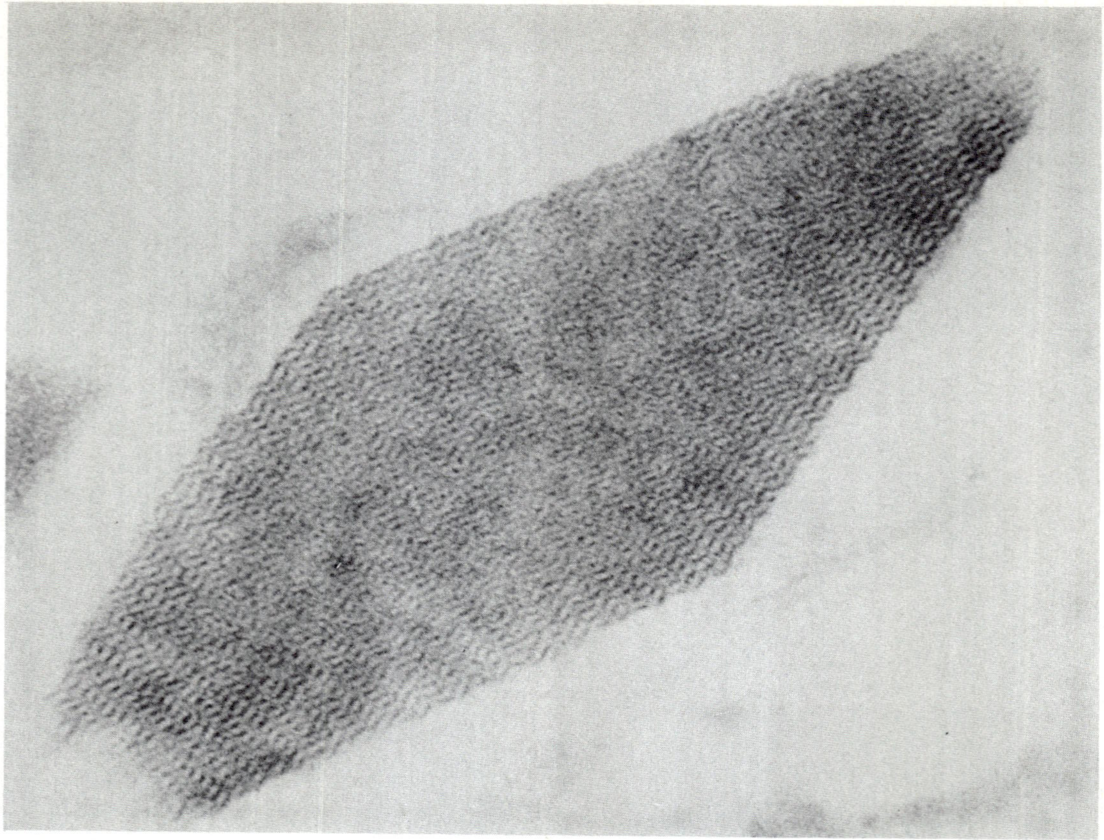

(b)

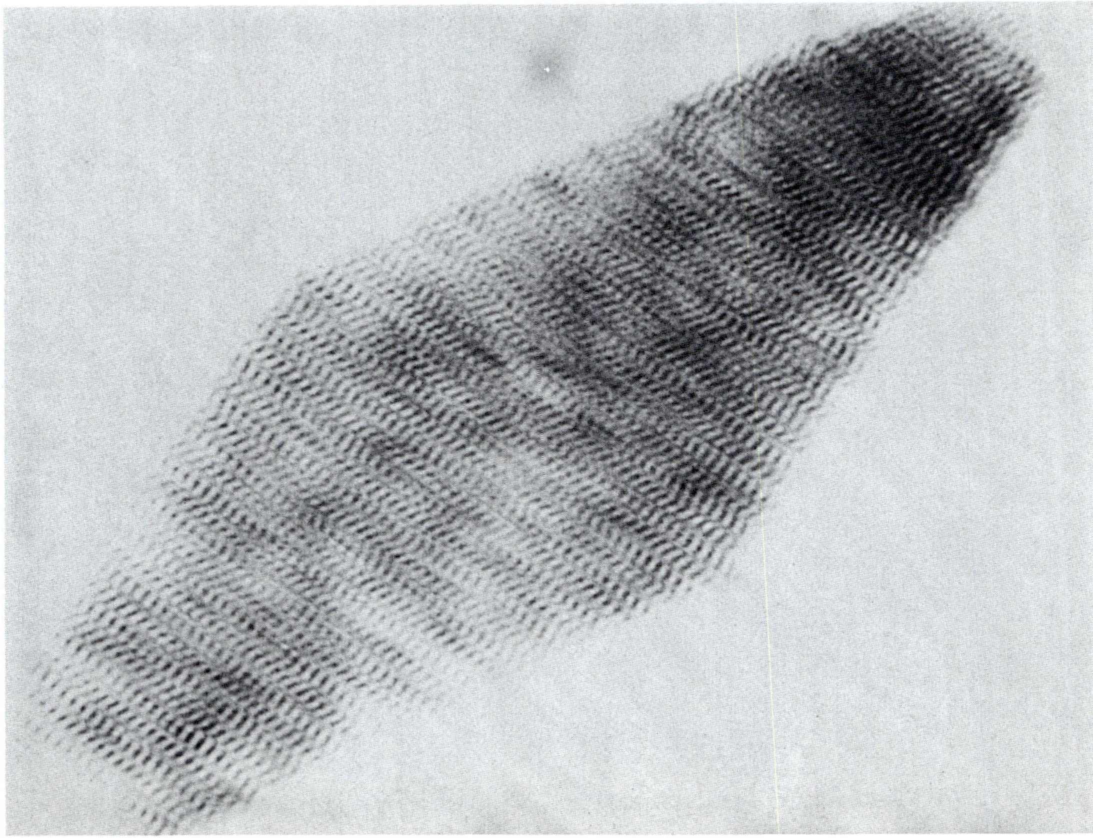

Fig. 2. Electron micrograph of a thin section through a crystal parallel to the long axis. (x256,000.) (a) Direct print from the electron micrograph negative; (b) Superimposition print from multiple negatives. (See text for details.)

Fig. 3. Superimposition print of an electron micrograph of a thin section through a crystal parallel to the base plane. (×256,000.)

partially enclosed in the forespore by invagination of the cytoplasmic membrane. Envelopment of the forespore by the invaginated membrane occurs in the usual way and this is followed by cortex and spore wall formation. In the phase contrast microscope the first sign of crystal formation, the appearance of a small rather refractile granule, is seen at an early stage in spore formation and this is confirmed in the electron microscope; this first sign of crystal material appears shortly after the cytoplasmic membrane has completed envelopment of the forespore.

With the majority of varieties of *B. thuringiensis,* spore and crystal formation are followed by lysis of the remnant of the sporangium wall releasing the spore and crystal separately into the growth medium (Norris and Watson, 1960). Several studies have confirmed that the crystal is outside the delicate exosporium which surrounds the spore itself (Fig. 4). With one organism however, *B. thuringiensis* var. *finitimus* (serotype II), the situation is different;

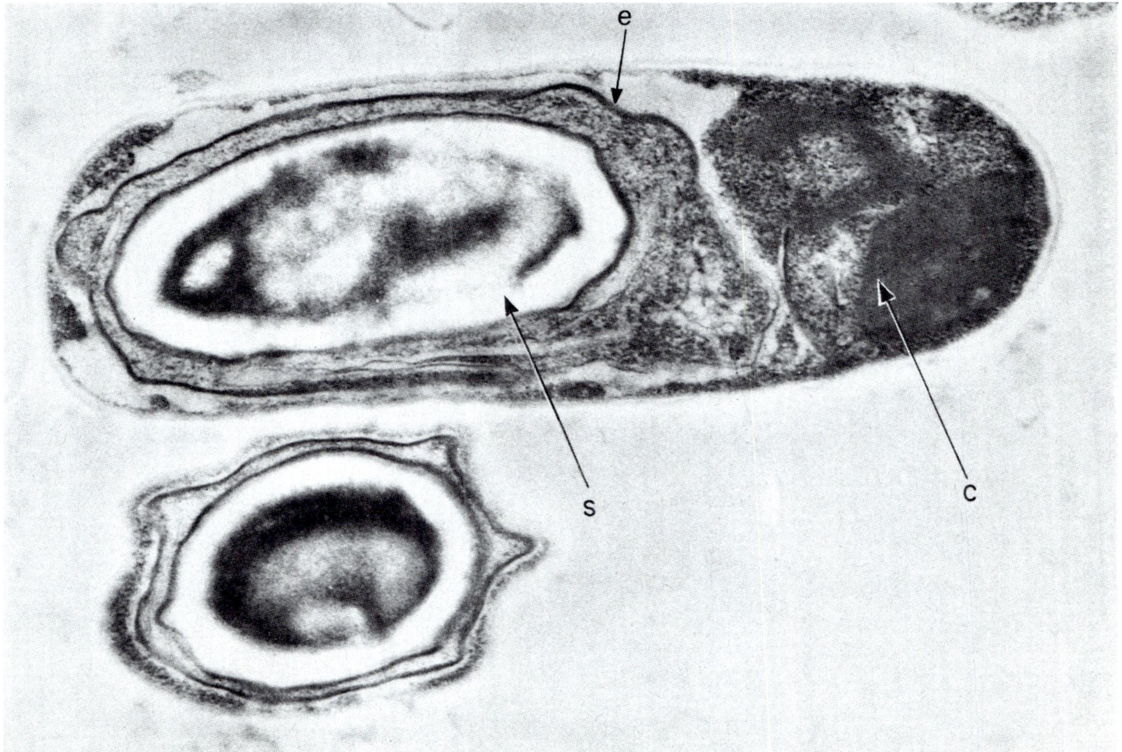

Fig. 4. Electron micrograph of a thin section through a sporangium of *Bacillus thuringiensis.* (×44,800.) s = spore; c = protein crystal; e = exosporium.

the spore and crystal do not separate from one another and are released from the disintegrated sporangium as a single entity. Electron microscope observation shows that in this bacterium the crystal forms within the exosporium and this membrane remains intact after release of the spore/crystal complex (Fig. 5).

In addition to following the production of the crystal visually by phase contrast or electron microscopy, it is possible to detect the formation of crystal antigens by harvesting cultures at various stages during sporulation, disintegrating the cells by ultrasonic irradiation in an alkaline buffer at pH 11 (or pH 10 in the presence of mercaptoethanol) and quantitatively determining, by titration against a specific crystal antiserum, the amount of antigen dissolved in the buffer (Norris, 1969). The appearance of crystal antigens in these extracts parallels the visual appearance of a discrete crystal. At no stage has it been possible to detect dissolved antigens in cell extracts at the lower pHs of the cell contents suggesting that the protein is not synthesized in soluble form prior to crystallization, but that the crystal begins to form as soon as protein appears in the cell—an important point when we consider the possible connection of the crystal protein with the sporulation process.

Several workers have studied crystal formation using the electron microscope and particularly significant are the recent observations of Somerville (personal communication), which suggest that the protein crystal develops in association with the exosporium of the developing forespore (Fig. 6, Somerville and James, personal communication). It is known that the exosporium has a complex structure with a degree of crystalline regularity in the basal membrane (Gerhardt and Ribi, 1964). Somerville and his co-workers have shown that the crystal protein is very similar in chemical nature to, and also shares antigenic determinants with, spore coat protein (Delafield *et al.*, 1968; Somerville *et al.*, 1968).

Aronson (1965) found that a substantial fraction of the RNA in sporulating cells is membrane-bound and suggested that this RNA may be a stable messenger for spore coat synthesis. These various observations could mean that the exposporium plays an important role in spore coat synthesis and that *B. thuringiensis* crystals arise as a result of a breakdown in the normal processes regulating synthesis of spore components.

V. Structure of the Crystal

Hannay's early electron micrographs of the crystal showed it to be a bi-pyramid with prominent surface striations spaced at approximately 29 nm. With the realization that this was a somewhat unique protein crystal it was natural that considerable interest should be generated in its physical structure. The carbon replica pictures of the crystal surface, published by Labaw (1964), revealed more detailed structure on the surface and he concluded that the basic protein sub-unit was a sphere approximately 8.7 nm in diameter. In a different

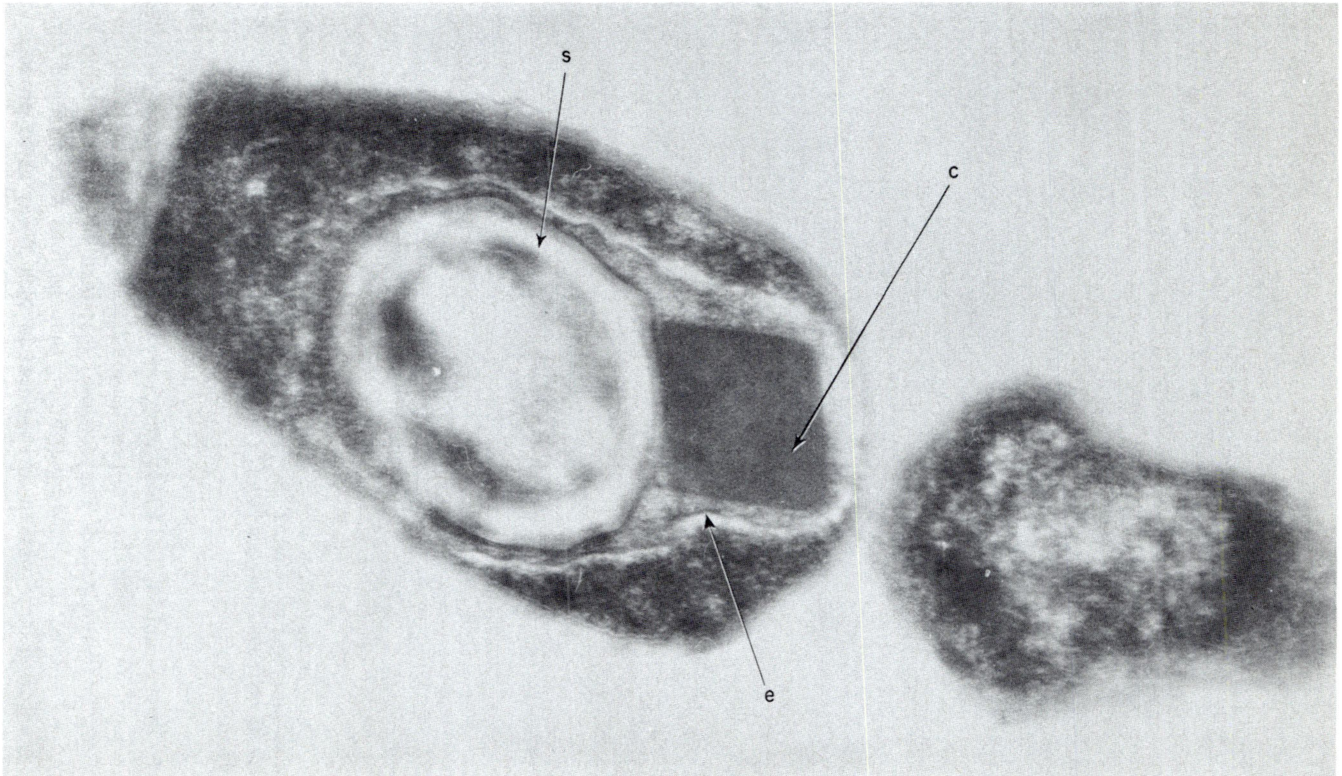

Fig. 5. Electron micrograph of a thin section through a sporangium of *Bacillus thuringiensis* var. *finitimus.* (×80,000.) s = spore; c = protein crystal; e = exosporium.

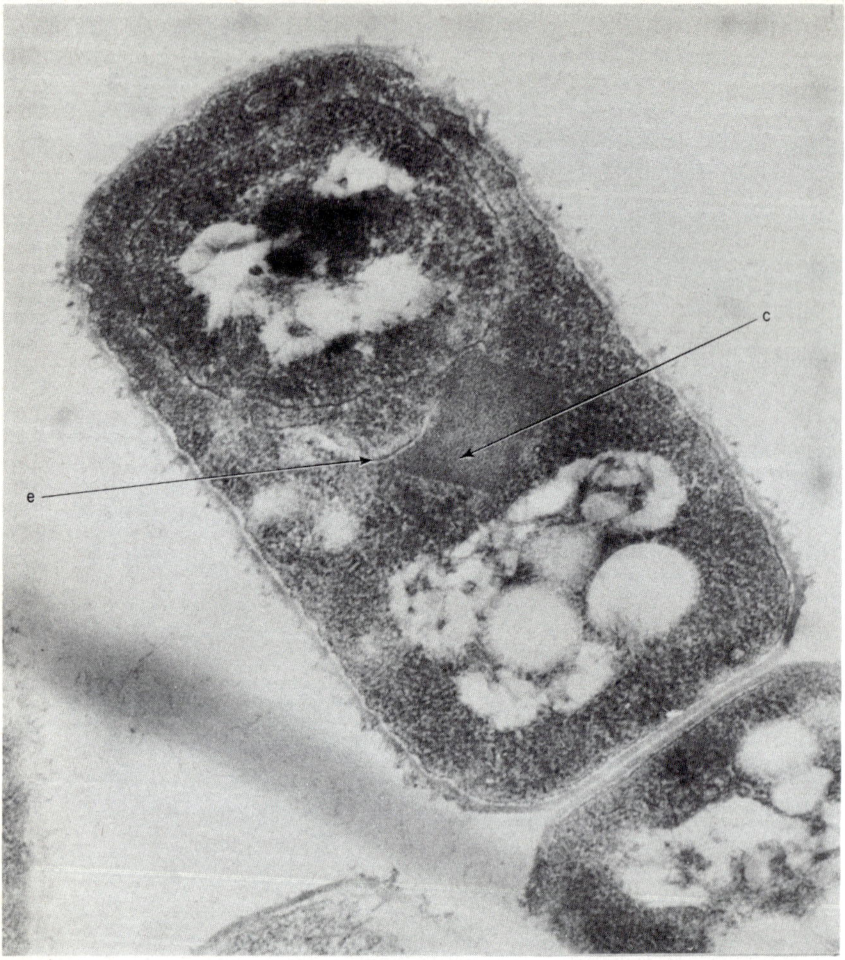

Fig. 6. Electron micrograph of a section through a developing sporangium of *Bacillus thuringiensis* showing association of the protein crystal with the exosporium. (×80,000.) Micrograph by H. J. Somerville and Mrs. C. James. c = protein crystal; e = exosporium.

approach, Holmes and Monro (1965) used X-ray diffraction methods to examine the crystal and interpreted the results as demonstrating that the protein sub-unit was rod- or dumb-bell-shaped. They claimed that their observations could be reconciled with those of Labaw by assuming that the rods were arranged with their centres on a close packed arrangement in such a way as to produce a four-fold screw symmetry. Figure 7 shows a model of a crystal built on a basis of

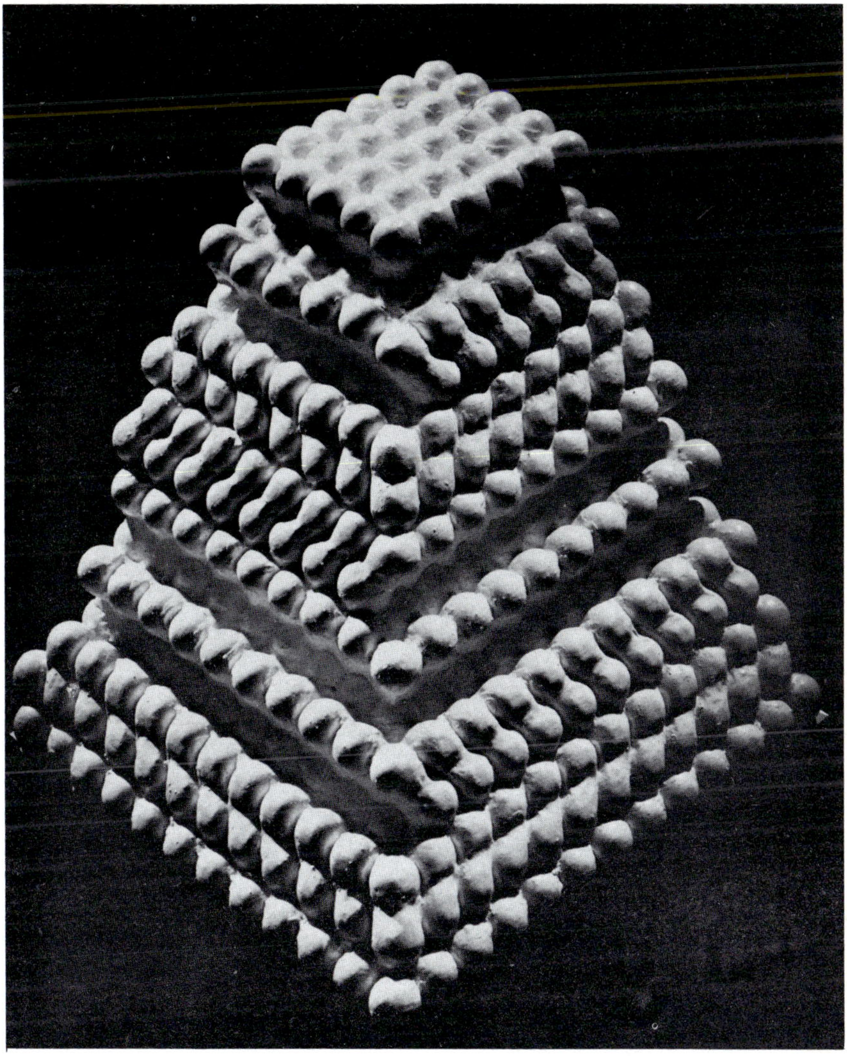

Fig. 7. Model of *Bacillus thuringiensis* protein crystal constructed on a basis of X-ray diffraction data.

the X-ray data as interpreted by Holmes and Monro (1965). It is evident from this model that the surface of the crystal should have certain characteristic features and that sections cut through the crystal, parallel to the longitudinal axis or parallel to the base plane, should show characteristic arrangements of the sub-units.

A. INTERNAL STRUCTURE

Norris (1969) obtained electron micrographs of thin sections through crystals either within cells or free lying (Figs 2 and 3). These suggested that the protein sub-unit was a rod shaped body, approximately 4.7 nm by 11.8 nm, and that the arrangement was compatible with the model based on X-ray diffraction data (Fig. 7).

B. SURFACE STRUCTURE

The crystal, particularly the fully formed crystal after release from the sporangium, is too thick to allow penetration by the electron beam in the electron microscope and special techniques must be employed to reveal the details of the surface structure of the crystal. The excellent pictures of Labaw (1964) reveal a very high degree of technical skill in their preparation; but the carbon replica method is relatively coarse and, although the results obtained at that stage were highly informative, they were not sufficiently detailed for reliable interpretation.

One of the problems with electron microscopy of the crystal surface is the nature of the preparative treatments. Extensive washing of the crystal certainly leads to erosion of the surface but detail on an unwashed crystal surface is probably masked by adsorbed protein from culture fluids and cell breakdown products. There is some variation in the behaviour of crystals from the different varieties and our present knowledge of the fine structure of the crystal surface is obtained by analysing pictures of crystals of different varieties. Nevertheless, there is ample evidence that the basic structure is similar in the different varieties and all of the techniques have been checked on several varieties.

Negative staining with phosphotungstic acid, which is often used to reveal the finest of detail in biological structures, would seem to hold little prospect of success for work on the large electron-opaque crystals, but in fact the tips of some crystals are sufficiently electron-transparent for negative staining and some of the most informative pictures have been produced by this method (Fig. 8). The best negative stained pictures to date have been obtained using crystals from *Bacillus thuringiensis* var. *finitimus.* It may be significant that these crystals are formed within the exosporium of the developing spore and it is possible that this delicate membrane protects the surface from masking or erosion effects. Similar, but less distinct structure, has been observed on the surface of crystals of other varieties.

Negative staining is not an easy technique and the operator is advised to practise for a considerable period of time before rejecting the method as unproductive. For examining *B. thuringiensis* crystals, freshly harvested bacteria (preferably grown on solid media) are washed in buffer and suspended in distilled water. The suspension is allowed to dry on formvar-coated electron microscope grids stained for 15 sec with 2% phosphotungstic acid in water at

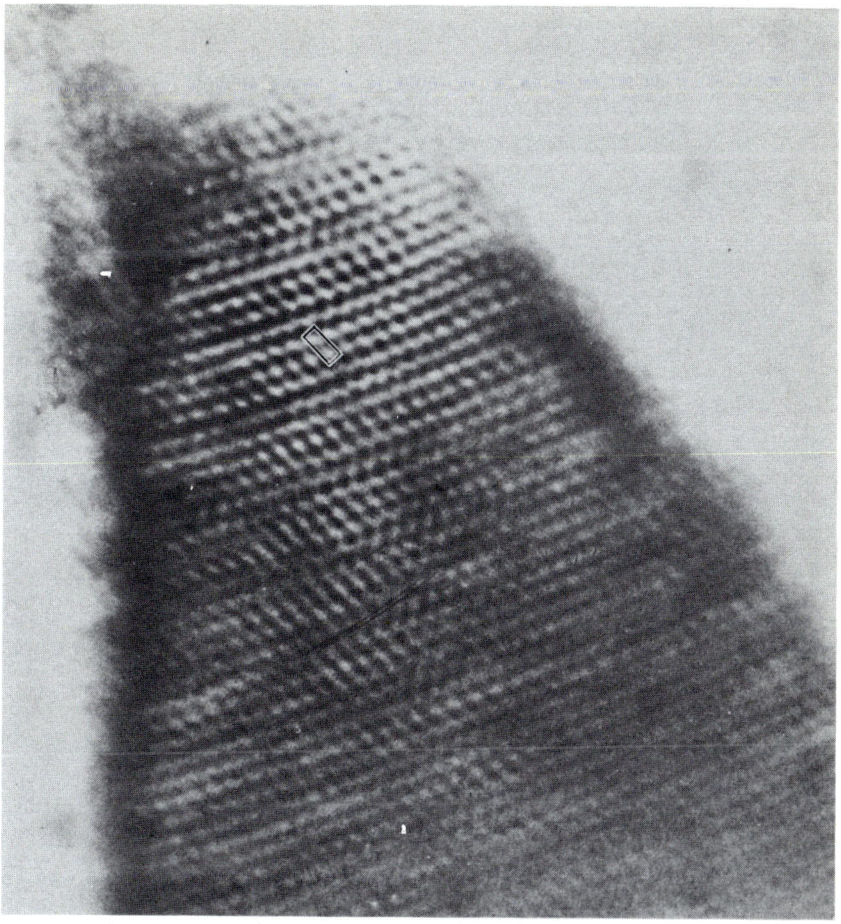

Fig. 8. Superimposition print from three negatives of an electron micrograph showing surface structure on a protein crystal of *Bacillus thuringiensis* var. *finitimus* revealed by negative staining with phosphotungstic acid. (See text for details of of photo/optic technique.) (x400,000.) Rectangle indicates a proposed dumb-bell-shaped sub-unit. Original photomicrograph by H. J. Somerville.

pH 7.0, and finally allowed to air dry. Preparations deteriorate rapidly in the electron microscope and photomicrographs are taken as quickly as possible after the grid is introduced.

Probably the recently introduced technique of freeze etching will yield highly informative pictures of surface structure of the crystals. This technique has the advantage that fresh material is rapidly frozen at the beginning of the preparative stage and that there will be little or no distortion due to fixation or drying.

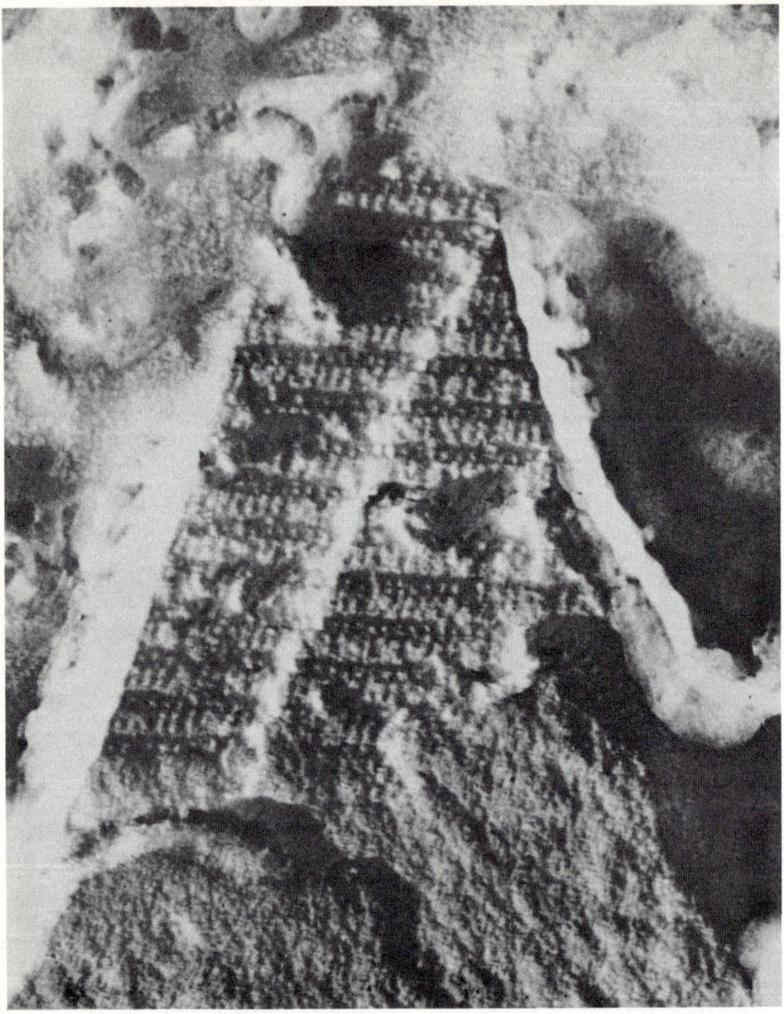

Fig. 9. Electron micrograph of a freeze-etched preparation showing part of one face of a *Bacillus thuringiensis* protein crystal. (×220,000.) Micrograph produced in co-operation with Dr. P. D. Walker.

Fig. 9 shows part of one face of a freeze etched crystal of *B. thuringiensis* var. *Tolworthi* (serotype IX).

Interpretation of electron micrographs is rarely simple. Even the mildest preparative techniques subject biological material to relatively harsh treatment and artifacts are common and sometimes subtle. Magnifications with the electron microscope reveal structure that cannot readily be checked by other means and it is important that as many different techniques as possible should be employed to prepare material for fine structure determinations. This is particularly true for the study of fine structure of the type present in the crystals of *B. thuringiensis.* Comparison of Figs 8 and 9 with the surface structure of the model in Fig. 7 shows that there is considerable similarity between the surface structure of the crystal and the model. At present, electron microscope evidence is not sufficiently strong to categorically confirm the structure described by Holmes and Monro (1965), but it is quite clear that if the structure of the actual crystal is not identical with the postulated structure it is certainly very similar to it. If the sub-unit indicated in Fig. 8 is indeed the basic protein sub-unit of the crystal, then it can be described as a dumb-bell-shaped structure measuring roughly 5.0 by 15.5 nm. These dimensions are compatible with those for the rod-shaped sub-unit seen in thin sections when account is taken of the shrinkage involved in fixation and embedding for microtomy.

VI. Future Developments

Knowledge of the synthesis and structure of the *Bacillus thuringiensis* crystal is today at an intriguing stage. After an initial period during which the technical problems associated with handling the crystal prevented a great deal of progress, the last few years have seen rapid developments in the subject. We can today present with some confidence a picture of a spore component over-produced, perhaps as a result of disturbance in control processes, and resulting in the crystallization within the cell of rod- or dumb-bell-shaped protein molecules in the form of crystal. It is clear that at least part of this molecule shares antigenic determinants with spore coat protein but several questions remain unanswered. Is the protein molecule completely homologous with a spore component or is only part of it derived from spore material? When dissolved in alkaline buffer the molecule clearly splits into several components (Chapter 11). Not all of the resulting fragments are toxic for caterpillars. What is the significance and relationship of the different toxic and non-toxic fragments in the original molecule? Are there bacterial strains which synthesize only part of the molecule and, if so, in what form do the molecular fragments accumulate? There is ample evidence that the crystal protein must be activated in some way, probably by digestion by the enzymes of the caterpillar gut, before it has a toxic action on the larva. It is most important that the full details of this activation process should be worked out and that the details should be related to what we know of the basic protein structure. Undoubtedly the most important question to be answered is the mode of action of the toxic fragment or fragments of the molecule in the caterpillar.

One striking feature of this work which must attract the attention of microbiologists and biochemists is the apparent similarity of the fine structure of the crystals of all the different bacteria and the marked differences in the toxicity of the proteins for various insect species. *B. thuringiensis* var. *finitimus* protein, for instance, is scarcely toxic at all for most insect species and *B. thuringiensis* var. *entomocidus* is many times more toxic for the silkworm, *Bombyx mori*, than is the closely related var. *subtoxicus*. There are numerous examples of these marked differences in toxicity (Table I in Chapter 13) and when we are able to explain them we shall be very much nearer to understanding the biological significance of the protein toxin.

The problems are, of course, formidable but they are receiving a great deal of attention and progress is rapid. We may confidently look forward to the solution in the near future of many problems concerning the fine structure and mode of action of *B. thuringiensis* crystal toxin. The topic is an important one for the person interested in insect control. We know little or nothing about the target site for this toxin in the insect. But we do know that the crystal has no detrimental effect on other life forms, including the majority of insects outside the order Lepidoptera. When we understand the nature of this target site and the way in which the *B. thuringiensis* protein toxin attacks it, we may well be in a position to synthesize novel types of insecticidal molecule capable of attacking a uniquely vulnerable site in the bodies of a number of important pest insects. We shall certainly have added a most fascinating and valuable chapter to the study of bacterial pathogenicity.

References

Arescaldino, I. (1969). *C.r. hebd. Séanc Acad. Sci. Paris* **269,** 1132-1135.
Aronson, A. I. (1965). *J. molec. Biol.* **13,** 92-104.
Berliner, E. (1915). *Z. angew. Ent.* **2,** 29-56.
Delafield, F. P., Somerville, H. J. and Rittenberg, S. C. (1968). *J. Bact.* **96,** 713-720.
Fitz-James, P. I. and Young, C. E. (1969). *In* "The Bacterial Spore" (G. W. Gould and A. Hurst, eds), pp. 39-72. Academic Press, London.
Gerhardt, P. and Ribi, E. (1964). *J. Bact.* **88,** 1774-1789.
Hannay, C. L. (1953). *Nature, Lond.* **172,** 1004.
Hannay, C. L. and Fitz-James, P. C. (1955). *Can. J. Microbiol.* **1,** 694-710.
Holmes, K. C. and Monro, R. E. (1965). *J. molec. Biol.* **14,** 572-581.
Labaw, L. W. (1964). *J. Ultrastruct. Res.* **10,** 66-75.
Luft, J. M. (1961). *J. biophys. biochem. Cytol.* **9,** 409-414.
Mattes, O. (1927). *Sber. Ges. Beförd. ges Naturw.* Marburg **62,** 381-417.
Monro, R. E. (1961). *Biochem. J.* **81,** 225-232.
Norris, J. R. (1969). *In* "Spores IV" (L. L. Campbell, ed.), pp. 45-58. Am. Soc. Microb.
Norris, J. R. and Watson, D. H. (1960). *J. gen. Microbiol.* **22,** 744-749.
Pendleton, I. R. (1969). *Process Biochem.* Dec. 1969, 29-32.
Singer, S., Goodman, N. S. and Rogoff, M. H. (1966). *Ann. N.Y. Acad. Sci.* **139,** 16-23.
Singer, S. and Rogoff, M. H. (1964). *Bacteriol. Proc.* 1964, p. 8.
Singer, S. and Rogoff, M. H. (1968). *J. Invertebrate Path.* **12,** 98-104.
Smirnoff, W. A. (1963). *J. Insect Path.* **5,** 242-250.
Somerville, H. J., Delafield, F. P. and Rittenberg, S. C. (1968). *J. Bact.* **96,** 721-726.
Young, I. E. and Fitz-James, P. C. (1959). *J. biophys. biochem. Cytol.* **6,** 483-498.
Yousten, A. A., Fisher, J. F. and Rogoff, M. H. (1969). *Bact. Proc.* p. 21.

CHAPTER 11

The Protein Crystal Toxin of *Bacillus thuringiensis*: Biochemistry and Mode of Action

K. E. COOKSEY

Division of Functional Biology,
Rosenstiel School of Marine and Atmospheric Sciences,[1]
University of Miami, Virginia Key, Miami, Florida, U.S.A.

I. Introduction

Bacillus thuringiensis has been known for many years but it was not until Hannay (1953) rediscovered the crystal-shaped parasporal body, and with Fitz-James (1955) showed that it was composed of protein, that research on this remarkable structure proliferated. Angus (1954, 1956) demonstrated that it caused most of the symptoms of toxicosis seen in silk worm larvae. The crystal has since been shown to play a key role in most susceptible lepidopterous larvae.

---

[1] Contribution No. 1146.

For the last 15 years the crystal protein, which Heimpel (1967) has recently termed the δ-endotoxin, has been studied extensively all over the world. This chapter describes progress made in the chemistry of the crystal. Sections II to IV E deal with techniques used to study the properties of the crystal and pertinent experimental detail. The general reader should refer to Sections IV F to VII, where the results presented in earlier sections and their practical applications are discussed.

II. Techniques for Preparation of Spores and Crystals

Four basic properties of the spore and crystal can be used to separate them. These are relative density, surface properties, solubility and germination of the spore. Each property has been exploited alone or in combination with others to achieve preparations which contain less than 0.03% contamination with the other particle.

One of the most successful methods has been a two phase liquid/liquid separation. The original description is that of Angus (1959), but many variations have been published (Table I). Basically a paste of spores and crystals is suspended in an aqueous salt solution in a separating funnel, a non-polar phase is added and the funnel agitated. When the phases separate spores predominate in the interfacial layer, whilst crystals remain suspended in the aqueous phase. Retreatments of the interfacial layer yield further quantities of crystals and shaking the aqueous layer with fresh lots of non-polar phase gives purer crystal suspensions. The author has tried most of the published methods with the Mattés isolate of *B. thuringiensis* and has found that of Murray and Spencer (1966) to be most useful. Many of the published methods are tailored to suit particular strains of *B. thuringiensis*. A method successful with one strain will not necessarily be the best for another.

A further method found promising is the separation of spores and crystals by a combination of surface charge and density in the continuous electrophoresis apparatus described by Hannig (1958). This utilizes a buffer film flowing between glass plates and produces relatively pure spores and crystals (Norris, unpublished). If the crystals are not required intact, the protein they contain can be prepared by solution and reprecipitation, as described later in this chapter. If the method for solution of the crystal protein is mild, pure viable spores can be obtained from the pellet after centrifuging and repeated washing.

III. Serology of Crystal Protein

One of the techniques of major interest to the protein chemist is immunology. It is particularly useful in the study of the protein crystal, for the biological activity of the protein cannot be demonstrated simply. An immuno-

Methods for the purification of crystal and spores from mixtures

Author	General type of method	Purity of preparations	% yield[a]
Angus, T. A. (1959)[b]	2-phase system: trifluorotrichloroethane	98% crystals	–
Murray, E. D. and Spencer, E. Y. (1966)[c]	2-phase system: chloroform	99.97% crystals	20
Goodman, N. S. *et al.* (1967)[d]	2-phase system: polyethylene glycol and sodium dextran sulphate	99.94% crystals	about 20
Pendleton, I. R. and Morrison (1966), Pendleton (1969)[e]	2-phase system: carbon tetrachloride, or xylene	98-99% crystals 99-100% spores	–
Bateson, J. B. (1965)[f]	2-phase system: trifluorotrichloroethane	99% crystals	0.8
Lecadet, M. M. (1965a)[g]	2-phase system: tetrabromoethane	99% crystals	–
Burges, H. D. (personal communication)[h]	Spores germinated with L-alanine, vegetative cells killed with streptomycin, crystals separated by isopycnic centrifugation	98.5% crystals	–
Gingrich, R. E. (1968)[i]	Spores separated by air-flotation in a water column; useful with commercially formulated insecticidal preparations	100% crystals, author claims no viable spores by culture check	36-38
Delafield, F. P. *et al.* (1968)[j]	2-phase system: sodium dextran sulphate and polyethylene glycol	99.9% crystals 99.7% spores	35 35

[a] $\frac{\text{wt of product}}{\text{wt of starting material}} \times 100\%$, or by actual count. Assuming a spore and crystal have equal weight or numbers, theoretical yield is 50% for both spores and crystals.

[b] *B. thuringiensis* var. *sotto* used: method also applicable to *berliner, entomocidus* and *alesti* strains, but complicated in the final purification step by difficulty in germinating spores of these organisms.

[c] *B. thuringiensis* var. *berliner, sotto* and *entomocidus* were used. Factors, such as the degree of mixing of the two-phase system, which influence the reproducibility of the method, are stressed.

[d] Suitable for most strains and based on the technique of Albertsson (1960).

[e] Spores prepared by a simple flotation technique. The spore-depleted mixture was then subjected to a two-phase separation process.

[f] Tri-n-butyl citrate used as a wetting agent.

[g] Applicable to several strains of *B. thuringiensis.*

[h] Method slow for large amounts of material because of slow germination of spores. This method is best used after one of the other procedures mentioned here. Monro (1961) describes a similar method.

[i] This method promises to be the best for the preparation of large quantities of crystals.

[j] This method is very similar to that of Goodman *et al.* (1967), but was developed for *B. thuringiensis* var. *alesti* isolate anduze, grown on agar.

logical test for the toxic protein is quicker and requires less material than, for instance, a toxicological one.

A. RECOGNITION OF SEROTYPES

Review of the many papers concerning crystal serology is complicated by the different techniques in use for the study of precipitin reactions. Antisera to whole crystals can be prepared by standard procedures. Some workers used whole crystals as antigens (e.g. Pendleton and Morrison, 1966), whereas others used dissolved crystal preparations (e.g. Cooksey, 1968). These three authors used rabbits to prepare antisera, whereas Krywienczyk and Angus (1960) used Guinea pigs. Pendleton and Morrison (1966) found only one main precipitin line per strain of dissolved crystal challenged with homologous antiserum. They concluded that groups of *B. thuringiensis* isolates distinguished by flagellar antigens (Bonnefoi and De Barjac, 1963) and vegetative-cell esterases (Norris, 1964), could be further subdivided on the basis of crystal antigens. De Barjac

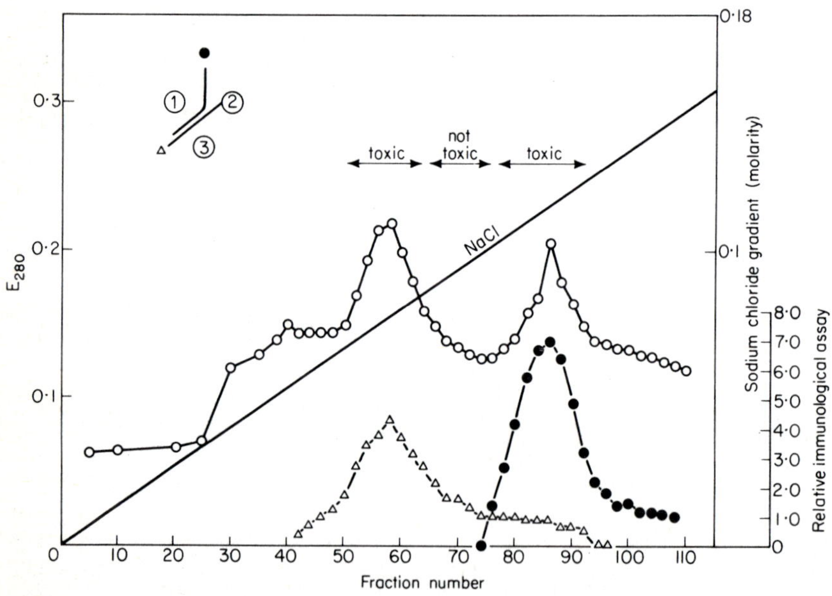

Fig. 1. Chromatography of undigested crystal protein on DEAE-cellulose at pH 9.0 in 0.05 *M*-glycine-NaOH buffer, with a gradient of 0 to 0.2 *M*-NaCl. ○, extinction at 280 nm. Diameter of precipitin circle in quantitative radial immunodiffusion assay: △, antigen characteristic of the Mattés isolate of *B. thuringiensis;* ●, second antigen of the Mattés isolate. Toxicity of fractions was measured by a feeding inhibition assay. Inset; Precipitin lines obtained when *B. thuringiensis* (Mattés isolate) dissolved crystal protein, (3), was challenged with homologous antiserum, (1). (2) is a control well, containing *B. thuringiensis* var. *tolworthi* soluble crystal protein (Cooksey, unpublished).

and Lecadet (1961) suggested that when alkali-dissolved crystal protein—as opposed to intact crystals—was used to immunize rabbits, the antisera reacted with soluble protein to give an increased number of precipitin lines. This may account for Pendleton and Morrison's detecting only one antigen per strain of crystal, although Cooksey, Kingham and Norris (unpublished) detected two major antigens with antisera produced with both crystal protein and intact crystals of the Mattés isolate of *B. thuringiensis*. This inconsistency could be explained by the fact that Pendleton and Morrison used 0.05*N*-NAOH (pH > 12) to dissolve crystals for immunodiffusion. Cooksey has shown, by means of a quantitative immunoassay, that power to react with antiserum is rapidly lost at pH 12 and above, therefore Pendleton and Morrison might have been measuring only the antigen most resistant to alkali or the one in highest concentration. This technical point however, does not detract from the conclusions of their paper. Cooksey (1968) found two major antigens in *B. thuringiensis*, Mattés isolate, when dissolved protein was challenged with homologous antiserum (Fig. 1). There was another faint line in Ouchterlony double diffusion tests that was not always seen. However, on occasion, the two single lines were seen to be double ones spaced very close together, making, in all, five lines. This total agrees with the results published by Krywienczyk and Angus (1967), although they used whole sporulated culture containing intact crystals emulsified in caterpillar gut secretion to challenge the antisera (Table II).

TABLE II

Cross reactions of crystal proteins from some strains of B. thuringiensis *and specific antibodies against crystal protein (Krywienczyk and Angus, 1967)*[a]

Crystal protein from:	No. of antigenic groupings shared using antisera:		
	sotto	*thuringiensis*	*entomocidus*
sotto	5	2	2
thuringiensis	3	5	3
entomocidus	4	2	5
finitimus	0	0	0
dendrolimus	1	3	2
subtoxicus	1	2	2
ashman	1	2	2
1-HA	4	2	4
morrison	2	3	2
alesti	3	2	1
tolworth	2	2	2
shvetsova	3	1	1

[a] Protein for immunization prepared by dissolving crystals in alkali followed by reprecipitation. Antigens obtained by emulsifying whole lyophyllised culture in *B. mori* gut secretion. (Copyright Academic Press.)

B. RELATION BETWEEN ANTIGENICITY AND TOXICITY

In view of the earlier remarks concerning the utility of immunology to detect crystal protein, it is particularly important to be sure that the antigenic property of the crystal is related to its toxic action. Any biochemical procedure for fractionation of the crystal protein utilizing an immunological assay system would not be valid if these two parameters were not related. Several workers have published papers in this field. One of the practical interests is in the replacement of a toxicological assay by an immunological assay. In order to examine the suitability of a crystalliferous insect pathogen for the control of an insect pest, a bioassay must be performed using the target insect and the insect pathogen. If the susceptibility of the insect to the various antigens contained in the strain described previously is known, then an immunological assay could replace the toxicological assay with a saving of time and effort. This idea depends on a greater knowledge of the crystal of *B. thuringiensis* than we have now. However, as we shall see, the relation between toxicity and antigen reaction is well documented. Krywienczyk and Angus (1960) showed that the three varieties of *B. thuringiensis,* var. *thuringiensis (berliner), sotto* and *entomocidus,* contained a common antigen. When this antigen was removed by precipitation with an antiserum, the supernatant protein was atoxic. They noted, however, that the strains were serologically quite different. A more recent study by Cooksey (1968) showed that there was a quantitative relation between the concentration of a particular antigen in a dissolved crystal preparation from the Mattés isolate of *B. thuringiensis* and the toxic properties of the same preparation. The quantitative immunoassay was based on the single diffusion method of Mancini *et al.* (1963). There have been several other quantitative immunological assays which could be applied to the analysis of the crystal antigen.

The serology of crystal protein-fractions prepared by proteolysis has attracted less attention than has serology of the undigested crystal protein. Pendleton and Morrison (1967), in addition to scanning 93 isolates of *B. thuringiensis* for intact crystal serotype, compared the same isolates on the basis of the serology of digested crystals. The crystals were digested *in vitro* with regurgitated gut enzymes of *Pieris brassicae* and used to challenge antisera prepared against purified intact crystals. Many of the antigenic patterns were found to change when compared with undigested crystals. Some antigens were lost, others were gained and the '*i*' antigen was a very frequent component of the digested crystal serotype. Krywienczyk and Angus (1967) on the other hand found many more antigens than Pendleton. They found five precipitin lines when soluble crystal protein was challenged with homologous antiserum. When heterologous antisera were used, a lesser number of precipitin lines were found, e.g. *B. thuringiensis* var. *sotto* soluble protein challenged with homologous antiserum gave five lines, whereas, when *B. thuringiensis* var. *thuringiensis (berliner)* crystal protein antiserum was used, only two antigens were detected (Table II).

IV. Biochemistry of the Crystal Protein

A. SOLUBILITY

Proteins are composed of amino acids joined in peptide linkage, so an obvious first approach in the study of the crystal protein was to analyse for amino acid content (Table III). No unusual amino acids were detected. It must be assumed that the amino acids are in their natural L-form since their configuration has not been described. Nothing in the primary structure of the protein accounts for its toxic properties. Some properties can be explained, however. The low pK (pH 4.4), is caused by the large number of dicarboxylic acids not in the form of amides (about half of them). The insolubility of the crystal cannot be attributed to a high number of -S-S-bridges in the protein, as the cystine content of the protein is not high enough.

The claim of Faust and Estes (1966) to explain the insolubility of the crystal, needs careful consideration. They analysed specially cleaned crystals from three strains of *B. thuringiensis* and found an average of 0.36% silicon (by weight). Although this has yet to be confirmed in the literature, the idea that the crystal has a silicaceous framework offers an attractive explanation for its insolubility.

In order to study the structure of the crystal protein by the usual methods of the protein chemist, it is essential to dissolve it. This requirement poses a thorny problem. The published methods of solution achieve their result by chemical modification of the crystal protein structure. The use of high pH and reducing agents to break -S-S-linkages, liberates more free polypeptide chains than are present in the original crystal. As it is not possible to study an insoluble protein, workers in the field must treat the dissolved protein as the starting point for their studies, even though it is in effect, an artifact. It is particularly important not to break carbon-carbon bonds during solution, so the mildest method should be used. In studies of the protein as a toxin, the method of choice should also preserve the toxicity.

Angus (1956) investigated the dissolution of protein crystals, by alkaline buffers, then Lecadet (1966) showed the effect of the concentration of reducing agents on the rate of dissolution. She measured this rate by the fall in turbidity of a suspension of crystals. One of the most conclusive facets of this work, which demonstrated the role of the reducing agent, was the inhibition of the dissolution rate of crystal protein by cystine—the disulphide of cysteine. Lecadet also used urea, a protein denaturant known to be effective in "unwinding" the secondary structure of a protein by breaking hydrogen bonds. Anderson and Rogoff (1966) used urea in the presence of sodium borohydride; a procedure not recommended because of the danger of destroying peptide bonds. Crystals were not completely solubilized, even in the presence of high concentrations (0.1 *M*) of reducing agent at neutral pH (Lecadet, 1967a).

Disc electrophoresis gives a largely qualitative picture of the molecules present in solutions of the crystal. The patterns obtained from crystal solution in high pH buffers (up to pH 12) had no major differences from the pattern in a

TABLE III

Amino acid analyses of B. thuringiensis *crystals: grams of amino acid residues/100 g*

Reference	Somerville *et al.* (1968)	Angus (1956)	Lecadet (1965a)		Holmes and Monro (1965)	Spencer (1968)			Cooksey (unpublished)			
Esterase type[a]	*alesti*	*sotto*	*berliner*	*anduze*	*berliner*	*entomocidus*	*alesti*	*galleriae*	*kenya*	*kenya*	*berliner*	*berliner*
Crystals	+		+	+	+	+	+	+	+		+	
Protein		+								+		+
Aspartic Acid	10.7	9.6	12.6	11.0	11.9	14.0	13.0	15.5	12.4	13.2	12.7	11.2
Threonine	4.8	4.5	5.8	5.1	5.2	6.8	7.0	7.0	6.3	6.4	6.3	5.6
Serine	4.8	4.8	4.4	5.6	5.4	6.0	6.5	6.2	5.3	5.9	5.0	4.2
Glutamic Acid	11.6	11.8	12.0	14.3	12.5	16.0	17.0	14.5	13.7	14.1	13.0	13.2
Proline	3.5	7.5	4.4	4.9	4.0	4.4	4.3	4.7	3.4	3.9	3.8	3.4
Glycine	3.3	3.2	4.3	4.5	3.0	4.8	4.8	4.2	3.6	4.5	3.4	4.0
Alanine	2.9	2.8	3.8	4.1	3.1	4.8	5.0	5.0	4.0	5.0	3.9	4.7
Cystine	1.2	1.2	1.4	1.3	0.3	1.4	1.9	1.5	2.0	N.D.	N.D.	N.D.
Valine	6.0	5.3	5.0	5.1	5.7	7.8	7.4	6.4	5.8	6.8	6.0	6.1
Methionine	0.9	1.3	1.5	1.7	1.6	0.7	0.2	0.8	0.4	2.0	1.1	1.8
Iso-leucine	5.1	11.2[b]	4.4	5.1	6.3	6.6	6.4	6.3	5.6	6.7	5.6	5.4
Leucine	7.1		7.7	7.9	8.8	10.5	9.5	9.3	8.3	10.0	8.1	8.3
Tyrosine	5.9	6.8	6.6	5.9	7.0	6.5	6.7	6.7	5.8	6.6	6.9	5.7
Phenylalanine	5.7	8.6	6.8	5.2	8.1	6.7	6.8	6.6	5.9	7.0	5.6	5.8
Lysine	3.1	3.6	3.4	4.0	4.0	4.4	5.4	4.6	4.6	5.8	4.9	7.2
Histidine	2.2	2.7	2.7	3.3	2.5	2.8	2.8	2.8	2.8	2.4	2.5	2.2
Arginine	7.5	9.6	7.8	7.5	8.5	9.0	10.4	9.9	8.6	7.5	7.6	5.2
Tryptophan	1.9	2.6	2.1	1.8	5.2	2.3	2.3	1.9	N.D.	N.D.	N.D.	N.D.
Ammonia	1.9	N.R.	N.R.	N.R.	2.0	N.R.	N.R.	N.R.	1.9	2.3	1.6	1.4
Total recovered	97.1	96.6	98.3	105.1	105.5	117.4	113.9	90.1	100.4	98.0	110.1	95.4

[a] Norris (1964).
[b] Angus (1956) used a paper chromatographic method incapable of resolving iso-leucine and leucine.
N.D. not determined.

milder solvent (pH 9.5, β-mercaptoethanol, urea) (Cooksey, 1968). A similar solvent was also used by Delafield *et al.* (1968). However, a quantitative loss of the toxic fraction occurred at high pH (Table IV).

A systematic examination of the conditions, using the quantitative radial immunodiffusion assay (Chapter 27), showed that although urea was necessary for a complete solubilization of crystal protein, a higher specific toxin activity (i.e. toxic units/mg protein) was obtained without urea. The 0.05 *M*-carbonate buffer, pH 9.5, containing 0.05 *M*-β-mercaptoethanol, was chosen as a solvent for routine use after examination of buffers with pH values from pH 8 to 9.5, buffer ions *tris*-hydroxymethyl amino methane *(tris),* borate, phosphate and carbonate; reducing agents, thioglycollate (mercaptoacetate), β-mercaptoethanol, dithiothreitol; with and without urea.

TABLE IV

Toxicity of dissolved protein compared with that of intact crystals (Cooksey, unpublished)

Preparation[a] (Mattés isolate)	ED_{50}[b] (μg protein)	
	Expt. 1	Expt. 2
Intact crystals	0.027	0.033
Protein extracted at pH 12.0	0.063	0.057

[a] A suspension of crystals of known concentration was divided into two parts. One part was brought to pH 12 with 2 *N*-NaOH. After centrifugation the supernatant solution containing soluble protein was removed and titrated to pH 9.0 with 2 *N*-acetic acid. The other part was adjusted to the same protein concentration as the dissolved protein. Protein determination: Lowry *et al.* (1951).

[b] Toxin concentration was measured by bioassay, using inhibition of feeding of *Pieris brassicae* larvae (Cooksey, 1968).

B. PHYSICAL TECHNIQUES AND CHEMICAL MODIFICATION OF THE PROTEIN

One of the difficulties of working with a solution of crystal protein is keeping it in solution. The protein is known to undergo reversible subunit aggregation (Somerville *et al.*, 1968; Cooksey, unpublished). This means that the protein chains, liberated by hydrogen bond and disulphide bond breakage, reaggregate to form larger entities which finally precipitate. This may explain the author's original difficulty in ion-exchange chromatography (Cooksey, 1968). Lecadet (1966) has overcome this problem of reaggregation to some extent by alkylation of the free sulphydryl linkages with *p*-chlormercuribenzoate. Cooksey has used iodoacetamide for the same purpose. It is interesting to note that alkylated protein, free from unalkylated protein, reacts with antiserum prepared against unalkylated soluble protein.

With the ultracentrifuge, Lecadet (1966) found four components in alkylated protein, the ratios of which changed with the pretreatment of the preparations—a result which may possibly be explained by the reversible association-dissociation phenomenon. The sedimentation coefficients were approximately 0.8 *S*, 5 *S*, 9 *S* and 27 *S*. In general, the proportion of slow sedimenting peaks was greater when the crystals were treated with reducing agent for a longer time. A coefficient of 0.83 *S* corresponds to a polypeptide with a molecular weight of about 10,000. Holmes and Monro (1965) found similar fractions (0.8 *S* and 4.1 *S*) as did Cooksey (1.1 *S* and 5.0 *S*). Watanabe *et al.* (1967) had slightly different results, 2.8 *S* and 3.8 *S*, with *B. thuringiensis* var. *sotto* as opposed to the var. *thuringiensis* isolates used by the other workers. Only Lecadet reported significant quantities of material with sedimentation coefficients greater than 5 *S*. These differences are probably partly explained by the use of different solvents. Watanabe *et al.* dissolved the crystal in sodium hydroxide, whereas Lecadet and Cooksey used carbonate buffers with reducing agents. Watanabe *et al.* used phosphate buffer at pH 7.8 with 0.5 *M*-urea in the ultracentrifuge tube in which some reassociation of the protein subunits must have occurred. This probably explains the absence of a 1 *S* component in his system.

C. CHROMATOGRAPHIC TECHNIQUES FOR SEPARATION OF THE POLYPEPTIDES OF CRYSTAL PROTEIN

Molecular exclusion chromatography or gel-filtration has been used to prepare protein fractions of restricted molecular weight range. Watanabe *et al.* (1967) found that crystals in solution at pH 11.5 and chromatographed at pH 7.8 in 0.1 *M*-phosphate buffer, separated into two toxic components. These were, however, minor rather than major components of the original solution. They studied *B. thuringiensis* var. *sotto*. Cooksey (1968) found similar results, with the Mattés isolate, except that the toxic components were major ones and immunologically distinct. Somerville *et al.* (1968), working with *B. thuringiensis* var. *alesti* (anduze isolate), found that the protein was excluded from Sephadex G-100 and G-200 (no biological activity of the fractions was reported). DEAE-cellulose was tried in all three studies as a subsequent purification step. The results of Somerville *et al.* (1968) demonstrate the difficulty in working with dissolved crystal protein. They attempted to chromatograph crystal protein on DEAE-cellulose which had been equilibrated with 0.01 *M*-*tris*-HCl, pH 8.3. A fraction (I) of the protein was eluted by 0.4 *M*-$(NH_4)_2CO_3$ in 0.01 *M*-*tris*-HCl and a second fraction (II) by 0.1 *N*-NaOH. After concentration by lyophilization and rechromatography each fraction gave the same elution profile. Both original fractions, and the fractions derived from them by rechromatography, behaved similarly in an immunodiffusion test. This behavior is good evidence of reversible aggregation. The elution profile was very similar to that published by Watanabe *et al.* (1967) and did not appear to represent true ion-exchange chromatography, but rather a total desorption of protein following the application of each eluant. Recently Cooksey (unpublished) has separated the two major antigens of *B. thuringiensis* var. *thuringiensis*, Mattés isolate, crystal protein on DEAE-cellulose at pH 9.0 in 0.05 *M*-glycine-NaOH containing 10^{-3} *M*-β-mercaptoethanol with a gradient of 0 to 0.2 *M*-NaCl (Fig. 1). The antigen characteristic of the Mattés strain was completely free from the second antigen. Both fractions were toxic when fed to *P. brassicae* larvae. The method offers possibilities for studying the individual antigens of the crystal as separate proteins.

D. OTHER TECHNIQUES

There have been few other reports of methods for the purification of the crystal protein polypeptide chains. Dissolved protein has been separated into several fractions by Norris and coworkers (unpublished) using electrophoresis on a moving buffer film in the apparatus developed by Hannig (1958). The results of several investigators with disc electrophoresis on an analytical scale, suggest that a preparative apparatus (Gordon, 1968) could be used with advantage to separate usable quantities of the antigens of the crystal.

The only other method described depends on the use of purified specific antisera. Although this technique cannot be used easily on a large scale, it is of value for precipitating unwanted antigens from mixtures. Each antiserum should be purified first by ammonium sulphate precipitation and Sephadex G-50 chromatography, so that only the gamma-globulin fraction of the serum is used. This facilitates subsequent purification of the unprecipitated antigen (e.g. Pendleton, 1968).

E. PROTEOLYSIS OF THE TOXIC PROTEIN

It is well established that the crystal is in fact a protoxin, and that the true toxin is a smaller molecule produced by proteolysis in the insect gut, e.g. Angus (1956), Lecadet and Martouret (1962), Pendleton (1968), and Cooksey (1968). Martouret (1960) described the appearance of the crystals as they dissolved over about half an hour in the chyle of *P. brassicae.* The crystals at first lost birefringence, swelled, distorted and finally dispersed. Faust *et al.* (1967) have examined the dissolution of crystals of *B. thuringiensis* var. *pacificus* in the mid-gut secretion of *Bombyx mori* in some detail. Their evidence suggests that, *in vivo,* the first event inside the insect gut is a partial solution of the crystal as a result of the high local pH, rather than proteolysis. According to Faust *et al.*, this first step probably involves the breakage of silicon-protein bonds, and it is only then that the gut proteases can act. One of the experiments they described in support of their idea concerned the activity of the gut proteases in borate buffer. At pH 9.0 in 0.05 *M*-borate or in 0.05 *M*-carbonate, the gut proteases had similar activity when azoalbumin, blood fibrin, or casein were used as substrates.

When the same conditions were used to hydrolyze intact crystals, only the carbonate buffered enzyme appeared to be active. Crystals suspended in carbonate buffer alone were dissolved to the extent of 14%, whereas in borate buffer, no protein was dissolved. In contrast, Lecadet and Martouret (1967b) found the gut enzymes of *B. mori* in borate buffer able to hydrolyze crystals, although borate at pH 10 was used. Trypsin, chymotrypsin, papain and pronase did not hydrolyze native (i.e. in no way denatured) protein crystals at pH 8.0-9.5 (Lecadet, 1965b; Faust and Estes, 1966). The gut enzymes of both *P. brassicae* and *B. mori* were able to hydrolyze native crystals (Lecadet and Martouret, 1967a, b). It was shown by Cooksey (1968) that chymotrypsin, trypsin, subtilisin as well as *P. brassicae* enzymes, were able to hydrolyze dissolved and reprecipitated crystal protein in carbonate buffer, pH 9.5, to yield toxic fragments of a similar size distribution, as judged by Sephadex G-200 chromatography (Fig. 3, see also Fig. 2). This was to be expected, as Lecadet and Dedonder (1966) showed that two gut proteases purified from *P. brassicae* chyle had specifities similar to, although somewhat wider than, trypsin and chymotrypsin. Disc electrophoretic examination of the process of proteolysis of

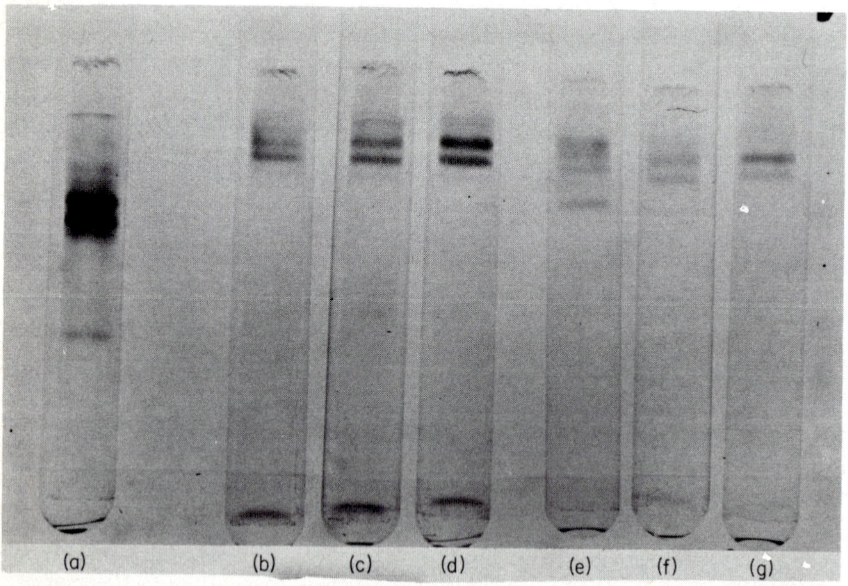

Fig. 2. Disc electrophoretic patterns of undigested and digested crystal protein of *B. thuringiensis*, Mattés isolate. (a) Protein extracted from a spore-crystal mixture at pH 9.5 in 0.05 *M*-carbonate buffer +0.05 *M*-β-mercaptoethanol. (b), (c) and (d), protein in sample (a) after 1, 2 and 3 hr incubation at pH 9.5 and 30°C with regurgitated gut enzymes from *Pieris brassicae*. (e), (f) and (g) purified crystals after 1, 2 and 3 hr incubation with gut enzymes. It can be seen that the patterns in tubes (d) and (g) are very similar. The disc electrophoretic method was that of Jovin *et al.* (1964) as modified by Cooksey (1968).

the intact crystals and dissolved protein with *P. brassicae* gut proteases showed that the two reactions were similar. Although at intermediate times the composition of the lysates differed, their final compositions were identical within the limits of the method. A preliminary fractionation of the lysate could be obtained by dialysis. Thus Lecadet and Martouret (1967a) showed that both dialysable and undialysable fractions were toxic both *per os* and by injection into

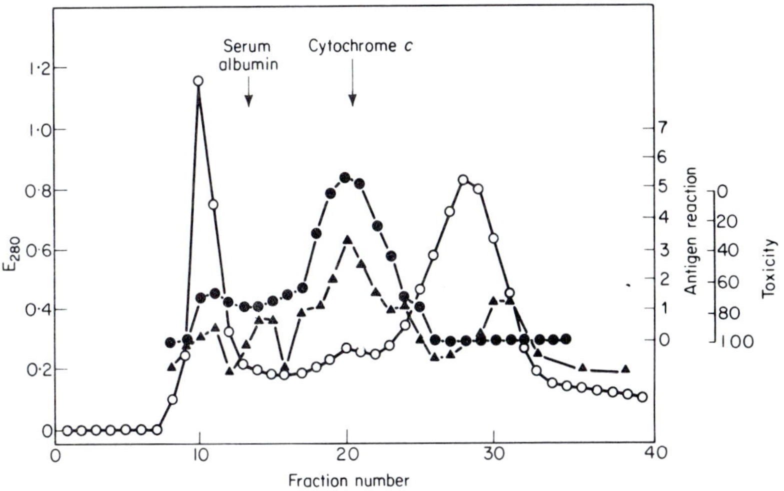

Fig. 3. Elution profile of products from purified crystal protein when digested with *P. brassicae* gut proteases. Purified protein was digested at pH 9.7 and 30°C with regurgitated gut enzymes and chromatographed on a Sephadex G-200 column equilibrated with 0.05 *M*-carbonate-bicarbonate buffer, pH 9.7. Antigen reaction (●) was measured by a radial immunodiffusion method. Toxicity (△) was measured by a feeding inhibition assay (scale: % leaf eaten). E represents extinction at 280 nm (o). The elution positions of Bovine serum albumen and Cytochrome C are included as reference proteins. (Cooksey, 1968, reprinted with permission from the Biochemical Journal.)

the hemocoel of *P. brassicae* larvae. A better fraction was obtained on Sephadex G-75. That part of the digest excluded from G-75 was termed the proteinaceous fraction of molecular weight (MW) about 50,000 and that part which was included, the peptide fraction (MW about 5000). The proteinaceous fraction could be reduced in quantity by a longer incubation with a concommitant increase in the peptide fraction. The proteinaceous fraction was not a single entity, as other molecules of MW about 13,000 were found (Lecadet and Dedonder, 1967). The fraction gave rise to six amino-terminal amino acids and six bands in starch gel electrophoresis. From this evidence, Lecadet and Dedonder concluded that there were six proteinaceous components of the lysate.

The peptide fraction contained free amino acids as well as four peptides. These peptides were purified on DEAE-Sephadex in 1% collidine-acetic acid. All four peptides were toxic by injection into *P. brassicae* larvae, but much less so than the lysate from which they were purified. As the fractionation was carried out at 35° C, the peptides may have been thermally damaged, because, if the unfractionated peptide mixture was incubated at 25° C for the time of the fractionation procedures, it lost activity significantly. However, the whole lysates could be stored for at least three years at −22° C, and lyophilized lysates or ammonium sulphate precipitates at 4° C. Cooksey (1968) published results that parallel those of Lecadet, although the fractionation was less complete. The fractionation of a lysate on Sephadex G-200 is shown in Fig. 3. The larger antigen peak (filled circles) represents a MW about 40,000 and coincides with a peak of toxin (triangles). The second toxin peak (triangles), eluted about fraction no. 30, did not react to give a precipitate in the quantitative immunoassay (filled circles). It is possible that the peptides in the second peak reacted with the antiserum but that the product was too small to precipitate. Pendleton (1968) confirmed and considerably extended the findings of Lecadet and Cooksey. Initially he found similar elution profiles when he fractionated lysates on Sephadex G-200. The first peak eluted was, almost certainly, undigested crystal protein. It could be eliminated by adding more of the same gut enzymes and incubating the lysate a second time. After 4 hr incubation the mixture contained only small peptides of MW about 5000. In contrast to Cooksey, Pendleton found no material of MW 40,000. However, Lecadet and Dedonder (1967) found the proteinaceous part of their digest to be relatively resistant to further proteolysis. Pendleton (1968) fractionated his digest further by the use of specific antisera. He was able to mask, rather than separate, the three antigens he detected in the lysate. The antigens could be masked individually or in pairs. Toxicity measurements on each fraction showed that only one of the antigenic determinants was toxic; however, the antigen which Pendleton calls 'h' and which was present in a large portion of the lysates of crystals from 93 strains (Pendleton and Morrison, 1967), appeared to be only slightly toxic when it alone was left unmasked by antibody. When combined with either of the other two antigens, the combination was as toxic as the untreated peptide fraction. The molecule must need at least two antigens unmasked for one to act as a cooperator in the active site of the toxin. The idea was advanced by Pendleton (1968) that the three antigenic sites were on one molecule as they migrated together on electrophoresis in polyacrylamide gel. When antiserum specific to one site (high molecular weight gamma-globulins), was reacted with the molecule and the mixture was passed through a Sephadex G-50 column, the other two antigenic determinants followed the reacted one and appeared in the excluded, high MW fraction. This was further evidence that all three antigenic sites were on the same molecule.

F. NUMBER OF POLYPEPTIDES AND SEPARATE TOXIC MOIETIES IN THE PROTEIN MOLECULE

This section will be used to interpret the evidence concerning the number of polypeptide chains in the crystal, how these chains are organized, and how the crystal is digested to yield smaller toxic fragments.

It is established that the crystal is composed of individual subunits (Norris, Chapter 10). These crystal subunits are, in turn, composed of one or more proteins which themselves are probably built from polypeptide chains covalently linked by disulphide bridges, and which may or may not be the protoxins mentioned later. The ultimate toxic molecule may be a whole chain or a part of a chain. Toxic molecules may be produced from different polypeptide chains and may differ in their toxicity. A precipitin reaction with an antiserum to the intact crystal may be produced by any of the building blocks of the crystal.

The evidence is overwhelming in favor of the thesis that the crystal contains several different polypeptide chains linked by disulphide bridges and hydrogen bonds. The questions of their number, and how many are toxic, are still open. The answers are clouded by the tendency of the polypeptides to associate. Evidence from the ultracentrifuge is of little help, because the experimental conditions used do not prevent association. Lecadet (1966) showed four differently sedimenting fractions in alkylated protein and four amino-terminal amino acids in significant quantities, which is evidence of at least four chains. Anderson and Rogoff (1966) found five different zones from partially solubilized crystal protein by paper electrophoresis. By reduction of crystals and electrophoresis in the presence of sodium dodecyl sulphate (S.D.S.), which should have prevented association, Cooksey found six distinct bands (Fig. 4(a)). Individual chains were therefore separated on the basis of molecular size (Shapiro *et al.*, 1967). The electrophoretic mobility of the smallest was comparable to that of Cytochrome C (MW = 13,000). Again disc electrophoretic examination of crystal protein, alkylated by the method of Anfinsen and Haber (1961), demonstrated six bands (Fig. 4(b)). We do not know how the chains are organized into the subunits which make up the crystal. It seems likely that the subunit MW will be about 200,000 (Holmes and Monro, 1965; Watanabe *et al.*, 1967; Cooksey, 1968; Pendleton, 1968). The organization of the subunits into the crystal is discussed in Chapter 10 and by Holmes and Monro (1965).

Examination of the antigenic composition of the crystal throws some light on the number of chains. Pendleton and Morrison (1967) found a maximum of five antigens in the crystal of a particular isolate of *B. thuringiensis*. This could be evidence in favor of multiple antigenic sites on one protein or single sites on several proteins, but equally it could be misleading since the antiserum was prepared against whole crystals. We do not know the state of the protein when the antibodies are formed. Antibodies may be elicited to proteins in different

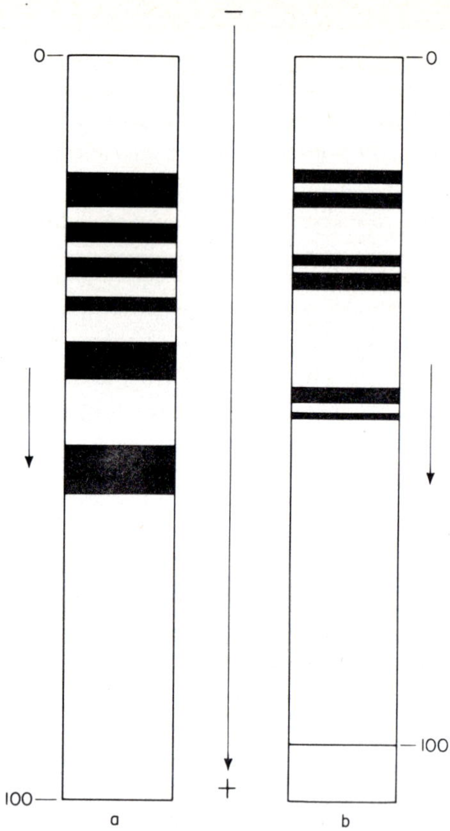

Fig. 4. Disc electrophoresis of dissolved crystals of the Mattés isolate of *B. thuringiensis* (Cooksey, unpublished). (a) Solution in 1% S.D.S. +0.4 *M*-β-mercaptoethanol, buffered at pH 9.5 with 0.05 *M*-carbonate. The soluble protein was dialyzed against 0.01 *M*-phosphate buffer, pH 7.1, containing 0.1% S.D.S. and separated on phosphate-buffered polyacrylamide gel containing S.D.S. (electrophoresis method: Shapiro *et al.,* 1967). (b) Solution in 8 *M*-urea containing 0.05 *M*-β-mercaptoethanol buffered with 0.1% methylamine and alkylated with iodoacetamide (alkylation method: Anfinsen and Haber, 1961; electrophoresis method: Jovin *et al.,* 1964, modified by Cooksey, 1968).

states of association and this may give a false idea of the number of distinctly different proteins present. Against the hypothesis that the multiplicity of antigens merely being reflects of association phenomena, is the fact that the crystal antigens are synthesized at different stages in the sporulation of the cell (Lecadet, Norris, personal communications). Further evidence against this is the separate genetic control of synthesis of two toxic antigens in mutants of *B. thuringiensis* (Rogoff, 1966). It is possible to select a strain of *B. thuringiensis* that is many times more toxic for a particular insect than the wild type strains. Such a strain is not necessarily highly toxic for another susceptible insect species

(Chapter 13). The reverse is also true. Mutants less toxic than the wild type strain do not lose their toxicity to separate insect species in parallel (Rogoff *et al.*, 1969). If only one toxic molecule was produced per cell, the ratios of susceptibilities of the various insects would always vary in the same manner. This too, is evidence for the presence of more than one toxic molecule in the same crystal.

The evidence available supports the idea that the crystal is a protoxin, which is activated in the insect gut to produce toxic molecules of about MW 5000. The number of different toxic molecules present in a crystal proteolysate has not been sufficiently studied. Pendleton (1968) calculated that 85% of the undigested protoxin molecule gave rise to a series of identical toxic molecules of low molecular weight and with several antigenic determinants on them. Lecadet and Dedonder (1967) found four different peptides of low molecular weight in their peptide fraction. All four were toxic and two of them, together, represented about 80% of the total peptide fraction. Unfortunately they did not report on the reactions of the fractions with crystal antisera, so a direct comparison of their work with Pendleton's is difficult. It is also difficult to equate Pendleton's or Lecadet and Dedonder's work with the idea that there are at least two different toxic proteins per crystal. Work in both treatises should be repeated using a different insect as test species. Pendleton (1969) has found more antigens than he originally reported, and one of these was particularly associated with toxicity of *B. thuringiensis* to *Philosamia cynthia* var. *ricini.* In the expansion of this work, it will be very interesting to see whether a different antigen will be involved in the toxic reaction in other insect species.

G. SIGNIFICANCE OF THE CRYSTAL PROTEIN TO THE BACTERIUM

The crystal is a stable feature of *B. thuringiensis,* and important in its pathogenicity. Even though some isolates have been cultured on artificial media for over 50 years (Heimpel and Angus, 1960) they still produce the toxic crystal. What use is this body to the organism when it is growing saprophytically? This question is hard to answer. Heimpel and Angus (1960) suggested that the crystal is a waste depository for unwanted metabolites. This is highly unlikely and difficult to test. It is much more reasonable to believe that the crystal arises from some sort of unregulated or poorly regulated biochemical event in the cell. This idea, however, makes it difficult to understand the evolutionary significance of the crystal in the role of the bacterium as an insect pathogen.

Somerville *et al.* (1968) have accumulated considerable evidence to support a suggestion that the crystal is a result of over-production of spore-coat protein. They showed an immunological similarity between crystal protein and this spore fraction. When antiserum to dissolved crystals was challenged with the spore fraction, four precipitin lines were observed, of which two were common to both spore-coat protein and crystal protein. The precipitin lines of identity were minor crystal antigens. However, the fraction of the spores extracted with urea and β-mercaptoethanol had the same iso-electric point, same precipitability by cations, and same amino acid analysis as crystal protein. The peptide maps formed from a tryptic digest of the two proteins were similar, as were the disc electrophoretic patterns. However, the conclusions drawn were not entirely justified by the published results. The peptide maps showed similarities, but in the electrophoretic procedure for the development of the maps, material remaining near the origin could represent another fraction of the spore. Again, disc electrophoresis left on the surface of the gel, material which did not enter the gel at pH 9.5. At pH 12 the bands of spore and crystal protein ran just behind the salt front, indicating both high charge and low molecular weight. This procedure would not resolve proteins of moderate dissimilarity and particularly proteins highly charged at this pH (proteins have pI = 4.4-4.6). The toxicity of the spore fraction for lepidopterous larvae, the ultimate test of similarity, was not reported.

The kinetics of synthesis of crystal antigens is reviewed in Chapter 10. Lecadet (1967b) has shown that the several crystal antigens of *B. thuringiensis* are not synthesized concurrently. One was synthesized in the first step of sporulation after septum formation but before the crystal was visible. Aronson and Fitz-James (1968) found that spore-coat precursor protein, was synthesized during forespore development, i.e. at about the same time as the "early" crystal antigen reported by Lecadet. Later, this spore protein incorporated cysteine by sulphydryl exchange and became considerably more insoluble, requiring a denaturant such as sodium dodecyl sulphate for solution. I suggest that this second spore fraction was present in the soluble spore fraction of Somerville *et al.* (1968). It is possible that closer homology between the more soluble fraction of spore-coat protein and crystal protein would have been obtained, if the broken-spore preparation had been extracted with sodium thioglycollate, buffered at pH 10.5, the reagent used by Aronson and Fitz-James to dissolve the more soluble part of the spore-coat. It is probable, therefore, that at least one antigen (or polypeptide chain) of the crystal is similar to spore-coat precursor protein. The other antigens (or polypeptide chains) represent more of a mystery.

Recently Banks *et al.* (1969) have suggested that the synthesis of penicillin does not occur in *Penicillium* sp. without the presence of a virus genome in the cell. The synthesis of diphtheria toxin is related to bacteriophage infection of the bacterial cell. Could there be a similar situation in *B. thuringiensis*? Perhaps the crystal is a co-crystallization of unregulated spore protein and a protein of a degenerate bacteriophage. Temperate phages of *B. thuringiensis* have been isolated (Colasito *et al.*, 1968; Colasito and Rogoff, 1969), also Aizawa and Fujiyoshi (1967) referred to possible phage conversion to increase pathogenicity of particular strains of *B. thuringiensis*. If phage conversion occurred in *B. thuringiensis*, an organism from which the phage genome had been removed would be very similar to *Bacillus cereus.* Removal or inactivation of the phage genome may allow the spore-related-protein to be formed giving rise to a degenerate protein crystal, which may or may not be toxic. This area of molecular biology warrants much more study.

V. Stability of the Crystal

The crystal protein is denatured by heat, although it is more stable than solubilized toxin. For example, 1 hr at 65°C did not inactivate intact crystals of *B. thuringiensis* var. *sotto,* whereas amorphous protein was totally inactivated by this exposure (Watanabe *et al.,* 1967). Crystals were not inactivated, even by treatment at 80°C for 20 min. Microbial degradation is possible at moderate temperatures. Moulds which produce extracellular proteases grow at temperatures as low as 10°C.

Many organic solvents are not compatible with the crystal. Chloroform, methanol, and acetone inactivated dissolved crystal protein but not intact crystals (Watanabe *et al.,* 1967; Angus, 1956).

Intact crystals and dissolved crystal protein were inactivated by common protein precipitants such as trichloracetic acid and mercuric chloride. Some compounds capable of reaction with proteins also inactivated the crystal, e.g. 2% formaldehyde (Angus, 1956; Watanabe *et al.,* 1967), as did extremes of pH. The toxicity and ability to react as an antigen was destroyed by exposures above pH 12 and below pH 3.3 (Angus, 1956; Cooksey, 1968). Although detergents, such as sodium dodecyl sulphate and Triton X-100, do not inactivate the crystal, they open up its structure and make it more sensitive to destruction by other means. Spores of *B. thuringiensis* are inactivated by ultraviolet light (sun-light). One hour in direct sunlight at 3200 ft candles inactivated over 80% of spores but crystals retained their toxicity after this and longer exposures (Cantwell and Franklin, 1966; Cantwell, 1967).

VI. Mode of Action and Toxicity of the Crystal

The effect of the crystal on lepidopterous larvae has been well studied and has been reviewed by Heimpel and Angus (1960). Heimpel and Angus (in press) demonstrated gut paralysis with a series of X-ray pictures of larvae which had ingested barium sulphate and *B. thuringiensis* crystals. Buccal and gut paralysis occurs in many species. They also demonstrated a general paralysis of the body, 1-7 hr after ingestion of crystals by *Bombyx mori* larvae, an effect which proved to be restricted to a few species.

Extensive changes in the gut epithelium accompanied the gut paralysis. White (1968) showed that immunofluorescent crystals are attracted to the epithelial cells within minutes of reaching the midgut and intense secretory activity is evoked in *P. brassicae.* Broersma and Buxton (1967) found that the epithelial

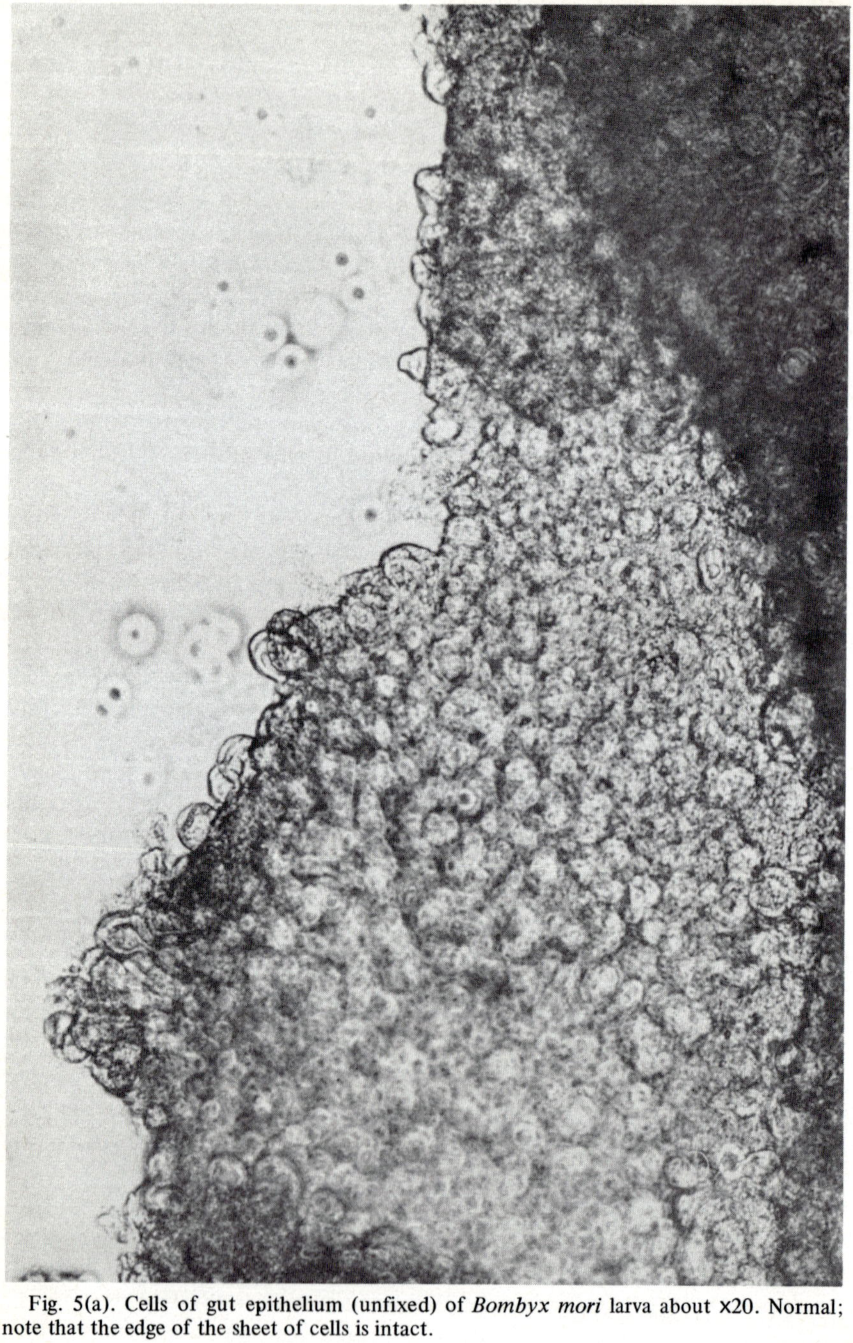

Fig. 5(a). Cells of gut epithelium (unfixed) of *Bombyx mori* larva about ×20. Normal; note that the edge of the sheet of cells is intact.

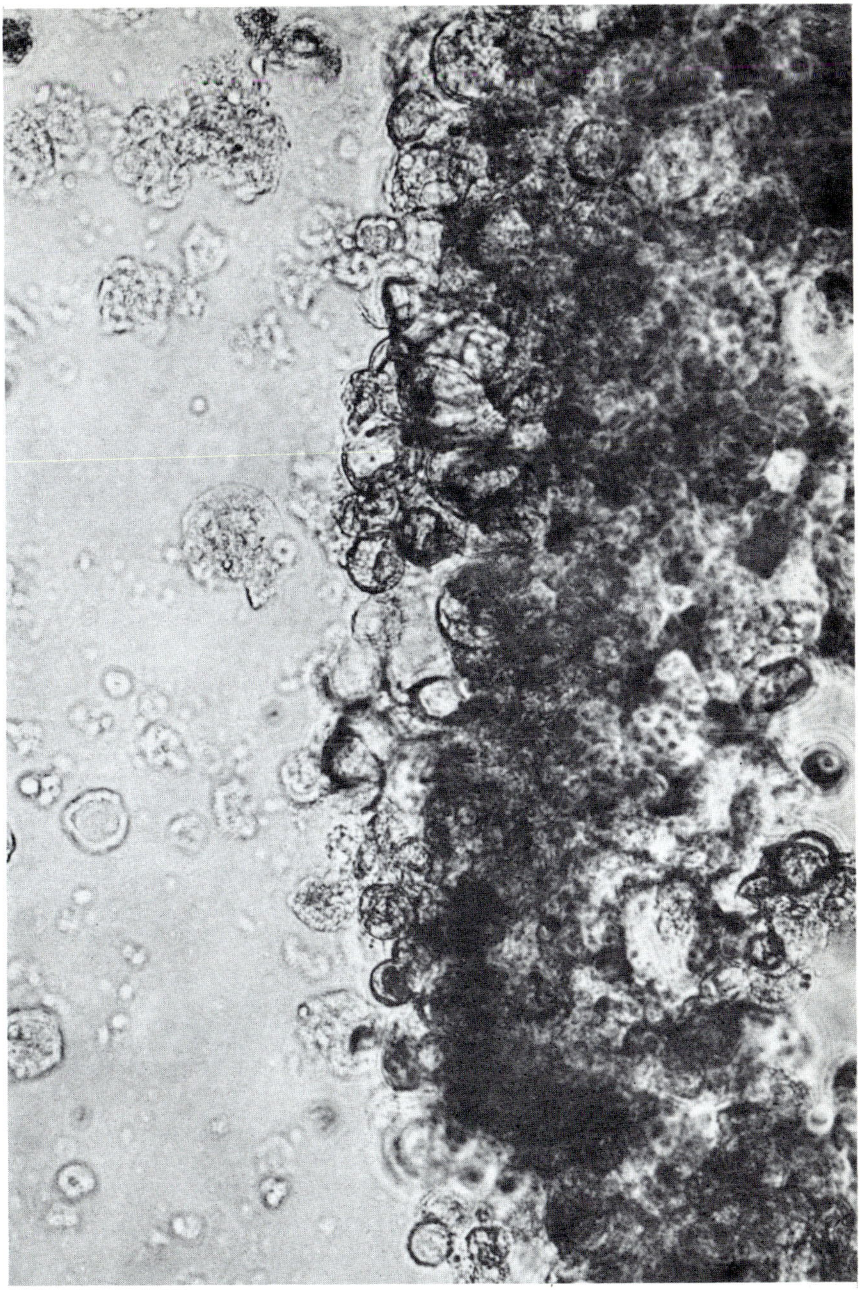

Fig. 5(b). Cells of gut epithelium (unfixed) of *Bombyx mori* larva about ×20, 2 hr after being fed *B. thuringiensis* var. *sotto* crystals. Edge of the sheet of cells is not intact. Cells have sloughed off from the main sheet and many cells have lost their contents. (Angus, in press).

cells of the midgut of the cabbage looper *(Trichoplusia ni)* assumed the appearance of being dehydrated and became eroded. The cells separated from one another and then from the basement membrane. Some of the cells became distorted, lost their ability to stain, and finally the cell contents leaked out. Sutter and Raun (1967) found a similar effect in the European corn borer, *Ostrinia nubilalis.* In addition, vegetative rods of *B. thuringiensis* attacked the disorganized midgut epithelium and penetrated the basement membrane. When the gut contents mixed with the hemolymph, the larvae died, but bacteremia was not necessary to cause death. Angus (in press) examined the gut epithelium of *B. mori* larvae in an unfixed and unsupported state. After immersion of larvae in water for 10 min to produce anoxia, sheets of cells were dissected from the midgut and examined with phase optics in isotonic Locke's saline. The cells from the control larvae held together in a coherent sheet (Fig. 5(a)) and the cell membranes appeared intact. In contrast, sheets of cells from treated larvae (Fig. 5(b)) contained cells with disrupted membranes. Many cells had released their contents into the suspending fluid (Fig. 6). White (1968) demonstrated aggregation of radioactive particles from tritium-labeled crystals at the base of disrupted epithelium 18 hr after *P. brassicae* caterpillars had ingested the crystal.

Early ideas about the precise nature of the effect on the midgut epithelium involved dissolution of the cell-cementing substance of the basement membrane by a hyaluronidase-like substance present in the crystal. There is no evidence for this other than the separation of the cells of the epithelium from one another. By feeding larve with crystals and $Na_2{}^{14}CO_3$ or U-^{14}C-glucose, Fast and Angus (1965) showed that the carbonate-^{14}C ion concentration in the hemolymph rose more quickly than that in the control larvae without protein crystals. This indicated an increased permeability of the gut wall—the first biochemical lesion attributable to the protein toxin. A more significant finding was the slower rise in hemolymph glucose compared with the control. Glucose usually enters the gut cells by an active transport system in the cell membrane and the slower rise in concentration in the hemolymph showed that this metabolically controlled system was impaired.

When *B. mori* larvae ingested valinomycin-treated foliage, they were affected in a similar way to larvae which had ingested crystals (Table V). Valinomycin increases the potassium permeability of the mitochondrial membranes (Harris *et al.*, 1966). In the larvae of *Cecropia* sp. (silkmoth) the midgut is a primary site of ion regulation, with K^+ moving from the hemocoel to the gut lumen by an active process (Haskell *et al.*, 1968). Disruption of K^+ regulation could account for the cell damage caused by the crystal.

Within 1-7 hr of a meal containing crystals, the blood pH of *B. mori* larvae rose from its normal 6.8 and the pH of the gut fell concomitant with general paralysis of the larvae. Injections of non-toxic alkaline buffer into the hemocoel of untreated insects also caused paralysis, which suggests that paralysis of larvae

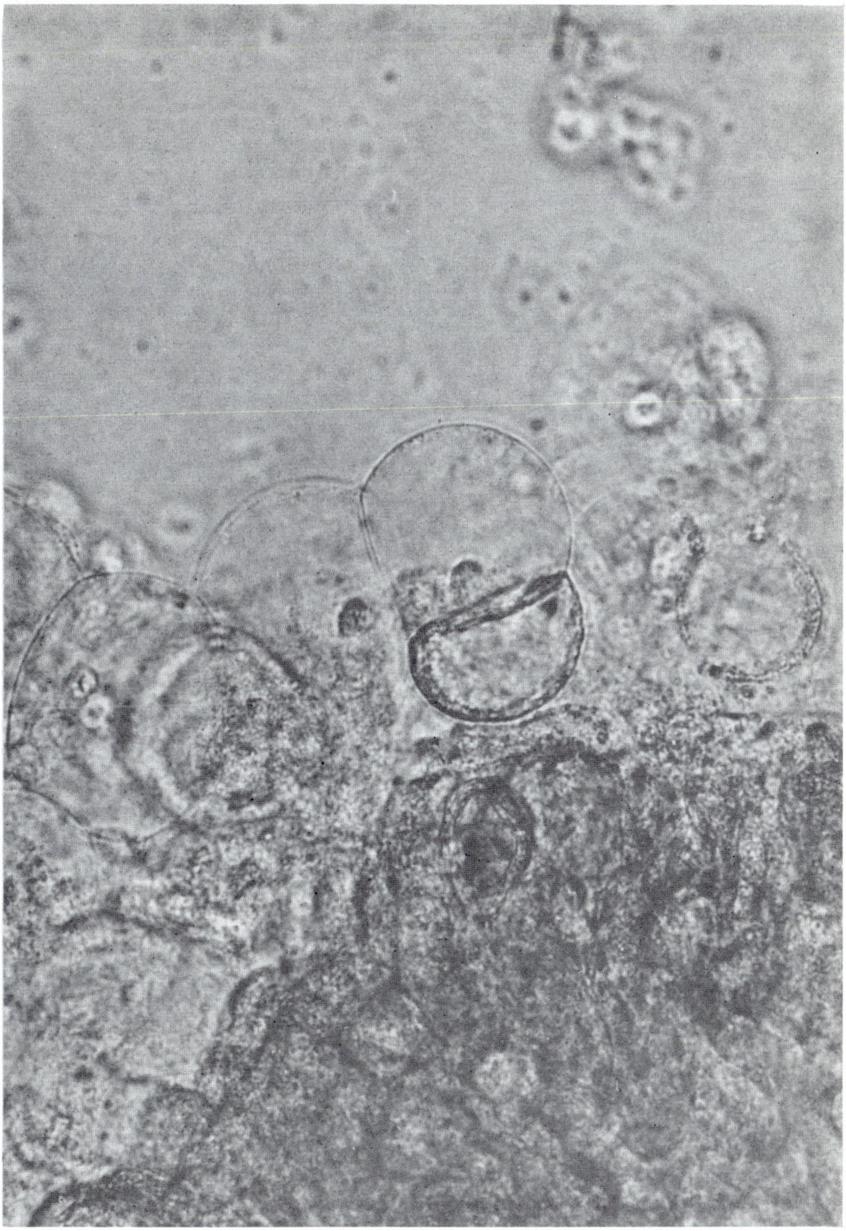

Fig. 6. Epithelial cells from the gut of a *B. mori* larva fed crystals of *B. thuringiensis.* About ×50. Some of the cells have become bubble shaped ("soap-bubble" appearance, Angus, in press) and many have burst.

TABLE V

Symptoms in larvae of Bombyx mori *fed valinomycin (Angus, 1968a)*[a]

Min after feeding	Behaviour and symptoms
20-45	Larvae fed normally
45-60	Feeding ceased; untreated foliage not eaten; blood pH 6.8-7.0
60-90	Insects sluggish, otherwise normal
90-180	Insects became paralysed; blood pH rose to pH 7.8-8.0

[a] Dissolved in ethanol and applied to foliage, which was allowed to dry and then fed to insects. (Copyright, Academic Press.)

poisoned by the crystals was caused by the increase in blood pH (Heimpel and Angus, 1959). Ramakrishnan (1968) showed that the hemolymph level of K^+ rose five-fold after larvae of *B. mori* had fed on foliage treated with crystals and proposed that this increase in K^+ in the hemolymph was responsible for the paralysis. Cooksey *et al.* (1969) showed that digested, but not undigested, crystal protein blocked nervous conduction in a preparation from the American cockroach, *Periplaneta americana* (Table VI). The test preparation was a cercal nerve and abdominal ganglia V and VI isolated from adult cockroaches. Nerve fibers in the cercal nerves synapse with giant fibers in ganglion VI, so that stimulation of the cercal nerve and the detection of the efferent response from the corresponding nerve cord above ganglion VI, can be used to study the synapses. A disruption of K^+ regulation at the synapse would certainly affect conduction of impulses. These various lines of evidence suggest that the mode of action of the crystal is to impair membrane permeability by a disruption in potassium ion regulation. However, more work is needed to prove this theory.

TABLE VI

Action of B. thuringiensis *crystal protein on a desheathed spinal gangliar preparation of* Periplaneta americana *(Cooksey* et al., *1969)*

Crystal protein in solution	Concentration (μg/ml)	Time of treatment (min)	Effect
Unhydrolyzed	24.0	60	None
Hydrolyzed by *P. brassicae*	2.4	45	Complete blockade
gut enzymes	24.0	12	Complete blockade

In a different approach Faust (1968) discovered that dissolved crystal protein formed a complex with protein of high isoelectric point *in vitro*. Several proteins important to cell metabolism fall into this category, e.g. cytochrome C and glyceraldehyde-3-phosphate dehydrogenase. Near pH 7 the protein-protein complex precipitated, and the biological activity of the cell-derived protein was masked. The crystal protein may thus inhibit important cell functions. However, *in vivo* the active principle of the crystal is the digested protein. Until the crystal is totally digested in the gut, some exists free and could inhibit enzymes in membranes of the epithelial cells. An important control experiment would have enhanced the value of this work. Reaction of another protein of low isoelectric point, e.g. ovalbumen, with the enzymes tested by Faust would have revealed whether formation of the complex was specific. The crystal protein also precipitates hemolymph protein (Faust and Dougherty, 1968), although this is not likely to be related to the mode of action of the toxic molecules released by digestion of the crystal protein.

With so many physiological effects in the insect, it is indeed fortunate that the crystal is not toxic to mammals. One of the reasons for this lack of toxicity is that, in mammals, primary digestion of proteins is at low pH. The stomach enzyme pepsin, which has its pH optimum at pH 2, degrades the crystal to an atoxic state.

B. thuringiensis crystal is a very toxic substance to Lepidoptera larvae (Table VII). Cooksey's assays were performed with one batch of insects, so the figures for dissolved protein and intact crystals can be compared. It is evident

TABLE VII

Toxicity of crystals and protein from B. thuringiensis

Author	Strain	Form of crystal protein	Test insect	LD50 (μg toxin/g larva)
Watanabe	*sotto*	dissolved	*Bombyx mori*	1.2
et al. (1967)	*sotto* (T84A-1)	dissolved	*B. mori*	0.8
	sotto (T84A-1)	digested	*B. mori*	0.072
Martouret *et al.* (1965)	*Berliner*	intact crystals	*Pieris brassicae*	0.25
Cooksey	*Berliner*	intact crystals	*P. brassicae*	0.30
(unpublished)	*Berliner*	dissolved	*P. brassicae*	0.60
Angus	*thuringiensis*	dissolved	*B. mori*	5.0
(1967)	*sotto*	dissolved	*B. mori*	0.015
	entomocidus	dissolved	*B. mori*	0.025
Faust (1968)	*dendrolimus*	dissolved	*B. mori*	6.2

that the solution procedure, as has been discussed in Section IV-A, must in someway damage the structure of the crystal protein, or lower the final yield of active toxic molecules produced by proteolysis. It cannot be decided from Table VII whether the protein digested *in vitro,* is more toxic than the intact crystal.

TABLE VIII

Relative toxicities of spore-crystal mixtures of B. thuringiensis *strains for two species of insects (Burges, 1967)*

Strain and serotype	Relative toxicity in units/mg preparation with 95% fiducial limits	
	Ephestia (Anagasta) kuehniella	*Galleria mellonella*
Berliner, I	1000	1000
Galleriae, V	3662 (2321-5778)	89,373 (69,566-114,820)

In diverse strains of *B. thuringiensis* the toxicity of dissolved crystal proteins (Table VIII) and pure crystals (Chapter 13, Table I) varies greatly in different insects, showing that the insects may be susceptible to different toxic moieties in the crystal. It is possible that variation in gut pH and enzyme content between species affects yields of the same toxic molecules. Even different rates of proteolysis in the guts of two insects could effect the rates of production of toxin from protein and thus the absolute toxin concentration at a particular time. Crystals of *B. thuringiensis* var. *thuringiensis* are more easily lysed by *Pieris* gut proteins than are crystals from *B. thuringiensis* var. *entomocidus* (Lecadet, personal communication). It is possible that two or more structures need to be present on the toxic molecule in order to obtain biological activity, or alternatively that two or more distinct peptides are required for full activity (see pp. 261 and 263). Differences in the crystal's structure and differences in the insect species must be used to explain the variations in toxicity of the crystal between bacterial strains with one insect, and between insect species with the crystal of one bacterial strain. The susceptibilities of different insect species to spore-crystal mixtures are discussed fully in Chapter 13.

VII. Conclusions and Future Research

I have attempted to present a biochemical picture of the protein crystal of *B. thuringiensis* with sufficient details of the experimental procedures to stimulate the interest of the reader. In the course of this account, opportunities have been taken to point out particular aspects requiring research. In general, future work should examine the structure of the smallest toxic fragment(s) and elucidate the precise mode of action of the crystal. At present, all commercial preparations of *B. thuringiensis* depend for their action on the intact crystal. In the future, it is possible that insecticides based on digested crystal may be produced. Even synthetic derivatives of the digested crystal may be manufactured. These will need to be carefully selected as the toxic peptides produced by proteolysis are much less thermostable than the whole crystal (Lecadet and Martouret, 1967a). A further word of caution is necessary. The remarkable specificity of the crystal may depend on the necessary activation step which occurs in the insect gut. Derivatives, especially those related to the digested crystal, may be more toxic to other insect species or even mammals, than the intact-crystal.

Research in the areas I have indicated may allow us to develop better microbial, and hopefully, better synthetic insecticides.

References

Aizawa, K. and Fujiyoshi, N. (1967). Proc. Joint U.S.-Japan Semin. Microbial Control Insect Pests. U.S.-Japan Committee Sci. Cooperation. Panel 8. Fukuoka, pp. 29-30.

Albertsson, P. A. (1961). "Partition of Cell Particles and Macromolecules". John Wiley, New York.

Anderson, R. F. and Rogoff, M. H. (1966). *In* "Advances in Chemistry", Vol. 53. "Natural Pest Control Agents" (D. G. Crosby, ed.), pp. 65-79. American Chemical Society, Washington, D.C.

Anfinsen, C. B. and Haber, E. (1961). *J. biol. Chem.* **236,** 1361-1363.

Angus, T. A. (1954). *Nature, Lond.* **173,** 545-546.

Angus, T. A. (1956). *Can. J. Microbiol.* **2,** 416-426.

Angus, T. A. (1959). *J. Insect Path.* **1,** 97-98.

Angus, T. A. (1967). *J. Invertebrate Path.* **9,** 256-260.

Angus, T. A. (1968a). *J. Invertebrate Path.* **11,** 145-146.

Angus, T. A. (in press). Proc. XIII Int. Congr. Ent. Moscow, 1968.

Angus, T. A. and Norris, J. R. (1968). *J. Invertebrate Path.* **11,** 289-295.

Aronson, A. I. and Fitz-James, P. C. (1968). *J. molec. Biol.* **33,** 199-212.

Banks, G. T., Buck, K. W., Chain, E. B., Darbyshire, J. E. and Himmelweit, F. (1969). *Nature, Lond.* **222,** 89-90.

Barjac, H. de and Lecadet, M. M. (1961). *C.r. hebd. Séanc Acad. Sci. Paris.* **252,** 3160-3162.

Bateson, J. B. (1965). *Nature, Lond.* **205,** 622.

Bonnefoi, A. and de Barjac, H. (1963). *Entomophaga* **8,** 223-229.

Broersma, D. B. and Buxton, J. A. (1967). *J. Invertebrate Path.* **9,** 58-69.

Burges, H. D. (1967). *Nature, Lond.* **215,** 664-665.

Cantwell, G. E. (1967). *J. Invertebrate Path.* **9,** 138-140.

Cantwell, G. E. and Franklin, B. A. (1966). *J. Invertebrate Path.* **8,** 256-258.

Colasito, D. J., Anderson, R. F. and Rogoff, M. H. (1968). *Bact. Proc.* pp. 6-7.

Colasito, D. J. and Rogoff, M. H. (1969). *J. gen. Virol.* **5,** 275-281.

Cooksey, K. E. (1968). *Biochem. J.* **106,** 445-454.

Cooksey, K. E., Donninger, C., Norris, J. R. and Shankland, D. (1969). *J. Invertebrate Path.* **13,** 461-462.

Delafield, F. P., Somerville, H. J. and Rittenberg, S. C. (1968). *J. Bact.* **96,** 713-720.

Fast, P. G. and Angus, T. A. (1965). *J. Invertebrate Path.* **7,** 29-32.

Faust, R. M. (1968). *J. Invertebrate Path.* **11,** 465-475.

Faust, R. M., Adams, J. R. and Heimpel, A. M. (1967). *J. Invertebrate Path.* **9,** 488-499.
Faust, R. M. and Dougherty, E. M. (1968). *J. Invertebrate Path.* **13,** 155-157.
Faust, R. M. and Estes, Z. E. (1966). *J. Invertebrate Path.* **8,** 141-144.
Gingrich, R. E. (1968). *J. Invertebrate Path.* **10,** 180-184.
Goodman, N. S., Gottfried, R. J. and Rogoff, M. H. (1967). *J. Bact.* **94,** 485.
Gordon, A. H. (1968). *In* "Electrophoresis of Proteins in Polyacrylamide and Starch Gels". North Holland Publ. Co., Amsterdam.
Hannay, C. L. (1953). *Nature, Lond.* **172,** 1004.
Hannay, C. L. and Fitz-James, P. C. (1955). *Can. J. Microbiol.* **1,** 694-710.
Hannig, K. (1958). *Hoppe-Seylers Z. Physiol. Chem.* **311,** 63-78.
Harris, E. J., Cockrell, R. and Pressman, B. C. (1966). *Biochem. J.* **99,** 200-213.
Haskell, J. A., Harvey, W. R. and Clark, R. M. (1968). *J. exp. Biol.* **48,** 25-37.
Heimpel, A. M. (1967). *J. Invertebrate Path.* **9,** 364-375.
Heimpel, A. M. and Angus, T. A. (1959). *J. Insect Path.* **1,** 152-170.
Heimpel, A. M. and Angus, T. A. (1960). *Bact. Rev.* **24,** 266-288.
Holmes, K. C. and Monro, R. E. (1965). *J. molec. Biol.* **14,** 572-581.
Jovin, T., Chrambach, A. and Naughton, M. A. (1964). *Analyt. Biochem.* **9,** 351-369.
Krywienczyk, J. and Angus, T. A. (1960). *J. Insect Path.* **2,** 411-417.
Krywienczyk, J. and Angus, T. A. (1967). *J. Invertebrate Path.* **9,** 126-128.
Lecadet, M. M. (1965a). *C.r. hebd Séanc. Acad. Sci. Paris* **261,** 5693-5696.
Lecadet, M. M. (1965b). Ph.D. Thesis: Etat Faculté des Science, Paris.
Lecadet, M. M. (1966). *C.r. hebd Séanc. Acad. Sci. Paris* **262,** 195-198.
Lecadet, M. M. (1967a). *C.r. hebd Séanc. Acad. Sci. Paris* **264,** 2847-2850.
Lecadet, M. M. (1967b). Colloq. Mol. Biology, October, Orsay, France.
Lecadet, M. M. and Dedonder, R. (1966). *Bull. Soc. chim. Biol.* **48,** 631-660.
Lecadet, M. M. and Dedonder, R. (1967). *J. Invertebrate Path.* **9,** 310-321.
Lecadet, M. M. and Martouret, D. (1962). *C.r. hebd Séanc. Acad. Sci. Paris* **254,** 2457-2459.
Lecadet, M. M. and Martouret, D. (1967a). *J. Invertebrate Path.* **9,** 322-330.
Lecadet, M. M. and Martouret, D. (1967b). *C.r. hebd Séanc. Acad. Sci Paris* **265,** 1543-1546.
Lowry, O. H., Rosebrough, N. J., Farr, A. L. and Randall, R. J. (1951). *J. biol. Chem.* **193,** 265-275.
Mancini, G., Vaerman, J. P., Carbonara, A. O. and Heremans, J. F. (1963). *In* "Protides of the Biological Fluids" (H. Peeters, ed.), p. 370, Elsevier Publ. Co., Amsterdam.
Martouret, D. (1960). *In* "Proc. 11th Int. Congr. Ent. Vienna", pp. 849-855.
Martouret, D., Lhoste, J. and Roche, A. (1965). *Entomophaga* **10,** 349-365.
Monro, R. E. (1961). *J. biophys. Biochem. Cytol.* **11,** 321-331.
Murray, E. D. and Spencer, E. Y. (1966). *J. Invertebrate Path.* **8,** 418-420.
Norris, J. R. (1964). *J. appl. Bact.* **27,** 439-447.
Pendleton, I. R. (1968). *J. appl. Bact.* **31,** 208-214.
Pendleton, I. R. (1969). *J. Invertebrate Path.* **13,** 423-428.
Pendleton, I. R. and Morrison, R. B. (1966). *Nature, Lond.* **212,** 728-729.
Pendleton, I. R. and Morrison, R. B. (1967). *J. appl. Bact.* **30,** 402-405.
Ramakrishnan, N. (1968). *J. Invertebrate Path.* **10,** 449-450.
Rogoff, M. H. (1966). Verbal Statement at the "Int. Coll. Insect Path. Microbial Control". Wageningen, The Netherlands (1966).
Rogoff, M. H., Ignoffo, C. M., Singer, S., Gard, I. and Prieto, A. P. (1969). *J. Invertebrate Path.* **14,** 122-129.
Shapiro, A. L., Vinuela, E. and Maizel, J. V. (1967). *Biochem. biophys. Res. Comm.* **28,** 815-820.
Somerville, H. J., Delafield, F. P. and Rittenberg, S. C. (1968). *J. Bact.* **96,** 721-726.
Spencer, E. Y. (1968). *J. Invertebrate Path.* **11,** 444-445.
Sutter, G. R. and Raun, E. S. (1967). *J. Invertebrate Path.* **9,** 90-103.
Watanabe, T., Tsutsui, R. and Iwahana, H. (1967). Proc. Joint U.S.-Japan Semin. Microbial Control Insect Pests. U.S.-Japan Committee Sci. Cooperation. Panel 8. Fukuoka, pp. 71-78.
White, A. G. (1968). Ph.D. Thesis, University of Leeds, 110 pp.

CHAPTER 12

The Thermostable Exotoxin of *Bacillus thuringiensis*

R. P. M. BOND, C. B. C. BOYCE

Shell Research Limited, Milstead Laboratory of Chemical Enzymology, Sittingbourne, Kent, England

and

M. H. ROGOFF, T. R. SHIEH

International Minerals and Chemical Corporation, Libertyville, Illinois, U.S.A.

I. Introduction

An interesting development in the study of the insect pathogen *Bacillus thuringiensis* took place in 1959 and 1960 when several independent reports were made that certain strains of this bacterium produced a heat-stable toxin which was insecticidal to species from several orders of insects. At least four facts readily distinguished the activity observed from that produced by the well known crystal protein (Chapter 10): the activity survived autoclaving at 120° for 15 min; the spectrum of insect species affected was quite different; the symptoms were different, and finally some serotypes which do not produce the crystal protein were shown to produce the heat-stable toxin.

---

[1] Only Section VI was written by M. H. Rogoff and T. R. Shieh.

By injecting the autoclaved supernatant from centrifuged bacterial cultures into the posterior pleural region of *Galleria mellonella* larvae, McConnell and Richards (1959) showed that the activity began to appear during the active phase of bacterial growth, before sporulation. At its maximum the LD_{50} value was 0.36 μl of supernatant per larva. In limited tests with other species, the corn borer *(Ostrinia nubilalis)*, a blow fly larva *(Sarcophaga bullata)*, and two cockroaches *(Periplaneta americana* and *Blatta orientalis)* were equally susceptible. However, none of these insects was affected when the bacterial supernatant was included in their diet. *G. mellonella*, for example, was not affected when fed a diet containing 16% w/v of supernatant. In addition McConnell and Richards successfully reared the yellow fever mosquito *(Aedes aegypti)* in water containing 10% v/v of supernatant in contrast to the results of Lilles and Dunn (1959) who found that the spray-dried total fermentation solids of a commercial *B. thuringiensis* preparation caused high mortality of *A. aegypti* when applied at a concentration of 0.4 g/litre. The fact that death did not occur for several days was similar to the findings of McConnell and Richards (1959) with *G. mellonella.*

In 1960, Burgerjon and de Barjac found that the autoclaved supernatant was toxic to several other Lepidoptera including: *Bombyx mori, Pieris brassicae, Malacosoma neustria* etc. and to single species of the Coleoptera *(Leptinotarsa decemlineata)* and Hymenoptera *(Pristiphora pallipes)*. The characteristics of the toxicity and of its production were similar to those described by McConnell and Richards in all but one respect—they were apparent when the supernatant was administered orally.

Hall and Arakawa (1959) found that when preparations of *B. thuringiensis*, containing viable spores and protein crystals were added to the larval medium of house flies *(Musca domestica)* the development of the larvae was markedly inhibited although there was little effect on treated adults. The effect was attributed to the protein crystals which is almost certainly incorrect because Briggs (1960) showed that the sterile supernatant from a filtered bacterial culture had a similar effect on house fly larval development. The term "fly factor" was subsequently introduced to describe the entity responsible.

In each of these studies the recorded symptoms are very similar. The effects develop slowly and are seen only at a moult or at metamorphosis. In sharp contrast, the protein toxin elicits a relatively rapid response. At the lowest effective doses, larval development proceeds normally and the insects pupate although some fail to emerge to the adult stage. A significant proportion of adults is often deformed, for example, by having only vestigial wings. At high doses pupariae are often deformed and at still higher doses death may occur at a larval moult. Death is never sudden but the larvae gradually become increasingly lethargic and pass through a prolonged moribund state before dying.

These early results, together with others we shall briefly mention, provided a considerable incentive for further work. The symptoms leading to death of insects suggested a very real prospect of a mode of action entirely different from those of the commonly used classes of insecticides, e.g. organophosphorus compounds, carbamates and chlorinated hydrocarbons. There were indications that the activity could be exploited under field conditions, e.g. for the control of house flies (Briggs, 1960; Dunn, 1960) and the pine moth, *Diprion pini* (Burgerjon and Biache, 1964). Finally, the studies of Briggs (1960) with hens, Dunn (1960) with cows and Krieg and Herfs (1963) with mice, suggested an acceptable oral tolerance of warm-blooded animals to *B. thuringiensis* preparations capable of controlling fly larvae. From a more basic point of view there were many interesting questions to answer: is more than one toxin involved?; what is its (their) nature?; what is the biochemistry of the toxic effect(s)?; what precisely is the(ir) toxicity to insects, mammals and other organisms?; and what is the role of the(se) toxin(s) in the pathogenicity of *B. thuringiensis*?

The progress that has been made in answering these questions in the 10 years since the discovery of the heat-stable toxins is the subject of this chapter.

II. Early Controversies Regarding the Thermostable Exotoxin

The activity detected by McConnell and Richards (1959) and that found by Burgerjon and de Barjac (1960) are often regarded as being identical despite the difference in the effective routes of administration. Also, it is often taken for granted that the inhibition of fly larval development caused by autoclaved *B. thuringiensis* supernatant also results from the same toxin. Consequently, names such as McConnell and Richards' factor, heat-stable toxin, thermostable toxin, *B. thuringiensis* exotoxin, fly factor, fly toxin etc., tend to be used as synonyms.

The evidence for the identity, or otherwise, of these materials can be considered under three headings: quantitative bioassay data, qualitative assay results and chemical results. The assertions in the literature depend almost entirely on the first of these but are not convincing because little, if any, attempt has been made to standardize conditions so as to permit a valid quantitative comparison of the various results. All too often the strain of the bacterium, the details of fermentation, the assay insect and the route of administration have been varied simultaneously. Quite frequently the test materials and the assay procedure have been ill-defined and on several occasions even such basic data as the dose used and the exposure time were omitted. Illustrating these many pitfalls is the apparent insensitivity of *G. mellonella* to oral administration of the supernatant (McConnell and Richards, 1959; Heitor, 1962; Cantwell *et al.,* 1964). As only a very limited range of doses was used in each case, it is possible that the doses applied were insufficient to elicit a response. That this must be so can be deduced from the results of Vaňková

(1966), Kreig (1967) and Schmid and Benz (1969) who have shown that the larval stage of this species is affected by oral application.

Using a considerably purified "exotoxin" and an elegant *Drosophila melanogaster* bioassay procedure, Schmid and Benz found that, when fed to *G. mellonella* larvae, the exotoxin was extensively de-activated in the larva and that the oral dose for *G. mellonella* was 247 times the injected dose. This would mean that the estimated oral LD_{50} for McConnell and Richards' supernatant would be 0.36 x 247 μl, or 89 μl/larva. Unfortunately, it is not possible to decide whether or not this dose was given as McConnell and Richards state the concentration of supernatant given in the food but omit to say how much food was eaten. It would appear that Heitor (1962) did not give more than 15 μl of supernatant (5 μl of 3 x concentrated supernatant) which would not be expected to produce a noticeable effect.

Cantwell *et al.* (1964) used up to 50 mg of a semi-purified toxin in an attempt to affect *G. mellonella* by the oral route. Their toxin was derived from a commercial preparation of *B. thuringiensis,* Parasporin, and so there is doubt about precisely what this material contained and what amount of supernatant was represented by the maximum dose of 50 mg used. However, it can be calculated to be less active than the completely unpurified, freeze-dried, sterile *B. thuringiensis* supernatant used by us and others. This doubt also weakens the argument of Cantwell *et al.* that:

> "since Burgerjon and de Barjac, and Krieg and Herfs found that their culture filtrates were effective against Lepidoptera, it is reasonable to propose that perhaps they were measuring the effect of yet another toxin since we have not been able to obtain any mortality in *Estigmene acrea, Plodia interpunctella* or *G. mellonella,* fed up to 50 mg of semi-purified toxin".

In any case their argument is already very dubious because although Burgerjon and de Barjac (1960) and Krieg and Herfs (1963) had worked with several species of Lepidoptera they did not use these three particular species.

More recently, without a great deal of supporting evidence, Heimpel (1967a) has taken the position that all the various observations referred to above are attributable to one toxin. We would agree that the balance of evidence favours this conclusion.[1] We base this on the following evidence.

First, in all the various observations of toxicity caused by the autoclaved *B. thuringiensis* supernatant the symptomology is very similar, an argument which seems to have been strangely neglected in spite of its freedom from many of the objections that apply to the existing quantitative data.

Second, we have recently obtained quantitative data which link the results of McConnell and Richards (1959) using *G. mellonella* with results of various authors, including Cantwell *et al.* (1964), who used *M. domestica* to detect

---

[1] Editor's note: see contrasting view in Chapter 9, p. 214).

TABLE I

The relative potencies of B. thuringiensis *exoculture and pure exotoxin (J. D. Tipton, Bond and Boyce, unpublished)*

Species	LD_{50} and 95% confidence limits (μg)		Slope (*b*)	Potency ratio and 95% confidence limits
	Supernatant[a]	Exotoxin		
Musca domestica (oral)	2710 (2160-3370)	10.6 (8.52-13.3)	−1.93	255 (185-348)
Galleria mellonella (injection)	2.78 (2.27-3.38)	0.00944 0.00774-0.0115)	−4.69	294 (222-389)

[a] Freeze dried exoculture of *B. thuringiensis* var. *thuringiensis* (same batch for both insect species) see Bond *et al.* (1969) for details of culture. N.B. the same conditions were used throughout but different batches of supernatant are referred to in other assays.

activity. We found that the LD_{50} obtained by injecting our sterile supernatant bacterial culture (see Bond *et al.,* 1969 for details of the culture) into *G. mellonella* is 0.17 μl/larva (equivalent to 2.8 μg of freeze-dried fermentation solids) in good agreement with McConnell and Richards who give an LD_{50} of 0.36 μl/larva for their supernatant. When we purified our supernatant using a *M. domestica* assay to monitor the procedure (Bond *et al.,* 1969) the total increase in potency was 255 times, in excellent agreement with the factor of 294 we found using *G. mellonella* as assay organism (Table I). Had the two species responded to different toxins the factor would probably have differed in each case. Results presented in Table II show that this same purified material is orally

TABLE II

Activity of exotoxin against insect larvae (J. D. Tipton, Bond and Boyce, unpublished)

Species	Method	LD_{50}	LD_{50} standard
Musca domestica	Treated medium	1 p.p.m.	10 p.p.m. Dieldrin
Drosophila melanogaster	Treated medium	1 p.p.m.	85 p.p.m. Imidazolidin-2-one
Aedes aegypti	Treated medium	1.9 p.p.m.	0.004 p.p.m. Baytex
Phaedon cochleariae	Sprayed foliage[a]	0.0035%	0.00073% Ethyl parathion
Plutella maculipennis	Sprayed foliage	0.0033%	0.00037% Ethyl parathion
Pieris brassicae	Sprayed foliage	0.0052%	0.00016% Ethyl parathion
Galleria mellonella	Injection	0.055 μg/g	74.2 μg/g DDT[b]

[a] % w/v solution sprayed to "run-off".
[b] Beard (1949).

active against a wide range of insects including *Pieris brassicae,* one of the Lepidoptera found to be susceptible by Burgerjon and de Barjac (1960). Furthermore, using assay techniques similar to those described by Cantwell *et al.* (1964) we find a factor of 1.9 for the concentrations required in the culture media of *Aedes aegypti* larvae and *M. domestica* larvae (LD_{50}s of 1.9 p.p.m. and 1.0 p.p.m. respectively). This is in excellent agreement with the factor of 2.1 which can be deduced from the results of Cantwell *et al.* (850 p.p.m. and 400 p.p.m.) for a similar response.

Third, only one toxin has been isolated in each of the four published purification procedures *(vide infra).* Furthermore, Bond *et al.* (1969) showed that, after a six-stage purification procedure, their purified fraction represented 36% of the original activity in the autoclaved supernatant. By recycling a known amount of pure material through the purification procedure, they showed that the major losses were mechanical (in particular from irreversible adsorption onto charcoal) and not by separation from other toxic materials.

Finally, as we shall discuss in detail later, the physical and chemical properties of the toxins that have been isolated and studied independently by three groups (de Barjac and Dedonder, 1965, 1968; Bond, Boyce and French, 1969; and Šebesta, Horská and Vaňková, 1969a) are all in good agreement despite the fact that two different bacterial strains of *B. thuringiensis* and completely different bioassay procedures were used.

We shall, therefore, adopt the term "exotoxin" for the heat-stable toxin (120°/15 min) released into the culture liquid by some strains of *B. thuringiensis.*

III. Bioassay Procedures

A comprehensive list of insect species reported to be susceptible to crude, sterile *B. thuringiensis* centrifuged supernatant is given in a recent review by Heimpel (1967a). Of these *Mamestra brassicae, Galleria mellonella, Drosophila melanogaster* and *Musca domestica* have been used most extensively for quantitative assays and were used to monitor the four reported purifications of the exotoxin *(vide infra).* Some of the important features of each assay method are summarized below.

Mamestra brassicae is often bred on cabbage plants in the glasshouse though it can be bred on the synthetic diet developed for *Pieris brassicae* (David and Gardiner, 1965). The test method described by Burgerjon and de Barjac (1964) involves spraying the material on to discs of cabbage leaf and exposing instar III larvae for two days. Deaths are counted after at least eight days. The control mortality is about 10%.

Galleria mellonella can be bred in the laboratory on a synthetic diet (Haydak medium), an advantage stressed by McConnell and Richards (1959) and by

Šebesta, Horská and Vaňková (1969b). An assay method which involves injecting mature larvae (instar V or VI) with up to 10 μl of test solution is described by both groups as well as by Vaňková (1966) and Schmid and Benz (1969). A second method which involves including the exotoxin in Haydak medium and feeding this to the larvae has been described by several authors including: Vaňková (1966), Krieg (1967) and Schmid and Benz (1969). The results of the last authors clearly demonstrate that injection is much more sensitive (by a factor of approximately 250) and has the advantage that the dose administered per larva is defined, though obviously this does not mean that the estimated lethal dose is necessarily precisely defined. It is not easy to decide exactly how much time need elapse before the assay can be read. Most authors observe for up to 14 days but Šebesta, Horská and Vaňková (1969b) state that this can be reduced to 48 hr. The control mortality in the injection method is very favourable and does not exceed 5-10% but the method does require a little skill. This species, like *M. brassicae,* is very susceptible to the crystal toxin of *B. thuringiensis* which, therefore, must be carefully excluded from test materials. Fortunately, this is easily achieved by autoclaving or membrane filtration.

Drosophila melanogaster, which is very easy to breed, can be used as assay subject and suitable techniques have been well described by Krieg (1966) and by Benz and Perron (1967). The exotoxin is incorporated in the larval medium which can be of the corn-yeast-agar type or the synthetic medium of Sang (1956). Benz and Perron note that care should be taken with the synthetic medium because some commercial brands of one of the ingredients, casein, are lethal. The best media resulted in only 5% control mortality. They also showed that yeast can reduce the effectiveness of exotoxin. This is not important in relative potency experiments but may lead to variation in absolute potency. The required exposure time is not specifically stated.

Musca domestica is also easily bred and is very widely available. Early workers exposed fly larvae to cattle faeces, which has the merit of assessing the practical value of exotoxin, but a much more convenient bioassay has been reported by Cantwell *et al.* (1964). The method involves exposing a known number of instar III larvae to a medium consisting of 1 : 1 milk-water, 2% w/v of yeast and a known amount of crude exotoxin, all of which is absorbed on to cotton. Again the exposure time is not given but, using a similar method, we have based our reading on the total number of adults to emerge after seven days at 30° (Bond *et al.,* 1969). The average control response is only 2%. We have also described a quicker method which involves exposing *M. domestica* eggs on a yeast-milk-agar medium treated with exotoxin. The response is based on the inhibition of development to the larval instar III after 48 hr. The method suffers from relatively poor reproducibility and sometimes from high control mortality and it is, therefore, best used only for semi-quantitative results.

In all of these assay methods the response of the insect follows a linear probit response–log dose relationship from which LD_{50} values or potency ratios can be calculated by well known methods (Chapter 27). Alternatively, computer programmes are available for a full statistical analysis of the results giving LD_{10}, LD_{50}, LD_{90} etc. and their fiducial limits, the slope β, and χ^2.

It is not yet possible to compare the precision of the various assays as very few results have been reported. Bond *et al.* (1969) found that the absolute LD_{50} value of exotoxin solution varied by a factor of almost 2 when assayed on four separate occasions by the longer, quantitative *M. domestica* method. The relative potency of this same solution, in comparison with a standard solution of pure exotoxin, gave better reproducibility (Table III). We also calculated the number

TABLE III

Potencies and confidence limits for the quantitative Musca domestica *assay with two solutions of exotoxin*[a]

	Occasion	Dose for 50% inhibition (μg)		Potency ratio A/B	95% confidence limits for A/B
		Supernatant (A)	Exotoxin (B)		
Based on all	1	2336	5.3	443	344-569
adults to emerge	2	1501	4.8	313	220-447
including	3	1128	2.9	386	270-550
deformed ones	4	1206	3.3	361	253-514
Based on	1	1382	2.9	476	344-659
normal	2	821	3.0	278	176-440
adults	3	876	2.0	447	282-706
only	4	808	2.3	349	221-552

[a] Solutions A and B were assayed together, with three replicates of each, on four separate occasions.

of replicates needed to detect various differences in potency ratios. For example, four replicates of six doses with 20 larvae/dose were required to detect a 30% difference in activity between solutions and to show which was the more active. Data for other potency ratios are given in Table IV.

Future bioassay work with exotoxin will benefit greatly if some form of standardization can be introduced to avoid a great deal of controversy and ambiguity which has been a feature of the early work on exotoxin. We heartily endorse the recommendation of Burgerjon (1965) and the resolution of Burges *et al.* (1967) made at the International Colloquium on Insect Pathology and Microbial Control, Wageningen, in 1966, to use a standard and to express results as relative potencies. This has the advantages over a standard bioassay method that many problems inherent in standardizing an assay are avoided and, when only one toxin is involved, the results are independent of the method used, so

TABLE IV

Number of replicates (of 6 doses: 20 larvae/dose) required in the Musca domestica *assay to detect potency differences at the 5% level of significance*

	All larvae			Normal larvae only		
Potency ratio	1.1	1.2	1.3	1.1	1.2	1.3
2 sided test[a]	29	8	4	47	13	6
1 sided test[a]	20	6	3	34	9	4

[a] The two-sided test is used when one wants to know if two ED_{50}s are significantly different from each other, e.g. if the two ED_{50}s are A and B and one is testing whether either of the situations A>B or B>A is significant. The one sided test is used when only one of these situations is of interest, e.g. when one is testing if A>B but it is of no interest if B>A however large this difference may be.

that the details of technique are left open for whatever is considered to be the most convenient. Now that the pure exotoxin is available, it is the obvious reference material and we have set aside a quantity for use as a bioassay standard. We shall be pleased to make this available in 1 mg samples to anyone interested.

IV. Purification

The purification of the exotoxin is simplified by the remarkably high concentration of the material present in the supernatant of centrifuged liquid cultures. A normal *B. thuringiensis* var. *thuringiensis* strain, grown without any attempt to increase the yield, produces a concentration of 50 mg/litre in the supernatant (Bond *et al.*, 1969). However, it is very difficult to establish that the exotoxin is chemically homogeneous. For the most part, this difficulty has been ignored.

The most important step in all the published purifications (de Barjac and Dedonder, 1965, 1968; Bond *et al.*, 1969; Šebesta *et al.*, 1967, 1969a), except that of Benz (1966), is adsorption onto and elution from charcoal. The possibility that this process would provide a means of partially purifying or of concentrating the exotoxin was first mentioned, somewhat obliquely, by Drake and Smythe in 1961 in a patent in which it was also indicated that the salts of certain metals could precipitate the exotoxin directly from the bacterial supernatant. Magnesium, calcium and barium were specifically mentioned. The manipulations described by Drake and Smythe were not directed toward a purification of the exotoxin, but were intended to describe a number of ways by which the toxin could be concentrated from the supernatant in a form convenient for use as an insecticide.

In the first purification attempted by de Barjac and Dedonder (1965) the bacterial supernatant was freed of cells, spores and other solid matter, concentrated six times by evaporation at low pressure and autoclaved at 120° for 15 min. The concentrate was adsorbed onto acid-washed charcoal which was washed with 0.01 *M*-EDTA (ethylene diamine tetra-acetic acid) and distilled water. A fraction toxic to *Mamestra brassicae* was eluted from the washed charcoal with 50% aqueous ethanol. This fraction, after concentration, was chromatographed on Whatman No. 1 paper in the system ethanol : *M*-ammonium acetate at pH 3.8. The band of $R_{\text{adenosine}}$ 0.13[1] was excised and eluted from the paper with distilled water. Paper chromatography of the toxic eluate in four other systems gave rise in each case to only one spot absorbing ultra-violet light (UV) at *ca* 260 nμ. The UV spectral characteristics of the eluate were interpreted as indicating an adenine nucleotide. Further, the eluate gave a positive test (the details of which were not specified) for phosphate and gave, on hydrolysis (no conditions given), a compound with spectral and chromatographic properties identical with those of adenine. Very mild hydrolyses of the toxic eluate (0.1 N-H_2SO_4 : 20 min at 100°) yielded a fragment which chromatographed with, and gave similar colour reactions to, ribose. de Barjac and Dedonder showed that in the toxic eluate the adenine, phosphate, ribose (estimated by the orcinol method which measures both bound and free ribose) and, after hydrolysis, the "reducing groups" were present in the molar ratio 1 : 1.2 : 1.4 : 1.4. The conditions required to release the 1.4 moles of "reducing groups" (0.1 N-HCl : 60 min at 100°) suggest that the yield of the free ribose identified chromatographically probably fell short of quantitative.

A few months after de Barjac and Dedonder's note, Benz (1966) described a purification which remains unique in that it uses neither charcoal adsorption nor precipitation by heavy metal salts. The supernatant from a centrifuged liquid culture of *B. thuringiensis* was concentrated to one-tenth by boiling. This is a rigorous test of the thermostability of the exotoxin and it is to be regretted that Benz did not quantitate the survival of toxicity. Successive amounts of ethanol were added to the concentrate and the resulting precipitate was removed and discarded. Finally, at an alcohol concentration of 90% v/v, a toxic fraction was precipitated. This was separated and re-dissolved in water and further purified either by chromatography on a cellulose column eluted with 80% ethanol in water or by ion exchange fractionation on Dowex-2 resin (the form of the resin was not specified) which was eluted successively with water, 10% acetic acid in water, and 5% KOH.

The toxic fractions isolated by the methods of de Barjac and Dedonder, and of Benz, had similar UV spectra. Colour tests suggested that Benz's toxin contained an aldopentose.

---

[1] Paper chromatographic mobility of a compound relative to the solvent front is represented as R_f and relative to a standard compound, *X*, as R_x.

The purification of Šebesta *et al.* (1967) involved adsorption onto charcoal from the centrifuged bacterial supernatant, elution from the charcoal with aqueous ethanol and subsequent fractionation on Dowex-1 formate eluted with 0-1.5 *M*-ammonium formate buffer. The material so isolated was shown to contain adenine and phosphate in a ratio of 1 : 1.2 by methods similar to those already described. However, Šebesta *et al.* detected no ribose as a hydrolysis product of their toxin. The chromatographic behaviour of their exotoxin in the system isobutyric acid : water : ammmonia was unusual. We have observed and attempted to explain similar behaviour with our exotoxin in the system ethanol : *M*-ammonium acetate at pH 3.8 (Bond *et al.*, 1969) but de Barjac and Dedonder (1965, 1968) did not record anomalous behaviour in this system.

In 1968 de Barjac and Dedonder published their second purification which involves precipitation (with mercury salts), charcoal adsorption and ion-exchange chromatography on Dowex-1 (chloride). A curious feature of this new work by the French group is that, whereas previously their toxin was eluted from charcoal with 50% aqueous ethanol, they now use this eluent to wash out impurities and then elute the toxin with "ammoniacal ethanol". Charcoals are, of course, notoriously variable in their properties. In this second paper the molecular weight of the exotoxin was found to lie between 700 and 800. The exotoxin took up two moles of periodate.

Šebesta *et al.* (1969a) have now given a more detailed description of their purification, together with some minor modifications.

The purification of Bond *et al.* (1969) used precipitation with barium, adsorption onto charcoal at a pH of approximately 1, elution therefrom with 50% aqueous ethanol containing 1% of concentrated ammonia, adsorption onto a Dowex-1 (Cl^-) or Permutit FFIP (Cl^-) resin, elution with 0.1 *N*-HCl containing 0.1 *M*-NaCl and desalting of the neutralized (with ammonia) eluate on Sephadex G-10. Remaining impurities are then removed either by preparative layer chromatography on cellulose and silica gel or by chromatography on DEAE cellulose. The combination of the barium precipitation with charcoal adsorption steps is rapid and convenient giving a 100-fold purification. The initial concentration of exotoxin in the bacterial supernatant is approximately 50 μg/litre and the overall yield is 36%. The quantitative data for this purification are given in Table V. Unfortunately no comparable figures for the other procedures are available.

Our purification requires little skill and virtually no experience up to the point of Sephadex G-10 desalting. This was completed in our laboratory, by an experienced technician in three days at his first attempt, starting with 120 litres of culture medium. Following the experimental procedure from our paper, an intelligent, but inexperienced, beginnner was able to undertake these stages of the purification after two weeks training. The preparative layer chromatography, however, requires a fair degree of skill and experience. The DEAE cellulose step

TABLE V

Summary of the data of Bond et al. *(1969) for purification of the exotoxin of* B. thuringiensis

Stage	Volume (litre)	Weight of solid fraction (g)	LD_{50} and 95% limits (μg)	Specific activity	Total activity (units) $\times 10^{-3}$	Overall % recovery and 95% confidence limits	$E^{1\%}_{1\,cm}$ max 260 nμ
Exoculture	110	1870	804 (679-951)	1.23	2300	–	slight[a]
Barium precipitate	–	1100	–	–	–	–	–
Charcoal eluate	4	8.5	6.4 (5.4-7.6)	156.2	1328	57 (46-71)	0.9×10^2
Dowex-1/ G10 Sephadex	0.2/0.06	4.0	3.8 (3.2-4.5)	263	1052	46 (37-56)	1.58×10^2
Pure	–	2.5	3.0 (2.5-3.5)	333	820	36 (29-44)	1.66×10^2

[a] End absorption, slight shoulder at 260 nμ..

is less exacting, particularly if the loading is kept low, and can be used by anyone familiar with general chromatographic procedures.

The method of Šebesta *et al.* (1969a) is also simple and straightforward, but there is one possible complication which may not be obvious. The purification relies on good resolution during Dowex-1 chromatography. Because of the molecular size of the exotoxin, resins of low cross-linking are best. The use of eluents of increasing ionic strength can result in the resin contracting and expanding and care is necessary for resolution to be maintained.

V. Chemistry

The exotoxin purified by de Barjac and Dedonder (1965, 1968), Šebesta *et al.* (1967, 1969a) and Bond *et al.* (1969) contains adenine substituted at the 9 position. The evidence for its presence comes from chromatography and ultra-violet spectroscopy (de Barjac and Dedonder, 1965, 1968; Šebesta *et al.*, 1967), isolation of the picrate and mass spectroscopy (Bond *et al.*, 1969). The arguments for the position of substitution and the references relevant thereto are given by Bond *et al.* (1969).

All the purified materials contain phosphate. The adenine: phosphate ratio has been variously given at 1 : 1.2 (de Barjac and Dedonder, 1965; Šebesta *et al.*, 1967), 1 : 0.98 (Bond *et al.*, 1969) and 1 : 1.04 (Šebesta *et al.*, (1969a). The latter two values are confirmed by elemental analysis for the free acid of the exotoxin. Assuming that all of the nitrogen is present in the adenine, these lead to values of 1 : 1.06 (Bond *et al.*, 1969) and 1 : 1.08 (Šebesta *et al.*, 1969a) for the ratio.

Molecular weight values from 707 (de Barjac and Dedonder, 1968) to 850 (Bond *et al.*, 1969; Šebesta *et al.*, 1968a) have been estimated for the exotoxins from the three laboratories. The value of 707 is very close to that required for the structure advanced by Šebesta's group (Farkas *et al.*, 1969). However, nitrogen analysis of the same material leads to a molecular weight of 795 (de Barjac and Dedonder, 1968). The precise method by which the value 707 is obtained is not made clear in the French paper. Their reference 10 to "Methods in Enzymology III" we presume refers to Bendich (1957). The differential extinction technique described there is applicable to free adenine in acid solution. Since de Barjac and Dedonder make no reference at the relevant point to any hydrolysis or subsequent chromatography, they appear to be applying the technique directly to the free acid of their exotoxin. If this is so, the method, as applied, is invalid. From their value of the adenine content, it is possible to calculate the $(\epsilon_{262.5}-\epsilon_{290})$[1] of their solution. If this is then used with the $(\epsilon_{262.}-\epsilon_{290})$ for a 10 γ/ml solution of adenosine (Bendich, 1957) their adenine content becomes 166 γ per 1000 γ of exotoxin, leading to a molecular weight of 810, in good agreement with their value for nitrogen analysis. With this new interpretation, the estimated values of the molecular weight fall in the range 730-850 and the two extreme values originate from the same laboratory (Šebesta *et al.*, 1968a, 1969a).

The ^{1}H n.m.r. (nuclear magnetic resonance) spectrum of the exotoxin isolated in our laboratory is shown in Fig. 1. The low field region of the

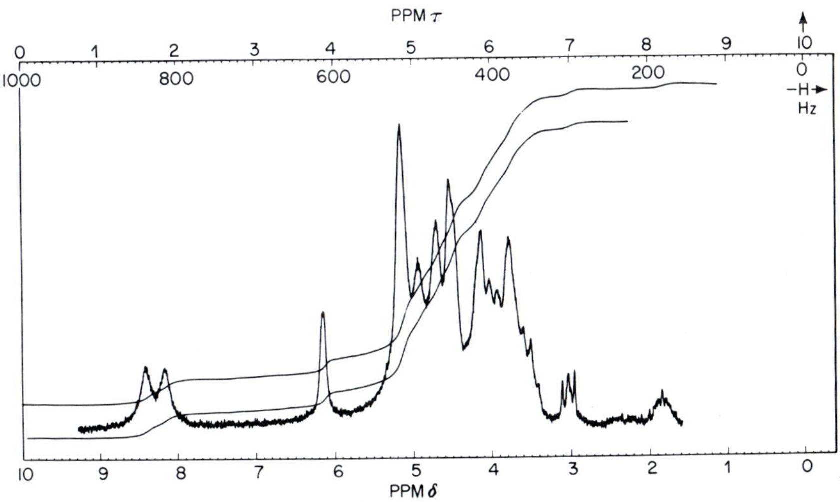

Fig. 1. ^{1}H n.m.r. of exotoxin.

[1] $\epsilon_{262.5}$ is the molar extinction coefficient at a wavelength of 262.5 nm.

spectrum, which includes singlets at 8.4 δ and 8.2 δ and a doublet at 6.13 δ, is almost identical with the equivalent region in the spectrum of adenosine (Fromageot *et al.*, 1966) and similar to that for AMP (Feldman and Agarwal, 1968). This, together with data on the hydrolytic cleavage of the adenine residue *(vide infra)*, establishes that the substitution at the 9 position of the adenine is by a moiety possessing an anomeric proton, whose magnetic environment is similar to that in adenosine, AMP, ADP and ATP. There is no signal at higher field than 3.4 δ, the absorptions centred around 1.8 δ and 3.0 δ being due to the internal lock compound, 3-(trimethylsilyl)-propane sulphonic acid sodium salt. It follows that all protons in the exotoxin, not exchangeable for deuterium, are attached to carbon atoms bound to electronegative substituents. For a natural product, this limits the chemical class of the unidentified groupings to either carbohydrates or certain amino acids. Since neither the exotoxin nor any of its hydrolysis products react with ninhydrin, the portion of the molecule still to be identified must be carbohydrate in nature.

The ^{31}P n.m.r. spectrum of the magnesium salt of the exotoxin is shown in Fig. 2. The spectrum was obtained with aid of a computer of average transients and shows a shift of +0.3 p.p.m. with respect to 85% H_3PO_4 as an external standard. The magnesium salt of AMP has a ^{31}P shift of –0.1 p.p.m. Data of ^{31}P shifts for phosphate esters are scanty (Clarke and Lyons, 1966). Such as exist (Nielson *et al.*, 1964) show that there is little difference between the value given above and those for phosphodiesters. Enzymic and chemical hydrolysis experiments (see below) define the exotoxin as a phosphomonoester, however, and the ^{31}P shift does not contradict these results. Unfortunately, the multiplicity could not be resolved.

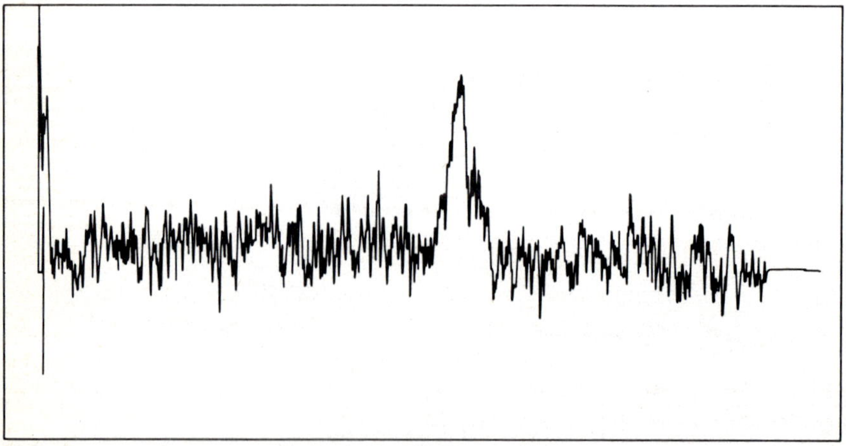

Fig. 2. ^{31}P n.m.r. of exotoxin.

The exotoxin can be dephosphorylated with acid or alkaline phosphomonoesterases (EC[1] 3.1.3.1 and EC 3.1.3.2) (Bond *et al.*, 1969; Šebesta *et al.*, 1969). This provides a dephosphorylated exotoxin which has been used in the structural studies of Šebesta *et al.* and Bond *et al.* The same dephosphorylated exotoxin is produced during hydrolysis of the exotoxin in acetate buffer at pH 4.0 (Bond *et al.*, 1969) at a rate which defines the phosphate moiety as a phosphomonoester (Vernon, 1957).

From the dephosphorylated exotoxin, allomucic acid has been obtained by acid hydrolysis (*N*-H_2SO_4 at 100° for 2 hr) and identified by comparison with authentic material (Bond, 1969). Prolonged hydrolysis (Dowex-50[H^+] at 100° for 14 hr) of the dephosphorylated exotoxin gave a 5.0% yield of D-glucose, identified and quantified with glucose oxidase.

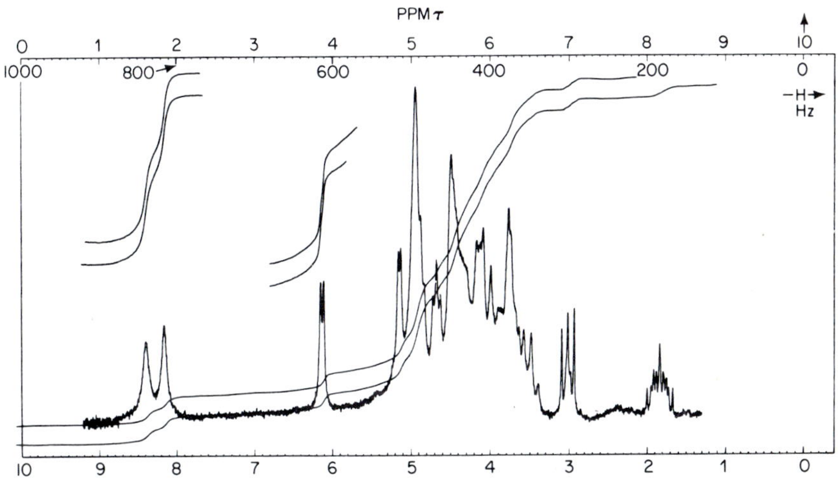

Fig. 3. [1]H n.m.r. of dephosphorylated exotoxin.

The [1]H n.m.r. spectrum of the dephosphorylated exotoxin, shown in Fig. 3 is similar to, but not identical with that of the exotoxin. The comments made earlier about the adenine protons and the anomeric proton apply here also and it should be noted that these three protons appear at almost exactly the same chemical shift in the two compounds. The shift of the anomeric proton indicates a trans-relationship between $H_{1'}$ and $H_{2'}$ (Nishimura and Shimizu, 1965). There is also a doublet at 5.17 δ which can, from the above hydrolysis result, be ascribed to the anomeric proton of glucose. The chemical shift and coupling constant *ca.* 3 cps (cycles per sec.), are compatible with an α-D-glucopyranose configuration (ver der Veen, 1963; Rao and Foster, 1963).

---

[1] EC = Enzyme Commission Report nomenclature.

The similarity between the exotoxin and the adenine nucleotides in respect of the immediate molecular environment of the adenine, suggested by the n.m.r. spectra, is further confirmed by the optical rotary dispersion (ORD) spectra and by studies of the rates of acid catalyzed cleavage of the *N*-glycosidic linkage. The ORD curves of the exotoxin and its magnesium salt are shown in Fig. 4, together with the curve for ATP. The similarity of shape is obvious. It can be concluded

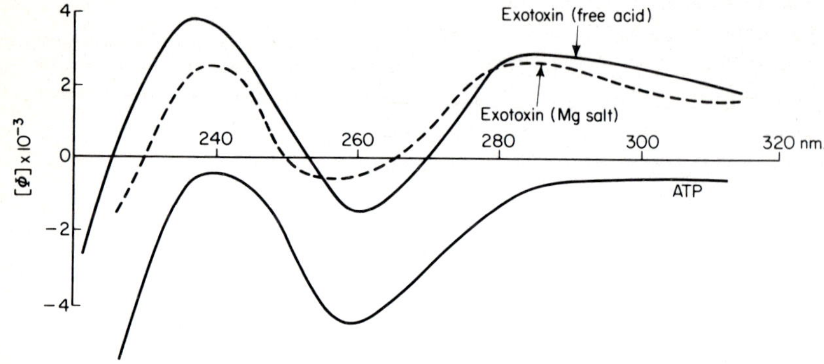

Fig. 4. Optical rotary dispersion curves of exotoxin and ATP in 0.1 *N*-HCl.

that, if the anomeric bond to adenine is from a pentofuranose, it has the β-configuration (Ulbricht *et al.*, 1964). The rates of hydrolysis of the exotoxin in N-H_2SO_4 at 100° were measured by following the appearance of a reducing function and of adenine. The first order rate constant has a value of 10^{-3} sec^{-1} identical with that for AMP (Bond *et al.*, 1969).

The data from UV and n.m.r. spectra, ORD curves and rates of hydrolysis all indicate that adenine is substituted at position 9 with a ribofuranose moiety in the β-configuration.

Acid hydrolysis of the dephosphorylated exotoxin produced, in addition to adenine and allomucic acid, a neutral sugar which had the molecular dimensions of a disaccharide, but which was stable to acid under conditions expected to cleave a disaccharide. The chemical nature of this fragment has been neatly clarified in a recent paper by Farkas *et al.* (1969). The reactions carried out and the significant measurements made on the various compounds are summarized in Schemes 1 and 2.

The molecular weights IV and VII, obtained by mass spectroscopy (scheme 2 for IV), indicate that the disaccharide arises by fusion of a hexose and a pentose unit. The hexose can be identified as glucose, which is a product of vigorous acid hydrolysis (*cf.* p. 289) of III (R = Me). The ORD curve of VI makes it likely that the pentose is ribose. The ability of III (R = Me) to form the acetonide IV supports the identity of the pentose and, given this identity, requires that it be substituted at position 5′. The Czechoslovak workers also mention evidence,

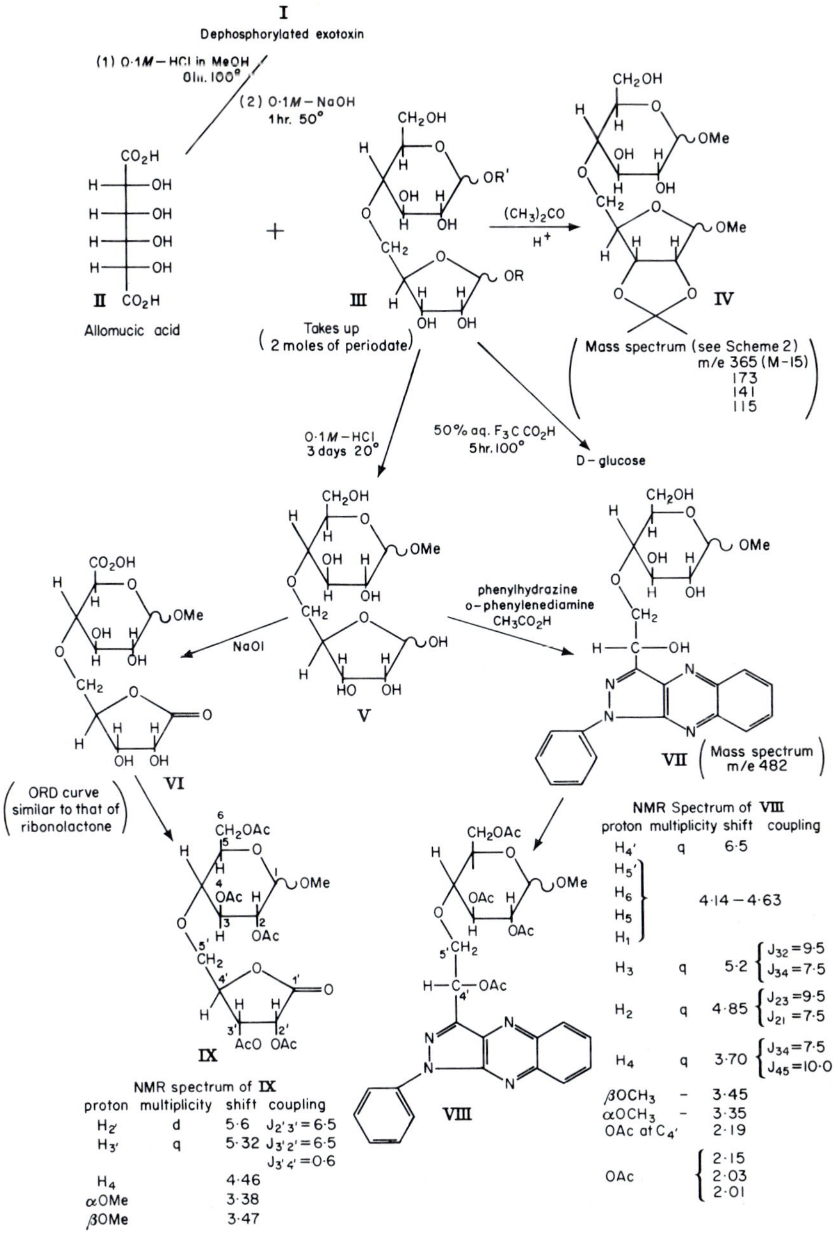

Scheme 1. Degradation of dephosphorylated exotoxin.

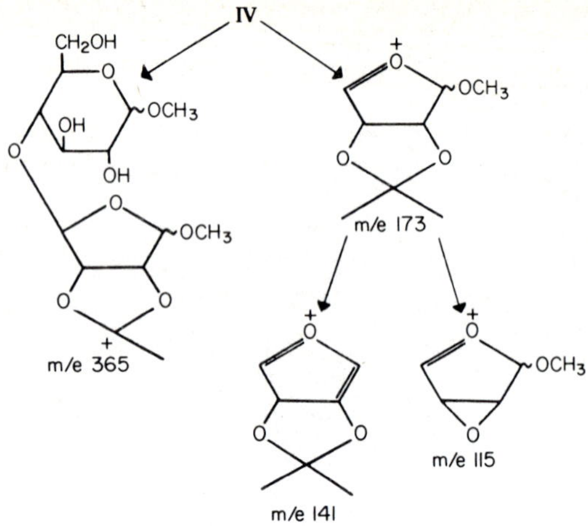

Scheme 2. Suggested fragmentation of IV by mass spectroscopy (Farkas *et al.*, 1969).

similar to our own outlined above, to indicate that the adenine is substituted by ribose.

The position of substitution of the glucose hangs, perhaps a little heavily, on the chemical shift of the 4 proton in compound VIII. The shift is in excellent agreement with that of the 3 proton in compound X, 3-0-methyl β-D-glucopyranose tetracetate (Lemieux and Stevens, 1965). It is therefore unfortunate that in IX, which is more closely analogous to X, the 4 proton has shifted up

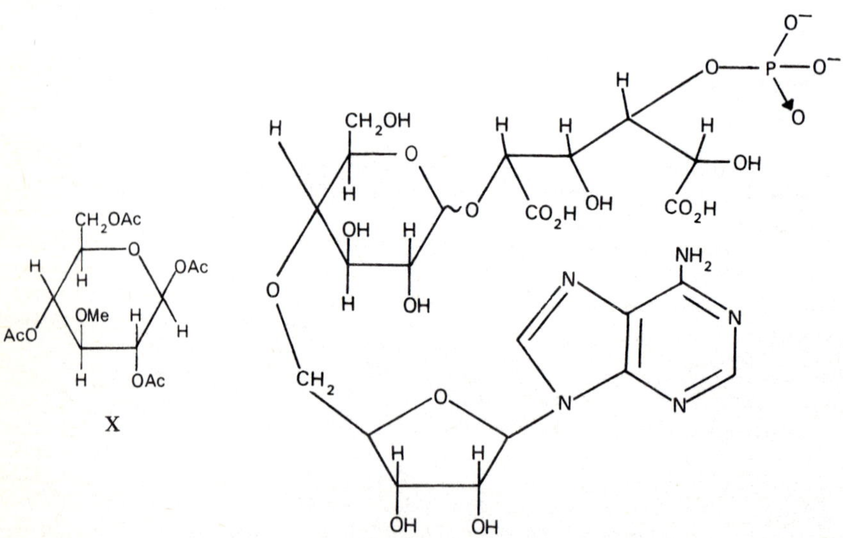

X

XI Structure of exotoxin proposed by Farkas *et al.* (1969).

field from its value in VIII. With a very small reservation concerning the position of substitution of glucose, then, structure III can be accepted as representing the product of acid catalyzed hydrolysis (R = H) or methanolysis (R = Me) of the dephosphorylated exotoxin.

Farkas *et al.* (1969) then use the structure of III, together with other evidence which we shall discuss presently to propose XI as the structure of the exotoxin.

For the placement of groups on the allomucic acid residue, Farkas *et al.* have relied on infra-red evidence which indicates that the exotoxin, on very mild acid treatment, forms a γ-lactone while the dephosphorylated exotoxin forms 2 γ-lactones. From the ion exchange behaviour of the various compounds, however, it is unlikely that the equilibrium involved is that between a hydroxy-acid and its γ-lactone, because the "lactones" have a higher affinity for a basic ion exchange column than have the hydroxy-acids from which they are derived. This is shown not only by the positions of elution but also by the widths of the peaks involved. There is no reason to accept the infra-red data and reject that from ion exchange yet, as presented, they are incompatible. A possible synthesis of the two results is that lactonization, if it is to occur, occurs during the evaporation of the fractions from the ion exchange column. On this hypothesis, using the nomenclature of Šebesta *et al.* (1969a), the desphosphorylated exotoxin and lactone B, as they elute from the column, are monocarboxylic acids. During the subsequent evaporation, the carboxyl group of lactone B lactonises while that of dephosphorylated exotoxin does not. Lactone A, as it elutes from the column, is a dicarboxylic acid, one of whose carboxyl groups lactonises during the subsequent evaporation. It follows that one carboxyl group is already masked in the dephosphorylated exotoxin.

We see in our laboratory a very similar pattern when dephosphorylated exotoxin is treated with acid under mild conditions and then analysed by ion exchange chromatography. None of the components when isolated has an infra-red peak at 1770 cm^{-1}, a circumstance which finds a ready explanation in our use of a buffer of higher pH (8.5) than that favoured by Šebesta *et al.* (1969a).

This explanation of the ion exchange and infra-red data could be accommodated in the structural proposal of Farkas *et al.* (XI) but would require some further information on the nature and extent of the masking of a carboxyl group in dephosphorylated exotoxin *as it is eluted from the column.* This in fact will not be easy to obtain because it is always necessary somehow to remove the buffer constituents.

The structure (XI) proposed by Farkas *et al.* (1969) permits no explanation of the isolation of ribose by de Barjac and Dedonder (1965).

In our laboratory, we have recently isolated adenosine as a hydrolysis product of dephosphorylated exotoxin. The conditions of its production are precisely defined and help to explain both the original observation of ribose as a hydrolysis product of exotoxin by de Barjac and Dedonder (1965) and the subsequent failure of Šebesta *et al.* (1967) to reproduce this result. Its isolation provides definitive chemical evidence for the adenine-ribose linkage in exotoxin and also necessarily casts doubt on the nature of the ribose-glucose linkage suggested in the structural proposal (XI) of Farkas *et al.* (1969).

The structure proposed by Farkas *et al.* (1969) (XI) summarises our knowledge of the chemistry of the exotoxin fairly well but it must be treated with circumspection for the moment. More evidence is needed on the mode of attachment of glucose to allomucic acid and on whether the disaccharide (III) represents a true structural component or an artifact.

One important feature of exotoxin has been and is its failure to crystallize. This eliminates the use of X-ray crystallography from consideration in structural work. It also leaves a residual uncertainty about the identity of the exotoxins produced in different laboratories. The reviewers have exchanged exotoxin samples with Šebesta's group and with H. T. Huang of International Minerals Corporation (Illinois). Insofar as chromatography, electrophoresis and ion exchange can be regarded as reliable criteria, all three samples are identical.

VI. Microbiology

As with most other aspects of *B. thuringiensis* metabolism, the biosynthetic and regulatory phenomena associated with exotoxin accumulation have received scant attention. Aside from the attractively unusual metabolism which may be involved in the biosynthesis of the compound, its accumulation at a commercially interesting level should warrant thorough investigation. To date only certain of the microbiological aspects have been explored.

The exotoxin has been reported to be biosynthesized mainly by strains of serotype I (Cantwell *et al.*, 1964; Krieg, 1966; Vaňková, 1966; de Barjac *et al.*, 1966). Strains of serotypes IVa and IVc (Burgerjon and de Barjac, 1967), V and VII (Heimpel, 1967b). IX (de Barjac *et al.*, 1966) and X (Krieg *et al.*, 1968) have also been reported to synthesize the compound. Of the preceding serotypes, confirmation of the exotoxin synthesis has been forthcoming for serotypes I (Rogoff *et al.*, 1969), IVa and IVc (Krieg, 1968a) and V (Krieg, 1968a; Rogoff *et al.*, 1969). Various laboratories have been unable to confirm exotoxin accumulation by serotype VII (Burgerjon and de Barjac, 1967; Krieg, 1968a; Rogoff *et al.*, 1969). Strains of serotype VIII have also been reported to elaborate a substance, or substances, toxic for flies (de Barjac *et al.*, 1966; Rogoff *et al.*, 1969). The activity, however, is apparently not due to the exotoxin. The former authors report no heat-stable toxin spot on paper chromatograms prepared from serotype VIII broths. The latter report different toxicity pattern characteristics of serotype VIII broths for *Heliothis zea* and *Trichoplusia ni* from those normally encountered with broths obtained from exotoxin-producing strains.

It has been suggested (Heimpel, 1967a) that production of exotoxin by strains of *B. thuringiensis* might prove a suitable characteristic for use as a taxonomic criterion. The suggestion, although constructive, has been subjected to valid criticism (Krieg, 1968a; Rogoff, 1968; Rogoff and Yousten, 1969). The main objection centres on the necessity for use of indirect evidence, mortality of flies, as an indication of the presence of exotoxin. Bacterial species which do not produce exotoxin can also kill flies (Aizawa and Fujiyoshi, 1968; Rogoff *et al.*, 1969). At this juncture it would seem that lacking an acceptable specific and sensitive chemical test for the full, active, defined exotoxin moiety, its production is not a suitable taxonomic criterion. The characteristic should, however, be re-evaluated for this purpose, should a satisfactory test be proposed.

Extracellular accumulation of purine bases, nucleosides or nucleotides by spore-forming bacilli is well documented (Nakayama *et al.*, 1964; Demain *et al.*, 1964; Fujimoto and Uchida, 1965). The accumulations are based on one, or a combination of three, types of metabolic activity. *De novo* synthesis of the purine moiety is involved in all (Fig. 5). The first system is common to most accumulating strains. These are various types of auxotrophic mutants, usually purine-requiring, preferably purine plus amino acid. The amino acid auxotrophy is usually for histidine, an amino acid known to play a regulatory role in the purine nucleotide interconversion cycles. The purine auxotrophy is selected so that the compounds accumulated represent intermediates preceding a point of enzymatic defect, dephosphorylated derivatives of the intermediates, or compounds accumulated as a result of blockage of one side of a branched metabolic path (e.g. IMP → XMP or AMP). Such metabolic patterns may be combined with the so-called "salvage enzyme" synthesis. The salvage enzyme functions in the pathway of resynthesis of nucleotides from catabolically-derived purine bases. The last accumulation pattern, reported for guanosine-5′-monophosphate (Demain *et al.*, 1964) results from extracellular enzymatic hydrolysis of excreted RNA.

The exotoxin accumulation in *B. thuringiensis* has only the fact of *de novo* synthesis of the purine moiety in common with the above systems. The accumulating strains are not purine auxotrophs (Conner and Hansen, 1967b; Shieh *et al.*, 1968), although certain of the strains do require amino acids for growth (Shieh *et al.*, 1968). Experiments by these authors (Table VI) indicate that the accumulation may not result from RNA degradation. In this way the unusual phenomenon of nucleotide accumulation by wild-type strains may be expressed. A second point of interest, pertinent to the accumulation, is that it occurs under conditions in which the normal feedback regulation of nucleotide synthesis would be expected to limit the accumulation of such compounds. Shieh *et al.* (1968) studied nucleotide metabolism in an exotoxin-accumulating strain of serotype I. In these studies certain purine derivatives, which play regulatory roles in the biosynthetic pathways (Fig. 5), were added to culture media of the serotype I strain (Table VI). They found that such additions

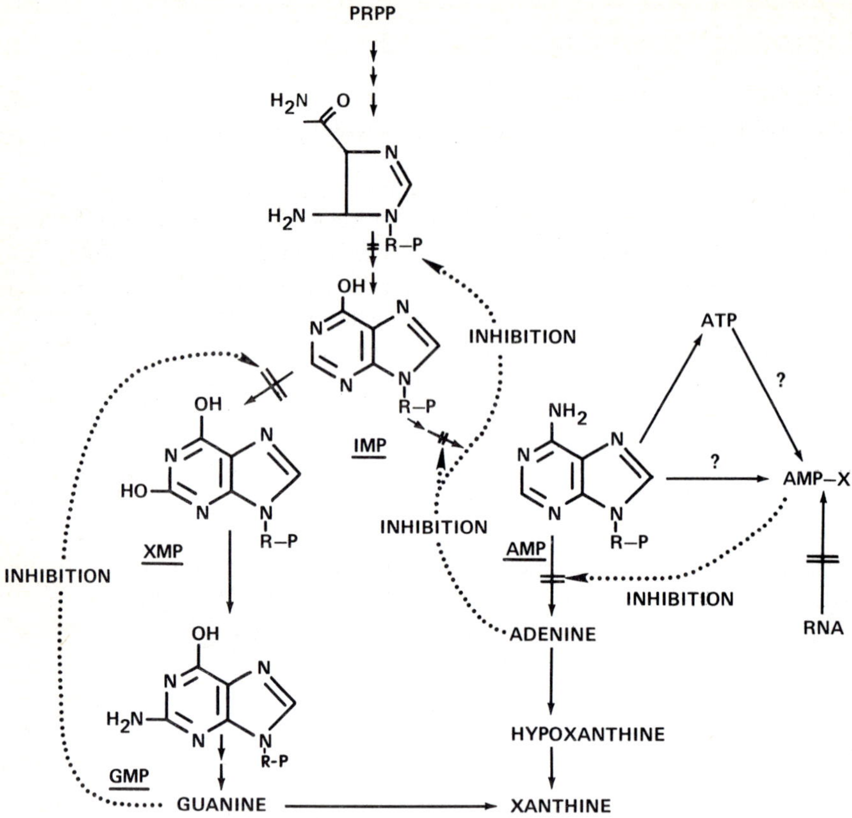

Fig. 5. Possible metabolic pathways involved in exotoxin synthesis.

resulted in a decrease in exotoxin accumulation. Thus, the normal feedback controls are operating in the strain, at least under imbalanced conditions. Their study gave further insight into the nucleotide metabolism of the strain. They demonstrated that the normal catabolic pathways involved in degradation of nucleotides were operating in the strain studied (Table VII).

It would be expected that accumulation of a nucleotide would not take place in a system of the type observed, where normal catabolism, i.e. nucleotidase activity, is present. Their experiments indicated that the exotoxin itself may be resistant to nucleotidase activity. Further, the exotoxin itself was shown to inhibit nucleotidase activity. This was demonstrated by the addition of exotoxin to suspensions of resting cells incubated with either AMP or IMP. Release of inorganic phosphate (P_i) from the compounds was measured (Table VIII). It was observed that inhibition of release of P_i from AMP was almost completely prevented; release of P_i from IMP was only partially inhibited.

TABLE VI

Inhibitory effect of purine derivatives on exotoxin accumulation by B. thuringiensis[a]

Purines	% inhibition
Adenine	50
Guanine	56
Xanthine	30
Hypoxanthine	45
Adenosine	68
Guanosine	61
Inosine	40

[a] Shaken flasks (500 ml) containing 100 ml of a casein/sucrose medium plus 0.1% of the appropriate purine were inoculated with a logarithmically growing bacterial culture. Exotoxin accumulated after 48 hr of incubation was determined from the optical density (OD) of suitably prepared samples at 258 nm. Corroboration of exotoxin identity was made by thin layer chromatography using a solvent system: *n*-butanol : acetone : glacial acetic acid : 5% ammonia at 9 : 3 : 3 : 2. % inhibition = 100(exotoxin, test flask): (exotoxin, control).

TABLE VII

Metabolism of purines by B. thuringiensis[a]

Purines	Zero time		16 hr incubation	
	λ max	Δ o.d.	λ max	Δ o.d.
Adenine	260	0.62	253	0.29
Guanine	272,250	0.29,0.27	268	0.10
Hypoxanthine	250	0.58	252	0.49
Xanthine	270	0.32	268	0.19

[a] Experiments by T. R. Shieh, R. F. Anderson and M. H. Rogoff. A wet paste of cells (2 g) harvested during logarithmic growth on casein/sucrose medium was made up to 100 ml in a 500 ml flask with 0.2 *M*-phosphate buffer, pH 7.0, containing sufficient purine base to make a final purine concentration of 0.1 mg/ml (w/v). The flasks were shaken at 30°C. Periodic samples, diluted 1 : 10 with 0.1 *M*-phosphate buffer, pH 7.0, were analysed spectrophotometrically.

Shieh *et al.* (1968) partially explain exotoxin accumulation by exotoxin-synthesizing strains of *B. thuringiensis* on the basis of these observations. The compound is accumulated neither as a result of mutational blockage of an enzymatic step in the nucleotide biosynthetic pathway, nor lack of enzymes involved in normal catabolism of the nucleotides. The exotoxin itself may be resistant to nucleotidase activity and may act as a competitive inhibitor of

TABLE VIII

Effect of growth medium and presence of exotoxin on the dephosphorylation of IMP and AMP (mg-P/ml/90 min)[a] *by* B. thuringiensis[b]

Substrate	Casein medium	Bacto-casitone	
	not treated	not treated	exotoxin treated
IMP	0.015	0.022	0.019
AMP	0.002	0.018	0.004
Exotoxin	0	0	0

[a] P estimation by the methods of Fiske and Subbarow (1925).

[b] Experiments by T. R. Shieh, R. F. Anderson and M. H. Rogoff. Each reaction vessel (250 ml flask) contained 40 ml of 0.2 *M*-tris buffer, pH 8.5, 10 ml of (each) substrate solution containing 3 mg/ml and 1.0 g of wet cell paste harvested during logarithmic growth from the appropriate medium.

nucleotidases. This nucleotidase inhibition would result in a decrease in the rate of catabolic formation of the purine bases adenine and guanine. These purines regulate IMP, AMP and XMP formation (Fig. 5). Low intracellular concentrations of these bases allow XMP and AMP synthesis to take place more or less continually. The major portion of IMP is probably channeled through the AMP branch of the biosynthetic path since the synthesis of exotoxin would rapidly remove AMP, a reaction product, from the system, shifting equilibrium towards this reactant. This is based on the assumption that AMP is an exotoxin precursor. The exotoxin-accumulating cell then mimics a catabolically blocked mutant. This might explain exotoxin accumulation by cells normally sensitive to the regulatory feedback mechanisms known to be operative in these bacilli. Competition by exotoxin for active enzyme sites involved in ATP metabolism in an *Escherichia coli* enzyme system (DNA dependent RNA polymerase) has also been observed by Šebesta and Horská (1968b). Their observations tend to support the role of the compound in the foregoing metabolic scheme. It might also merit some extrapolation to mode of action.

The literature offers little else of microbiological import. A correlation between exotoxin accumulation and physiological state as measured by growth could be deduced from the studies of Conner and Hansen (1967a, b). No indication of effects of single amino acid additions could be extrapolated to a single producing unit basis. Effects of single amino acids, specifically on the exotoxin synthesis rather than on growth, are therefore not indicated.

From the preceding, it is obvious that many gaps exist in our knowledge of the biosynthetic pathways and regulatory systems involved in the synthesis of the exotoxin. These systems evoke considerable interest and hopefully some light will be shed on the mechanisms involved in future.

VII. The Biological Activity of Thermostable Exotoxin

It is difficult to evaluate many of the results of experiments on the biological activity of the unpurified, sterile, bacterial supernatant for the reasons stated earlier and, as they give no idea of the absolute toxicity of the pure toxin we shall concentrate where possible on results with pure exotoxin. Although these are relatively few, some conclusions can be drawn already.

A. INSECTICIDAL ACTIVITY

The inherent insecticidal activity of the exotoxin is considerable and it appears to be effective against a wide range of insect species.

The LD_{50} for *Galleria mellonella* by injection is 0.5 μg/g (Šebesta *et al.*, 1969b). Our value, 0.01 μg/larva (Table I) or 0.055 μg/g, is probably lower because it was based on the inhibition of emergence of adults from treated larvae, whereas the Czechoslovakian workers based their result on larval mortality. In our experience the latter method always requires higher doses of exotoxin. Even with the higher figure, the toxicity of exotoxin is very much greater (approximately 1000 times) than DDT injected into *G. mellonella* larvae, as Schmid and Benz (1969) have already pointed out.

In assays of more practical significance exotoxin still compares favourably with commercially useful insecticides against some species. The first results were reported by de Barjac and Dedonder (1965), who found an LD_{50} of approximately 6 μg/g for *Mamestra brassicae* larvae fed on treated cabbage. Results shown in Table II illustrate particularly noteworthy activity against *Musca domestica* and *Drosophila melanogaster* larvae. The activity against larvae of another dipteran, *Aedes aegypti,* is similar but compares poorly with standard larvicides of which there has been far greater development than of materials for control of house fly larvae. Baytex, for example, is more than 400 times as active as exotoxin under the same conditions against *A. aegypti* larvae. The activity of exotoxin against three foliar insects: *Phaedon cochleariae, Plutella maculipennis* and *Pieris brassicae* compares more favourably with the standard (ethyl parathion) and has a similar level of basic activity to some compounds which are used commercially.

The activity of exotoxin against insect ova is unknown but it is well recognized that exotoxin is not toxic to adults of a wide range of insect species at larvicidal dose levels.

It is of interest that Šebesta *et al.* (1969) find that the dephosphorylated exotoxin is not effective against *G. mellonella.* They do not give dose levels but we have confirmed their observation with *M. domestica* using 100 times the larval LD_{50} dose of exotoxin.

B. MAMMALIAN TOXICITY

Toxicity data with pure exotoxin against mammals are extremely limited.

Šebesta *et al.* (1969) found an LD_{50} value of 18 μg/g for mice by intraperitoneal injection. They state that death always occurred on the third day after treatment and they point out that even though *G. mellonella* is substantially more susceptible than mice to exotoxin (0.5 μg/g compared with 18 μg/g) their results place exotoxin in the category of mammalian toxic materials. They found no pathological effects on the brain, liver, lymphatic system or bone marrow by histological studies. de Barjac and Riou (1969) found an LD_{50} of 13.3 μg/g for mice by intraperitoneal and 16.6 by subcutaneous injection. They found hepatic necrosis and often injuries to the kidney and spleen. Sublethal doses showed no cumulative effects. These LD_{50} values have been confirmed by E. Thorpe (unpublished).

The contrast of these results with earlier results using crude bacterial supernatant (Krieg and Herfs, 1963) calls for comment. Once again this can be explained by assuming that the doses used in the early work were inadequate for an effect. Krieg and Herfs gave young mice three intraperitoneal injections of up to 1 ml of supernatant; assuming for the sake of argument a concentration of 50 μg of exotoxin per ml of supernatant, as we find, and a weight of 20 g per animal, each injection is equivalent to only 2.5 μg/g. With the same assumptions their oral administration of 50 ml of *B. thuringiensis* supernatant, over 10 days, is the equivalent of 2.5 mg exotoxin per mouse or a dose of 125 μg/g. As no effects were seen, these results are encouraging. Further studies for acute and chronic effects are obviously needed if exotoxin is to be considered for practical use and to ensure that use of viable spores, in commercial preparations of *B. thuringiensis* that contain strains known to produce exotoxin, is safe. This is particularly necessary because of the nucleotide nature of exotoxin and the possibility of mutagenic effects.

C. OTHER BIOLOGICAL EFFECTS

The only arthropod, other than insects, reported susceptible is the two-spotted spider mite, *Tetranychus telarius* (Krieg, 1968b). Gevrey and Euzéby (1966) have reported a preliminary study of the effect of *B. thuringiensis* var. *thuringiensis* supernatant on the development of mixed cultures of several nematode parasites of animals. These included: *Haemonchus contortus, Ostertagia* sp., *Trichostrongylus* sp., *Bunostomum trigonocephalum, Cooperia* sp., *Oesophagostomum venulosum* and *Chabertia ovina.* When ova were exposed to media containing concentrated supernatant (6-24 times) development was inhibited but it is not clear whether the various species were equally susceptible. Benz (1966) found no effects when fish or *Tubifex* sp. (oligochaete annelids) were exposed to a concentration of supernatant which was toxic to

D. melanogaster, but the species used were not defined nor were the precise conditions of treatment. No effects against micro-organisms have been reported.

VIII. Biochemistry and Mode of Action

Our present knowledge of the mode of action of the exotoxin is due exclusively to the recent work of Šebesta and Horská (1968b)[1] and of Šebesta *et al.* (1969b).

Their approach to the problem was conditioned by the pattern of mammalian toxicity which they observed in mice. Specifically, death occurred in the test animal on the third day after injection which led them to investigate the effect of the exotoxin on DNA, RNA and protein synthesis.

A dose corresponding to 10 times the LD_{50} did not affect either the incorporation of randomly labelled ^{14}C thymidine into DNA or randomly labelled ^{14}C L-leucine into protein but a dose representing one-third of the LD_{50} resulted in a 60% inhibition of the incorporation of 6-^{14}C orotic acid into RNA. The incorporation of randomly labelled ^{14}C cytidine was similarly affected. These observations require that, if the exotoxin has only one site of action, this lies between cytidine triphosphate and RNA. From this it would appear most probable that the polymerase system is affected. For confirmation of this Šebesta and Horská used a bacterial system and showed that the DNA-dependent RNA polymerase (EC 2.7.7.6), from *Escherichia coli* A 19 ($RNase^-$), was inhibited by the exotoxin.[1]

The inhibition is competitive with ATP in the sense that it is partly reversed by addition of ATP but not by the other ribonucleotide triphosphates. However, the degree of inhibition is controlled by the ratio of exotoxin to ATP rather than by their absolute values. Inhibition occurs whether the exotoxin is added before or after the onset of polymerization. From this observation, it follows that the exotoxin must inhibit the polymerization step. Inhibitory action solely on the process of association (with DNA) and initiation is excluded, although on rigorously logical grounds the evidence does not exclude a combined effect on polymerization and one, or both, of the other processes.

It will be of interest to have more quantitative data on the partial reversal of inhibition by ATP. The partial reversibility could result from the high affinity of the enzyme for exotoxin or from the exotoxin interfering with the enzymatic mechanism in a two-step process involving reversible and irreversible stages.

---

[1] The comments of Rogoff and Yousten (1969) regarding the results of Šebesta and Horská (1968b) arise because of a misprint in which the concentrations of columns 2, 3 and 4 of Table I of Šebesta and Horská (1968b) and of [^{14}C] UTP were quoted in μ mol in error. They should of course be in mμ mol. (K. Šebesta, personal communication; Errata, 1969, *Biochem. Biophys. Acta* **174**, 793).

References

Aizawa, K. and Fujiyoshi, N. (1968). Abstr. Joint U.S.-Japan Semin. Microbial Control Insect Pests. U.S.-Japan Committee Sci. Cooperation. Panel 8. Fukuoka, 29-30.

Barjac, H. de, Burgerjon, A. and Bonnefoi, A. (1966). *J. Invertebrate Path.* **8,** 537.

Barjac, H. de, and Dedonder, R. (1965). *C.r. hebd. Séanc. Acad. Sci. Paris* **260,** 7050-7053.

Barjac, H. de, and Dedonder, R. (1968). *Bull. Soc. chim. Biol.* **50,** 941-944.

Barjac, H. de, and Riou, J.-Y. (1969). *Revue Path. comp. Méd. exp.* **6,** 367-374.

Bendich, A. (1957). *In* "Methods in Enzymology" (S. P. Colowick and N. O. Kaplan, eds), Vol. III, p. 722. Academic Press, New York.

Beard, R. L. (1949). *J. econ. Ent.* **42,** 292-300.

Benz, G. (1966). *Experientia* **22,** 81-82.

Benz, G. and Perron, J-M. (1967). *Experientia* **23,** 871-872.

Bond, R. P. M., Boyce, C. B. C. and French, S. J. (1969). *Biochem. J.* **114,** 477-488.

Bond, R. P. M. (1969). *Chem. Communs.* 338-339.

Briggs, J. D. (1960). *J. Insect Path.* **2,** 418-432.

Burgerjon, A. (1965). *Entomophaga* **10,** 55-65.

Burgerjon, A. and de Barjac, H. (1960). *C.r. hebd. Séanc. Acad. Sci. Paris* **251,** 911-912.

Burgerjon, A. and de Barjac, H. (1964). *Mém. hors. Sér. Entomophaga* No. 2, 221-225

Burgerjon, A. and de Barjac, H. (1967). *J. Invertebrate Path.* **9,** 574-577.

Burgerjon, A. and Biache, G. (1964). *J. Insect Path.* **6,** 538-541.

Burges, H. D. *et al.* (1967). *In* "Insect Pathology and Microbial Control" (P. A. van der Laan, ed.), pp. 314-338. North-Holland Publ. Co., Amsterdam.

Cantwell, G. E., Heimpel, A. M. and Thompson, M. J. (1964). *J. Insect Path.* **6,** 466-480.

Clarke, F. B. and Lyons, J. W. (1966). *J. Am. chem. Soc.* **88,** 4401-4405.

Conner, R. M. and Hansen, P. A. (1967a). *J. Invertebrate Path.* **9,** 12-18.

Conner, R. M. and Hansen, P. A. (1967b). *J. Invertebrate Path.* **9,** 114-125.

David, W. A. L. and Gardiner, B. O. C. (1965). *Nature, Lond.* **207,** 882-883.

Demain, A. L., Vitali, R. A., Wilker, B. W. and Rothrock, J. W. (1964). *Biotechnol. Bioeng.* **6,** 361-365.

Drake, B. B. and Smythe, C. V. (1961). U.S. Patent 3,087,865.

Dunn, P. H. (1960). *J. Insect Path.* **2,** 13-16.

Farkas, J., Šebesta, K., Horská, K., Samek, Z., Dolejš, J. and Šorm, F. (1969). *Colln Czech. chem. Commun. Engl. Edn* **34,** 1118-1119.

Feldman, I. and Agarwal, R. P. (1968). *J. Am. chem. Soc.* **90,** 7329-7333.

Fiske, C. H. and Subbarow, Y. (1925). *J. biol. Chem.* **66,** 375-400.

Fromageot, H. P. M., Griffin, B. E., Reese, C. B., Sulston, J. E. and Trentham, D. R. (1966). *Tetrahedron* **22,** 705-710.

Fujimoto, M. and Uchida, K. (1965). *Agr. Biol. Chem.* **29,** 249-259.

Gevrey, J. and Euzéby, J. (1966). *Bull. Soc. Sci. vet. Méd. Comp. Lyon* **68,** 111-119.

Hall, I. M. and Arakawa, K. Y. (1959). *J. Insect Path.* **1,** 351-355.

Heimpel, A. M. (1967a). *A. Rev. Ent.* **12,** 287-322.

Heimpel, A. M. (1967b). *J. Invertebrate Path.* **9,** 364-375.

Heitor, F. (1962). *XI Int. Congr. Ent. Wien 1960,* **2,** 845-849.

Krieg, A. (1966). *Entomologia exp. appl.* **9,** 185-190.

Krieg, A. (1967). *Anz. Schädlingsk.* **40,** 8-9.

Krieg, A. (1968a). *J. Invertebrate Path.* **12,** 366-378.

Krieg, A. (1968b). *J. Invertebrate Path.* **12,** 478.

Krieg, A. and Herfs, W. (1963). *Z. PflKrankh. PflPath. PflSchutz* **70,** 11-21.

Krieg, A., de Barjac, H. and Bonnefoi, A. (1968). *J. Invertebrate Path.* **10,** 428-430.

Lemieux, R. U. and Stevens, J. D. (1965). *Can. J. Chem.* **43,** 2059-2070.

Lilles, J. N. and Dunn, P. H. (1959). *J. Insect Path.* **1,** 309-310.

McConnell, E. and Richards, A. G. (1959). *Can. J. Microbiol.* **5,** 161-168.

Nakayama, K., Suzuki, T., Sato, Z. and Kinoshita, S. (1964). *Amino Acid Nucleic Acid (Tokyo)* **9,** 7-13.

Nielson, M. L., Pustinger, J. V. and Strobel, J. (1964). *J. chem. Engng Data* **9,** 167-170.

Nishimura, T. and Shimizu, B. (1965). *Chem. pharm. Bull., Tokyo* **13,** 803-810.
Rao, V. S. R. and Foster, J. F. (1963). *J. phys. Chem. Ithaca* **67,** 951-952.
Rogoff, M. H. (1968). *J. Invertebrate Path.* **10,** 453-454.
Rogoff, M. H. and Yousten, A. A. (1969). *Ann. Rev. Microbiol.* **23,** 357-386.
Rogoff, M. H., Ignoffo, C. M., Singer, S., Gard, I. and Prieto, A. P. (1969). *J. Invertebrate Path.* **14,** 122-129.
Sang, J. H. (1956). *J. exp. Biol.* **33,** 45-72.
Šebesta, K. and Horská, K. (1968b). *Biochim. biophys. Acta.* **169,** 281-282.
Šebesta, K., Horská, K. and Vaňková, J. (1967). *In* "Insect Pathology and Microbial Control" (P. A. van der Laan, ed.), pp. 238-242. North-Holland Publ. Co., Amsterdam.
Šebesta, K., Horská, K. and Vaňková, J. (1968a). Abstracts, 5th Meeting FEBS, Prague, p. 250, Czechoslovak Biochem. Soc.
Šebesta, K., Horská, K. and Vaňková, J. (1969a). *Colln. Czech. chem. Commun. Engl. Edn.* **34,** 891-898.
Šebesta, K., Horská, K. and Vaňková, J. (1969b). *Colln Czech. chem. Commun. Engl. Edn.* **34,** 1786-1791.
Schmid, E. and Benz, G. (1969). *Experientia* **25,** 96-98.
Shieh, T. R., Anderson, R. F. and Rogoff, M. H. (1968). *Bact. Proc.* p. 6.
Ulbright, T. L. V., Jennings, J. B., Scopes, P. M. and Klyne, W. (1964). *Tetrahedron Lett.* 695-698.
van der Veen, J. M. (1963). *J. org. Chem.* **28,** 564-566.
Vaňková, J. (1966). *Acta bohemoslov* **63,** 10-16.
Vernon, C. A. (1957). Chemical Society, Special Publication, No. 8, p. 17.

CHAPTER 13

Determination and Significance of the Host Spectrum of *Bacillus thuringiensis*

A. BURGERJON and D. MARTOURET

Station de Recherches de Lutte Biologique et de Biocoenotique, I.N.R.A., La Minière par Versailles, France

I. Introduction and Definition of Susceptibility

Under natural conditions, epizootics due to *Bacillus thuringiensis* are infrequent and limited to septicaemia in populations of a few species such as *Dendrolimus sibericus* (Talalaev, 1958, 1961), *Ephestia (Anagasta) kuehniella* (Kurstak, 1964), and *Selenephera lunigera* (Kulagin, in Talalaeva, 1967). On the other hand, the isolation of currently known strains from naturally infected insects indicates the persistence of the bacterium in the natural environment and its potential as an entomopathogen. As a native strain is most frequently isolated from only a few dead or dying insects in a population *B. thuringiensis* is possibly a natural enzootic regulatory factor. Presumably its natural occurrence remains at a level below the minimum concentration required for the build up of an epizootic (compared by Franz (1961) with Liebig's minimum law) because the lethal bacterial agents, spores and crystals, appear only in very small numbers in the host's cadaver, as suggested by Angus (1968).

Interest in *B. thuringiensis* during the last 15 years is, therefore, due not to its power of contagion but to its selective killing of insects when applied as microbial insecticide. Another remarkable property is that it can easily be produced saprophytically on an industrial scale. Consequently, it is now the object of much encouraging research throughout the world.

We cannot consider here the many environmental factors, both variable and provisional in character, whose effects on the pathogenicity of the bacillus and on the variability of the host introduce profound modifications in the germ-insect relationships. Our study of the host spectrum of *B. thuringiensis* is limited to the specificity of the micro-organism and the susceptibility of the host in the laboratory, under carefully controlled conditions. By susceptibility we mean the reaction of the insect, i.e. the abnormal or pathological effects of *B. thuringiensis,* or its lethal bacterial elements, alone or in association, and studied quantitatively.

II. General Characteristics of the Host Spectrum

Three main characteristics of the host spectrum can be summarized from the efforts of a few pioneer workers, first listed by Steinhaus (1957).

1. The entomopathogenic activity of a strain of *B. thuringiensis* differs in various insect species as has been shown among others by Angus (1956a) using var. *sotto,* Hall and Dunn (1958) using var. *berliner,* and finally by Burgerjon and Grison (1959) using using var. *alesti (anduze).* For each insect species the observed degree of entomopathogenic activity expresses the susceptibility to the particular bacterial strain, and for the whole set of species examined it defines the *specificity spectrum of the strain in question.*

2. Several different strains of *B. thuringiensis* exhibit different degrees of entomopathogenic activity, in the same host species as found by Vasiljević (1957) on *Hyphantria cunea,* Toumanoff and Vago (1955) on *Bombyx mori,* and Toumanoff (1955) on *Galleria mellonella* and *Pieris brassicae.* These differences in susceptibility shown by a single species to different strains of *B. thuringiensis* define the *susceptibility spectrum of the host species.*

3. Most susceptible species quoted by Steinhaus are Lepidoptera; a few are *Tenthredinidae* (Hymenoptera) (Heimpel, 1955b), Coleoptera (Steinhaus, 1951; Steinhaus and Bell, 1953) and Orthoptera.

These characteristics have since been elaborated and confirmed by many studies in many countries. Definition of the bacterial material was improved by advances in strain identification and knowledge of the active principles of the bacillus. Burgerjon (1962, 1964a, b), Wiegand (1963, 1968), Krieg (1965a, b),

Burges *et al.* (1967), and others have tried to standardize methods for measuring the activity of bacterial preparations. The relative sensitivity of a large number of harmful or useful insects have been compared using one or more strains of *B. thuringiensis* (Angus, 1956a; Watanabe, 1963; White and Briggs, 1964; Vaňková, 1964, 1966; Broersma and Buxton, 1967; Gukasian, 1967; Burgerjon and Biache, 1967a; Angus and Norris, 1968; etc.).

Three further characteristics became clear from one of these papers (Burgerjon and Biache, 1967a).

4. Strains belonging to the *same* H serotypes and recognized on other bacteriological characters have their own specific activity, just as those belonging to *different* serotypes, an idea already mooted by Grigorova (1964), and confirmed by Angus and Norris (1968) and illustrated in Fig. 1.

5. The ED_{50}s of different strains can appear in different sequences for different species, so that there are reversals of the sequences for a pair of species, termed "cross activity".

6. The activity spectra of bacterial strains are not correlated with the systematic relationships of the insect species.

These general characteristics of the host spectrum demonstrate the extreme diversity of the processes governing the relationships between the bacterial strains and the host species. They also show the impossibility of forecasting *a priori* the activity of strains on a given insect on the basis of the systematic relationships of the pathogen and of the insect. Determination of the host spectrum has no practical value for biological control unless it includes all the known strains and the species under discussion, although a knowledge of whether a strain produces the heat stable exotoxin helps to delimit the broad scope of the spectrum (p. 311).

III. The Role of the Active Principles of *B. thuringiensis* in the Host Spectrum

At present it is known that the differences in the reactions of insect species are controlled in two categories, specific either to the bacterium or to the insect, whose interplay determines the susceptibility of a given insect species.

The bacterial factors are the diverse bacterial elements active *per os,* which cause infection or toxaemia in the insect. Some of these elements, like the spore (Berliner, 1915), the crystal (Hannay, 1953), and thermostable exotoxin (Burgerjon and de Barjac, 1960, 1962), are present in the bacterial culture and can act as soon as they are ingested by an insect. Others, like proteinases of the phospholipase and lecithinase type (Toumanoff, 1953; Heimpel, 1955b) are produced only by the bacterium when an infection develops in the host organism. Factors peculiar to the insect host include all the physiological processes capable of favouring or inhibiting attack by the bacterial elements either alone or in associations. All known strains of bacteria and both categories of factors must be studied to appreciate fully the role played by each element in the determination of species susceptibility.

A. THE CRYSTALS OR PARASPORAL INCLUSIONS

The crystals consist of protein and are generally present in all strains of *B. thuringiensis* in which they are considered to be one of the taxonomic characteristics (Norris, 1964). Their toxic properties on ingestion have been demonstrated in *Bombyx mori* (Hannay, 1953; Angus, 1954; Fitz-James *et al.*, 1958) using var. *sotto* and var. *alesti.* The observations by Angus (1956b) and others have established that the crystal is active only in the majority of Lepidoptera. Ingestion of the crystals alone can kill susceptible species of this order. The first symptom is always cessation of feeding. Accompanying disorders are of two sorts. 1. Physiological, such as a change in permeability of the midgut, and changes in the pH of the haemolymph and of the alimentary canal, causing symptoms such as gut paralysis, lethargy, and general paralysis of the insect. 2. Pathological, such as increase of the intestinal microflora and destruction of midgut epithelial cells, developing into a "flaccidity" syndrome involving lethal escape of bacteria or "potential pathogens" from the intestinal flora into the haemocoel (Vago, 1959).

The development and the intensity of these toxic-septicaemic processes are extremely variable, depending both on the insect species and the bacterial strain involved.

1. Factors Related to the Species

In the gut of the host, the toxic activity of the crystal depends on certain intrinsic properties of the intestinal contents, such as the pH of the proteolytic enzyme secretion, and the presence of bacillary spores ingested simultaneously with the crystals.

a. Action of the pH. The crystal is active in those species of Lepidoptera in which the pH of both the foregut and the midgut is strongly alkaline and above 8.9, as in *B. mori, Malacosoma* spp., *Nymphalis antiopa, Lymantria (Porthetria) dispar* (Angus, 1956b; Heimpel and Angus, 1959), and *P. brassicae* (Martouret, 1962). Nevertheless, the absence of a toxaemia in other species whose intestinal pH is alkaline, e.g. in *Agrotis ipsilon* (pH 9.5) and *Agrotis (Euxoa) segetum* (pH 9.6), in which the crystal dissolves in the intestinal medium, and also in *Lycophotia saucia* (pH 9.9) and *Mamestra brassicae* (pH 10.2), in which the crystal does not dissolve, suggests that other factors condition or complement the action of the pH in the solution of the crystal and the manifestation of the toxicity (Martouret, 1961).

The Lepidoptera whose gut pH is alkaline can be divided into two categories, one including species sensitive and the other those resistant to the action of the crystal.

Among the sensitive species, Heimpel and Angus (1959) have distinguished two types with differing symptoms after the crystal is ingested. Type 1 is represented by *B. mori* L., *Protoparce* spp., *Antheraea pernyi* etc., in which feeding stops suddenly, then the body is generally paralysed, accompanied by an increase in the alkalinity of the haemolymph, a fall in the intestinal pH and destruction of the epithelium (Figs 5 and 6, Chapter 11). It is now believed that the permeability of the midgut is altered and the regulation of potassium ions impaired (Chapter 11). Type II includes such species as *Malacosoma* spp., *Hyphantria cunea, Datana* spp. (Angus and Heimpel, 1959) and *P. brassicae* (Martouret, 1962). In these, no general paralysis, nor sudden alteration in the haemolymph as feeding ceases, has ever been shown. Only in *P. brassicae* has lethargy been observed, accompanied by a lowering of the foregut and midgut pH, and followed later by a generalized paralysis (Martouret, 1962), and destruction of the intestinal epithelium (Martouret *et al.*, 1965). Probably the intestinal permeability is also modified in the species of type II, as has been shown by Benz (1966) in *P. brassicae*: the high buffering power of the haemolymph prevents a detectable change in its pH. The susceptibility of the Lepidoptera sensitive to the crystal and the severity of the symptoms in the different species appears to depend on this physiological upset.

b. Action of proteolytic enzymes. The foregut contents of caterpillars such as *P. brassicae* and *B. mori* have a characteristic enzyme system with a selective proteolytic activity in an alkaline medium (Lecadet and Dedonder, 1966a, b). These proteases, devoid of toxic activity (Lecadet and Martouret, 1965), hydrolyse the crystals and liberate several soluble substances of proteinic and peptidic nature (Dedonder and Lecadet, 1964; Lecadet and Dedonder, 1967). This has been confirmed recently by Watanabe *et al.* (1968) and by Faust *et al.* (1967).

While the intact crystal acts only *per os,* the products of enzymatic hydrolysis of the crystal are also toxic on parenteral injection. By both methods these products provoke the same symptoms (Martouret, 1964; Lecadet and Martouret, 1967a; Lhoste and Martouret, in press), not only on the caterpillars of *P. brassicae* and *B. mori,* but also on those of *E. kuehniella* (Lecadet and Martouret, 1962, 1967a, b), a species normally insensitive to the action of the intact crystals alone (Heimpel and Angus, 1959). Thus the insect's enzymes change the protoxin of the crystal into a directly acting true toxin. The differences in susceptibility of various insect species to the crystal are connected with the specificity of the gut proteases, which control the hydrolysis of the crystals *in vivo.*

c. Combined action of spores and crystals. Among the Lepidoptera insensitive to the crystal alone and not possessing the intestinal pH or set of enzymes necessary to activate the protoxin, some species, such as *E. kuehniella* and

Ostrinia nubilalis, show toxaemic symptoms only after eating both crystals and spores together (Heimpel and Angus, 1959; Burgerjon and Yamvrias, 1959; Raun *et al.*, 1966).

This corresponds to Heimpel and Angus' type III, in which spores or crystals eaten alone never cause marked lethal physiological reactions. An intestinal pH below 8.9 may not allow the crystal to dissolve but it does allow the spores to germinate. Nevertheless, Heimpel and Angus verified, in sublethally infected *E. kuehniella,* that the vegetative forms rapidly degenerated and disappeared from the intestines of insects transferred to fresh food not containing spores or crystals. In contrast, ingestion of the spore-crystal complex stopped feeding just as readily as the active toxin (cf. p. 309) from an enzymatic hydrolysate of the crystals (Yamvrias, 1962). There was no general paralysis or intestinal paralysis such as described for species of types I and II. The cessation of feeding was followed by a morbid state of varying duration, accompanied by fairly slow bacillary multiplication in the intestine and, according to Mattes (1927), a degradation of the epithelial cells, leading to a final lethal septicaemia.

In this complex intestinal disease caused by the combined effects of the toxin and the bacillary growth, the germination of spores, or the activity of the vegetative cells produced from them appears to establish conditions favourable to the action of the crystals, while the resulting toxaemia appears to increase the susceptibility of the insect to the bacterial infection.

2. Factors Associated with the Bacterial Strains

The crystals from various strains of *B. thuringiensis* exhibit appreciable differences in toxicity against the same host species. This has been shown by Lecadet and Martouret (1964) for var. *alesti (anduze)* and var. *berliner,* by Angus (1967) for var. *entomocidus, sotto* and *berliner,* and more recently by Martouret and Biache (in press) for var. *berliner, entomocidus* and *dendrolimus,* in *B. mori* and *P. brassicae* (Table I). Thus, the activity spectrum of the spore-crystal complex, seems to depend, in these species, on the action of the crystals alone.

The amino acid composition of the crystals of *B. thuringiensis* varies so little between the different strains (Table III, Chapter 11) that it does not seem possible that such slight variations could be responsible for the pronounced toxicity differences.

Serological studies on the crystal digested by gut juice are reviewed in Chapter 11 and confirm the idea expressed by Lecadet and Martouret (1964) when comparing the toxicity of the hydrolysis products of crystals from var. *alesti* and *berliner*: "The differences in toxicity can be explained by the manner in which the *in vivo* hydrolysis is effected, at the same degree of *in vitro* lysis the hydrolysates of the two strains have an equal protein content and a toxic activity of the same order." The differences observed between the two strains

TABLE I

Toxicity of intact crystals for two species of Lepidoptera[a]

Variety of *B. thuringiensis*	*Pieris brassicae* Instar V larvae		*Bombyx mori* Instar IV larvae	
	ED_{50}[b] (μg)	LD_{50}[b] (μg)	ED_{50}[b] (μg)	LD_{50}[b] (μg)
entomocidus (serotype VI)	0.021 0.000-0.083	0.082 0.045-0.148	0.17 0.08-0.41	0.15 0.07-0.30
berliner, isolate 22 105 (serotype I)	0.045 0.034-0.059	0.074 0.057-0.099	0.45 0.34-0.59	0.31 0.23-0.41
dendrolimus (serotype IVa)	0.034 0.026-0.045	0.210 0.132-0.331	1.66 1.02-2.69	2.08 1.41-3.09

[a] Martouret and Biache, in press.
[b] Micrograms pure crystal per gram of larva–ED_{50} reduction of feeding in 24 hr; LD_{50}-death of larvae up to the time of pupation.

suggested differences in the structure of the crystals, some of whose bonds might be less accessible to the insect enzymes. Electron microscopic observations lend some support to this hypothesis, not only showing appreciable differences between the sizes of the protein molecules making up the crystals of various strains (Vaňková and Kralik, 1966), but also indicating some correlations between the molecular organization in the crystals and their degree of toxicity when reacted with proteases (Grigorova *et al.*, 1967).

There is no longer any doubt that knowledge of the sensitivity of the crystals of different strains to insect proteases will help to interpret differences between susceptibilities of the various Lepidoptera species to these crystals.

B. THE THERMOSTABLE EXOTOXIN

The vegetative stages of *B. thuringiensis* produce a thermostable exotoxin active *per os* (Burgerjon and de Barjac, 1960, 1962) and on injection (McConnell and Richards, 1959) into the haemolymph in larvae of Lepidoptera, Hymenoptera, Coleoptera and Diptera. This toxin has been isolated in pure form. Chapter 12 reviews the tests on different insects and concludes that, almost certainly, only one chemical compound is involved.

Burgerjon (1965) concludes that the activity of toxins other than the crystal and the thermostable exotoxin cannot be demonstrated in industrial products. The γ-exotoxin and the α-exotoxin (lecithinase C, phospholipase C) of Heimpel (1967a) do not appear to us to be active components affecting the host spectrum, since one is a still unidentified, atoxic enzyme, while the other (associated with the non-crystalliferous *B. cereus*) could have been confused with the thermostable exotoxin, now known to be produced in some acrystalliferous mutants of *B. thuringiensis* (de Barjac *et al.,* 1966). Smirnoff and Berlinguet's (1966) thermolabile toxin also requires caution, since it has been identified in only a single commercial product, more as the result of an industrial accident, in the same way as one of the two active thermostable principles found by Burgerjon (1964a). Experimental culture failed to reproduce the same results.

It is now possible to distinguish the thermostable exotoxin and to characterize its effects with certainty. Investigations on the chemical nature of the purified material from various sources, reviewed in Chapter 10, confirm that the active thermostable principle is a nucleotide-like material. In addition, recent work by Burgerjon and Biache (1967b, c) has enabled the exotoxin to be recognized by the symptoms which it produces in the insects, i.e. the specific delayed effect occurring at moulting, as pointed out by Burgerjon and de Barjac (1960) and the teratological effects in nymphs and adults developing from sublethally poisoned larvae. Such effects directly implicate the host spectrum. The least teratological effect appears to be atrophy of the mouth parts, the first part to be attacked being the proboscis of the pupal and adult Lepidoptera and the labrum of the house fly. In the Colorado beetle (Burgerjon *et al.,* 1969) the labial palps disappeared, the extremity of the glossa being prolonged in the centre into a unique appendage resembling the lost palps. Also claws, similar to those on the tarsi, developed on segments of the antennal clubs. These effects are hereditary (Burgerjon, in press). The consequences of these deformities depend on the buccal type to which the species belongs and the functions of the affected organs. While a Colorado beetle suffering fairly severe atrophy continues to feed with mandibles that remain almost intact, in *P. brassicae* atrophy of the proboscis prevents feeding (Burgerjon and Biache, 1967c).

There are also indirect repercussions on the reproductive function, and we suspect that the reproductive inhibitor described by Hitchings (1967) in the southern armyworm adults could be exotoxin, which prevents normal feeding. In addition, chronic poisoning due to ingestion of the toxin in the adult stage can produce morphophysiological changes in cogenesis, e.g. in Drosophila (David and Vago, 1967). Under the same conditions it appeared to kill worker bees (Martouret and Euverte, 1964).

Using *P. brassicae,* Burgerjon and Biache (1967c) compared the toxicity of the exotoxin from four H-serotypes of *B. thuringiensis,* I, VII, VIII and IX, and found the same teratological symptoms. Thus, in contrast to the crystal, the exotoxin from different strains shows identical properties and appears to influence the host spectrum only quantitatively in that different strains produce very different quantities of toxin. For example, strains of serotype VIII produced less toxin than did those of serotype I (de Barjac *et al.,* 1966), and certain strains produced only traces, which were, however, detectable by their very sensitive teratological activity (Burgerjon and de Barjac, 1967).

Autoclaving of the bacterial preparations is a convenient preliminary in the detection of the exotoxin, and should be carried out for better differentiation of the active principles involved in the experimental results. Thus, the precise relationship between the soluble factor used in experiments with termite species by Smythe and Coppel (1965) and the thermostable exotoxin would be better understood if autoclaved preparations had been used.

C. THE SPORES

In the determination of insect susceptibility to *B. thuringiensis,* the role played by ingested spores depends on the medium offered for the development of the bacillus in the host's gut. The composition of this medium is peculiar to the insect species, being composed of food in the process of digestion and enzymatic secretions, supporting a more or less varied and abundant microflora. It is also extremely variable, according to the diet and the physiological stage of the host. Since this medium is so complex, and since the results of spore action are often masked by the spectacular symptoms of the toxaemic activity of the crystal, our knowledge of the relationships between the gut contents and the infecting micro-organism has not been far advanced. To understand the consequences on the susceptibility of the insect, it is necessary to examine both the factors in the gut medium and the mechanisms of infection with *B. thuringiensis.*

1. Factors Controlling Germination of Spores and Activity of the Bacilli

Among the factors that could affect microbial development in the gut are the pH, the redox potential, the anaerobic rate, enzymes, antibiotics, antagonists and phages. The involvement of several of these has now been demonstrated.

a. The action of pH. As alkaline media of pH 9.0-9.5 are generally unfavourable for the development of *B. thuringiensis* (Kushner and Lisson, 1959) and for the retention of its virulence (Toumanoff and Vago, 1952), the gut pH is one of the more important factors. In a number of Lepidoptera whose gut pH is generally above 9.0 in the larval stage (Heimpel, 1955a, 1960), spore germination is inhibited and ingested vegetative cells are rapidly destroyed, e.g. in *B. mori* (Aoki and Chigasaki, 1915). Nevertheless, when bacteria do survive in these species they may commence growth and infect the host when the gut pH falls either naturally at moulting and pupation in some species, or during a period of inanition as in *Malacosoma disstria* (Heimpel, 1955a), or as a result of the toxaemic action of the crystal to which this category of insect is sensitive (cf. p. 309) (Heimpel and Harshbarger, 1965). In other Lepidoptera and phytophagous Hymenoptera whose gut pH remains below 9.0, and in the absence of other inhibitory factors, spores germinate and multiply in the gut, at different rates according to the host species. While the vegetative forms degenerate in *E. kuehniella* (cf. p. 310), in other species such as *Cydia pomonella* (Stephens,

1952) or *Pristiphora erichsonii* (Heimpel, 1955a), the bacilli multiply rapidly and invade the gut lumen. However, the greatest resistance to infection is shown by *E. kuehniella,* whose mesenteric pH is not significantly more alkaline than that of *C. pomonella,* suggesting to Angus (1964) that pH is not the only factor controlling the activity.

b. Action of antibiotic and bacteriostatic factors. Various strains of *B. thuringiensis* are sensitive to certain antibiotics (Toumanoff and Lapied, 1955; Afrikian, 1960; Ignoffo, 1963). Also development of the bacterium is inhibited by some other substances found in a number of plants eaten by the insects (Gukasian, 1958; Kushner and Harvey, 1960, 1962; Smirnoff and Hutchinson, 1965; Smirnoff, 1965, 1967, 1968). The inhibitory substances in plant food may oppose bacterial development within the gut and temporarily modify the host's susceptibility to the given strain or strains of *B. thuringiensis.* However, the bacterium may become pathogenic when ingestion of the inhibitor ceases, especially during the prenymphal stage. There are also many indications of other naturally occurring antibiotic substances in the intestinal contents and the haemolymph of arthropods (Heimpel and Harshbarger, 1965). Although no activity of this nature has so far been detected in *B. thuringiensis* infections, such phenomena might be responsible for the differences in sensitivity found between species.

c. Action of bacteriophages. Bacteriophages attack various strains of *B. thuringiensis* (Yoder and Nelson, 1960; Gochnauer, 1960; Khachatrian and Rautenstein, 1963; Schvetsova, 1963). Some have already been observed in the gut of several Lepidoptera (Schvetsova, 1964), where they might reduce the insect's susceptibility to infection by ingested spores, but there is no proof of this hypothesis.

2. *Mechanisms of Infection by the Spore and the other Bacillary Elements*

a. Toxico-infection. In Lepidoptera whose gut pH exceeds 9.0, as in *B. mori* and *P. brassicae,* etc., a simultaneous ingestion of spores and crystals is one of the conditions which enables the spore to play a part in infection. The secondary effects of toxaemia caused by the crystal, such as reduction of the gut pH to near neutral, allow germination of the spores and multiplication of the bacilli in the gut (Heimpel and Angus, 1959), while destruction of the peritrophic membrane and the midgut epithelium allows the infection to invade the haemocoel, causing death by septicaemia. In oligo-infections induced *per os* by small doses of the spore-crystal complex in *B. mori* (Vago, 1959) or in *P. brassicae* (Isakova, 1964), the subacute toxicosis usually induces a syndrome of bacterial dysentery, or "flaccidity", characterized by a predominance of the common species of the intestinal microflora (Chapter 21). These species are classified as potential pathogens (Bucher, 1960) and are normally avirulent. Among these, the growth of *B. thuringiensis* is only facultative and apparently inhibited, possibly due to the antagonistic action of the microflora or other unfavourable conditions in the gut medium (Chapter 21).

In a way, the orientation of the toxico-infection toward the fatal syndromes, septicaemia or "flaccidity" depends on the degree of initial poisoning of the host, and therefore not only on the ingested dose but also on the specific sensitivity to the crystal of the strain of *B. thuringiensis* in use. The role of the spores could thus, in part, explain discrepancies between mortality and the amount of reduction in food consumption, after the ingestion of the spore-crystal complex of different bacterial strains by different insect species (Burgerjon, 1962; Burgerjon and Biache, 1967a; Angus and Norris, 1968).

In the phytophagous Hymenoptera, and the Lepidoptera insensitive to the intact crystals owing to their intestinal pH, ingestion of the spores alone or with crystals can induce a bacillary infection in the gut, which rapidly develops into a lethal septicaemia. As shown by Heimpel (1955b) in *P. erichsonii* and by Mayas (1970) in *C. pomonella*, the syndrome is characterized by symptoms such as diarrhoea, lethargy, and atony, accompanied by a succession of histological lesions culminating in destruction of the peritrophic membrane and the midgut epithelial cells, together with cellular degeneration of organs such as the salivary glands, Malpighian tubules, muscles, nerve tissue, and hypodermis. This suggests secondary toxaemia after bacterial infection, somewhat distinct from that caused by the crystals. Heimpel (1955b) established a correlation between the pathogenicity of several strains of *B. cereus* and *B. thuringiensis* for *P. erichsonii*, and their respective abilities to produce a lecithinase. Kushner and Heimpel (1957) postulated that multiplication of the bacilli in the gut contents of the saw-fly produces a toxic enzyme, whose diffusion in the host's body causes the observed histological disorders. Heimpel noted that the pH of the midgut of *P. erichsonii* (7.1-8.4; Heimpel, 1955a) and that of *C. pomonella* (7.5-8.0; Stephens, 1952) are similar to the optimum range for the activity of lecithinase (6.6-7.4). However, according to Mayas (1970), the pathogenicity of several strains of *B. thuringiensis* in *C. pomonella* agrees neither with their lecithinase capacities nor with their proteolytic capacities. Thus, as reported by Rogoff (1966), the activity of bacterial enzymes in the mechanisms of susceptibility to infection by *B. thuringiensis* should not be disregarded, though their role should not be overestimated.

b. Postlarval septicaemia. Mortality following ingestion of *B. thuringiensis* occurs not only during the larval stages due to toxaemia, but also later as a septicaemia occurring during the weaving of the cocoon and at pupation in some species, such as *Malacosoma disstria, Sarrothripus cinereana, Nymphalis antiopa* (Angus, 1965), and *Choristoneura fumiferana* (Klein and Lewis, 1966). Similar results have been observed in *Spilonota ocellana* (Oatman and Legner, 1964) and in *Pectinophora gossypiella* (Ignoffo and Graham, 1967) at the end of the winter larval diapause. Kulagin (in Talalaeva, 1967), observed a natural epizootic of septicaemic character produced by crystal-forming bacteria in the last-stage larvae and pupae of a population of *Selenephera lunigera* (Lepidoptera, *Lasiocampidae*).

As in periods of physiological stress in larvae (pp. 313-314), post-larval septicaemia may be allowed to develop by the disappearance of inhibitory factors habitually present in the host's intestine. However, the bacillary elements alone may not always be responsible for the delayed septicaemia. Many of the results cited here have been obtained with commercial preparations in which neither the strain, nor the constituents, nor the method of preparation were precisely reported, and in which the presence of the thermostable exotoxin can be suspected as a contributory factor to the quasi-toxico septicaemic mortality. In contrast, one can be much more certain of the origin of the septicaemia observed by Tyumentsev (1963, 1966) in the pupae of *Dendrolimus sibiricus* developing from large larvae that had ingested spores of only one strain, *B. thuringiensis* var. *dendrolimus* (serotype IV), because this strain does not produce the thermostable exotoxin (Burgerjon and de Barjac, 1964).

Whatever the underlying mechanisms may be, a number of insect species show susceptibility to the spores of *B. thuringiensis* and to the bacterial infection caused by these spores, with or without the help of toxic processes.

IV. Bacterial Taxonomy and the Host Spectrum

This subject can be viewed from two aspects, the significance of classical bacterial taxonomy in determining host spectra and the value of host spectra as characters that help to distinguish bacterial strains.

For practical purposes the most useful approach to the classical taxonomy of *B. thuringiensis* is to distinguish the pathogen from *B. cereus* by the formation of the crystal, dividing the crystal-formers by their H-serotypes and sometimes further by sub H-serotypes, together with biochemical characters and esterase patterns (de Barjac and Bonnefoi, 1962, 1967).

It has now been established that the host spectra of the spore-crystal complex are different for strains belonging to different H-serotypes, and for strains of the same serotype, such as *sotto* and *dendrolimus* (serotype IV), or *entomocidus* and *subtoxicus* (serotype VI) (Burgerjon and Biache, 1967a), but we do not yet know of any experimental results revealing the existence of different host spectra for strains recognized as taxonomically identical by bacteriologists. Even strain 562-5A, described by Bucher *et al.* (1966) as characteristic of serotype I, possesses some bacterial characteristics anomalous for this group; for instance the morphology of its crystal is different, it produces acid from galactose and, in broth culture, it does not form a pellicle but produces turbidity like the *alesti* (III) and *sotto* (IV) serotypes. The spore-crystal complex of this strain has its own spectrum of activity, as shown by the experiments of Bucher *et al.* and the results for the two crystal-sensitive species in Fig. 1, *P. brassicae* and *B. mori.* The activities of the whole cultures A and B, of different strain, are similar in *P. brassicae,* and A is almost 10 times as active as B in *B. mori,* both on the evidence of mortality and of reduction in feeding. Their corresponding activities against E, x4 and x40, are in corresponding ratios. Thus the strains of *B. thuringiensis* classified on the above bacteriological characters form a basis for distinguishing host spectra of the spore-crystal complex.

The exotoxin, however, is produced in variable quantity by otherwise identical isolates of the same strain (see below). Thus bacterial taxonomy does not form a basis for determining host spectra that are dependent on the action of the exotoxin.

If the host spectrum is to be of value in the taxonomy of *B. thuringiensis,* the spectrum of the spore-crystal complex of a given strain must be an irreversible and intrinsic characteristic of the strain, following Heimpel's (1968) and not Rogoff's (1968) conception. For instance, Heimpel (1967b) distinguished var. *subtoxicus* and var. *entomocidus* in serotype VI by differences in their activity against *P. brassicae* and *B. mori.* However, 779 cases of cross-activity, i.e. reversal of susceptibility of a pair of species to two different strains, could also be considered (Burgerjon and Biache, 1967a) and so the use of these host spectra seem impractical in a taxonomic key.

The production of exotoxin is not absolutely dependent on the serotype or other bacteriological characteristics, as has been shown for the strain *B. thuringiensis* 058 (serotype I) isolated in Czechoslovakia, which does not produce the thermostable toxin (Burgerjon and de Barjac, 1962), and the same is true for several other strains within the serotype IV, IVa, and IVc (Burgerjon and de Barjac, 1967). Also different strains produce the toxin in greatly different amounts (p. 312). Thus the production of exotoxin is not a good taxonomic character and we must agree with Rogoff's criticism of its use by Heimpel. Not only is the use of exotoxin impractical and unsound, but also his nomenclature is one of the most confused because it changes names established through usage, e.g. the designation of strain 058 serotype I as *B. thuringiensis* var. *amuscatoxicus.* This is an illogical and fallacious name, since this strain has already shown its inability to produce the thermostable exotoxin in bioassays on *Lymantria dispar* (Burgerjon and de Barjac, 1964) and *Locusta migratoria* (Burgerjon *et al.,* 1964), and the identity of the specific fly toxin with the thermostable exotoxin can no longer be contested. Following the proposition put forward by Heimpel, this strain, like all the others not producing the thermostable toxin in appreciable quantities should be designated at the same time as *amuscatoxicus, alocustatoxicus* etc. A recent taxonomic review by Krieg (1968), which came to our attention after this chapter has been prepared, contains a discussion of the taxonomic considerations concerning the host spectrum.

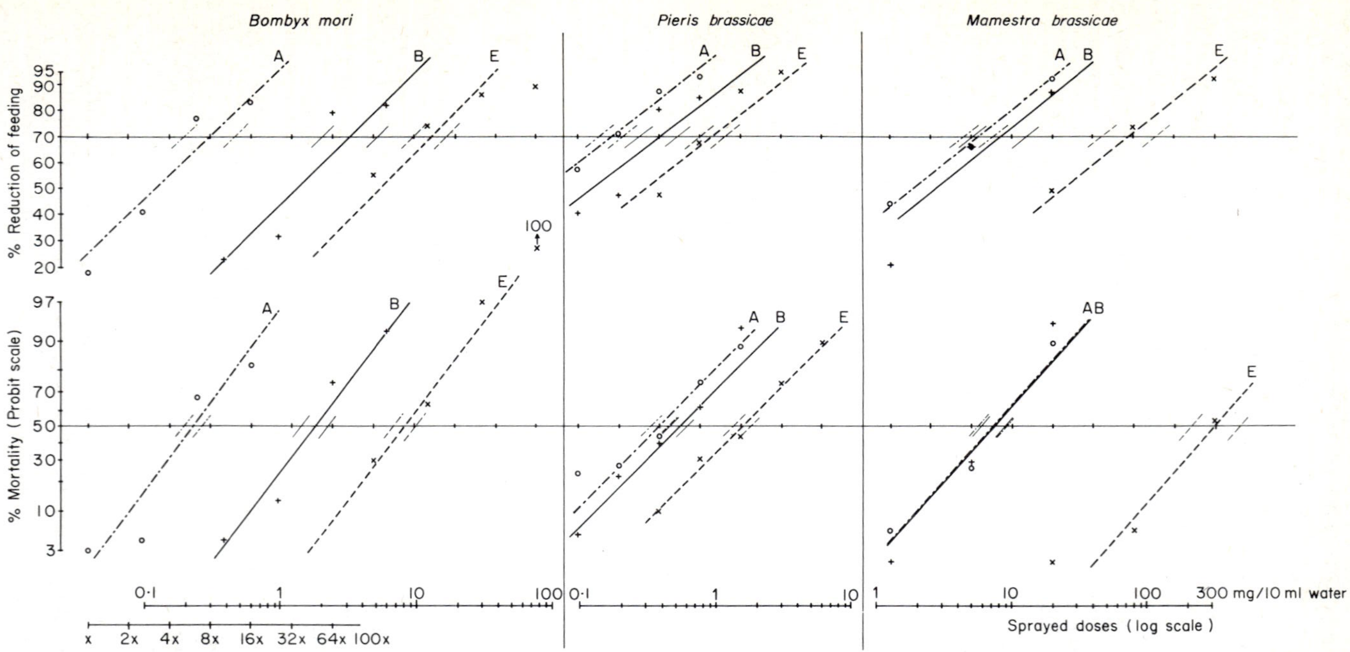

Fig. 1. Three preparations of serotype I; bioassayed against three Lepidoptera (Burgerjon and de Barjac, unpublished). E = international standard preparation E 61. B = a laboratory preparation of the same strain as E but obtained by evaporating the total culture (spores, crystals, thermostable exotoxin). A = a preparation of strain 562-5A (Bucher *et al.*, 1966) obtained simultaneously with and under the same conditions as B. Larvae were allowed to feed freely on treated mulberry or cabbage leaves (Burgerjon, 1956). Measurement of the amount of treated foliage eaten in 24 hr (Burgerjon, 1962) and counting the subsequent deaths permitted the reduction in feeding and the final mortality to be established. The difference in the results obtained with *Pieris* and with *Bombyx* demonstrates the specificity of the action of the spore-crystal complexes of strains in cultures A and B. The difference between the reduction of feeding and the mortality in *Mamestra* is explained by A and B being total cultures, in which the exotoxin remained present, while the centrifugation residue E did not contain it. In *Mamestra* the effect of the exotoxin is manifested not because this species is more sensitive to it, but because it is less sensitive to the spore-crystal complex, as shown by the increased doses used. The presence of the exotoxin in preparations A and B was demonstrated in another experiment by bioassay of the autoclaved preparations with *Mamestra.* Both preparations caused 100% mortality at the larval moult. There is no difference between A and B in *Mamestra,* although Bucher *et al.* (1966) found a much higher activity for A against another Noctuid. Without the comparison with the international standard E61 it is difficult to judge the "typical" strain (B) used by Bucher *et al.*

V. Experimentation and the Host Spectrum

In view of the great diversity of the processes governing the relationships between the strains and the host species, an interpretation of the susceptibility differences observed between different species is extremely complex and delicate in an experimental determination of the host spectrum of *B. thuringiensis.* We shall examine the factors that influence the comprehension of the host spectrum; above all, we wish to emphasize the ease with which apparently contradictory results can be obtained in the course of this experimentation.

A. NATURE OF THE PREPARATION

Beginning with a given strain, the seven combinations of the three active principles whose role has already been examined would form seven preparations differing both in their nature and in their host spectrum, i.e.:

1	2	3	4	5	6	7
Spore	Spore	–	Spore	–	–	Spore
Crystal	Crystal	–	–	Crystal	Crystal	–
Exotoxin	–	Exotoxin	Exotoxin	–	Exotoxin	–

While 1-3 are obtained industrially by different methods of harvest, 4 corresponds to a mutant form of *B. thuringiensis,* which, having lost the ability to form the crystal, remains serologically distinct from *B. cereus* and may still produce the exotoxin (de Barjac *et al.,* 1966). Preparations 5, 6 and 7, appear at present to belong exclusively to the realm of laboratory experimentation. Variation in the proportions of the constituents, produces intermediates between the seven types, especially in commercial preparations, where the degrees of retention of the active principles will depend on the mode of the harvest. This is illustrated by different results with *Mamestra brassicae* and the two crystal-sensitive species in Fig. 1. The viability of the spores may be lowered more rapidly than the toxicity of the crystals, a difference expressed by different effects on *Ephestia kuehniella* and *Pieris brassicae* (Burgerjon and Yamvrias, 1959). The significance of the variations in crystal content and the spore count of different batches are discussed further in Chapter 27. It is thus important, before undertaking any experimental work on the host spectrum of a preparation of *B. thuringiensis,* to determine precisely the nature of the preparation.

B. EXPERIMENTAL TECHNIQUES

Administration by injection into the haemocoel or by ingestion are fundamentally different, and may give very different results, according to whether the preparation contains the crystal, the exotoxin, the spore or any combination of these three elements (Martouret, 1961). The resulting ED_{50} or LD_{50} values, related to the weight of the test insect, can be considered as objective criteria of activity only to the extent that they are accompanied by a detailed description of the technique and are reproducible.

For the same reasons, forced ingestion by syringe and free ingestion of treated foliage do not necessarily lead to identical results. In particular, when comparing the action of the crystal to that of the exotoxin by means of free ingestion, the quantities of the crystal eaten by the insect are not in the same ratio as that in the serial concentrations applied to the leaves, because the arrest in feeding caused by the crystals prevents further intake by the insect, the effect being more rapid with high concentration on the foliage. This does not happen with the exotoxin, whose ingestion continues until the toxic effects intervene at the next moult (Burgerjon and Biache, 1967c).

After free ingestion of mixtures of the two toxins, the action of the exotoxin is manifested only in species, such as the Noctuidae *(Mamestra brassicae* in Fig. 1), showing little sensitivity to the activity of the crystal (Burgerjon and de Barjac, 1962), since for crystal-sensitive species ingestion of the exotoxin is rapidly interrupted by the arrest in feeding caused by the crystal.

C. EXPERIMENTAL CONDITIONS

The reactions of insects to the strains and the active elements of *B. thuringiensis* are so diverse that the choice of experimental conditions such as the criteria of interpretation, the doses used, and the age of the test insects can have profound effects on the results. These factors must therefore be borne in mind in evaluation of the work.

Thus, when comparing the activity of the spore-crystal complex in certain strains, such as var. *alesti* (serotype III) and var. *berliner* (serotype I), the ratio of observed reduction in feeding is often different from that of mortality evoked by the same doses of these strains in the same individuals (Burgerjon, 1962). Whatever criterion is adopted, the slopes of the dose-effect regression curves are different for each strain, and comparison of the effects of the two strains on one host species depends on judicious choice of the doses tested.

With the exotoxin, whatever activity criterion is selected–teratological symptoms or death–it should be remembered that the intensity of the effect decreases with increasing proximity of ingestion to the beginning of a larval instar. The opposite is observed with the crystal (Burgerjon and Biache, 1967c; Burgerjon, in press). A preparation containing the spore-crystal complex and one containing only the thermostable toxin will therefore exhibit essentially opposite behaviour, depending on the stage in the instar at which they are eaten. Consequently a comparison between the activity of the crystal and that of the exotoxin is more dependant on the experimental conditions than a comparison of crystal from two different strains. It would thus be difficult and not very useful to recommend here standardization of experimental methods aimed at establishing the host spectrum of preparations as variable in nature and effects as those based on *B. thuringiensis*. It is rather a diversity of experimental methods that can, at present, increase the probability of demonstrating the various properties of the bacterial preparations.

VI. Significance of the Host Spectrum in Applied Pathology

To attain satisfactory control of one or more pest species in a given environment, it is necessary, among other problems, to select a bacterial preparation effective against the pests but harmless as far as possible to the useful insect population. Knowledge of the potentialities of the available strains of *B. thuringiensis* increases the precision with which this selection can be made (Martouret, 1967). However, the host spectrum established in the laboratory shows the species susceptible under conditions that favour the bacterium. Practical pest control must take into consideration the many interactions exerted by various natural ecological and ethological factors on the host-parasite relationships, e.g. the feeding of caterpillars protected in buds, the effect of temperature, weathering etc. (Chapters 3 and 19). The impact of such natural factors limits to some extent the agricultural significance of the host spectrum of *B. thuringiensis*. The selection of the best strain is also governed by its suitability for industrial production (Chapter 24) and, as emphasized by Ignoffo (1967), by the width of its effective host spectrum, i.e. the number of pests that it will control, which determines its commercial potential. For forecasting in the realm of applied insect pathology, the host spectrum inherent in the various available industrial products, and the bacterial elements that they contain, should be characterized at the stage of industrial production (Chapter 27; Burgerjon, 1964b).

VII. Discussion, Conclusions and Future Research

The present contribution on the host spectrum of *B. thuringiensis* aims at an objective analysis, permitting an appreciation and assessment of the copious literature devoted to the subject, so that further experimental work can be placed on a rational and rigorous basis. The still insufficient knowledge of the roles and interactions between the various ethological, ecological, technological and economic factors explains the gap existing between the wide perspectives already offered by the host spectrum of *B. thuringiensis* and the very limited number of pests so far effectively combated with the aid of industrial preparations. More than a thousand investigations on *B. thuringiensis* have been published, a number of them being concerned with the role of the micro-organism and its toxins in different arthropods; the susceptibility of around 400 species has been confirmed. Among these:

1. Numerous Lepidoptera are more or less sensitive to the toxic action of the crystal alone, according to the strains considered.

2. Certain Lepidoptera are susceptible only to the combined action of the spores and the crystals, which is manifested by chronic toxaemia and an atypical dysentery.

3. Others, comprising several Lepidoptera and several phytophagous Hymenoptera, are susceptible only to the action of the bacillary spores, whose germination and vegetative multiplication produces toxaemic effects comparable to those evoked by certain enzymes, and sometimes also delayed septicaemia in the post-larval stages.

4. Many at least of these species, and a large number of others in various orders of insects, can be affected by the exotoxin, when the toxin is present in effective amounts in the bacterial preparation.

The results already obtained from fundamental investigations help us to understand the host spectrum of *B. thuringiensis.* There is no doubt that the perspectives offered by future research on the development of our knowledge of the host spectrum, will have both theoretical and practical implications.

We shall not discuss here the plans for fundamental research on *B. thuringiensis* proposed in Chapters 10, 11 and 12, with which we concur. On the other hand, the opportunities offered by strains other than those currently industrialized should be examined for practical pest control of a range of economically important pests. In the near future, this research should not only define experimental conditions particularly adapted to the biology of each of the pests under consideration, but also precisely establish the characteristics of the particular microbial material. To ensure information of this quality, without which experimental results have only mediocre value and a limited range, studies of the host spectrum of strains of *B. thuringiensis* should utilize the principles and techniques already developed for the characterization of industrial products, which have been presented at several international colloquia devoted to standardization (Chapter 27). In particular, it will be necessary to determine quantitatively in each case, in relative or absolute values, the active principle or principles present in taxonomically well defined bacterial preparations.

General application of standard reference preparations based on different strains of *B. thuringiensis* and their toxins would be a first step in facilitating world wide interpretation of the results obtained in the domain of the host spectrum and in making such results useful for practical pest control and invertebrate pathology.

References

Afrikian, E. G. (1960). *J. Insect Path.* **2,** 299-304.
Angus, T. A. (1954). *Nature, Lond.* **173,** 545.
Angus, T. A. (1956a). *Can. J. Microbiol.* **2,** 111-121.
Angus, T. A. (1956b). *Can. Ent.* **88,** 280-283.
Angus, T. A. (1964). *Entomophaga Mém. hors Sér.* **2,** 165-173.

Angus, T. A. (1965). *Proc. ent. Soc. Ont.* **95,** 133-134.
Angus, T. A. (1967). *J. Invertebrate Path.* **9,** 256-260.
Angus, T. A. (1968). *Wldl Rev. Pest Control* 7, 1.
Angus, T. A. and Heimpel, A. M. (1959). *Can. Ent.* **41,** 352-358.
Angus, T. A. and Norris, J. R. (1968). *J. Invertebrate Path.* **11,** 289-295.
Aoki, K. and Chigasaki, Y. (1915). *Mett. Med. Fak. Kais Univ. Tokyo* **13,** 419-440.
Barjac, H. de and Bonnefoi, A. (1962). *Entomophaga* 7, 6-61.
Barjac, H. de and Bonnefoi, A. (1967). *C.r. hebd. Séanc Sci., Paris* **264,** 1811-1813.
Barjac, H. de, Burgerjon, A. and Bonnefoi, A. (1966). *J. Invertebrate Path.* **8,** 537-538.
Benz, G. (1966). *J. Insect Physiol.* **12,** 137-151.
Berliner, E. (1915). *Z. Angew. Ent.* **2,** 29-56.
Broersma, D. B. and Buxton, J. A. (1967). *J. Invertebrate Path.* **9,** 58-69.
Bucher, G. E. (1960). *J. Insect Path.* **2,** 172-195.
Bucher, G. E., Angus, T. A. and Krywienczyk, J. (1966). *J. Invertebrate Path.* **8,** 485-491.
Burgerjon, A. (1956). *Annls Épiphyt.* **7,** 675-684.
Burgerjon, A. (1962). *Annls Épiphyt.* **13,** 59-72.
Burgerjon, A. (1964a). *Entomophaga Mém. hors Sér. No. 2, 227-239.*
Burgerjon, A. (1964b). *Entomophaga Mém. hors Sér. No. 2, 255-261.*
Burgerjon, A. (1965). *Entomophaga* **10,** 55-65.
Burgerjon, A. (In press). *Congr. Int. Microbiol., Mexico* (1970).
Burgerjon, A. and de Barjac, H. (1960). *C.r. hebd. Séanc. Acad. Sci., Paris* **251,** 911-912.
Burgerjon, A. and de Barjac, H. (1962). *Proc. 11th Int. Congr. Ent. Vien* (1960). **2,** 835-839.
Burgerjon, A. and de Barjac, H. (1967). *J. Invertebrate Path.* **9,** 574-577.
Burgerjon, A. and Biache, G. (1967a). *Entomologia exp. appl.* **10,** 211-230.
Burgerjon, A. and Biache, G. (1967b). *C.r. hebd. Séanc. Acad. Sci., Paris* **264,** 2423-2425.
Burgerjon, A. and Biache, G. (1967c). *Ann. Soc. Ent. Fr. N.S.* **3,** 929-952.
Burgerjon, A. and Grison, P. (1959). *Entomophaga* **4,** 205-209.
Burgerjon, A. and Yamvrias, C. (1959). *C.r. hebd. Séanc. Acad. Sci., Paris* **249,** 2871-2872.
Burgerjon, A. and Yamvrias, C. (1962). *Proc. 11th Int. Congr. Ent. Wien (1960).* **2,** 842-844.
Burgerjon, A., Biache, G. and Cals, P. (1969). *J. Invertebrate Path.* **14,** 274-278.
Burgerjon, A., Grison, P. and Kachkouli, A. (1964). *J. Insect Path.* **6,** 381-383.
Burges, H. D. *et al.* (1967). *In* "Insect Pathology and Microbial Control" (P. A. van der Laan, ed.), pp. 306-338. North Holland Publ. Co., Amsterdam.
David, J. and Vago, C. (1967). *Entomophaga* **12,** 153-159.
Dedonder, R. and Lecadet, M-M. (1964). *Entomophaga Mém. hors Sér.* No. 2 197-203.
Faust, R. M., Adams, J. R. and Heimpel, A. M. (1967). *J. Invertebrate Path.* **9,** 488-499.
Fitz-James, P. C., Toumanoff, C. and Young, E. I. (1958). *Can. J. Microbiol.* **4,** 385-392.
Franz, J. M. (1961). *Handb. Pflkrankh.* **6,** 1-302.
Gochnauer, T. A. (1960). *Bact. Proc.* **60,** 79-80.
Grigorova, R. (1964). *Entomophaga Mém. hors Sér.* **2,** 179-191.
Grigorova, R., Kantardgieva, E. and Pashov, N. (1967). *J. Invertebrate Path.* **9,** 503-509.
Gukasian, A. B. (1958). *Rep. Siberian Branch Acad. Sci. USSR* **7,** 85-101.
Gukasian, V. M. (1967). *Acad. Sci. URSS Fil. de Sibérie. Moscou,* 136-139.
Hall, I. M. and Dunn, P. H. (1958). *J. econ. Ent.* **51,** 296-298.
Hannay, C. L. (1953). *Nature, Lond.* **172,** 1004.
Heimpel, A. M. (1955a). *Can. J. Zool.* **33,** 99-106.
Heimpel, A. M. (1955b). *Can. J. Zool.* **33,** 311-326.
Heimpel, A. M. (1960). *Proc. ent. Soc. Ont.* **91,** 52-76.
Heimpel, A. M. (1967a). *Ann. Rev. Ent.* **12,** 287-322.
Heimpel, A. M. (1967b). *J. Invertebrate Path.* **9,** 364-375.
Heimpel, A. M. (1968). *J. Invertebrate Path.* **10,** 454-456.
Heimpel, A. M. and Angus, T. A. (1959). *J. Insect Path.* **1,** 152-170.
Heimpel, A. M. and Harshbarger, J. C. (1965). *Bact. Rev.* **29,** 397-405.
Hitchings, D. L. (1967). *J. econ. Ent.* **60,** 596-597.

Ignoffo, C. M. (1963). *J. Insect Path.* **5**, 395-397.
Ignoffo, C. M. (1967). *In* "Insect Pathology and Microbial Control" (P. A. van der Laan, ed.), pp. 91-117. North-Holland Publ. Co., Amsterdam.
Ignoffo, C. M. and Graham, H. M. (1967). *J. Invertebrate Path.* **9**, 390-394.
Isakova, N. P. (1964). *Entomophaga Mém. hors Sér.* No. 2, 175-178.
Khachatrian, L. S. and Rautenstein, Y. I. (1963). *Microbiology USSR* **32**, 813-818.
Klein, W. H. and Lewis, F. B. (1966). *J. Forestry July,* 458-462.
Krieg, A. (1965a). *Entomophaga* **10**, 3-20.
Krieg, A. (1965b). *Entomophaga* **10**, 49-54.
Krieg, A. (1968). *J. Invertebrate Path.* **12**, 366-378.
Kurstak, E. S. (1964). *Entomophaga Mém. hors Sér.* No. 2, 245-247.
Kushner, D. J. and Harvey, G. T. (1960). *Can. Sci. Serv. Div. For. Biol. Bi-monthly. Progr. Rep.* **16**, 5.
Kushner, D. J. and Harvey, G. T. (1962). *J. Insect Path.* **4**, 155-184.
Kushner, D. J. and Heimpel, A. M. (1957). *Can. J. Microbiol.* **3**, 547-551.
Kushner, D. J. and Lisson, T. A. (1959). *J. gen. Microbiol.* **21**, 96-108.
Lecadet, M-M. and Dedonder, R. (1966a). *Bull. Soc. Chim. biol.* **48**, 631-660.
Lecadet, M-M. and Dedonder, R. (1966b). *Bull. Soc. Chim. biol.* **48**, 661-691.
Lecadet, M-M. and Dedonder, R. (1967). *J. Invertebrate Path.* **9**, 310-321.
Lecadet, M-M. and Martouret, D. (1962). *C.r. hebd. Séanc Acad. Sci., Paris* **254**, 2457-2459.
Lecadet, M-M. and Martouret, D. (1964). *Entomophaga Mém. hors Sér.* **2**, 205-212.
Lecadet, M-M. and Martouret, D. (1965). *J. Invertebrate Path.* **7**, 105-108.
Lecadet, M-M. and Martouret, D. (1967a). *J. Invertebrate Path.* **9**, 322-330.
Lecadet, M-M. and Martouret, D. (1967b). *C.r. hebd. Séanc Acad. Sci., Paris* **265**, 1543-1546.
Lhoste, J. and Martouret, D. (In press). *Proc. 13th Int. Congr. Ent. Moscow.* 1968.
McConnell, E. and Richards, A. G. (1959). *Can. J. Microbiol.* **5**, 161-168.
Martouret, D, (1961). *C.r. 13th Symp. Phytia. Phyto. Gand.* 1116-1126.
Martouret, D. (1962). *C.r. 11th Congr. Int. Ent. Wien* (1960) No. 2, 849-855.
Martouret, D. (1964). *Entomophaga Mém. hors Sér.* **2**, 213-220.
Martouret, D. (1967). *C.r. hebd. Séanc. Acad. Agric. Fr.* **53**, 154-159.
Martouret, D. and Biache, G. (In press.)
Martouret, D. and Euverte, G. (1964). *J. Insect Path.* **6**, 198-203.
Martouret, D., Lhoste, J. and Roche, A. (1965). *Entomophaga* **10**, 348-365.
Mattés, O. (1927). *Gesel. f. Geford. Ges. Natur. Sitzberg Marburg.* **62**, 381-417.
Mayas, I. (1970). *Thèse Fac. Sci., Paris,* 92 pp.
Norris, J. R. (1964). *J. appl. Bacteriol.* **27**, 439-447.
Oatman, E. R. and Legner, E. F. (1964). *J. econ. Ent.* **57**, 294.
Raun, E. S., Sutter, G. R. and Revelo, M. A. (1966). *J. Invertebrate Path.* **8**, 365-375.
Rogoff, M. H. (1966). *Adv. appl. Microbiol.* **8**, 291-313.
Rogoff, M. H. (1968). *J. Invertebrate Path.* **10**, 453-454.
Schvetsova, O. I. (1963). *Méthods de Lutte Microbiologiques contre les Insectes Nuisibles Acad. Sci. URSS.* Moscou. 44-48.
Schvetsova, O. I. (1964). *URSS Acad. Sci. Invest. Méthods Biol. Control agric. forest Pest Moscow* (1964). 113-116.
Smirnoff, W. A. (1965). *J. Invertebrate Path.* **7**, 71-74.
Smirnoff, W. A. (1967). *Phytoprotection* **48**, 119-127.
Smirnoff, W. A. (1968). *J. Invertebrate Path.* **11**, 513-515.
Smirnoff, W. A. and Berlinguet, L. (1966). *J. Invertebrate Path.* **8**, 376-381.
Smirnoff, W. A. and Hutchinson, P. M. (1965). *J. Invertebrate Path.* **7**, 273-280.
Smythe, R. V. and Coppel, H. C. (1965). *J. Invertebrate Path.* **7**, 423-426.
Steinhaus, E. A. (1951). *Pacific Sea Board mimeographed,* 16.
Steinhaus, E. A. (1957). *No. 4 mimeographed series Lab. Path. Dep. Biol. Control Univ. California Berkeley,* 24.
Steinhaus, E. A. and Bell, C. R. (1953). *J. econ. Ent.* **46**, 582-598.
Stephens, J. M. (1952). *Can. J. Zool.* **30**, 30-40.
Talalaev, E. V. (1958). *Ent. Obozr.* **37**, 641-652.

Talalaev, E. V. (1961). *Vest. sel.'-khoz. Nauki, Alma-Ata* **6**, 100-105.
Talalaeva, G. B. (1967). *Ent. Obozr.* **66**, 319-321.
Toumanoff, C. (1953). *Annls Inst. Pasteur, Paris* **83**, 85-90.
Toumanoff, C. (1955). *Annls Inst. Pasteur, Paris* **89**, 644-653.
Toumanoff, C. and Lapied, M. (1955). *Annls Inst. Pasteur, Paris* **87**, 370-374.
Toumanoff, C. and Vago, C. (1952). *C.r. hebd. Séanc. Acad. Sci., Paris* **235**, 1715-1717.
Toumanoff, C. and Vago, C. (1955). *Annls Inst. Pasteur, Paris* **88**, 388-392.
Tyumentsev, S. N. (1963). *Mikrobiologija,* **32**, 879-884.
Tyumentsev, S. N. (1966). *Conférence Samarkand-Tachkent.* 179-181.
Vago, C. (1959). *Annls Épiphyt. hors Série,* No. 10, 181 pp.
Vaňková, J. (1964). *Entomophaga Mém. hors Sér.* No. 2, 271-291.
Vaňková, J. (1966). *Acta Bohemoslov.* **63**, 10-16.
Vaňková, J. and Kralik, O. (1966). *Zentbl. Bakt. ParasitKde* 380-390.
Vasiljević, L. A. (1957). *Mem. Inst. Plant. Prot. Beograd.* **7**, 79 pp.
Watanabe, M. (1963). *Ann. Sankyo Res. Lab.* **15**, 156-159.
Watanabe, T., Tsutsui, R., Iwahana, H. and Abe, K. (1968). Proc. Joint U.S.-Japan Semin. Microbial Control Insect Pests. U.S.-Japan Committee Sci. Cooperation. Panel 8. Fukuoka, pp. 71-78.
White, C. A. and Briggs, J. D. (1964). *Entomophaga Mém. hors Sér.* No. 2, 305-308.
Wiegand, H. (1963). *Entomophaga* **8**, 35-41.
Wiegand, H. (1968). *Bioma. Z.* **10**, 34-43.
Yamvrias, C. (1962). *Entomophaga* **7**, 101-159.
Yoder, P. E. and Nelson, E. L. (1960). *J. Insect Path.* **12**, 198-200.

CHAPTER 14

Synergism of Micro-organisms and Chemical Insecticides

GEORG BENZ

Department of Entomology, Swiss Federal Institute of Technology, Zurich, Switzerland

I. Introduction

Integrated control of insects is one way of lessening the severe impact of pesticides on the ecosystem. It is already more or less established and has sometimes led to the simultaneous application of biological and chemical agents. Another approach is based on the observation made by insect pathologists that insects, like other organisms, are more susceptible to disease when under the influence of stress produced by crowding, malnutrition, and other environmental factors (Steinhaus, 1958; Vago, 1959). It was thought by some workers that chemical insecticides might act as stressors and thus promote contraction or activation of infectious diseases or make insects more susceptible to the action of microbial toxins. This approach was supported by observations made in the field after insect populations had been treated with insecticides (Schaefer, 1936; Fankhaenel, 1957; Kovačević, 1958). Of particular interest is the report of Telenga and Dyadechko (1957) that healthy larvae of the codling moth, *Cydia*

(Carpocapsa) pomonella, the tent caterpillar, *Malacosoma neustria,* and some other species could not be infected with spores of the muscardine fungus, *Beauveria bassiana* unless the insects had first been treated with weak doses of DDT or HCH.

In this chapter reported synergism of micro-organisms and chemical substances will be reviewed and the significance of the findings discussed. Viruses, although not organisms, will be included in the term micro-organism. The discussion and evaluation of synergism between such unlike pairs of agents is not easy, because little systematic and basic research on this subject has been published so far. Most reports give results of empirical experiments in the field, and often necessary controls are missing or the results have not been reproduced. Reports on virus-insecticide combinations are particularly scarce. Some unpublished data by Schnyder and Benz are therefore included. The evaluation of synergism of micro-organisms and insecticides is further complicated by the predominance of reports in the Slavic languages; the original literature was rarely available to the author.

Since this book deals mainly with practical insect pathology and control, it was felt that the absence of synergism and antagonism should be discussed as well. Such cases demonstrate the fact that synergism and antagonism are sometimes rather a question of concentrations than of which micro-organism is combined with which insecticide. Synergism of pathogens and acaricides is described in Chapter 15.

II. Terminology and Classification

A. THEORETICAL ASPECTS

1. Definition of Synergism and Antagonism

The use of the term synergism is not uniform. It is derived from the Greek *synergos* and means working together. Most treatises on synergism are concerned with the synergism of insecticides, i.e. the combination of two insecticides or an insecticide and a non-toxic substance. If the latter has the ability to enhance the action of the toxicant it is called a synergist, if it reduces the toxic effect it is an antagonist (from Greek *antagonizesthai* = to struggle against). The same distinction can be used to describe the combined actions of micro-organisms and non-lethal[1] doses of insecticides. In this case, however, missing synergism and

[1] The meanings of the terms sublethal and lethal in connection with doses of toxicants are ambiguous. By definition an LD_{50} kills 50% of the treated individuals, whereas 50% survive. Thus the same dose is lethal for the individuals which die and sublethal for the survivors. To avoid any ambiguity the term non-lethal is applied to doses and concentrations which cause no significant mortality, whereas the term lethal is applied to all doses or concentrations causing significant mortality from 1 to 100%. Specific indications are given as percentage mortality or as LD and LC values respectively, e.g. LD_{30}, LC_{70}, etc. The unspecific indication "slightly toxic" is sometimes used when corrected mortality does not exceed 10%.

antagonism may sometimes not be distinguishable by the simple evaluation of the death rate (see Inapparent antagonism).

The situation is also clear when two insecticides, such as organophosphates are combined. Since both agents may act on the same target within the insect, i.e. acetylcholinesterase, the molecules of one compound may replace the molecules of the other. If no interaction between the two types of molecules occurs, an additive effect is expected, i.e. the combination of half the LD_{50} of each component should produce the same effect as an LD_{50} of either compound. A less than additive effect indicates antagonism and a greater effect synergism. However, if a micro-organism and a lethal dose of an insecticide are combined the latter can rarely be expected to hit the same target as the micro-organism. Assuming completely independent action of the two agents the combination of half the LD_{50} of each can give much less to more than 50% mortality, depending on the slopes of the respective curves. The combination of the two LD_{50}s, on the other hand, would always result in 75% mortality. It is not even important whether or not the two independent components act simultaneously. Independent action resembles the situation met in an experiment where a pathogen or an insecticide is tested and in which natural mortality occurs. The latter may be regarded as the independent substitute for one of the two components in a combination experiment. Applicability of Abbot's formula is therefore a test for independent action. The combined effect of a micro-organism and an independently acting chemical substance can be calculated if the effect of each agent alone is known. A significantly smaller effect indicates antagonism and a significantly larger effect true synergism. Co-operation by means of independent action is purely accidental, achieved solely by the fact that both agents produce the same effect, i.e. death. Independent action therefore does not represent true synergism. However, for the sake of simplicity and in order to take a practical point of view, independent action will be considered in this chapter as the elementary form of synergism (in analogy to commensalism as the simplest form of symbiosis).

2. Dose-Mortality Effects

a. Synergism. Theoretically, co-operation (if it occurs) between dissimilar agents such as micro-organisms and lethal doses of insecticides is expected in the form of independent synergism (see Section II C 1a). Higher levels, i.e. potentiation of a micro-organism by an insecticide, are probably restricted to certain dose-ranges of the toxicant. An example in Fig. 1 illustrates the effects of combining the nuclear polyhedrosis virus of the looper *Idaea (Sterrha) seriata* with orally applied DDT. In these combinations, low doses of DDT up to 2 p.p.m. had no effect on mortality. However, more than an additive effect was reached at the concentration of 5 p.p.m. At 10 p.p.m. the synergistic effect was reduced, but was still higher than could be expected from independent action.

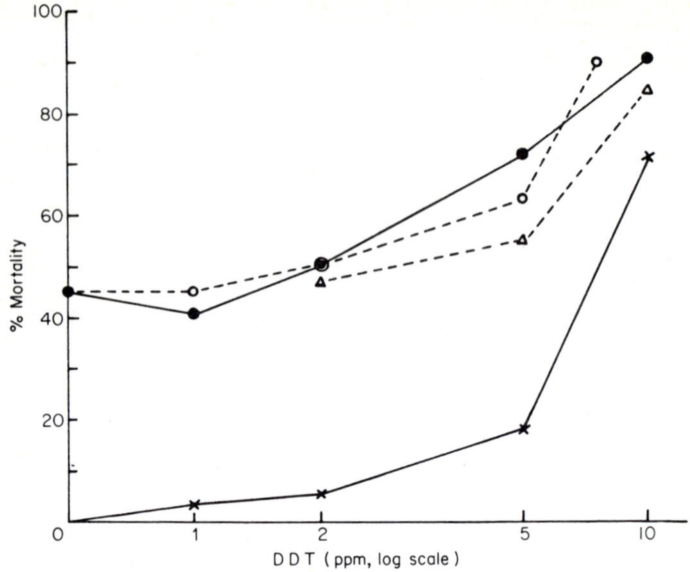

Fig. 1. Synergistic action of DDT and nuclear polyhedrosis virus of *Idaea seriata.* Each point represents 60-80 larvae in replicates of 20. Variation between the upper three concentrations exceeds variation within concentrations (Schnyder and Benz, unpublished). ● = total mortality in combination; x = mortality caused by DDT alone. The broken lines indicate theoretical mortalities expected from independent action (△), and additive effect (○).

The dose dependence may be even better exemplified by the combined action of *Bacillus thuringiensis* (BT) and DDT on sixth instar larvae of the moth *Agrotis ipsilon* (Fig. 2). The graph shows that BT alone has little pathogenic potency in this noctuid species. However, a low dose of BT combined with a relatively low dose of DDT produced a good synergistic effect (combination I). Synergism was less pronounced when BT was applied at a higher concentration (combination II), but better again when DDT too was used at a higher concentration (combination III). Similar combinations in other developmental stages may result in clear antagonism (combination IV and Table III). A further example is given below (Shekhurina, 1959).

b. Antagonism. (i) Apparent antagonism. Antagonism is often found when micro-organisms and insecticides are combined. In its simplest form it is the result of incompatibility of the micro-organism and the insecticide. This can be easily tested *in vitro* for bacteria and fungi. Incompatibility produces an antagonism increasing with the dose of the toxicant, and synergism may be completely absent. However, if the insect is far more sensitive than the micro-organism to the toxicant, independent action may be found with lethal, and true synergism with non-lethal, doses. The latter is well illustrated by the

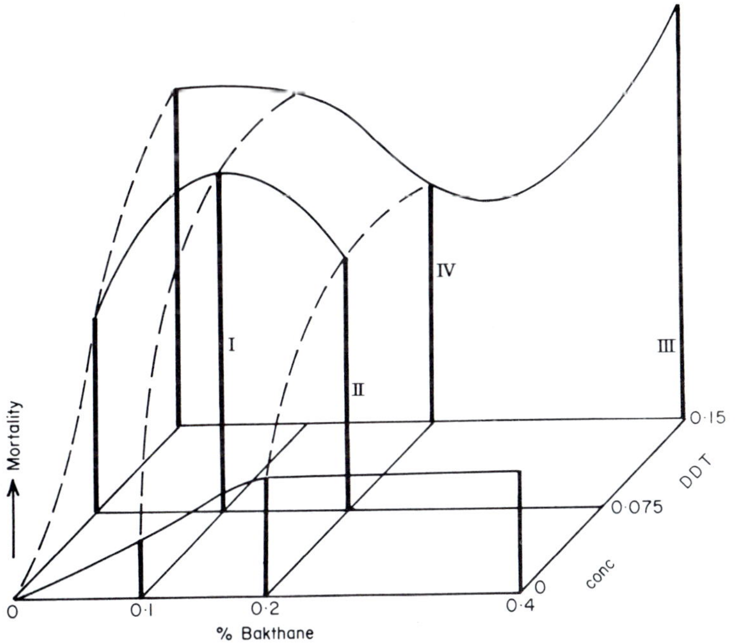

Fig. 2. Three-dimensional representation of mortality effects in sixth instar larvae of *Agrotis ipsilon* caused by three concentrations of *Bacillus thuringiensis,* two concentrations of DDT, and their combinations (after Haenggi, 1965). The roman numbers indicate different combinations mentioned in the text.

work of Shekhurina (1959), who treated the wheat bug *Eurygaster integriceps* with the fungus *Beauveria bassiana.* Although the fungus alone caused only 22.5% mortality, its effect was more than tripled (73.7%) in combination with non-lethal to slightly toxic doses of Wofatox (a mixture of methylparathion and parathion) causing 0-9% mortality. But in combination with a lethal dose of the insecticide, which alone caused 46.2% mortality, only 32.6% of the bugs died. This antagonism is partly due to the incompatibility of *B. bassiana* and methylparathion, as reported by Dirimanov and Angelova (1962). Since mortality in the combination was reduced to less than 46.2% the results of Shekhurina may indicate mutual incompatibility, i.e. the fungus was inhibited by the toxicant but in turn detoxified the latter.

Although the antagonistic effect mentioned above may be explained in terms of incompatibility, other mechanisms exist. Schnyder and Benz (unpublished) combined the granulosis virus of *Zeiraphera diniana* with non-lethal doses of Nirosan (tetranitrocarbazole) and found an antagonistic effect for the lowest dose of the insecticide, but none with a four times higher concentration (Fig. 3).

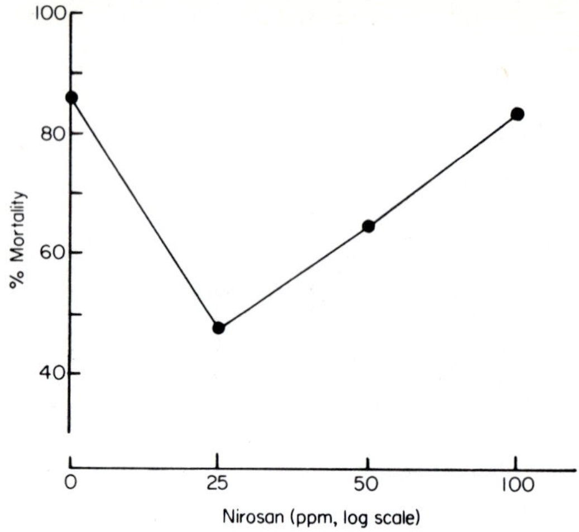

Fig. 3. Antagonistic action of non-lethal doses of Nirosan on the granulosis virus of *Zeiraphera diniana*. Antagonism shows negative correlation with dose of insecticide. Each point represents 4 x 25 larvae. Results are reproducible (Schnyder and Benz, unpublished).

(ii) Hormoligosis. The antagonistic effect in Fig. 3 may be due to hormoligosis (Luckey, 1968). This author has demonstrated that non-lethal doses of insecticides may stimulate the growth of the cricket *Acheta domesticus.* Schnyder and Benz could not verify the hormoligant nature of Nirosan in *Z. diniana,* but found non-lethal concentrations of this insecticide and of derris to reduce natural mortality in *I. seriata* significantly and reproduceably (3 and 2 experiments respectively). Non-lethal doses of carbaryl (Sevin), on the other hand, reduced natural mortality in larvae of *Z. diniana* from natural populations in the phase of the highest density. This effect of carbaryl was not found in *I. seriata.*

(iii) Inapparent antagonism. Antagonistic effects, although present, may not always become apparent. A good example is found in the combination of the granulosis virus of *Z. diniana* with non-lethal concentrations of derris (Schnyder and Benz, unpublished). In this case the virus alone and all the combinations produced about 84% total mortality (Fig. 4), i.e. neither synergism nor typical antagonism was present. However, diagnosis of the dead larvae showed that death caused by acute virosis was negatively correlated with the dose of the insecticide. The experiment has been reproduced with the same result. Obviously, two-thirds to three-quarters of the potential virus production were lost, possibly because the hosts died before the virus capsules were formed. The same was found in two experiments where a high dose of the nuclear polyhedrosis virus of *I. seriata* was combined with orally applied non-lethal to highly lethal concentrations of DDD (Fig. 5).

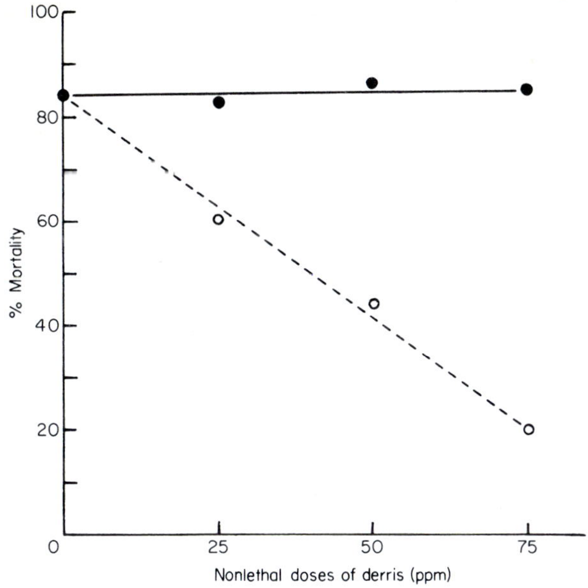

Fig. 4. Inapparent antagonism of non-lethal doses of derris to a dose of the granulosis virus of *Zeiraphera diniana*. Each point represents about 50 larvae. Results reproduced in two further experiments (Schnyder and Benz, unpublished). ● = total mortality; ○ = cases of acute virosis.

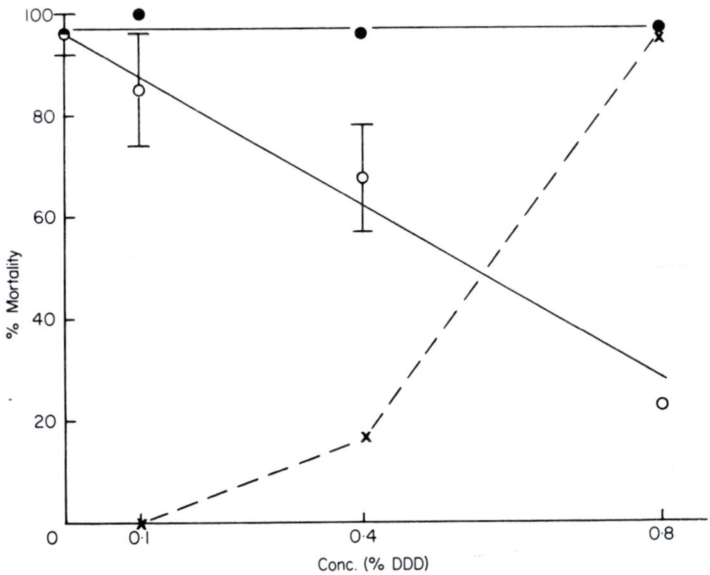

Fig. 5. Inapparent antagonism of orally applied non-lethal and lethal doses of DDD to a high dose of the nuclear polyhedrosis virus of *Idaea seriata*. Two experiments; each point 100 larvae; acute virosis with variation of the two experiments. Other experiments with lower doses of virus gave similar results (Schnyder and Benz, unpublished). ● = total mortality; ○ = cases of acute virosis; x = DDD alone.

c. Detachment of an antagonistic relation. Schnyder and Benz (unpublished) combined a dose of the polyhedrosis virus of *I. seriata,* causing 83% larval mortality, with different doses of topically applied DDD. The combinations with non-lethal and slightly lethal doses of the insecticide gave inapparent antagonism as discussed above (Fig. 6). Mortality from acute virosis dropped as low as 56% with 40 p.p.m. of DDD. However, the lethal dose of 50 p.p.m. of the toxicant, which alone caused 61% mortality, raised the total mortality to 97% and restored incidence of acute virosis to 80% (see also Table IV, E2). These findings of five independent experiments indicate that DDD antagonized the virus at low doses, but not at the highest dose. Obviously the antagonistic relation changed to independent action at doses above 40 p.p.m. It should be noted that combinations of the same virus with the same insecticide may lead to true synergism (Table IV, E3).

Detachment of an antagonistic relation can also be deduced from results of Shekhurina (1958), who treated fifth instar larvae of *Eurygaster integriceps* with *B. bassiana* in combination with relatively low doses of DDT. The insecticide had an antagonistic effect as long as the toxicant alone did not cause more than 40% mortality. However, an LD_{80} of DDT combined with the fungus gave 100% mortality in the laboratory, i.e. synergism.

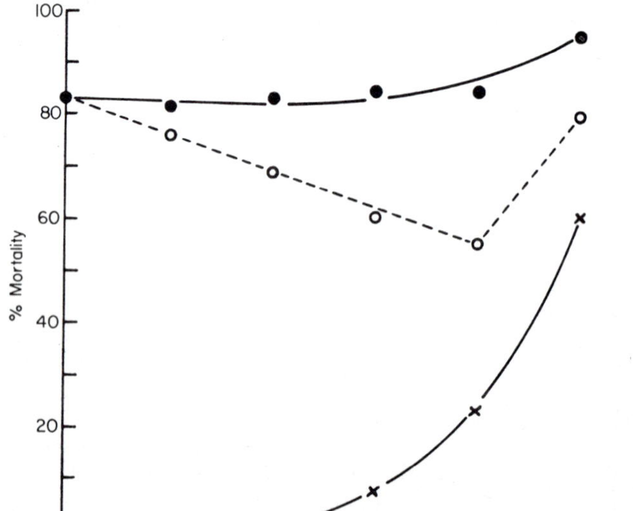

Fig. 6. Inapparent antagonism of non-lethal and lethal doses of topically applied DDD to nuclear polyhedrosis of *Idaea seriata,* and detachment of antagonistic relation at high dose of the insecticide. Two experiments; each point represents 4 x 25 larvae. Reproducible in three further experiments (Schnyder and Benz, unpublished). Symbols as in Fig. 5.

3. Simultaneous and Sequential Application

The same dose of an insecticide may have quite different effects when applied at different times after infection. Schnyder and Benz (unpublished) found that a dose of 0.1% Nirosan applied at a certain date to larvae of *I. seriata* produced 92% mortality, but only 29% when applied nine days later (Fig. 7). Simultaneous application of this dose of the insecticide with an LD_{75} of the

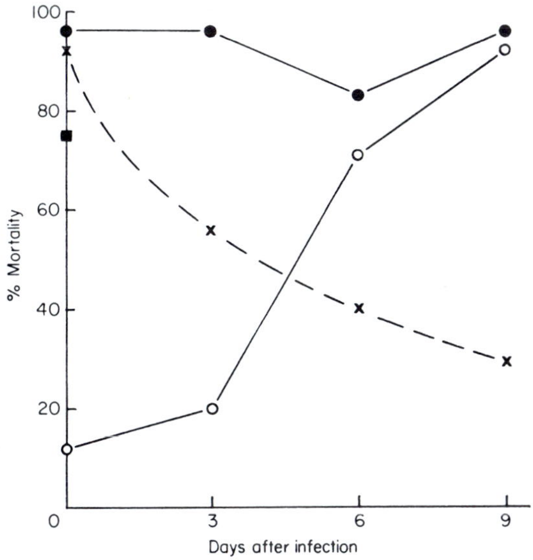

Fig. 7. Inapparent antagonism of lethal dose of Nirosan (0.1%) applied at 0 and 3 days after infection with nuclear polyhedrosis virus of *Idaea seriata,* and loss of antagonism at six and nine days after infection. Each point represents 50 larvae (Schnyder and Benz, unpublished; compare also Table IV, E7, where 0.1% Nirosan gave only 48% mortality). ■ = virus alone; x = insecticide alone; ● = total mortality in combinations; ○ = acute virosis in combinations.

polyhedrosis virus of *I. seriata* resulted in a strong inapparent antagonism. This antagonism was practically lost when the insecticide was applied six days after infection. Application of Nirosan nine days after infection resulted in 96% mortality. Since at this date the insecticide alone would have killed only about 30% of the larvae we may, theoretically, speak of synergism (subadditive synergism, see II C 1), though the same effect could have been obtained with the insecticide alone, if applied nine days earlier.

It has been shown in Fig. 5 that the simultaneous application of a relatively high dose of the same virus and certain concentrations of DDD lead to inapparent antagonism. This antagonism becomes much reduced, if the toxicant is applied 3-9 days after infection (Schnyder and Benz, unpublished). Moreover, in one experiment in which the larvae had been infected with a relatively low dose of the virus, its suppression was lost when 0.1 or 0.4% of DDD were applied six days after infection (Fig. 8(a)). In addition, virus incidence was highly synergized when the same doses of DDD were applied nine days after infection. However, such results are difficult to reproduce. Fig. 8(b) gives the results of a repetition of the experiment a few weeks later. In this case both insecticide concentrations gave a pronounced antagonistic effect when applied six days after

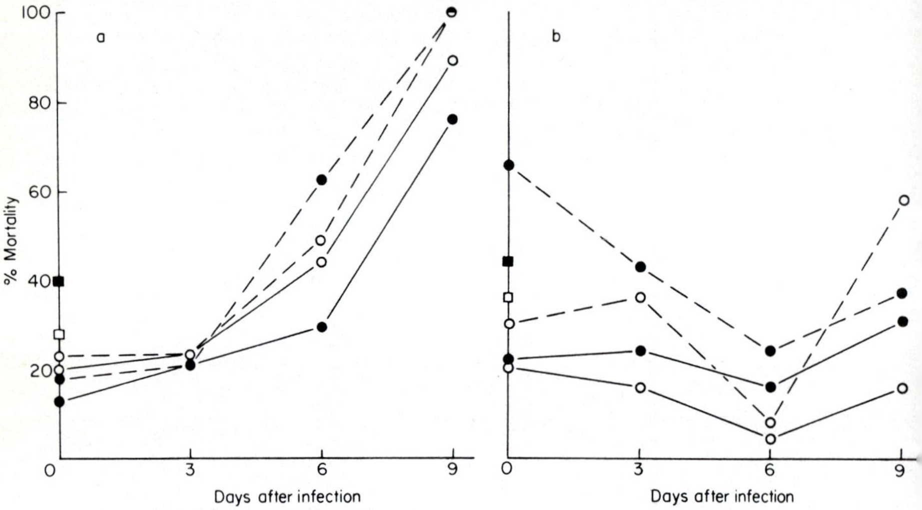

Fig. 8. Effect of two doses of DDD (○ = 0.1%; ● = 0.4%) applied at 0-9 days (abscissa) after infection of larvae of *Idaea seriata* with a low dose of nuclear polyhedrosis virus. Each point represents 50 larvae. a = first experiment with typical synergism; b = repetition of same experiment seven weeks later (Schnyder and Benz, unpublished). ■ = total mortality caused by application of virus alone; □ = acute virosis after virus alone; solid lines = cases of virosis in combinations; broken lines = total mortality in combinations.

infection. Some synergism, though less pronounced, occurred after the simultaneous application of the higher dose of DDD, whereas the lower dose was synergistic when applied nine days after the infection. The results are difficult to understand.

Girardeau and Mitchell (1968) infected larvae of the cabbage looper *Trichoplusia ni* with a sub-acute dose of a nuclear polyhedrosis virus (about 50 polyhedra/larva, producing less than 10% mortality). They could not reduce the LD_{50} for endrin, endosulfan or trichlorfon, if the insecticides were applied simultaneously with the virus, but found much reduced LD_{50}s when endrin and endosulfan were applied 24 hr and trichlorfon 48 hr after infection.

4. *Mortality-time*

Schnyder and Benz (unpublished) combined an LD_{90} of the granulosis virus of *Z. diniana* with an LD_{70} of Nirosan. Both the virus and the combination caused 90% mortality, i.e. less than expected from independent action. However, the curves of mortality-time being nearly identical for the virus and the insecticide respectively, time until death was much reduced when the two agents were combined (Fig. 9). Thus, although the combined action of the virus and Nirosan indicated an antagonistic relation concerning the rate of mortality, synergism must be postulated concerning the time of death. This synergism was

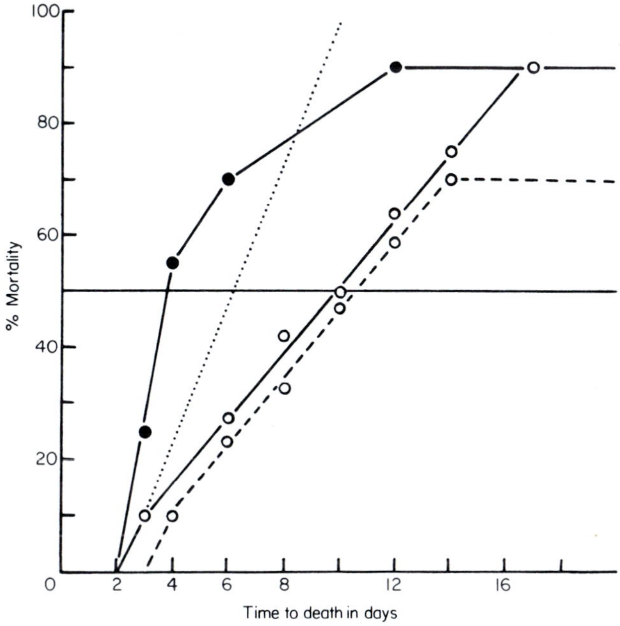

Fig. 9. Temporal synergism of granulosis virus of *Zeiraphera diniana* and Nirosan (Schnyder and Benz, unpublished). —○— = virus alone; – – ○ – – = insecticide alone; ● = combined effect. The dotted line would be expected if synergism was only additive.

more than additive up to eight days after treatment. No such synergism has been found in combinations of the nuclear polyhedrosis virus of *I. seriata* with DDT and DNOC (Schnyder, 1967).

B. PRACTICAL ASPECTS

Mortality-time may be far more important from a practical point of view than total mortality. Since the plant producer wants to grow commercially acceptable crops, he is mainly interested in reduced damage. The work of Getzin (1962) demonstrates clearly that the estimation of reduction of damage gives more practical information than the most exactly determined mortality rates. Thus cauliflower has its full commercial value only when the head and the wrapper leaves are intact. If treatment with a suspension of polyhedrosis virus against the cabbage looper *Trichoplusia ni* results in high larval mortality, but no heads with acceptable wrapper leaves can be harvested, the treatment is practically lost. Field experiments should therefore always include data on crop damage. Whether or not the term synergism should be applied if reduced damage is caused by the combination of two agents is merely a semantic problem. Since induced stoppage of feeding is a well defined biological effect the use of the word in the term *economic synergism* can be justified.

A further practical point to be considered is the simultaneous damage caused by more than one insect species. If one agent gives satisfactory control for only one of the pest species, whereas the combination of two agents leads to satisfactory control of all species involved (e.g. in the combination of the nuclear polyhedrosis virus of *T. ni* and insecticides, as indicated by Hofmaster and Ditman, 1961), it might be acceptable to speak of *interspecific economic synergism*.

C. CLASSIFICATION OF SYNERGISMS

1. Classification by Simple Mortality Data

a. Independent synergism (= independent action with zero correlation). A system of two components acting independently and not interfering with each other. If P_M is the probability of death by the micro-organism taken alone, and P_I the corresponding value for the insecticide, the probability of death by the combined action is $P_{M+I} = P_M + P_I(1-P_M)$ or, if the corresponding values of mortality in % are used: $M_{M+I} = M_M + M_I(1-M_M/100)$.

b. Subadditive synergism. A system of two components which together produce an effect greater than independent synergism but less than the algebraic sum of the two single effects. A weak potentiating effect is necessary to produce such a result.

c. Supplemental synergism. A system of two effective components which together produce an effect greater than the algebraic sum of the single effects ($M_{M+I} > M_M + M_I$).

d. Potentiating synergism. A system of a component A causing the effect M_A and a synergist (S) which alone causes no effect ($M_S = 0$), but which in combination produce an effect which is significantly greater than M_A. This type of synergism may be found when non-lethal concentrations of an insecticide are combined with a micro-organism.

e. Coalitive action. A system of two components of which each alone causes no measurable effect but which together produce a significant effect. Such a system may be found when an inapparent infectious disease becomes acute under the influence of a chemical stressor in sublethal concentration (Kovačević, 1958) or when infection with an externally applied micro-organism is possible only in combination with non-lethal or sublethal doses of an insecticide (examples in Tables II and III).

2. *Other Types of Synergism*

Other types of synergism have been discussed above. *Temporal synergism* occurs when two components together kill insects quicker than either component alone. This synergism may be included in *economic synergism,* i.e. a system of two components which together reduce damage more than each component alone. Intraspecific and interspecific economic synergism can be differentiated.

III. Review of Cases of Synergism and Failure

A. GENERAL REMARKS

In the following section the amounts of insecticides applied per hectare (1 ha = 2.471 acres) are usually indicated as amounts of the pure substance, e.g. 8 kilos (kg) of a 5% preparation of DDT will be indicated as 400 g DDT/ha.

The evaluation of the success of a combination of a micro-organism with an insecticide is only possible when all mortality factors are estimated separately, i.e. a report should always give information on natural mortality (M_N), mortality caused by the micro-organism alone (M_M, i.e. M_F, M_B, M_V for fungi, bacteria or viruses), the insecticide alone (M_I), and the combination of the two agents (M_{M+I}). It has been pointed out in the introduction that often some of the controls are missing. Many examples given by Russian workers are of this type. Since such experiments do not withstand proper analysis they are only mentioned in the following review, but not further discussed.

B. SYNERGISM OF MICROSPORIDA AND INSECTICIDES

Very little information is available on synergistic combinations of microsporida and insecticides. However, an example of such synergism has been published by Rosicky (1951) and Weiser (1961). It was shown that infection of the weevil *Otiorrhynchus ligustici* with the microsporidan *Nosema otiorrhynchi* accelerated death caused by arsenate of lime and knockdown as well as death caused by DDT and an unknown fumigant with contact effect. In the latter case nosematosis increased total mortality by preventing revival after knockdown. The death rates (Table I) indicate independent action and temporal synergism. Strangely enough the micro-organism seems to be the synergist of the insecticides and not vice versa.

Food consumption in healthy and diseased weevils was much reduced by arsenate or DDT. This effect was less pronounced in the case of the fumigant which reduced it by two-thirds in healthy beetles, but showed synergism in diseased insects, in which food consumption was 5% of the controls.

C. SYNERGISM OF FUNGI AND INSECTICIDES

1. *Compatibility of Fungi and Pesticides*

Fungicides reduce germination and growth of entomopathogenic fungi

TABLE I

Percent mortality of Otiorrhynchus ligustici *(non-infected and infected by* Nosema otiorrhynchi *) caused by different insecticides (after Rosicky, 1951)*

	Non-infected					Infected				
Days after treatment	2	4	6	9	14	2	4	6	9	14
Controls	0	3	15	25	32	17	20	33	40	72
Arsenate of lime	0	67	85	95	100	91	98	100	100	100
DDT 5%	–	3	75	84	96	–	76	78	98	100
DDT 10%	–	6	97	100	100	–	78	82	97	100
Fumigant 5%	–	0	40	63	80	–	68	73	94	95
Fumigant 10%	–	2	63	74	86	–	83	86	97	97

considerably (Fisher and Griffiths, 1950; Griffiths and Fisher, 1950; Pickett and Patterson, 1953; Hall and Dunn, 1959; Yendol, 1968). This is not generally true for insecticides (Kral and Neubauer, 1953; Kerner, 1958; Telenga *et al.*, 1959). Dirimanov and Angelova (1962) tested 22 insecticides on *Beauveria bassiana.* They found DDT, diazinon, dieldrin and toxaphene to be harmless, whereas some inhibited growth of the fungus strongly (e.g. methylparathion, parathion, Systox) and some absolutely (e.g. malathion). Fungi of the genus *Entomophthora* are probably more susceptible to insecticides. Vegetative growth of *E. exitialis* and *E. obscura* is impaired by DDT, demeton, malathion, parathion and trithion (Hall and Dunn, 1959; see also Yendol, 1968). However, the tests mentioned have been performed on artificial media and may not give more than tentative answers concerning the influence of insecticides in the living insect system.

2. *Reports of Synergism*

a. Mortality data. A fairly comprehensive review of cases of simultaneous application of fungi with insecticides has been given by Müller-Kögler (1965). Biopreparations of the white muscardine fungus *B. bassiana,* together with DDT, HCH or Wofatox have been used extensively, whereas green muscardine, *Metarrhizium anisopliae,* together with HCH was used only for the control of the sugar beet weevil *Cleonus punctiventris.* Some typical results are compiled in Table II. Of all the other insect pathogenic fungi only *Aspergillus repens* has been combined with HCH, but did not give satisfactory control of *C. punctiventris* (Kruel, 1958).

The experiments on *C. punctiventris* in southern Russia reported by Telenga (1958c) deserve some comment. The populations of the weevil in the region of Kiev were naturally attacked by *B. bassiana* and *M. anisopliae.* In 1956 natural mortality was 62-72% and incidence of mycoses 47-55%. Treatment of the soil with HCH caused little additional mortality (75%) but incidence of mycoses increased by 15-23%. In 1957 natural mycoses killed 34-43% of the beetles on

TABLE II

Synergism of fungi and insecticides. Mortality (M) in %: M_N = untreated (natural mortality), M_F = fungus alone, M_I = insecticide alone, M_{F+I} = combination. Figures in italics are mortalities corrected for natural mortality

Fungus, and amount/ha or concentration	Insect species (laboratory tests = (L); gen. I or II = generations)	Insecticide (amount/ha or concentration)	M_N	M_F	M_I	M_{F+I}	Effect	Literature
B. bassiana	*M. neustria*	DDT 0.5%	36.4	52.3	24.0	60.1		
			–	*25.0*	*–12.4*	*37.4*	weak potentiation[a]	Telenga *et al.* (1959)
0.8%	*M. neustria* (L)	DDT 0.05%	?	88	79	97	independent	Zigaev (1961)
0.8%	*M. neustria*	DDT 0.05%	?	80	80	83.9	weak antagonism	Zigaev (1961)
2 kg	*C. pomonella* (1957)	DDT 1%	2.8	10.9	8.8	71.7	supplemental[b]	Telenga (1958c)
	C. pomonella, gen. I	DDT 1%	?	5.8	5.8	61.2	coalitive action	Telenga (1959)[c]
	C. pomonella, gen. II	DDT 1%	?	1.3	0	66.7		
1%	*Hyphantria cunea*, gen. I	DDT 0.1%	22.2	?	20.3	81.0	coalitive action	Sikura (1959)
	Hyphantria cunea, gen. II	DDT 0.1%	3.5	?	18.4	62.8		
10 kg	*E. integriceps*	Wofatox 10 kg	10.0	32.5	18.7	83.7		
			–	*25.0*	*9.7*	*81.9*	potentiation[d]	Shekhurina (1959)
	E. integriceps (L)	DDT 0.05%	–	90.1	80.2	100	independent?	Shekhurina (1958)
22×10^6 spores	*L. decemlineata*	DDT 100 g	20.6	64.6	71.7	98.6		
			–	*55.4*	*64.3*	*98.2*	subadditive	Telenga (1964)
5 kg	*C. punctiventris* (1956)	HCH 210 g	46.6	65.7	76.0	83.9		
			–	*35.8*	*55.1*	*69.9*	independent	Telenga (1957, 1958a, b)
5 kg	*C. punctiventris* (1957)	HCH 210 g	34.5	32.0	39.4	65.4		
			–	–	*7.5*	*47.1*	potentiation	Telenga (1957, 1958a, b)
M. anisopliae	*C. punctiventris* (1956)	HCH 210 g	33.3	76.8	53.6	85.7		
5 kg			–	*65.2*	*30.4*	*78.6*	independent	Telenga (1957, 1958a, b)

[a] Negative M_I indicates hormoligosis.
[b] Earlier results in 1956 irregular (see text).
[c] Control unsatisfactory; similar experiments in Moldavia even worse (Petrukhina, 1961).
[d] Doses of 1-10 kg of Wofatox, same mortality; probably non-lethal; smaller doses, little effect; larger doses, antagonistic (see II.A.1).

untreated control plots and 58% of those with the application of HCH. These are clear cases of synergism with a natural pathogen. Application of 5 kg/ha of a preparation of *B. bassiana* alone did not increase mortality by mycosis in 1956, but raised the incidence of mycosis to 80% in 1957. However, the combination of the biopreparation with HCH had a synergistic effect in 1956 (83% mycoses, 91-96% total mortality) but not in 1957.

Besides the cases mentioned in Table II a number of other experiments could be cited in which *B. bassiana* has been combined with insecticides and where synergism has been claimed. Unfortunately the controls with the fungus or the insecticide alone or both are missing. They are compiled in the list below. Coleoptera: *Galerucella luteola*/DDT with nearly 100% mortality (Dyadechko, 1957); *Cleonus punctiventris*/HCH or Wofatox (Bogdanov, 1961); *Leptinotarsa decemlineata*/DDT (Dyadechko, 1959; Kaytazov, 1962; Telenga and Dyadechko, 1957; Telenga *et al.*, 1959). Hymenoptera: *Caliroa cerasi*/DDT, about 100% mortality (Dyadechko, 1957 cit. Telenga, 1958a, 1964). Lepidoptera: *Cydia (Carpocapsa) pomonella*/DDT (Balevskji, 1962); *Tortrix viridana*/DDT, 100% mortality (Dyadechko and Sikura, 1961).

b. After-effects. Telenga (1958a, c) found 40% natural mortality in caterpillars of *Euproctis chrysorrhoea* and 89.5% mortality after treatment with *B. bassiana* and a low dose of DDT. Surviving moths from treated and untreated plots laid eggs with 52.2 and 7.1% embryonic mortality. The winter nests on treated plots contained an average number of 4.2 full grown larvae, those of the controls 189 larvae. The results indicate an after-effect with 97.8% control in the second generation.

Another interesting after-effect has been investigated by El-Tahtaqui (1964) in *L. decemlineata.* Whereas 16.6% of untreated females entered diapause none did so after L3 had been treated with *B. bassiana,* and 31.2% after treatment of L4. Since most non-diapausing beetles die in winter, *B. bassiana* alone has a positive control effect on L3 and a negative after-effect on L4. However, when L4 were treated with a combination of the fungus and a non-lethal dose of DDT none of the surviving females entered diapause.

The same author found that the egg production of *L. decemlineata* was stimulated 1.3 times by *B. bassiana* and 1.8 times by a non-lethal dose of DDT. The stimulating effect was completely lost when the fungus and DDT were applied simultaneously.

3. Reports of Failure and Antagonism

Failure may occur if synergism is absent or too weak. Thus treatment of *C. pomonella* with *B. bassiana* and DDT in 1956 gave only 20 and 50% control after respectively one and two treatments (Telenga, 1958b), i.e. much less than in 1957 (Table II). The same treatment in Moldavia gave no satisfactory results at all (Petrukhina, 1961). Failure of a combination of *B. bassiana* and HCH against the beetle *Phytodecta fornicata* was reported by Dirimanov and Angelova (1961). Treatment of *Eurygaster integriceps* with *B. bassiana* and low doses of DDT in the field even resulted in antagonism (Shekhurina, 1958). The same was found for the combination with 15 kg/ha of Wofatox, whereas 10 kg/ha of this insecticide gave a synergistic effect (Shekhurina, 1959).

D. SYNERGISM OF BACTERIA AND INSECTICIDES

1. General Remarks

Reports indicating increased mortality of insects by bacterioses following low doses of DDT suggest that toxicants may have synergistic effects on many bacteria (Fankhaenel, 1957; Pristavko, 1963a, b; Spaić, 1960; Telenga, 1958c). However, all studies on synergism of bacteria with chemical substances have been performed with *Bacillus thuringiensis* (BT). Commercial preparations of BT can be mixed with most insecticides, fungicides, spreaders, stickers, and other adjuvants without serious loss in activity. Of 14 fungicides, including copper oxychlorine, only the Bordeaux mixture of copper sulphate with lime reduced the effect of BT. Of 17 insecticides, including eight organophosphates, only technical HCH (but not the gamma isomer lindane), malathion, and TEPP have been reported as antagonists of BT (McEwen *et al.*, 1960; Godavaribai *et al.*, 1962; Fedorintchik, 1964; Sandner and Kot, 1964). The interested reader is referred to the paper by Herfs (1965) which contains a fairly complete bibliography.

2. Cases of Synergism

Mortality data derived from combinations of BT and chemical substances are compiled in Table III. In all cases cited, sublethal doses of DDT resulted in potentiating synergism. Field experiments by Petrukhina (1961) and Vasiljević (1961) gave very good results against *Aporia crataegi* and *Hyphantria cunea*, but mortality caused by DDT alone has not been determined. Mortality of *A. crataegi* was so high that supplemental or potentiating synergism is indicated. In the case of *H. cunea* potentiation remains questionable.

Boric acid, which has some insecticidal potency, also potentiated the action of BT in *Lymantria (Porthetria) dispar* at an almost non-lethal concentration. This effect was not found with other acids (Doane and Wallis, 1964). The case is remarkable because 1% boric acid increased the death rate in all but the first combination by about 31%, indicating an additive effect depending almost solely on the concentration of the boric acid. It is unlikely, however, such high concentrations of borate could be used in the field.

Combinations of BT and lethal concentrations of DDT gave the whole spectrum from antagonism to supplemental synergism in laboratory tests with *A. ipsilon* (Haenggi, 1965), and independent synergism when applied in the field against *Z. diniana* (Benz and Auer, unpublished). Field experiments against *T. ni*

TABLE III

Mortality data (corrected for natural mortality) on synergism and antagonism of Bacillus thuringiensis *(BT) and insecticides*

Insect species	BT preparation, amount/ha or concentration	Insecticide, amount/ha or concentration	M_I	M_B	M_{I+B}	Effect	Reference
Agrotis ipsilon (L1/L2)	Bakthane 0.1%	DDT 0.0125%	60	33	60	antagonism	Haenggi (1965)
		0.025%	70	33	67	antagonism	
		0.05%	70	33	90	subadditive	
Agrotis ipsilon (L4)	Bakthane 0.1%	DDT 0.0125%	0	3	57	coalitive action	
		0.025%	53	3	53	–	
		0.05%	63	3	90	potentiation	
Agrotis ipsilon (L6)	Bakthane 0.1%	DDT 0.075%	45.4	14.4	79.4	supplemental	
	0.2%	0.075%	45.4	27.8	58.8	independent	
	0.2%	0.15%	79.3	27.8	55.7	antagonism	
	0.4%	0.15%	79.3	27.8	96.9	subadditive	
Aporia crataegi	Entobacterin-3 1%	DDT 0.002%	?	69.3	100	potentiation	Petrukhina (1961)
Hyphantria cunea	40 x 10^9 spores	DDT 0.025%	?	56	91	potentiation?	Vasiljević (1961)
Hyponomeuta malinellus	Entobacterin 0.1%	DDT 0.002%	–	6.3	55.8	potentiation	Petrukhina (1959)
	0.25%		–	7.2	90.7	potentiation	
	0.5%		–	87.6	98.6	potentiation	
	1.0%		–	92.2	100	potentiation	
Lymantria dispar	Thuricide–90T 0.016%	Boric acid 1%	–	3.1	18.4	potentiation	Doane and Wallis (1964)
	0.032%		–	3.1	33.7	potentiation	
	0.062%		6	35.4	66.6	potentiation	
	0.125%		6	50.5	81.8	potentiation	
Trichoplusia ni	Biotrol 1 lb	Parathion 0.25 lb	63.5	77.9	92.4	independent[a]	McEwen *et al.* (1960)
			76.2	71.7	89.6	independent	
		Carbaryl 0.5 lb	51.2	77.9	90.7	independent[a]	
		Demeton 0.5 lb	29.1	77.9	81.4	independent	
Trichoplusia ni	Bakthane 2 lb	Naled 2 lb	54.4	16.0	67.6	independent	Creighton *et al.* (1964)
Zeiraphera diniana	Thuricide–90T 7L	DDT 250 g	57.4	53.2	83.0	independent	Benz and Auer (unpublished)

[a] Weak antagonism after standing of mixture for 3 hr.

by McEwen *et al.* (1960) with lethal doses of parathion, carbaryl and demeton, as well as by Creighton *et al.* (1964) with Naled indicated independent action.

Other positive results have been reported by Fankhaenel (1962) for the combination with Wofatox against the looper *Bupalus piniarius,* and by Hudon (1962) for combinations of BT and DDT or carbaryl against the corn borer *Ostrinia nubilalis.* However, the combination of BT and DDT failed one and two years later (Hudon, 1963). The results of Genung (1960) with BT and toxaphene against *T. ni* may be evaluated as slightly positive.

3. *Reports of Failure and Antagonism*

Reports of failure range from missing synergism to straight antagonism. Some antagonistic combinations have been mentioned above and in Table III. The results of Creighton *et al.* (1961) with Thiodan and Shell SD-4402 against the tobacco budworm *Heliothis virescens* and the hornworm *Protoparce sexta* indicate antagonism, since the combinations with BT gave neither higher mortality nor reduction of damage, compared with the single components. Missing synergism of BT and DDT in caterpillars of *Leucoma salicis* has been reported by Kudler and Lysenko (1963). Similarly no synergism of BT and HCH was found in the moth *Sitotroga cerealella* (Sandner and Kot, 1964). This case may be regarded as double failure since the same combination gave a small synergistic effect in *Trichogramma cacoeciae,* an egg parasite of *S. cerealella.*

E. SYNERGISM OF VIRUSES AND INSECTICIDES

1. *Compatibility of Viruses and Insecticides*

The compatibility of the granulosis virus of the red-banded leafroller *Argyrotaenia velutinana* with six fungicides has been studied by Glass (1958). Only Glyodin (36%, 2 qt/100 gal) reduced mortality significantly (50% instead of 80%). All adjuvants so far tested are compatible with nuclear polyhedrosis viruses (Clark and Reiner, 1956; Smirnoff, 1961; Wolfenbarger, 1964; Ignoffo and Montoya, 1966). The detergent Teepol reduced the pathogenicity of the nuclear polyhedrosis virus of *Idaea seriata* (Schnyder, unpublished).

Ignoffo and Montoya (1966) treated nuclear polyhedra from the corn ear-worm *Heliothis zea* with DDT, endrin, carbaryl, toxaphene, and methyl-parathion. Only methylparathion reduced the pathogenicity of the virus ($M_V = 61\%, M_{V+I} = 42\%$).

2. *Studies on Granuloses*

No systematic studies on synergism between granulosis viruses and insecticides have been published so far. Schnyder and Benz (unpublished) combined the granulosis virus of *Zeiraphera diniana* and different insecticides in the laboratory. Results with DDD, derris, lindane, and Nirosan are discussed in Section II of this chapter. Other insecticides tested were carbaryl, DDT and pyrethrum. None was able to potentiate a weak dose of the virus producing 0-3% granulosis. Lethal doses of all insecticides tested suppressed acute virus disease. Antagonism of non-lethal doses has been found with derris (Fig. 4), and Nirosan (Fig. 3). However, the latter gave temporal synergism (Fig. 9). Sublethal doses of carbaryl and DDT had neither antagonistic nor synergistic effects, whereas DDD can synergize the virus (Table IV, E1).

It has been mentioned by Kovačević (1958, 1962) that sublethal doses of DDT and lindane activate granulosis of *Hyphantria cunea.* Sublethal doses of DDT (5-100 p.p.m.) produced 60-85% larval mortality (mainly granulosis, but also bacterioses), compared with 55% mortality in the controls (Kovačević, 1962).

3. Nuclear Polyhedroses

a. Laboratory investigations. Schnyder (1967) and Schnyder and Benz (unpublished) studied synergism of the nuclear polyhedrosis virus of *I. seriata* and the insecticides carbaryl, derris, DDD, DDT, Nirosan, imidazole, pyrethrum, methoxychlor, and toxaphene. The last three compounds had only antagonistic properties, mainly because they inhibited uptake of virus treated food (except for imidazole which exhibited metabolic antagonism). None of the insecticides tested was able to potentiate nonlethal doses of the virus.

Data on DDD, DDT and Nirosan are given in Table IV, and Figs 1 and 5-8. The three substances may synergize or antagonize the virus, depending on the doses of each agent. The experiments are not easy to reproduce, since no clear borderline exists between non-lethal and lethal doses. The weight and the physiological condition of the insects is of great importance. For instance, experiments with orally applied DDD (Table IV, E3) indicate that synergism of a low dose of the virus (8-11% mortality) and 0.1% of the insecticide is reproducible, whereas 0.4% of DDD may potentiate the virus if this dose of DDD by itself is non-lethal, and antagonize the virus if it is lethal. High doses of the virus are antagonized by 40 p.p.m. of DDD, but gave independent action with 50 p.p.m. (Table IV, E2, and Fig. 6). Infection of the larvae with 4×10^5 polyhedra led to 12%, 28% and 57% mortality in the experiments E4, E8 and E9 respectively (Table IV). Four topical applications of DDT on the days 1, 3, 6 and 9 of infection produced a synergistic effect in E8, but antagonism in E9. Synergism was less pronounced when the applications began on day 3 or 6 of infection. The same was true for hidden antagonism of Nirosan and DDD (Fig. 6). A non-lethal dose of Nirosan potentiated mortality and incidence of virosis, whereas higher doses of the insecticide had a synergistic effect concerning mortality, but antagonized the incidence of acute virosis (Table IV, E5).

Ignoffo and Montoya (1966) found that carbaryl slightly synergized the polyhedrosis virus of *H. zea* ($M_V = 61\%, M_{V+I} = 79\%$). Activation of the nuclear

TABLE IV

Combined effects of insecticides and viruses[a]

E	Virus	Insecticide; relative conc.; application	M_V	M_I	M_{V+I}	total virus	Effect
1	G	DDD 25 p.p.m. oral/topical	58	0	70	66	weak subadditive
			69	0	78	71	weak subadditive
		50 p.p.m. oral/topical	69	0	93	75	potentiation
		100 p.p.m. oral/topical	58	0	87	74	potentiation
			69	0	93	82	potentiation
2	PS	DDD 40 p.p.m. topical	83	24	57	56	antagonism
		50 p.p.m. topical	83	61	97	80	independent
3	PS 3×10^5	DDD 0.1% oral	8	0	49		potentiation
			10	0	39		potentiation
			11	4	22		supplemental
			10	8	17		additive
		0.4% oral	8	0	42		potentiation
			10	0	17		potentiation
			11	22	25		antagonism
			10	47	44		antagonism
4	PS 4×10^5	Nirosan 0.05% oral	12	40	55	34	additive
5	PS 3×10^5	Nirosan 0.05% oral	12	0	46	34	potentiation
	6×10^6	0.10% oral	75	48	96	12	synergism, but virus
	6×10^6	0.15% oral	75	94	100	5	development inhibited
6	PS	Imidazole 5% oral	16	62	63	4	inapparent antagonism
7	PS 1×10^7	DDT 0.03% topical, 6 d	86	5	100	92	supplemental
		0.06% after	86	40	100	86	supplemental
		0.12% infection	86	83	100	48	supplmental (virus antag.)
8	PS 4×10^5	DDT 1,3,6,9 d post infect.	28	6	80		potentiation
		3,6,9 d post infect.	28	6	67		potentiation
		6,9 d post infect.	28	6	49		potentiation
9	PS 4×10^5	DDT 1,3,6,9 d post infect.	57	8	15		antagonism
		3,6,9 d post infect.	57	0	32		antagonism
		6,9 d post infect.	57	0	27		antagonism
10	PT 15×10^{10}/ acre	Parathion 0.5 lb/acre	53	71	82		independent
		Toxaphene 2 lb/acre	53	46	67		weak antagonism

[a] Granulosis virus of *Z. diniana* (G) or nuclear polyhedrosis viruses of *I. seriata* (PS), and *T. ni* (PT). Relative dose of virus (polyhedra/ml) is given where necessary for understanding. Experiments (E) 1-6 by Schnyder and Benz (unpublished), 7-9 by Schnyder (1967), and 10 by Getzin (1962).

polyhedrosis of larvae of *Lymantria dispar* by sublethal doses (5-10 p.p.m.) of DDT or lindane leads respectively to 100% and 70-100% mortality (mainly by polyhedrosis) when natural mortality reaches only 25-55% (Kovačević, 1960, 1962). The disease is also activated by sublethal doses of aldrin, dieldrin and endrin (Schmidt, 1959). Activation of latent viroses by other chemicals such as NaF, KNO_2, H_2O_2, hydroxylamine and others has been reported by many authors (see Aruga, 1963).

Girardeau and Mitchell (1968) working with *T. ni* found much reduced LD_{50}s for endrin, endosulfan and trichlorfon if the larvae had been infected previously with a sub-acute dose of a nuclear polyhedrosis virus (see II.A.3). The LD_{50}s, expressed as μg/larva, for normal and infected insects respectively were 7.6 and 2.2 with endrin, 13.0 and 2.2 with endosulfan, and 9.4 and 2.5 with trichlorfon. Thus the sub-acute infection increased the susceptibility to the three insecticides by a factor of 3.3-5.7.

b. Field experiments. Field experiments with the nuclear polyhedrosis virus of *T. ni* and insecticides have been reported by many authors. McEwen and Hervey (1958) found TEPP ineffective. Genung (1960) reported control of *T. ni* by a virus-toxaphene combination to be far superior to that with either agent alone (economic synergism). Hofmaster and Ditman (1961) found interspecific economic synergism of the virus with dibrom, mevinphos, endrin-parathion, toxaphene-parathion, and malathion-Perthane. A three-fold increase in virus dosage was significantly inferior to a virus-oil-endrin combination (Wolfenbarger, 1965). In other experiments the virus was combined with DDT, endrin, mevinphos, parathion, toxaphene, and DDT-toxaphene. Looper control was good with all combinations, but data on the effect of the virus alone are not given.

The best analyzed field tests have been reported by Getzin (1962). Some of the data are given in Table IV. The tests with parathion and toxaphene indicate independent synergism (or weak antagonism) and good economic synergism.

It has been stated by Kovačević (1958, 1960) that sublethal doses of DDT induce the outbreak of the latent polyhedrosis of *L. dispar* in the field.

4. Cytoplasmic Polyhedroses

Vasiljević (1967) tested three doses of the cytoplasmic polyhedrosis virus of *L. dispar* with three toxic concentrations of DDT and a toxic and two subtoxic doses of lindane. DDT gave independent synergism in most cases. Lindane, even at toxic concentrations, had no effect on the rate of mortality ($M_V = M_{V+I}$). Some antagonistic effect of the toxic dose is therefore indicated. Temporal synergism was never found.

IV. Discussion

A. SIGNIFICANCE OF THE REPORTS

Synergism between insect pathogens and insecticides has been investigated mainly in Coleoptera and Lepidoptera. Of all other insects only two examples of Hymenoptera and one of Heteroptera are known. The spectrum of the micro-organisms studied is also rather limited: one microsporidan, three fungi, one bacterium, and six viruses. From the large number of insecticides four have been tested most extensively, i.e. DDT, HCH (particularly the gamma isomer lindane) and the mixture of methylparathion and ethylparathion. Subtoxic doses of these insecticides may have potentiating or activating effects on micro-organisms in insects. Lethal concentrations, on the other hand, tend to produce independent synergism or antagonism. True synergism, i.e. subadditive and supplemental synergism of toxic concentrations is not frequent. Other chemicals reported to have potentiating effects or give coalitive action are boric acid, DDD, Nirosan or aldrin, dieldrin and endrin. Independent synergism of *B. thuringiensis* or a virus has been found with toxic doses of carbaryl, demeton, naled, and parathion. Derris, imidazole, methylparathion, malathion, and TEPP are as a rule antagonists. However, it is clear that synergism or failure of some combinations is more dependent on quantitative than qualitative factors, i.e. the same combination may produce a synergistic, an antagonistic or no effect. The same combination may also give a positive result in one species but not in another and a positive result in one year but not in another. Even the time of application (simultaneous or in a sequence) may have an influence.

Evaluation of success depends largely on the type of analysis applied to the experiment. Total mortality is only one aspect; time of mortality or reduction of damage may be of more significance. Missing synergism, as measured by total mortality, may be synergism if mortality-time or reduction of damage are estimated. After-effects have rarely been studied although they may be important for insect control.

B. MECHANISMS INVOLVED

Antagonism is more easily explained than synergism. One mechanism that may cause antagonism is simple incompatibility of micro-organisms and insecticides. However, incompatibility may sometimes be caused by impurities in technical grade insecticides rather than by the active substance itself (e.g. technical HCH versus lindane). Basic experiments should therefore always be conducted with pure and technical grade substances.

A second mechanism may be the prevention of food uptake. If low doses of insecticides have a strong repellent effect (e.g. derris in *Z. diniana* or methoxychlor and toxaphene in *I. seriata*) or too strong a knockdown effect (like pyrethrum) the test insects may be prevented from taking up an effective dose of the micro-organism or a lethal dose of the insecticide itself.

Toxic doses of insecticides can act antagonistically on viruses since these microbes depend on viable cells. If the insecticide alters the cell metabolism too strongly, multiplication of viruses may be blocked. Contrary to this, antagonism may result when a micro-organism (e.g. a fungus) has the ability to detoxify the insecticide metabolically.

Hormoligosis may be a further cause of antagonism. If subtoxic doses of an insecticide stimulate the metabolism of an insect instead of weakening it, susceptibility to microbial attack may be reduced.

Hormoligosis in the micro-organism, on the other hand, may result in synergism. It is well known that DDT can stimulate the metabolism of plants. There is no argument against the hypothesis that the same may be true in micro-organisms. Unfortunately no systematic investigations in this direction have been undertaken. The hormoligant character of some insecticides may be responsible for the fact that the same combination of agents can produce different results in different insect species and in different populations of the same species. Even in carefully controlled experiments conditions may be so variable that the insecticide may be a hormoligant for the insect and/or the micro-organism.

Some of the synergistic effects of insecticides are the result of physiological stress. DDT and some other insecticides act probably via the central and sympathetic nervous systems on the hormonal system of insects. Such a mechanism may cause the after-effects in *Leptinotarsa decemlineata,* studied by El-Tahtaqui (1964). Neurohormones and other pharmacologically active substances are released into the blood after treatment with DDT and organophosphates, but also after physical stress (review of literature by Sternburg *et al.*, 1959 and Davey, 1963). Thus the same basic mechanism may be involved when the susceptibility to virus infection is increased by a mechanical stressor in *T. ni* (Jacques, 1961) or sublethal doses of DDT in *L. dispar* (Kovačević, 1960).

Treatment of insects with some insecticides reduces the number of haemocytes (Telenga, 1957, 1958c; Sirotina, 1961). Since phagocytosis is an important defence mechanism, such reduction can increase the susceptibility of insects to infection with micro-organisms. Sublethal doses of DDT seem to cause leakage of the gut in *L. decemlineata* since intestinal bacteria enter the haemocoel within 24 hr (Pristavko, 1963a, b). This effect of DDT may be responsible for its synergism with BT in *A. ipsilon,* in which the gut proteases are not able to activate the *Bacillus*-endotoxin.

In some synergistic combinations the micro-organism seems to be the synergist of the insecticide and not vice versa. This may be the case when the micro-organism slows down the detoxication of the insecticide. Infection of Malpighian tubules of *O. ligustici* by *N. otiorrhynchi* (Table I) probably reduces the excretory functions so much that toxic levels of insecticides are reached quicker than in healthy beetles.

Synergism of BT and boric acid is intriguing because a certain sublethal dose of the chemical, when combined with different doses of the *Bacillus,* increases mortality by a fixed percentage. This might indicate that low doses of boric acid can enter the haemocoel only in caterpillars where the gut wall has been made permeable by the action of BT, but not in healthy insects. This hypothesis, however, needs experimental proof.

C. PRACTICAL USES AND RECOMMENDATIONS

1. Sublethal Doses of Insecticides

The reports discussed in this chapter show that combinations of micro-organisms and nonlethal doses of insecticides do not always give consistent results. Synergism of nonlethal concentrations of insecticides and viruses is rare; their combination cannot be recommended. The combination of fungi and nonlethal doses of insecticides gives intriguing results. Such combinations are not commendable for the control of *M. neustria* and *H. cunea,* since these species can be controlled by BT, alone, or in combination with low doses of DDT (Table III). Fungi are also unsatisfactory for the control of *C. pomonella.* The simultaneous application of *B. bassiana* and 10 kg/ha of Wofatox gave good control of *E. integriceps* (Table II). However, since the dose of the insecticide needed is very high, this combination can be recommended only if other control measures fail.

B. bassiana combined with sublethal doses of DDT (but not HCH) for the control of coleopterous insects seems to give consistent results, i.e. all authors working with this combination reported positive results. The addition of sublethal concentrations of DDT to BT can be recommended for the control of susceptible species such as *A. crataegi, Hyphantria cunea* and *Hyponomeuter malinella* on fruit trees. The low doses of the insecticide will not leave undesirable residues but may potentiate the *Bacillus* considerably (Table III).

It has been mentioned before that the potency of sublethal doses may vary under different circumstances. Although a sublethal dose of an insecticide may help to save part of the more expensive biopreparation, it is not safe to make a prediction in most cases. Experiments will always be necessary, i.e. such combinations may be of practical value only for trained personnel, not for the layman.

2. Toxic Doses of Insecticides

Although the combined application of microbial control agents and toxic doses of insecticides rarely produces effects which are better than independent synergism, such combinations may be advantageous in those cases where ecological synergism occurs and where the action of the micro-organism alone is not fully satisfactory. An example is the control of *T. ni* by the nuclear polyhedrosis virus and parathion (Getzin, 1962). Since parathion also gives independent synergism with BT (McEwen *et al.,* 1960) one might expect good control of all cabbage feeding insects by the simultaneous application of parathion, BT, and virus (nuclear polyhedrosis virus of *T. ni* in North America; nuclear and cytoplasmic polyhedrosis virus of *Mamestra* in Europe). However, insecticides with a long half-life should be avoided.

Combinations of micro-organisms with toxic doses of chlorinated insecticides can be recommended only if control by the micro-organism alone is unsatisfactory and a relatively low dose of the insecticide is needed. Thus damage to larch forests caused by *Z. diniana* can be prevented within 8-9 years by one or two applications of 1.25 kg/ha of DDT (Auer, unpublished). One-fifth this dose of DDT is sufficient if combined with BT (Benz and Auer, unpublished). Such a small amount of DDT will not disturb the ecosystem and should not leave undesirable amounts of residues.

If field tests confirm the control of *A. ipsilon* by BT and low doses of DDT (Haenggi, 1965), and if the same effect could be found in *Mamestra brassicae,* another pest of cruciferous crops in Europe, this combination might be used for the simultaneous control of *Pieris brassicae, P. rapae, Plutella maculipennis* (Krieg, 1967), and the noctuids mentioned above. However, an alternative method not including chlorinated insecticides has already been mentioned above.

The combination of *B. bassiana* with low doses of DDT for the control of *Euproctis chrysorrhoea,* or with HCH against *Cleonus punctiventris,* has been recommended by Telenga in many papers. However, HCH cannot be recommended by the author, since the leaves of sugar beet are usually ensilaged for cattle and HCH (even if applied only in the ground) might appear in milk.

D. FUTURE LINES OF RESEARCH

Chlorinated insecticides, particularly DDT and DDD, seem to have the greatest ability to synergize micro-organisms and viruses. These insecticides are renowned for their ability to stimulate the microsomal enzyme systems of living cells (see O'Brien, 1967). It is possible that this mechanism is involved in synergism. However, chlorinated insecticides should be avoided because they leave undesirable residues. DDE and dicofol, on the other hand, are non-toxic for vertebrates and insects, but have similar inductive properties as insecticides. It might be worth while to test whether or not these compounds could replace DDT, DDD and HCH as synergists.

Organophosphates and carbamates have almost exclusively been used at toxic concentrations. Research is needed on their effects at sublethal dosage.

A further line of research should follow the hypothesis presented in connection with the combination of BT and boric acid. Since BT causes leakage of the gut in susceptible insects it might be possible to replace boric acid by other, less toxic substances which ordinarily cannot enter the haemocoel (see Benz, 1962, 1966). Such substances might be added to commercial preparations of BT in order to increase their efficacy.

The problem of resistance to insecticides is becoming more and more important. Studies should be conducted with the aim of overcoming resistance with the help of micro-organisms. The question of whether or not insecticide resistance may reduce the effects of synergistic combinations should also be studied.

References

Aruga, H. (1963). *In* "Insect Pathology, an Advanced Treatise" (E. A. Steinhaus, ed.), Vol. I, pp. 381-412. Academic Press, New York.

Balevskji, A. D. (1962). *Zesz. probl. Postep. Nauk roln.* **35**, 69-78. (In Russian; Polish and German summary.)

Benz, G. (1962). *J. Insect Path.* **4**, 492-495.

Benz, G. (1966). *J. Insect Physiol.* **12**, 137-151.

Bogdanov, V. (1961). *Rastit. Zasht.* **9**, 64-71. (Bulgarian with English summary.)

Clark, E. C. and Reiner, C. E. (1956). *J. econ. Ent.* **49**, 703-704.

Creighton, C. S., Kinard, W. S. and Allen, N. (1961). *J. econ. Ent.* **54**, 1112-1114.

Creighton, C. S., Cuthbert, F. P., Jr. and Reid, W. J., Jr. (1964). *J. Insect Path.* **6**, 102-110.

Davey, K. G. (1963). *J. Insect Physiol.* **9**, 375-381.

Dirimanov, M. and Angelova, R. (1961). *Priroda, Sofia* **10**, 58-61. (Bulgarian, cited by Müller-Kögler, 1965).

Dirimanov, M. and Angelova, R. (1962). *Rastit Zasht.* **10**, 63-67. (Bulgarian with English summary.)

Doane, C. C. and Wallis, R. C. (1964). *J. Insect Path.* **6**, 423-429.

Dyadechko, N. P. (1957). *Les. Khoz.* **10**, 27-28. (In Russian.)

Dyadechko, N. P. (1959). *Naučn. Trudy Ukrainsk. naučn.-issled. Inst. Zašč. Rast.* **8**, 221-223. (In Russian.)

Dyadechko, N. P. and Sikura, A. I. (1961). *Les. Khoz.* **10**, 56-57. (In Russian.)

El-Tahtaqui, M. M. (1964). *Entomophaga, Mém. hors Sér. No. 2,* pp. 549-553.

Fankhaenel, H. (1957). *Ber. 8. Wanderversamml. dtsch. Ent. (München, 1957),* pp. 105-119.

Fankhaenel, H. (1962). *Pflanzensch.-Dienst* (N.F.) **16**, 121-127.

Fedorintchik, N. S. (1964). *Entomophaga, Mém. hors Sér. No. 2,* pp. 51-61.

Fisher, F. E. and Griffiths, I. I., Jr. (1950). *J. econ. Ent.* **43**, 712-718.

Genung, W. G. (1960). *Florida Ent.* **43**, 65-68.

Getzin, L. W. (1962). *J. econ. Ent.* **55**, 442-445.

Girardeau, J. H., Jr. and Mitchell, E. R. (1968). *J. econ. Ent.* **61**, 312-313.

Glass, E. H. (1958). *J. econ. Ent.* **51**, 454-457.

Godavaribai, S., Krishnamurthy, K. and Majumder, S. K. (1962). *Pest Technol.* **4**, 155-158.

Griffiths, J. T., Jr. and Fisher, F. E. (1950). *J. econ. Ent.* **43**, 298-305.

Haenggi, A. (1965). *Entomophaga* **10**, 343-348.

Hall, I. M. and Dunn, P. H. (1959). *J. econ. Ent.* **52**, 28-29.

Herfs, W. (1965). *Z. PflKrankh.* **72**, 584-599.

Hofmaster, R. N. and Ditman, L. P. (1961). *J. econ. Ent.* **54**, 921-923.

Hudon, M. (1962). *J. econ. Ent.* **55**, 115-117.

Hudon, M. (1963). *J. econ. Ent.* **56**, 804-808.

Ignoffo, C. M. and Montoya, E. L. (1966). *J. Invertebrate Path.* **8**, 409-412.

Jaques, R. P. (1961). *J. Insect Path.* **3**, 47-54.

Kaytazov, A. (1962). *Priroda, Sofia* **11**, 103-105. (In Bulgarian.)

Kerner, G. (1958). *Trans. 1. Int. Conf. Insect Path. Biol. Control, Praha, 1958,* pp. 169-176.

Kovačević, Z. (1958). *Trans. 1. Int. Conf. Insect Path. Biol. Control, Praha, 1958,* pp. 115-119.

Kovačević, Z. (1960). *Verhandl. XI. Int. Kongr. Ent., Wien* **2**, 796-801.

Kovačević, Z. (1962). *Yugoslav. Plant. Prot. Symp. Zagreb, 1961. Agron. Glasn. 1962,* 520-528. (In Serbocroat, with German summary.)

Král, J. and Neubauer, Š. (1953). *Zool. ent. Listy, Brno* **2**, 241-250. (In Czech, with German and Russian summaries.)

Krieg, A. (1967). "Neues über *Bacillus thuringiensis* und seine Anwendung". *Mitt. biol. BundAnst. Ld- u. Forstw.* No. **125**, 106 pp.

Kruel, W. (1958). *Verh. dtsch. Ges. angew. Ent., 14. Mitgl. Versamml., Göttingen, 1957,* pp. 28-36.

Kudler, J. and Lysenko, O. (1963). *Lesn. Casopis, Praha* **9**, 787-798.

Luckey, T. D. (1968). *J. econ. Ent.* **61**, 7-12.

McEwen, F. L. and Hervey, G. E. R. (1958). *J. econ. Ent.* **51,** 626-631.

McEwen, F. L., Glass, E. H., Davis, A. C. and Splittstoesser, C. M. (1960). *J. Insect Path.* **2,** 152-164.

Müller-Kögler, E. (1965). "Pilzkrankheiten bei Insekten". Paul Parey, Berlin and Hamburg, 444 pp.

O'Brien, R. D. (1967). "Insecticides, Action and Metabolism", 332 pp. Academic Press, New York.

Petrukhina, M. T. (1959). *In* "Biol. Metod Borby s Vredit. Rast., Kiev" (N. A. Telenga, N. S. Shcherbinovskij and N. P. Dyadechko, eds), pp. 101-105.

Petrukhina, M. T. (1961). *Trud. Moldavsk. nauchno-issled. Inst. Sadovod. Kišinev* 7, 79-92.

Pickett, A. D. and Patterson, N. A. (1953). *Can. Ent.* **85,** 472-478.

Pristavko, V. P. (1963a). *Nauk. praci. Ukr. nauk.-dosl. inst. zakhistu roslin* **12,** 95-98. (In Ukrainian, cit. *Document. Oosteurop. landbouwk. lit.* **5,** 79 (1964).)

Pristavko, V. P. (1963b). *Sbornik: 5. sovešč. Vses. ent. obšč., 1963, Moskva-Leningrad,* pp. 110-111. (In Russian.)

Rosicky, B. (1951). *Věst. čsl. Spol. zool.* **15,** 219-234.

Sandner, H. and Kot, J. (1964). *Entomophaga, Mém. hors Sér. No. 2,* pp. 545-547.

Schaefer, E. E. (1936). "The White Fungus Disease *(Beauveria bassiana)* Among Red Locusts in South Africa, and Some Observations on the Grey Fungus Disease *(Empusa grylli)*". Sci. Bull. Dep. Agric. South Afr., No. 160, 28 pp.

Schmidt, L. (1959). *Plant. Prot. Beograd* **56,** 45-51.

Schnyder, U. (1967). "Untersuchungen einer Kernpolyedrose von *Sterrha seriata* Schrk. (= *Ptychopoda seriata* Schrk., = *Acidalia virgularia* Hb.) (Geometridae, Lepidoptera) und deren Beeinflussbarkeit durch Hunger, DDT, DNOC and Farnesylmethyläther". Thesis ETH, Zurich, 60 pp.

Shekhurina, T. A. (1958). *In* "Biologiczeskiy Metod Borby s Vreditelyamy selskhozya Astvennikh Kultur y lesnykh nasashdeniy". Izdanie Ministerva selkogo Khozyaystva Moldavskoi SSR, pp. 55-56. (In Russian.)

Shekhurina, T. A. (1959). *In* "Biologiczeskiy Metod Borby s Vreditelyamy Rasteniy". Izdat. Akad. Nauk Ukrainskoy SSR, Kiev, pp. 202-206. (In Russian.)

Sikura, A. I. (1959). *In* "Biologiczeskiy Metod Borby s Vreditelyamy Rasteniy". Izdat. Akad. Nauk Ukrainskoy SSR, Kiev, pp. 126-140. (In Russian.)

Sirotina, M. I. (1961). *Dokl. Akad. Nauk S.S.S.R.* **140,** 720-723. (In Russian.) Cit. *Rev. appl. Ent. A.* **50,** 447 (1962).

Smirnoff, W. A. (1961). *J. Insect Path.* **3,** 29-46.

Spaić, I. (1960). *Plant Prot., Beograd* **57/58,** 215-224.

Steinhaus, E. A. (1958). *10th Int. Congr. Ent., Montreal, 1956* **4,** 725-730.

Sternburg, J., Chang, S. C. and Kearns, C. W. (1959). *J. econ. Ent.* **52,** 1070-1076.

Telenga, N. A. (1957). Publ. Akad. Nauk S.S.S.R., Leningrad. (In Russian.) Cit. Müller-Kögler (1965).

Telenga, N. A. (1958a). "Biologische Schädlingsbekämpfung an den landwirtschaftlichen Kulturen und Forstpflanzungen in der UdSSR". 9. Int. Konf. Quarant., Pflanzenkrankh., Pflanzenschutz, Moskau, 1958, 17 pp. (German edition.)

Telenga, N. A. (1958b). Bjull. nauczno-tekhn. Inf. URSR nauzcno-issled. Inst. Zashcz. Rast. No. 4, 21-38. (In Ukrainian.)

Telenga, N. A. (1958c). Trans. 1. Int. Conf. Insect Path. Biol. Control, Praha, 1958, pp. 155-168.

Telenga, N. A. (1959). *In* "Biologiczeskiy Metod Borby s Vreditelyamy Rasteniy". Izdat. Akad. Nauk Ukrainskoy SSR, Kiev, pp. 147-158. (In Russian.)

Telenga, N. A. (1964). *Entomophaga, Mém. hors Sér. No. 2,* pp. 531-544.

Telenga, N. A. and Dyadechko, N. P. (1957). Manuscript Coll. C.I.L.B. on the population dynamics and biological control of the potato beetle *(Leptinotarsa decemlineata),* Hamburg, 1957. Cit. Müller-Kögler (1965).

Telenga, N. A., Dyadechko, N. P. and Sikura, A. I. (1959). *Dopov. Ikrainsk. Akad. sels-kokh. Nauk* **2,** 27-29. (In Ukrainian.) Cit. *Rev. appl. Mycol.* **39,** 661 (1960).

Vago, C. (1959). "L'enchaînement des maladies chez les insectes". *Annls Epiphyt.* 1959, thèse, 181 pp.
Vasiljević, L. A. (1961). *Arh. poljopr. Nauke* **14,** 133-149. (In Serbocroat, English summary.)
Vasiljević, L. A. (1967). *Plant Prot. Beograd* **96/97,** 323-332.
Weiser, J. (1961). "Die Mikrosporidien als Parsiten der Insekten". Monogr. angew. Ent. No. 17. Paul Parey, Hamburg and Berlin, 149 pp.
Wolfenbarger, D. A. (1964). *J. econ. Ent.* **57,** 732-735.
Wolfenbarger, D. A. (1965). *J. Invertebrate Path.* **7,** 33-38.
Yendol, W. G. (1968). *J. Invertebrate Path.* **10,** 116-121.
Zigaev, G. N. (1961). *Les. Khoz.* **14,** 47-48. (In Russian.) Cit. Müller-Kögler (1965).

CHAPTER 15

Microbial Control of Mites and Ticks

JERZY J. LIPA

Laboratory of Biological Control, Institute of Plant Protection, Poznań, Poland

I. Introduction

Mites (Acarina) are serious pests of plants, as well as parasites of man and animals. Our interest in their pathogens, therefore, has not only theoretical but also practical implications of value in the control of noxious mites. In fact, cases where naturally occurring pathogens greatly reduced populations of mites have been described. Furthermore, promising results have been obtained in field experiments using pathogens to control mites. In general, however, our knowledge of micro-organisms associated with mites is very incomplete compared with that of insect pathogens. For example, no specific bacterial diseases of mites have so far been recorded.

This treatise will review the diseases of mites and examine the possibilities of microbial control. The interested reader is advised to consult an earlier, and in some respects, more complete paper on this subject (Lipa, 1962b).

II. Viral Diseases

Few viral diseases of mites are known and all belong to the non-inclusion group. Some of these viruses have been photographed and to some extent biochemically characterized. However, they have not so far been described taxonomically.

A. VIROSIS OF *PANONYCHUS CITRI*

The earliest record of a virus infection of a mite was made by Muma (1955) who observed specimens showing low activity and diarrhoea in a population of citrus red mite *P. citri* in Florida. The occurrence of virus infection in *P. citri* was experimentally proved by Munger *et al.* (1959) and Smith *et al.* (1959) who showed that the infection could be easily transmitted to healthy populations.

Symptoms and signs of infection by the disease in *P. citri* are complex and characteristic. The most striking symptoms are complete immobilization of the mite with stiffened legs. Diarrhoea frequently occurs and dead mites are often fixed to the feeding surface by faeces. A very characteristic feature, numerous birefringent crystals accumulated in the haemocoel of sick mites, was reported by Smith and Cressman (1962). The presence of crystals is a sign of infection, and they are apparently a result of metabolic disturbances. In laboratory rearing 84% of paralysed, or dying, females of *P. citri* and 54% of their active stages contained crystals (Fig. 1). The crystals are useful in determining the presence or absence of virus diseases in field populations of *P. citri*.

The etiological agent was demonstrated by Smith *et al.* (1959) who found oval, free virus particles, 35 mμ in diameter, located in the cytoplasm of body cells of diseased mites. Estes and Faust (1965) showed that the virus particles contained DNA.

The virus is not transmitted transovarially, but is easily disseminated artificially by spray applications or by an introduction of diseased mites into healthy populations.

B. VIROSIS OF *PANONYCHUS ULMI*

The European red mite *P. ulmi* is now a cosmopolitan species that has spread from Europe to other continents. Individuals with virus disease were first reported by Steinhaus (1959) in California and later by Bird (1967) in Canada.

Symptoms and signs of infection of *P. ulmi* are variable and depend on the

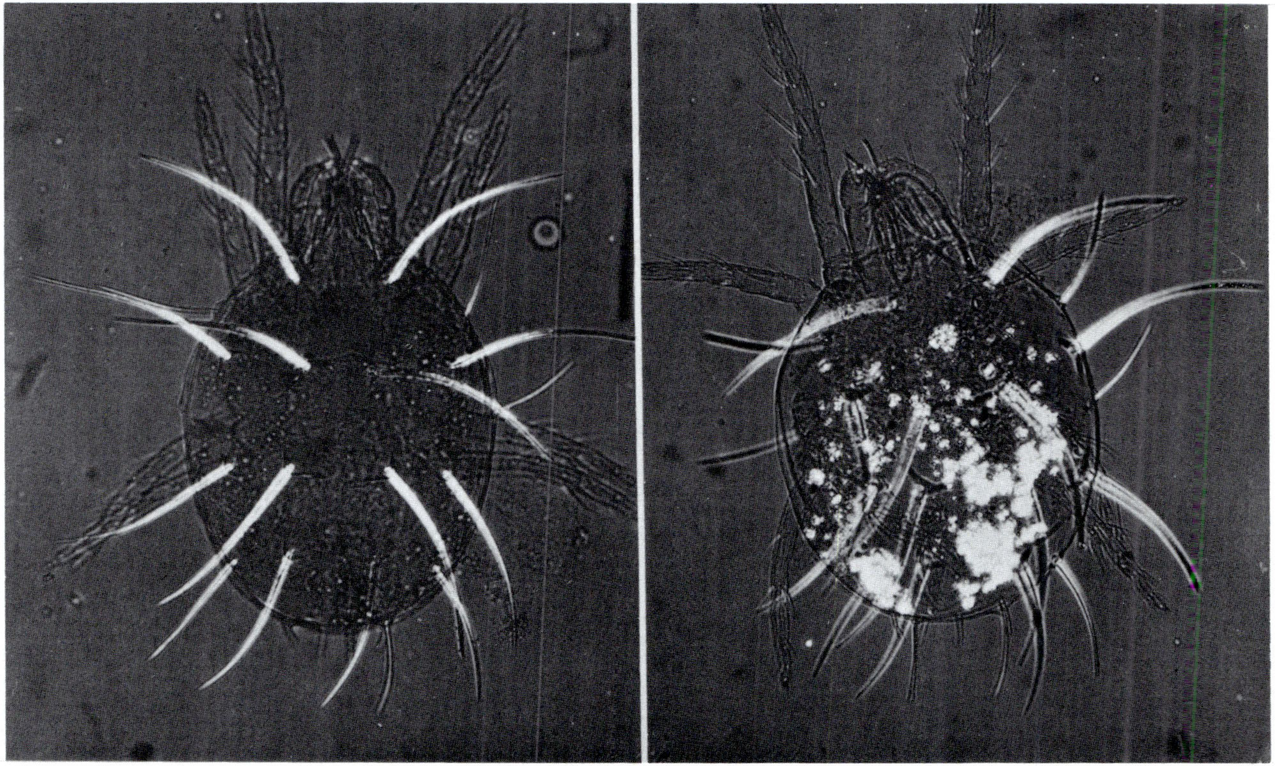

Fig. 1. Healthy mites, *Panonychus citri* (left) and mites infected with non-inclusion virus with characteristic crystals (right) as seen under polarized light (600x). (Courtesy of J. E. Gilmore.)

stage of infection. Diseased mites are dark red and have black spots on their backs. They gradually become immobile and when put on their backs they cannot return to their normal position. Mites in the last stage of infection exhibit diarrhoea and become fixed to the surface by faecal material.

In the bodies of dead mites, Steinhaus (1959) demonstrated oval, virus-like particles 40 mμ in diameter. Bird (1967) found rod-shaped virus particles, 200 x 90 mμ, in the nuclei of fat cells. These observations suggest that two viral diseases may affect *P. ulmi*.

C. VIROSIS OF *TETRANYCHUS* SPP.

Boudreaux (1959) described virus-like substances transmitted to the offspring of *Tetranychus cinnabarinus* and *T. telarius*. These substances were responsible for the absence of certain chemosensory setae on forelegs of females, but otherwise seemed to have no detectable effect on the host organism. The etiological agent has not been described morphologically or biochemically.

III. Fungal Diseases

A. INFECTIONS CAUSED BY PHYCOMYCETES

Fungi of the order Entomophthorales appear to be important pathogens of mites. The species recorded, so far, on mites belong to the genus *Entomophthora,* which has recently been split to include the genera *Entomophthora, Triplosporium* and *Conidiobolus,* a change that has not so far become common usage among experimental mycologists (see Ch. 5).

Petch (1940) was the first to report an entomophthoraceous infection on a mite, *Halotydeus destructor,* and described the fungus involved as *Entomophthora acaricida.* Later, Petch (1944) described a second species, *E. acaridis,* from other Acarina.

Entomophthoraceous diseases of mites infesting citrus are relatively well known. Fisher (1951) reported *Entomophthora* sp. on *Panonychus citri* and this pathogen was responsible for a high mortality of the mite ranging from 32% to 95%. The bodies of mites killed by the fungus were somewhat distended, cheesy in consistency and dark red or dark purple in colour. At high humidities large numbers of conidiophores were produced on the surface of the body which became greyish in colour.

A fungus attacking *Eutetranychus banksi* was first observed by Fisher (1954) and later described as *Entomophthora floridana* by Weiser and Muma (1966). This fungus produces single conidiophores with pyriform conidia averaging 12 x 15 μ.

Selhime and Muma (1966), while studying the biology of *E. floridana,* found that this pathogen had a 5-6-day life-cycle. The death of the mite was caused by dense hyphal growth inside the body (Fig. 2). These authors observed that

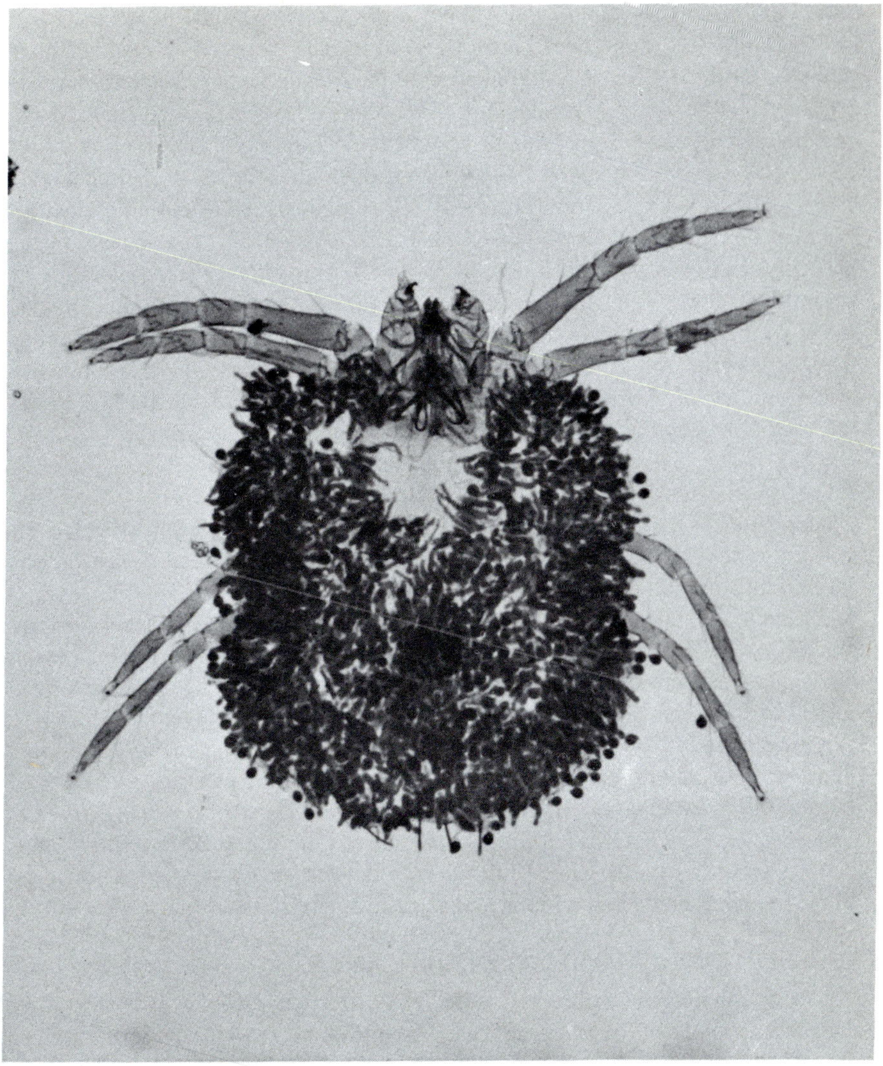

Fig. 2. *Eutetranychus banksi* infected with *Entomophthora floridana*, stained with cotton blue in Amman's solution (600x). (Courtesy of J. Weiser.)

E. floridana also attacked *P. citri* and *Eutetranychus sexmaculatus*, but the rate of infection was much lower than in *E. banksi*. As shown by Muma (1969), *E. floridana* is a very common pathogen of *E. banksi* especially in southern Florida infecting up to 100% of adult females of this mite.

Carner and Canerday (1968) observed an entomophthoraceous fungus infecting *Tetranychus telarius* and *T. urticae*. They identified it as

Entomophthora fresenii, a well-known pathogen of aphids. However, this identification has been questioned by Wilding and Weiser (Carner, personal communication, 1969). Mites infected with the fungus become swollen, sluggish and lighter in colour. After death, conidiophores developed producing round conidia. Mean sizes are: hyphal bodies (late infection) 25 x 7.3, conidia 13.1 x 12.0, secondary spores 16.1 x 12.6 μ (Carner, personal communication, 1969). The fungus was not observed in *T. atlanticus* collected in the same localities.

Triplosporium tetranychi killed 80-85% of *Tetranychus urticae (althaeae)* in autumn (Weiser, 1968). This fungus produces broad pyriform conidia, 15-17 x 12-15 μ. The black resting spores occur in almost every infected mite; they are pyriform, 20-23 x 16-19 μ. Steinhaus and Marsh (1962) observed resting spores of *Entomophthora* sp. in *Tetranychus pacificus*. Batko (1965) recorded *Conidiobolus brefeldianus* from *Tyrophagus perniciosus*.

B. INFECTIONS CAUSED BY ASCOMYCETES

Members of the genera *Penicillium* and *Aspergillus* have been recorded on mites. Charles (1941) reported *Aspergillus depauperatus* on dead *T. urticae* but gave no information on its pathogenicity.

Kolomiec (1950) observed that *Aspergillus fumigatus* caused mortality among laboratory cultures of the ticks *Hyalomma scupense* and *Dermacentor marginatus*. Infected females died before, or just after, laying eggs. Kolomiec suggested that there are special strains of *A. fumigatus* parasitic on mites.

Čerepanova (1964) isolated members of 15 genera of fungi from eggs, larvae, nymphs and adults of nine species of ticks: *Argas persicus, A. reflexus, Dermacentor marginatus, Hyalomma detritum, Ixodes persulcatus, I. ricinus, Ornithodorus papillipes* and *Ehipicephalus bursa*. She found *A. fumigatus* and a distinctly pathogenic species, *Penicillium insectivorum*, on the first six species. These fungi infected all developmental stages of their hosts.

C. INFECTIONS CAUSED BY BASIDIOMYCETES

An eriophyid, the citrus rust mite *Phyllocoptruta oleivora*, is attacked by *Hirsutella thompsonii* (Fisher, 1950a). The mycelium is white at first, but later becomes greyish. Hyphae and shortseptate, 1.7-3.3 μ in diameter. Conidiophores are rigid and hyaline, producing oval to round conidia, 2.1-3.3 x 2.1-3.3 μ. Infected mites are sluggish and yellow to tan as compared to the pale lemon-yellow typical of healthy adults; dead mites are tan to light brown (Fisher, 1950a; Burditt *et al.*, 1962). *H. thompsonii* caused a high mortality in wild populations of *P. oleivora* and seems to be a key factor in natural control of this pest (Fisher *et al.*, 1949; Fisher, 1950b; Muma, 1955, 1958).

Although *P. oleivora* seems to be the chief host of *H. thompsonii* this fungus also attacks other mites. It caused relatively high mortality of the eriophyid,

Aceria vaccinii, infesting the blueberry (Baker and Neunzig, 1968). Healthy mites are whitish but when infected they darken, become moribund and die. Hyphae of *H. thompsonii* filled the abdomen of *A. vaccinii* and protruded from legs and genital and anal openings (Fig. 3).

A few unidentified *Hirsutella* spp. were reported by Muma *et al.* (1961) on *Eutetranychus banksi, E. sexmaculatus* and *P. citri.*

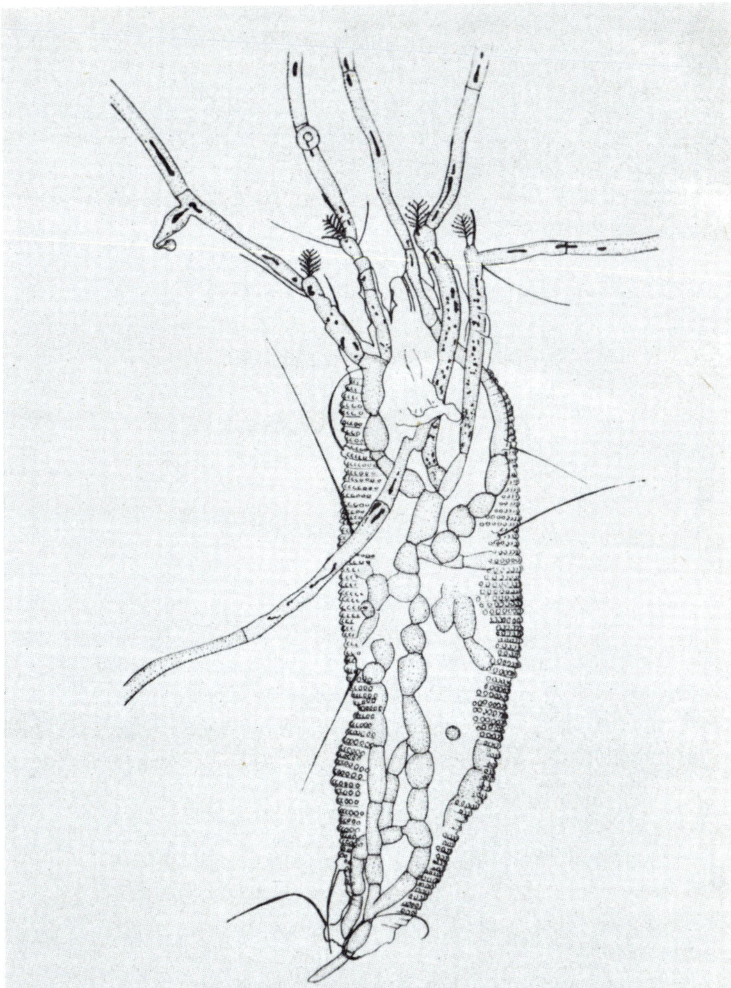

Fig. 3. Adult *Aceria vaccinii* infected with *Hirsutella thompsonii.* (Courtesy of Baker and Neunzig, 1968.)

D. INFECTIONS CAUSED BY FUNGI IMPERFECTI

The most important are species belonging to the genus *Beauveria*. Oudemans (1915) first observed that *Beauveria bassiana (Sporotrichum globuliferum)* killed *Tarsonemus spirifex*. It has been proved that this fungus caused mortality of *Tetranychus urticae* (Dresner, 1949) and of *Bryobia rubrioculus (redikorzevi)* (Dyadecho, 1958, 1959a, b). A number of authors have observed *B. bassiana* infecting ticks (Ixodidae). A female *Ixodes ricinus* brought from field to laboratory did not lay eggs and was killed by *B. bassiana*, hyphae protruding through the mouth (Samšinakova, 1957). Gorškova (1967) studied the histopathological changes in larvae of *I. ricinus* infected with various strains of *B. bassiana*. Boyčev and Rizvanov (1960) observed that *Botrytis cinerea* (evidently *B. bassiana*) killed eggs of *I. ricinus*.

Leatherdale (1965) found that *Paecilomyces eriophytis (Botrytis eriophytis)*, originally described from an eriopyhyid *Cecidophyopsis ribis*, was infective to *Eriophyes padi, Aceria hippocastani* and *Panonychus ulmi*. The conidia of the fungus are cylindrical with rounded ends, 4-6 x 1.5-2.5 μ.

Petch (1926) described *Moniliopsis rigida* from *Phyllostachys bambusoides* and Charles (1941) observed this fungus on unidentified Acarina.

IV. Protozoan Diseases

A. GREGARINE INFECTIONS

Nicollet (1855) was the first to record gregarine infection in mites, describing *Gregarina oribatarum* from an unidentified mite. Michael (1884) observed unidentified *Gregarina* sp. in *Damaeus oblongus* as did Wellmer (1911) in *D. geniculatus*. Erhardova (1955) described *Gregarina corolla* and *G. scutovertexi* from *Schutovertex minutus*, a well-known vector of a cestode, *Moniezia expana*. Issi and Lipa (1968) recorded an unidentified gregarine developing in the midgut epithelium of *Limnochares aquaticus*. Nothing, however, is known about the pathogenicity of gregarines parasitic in mites.

B. MICROSPORIDAN INFECTIONS

Although we know more than 250 species of microsporidans in insects only three have been recorded in mites. Weiser (1956) reported the first case of microsporidosis in mites and described *Nosema steinhausi* from *Tyrophagus putrescentiae (noxius)*.

Lipa (1962a) described *Nosema sperchoni* from the water mite, *Sperchon* sp. Issi and Lipa (1968) described *Gurleya sokolovii* causing general infection in another water mite, *Limnochares aquaticus*. This parasite damaged various tissues of the host (Fig. 4) and caused high mortality in a natural population. In some years all mites examined were infected with the pathogen.

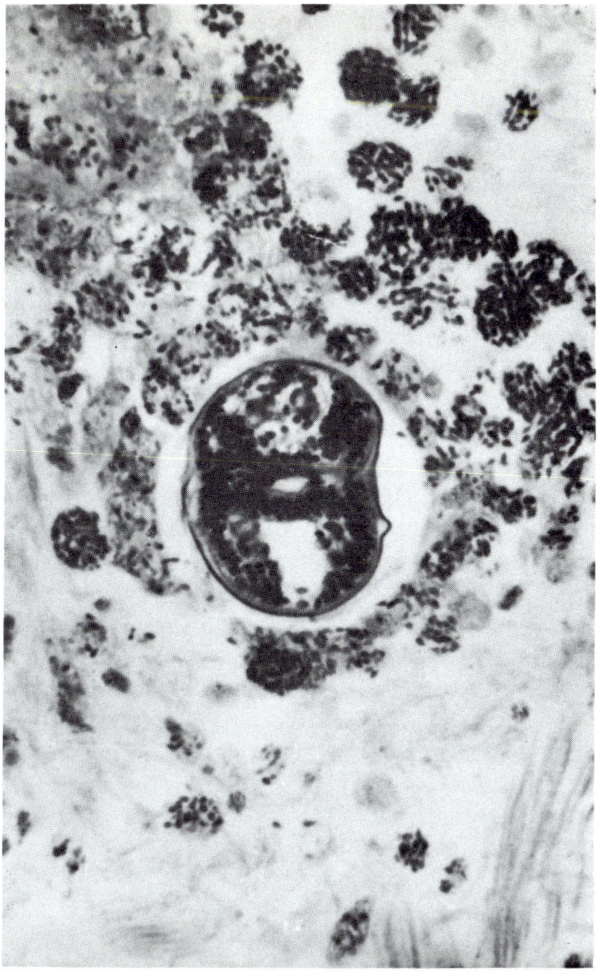

Fig. 4. Cross-section through the body of *Limnochares aquaticus* infected with microsporidan *Gurleya sokolovii*; notice black spores in the fat body and in the nerve cord stained with Heidenhain's haematoxylin (1200x).

C. OTHER PROTOZOAN INFECTIONS

Keilin (1921) described *Helicosporidium parasiticum* (order Helicosporida) from the mite *Hericia hericia* which is associated with sap exuding from trees. This protozoan also parasitizes the flies *Dasychylea obscura* and *Mycetobia pallipes*.

Thor (1930a, b) described several micro-organisms, which he placed in the Haplosporida, from Oribatid and Mesostigmatid mites, including members of the family Gamasidae. After a careful analysis of the descriptions and illustrations presented by Thor, one can conclude that many of these micro-organisms are, in fact, members of the Entomophthorales (Lipa, 1962b). Similar micro-organisms were observed by Lindquist (1961) in *Arctoseius* spp.

V. Natural Control

The importance of pathogens in the natural control of mites has been demonstrated by several authors. In fact, heavy epizootics are caused by viruses and fungi, which frequently lower the density of various mites below that causing economic damage.

A. ROLE OF VIRUSES

The non-inclusion virus affecting *Panonychus citri* has frequently been observed in the field, but only once as heavy epizootic. Tashiro and Beavers (1966) found a heavy infestation of *P. citri* on California citrus trees, with 40-50 motile forms per leaf, birefringent crystals being typical of this virus infection in 54% of the live mites and 77% of the dead ones. Population densities of *P. citri* on sample trees rapidly decreased and by mid-April were considered to be below economic levels. This situation lasted for the first half of 1965 and was attributed to the mortality caused by the virus. A similar suppression of the mite populations by this virus was also observed in April 1966.

Shaw *et al.* (1968b) also observed that virus epizootics affect the population density of *P. citri.* In Tulare county of central California the average population of mites for all groves rose to nearly one adult female per leaf during April 1966. The incidence of virus increased in parallel and mite populations decreased rapidly until they practically disappeared (Fig. 5). The authors considered that temperature and disease play major roles in summer declines of mite density.

B. ROLE OF FUNGI

Even more striking suppression of populations of various mites have been caused by fungus diseases. Fisher *et al.* (1949) and Fisher (1950b) observed a heavy epizootic in a grapefruit grove caused by *Hirsutella thompsonii* in populations of *Phyllocoptruta oleivora.* The mite populations, which were high in July and August, began to decrease in September and by October were very low. In parallel, the percentage of infested fruits decreased from 96% in August to 16% in November. Similar reductions of populations of *P. oleivora,* probably caused by the same fungus, were observed by Speare and Yothers (1924) and Yothers and Mason (1930).

Significant reductions in populations of *P. citri* were caused by *Entomophthora* sp. (Fisher, 1951). During September and October 1950 the adult mortality ranged from 32% to 95%.

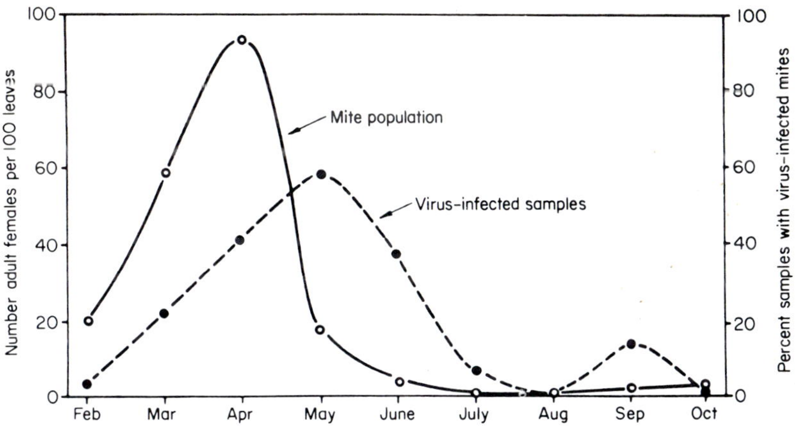

Fig. 5. Population of *Panonychus citri* and incidence of virus disease in Tulare county (central California) groves in 1966. (Courtesy of Shaw *et al.*, 1968b.)

Muma (1955, 1958) demonstrated that fungi played a major role in the natural control of *P. oleivora* and *P. citri,* while predatory and parasitic arthropods appeared to play only a minor role. Large reductions in populations of *P. oleivora,* in late summer and early autumn, were always associated with a high incidence of infection by *H. thompsonii.* Similar reductions in numbers of *P. citri* were caused by *Entomophthora* sp. (Fig. 6), and some populations were wiped out. In all these cases, epizootics occurred after heavy rains, which favoured the development of fungi. Epizootics are host-density dependent for, the greater the mite density, the greater the degree and duration of population reduction.

During a four-year study, Muma (1969) demonstrated the role of *Entomophthora floridana* in the natural control of *Eutetranychus banksi.* Data from six citrus groves indicated that epizootics of *E. floridana* killed from 36.8% to 86.3% of *E. banksi.*

Carner and Canerday (1968) observed mortality ranging from 0% to 90% caused by *Entomophthora (?fresenii)* in *Tetranychus urticae* and *T. telarius.* Of field collected mites held in the laboratory, 72% died after one and 88% after two days.

C. EFFECT OF CHEMICALS ON NATURAL CONTROL

The use of fungicides and some acaricides may interfere with natural control of mites as some of these preparations are detrimental to pathogenic fungi.

In a detailed study of this problem, Griffiths and Fisher (1950) found that on trees sprayed with zinc sulphate ($ZnSO_4$) and copper ($CuOH_2$ and $CuSO_4$), populations of *P. oleivora* were much higher than on untreated trees. On trees sprayed with pyrophyllite the increase was very small. The authors considered

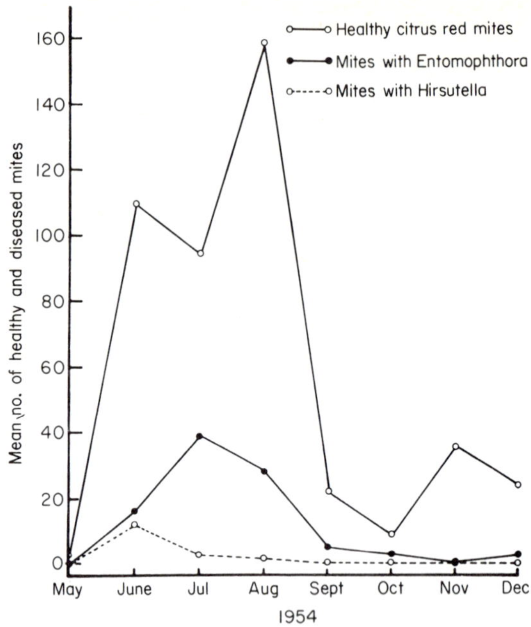

Fig. 6. A comparison of populations of *Panonychus citri* infected with *Hirsutella* and with *Entomophthora* in an orange grove not sprayed with chemicals in Florida in 1954. (Courtesy of Muma, 1955.)

that the increase in density of *P. oleivora* was due to decrease in the incidence of infection with *H. thompsonii* caused by cations of zinc and copper toxic to the fungus. Sulphur was also toxic to *H. thompsonii.*

On the other hand Dyadecho (1958, 1959a, b) reported using a mixed preparation of *Beauveria bassiana* and small dosages of acaricides with much better results in controlling *Tetranychus* spp. and *Bryobia rubrioculus* than with either agent alone. He explained that chemically treated mites were more susceptible to fungus infection so that higher mortality of the pest was obtained after such treatment. He also observed, however, that lime-sulphur was toxic to the fungus and suggested that *B. bassiana* should be used four days after lime-sulphur sprays.

VI. Microbial Control

A. USE OF VIRUSES

The non-inclusion virus of *Panonychus citri* has been intensively studied and used as a microbial control agent. Munger and Gilmore (1960) developed a method of producing large numbers of *P. citri* to obtain virus material. Later, Gilmore and Munger (1963, 1965) and Gilmore (1965) compared two methods of application of the virus: (1) spraying healthy colonies of *P. citri* with aqueous suspensions prepared from diseased mites; and (2) introducing active, infected mites into healthy colonies. Both methods were effective although, at lower population levels, the introduction of diseased mites transmitted the virus better than spraying.

The use of water suspensions of the virus creates some problems. The suspension must be prepared immediately before application (Gilmore, 1965) and the pH must be kept between 5.6 and 6.6 (Chambers, 1968). Alkaline water should not be used. Infectivity is rapidly lost on exposure to sunlight (Gilmore and Munger, 1963).

Dried deposits of aqueous suspensions of the virus generally remain infective only a few hours. On the other hand, natural deposits from diseased mites remain infective for a long time. The best method, therefore, is to store dead mites in loosely stoppered vials kept in jars with desiccants at –23.3° C. Virus stored in this manner retains high infectivity for six months or longer (Gilmore and Munger, 1963).

Several authors studied the possibility of virus controlling *P. citri* under laboratory and field conditions. In laboratory experiments, Gilmore and Munger (1965) observed that epizootics were influenced by population density and the method of virus application. When the pathogen was sprayed, the number of diseased mites increased progressively with densities of 1, 5, 20 and 80 mites caged on 45-75 cm^2 surface area of lemon. When single, infected mites were introduced into populations at the same levels, there was a 10-fold increase over the spray transmission at the lowest level.

The best way to apply the virus appears to be the introduction of infected mites to native, healthy populations of *P. citri.* Gilmore and Tashiro (1966) discussed methods and general problems of the use of inoculated mites. The mites should be infected in the protonymph stage and incubated for five days, by which time about 93% of mites become infected. These mites are released in the groves and so spread the disease among the pest populations. The incubation period required for transinfectivity is very short, ranging from three to five days.

Gilmore (1965) did two-year field experiments on the use of the virus to control *P. citri.* Sprays at a concentration of 0.1 g/litre and dosages from 2 to 6 litres/tree were compared with the release of laboratory infected mites at the rate 100, 1000, 5000 and 10,000 mites/tree. Both methods of treatment were applied either simultaneously or at a few days' interval. Treatments continued for a few months at six-week intervals. Within a month very heavy mite populations were reduced to well below economic level and maintained there for one year in all experimental plots. This was the first evidence that a heavy virus epizootic may be induced in natural populations of *P. citri* under field conditions.

In similar field experiments, Shaw *et al.* (1968a) found that a 0.01% virus suspension produced the same incidence of disease as one of 0.1%. When suspensions were buffered at pH 6.0, the incidence of infection was twice as high as that with unbuffered suspensions. The release of infected mites, collected from naturally infected populations, into citrus groves with healthy populations of *P. citri* produced an incidence of infection more than twice that obtained after the release of mites reared and infected in the laboratory. In all experimental groves an epizootic of the disease and a significant reduction of the mite population were observed.

Tashiro (1966) observed that *P. citri* inoculated with the virus dispersed as rapidly, and as far as, virus-free mites. Furthermore, it may be supposed that wind plays an important role in dispersing infected mites.

Gilmore and Tashiro (1966) showed that the release of infected mites did not add to the feeding damage of healthy mites nor to the biotic potential of wild populations of *P. citri.* Moreover, as demonstrated by Shaw *et al.* (1967), the biotic potential and beneficial activity of three phytoseid mites, *Amblyseius hibisci, A. limonicus* and *Typhlodromus occidentalis* were not reduced when fed with virus-infected *P. citri.* We may, therefore, conclude that the non-inclusion virus has all the necessary features to become a valuable agent for biological control of *P. citri.*

B. USE OF FUNGI

Dresner (1949) found that a 0.5% spore preparation of *Beauveria bassiana* was effective against *Tetranychus telarius (bimaculatus)* on beans. The experiments were carried out in July in very favourable weather for infection and development of the fungus; the air humidity early in the morning was 91.3% R.H. and the temperature 23.3°C. Mortality of mites on treated plots was 71.1%, that is, three times higher than on untreated plants.

Dyadecho (1958, 1959a) sprayed apple trees with spores of *B. bassiana* at unknown concentration and a dosage of 4 kg/acre and/or demeton methyl at 0.025% and lime-sulphur against *Bryobia rubrioculus (redikorzevi).* Chemical acaricides and *B. bassiana* applied alone were moderately effective. However, when *B. bassiana* was applied together with demeton methyl or four days after spraying with lime-sulphur (at half of the recommended dosage), results were excellent. Microscopic examination of haemolymph of dying mites revealed the fungus in only 17% while bacterial septicaemia was observed in others. One to two months after treatment no mites were observed on treated trees, but heavy mite populations developed on untreated trees.

In a later paper, Dyadecho (1959b) reported that similar results were obtained when 4 kg/acre of *B. bassiana* preparation was used together with 0.025% fenthion against *B. rubrioculus, Tetranychus urticae* and *T. viennensis.*

Čugunin (1959) used an unidentified microbial preparation containing fungi, bacteria, *Nosema* (protozoan) and polyhedrosis virus against *B. rubrioculus.* This preparation, originally prepared to control the gypsy moth, *Lymantria dispar,* was used against *B. rubrioculus* and the codling moth *Cydia (Carpocapsa) pomonella.* Čugunin reported a significant reduction of the mite population.

Boyčev and Rizvanov (1960) infected eggs of *Ixodes ricinus* with *Botrytis cinerea* (evidently *Beauveria bassiana*). A culture of the fungus was added to ovipositing females in conical flasks and incubated at 25° C and 90% R.H. Twenty days later all females had died after laying on average 700-800 eggs. The first larvae from untreated eggs were observed 27 days after laying. However, only an average of 6-7% of the treated eggs hatched after 40 days. Gorškova (1967) infected starved larvae of *I. ricinus* in the laboratory with spores of *B. bassiana* and observed mortality of 86, 94 and 100%, depending on the fungal strain.

Köhler and Fritzsche (1956) observed that filtrates of *Streptomyces albus* and other species were toxic to *Panonychus ulmi* and *Bryobia praetiosa.* Apparently, antibiotic substances have a toxic effect on some mites.

TABLE I

Selected combinations of mite and pathogen species most promising for research on natural control and applied microbial control

Host	Pathogen	Crop	Key reasons
Panonychus citri	Non-inclusion virus	Citrus	Ease of preparation and application of the virus by spraying or colonization of diseased mites
Eutetranychus banksi	*Entomophthora floridana*	Citrus	The pathogen readily attacks all instars and eliminates host populations
Phyllocoptruta oleivora	*Hirsutella thompsonii*	Citrus	Reduction in mite populations is always associated with epizootics
Tetranychus urticae	*Triplosporium tetranychi*	Various including glasshouse crops	The fungus causes severe epizootics and mortality of 85% of hosts
Panonychus ulmi	Non-inclusion virus	Orchards	To examine whether the virus occurs over the whole of the host's distribution range
Ticks	*Beauveria bassiana*	–	To collect information on susceptibility of ticks and host range of the fungus

VII. Conclusions

Disease of mites (Acarina) is a neglected area of research, a situation which should be improved. Studies in comparative invertebrate pathology are necessary as a basis for the microbial control of mites noxious to plants, animals and man.

Several authors have demonstrated that some pathogens of mites are major factors in the natural control of phytophagous mites in warm and humid climates. It is necessary, therefore, to study which micro-organisms should be used, and under what conditions, to control mites and to cause epizootics.

Any research on micro-organisms of mites and ticks can have practical implications. However, some projects seem to be of special importance and they should be urgently studied. Table I gives some examples of mites, pathogens and crops where research could most usefully be applied. Of utmost importance are studies on the effect of chemicals on natural control of mites. Pesticides used on crops commonly attacked by mites should be tested for toxicity against pathogenic micro-organisms that govern the mite populations. Whenever possible, only pesticides atoxic to fungi and other pathogens infecting mites should be used, especially in citrus groves where fungi play a major role in the natural control of tetranychid mites.

References

Baker, J. R. and Neunzig, H. H. (1968). *J. econ. Ent.* **61,** 1117-1118.

Batko, A. (1965). Monograph of Polish Entomophthoraceae. Ph.D. Thesis. Inst. Botany, Warsaw Univ.

Bird, F. T. (1967). *J. Insect Path.* **1,** 270-280.

Boudreaux, H. H. (1959). *J. Insect Path.* **1,** 270-280.

Boyčev, D. and Rizvanov, K. (1960). *Zool. Zh. Ukr.* **39,** 460.

Burditt, A. K., Reed, D. K. and Christensen, C. M. (1962). *Florida ent. Soc.* **46,** 1-5.

Carner, G. R. and Canerday, T. D. (1968). *J. econ. Ent.* **61,** 956-959.

Chambers, D. L. (1968). *J. Invertebrate Path.* **10,** 245-251.

Charles, V. K. (1941). *Insect Survey Bull.* **21,** Suppl. to No. 9, 707-785.

Čerepanova, N. P. (1964). *Bot. Zh., Kiev* **49,** 696-699.

Čugunin, J. V. (1959). *In* "Biologičeskij Metod Borby s Vrediteljami Rastenij" (N. A. Telenga, ed.), pp. 163-173. Izdatelstvo Ukrainskoj Akad. Selsk. Nauk, Kiev.

Dyadecho, N. P. (1958). *In* "Biologičeskij Metod Borby s Vrediteljami Selskochozjastvennych Kultur i Lesnych Nasaždenij" (V. P. Vassiliev *et al.,* eds), pp. 14-16. Izdatelstvo Min. Selsk. Choz. Moldavskoj SSR, Kišinev.

Dyadecho, N. P. (1959a). *In* "Biologičeskij Metod Borby s Vrediteljami Rastenij" (N. A. Telenga, ed.), pp. 35-41. Izdatelstvo Ukrainskoj Akad. Selsk. Nauk, Kiev.

Dyadecho, N. O. (1959b). *Zashch. Rast.* No. 5, 36-37.

Dresner, E. (1949). *Contr. Boyce Thompson Inst. Pl. Res.* **15,** 319-335.

Erhardova, B. (1955). *Čslká. Parasit.* **3,** 35-37.

Estes, Z. E. and Faust, R. M. (1965). *J. Invertebrate Path.* 7, 259-260.

Fisher, F. E. (1950a). *Mycologia* **42,** 290-297.

Fisher, F. E. (1950b). *J. econ. Ent.* **43,** 305-309.

Fisher, F. E. (1951). *Florida Ent.* **34,** 83-88.

Fisher, F. E. (1954). *Florida Agric. exp. Stn. Ann. Rep. 1953,* p. 191.

Fisher, F. E., Griffiths, J. T., Jr. and Thompson, W. L. (1949). *Phytopath.* **39,** 510-512.

Gilmore, J. E. (1965). *J. econ. Ent.* **58,** 1136-1140.
Gilmore, J. E. and Munger, F. (1963). *J. Insect Path.* **5,** 141-151.
Gilmore, J. E. and Munger, F. (1965). *J. Invertebrate Path.* **7,** 156-160.
Gilmore, J. E. and Tashiro, H. (1966). *J. Invertebrate Path.* **8,** 334-339.
Gorškova, G. J. (1967). *Vestnik Leningradskogo Univ.* **9,** 25-32.
Griffiths, J. T. and Fisher, F. E. (1950). *J. econ. Ent.* **43,** 298-305.
Issi, I. V. and Lipa, J. J. (1968). *J. Invertebrate Path.* **10,** 165-175.
Keilin, D. (1921). *Parasitol.* **13,** 97-113.
Köhler, F. and Fritzsche, R. (1956). *Anz. Schädlingsk.* **29,** 65-68.
Kolomiec, J. S. (1950). *Priroda* No. 4, 7.
Leatherdale, D. (1965). *J. Invertebrate Path.* **7,** 325-328.
Lindquist, F. E. (1961). *Hilgardia* **30,** 301-350.
Lipa, J. J. (1962a). *Bull. Acad. Sci. Polonaise, Ser. Biol. Sci.* **10,** 435-437.
Lipa, J. J. (1962b). *Biuletyn Inst. Ochrony Roślin* **18,** 175-202.
Michael, A. D. (1884). "British Oribatidae". Royal Society, London.
Muma, M. H. (1955). *J. econ. Ent.* **48,** 432-438.
Muma, M. H. (1958). *Proc. 10th Int. Congr. Ent., Montreal 1956,* **4,** 633-647.
Muma, M. H. (1969). *Florida Ent.* **52,** 107-112.
Muma, M. H., Selhime, A. G. and Denmark, H. A. (1961). *Florida Agric. Stn Tech. Bull.* **634,** 1-39.
Munger, F. and Gilmore, J. E. (1960). *J. econ. Ent.* **53,** 964-966.
Munger, F., Gilmore, J. E. and Davies, W. S. (1959). *Calif. Citrogr.* **44,** 190, 216.
Nicollet, H. (1855). *Archives Mus. Hist. Nat.* **7,** 351-481.
Oudemans, A. C. (1915). *Tijdschr. PlZeikt.* **21,** 111-123.
Petch, T. (1926). *Trans. Br. mycol. Soc.* **11,** 258-266.
Petch, T. (1931). *Trans. Br. mycol. Soc.* **16,** 55-75.
Petch, T. (1940). *Proc. Linnean Soc. N.S. Wales* **65,** 259-260.
Petch, T. (1944). *Trans. Br. mycol. Soc.* **27,** 81-93.
Samšinakova, A. (1957). *Zool. Listy* **6,** 329-330.
Selhime, A. G. and Muma, M. H. (1966). *Florida Ent.* **49,** 161-168.
Shaw, J. G., Chambers, D. L. and Tashiro, H. (1968a). *J. econ. Ent.* **61,** 1352-1355.
Shaw, J. G., Moffit, C. and Scriven, G. T. (1967). *J. econ. Ent.* **60,** 1751-1752.
Shaw, J. G., Tashiro, H. and Dietrick, E. J. (1968b). *J. econ. Ent.* **61,** 1492-1495.
Smith, K. M. and Cressman, A. W. (1962). *J. Insect Path.* **4,** 229-236.
Smith, K. M., Hills, G. J., Munger, F. and Gilmore, J. E. (1959). *Nature, Lond.* **184,** 70.
Speare, A. T. and Yothers, W. W. (1924). *Science (n.s.)* **60,** 41-42.
Steinhaus, E. A. (1959). *J. Insect Path.* **1,** 435-437.
Steinhaus, E. A. and Marsh, G. A. (1962). *Hilgardia* **33,** 349-490.
Tashiro, H. (1966). *Ann. ent. Soc. Am.* **59,** 1206-1210.
Tashiro, H. and Beavers, J. B. (1966). *Calif. Citrogr.* **51,** 503-506.
Thor, S. (1930a). *Z. Parasitenk.* **2,** 551-570.
Thor, S. (1930b). *Norges Svalbard-und Ishava-undersokelser* **27,** 1-157.
Weiser, J. (1956). *Čslkà. Parasit.* **3,** 187-192.
Weiser, J. (1968). *Folia Parasit.* **15,** 115-122.
Weiser, J. and Muma, M. H. (1966). *Florida Ent.* **49,** 155-159.
Wellmer, L. (1911). *Schr. Physik.-Ökon. Geselsch. Konigsberg* **52,** 103-164.
Yothers, W. W. and Mason, A. C. (1930). *U.S.D.A. Techn. Bull.* 176.

CHAPTER 16

Microbial Control of Aphids and Scale Insects

MAGNUS GUSTAFSSON

Vårdsaträvägen, Uppsala, Sweden

I. Introduction

Aphids and scales are serious enemies of many important cultivated plants throughout the world. Pathogens of these insects have been known for about a hundred years and several have been used for biological control since the beginning of this century. Before discussing the current and future possibilities of biological control the pathogens of these insects will be surveyed.

Virus infections have not been definitely demonstrated in aphids or scales though virus-like particles were found in aphids by Wayne and Briggs (1966). However, in this and similar cases, it is doubtful whether they were virus infections, natural cell components or plant viruses. Aphids are of great importance as vectors of plant viruses which may influence their reproduction (Laurema *et al.,* 1966).

Insect pathogenic bacteria occur very rarely in aphids and scales. A bacterium, *Bacillus* "C", was reported from red scale in California (Sokoloff and Klotze, 1942) and Fawcett (1944) attributed some practical importance to this bacterium. Steinhaus (1951) made infection experiments with the bacterium, a strain of *Bacillus cereus,* and found a non-specific toxic effect but no infectivity. A report of diagnostic findings by Steinhaus and Marsh (1962) includes a bacteriosis on *Therioaphis trifolii.*

The fungi are the prevailing disease-causing agents in aphids and scales. In aphids most of the diseases are caused by species of *Entomophthora.* The following 14 species occur on aphids: *E. aphidis, E. atrosperma* (Petch, 1932), *E. coronata, E. exitialis, E. fresenii, E. lageniformis, E. neri* (Rudraiah and Usman, 1955), *E. obscura, E. occidentalis, E. planchoniana (cromaphidis), E. pyriformis* (Thoizon, 1967a), *E. sphaerosperma, E. thaxteriana (ignobilis)* and *E. virulenta.* Those species for which no references are given are listed in the comprehensive work by Gustafsson (1965) with information on synonyms and literature.

Other fungi found on aphids include *Acrostalagmus aphidum* (Nolla, 1929), *Cephalosporium muscarium, C. aphidicola, Cladosporium aphidis, Hirsutella aphidis* and *Paecilomyces farinosus (Spicaria farinosa)* (Leatherdale, 1958). Burger (1926) found that *Cephalosporium* sp. could attack living insects but *Cladosporium* sp. could not. *A. aphidum* has been studied and tested for biological control (Nolla, 1929; Wolcott, 1955; Shands *et al.*, 1958).

MacLeod (1963) surveyed the biology of the Entomophthoraceae and Batko and Weiser (1965) proposed a new classification of the family. Gustafsson (1965, 1966) referred to much of the world literature on *Entomophthora,* especially on aphids. Species occurring on aphids have recently been studied by Shands *et al.* (1963), Ege (1965), Evlakhova and Voronina (1965), Voronina (1966), Thoizon (1967a, b), Prasertphon (1963, 1967a, b), Yendol (1968), Ramaseshiah (1967), Sahni (1968) and Gustafsson (1969). Lists of host aphids and pathogenic fungi were published by Steinhaus (1951), Steinhaus and Marsh (1962) and Leatherdale (1958).

Many pathogenic fungi occur on scales. The most important genera are: *Myiophagus*; *Cordyceps* with the conidial stages generally considered to be in *Spicaria (Isaria)*; *Botrytis*; *Hirsutella*; *Cephalosporium*; *Sphaerostilbe* with the conidial stage believed to be *Fusarium (Microcera)*; *Nectria*; *Podonectria*; *Hypocrella* (with conidial stage in *Aschersonia*); *Myriangium* and *Stemphylium. Septobasidium* species occur both as symbionts and parasites. Most genera have been treated taxonomically: *Myiophagus* (Karling, 1948), *Cordyceps* (Mains, 1958), *Spicaria (Isaria)* (Petch, 1925b; Mains, 1955), *Cephalosporium* (Petch, 1925a), *Hypocrella* and *Aschersonia* (Petch, 1921), *Myriangium* (Petch, 1924, 1946; Miller, 1940) and *Septobasidium* (Couch, 1938). Steinhaus (1949) surveyed the fungal diseases of scales and, from the pathological aspect, *Cordyceps* was treated by McEwen (1963), Hymenomycetes by Madelin (1963).

Several attempts have been made to control citrus scales microbially in Florida (Watson and Berger, 1937; Berger, 1942; Fawcett, 1948; Muma *et al.*, 1961). *Cephalosporium lecanii* has been used frequently for the biological control of scales and seems to have given good results all over the world, e.g. in the West Indies (Bovell, 1912), in Ceylon (Deutrom, 1918), in India (Anstead, 1920), in Guam (Vandenberg, 1928), in Puerto Rico (McCelland and Tucker,

1929), in the Seychelles (Sqibbs, 1934), in Brazil (Viergas, 1939), and in the U.S.S.R. (Evlakhova, 1941; Pospelov, 1940).

These and similar projects have several features in common. They have been largely empirical (cf. Beirne, 1962), the aim usually being to achieve a rapid practical result. The trials were made by direct application of field-collected diseased insects or by spraying spore suspensions from such material. The fungi were seldom isolated and cultivated. In some experiments it is not clear whether the fungus established itself permanently or if other pathogenic fungi occurred naturally. Facts about chemical treatments and weather conditions were also lacking and so it was not possible to determine whether an experiment had succeeded or failed. These earlier trials demonstrated the need for accurate and systematic planning in biological control.

II. Trials of Entomogenous Fungi: General Principles

A suitable working routine for the practical use of pathogens can be summarized:

1. Investigation into the ecology of the host insect, especially its natural enemies.
2. Choice of one or more pathogens based on these investigations.
3. A detailed study of the chosen pathogens including infectivity, cultivability and side-effects on people and animals.
4. Propagation of the organism (or organisms), storage, distribution and application.

It is essential that these investigations assess the effects of chemical treatments required for simultaneous use against other pests and against plant diseases. The depressing effects of fungicides on fungi pathogenic to scales have been studied by Osburn and Spencer (1938), Holloway and Young (1943) and Griffiths and Fisher (1949); the detrimental effects of fungicides and insecticides on *Entomophthora* species by Hall and Dunn (1959); the effects of some pesticides on the germination of *Entomophthora* conidia by Yendol (1968).

Numerous investigations of the ecology and population dynamics of aphids treat the effects of predators, parasites and weather conditions but several point to the great importance of the pathogenic fungi, though the species have rarely been classified. The fungi are usually species of *Entomophthora.* Animal enemies are frequently unable to prevent aphids from increasing in numbers, since they often occur too late in the season (Skuhravy and Novak, 1966; Bombosch, 1963; Hodek, 1967) though they can decrease the numbers of aphids the following year (Way, 1967).

The importance of entomogenous fungi in controlling aphids on potatoes has been studied by Shands *et al.* (1963) in a most comprehensive investigation. For over 11 years they identified all the fungi, predators and parasites found and recorded meteorological data. They found that, of all biological agents, the entomogenous fungi were outstanding in reducing the aphid population. The key species, *E. aphidis, E. thaxteriana* and *E. sphaerosperma,* are also the most common in other parts of the world. In Sweden, the author (Gustafsson, 1969) found the following species occurring in collections over a five-year period (expressed as percentage of all entomogenous species found): *E. aphidis* 45%, *E. thaxteriana* 19%, *E. fresenii* 18%, *E. planchoniana* 10%, *E. sphaerosperma* 6%, *E. exitialis* 1% and *E. virulenta* 1%. *E. coronata* was isolated from soil.

There is no definite correlation between the occurrence of these fungi and weather conditions. The amount and frequency of precipitation are not the only limiting factors, because the species react differently; *E. fresenii* occurred as frequently or even more frequently in dry and warm summers as in wet and cold; *E. aphidis* was more common in wet summers; *E. thaxteriana* replaces *E. aphidis* in drier regions (Rockwood, 1950). *E. virulenta* and *E. exitialis* are less common, but occur in different parts of the world. *E. exitialis* has recently been reported from India (Sahni, 1968), where work directed at using *Entomophthora* species in biological control has recently started.

Even though a fungal species occurs, it may develop naturally too late in the season though earlier, artificial introduction may have been successful. It may also be possible to introduce a more virulent strain which is better adapted to the environment (Evlakhova and Chvetzova, 1964). Some species, while very common, spread quite slowly, so that their introduction seems to be of little value.

Some species of *Entomophthora* attack only certain aphids and all species have specific host spectra. The detailed studies of the organisms previously suggested (2) are therefore most necessary and should include:

a. determination, isolation and cultivation;
b. investigation of physiology and sporulation;
c. investigation of infectivity and pathogenicity;
d. experiments for mass cultivation.

The author has tried to follow this programme in studying *Entomophthora* species (Gustafsson, 1966). Strains of 16 species were isolated and their physiology tested on various media (suitable C- and N-sources, pH and temperature optima). Great differences were found between, and within, species in sporulation and cultivation. As in other micro-organisms, these properties often changed after long periods of artificial cultivation. Species with rapid growth and abundant sporulation were selected for further studies by weighing the spores produced on various media (Gustafsson, 1969).

The germination capacity of spores is very important (Müller-Kögler, 1960, 1967b). Yendol (1968), investigating some of the factors that influence the germination of the conidia of *E. coronata, E. virulenta* and *E. apiculata,* showed that 95-100% R.H. was needed. At lower humidities the germination capacity is drastically reduced. Certain fungicides and insecticides inhibit germination.

III. Advances in Cultural and Application Techniques

The few infection experiments with entomogenous fungi on aphids have usually been made merely by inverting cultures. A more suitable method is by spraying suspensions of conidia (Gustafsson, 1969). The author used *Aphis fabae* and *Myzus persicae,* reared on sugar beet plants, as test insects. When the aphids had increased sufficiently, all leaves excepting two were removed, the plants placed at 100% R.H. and sprayed with a conidial suspension. The numbers of dead aphids were counted after two, four and six days, though they were not removed. In experiments with *E. virulenta* on *M. persicae,* mortality was only 6% after six days. In contrast, with *A. fabae,* 10-12% were dead after two days, 35-39% after four days and 84% after six days. The increasing mortality could be explained by the increasing numbers of conidia available as more aphids died. There were no differences in mortality between larvae and adults, and only small differences between *E. virulenta* and *E. coronata.* Maximum infection could be achieved after only 4 hr exposure at 100% R.H.

These experiments show that the infection time for these species is short, that the difference in mortality between adults and larvae is small and that the differences in susceptibility between species of aphids can be great. Clearly it is important to do the infection experiments on the insect species to be controlled. Such experiments with *Entomophthora* species on aphids have recently been carried out by Thoizon (1967b) and Ege (1965).

Fungi can be used in biological control in four ways (Franz, 1961), utilizing (1) naturally infected insects, (2) artificially infected insects, (3) fungal cultures, and (4) harvested fungus spores. Several application techniques exist depending on the crop to be treated, the organism involved and whether the aim is permanent or temporary control. Infected insects, (1) and (2), could be used directly or by preparing sprays. Cultures, (3), could be used as (a) foci of infection (solid cultures), (b) sprays (liquid cultures) or (c) applications to the soil. The spores, (4), could be used for dusting, spraying, seed treatment or application to the soil.

To introduce a pathogen as a permanent control all four principal methods, (1-4), can be used. For the control of scales, method (1) has been used frequently for artificial dissemination of *E. exitialis, E. virulenta* and *E. coronata.* Hall and Dunn (1958) used methods (1), (2) and (3).

For repeated treatment, on a larger scale, some methods are laborious and expensive. Beirne (1962) compared permanent and temporary biological control with chemical control. Temporary control has some disadvantages: the biological agents are more vulnerable to destruction by weather than insecticides, they require more careful application and they are relatively costly to prepare.

Isolation and cultivation of the fungus has many advantages, for various isolates can be tested, infectivity and growth can be investigated and mass production techniques on suitable media developed. Many of the fungi pathogenic on scales have long-lived conidia. For these species, cultivation on liquid media and preparation of powders or sprays seem the simplest procedures particularly as scales often infest trees. Application to the soil or seed treatment may be simple and inexpensive methods for protection of annual crops.

The conidia of *Entomophthora* species are very short-lived and therefore unsuitable for use as spore preparations. Some species, however, produce resting spores easily, e.g. *E. virulenta, E. coronata* and *E. exitialis.* The resting spores of *E. virulenta* and *E. coronata* germinate readily and can be produced on solid or liquid media with soya bean meal, cotton seed meal, glucose or maltose and corn steep liquor (Gustafsson, 1969). It is also possible to cultivate some other *Entomophthora* species on similar liquid media, though they do not produce resting spores. *E. coronata* has been cultivated as submerged cultures in a fermentor on low-cost media by Jönsson (1968).

Müller-Kögler (1967) discusses some of the problems of mass cultivation and the use of entomogenous fungi. Sabouraud agar and other expensive media have been used for the cultivation of *Entomophthora* species even on a larger scale (Hall and Dunn, 1958), but Evlakhova (1966) has cultivated *C. lecanii, Spicaria* sp. and other insect pathogenic species on media based on corn, wheat, potato, pumpkin and other vegetables. Martignoni (1964), who discussed mass cultivation methods in a survey on cultivation of insect pathogens, suggested that the future lies in submerged fermentation. MacLeod (1959a, b) has studied *Hirsutella* in submerged culture while the sporulation of other species in this technique has been studied by Vézina *et al.* (1965).

The author has tried a new method for the cultivation of *Entomophthora* species (Gustafsson, 1969) on soil media in air-tight tins as used for root nodule bacteria. The cultures were distributed directly to the growers. At first a soil medium was tested, then vermiculite, with the addition of essentially the same nutrients as previously used in cultivation on liquid media. The tins and the medium were autoclaved, incubated, inoculated, closed and stored at room temperature, where all the cultures of *E. virulenta* and *E. coronata* survived seven months. Cultures stored at –20° C survived six months. These periods were the longest tested. Other species *(E. aphidis, E. apiculata, E. culicis, E. sphaerosperma* and *E. thaxteriana)* cultivated in the same way survived 4-5 months. Prasertphon (1967) has shown that cultures of several *Entomophthora* species can survive for a long time in air-tight tubes on normal media.

The most important advantages of cultivation in air-tight tins are long storage without sub-culturing, ease of storage, distribution and application. The fungi can then be introduced into the soil early in the season at sowing. The method is probably also practicable with other fungi and with bacteria.

IV. Conclusions

The epizootology and other practical problems with entomogenous fungi are treated by Tanada (1963, 1964), Ferron (1967) and Müller-Kögler (1965, 1967b). Bombosch (1963) emphasized the similarity between a fungal epizootic and a fungal epiphytic. The main conditions for an epiphytic (cf. Gäumann, 1951) may be summarized:

1. A susceptible host in sufficient numbers.
2. Large epiphytic potential in the pathogenic organism.
   a. Presence of an aggressive pathogen.
   b. Large reproduction capacity in the pathogen.
   c. Good spreading capacity in the pathogen.
   d. Pathogen tolerant of variation in the environment.
3. Suitable environmental conditions, i.e. optimal climate and micro-climate.

If these conditions are compared with what is known of the ecology of *Entomophthora* species it will be seen that:

1. Only a few of the susceptible hosts are needed if the infectious material is present in sufficient quantities (Bombosch, 1963; Tanada, 1963; Shands *et al.*, 1963; Hall and Dunn, 1957). If few aphids were present in the preceding year (e.g. owing to the crop rotation) the infectious material may be too sparse. Early introduction of infectious material into the soil or as seed dressing may help an epizootic to develop earlier in the season. This is essential since the early part of the season is the most critical in the dynamics of aphid populations (Hodek, 1967).
2. a. If an aggressive pathogen is lacking it can be introduced.
   b. The reproductive capacity is good in most *Entomophthora* species and the life-cycle is short.
   c. Possibilities of spread are good. The conidia are dispersed by air currents and flying insects.
   d. The capacity for surviving periods of cold and drought is good (Bosch *et al.*, 1959).
3. Suitable climatic conditions are of the utmost importance for fungal epizootics. For the development of the infectious material in the soil, sufficiently high temperature and enough moisture are needed. The primary infection may need rainfall and irrigation practices could facilitate inoculation. For sporulation and spore germination, high humidity is necessary. For some species the infection time is short and even shorter periods of high humidity, e.g. dew (Hall and Dunn, 1957), can be sufficient. The micro-climate is most important and depends on

the soil, the climate and the plant stand. If the micro-climate is suitable, the fungi can develop even in regions with low precipitation (Tanada, 1963). The differences between various species have previously been mentioned.

It therefore seems quite feasible to initiate an epizootic under most field conditions. Some guiding principles and suitable methods for studying and utilizing pathogenic fungi on aphids and scales have been outlined. Planning of the work, ecological investigations and a thorough knowledge of the fungi are important. Secondary effects on man and animals may occur and should be considered (Müller-Kögler, 1967a). Infection experiments and methods for mass cultivation are essential while more fungal species should be isolated from both aphids and scales.

In an interesting discussion of the principal problems of biological control, Turnbull and Chant (1961) emphasize the danger that long-term projects drive one into basic ecology while shorter-term, applied projects lead away from science to empirical control. A balanced approach is essential. Perhaps the introduction of organisms for long-term control of aphids and scales is still the best method, but full use should be made of modern microbiological methods to facilitate temporary biological control.

References

Anstead, D. R. (1920). *Rep. Proc. 3. Ent. Meeting,* Pusa, pp. 328-332.

Batko, A. and Weiser, J. (1965). *J. Invertebrate Path.* **7,** 455-463.

Beirne, B. P. (1962). *Ann. Rev. Ent.* **7,** 387-400.

Berger, E. W. (1942). *Florida Ent.* **25,** 26-29.

Bombosch, S. (1963). *Z. angew. Ent.* **52,** 105-141.

Bosch, R. van den, Schlinger, E. I., Dietrick, E. J. and Hall, I. M. (1959). *J. econ. Ent.* **52,** 142-154.

Bovell, J. R. (1912). *West Indian Bull.* **12,** 399-402.

Burger, O. F. (1926). *Univ. Florida agric. exp. Stn. Rep. 1926,* 84R.

Couch, J. N. (1938). "The Genus Septobasidium". Univ. North Carolina Press, Chapel Hill.

Deutrom, H. A. (1918). *Tropical Agric. Mag. Ceylon agric. Soc.* **51,** 218-224.

Ege, O. (1965). *Arch. Microbiol.* **52,** 20-48.

Evlakhova, A. A. (1941). *Bull. Plant. Prot.,* Leningrad, 1941, 64-68 (*Rev. appl. Ent.* A **30,** 377, 1942).

Evlakhova, A. A. (1966). *Zashch. Rast.,* Moskva, 11, 43 (*Rev. appl. Mycol.* **46,** No. 1425, 273, 1967).

Evlakhova, A. A. and Chvetzova, O. I. (1964). *Entomophaga, Mém. hors Sér.* No. 2, 521-527.

Evlakhova, A. A. and Voronina, E. G. (1965). *Proc. 12 int. Congr. Ent. 1964,* p. 751.

Fawcett, H. S. (1944). *Bot. Rev.* **10,** 327-348.

Fawcett, H. S. (1948). *In* "The Citrus Industry" (H. Webber and L. Batchelor, eds), Vol. 2, pp. 627-664. Univ. California Press, Berkeley.

Ferron, P. (1967). *Annls Epiphyt.* **18,** 361-382.

Franz, J. M. (1961). *In* "Handbuch der Pflanzenkrankheiten" (H. Richter, ed.), Vol 6, 3. Lieferung, pp. 1-302. Parey, Berlin and Hamburg.

Gäumann, E. (1951). "Pflanzliche Infektionslehre". Birkhäuser, Basel.

Griffiths, J. T., Jr. and Fisher, F. E. (1949). *J. econ. Ent.* **42,** 829-833.

Gustafsson, M. (1965). *Lantbrukshögsk. Ann.* **31**, 102-212.
Gustafsson, M. (1966). *Lantbrukshögsk. Ann.* **31**, 405-457.
Gustafsson, M. (1969). *Lantbrukshögsk. Ann.* **35**, 235-274.
Hall, I. M. and Dunn, P. H. (1957). *Calif. Agric.* 11, 5, 14.
Hall, I. M. and Dunn, P. H. (1958). *J. econ. Ent.* **51**, 341-344.
Hall, I. M. and Dunn, P. H. (1959). *J. econ. Ent.* **52**, 28-29.
Hodek, I. (1967). *Entomophaga, Mém. hors Sér.* No. 3, 122-123.
Holloway, J. K. and Young, T. R., Jr. (1943). *J. econ. Ent.* **36**, 453-457.
Jönsson, A. G. (1968). *Appl. Microbiol.* **16**, 450-457.
Karling, J. S. (1948). *Am. J. Bot.* **35**, 246-254.
Laurema, S., Markkula, M. and Raatikainen, M. (1966). *Ann. Agric. Fenniae* **5**, 94-99.
Leatherdale, D. (1958). *Ent. mon. Mag.* **94**, 103-105.
MacLeod, D. M. (1959a). *Can. J. Bot.* **37**, 695-714.
MacLeod, D. M. (1959b). *Can. J. Bot.* **37**, 819-834.
MacLeod, D. M. (1963). *In* "Insect Pathology An Advanced Treatise" (E. A. Steinhaus, ed.), Vol. 2, pp. 189-231. Academic Press, New York and London.
Madelin, M. F. (1963). *In* "Insect Pathology An Advanced Treatise" (E. A. Steinhaus, ed.), Vol. 2, pp. 233-271. Academic Press, New York and London.
Mains, E. B. (1955). *Pap. Michigan Acad. Sci., Arts, Lett.* **40**, 23-32.
Mains, E. B. (1958). *Mycologia* **50**, 169-222.
Martignoni, M. E. (1964). *In* "Biological Control of Insect Pests and Weeds" (P. DeBach, ed.), pp. 579-609. Chapman and Hall, London.
McCelland, T. B. and Tucker, C. M. (1929). *Agric. Notes Porto Rico Exp. Stn.* **48**, 1-2.
McEwen, F. L. (1963). *In* "Insect Pathology An Advanced Treatise" (E. A. Steinhaus, ed.), Vol. 2, pp. 273-290. Academic Press, New York and London.
Miller, J. M. (1940). *Mycologia* **32**, 387-600.
Müller-Kögler, E. (1960). *Z. PflKrankh.* **67**, 663-668.
Müller-Kögler, E. (1965). "Pilzkrankheiten bei Insekten". Parey, Berlin and Hamburg.
Müller-Kögler, E. (1967a). *Entomophaga* **12**, 429-441.
Müller-Kögler, E. (1967b). *In* "Insect Pathology and Microbial Control" (P. A. van der Laan, ed.), pp. 339-353. North-Holland Publ. Co., Amsterdam.
Muma, M. H., Selhime, A. G. and Denmark, H. A. (1961). *Florida agric. exp. Sta. Tech. Bull.* **634**, 1-39.
Nolla, J. A. B. (1929). *J. Dep. Agric. Porto Rico* **13**, 59-72.
Osburn, M. R. and Spencer, H. (1938). *J. econ. Ent.* **31**, 731-732.
Petch, T. (1921). *Ann. R. Bot. Gard. Peradeniya* **7**, 167-278.
Petch, T. (1924). *Trans. Br. mycol. Soc.* **10**, 45-80.
Petch, T. (1925a). *Trans. Br. mycol. Soc.* **10**, 152-182.
Petch, T. (1925b). *Trans. Br. mycol. Soc.* **10**, 183-189.
Petch, T. (1932). *Trans. Br. mycol. Soc.* **17**, 170-178.
Petch, T. (1934). *Trans. Br. mycol. Soc.* **19**, 34-38.
Petch, T. (1946). *Trans. Br. mycol. Soc.* **29**, 74-77.
Pospelov, V. P. (1940). *Summary Sci. Res. Work. Inst. Plant Prot. for 1939.* **8**, 125-129. Leningrad Acad. Sci. (*Rev. appl. Ent.* A **29**, 582-584, 1941).
Prasertphon, S. (1963). *J. Insect Path.* **5**, 174-181.
Prasertphon, S. (1967a). *J. Invertebrate Path.* **9**, 140-142.
Prasertphon, S. (1967b). *J. Invertebrate Path.* **9**, 281-282.
Ramaseshiah, G. (1967). *J. Invertebrate Path.* **9**, 128-130.
Rockwood, L. P. (1950). *J. econ. Ent.* **43**, 704-707.
Rudraiah, M. P. and Usman, S. (1955). *Science and Culture* **21**, 158-159.
Sahni, M. L. (1968). *J. Invertebrate Path.* **10**, 425-426.
Shands, W. A., Simpson, G. W. and Hall, I. M. (1963). *Maine agric. Exp. Stn. Bull.* T.6 (Technical Ser.), 1-42.
Shands, W. A., Thompson, C. G., Simpson, G. W. and Wave, H. E. (1958). *J. econ. Ent.* **51**, 184-186.
Skuhravy, V. and Novak, K. (1966). *Z. angew. Ent.* **57**, 141-166.

Sokoloff, V. P. and Klotze, L. J. (1942). *Phytopathology* **32,** 187-198.
Sqibbs, F. L. (1934). *Rep. Dep. Agric. Seychelles for 1933,* p. 5.
Steinhaus, E. A. (1949). "Principles of Insect Pathology". MacGraw-Hill, New York, Toronto and London.
Steinhaus, E. A. (1951). *Hilgardia* **20,** 629-678.
Steinhaus, E. A. and Marsh, G. A. (1962). *Hilgardia* **33,** 349-490.
Tanada, Y. (1963). *In* "Insect Pathology An Advanced Treatise" (E. A. Steinhaus, ed.), Vol. 2, pp. 423-475. Academic Press, New York and London.
Tanada, Y. (1964). *In* "Biological Control of Insect Pests and Weeds" (P. DeBach, ed.), pp. 548-578. Chapman and Hall, London.
Thoizon, G. (1967a). *Entomophaga* **12,** 303-307.
Thoizen, G. (1967b). *C.r. hebd. Séanc. Acad. Sci. Paris* **265,** 2001-2003.
Turnbull, A. L. and Chant, D. A. (1961). *Can. J. Zool.* **39,** 697-753.
Vandenberg, S. R. (1928). *Ann. Rep. Guam agric. exp. Stn. for 1926,* pp. 15-19.
Vézina, C., Singh, K. and Sehgal, S. N. (1965). *Mycologia* **57,** 722-736.
Viergas, A. P. (1939). *Sao Paulo Inst. Café Rev.* **14,** 754-772.
Voronina, E. G. (1966). *Bot. Z.* **44,** 721-727.
Watson, J. R. and Berger, E. W. (1937). *Florida agric. Exten. Serv. Bull.* **88,** 1-135.
Way, M. J. (1967). *Ann. appl. Biol.* **59,** 175-188.
Wayne, B. P. and Briggs, J. D. (1966). *J. Invertebrate Path.* **8,** 122-123.
Wolcott, G. N. (1955). *Univ. Puerto Rico agric. exp. Stn. Bull.* **130,** 1-19.
Yendol, W. G. (1968). *J. Invertebrate Path.* **10,** 116-121.

CHAPTER 17

Microbial Control of Termites

ANDERS E. LUND

Texas Forest Products Laboratory, Lufkin, Texas, U.S.A.

I. Introduction

For a number of years chemical toxicants have been accepted as the standard control measure for termites (Isoptera) in many countries. However, during the last decade considerable effort has been devoted to the development of alternative procedures. Due to the cryptobiotic habits of most termites the development of these measures has been extremely slow.

II. Pathogen Studies

The Koppers Company, Inc. of Pittsburgh, Pennsylvania, U.S.A., conducted and evaluated laboratory studies of different organisms and the attractant, repellent, and pathogenic responses induced in subterranean termites (*Reticulitermes* spp.), beginning in the late 1950's. These studies led to the issuance of five U.S. patents (Lund, 1966). In the early 1960's this company also conducted a number of field tests with attractant-toxicant and pathogen combinations to control subterranean termites (Lund, 1969). *Aspergillus flavus* and *Serratia marcescens* were among the pathogens used. Strain selection was based on pathogenicity to termites in the laboratory. After eight years, field results were not encouraging though it was known that some possible sources of pathogen inactivation had been present initially in the test plots. Toumanoff and Toumanoff (1959) also studied the disease of termites caused by *S. marcescens.*

Though no field results were reported, a U.S. Patent was issued for the biological control of termites by spores of *Entomophthora virulenta* and *Bacillus thuringiensis* (Page, 1967). *Absidia coerulea* was reported to be pathogenic to subterranean termites by Lund and Engelhardt (1962), based on laboratory studies conducted at Duke University during 1955-58. The pathogenicity to *Reticulitermes flavipes* of certain externally occurring fungi was reported by Smythe and Coppel (1966). They concluded that seven fungal species were not significantly pathogenic to colonies. In a follow-up study at the U.S. Department of Agriculture, Wood Products Insect Laboratory, at Gulfport, Mississippi, Smythe (personal communication) concluded that none, of about 200 termite organism isolates, looked promising as microbial control agents.

The Bündensanstalt für Materialprüfung, Berlin, is initiating studies on the biological control of subterranean termites (G. Becker, personal communication) and the University of Hawaii is reported to be currently evaluating certain organisms as termite pathogens.

III. Conclusions

Laboratory studies have demonstrated the possibility of controlling subterranean termites using pathogens. However, of the hundreds of organisms evaluated, very few have shown sufficient activity to justify further testing under field conditions. In field trials no organism has demonstrated significant pathogenicity though the reported trials may have been improperly implemented. Within the last three years there has been a substantial increase in the number of institutions and investigators examining the possibilities of microbial control of termites and so it appears likely that within the next few years a more complete evaluation will be available.

References

Lund, A. E. (1966). *U.S. Patents* **3,** 249, 492; **3,** 249, 439; **3,** 249, 494; **3,** 249, 500; **3,** 249, 501.

Lund, A. E. (1969). *In* "B.W.P.A. Termite Symposium". British Wood Preserving Association, London, pp. 107-115.

Lund, A. E. and Engelhardt, N. T. (1962). *J. Insect Path.* **4,** 131-132.

Page, R. Z. (1967). *U.S. Patent* **3,** 337, 395.

Smythe, R. V. and Coppel, H. C. (1966). *J. Invertebrate Path.* **8,** 266-267.

Toumanoff, C. and Toumanoff, C. (1959). *C.r. hebd. Séanc. Acad. Agric. Fr.* **45,** 216-218.

CHAPTER 18

Microbial Control of Arthropods of Medical Importance[1]

MARSHALL LAIRD

Memorial University of Newfoundland, St. John's, Newfoundland, Canada

I. Trends in Biological Control of Medically Important Arthropods

No two persons compiling a bibliography on the biological control of "vectors" would be likely to achieve the same result. One would confine himself to the major groups of arthropods transmitting disease organisms to man and other vertebrates. Another would (as in this chapter and Appendix 7) deal with all arthropods of health interest. The latter approach entails including a wide range of nuisance species, such as many of the non-biting chironomid midges, as well as true vectors, such as many of the mosquitoes.

Again, one author might rely heavily upon titles and abstracts from an information storage and retrieval facility, able to yield only what had been fed into it in the first place. Another might at least skim through a wide range of publications—and thus chance across apposite sections, paragraphs, or brief observations not apparent from either title or abstract. It is noted

[1] Studies in Biology from the Memorial University of Newfoundland, No. 139.

in this context that of the 1973 references in the most exhaustive general compilation to date (Jenkins, 1964) some 650 titles (33% of the total) contain no clue to their relevance.

The coverage of Jenkins' bibliography is reasonably good up to and including 1960. It is rather less so from then until the end of 1962, and there are only a few random citations for 1963 and 1964. Now, with help from collaborators[1] in many countries, an additional 366 titles up to the end of 1962 can be listed (Appendix 7, Section 1). It might have been expected that the majority of these would have been articles including only chance remarks of biological control or invertebrate pathology interest. The reverse in fact proved true. Only 70 (19%) were in this category. Contributing factors here were a purposeful survey of Eastern European journals by Russian, Czech and other colleagues with directly pertinent articles primarily in mind, and the culling from the chironomid literature of many articles specifically concerning parasites or predators.

None of these previously-overlooked publications nor the 500 additional ones for 1963-67 (Appendix 7, Section 2) deal with larvivorous fish. The reason for this is the publication (Gerberich and Laird, 1966, 1968) of an annotated bibliography on mosquito-destroying fish, with rather more than 700[2] references (359 of them up to 1962 and not mentioned by Jenkins, 306 mentioned by him and 52 published from 1963 to 1967, coverage for the last two years being poor).

All told, some 3250 publications on the biological control or pathology of arthropods of public health interest are mentioned in these bibliographies. Allowing for articles that have appeared since the cut-off dates of the most recent lists, also for the inevitable material still overlooked, it is evident than an exhaustive bibliography on the overall subject would run to at least 3500-4000 references.

Larvivorous fish comprise the chief topic of the earlier contributions on biological control, as such, in medical entomology. Especially in the years between the two World Wars, there were some rather limited successes involving other types of naturalistic control. These included the manipulation of mosquito larval habitats to render them unattractive to particular vectors, through such devices as artificial shading or exposure to sunlight, and the deliberate increase of organic loading (Williamson, 1949). However, *Gambusia, Poecilia (Lebistes)* and here and there certain other larvivores,

[1] Who responded to a footnoted request for notice of omissions, on p. 6 of Jenkins' bibliography.

[2] Lack of editorial contact prevented the correction in the 1968 version issued by FAO of numerous errors carried over to the 1966 version earlier issued by WHO, from Gerberich (1946). For example, the double citation of two papers by Rao and Ramoo under "Bhasker, R. R." and "Rao, R. B.", also failure to recognize the recent synonymizing of *(Lebistes)* with *Poecilia reticulata.*

were the real mainstay. Lately there has been renewed interest in the control potentialities of fish, used very selectively in specific types of mosquito larval habitats in accordance with sound ecological principles (Gerberich and Laird, 1966, 1968). The integrated use of fish and chemical larvicides has also been studied, due attention being given to the effects of these compounds on the chosen larvivores (Boyd and Ferguson, 1964a, b). In particular, "annual" cyprinodonts of the genera *Cynolebias* and *Nothobranchius* have been attracting considerable attention by their suitability for establishment in pools too short-lived to support permanent populations of "classical" larvivores–the latter bear living young, while "annual" fish lay desiccation-resistant eggs.

However, while much of what has been published on larvivorous fish describes work undertaken with practical biological control in view, this is not so with the rest (and much the greater part) of the literature relevant to biological control in medical entomology. The bulk of this concerns taxonomy, notably the description of new parasites and pathogens from vectors; fundamental studies of population dynamics, e.g. many papers on Hymenoptera from muscoid fly hosts; laboratory feeding experiments with aquatic predators such as water beetles and dragonfly nymphs; field experiments along similar lines; biochemical studies, e.g. involving *Crithidia* flagellates; and random observations–whether of field events or accidental mortalities in laboratory colonies. Still omitting fish from consideration, the number of pertinent articles published in the years indicated, corrected upwards to the nearest 10 and probably somewhat below the actual figure at that, were:

1910	10
1920	30
1930	30
1940	20
1950	20
1960	110

The more than five-fold increase between 1950 and 1960 obviously merits closer examination. As there is no marked surge for the first half of the 'fifties, and the annual total has regained its 1930 level of 30 only by 1955, that year is a convenient starting point for a more detailed breakdown:

1955	30
1956	40
1957	40
1958	50
1959	70
1960	110

Clearly, then, something was happening in the second half of the 1950's to stimulate interest in invertebrate pathology, biological control and ancillary topics as they concern public health entomology.

That "something" was the insecticide resistance problem, then coming into focus as "the most important single problem facing vector-control programmes" (WHO, 1958). This phenomenon clearly prejudiced the successful conclusion of widespread activities then being developed under WHO's malaria eradication programme, based upon the interruption of transmission by the massive use of residual compounds, notably DDT, applied to the inner walls of dwellings. It was realized, therefore, that available chemical control procedures might soon need support from conventional and/or novel biological techniques in altogether new integrated control methodologies practised upon a foundation of detailed ecological knowledge of the specific vectors under attack (Laird, 1959, 1963). Linked with this was the start, in 1958, of WHO's pilot project assessing the comparative merits of a microbial control agent (a *Coelomomyces* fungal pathogen) and larvicidal dieldrin-cement briquettes against isolated atoll populations of the filariasis vector, *Aedes (Stegomyia) polynesiensis,* in the Tokelau Islands (see also p. 393) (Anon., 1958; Laird and Colless, 1962; Laird, 1967).

WHO's long-term biological control investigations, forming part of the Organization's comprehensive vector biology and control programme, began in earnest in 1961/62. Against this background, it is interesting to summarize the continuing output of relevant papers since 1960:

1961	80
1962	80
1963	90
1964	120
1965	120
1966	120
1967	80

(last record probably less complete than earlier years)

Thus since 1957, in which the record annual total of pertinent contributions achieved in 1956 was equalled, the annual output has in three years (1964, 1965, 1966) tripled the 1957 one. Since 1959, it has never less than doubled the 1957 output.

How much of the greatly increased yield is directly referable to biological control as distinct from topics in one way or another germane to the subject? Perhaps the best way of estimating this is to return for a moment to the matter of larvivorous fish. The Gerberich and Laird bibliography being reasonably complete through 1965, that year (well into the recent upsurge of interest in biological control in medical entomology) is arbitrarily selected as the cut-off date. In five-year spans from 1951, the following output (figures to the nearest 10 upwards) held good for larvivorous fish articles, and papers on other topics in one way or another relevant to biological control in medical entomology:

Period	Larvivorous fish articles	Papers on other relevant topics
1951-55	20	150
1956-60	30	280
1961-65	40	460

The rate of increment is significantly greater in the "other topics" column, an overall tripling of output in 15 years having taken place, as compared with a doubling of interest in larvivorous fish.

What about the balance between mission-oriented and general interest papers in the second column? In 1951-55 some 6% of the relevant output was mission-oriented; in 1956-60 the figure had only risen to 7%; but in 1961-65 it was 18%. Once again the data reveal a tripling of interest over a 15-year period in which it was becoming steadily more evident that the modern synthetic organic pesticides were not of themselves the panacea hailed by many in the 1940's.

And (still setting the larvivorous fish literature aside), what about the relative output of publications on microbial control of vectors by comparison with those on, for instance, entomophaga? In 1951-55 none of the mission-oriented papers in the second column concerned microbial control; in 1956-60 just under half of them did; and in 1961-65 some two-thirds of them did. Moreover, reference to the 1963-67 bibliography in Appendix 7 will show that only about 14% of the contributions listed did not deal primarily with biological control or invertebrate pathology and indicate this in their titles.

Here, it is submitted, are trends of major importance that were not considered at all by Rothman and Woodhead (1968) in their synopsis of "publication trends in biological control". Based on classified bibliographies on this general subject appearing in *Entomophaga* from time to time, this synopsis sought to classify its subject matter under nine broad headings employed by Franz (1956). These headings lump together economic and medical entomology. The authors were apparently unaware of the important dichotomy through lacking any personal involvement in the specialty they were writing about. They were simply endeavouring to analyse "the relative growth rates of various topics within a restricted field" and used this one as an example of their technique, "In view of the interest generated by the pesticides controversy in the United States and elsewhere." In doing so (quite validly in so far as Franz's nine broad headings are concerned) they altogether overlooked the facts that (a) over the past decade or so medical entomologists have belatedly begun to pay serious attention to the feasibility of developing practical microbial control procedures as effective as those already being used to good effect in economic entomology; and (b) contributions concerning the microbial control of vectors are becoming steadily more numerous than those on larvivorous fish, and other candidate biological control agents such as entomophaga.

Rothman and Woodhead correctly observed that from the mid-1950's to the mid-1960's the three maximum growth rates among the major headings referred to were in (a) fundamental research on the utilization of entomophagous arthropods (without taxonomy); (b) fundamental research on micro-organisms as pathogens of arthropods (but not aiming at complete coverage of the specialized topic of diseases of honey-bees and silkworms); and (c) autocidal control.

The last-named topic is of considerable current interest to medical entomologists. Striking successes with radiation-induced male sterility in screwworm control have led to laboratory and field experiments against other vectors (e.g. tsetse flies, mosquitoes), sometimes with novel genetically based procedures (e.g. cytoplasmic incompatibility). Entomophagous arthropods, though, have been very much less used in medical entomology than in agricultural entomology. Indeed, the only widespread use of entomophaga against disease vectors has involved a few hymenopterous parasites. These include *Mormoniella (Nasonia), Spalangia,* and certain other enemies of muscoid flies (Bennett, 1966; Bennett and Legner, 1967; Legner *et al.,* 1967; Whiting, 1967), *Hunterellus* tick parasites (Cole, 1965), and certain enemies of cockroaches and black widow spiders (Jenkins, 1964).

Due largely to the failure to collect adequate baseline data against which to monitor the results of introductions, none of these efforts to date have shown convincing evidence of the achievement of significant lasting control, so frequently described in the far more extensive literature on the practical use of entomophaga in economic entomology. In any case, only a tiny fraction of the known entomophaga are applicable to the control of insects of health importance. The most important of all vectors (the diverse mosquitoes transmitting malaria, filariasis, yellow fever, dengue and a varied assortment of other arboviruses) are not certainly known to harbour even a single species of insect endoparasite, although an inadequately known egg parasite of *Anopheles* spp. in the Philippines (Pagayon, 1963) is probably a helminth but might be a hymenopteran. In so far as practical biological control is concerned, the larvivorous fish are the closest equivalent of entomophaga in the control of medically important arthropods.

Recollecting that Rothman and Woodhead named microbial control-related research as the second most important trend in biological control from the mid-1950's to the mid-1960's, we may now recall the figures quoted earlier for mission-oriented as contrasted with other types of investigations. In 1961-65, of the approximately 500 papers on biological control and invertebrate pathology in medical entomology, 40 (8%) concerned larvivorous fish. Rather more than 80 (16%) described other types of mission-oriented work, almost two-thirds of these relating to microbial control. That is to say, of about 500 papers in the general field, 120 were mission-oriented; 40 of these related to larvivorous fish, 27 to, for instance, control by entomophaga and 53 (44% of the total) to microbial control.

Even so, few field trials of microbial agents have yet been undertaken against selected vector populations. Most of the mission-oriented work mentioned consists (1) of reviews advocating studies of aspects of invertebrate pathology out of which eventual practical microbial control procedures might be developed; (2) of such studies, so reported as to emphasize future control relevance; and (3) of field surveys aimed at either elucidating certain host-parasite relationships under natural conditions, or detecting candidate biological control material for laboratory assessment.

Over the past decade there have been localized assessments of candidate microbial agents against arthropods of health importance, for instance, with *Bacillus sphaericus* and *B. thuringiensis* against various Diptera (see p. 398). While so far, such studies have given rather contradictory results, they have included advanced developmental research involving the testing of commercial formulations of "microbial insecticides" against selected vectors (e.g. houseflies; Borgatti and Guyer, 1963). However, only two inter-country pilot projects have yet taken place. Both concerned isolated vector populations on small Pacific islands. WHO and the New Zealand Government jointly sponsored the first. In this venture, *Coelomomyces* fungi from Singapore were successfully established in an *Aedes polynesiensis* population on Nukunono Atoll, Tokelau Islands. The introduction took place in 1958, linked with a careful survey which confirmed the prior absence of these pathogens from the experimental site. Its results, and those of the parallel experiment with dieldrin-cement briquettes on the neighbouring atoll of Atafu, have been monitored over the succeeding years (see also p. 390). At the time of writing, February 1969, a recently-collected consignment of larvae obtained by a New Zealand expedition is being studied to determine the present level of fungal infection. The peak figure to date was recorded in 1965, when parasitized larvae were discovered in 13 (37.1%) of 35 habitats sampled (of course, no sample of parasitized larvae as such can show any evidence of that fraction of the population dying early and disintegrating). There was some (but nevertheless inconclusive) indication from certain Nukunono islets revisited in 1960 (since when no adult mosquito surveys have been conducted there) of a reduction in the incidence of female *A. polynesiensis* since 1958; but although these were the same islets from which *Coelomomyces*-positive larvae were recorded in 1960, it could not of course be claimed from the scanty field data available (Laird, 1967) that the introduction of the fungus had actually brought about an appreciable lowering of the mosquito population there. What can be said, is that a highly encouraging establishment of *Coelomomyces* was indeed achieved; and that evidence from elsewhere (Muspratt, 1963a) has linked high natural incidence of these fungi with excessive rarity of host adults. Furthermore, Umphlett (in Couch, 1968) has demonstrated average 50% infection rates *(Coelomomyces punctatus/Anopheles quadrimaculatus)* in University Lake, Chapel Hill, N.C., U.S.A., reportedly keeping this field population of the host "well under control".

The second inter-country pilot project was initiated (like the first with WHO support) in 1966, on another Pacific island, Nauru, where Chapman (1967) made a preliminary survey which indicated the apparent absence of significant pathogens or parasites from local populations of *Aedes aegypti* and *Culex pipiens fatigans.* In 1967, D. G. Reynolds[1] introduced mermithid nematodes originally derived from Zambian mosquitoes (Muspratt, 1963b, 1965), and the microsporidan protozoan *Plistophora culicis.* The latter was originally isolated from laboratory colonies of *Anopheles gambiae,* in which from 50 to 100% of the adults were infected (Canning, 1957; Garnham, 1956). In a major break-through this strain of *P. culicis* was afterwards transferred to a laboratory stock of *C. p. fatigans* in England (Reynolds, 1966). Natural and artificial larval habitats of *C. p. fatigans* at Nauru duly yielded larvae parasitized by *P. culicis* and mermithid infections were achieved in the same host and *A. aegypti* too. This introduction will, like the Tokelau one, be monitored by assessment surveys.

Perhaps the most encouraging aspect of all the varied work now under way in the field of microbial control of medically important arthropods, is the emergence of a definite pattern pointing towards eventual practical application. Thus, a continuing global survey for candidate biological control agents, based upon the use of a pocket collecting kit developed for the purpose (Cantwell and Laird, 1966), is bringing much valuable material into the WHO International Reference Centre for Diagnosis of Diseases of Vectors (Briggs, 1966, 1967). The organisms so obtained are being intensively studied by appropriate specialists.

An immediate dividend is that we already have a far clearer picture of

[1] Who conducted this project under United Kingdom auspices, and has kindly permitted my mentioning his preliminary and as yet unpublished results.

the taxonomy, distribution, hosts, and incidence of particular groups of candidate biological control agents than was available 10 years ago. For example, a monograph currently being prepared by J. N. Couch of the University of North Carolina and myself will contain information on about twice as many species of *Coelomomyces* as were known in the early 1960's. More important still, it will present a reasonably valid picture of the geographical and host distribution of these fungi–whereas a plot made less than a decade ago would simply have indicated the homes and travel itineraries of the handful of biologists interested in *Coelomomyces.* Our present information, though, is based upon a survey involving the sending of WHO collecting kits and background information to collaborating scientists all over the world. The scale of this survey is realized when one considers that by 31 July 1968 more than 800 kits had been given to investigators in upwards of 110 countries, 207 kits having by that date been returned with study material to the International Reference Centre already mentioned. The background information referred to notably includes specially prepared WHO mimeographed documents, distributed free (like the kits themselves) by the Vector Biology and Control Unit, WHO, Avenue Appia, 1211 Geneva-27, Switzerland. These documents include an illustrated guide to the recognition of diseased vectors (Weiser, 1968a). The same author (1963) published a useful account of diseases of European insects of medical importance. Of course, much relevant taxonomic, survey and experimental work in this field is carried on without any direct connection with WHO programme activities. Examples are the important research undertaken by the USDA's Lake Charles Laboratory (Chapman, 1964), comprehensive studies of octosporeosis of houseflies at Cornell University (e.g. Kramer, 1966), work on, for instance, microsporidans of blackflies and entomophthoraceous fungi of mosquitoes and muscoid flies in Eastern Europe (Weiser, 1964; Weiser and Batko, 1966), investigations of mermithids of chironomid midges in the Federal Republic of Germany (Wülker, 1965) and studies of mermithids of blackflies in Canada (Welch, 1964) and the U.S.S.R. (Rubtsov, 1963). However, each of the investigators just named has in recent years done consultant work for WHO and/or attended research planning meetings at WHO Headquarters, Geneva. Appendix 7, Section 1, shows that, like many other research workers in many different countries, they have all also collaborated in the global programme outlined above by permitting the pre-publication circulation of significant papers as WHO mimeographed "preprints".

This kind of widespread collaboration, with an international Specialized Agency of the United Nations as catalyst, clearly represents a highly encouraging trend conducive to the early development of practical microbial control procedures. The existence of such a programme, too, cannot help but arouse interest outside the ranks of those immediately concerned with it. By precept it encourages a logical sequence of events from preliminary surveys through purely taxonomic work to field ecological studies and indoor and outdoor laboratory experiments; and ultimately, to larger scale pilot projects along the lines of those in the Tokelaus and Nauru. These events should, of course, be accompanied by laboratory culture and commercial-level mass production activities (WHO, 1964), and should be followed by large-scale field establishments on the basis of which effective microbial control techniques can be developed for integration with other procedures (Jafri, 1965a; Laird and Wright, 1966).

There are encouraging signs from many directions that practical microbial control techniques will indeed be added to our overall armoury of vector control measures in the rather near future. Nevertheless, the fact must be faced that as of February 1969 we still lack even a single such technique involving an agent commercially available in standardized formulations properly cleared by agricultural and health authorities, and giving a predictable level of control against a specific vector.

What, then, are the directions that seem most promising at this stage? Which groups of pathogens and parasites of invertebrates at present seem to offer the most encouraging prospects for biological control? What further steps are indicated before such organisms, once developed to the point of commercial exploitation, can be cleared for general use, and what action might best transfer microbial control from the position of obvious desirability to that of practicality in vector control? The remainder of this chapter will attempt to answer these questions.

II. Promising Candidate Microbial Control Agents

A. VIRUSES

Rivers (1964), pointing out that virus diseases of insects show promise against certain economic pests, drew attention to the facts that these pathogens are cheap to produce, species-specific, spread by the hosts themselves, and harmless to all other forms of life. However, Jenkins (1964) was able to list only five published relationships between medically important arthropods and viral entities of uncertain nature in his Table IV, while recognizing that "this almost certainly reflects a lack of relevant research rather than of viral pathogens". Vago (1964a) cautioned that viral specificity among insects was beginning to prove less strict than had previously been suspected, infections with the same virus having been achieved in several different hosts. He felt, nevertheless, that this was not a serious hindrance, the point simply underlining the desirability of assuring that a target arthropod is at the centre of the spectrum of virulence of the pathogen chosen for use against it. Vago also drew attention to viral dynamism as a further factor of basic importance to microbial control, recollecting that when a species or population of insect is exposed to several viruses, one among them will predominate over the others and bring about the most intense infections.

In another contribution Vago (1964b) considered the future potentialities of viruses against arthropod disease vectors. He emphasized that this field had not even begun to be exploited by medical entomologists, although in economic entomology (thanks, e.g. to the prevalence of viral pathogens among pest Lepidoptera) large-scale applications against forest pests had already been carried out with very encouraging results in France, the United Kingdom and Canada.

Mentioning that a virus of the housefly, a possible virus of a chironomid, and polyhedral bodies in *Culex tarsalis* were under observation in his own laboratory, Vago (1964b) emphasized that the basis of microbial control is a knowledge of specific pathogens highly infectious for the target arthropods. He claimed that any work of practical importance in this context would have to await the discovery of such viruses, as yet unknown, in vectors of human diseases. He also recollected that viral material has to be ingested by insects before an infection can be produced. Thus, he submitted, the initial application of viruses against all stages of houseflies is easily accomplished, but in the case of haematophagous species (e.g. mosquitoes) only the non-bloodsucking larvae are directly vulnerable. However, it must be added that flower-feeding male or indeed female mosquitoes would be equally susceptible to topical applications of appropriate viruses. Furthermore, initial results from transmission experiments with the iridescent virus of *Aedes taeniorhynchus* (MIV) described from the U.S.A. by Clark *et al.* (1965) have indicated that when healthy larvae acquire, just before pupation, this pathogen from the bodies of dead ones, they give rise to diseased adults, which lay infected eggs. Larvae developing from these show disease symptoms (yellow to yellow-green iridescence, particularly in the thorax) in the early fourth instar and die without pupating (Linley and Nielsen, 1968a, b). It is noted, too, that Canadian investigations published as this goes to press (Harris *et al.*, 1969) have demonstrated that *Aedes aegypti* and *Culex tarsalis* females are attracted to, and will feed from certain larval Lepidoptera, Coleoptera and Hymenoptera. This opens up the possibility that mosquito adults may acquire infections in a hitherto unsuspected manner, besides perhaps even inoculating insect pathogens into vertebrates including man.

The discovery of MIV and of an iridescent virus in *Aedes annulipes* (Weiser, 1965), were soon followed by the reporting (Chapman *et al.*, 1966) and investigation (Woodard and Chapman, 1968) of MIV in other mosquito hosts as well as *A. taeniorhynchus.* It must be noted, though, that there are already indications that MIV induces disease in only a relatively small proportion of the larvae harbouring it (Linley and Nielsen, 1968a). Also, only 53 (10.6%) of 500 healthy, first generation larvae exposed to 10 virus-killed larvae in a laboratory pan, developed symptoms (Linley and Nielsen, 1968b). Nevertheless, the mere fact that we now know of viruses harmful to mosquitoes suggests that an intensified and really widespread search may eventually reveal related pathogens well suited to practical use against medically important insects.

B. RICKETTSIAE

Despite the occurrence of entomopathogenic rickettsiae among, e.g. scarabaeid beetles (Dutky and Gooden, 1950), craneflies (Müller-Kögler, 1958) and crickets (Vago and Martoja, 1963), Jenkins (1964) could list only 14 associations between this group of organisms and arthropod vectors. Nine of his associations involved lice, and rickettsiae of medical significance; two species caused relatively minor harm to mosquitoes; and one each occurred in sandflies, fleas and bedbugs. Vago (1964b) referred to his own experience in adapting a rickettsia of *Tipula paludosa* to *Aedes aegypti,* and suggested trying to adapt arthropod-pathogenic species to new hosts belonging to the same general taxonomic group as the natural host.

C. BACTERIA

Under this heading Jenkins (1964) listed 71 associations with medically important arthropods of all major groups except tabanids and spiders. Much of the relevant literature has concerned the normal microbial gut flora of the hosts investigated. In recent years, though, attention has been given to the feasibility of inhibiting muscoid fly production from the faeces of chickens and cattle by using *Bacillus thuringiensis* as a feed additive (Briggs, 1960; Burns *et al.,* 1961; Greenwood, 1964; Gingrich, 1965; Millar, 1965; Galichet, 1966). The active factor appears to be the thermostable exotoxin (Burgerjon and Galichet, 1965). Commercial preparations of this organism are now widely marketed, and the susceptibiility of various flies is being widely explored. Thus, Yendol and Miller (1967) have recently reported tests against face flies. The thermostable toxin is effective against other Diptera, including *Aedes aegypti.* Before leaving *B. thuringiensis,* it must be noted that housefly resistance to this species has been reported (Harvey and Howell, 1965).

Like *B. thuringiensis* (Briggs, 1964) *B. sphaericus* is easily mass-produced, flourishing and sporulating in both defined and complex media. Despite some discouraging early results against mosquitoes (Kellen *et al.,* 1965), it is currently giving rather more cause for optimism. Thus Singer *et al.* (1966)

found that a strain pathogenic for certain mosquito larvae grew poorly *in vitro* when first isolated, but that "suitable transfer and enrichment procedures soon resulted in satisfactory cultural conditions". They further pointed out that "the effectiveness of *B. sphaericus* against susceptible mosquito larvae depends on infection rather than any as yet identifiable toxic entity". Being able to survive as a saprophyte, *B. sphaericus* might, they considered, be able to maintain itself under field conditions for extended periods at sufficiently high population levels for effective control of susceptible mosquito larvae. However, noting that *B. sphaericus,* while ubiquitous, has not been shown to cause epizootics among mosquitoes in nature, they submitted that it might be necessary either to establish very high population levels of the pathogen or to select unusually virulent strains for field use.

The bacterial control of mosquitoes is now receiving widespread attention in the U.S.S.R. among other countries (Lavrentyev *et al.*, 1965). One thing is clear, a great deal of research (much of it broadly ecological) remains to be undertaken before bacterial pathogens can be considered ready for practical use against vectors. In particular, application techniques (cf. Grison and Bourguignon, 1965) must be perfected. Limited experience with synergistic effects in economic entomology to date, suggest that future joint application of bacterial pathogens and selective chemical pesticides, or the simultaneous use of such pathogens and, e.g. irradiation (Jafri, 1964, 1965a, b) merit thoughtful attention.

D. FUNGI

Many papers on *Coelomomyces* have appeared over the past decade. No longer thought to be restricted to mosquito hosts, the genus (now referred to the Chytridiomycetes) has been reported from sandflies (Leão and Pedroso, 1965), and possibly blackflies (Garnham and Lewis, 1959). Also, two long-overlooked references have been rediscovered by Weiser (Rašin, 1928, 1929) indicating its occurrence in chironomid midges. Many new host and locality records have been published, and new species described. Among these is *C. opifexi,* which in one particular pool has been recorded from 67% of the larvae of the host; the unique New Zealand brackish-water mosquito, *Opifex fuscus* (Pillai, personal communication, 1969).

Despite the encouraging outcome of the Tokelau Islands pilot project (Laird, 1967), and the evident effectiveness of certain of these fungi as natural controls of anopheline populations—Muspratt (1963) demonstrated up to 100% mortality in Zambian *A. gambiae* populations due to *C. indicus*—we are still very far from practical mass-production procedures. Madelin (1968) has devoted prolonged attention to the subject, and has obtained massive laboratory infections by the introduction into larval cultures of infective material derived directly from parasitized larvae. Also, Couch (1968) has followed the process of sporangial germination in *C. punctatus* and he and his associates have brought about both laboratory and field infections of *Anopheles quadrimaculatus* in North Carolina, U.S.A. However, no species of *Coelomomyces* has yet been cultivated on an artificial medium. This is an obvious prerequisite to the practical use of any members of the genus as biological control agents.

A number of workers have suggested the feasibility of employing *Entomophthora* spp. against, e.g. muscoid flies and mosquitoes. Although Madelin (1966) remarked that "the successful cultivation of entomophthoraceous fungi is still rather uncommon", Weiser (personal communication, 1966) has had success with species from both mosquitoes and muscoid flies. Field experiments involving *Entomophthora coronata* were in fact under consideration when work was suspended due to the realization that they might be a health hazard (see p. 403). In recent years there have been reports from many areas of heavy mortalities caused by *Entomophthora* in hibernating *Culex pipens* subsp. Pertinent observations have been published by Kuprijanova (1966) and Weiser and Batko (1966); van der Laan (personal communication, 1966) has informed me that large numbers of infected mosquitoes die while hibernating in caves in the Netherlands.

Trichomycetes of interest to us in the present context include members of the genera *Rubetella, Carouxella* and *Smittium.* Clark *et al.* (1963) established axenic cultures of two species of *Rubetella* from Californian mosquitoes and succeeded in infecting larvae in the laboratory. Coluzzi (1966) obtained experimental infections with a related organism in *A. gambiae,* and *Smittium* has been cultured too (Lichtwardt, 1964; Farr and Lichtwardt, 1967). However, much remains to be learnt about the complete life-cycles of these Trichomycetes, which are increasingly felt to be merely endocommensal or ectocommensal and not really injurious to the host.

Among the Deuteromycetes, or Fungi Imperfecti, *Beauveria bassiana* has received much attention (like *Bacillus thuringiensis*) as a broad-spectrum microbial control agent for use against economic insect pests. While, as Madelin (1966) emphasized, the genetics of virulence in this species "as indeed in all entomogenous fungi" are far from fully understood and merit critical study, preliminary experiments against vectors have not been encouraging (Clark *et al.*, 1967). An allied fungus *Metarrhizium anisopliae* can be artificially cultured, and its conidia may survive 16 years of lyophilized storage (Hesseltine *et al.*, 1960). Roberts (1967) has drawn attention to its possible usefulness against mosquitoes. Finally, it is noted that *Aspergillus* spp. are known to be pathogenic for certain arthropods of public health importance including bedbugs, houseflies, mosquitoes (Hati and Ghosh, 1965) and ticks (Kolomiyets, 1950). Amonkar (1965) reported that *A. flavus* causes high mortalities in houseflies, and the same species has been observed to destroy a *Cimex lectularius* colony in 18 days (Cockbain and Hastie, 1961). At least as interestingly, Beard and Walton (1965) have indicated that a toxin derived from *Aspergillus* is lethal to housefly larvae. Another fungus with a toxic extract showing some pathogenicity to mosquitoes and houseflies is a species of *Macrosporium* studied by Damodar *et al.* (1964) in India.

Mycological research topics meriting priority attention are the establishment of artificial cultures of the more promising candidates, studies of host specificity, and investigations into the genetic basis of virulence together with the prospect of increasing the virulence of selected species against target vectors. Roberts (1967), who advocated genetic manipulation (including somatic recombination) to produce desirable traits enhancing virulence, stressed that, "The genetics of entomogenous fungi is a virtually unexplored field."

E. PROTOZOANS

Of the many groups of Protozoa known to attack arthropod vectors–Jenkins (1964) listed 191 relationships involving all the main taxa of medically important insects–microsporidans include the more promising candidate biological control agents. While we still do not know nearly enough about the effects of many of the protozoans (especially various flagellates, gregarines and ciliates) on their vector hosts, and such knowledge is much to be desired because of its relevance to a proper understanding of both natural and laboratory mortalities, it is the Microsporida which cause the most spectacular epizootics. Not surprisingly, therefore, it is this group that has attracted the greatest attention in recent years. Comprehensive surveys (e.g. Chapman, 1964; Kellen, 1962, 1965) have yielded much new information. Many new species (especially of *Thelohania* from mosquitoes) have been described–although Weiser (1968b) has recently demonstrated that taxonomic criteria in these parasites are more plastic and subject to the influence of their host than some workers have appreciated. Appendix 7 contains many examples of vector/microsporidan relationships to supplement those published by Jenkins (1964). As one example of what is being accomplished in this field, the work of Kramer on octosporeosis of muscoid flies (1963-67) in Section 2 of Appendix 7 can be quoted. As regards field trials towards practical microbial control involving Microsporida, Reynolds' project on Nauru has already been mentioned.

F. NEMATODES

Dutky (1967) has claimed that *Neoaplectana carpocapsae* (DD 136) "and its associated bacterial insect pathogen" have great potentialities for the control of many insects, including certain vectors. This nematode is easy to propagate in very large numbers on easily maintained insect hosts, as well as on artificial media, and it remains viable in storage for long periods (Dutky, 1967). Welch and Bronskill (1962) demonstrated that larval *Aedes aegypti* infected by *N. carpocapsae* in the laboratory die within 1-1.5 days due to bacterial septicaemia. This same nematode/bacterial combination has also been field-tested against housefly larvae in chicken manure. It killed at least 40% of the maggots within two days of application and no fly breeding whatsoever remained three months later (Dutky, 1967).

In nature mermithid nematodes have sometimes caused considerable mosquito mortality. Thus Jenkins (1964) lists numerous papers reporting up to 100% infection of mosquitoes under field conditions, and a dramatic reduction in numbers of pest chironomid midges to a point not far short of eradication has been described by Wülker (1958, 1961). Parasite-induced intersexuality caused this population decline, and the same phenomenon has been noted for mermithids from other chironomids and *Culicoides* (Smith and Perry, 1967). Other vectors harbouring mermithids include tabanids in Alberta, Canada (Shamsuddin, 1966), and blackflies (Rubtsov, 1963; Welch, 1964).

Again, nematodes of the genus *Heterotylenchus* parasitize the face fly in the U.S.A. (Nickle, 1967; Stoffolano and Nickle, 1966), and cause parasitic castration of flea vectors of plague in the U.S.S.R. (Kurochkin, 1960). A diversity of other nematodes infect cockroaches (Roth and Willis, 1960; Kloss, 1966).

There is thus every likelihood that certain nematodes (among which *N. carpocapsae* is prominent on present evidence) will eventually be used against vectors as practical biological control agents. In this context Dutky (1967) has emphasized that *N. carpocapsae* is well suited to application in integrated control procedures, being resistant to most of the widely employed pesticides and applicable with conventional spraying equipment.

III. Possible Hazards of the Use of Microbial Agents in Vector Control

A. HYPERPARASITES AND PREDATORS

Even fungal pathogens are not without their own specific parasites, which might well reduce their efficiency in future commercially developed formulations unless adequate safeguards are ensured. Thus the ascomycete *Melanospora parasitica* attacks *Beauveria bassiana* in the U.S.S.R. (Shekhurina, 1960).

Tamashiro (1967) and Chapter 23 consider the deleterious and other possible effects of microbial pathogens on non-target arthropods of biological control value, the examples, however, being of economic and not health concern. This is a subject that deserves the attention of medical entomologists. It might be observed that the inadequately described *Coelomomyces notonectae* of backswimmers (Bogoyavlenskij, 1922; Keilin, 1927) could conceivably represent an infection derived from larval mosquito prey. Again, a microsporidan of the genus *Nosema* has been described from *Sperchon* watermites, predators on mosquito larvae in Ontario, Canada (Lipa, 1962).

In similar vein, if nematodes such as *N. carpocapsae* ever come into general use in spray preparations, it is possible that they will be vulnerable to various predators including protozoans and tardigrades (Doncaster and Hooper, 1961) as well as certain specialized nematode-trapping fungi (e.g. Cooke, 1963).

B. HEALTH HAZARDS

Details of this subject are given in Chapter 22. Present evidence suggests that entomopathogenic viruses are completely harmless to all vertebrates. Bacteria are another matter, though, and the exhaustive screening processes adopted in clearing *Bacillus thuringiensis* for commercial use might well be taken as a model in this context. As to rickettsiae, some species that are primarily pathogens of insects have also been shown in experiments to attack vertebrates (Vago, 1964a). There might be risks for man and other vertebrates in the practical use of insect-pathogenic fungi, too. Thus the muscoid fly pathogen *Entomophthora coronata* has been incriminated as a cause of phycomycosis in horses and man. Species of *Aspergillus* can cause serious infections in the lungs of various vertebrates; and as yet we have no way of knowing whether or not the future mass cultivation of such species as *Coelomomyces* might furnish a commercial product posing health risks ranging from allergies to infections like these.

As regards protozoans, species of *Nosema* have been described from rats and mice. Petri (1966) has shown that large doses of *N. culiculi* will kill mice. Finally, Foster (1963) has indicated that mermithid nematodes originating from *Glossina palpalis* may establish infections in man. While these infections are apparently benign when confined to the intestinal tract, they are severe if other organisms become involved.

In the light of these facts it is therefore urged that health hazards associated with the practical use of microbial control agents should be regarded as a major priority at this time. There would, thus, be everything to be said for establishing an appropriate International Reference Centre to play a leading role in the sequence of steps towards the practical use of pathogens for vector control.

References

Amonkar, S. V. (1965). *J. Invertebrate Path.* **7**, 513-514.

Anon. (1958). *Chronicle Wld Hlth Org.* **12**, 383.

Beard, R. L. and Walton, G. S. (1965). *J. Invertebrate Path.* **7**, 522-523.

Bennett, F. D. (1966). "Memorandum on the Possibilities of Biological Control of the Muscoid Flies by Hymenopterous Parasites", pp. 1-5. CIBC Report, Curepe, Trinidad. Mimeogr.

Bennett, F. D. and Legner, E. F. (1967). "Memorandum on the Possibilities of Biological Control of the Muscoid Flies by Hymenopterous Parasites". World Health Organization mimeographed document, WHO/VBC/67.22. 10 pp.

Bogoyavlenskij, N. V. (1922). *Arkh. russk. protist. Obschch.* **1**, 118-119.

Borgatti, A. L. and Guyer, G. E. (1963). *J. Insect Path.* **5**, 377-384.

Boyd, C. E. and Ferguson, D. E. (1964a). *Mosquito News* **24**, 19-21.

Boyd, C. E. and Ferguson, D. E. (1964b). *J. econ. Ent.* **57**, 430-431.

Briggs, J. D. (1960). *J. Insect Path.* **2**, 418-432.

Briggs, J. D. (1964). *Bull. Wld Hlth Org.* **31**, 495-497.

Briggs, J. D. (1966). "1965 Activities of the WHO International Reference Centre for Diagnosis of Diseases of Vectors". World Health Organization mimeographed document, WHO/EBL/66.73. 8 pp.

Briggs, J. D. (1967). "1966 Activities of the WHO International Reference Centre for Diagnosis of Diseases of Vectors". World Health Organization mimeographed document, WHO/VBC/67.8. 8 pp.

Burgerjon, A. and Galichet, P. F. (1965). *J. Invertebrate Path.* **7**, 263-264.

Burns, E. C., Wilson, B. H. and Tower, B. A. (1961). *J. econ. Ent.* **54**, 913-915.

Canning, E. U. (1957). *Riv. Malar.* **36**, 39-50.

Cantwell, G. E. and Laird, M. (1966). *J. Invertebrate Path.* **8**, 442-451.

Chapman, H. C. (1964). *Quarterly Reports, Insects Affecting Man and Animals Research Laboratory,* Lake Charles, Louisiana, U.S.A.

Chapman, H. C. (1967). "A Survey of Nauru Island for Mosquitoes and their Internal Pathogens and Parasites". Mimeographed document, World Health Organization, WHO/VBC/67.28. 11 pp.

Chapman, H. C., Clark, T. B., Woodard, D. B. and Kellen, W. R. (1966). *J. Invertebrate Path.* **8**, 545-546.

Clark, T. B., Kellen, W. R., Fukuda, T. and Lindegren, J. E. (1967). *Proc. Calif. Mosquito Contr. Ass.* **35**, 99.

Clark, T. B., Kellen, W. R. and Lindegren, J. E. (1963). *Nature, Lond.* **197**, 208-209.

Clark, T. B., Kellen, W. R. and Lum, T. M. (1965). *J. Invertebrate Path.* **7**, 519-521.

Cockbain, A. J. and Hastie, A. C. (1961). *J. Insect Path.* **3**, 95-97.

Cole, M. M. (1965). "Biological Control of Ticks by the Use of Hymenopterous Parasites. A Review". World Health Organization mimeographed document, WHO/EBL/43.65. 12 pp.

Coluzzi, M. (1966). *Proc. 1st Int. Congr. Parasitol.,* Rome, 1964 **I**, 592-593.

Cooke, R. C. (1963). *Ann. appl. Biol.* **51**, 295-301.

Couch, J. N. (1968). Proc. Joint U.S.-Japan Seminar on Microbial Control of Insect Pests, Fukuoka, April 21-23, 1967, pp. 93-105. U.S.-Japan Comm. Sci. Co-op. Panel 8, Inst. Biol. Control, Fukuoka, Japan.

Damodar, P., Perti, S. L. and Agarwal, P. N. (1964). *Indian J. Ent.* **26**, 110-112.

Doncaster, C. C. and Hooper, D. J. (1961). *Nematologia.* **6**, 333-335.

Dutky, S. R. (1967). *Abstr. Joint U.S.-Japan Semin. Microbial control Insect Pests. April 21-23, 1967,* pp. 49-50. U.S.-Japan Committee Sci. Cooperation, Panel 8, Fukuoka.

Dutky, S. R. and Gooden, E. L. (1950). *J. Bact.* **63**, 743-750.

Farr, D. F. and Lichtwardt, R. W. (1967). *Mycologia* **59**, 172-182.

Foster, R. (1963). *Ann. trop. Med. Parasit.* **57**, 347-358.

Franz, J. M. (1956-59). *Entomophaga* **1-14**, see Appendix 1F for pages.

Galichet, P. F. (1966). *Ann. Zootech.* **15**, 133-145.

Garnham, P. C. C. (1956). *Bull. Wld Hlth Org.* **15,** 845-847.
Garnham, P. C. C. and Lewis, D. J. (1959). *Trans. R. Soc. trop. Med. Hyg. Lond.* **53,** 12-40.
Gerberich, J. B. (1946). *Am. Midl. Nat.* **36,** 87-131.
Gerberich, J. B. and Laird, M. (1966). "Bibliography of Papers Relating to the Control of Mosquitoes by the Use of Fish. An Annotated Bibliography for the Years 1901-1966". *FAO Fisheries Technical Paper* No. 75, 1-70. Dec. 1968.
Gingrich, R. E. (1965). *J. econ. Ent.* **58,** 363-364.
Greenwood, E. S. (1964). *N.Z. Jl. Sci.* **7,** 221-226.
Grison, P. and Bourguignon, S. (1965). *C.r. hebd. Séanc. Acad. Agric. Fr.* **51,** 112-116.
Harris, P., Riordan, D. F. and Cooke, D. (1969). *Science,* **164,** 184-185.
Harvey, T. L. and Howell, D. E. (1965). *J. Invertebrate Path.* **7,** 92-100.
Hati, A. K. and Ghosh, S. M. (1965). *Bull. Calcutta Sch. trop. Med. Hyg.* **13,** 18-19.
Hesseltine, C. W., Bradle, B. J. and Benjamin, C. R. (1960). *Mycologia* **52,** 762-774.
Jafri, R. H. (1964). *Revue Path. vég. Ent. Agric. Fr.* **43,** 37-51.
Jafri, R. H. (1965a). *Proc. XII Int. Congr. Ent.,* London, July 1964, 747-748.
Jafri, R. H. (1965b). *J. Invertebrate Path.* **7,** 66-70.
Jenkins, D. W. (1964). "Pathogens, Parasites and Predators of Medically Important Arthropods". Annotated list and bibliography. Suppl. to Vol. 30, *Bull. Wld Hlth Org.* 150 pp.
Keilin, D. (1927). *Parasitology* **19,** 365-367.
Kellen, W. R. (1962). *Mosquito News* **22,** 87-95.
Kellen, W. R. (1965). *Proc. XII Int. Congr. Ent.,* London, July 1964, 728-729.
Kellen, W. R., Clark, T. B., Lindegren, J. E., Hoe, B. C., Rogoff, M. H. and Singer, S. (1965). *J. Invertebrate Path.* **7,** 442-448.
Kloss, G. R. (1966). *Pap. Avulsos Zool.,* São Paulo **18,** 147-188.
Kolomiyets, Y. S. (1950). *Priroda* (Mosk.) **39,** 64-65. (In Russian.)
Kramer, J. P. (1966). *Am. Midl. Nat.* **75,** 214-220.
Kuprijanova, E. S. (1966). *Zool. Zh.* **45,** 675-678. (In Russian.)
Kurochkin, J. V. (1960). *Dokl. Akad. Nauk. USSR* **135,** 1281-1284. (In Russian.)
Laird, M. (1959). *Acta trop. (Basel)* **16,** 331-355.
Laird, M. (1963). *Bull. Wld Hlth Org.* **29** (suppl.), 147-151.
Laird, M. (1967). *Chronicle Wld Hlth Org.* **21,** 18-26.
Laird, M. and Colless, D. H. (1962). *Proc. XI Int. Congr. Ent.,* Vienna, 1960 **2,** 867-868.
Laird, M. and Wright, J. W. (1966). *Proc. FAO Symposium on Integrated Pest Control,* Rome **3,** 77-79.
Lavrentyev, P. A., Salnikov, V. G. and Anisin, S. D. (1965). *Veterinariya* (Mosk.) **42,** 107-108. (In Russian.)
Leão, A. E. A. and Pedroso, M. C. (1965). *Mycopath. Mycol. appl.,* den Haag **26,** 305-307. (In Portuguese.)
Legner, E. F., Bay, E. C. and White, E. B. (1967). *Ann. ent. Soc. Am.* **60,** 462-468.
Lichtwardt, R. W. (1964). *Am. J. Bot.* **51,** 836-842.
Linley, J. R. and Nielsen, H. T. (1968a). *J. Invertebrate Path.* **12,** 7-16.
Linley, J. R. and Nielsen, H. T. (1968b). *J. Invertebrate Path.* **12,** 17-24.
Lipa, J. J. (1962). *Bull. Acad. polon. Sci.* **10,** 435-437.
Madelin, M. F. (1966). *Ann. Rev. Ent.* **11,** 423-448.
Madelin, M. F. (1968). *J. Elisha Mitchell Sci. Soc.* **84,** 115-124.
Millar, E. S. (1965). *N.Z. Jl. agric. Res.* **8,** 721-722.
Müller-Kögler, E. (1958). *Naturwissenschaften* **45,** 248.
Muspratt, J. (1963a). *Bull. Wld Hlth Org.* **29,** 81-86.
Muspratt, J. (1963b). "Progress Report (May, 1963) on Investigations Concerning Three Mosquito Pathogens at Livingstone, Northern Rhodesia". Mimeographed document, World Health Organization, WHO/EBL/12. 7 pp.
Muspratt, J. (1965). *Bull. Wld Hlth Org.* **33,** 140-144.
Nickle, W. R. (1967). *J. Parasit.* **53,** 398-401.
Pagayon, A. U. (1963). *Hlth. Dep. Bull. (Manila),* 1960-63, **32-35,** 41-45.
Petri, M. (1966). *Acta path. Microbiol. scand.* **66,** 13-30.

Rašin, K. (1928). *Věst. VI Sjezdu Česk. přirodozpytcu v Praze* **3,** 146.
Rašin, K. (1929). *Biol. Spis. Vys. Šk. Zvěrolék* **8,** 1-13.
Reynolds, D. G. (1966). *Nature, Lond.* **210,** 967.
Rivers, C. F. (1964). *Discovery* **25,** 27-31.
Roberts, D. W. (1967). *In* "Insect Pathology and Microbial Control" (P. A. van der Laan, ed.), pp. 243-246. North-Holland Publ. Co., Amsterdam.
Roth, L. M. and Willis, E. R. (1960). *Smithson. misc. Collns 141,* Publ. 4422, 470 pp.
Rothman, H. and Woodhead, M. *Nature, Lond.* **220,** 1053-1054.
Rubtsov, I. A. (1963). *Zool. Zh.* **42,** 1768-1784. (In Russian.)
Shamsuddin, M. (1966). *Quaest. ent.* **2,** 253-256.
Shekhurina, T. A. (1960). *Botan. Zh.* **45,** 606-608. (In Russian.)
Singer, S., Goodman, N. S. and Rogoff, M. H. (1966). *Ann. N.Y. Acad. Sci.* **139,** 16-23.
Smith, W. W. and Perry, V. G. (1967). *J. econ. Ent.* **60,** 1025-1027.
Stoffolano, J. G., Jr. and Nickle, W. R. (1966). *J. econ. Ent.* **59,** 221-222.
Tamashiro, M. (1967). *Abstr. Joint U.S.-Japan Semin. Microbial Control Insect Pests,* pp. 55-57. U.S.-Japan Committee Sci. Cooperation. Panel 8, Fukuoka.
Vago, C. (1964a). *Rev. Path. veg. Ent.* **43,** 101-111.
Vago, C. (1964b). *Bull. Wld Hlth Org.* **31,** 513-517.
Vago, C. and Martoja, R. (1963). *C.r. hebd. Séanc. Acad. Sci. Paris* **256,** 1045-1047.
Weiser, J. (1963). *Bull. Wld Hlth Org.* **28,** 121-127.
Weiser, J. (1964). *Bull. Wld Hlth Org.* **31,** 483-485.
Weiser, J. (1965). *Bull. Wld Hlth Org.* **33,** 586-588.
Weiser, J. (1968a). Guide to field determination of major groups of pathogens and parasites affecting arthropods of public health importance. Mimeographed document, World Health Organization, WHO/VBC/68.59. 11 pp. + 13 plates with 48 photographic illustrations.
Weiser, J. (1968b). *In* Abstracts, *XIII Int. Congr. Ent. Moscow, 1968,* p. 295.
Weiser, J. and Batko, A. (1966). *Folia Parasitol.* **13,** 144-149.
Welch, H. E. (1964). *Bull. Wld Hlth Org.* **31,** 857-863.
Welch, H. E. and Bronskill, J. F. (1962). *Can. J. Zool.* **40,** 1263-1268.
Whiting, A. R. (1967). *Q. Rev. Biol.* **42,** 333-406.
Williamson, K. B. (1949). *In* "Malariology" (M. F. Boyd, ed.), Vol. 2, pp. 1360-1384. Saunders, Philadelphia.
Woodard, D. B. and Chapman, H. C. (1968). *J. Invertebrate Path.* **11,** 296-301.
World Health Organization (1958). "Expert Committee on Insecticides, Eighth Report". *Wld Hlth Org. techn. Rep. Ser.* 153.
World Health Organization (1964). *Bull. Wld Hlth Org.* **31,** 433-622.
Wülker, W. (1958). *Gew. u. Abwässer,* **20,** 61-67.
Wülker, W. (1961). *Arch. Hydrobiol., Suppl.* **25,** 127-181.
Wülker, W. (1965). *Z.f. Parasitenkunde* **26,** 29-49.
Yendol, W. G. and Miller, E. M. (1967). *J. econ. Ent.* **60,** 860-864.

CHAPTER 19

Influence of Environment and Modern Trends in Crop Management on Microbial Control

J. M. FRANZ

Biologische Bundesanstalt für Land- und Forstwirtschaft, Institut für biologische Schädlingsbekämpfung, Darmstadt, Germany

I. Environment

The environment is considered here as the sum of all external factors that influence interaction between pathogen and host. The host is also part of the environment of the pathogen and vice versa. The activities of man are emphasized as environmental factors among the factors orientated in Fig. 1, which indicates the complexity of the interrelations to be considered, and the scheme to be followed in their study. One particular activity of man, the application of pathogens, is a vital environmental feature, ranging from the micro-aspect of perhaps a droplet of water in a spray bearing a formulated spore to its destination, to man's choice of strain, storage, timing, dosage, mode of application, formulation and integration. These aspects form the subjects of several chapters and will not be considered here in detail, but they must be borne in mind during this discussion. Rather, the other important form of man's activities—as architect of the crop—will be subjected to detailed analysis.

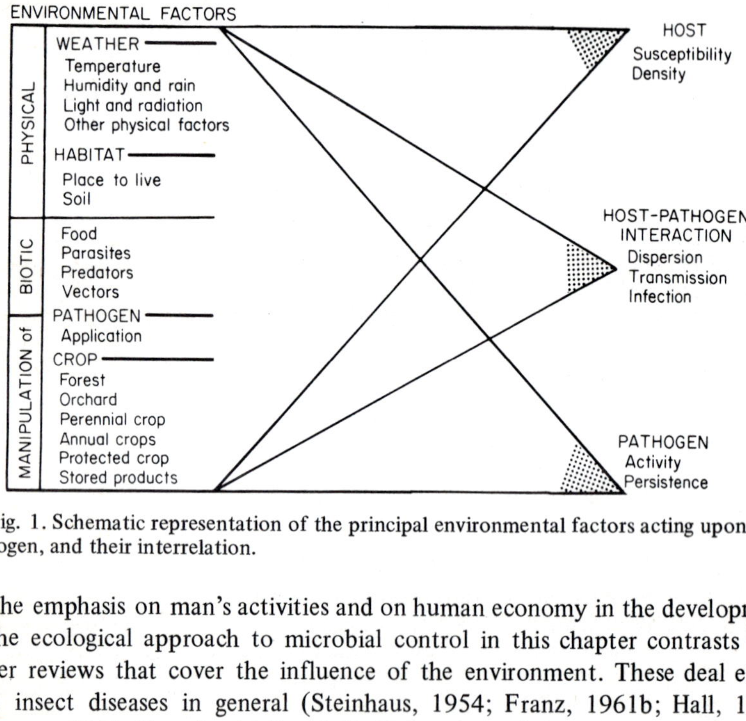

Fig. 1. Schematic representation of the principal environmental factors acting upon host, pathogen, and their interrelation.

The emphasis on man's activities and on human economy in the development of the ecological approach to microbial control in this chapter contrasts with earlier reviews that cover the influence of the environment. These deal either with insect diseases in general (Steinhaus, 1954; Franz, 1961b; Hall, 1961; Cameron, 1963; Tanada, 1963, 1967; Hurpin, 1967) or with diseases due to particular pathogen groups (Steinhaus, ed., 1963; van der Laan, ed., 1967; Weiser, 1961, on protozoans; Müller-Kögler, 1965, on fungi; Krieg, 1967a, on *Bacillus thuringiensis*).

II. Modern Trends in Crop Management

Crop management is understood here as the total of man's effort to produce organic matter, particularly to cultivate plants for food and fibre. Trends result primarily from attempts to improve the economic balance of this process and to achieve higher yields from lower energy input. Some common features are recognizable in the development of crop management in most technically advanced regions. These will serve as the basis for our discussion on the influence of this type of agriculture or silviculture on microbial control.

At least in agriculture, there is a trend towards intensive, large-scale, single crop units operated mechanically. This trend is usually only practicable in large-scale monoculture. The demand for particular commodities, or trade factors, may force farmers to cultivate plants or animals outside their optimum area. Traditional crop rotation is frequently sacrificed to the repetition of immediately profitable crops. Obviously, this trend influences pest control. Some contrasting side-tracks also appear, mainly in overpopulated areas like continental Europe: hobby gardening, where the occupation but not the yield is the main interest; orchards and fields not treated with synthetic chemicals but fertilized only with organic matter to produce plants intended to withstand pests naturally. Depending on the priority of profit, occupation, or emphasis on health, the choice of pest control measures will be different.

The situation in forestry and timber production is at least as variable as in agriculture. Only two extremes will be mentioned: (1) the monoculture of valuable tree species over large areas, usually preceded by the profitable exploitation of trees from more or less mixed and seemingly inexhaustible virgin stands; (2) in areas like Central Europe, where timber production now adds little to the national income, the forest cover is recognized as immensely valuable for more general reasons like water supply, oxygen production, nature conservation or protection against erosion, and where care is taken to preserve healthy and mixed forests as recreation areas. Obviously, the management of this "crop" will again depend on priorities set partially by the political or sociological situation. Where immediate profit ceases to be the overriding parameter, long-term, ecological viewpoints become acceptable to forest management in its effort to preserve the stability of the plant community; then, biological methods of pest control are more readily considered. Microbial control, thus, will be affected by environmental factors including those of human origin like crop management.

III. Microbial Control

Microbial control is part of biological control and is concerned with the employment of micro-organisms and/or their products by man for pest control. Nematodes and mites are included in this review only insofar as they act as vectors of pathogenic micro-organisms, as do many insects and other animals. The principal pathogens or germs of insects are bacteria, rickettsiae, fungi, protozoans and viruses. They are used in their natural status or, more frequently, as pathogen preparations or formulated pathogens. The term "microbial insecticide" is avoided here because it is likely to minimize the organismic nature of pathogens and the fundamental differences that exist between chemical insecticides and pathogens. In brief, these differences (Franz, 1964a) are:

(a) Pathogens approved for microbial control are harmless to vertebrates and more selective than chemicals (Chapters 22 and 23).
(b) The appearance of host strains resistant to pathogens is believed to be less likely than to chemicals (Chapter 20).
(c) Virulent strains of pathogens can be selected (Chapter 30).
(d) Pathogens can persist biologically by transmission from generation to generation of host.
(e) Pathogens can be dispersed by the release of contaminated or infected insects.
(f) Pathogens influence target insect populations more deeply than is indicated by simple mortality figures (see below).

Microbial control can be, admittedly, in some ways similar to chemical control if it is used only to achieve short-term effects as nowadays particularly with *Bacillus thuringiensis.* The degrees of permanency of control grade into a transition with the long-term effect. The latter begins when, in addition to the treated individuals, the subsequent generation is also affected, the ultimate degree being enzootic establishment of the pathogen.

Environmental factors usually influence short- and long-term control differently. Physical factors (Fig. 1) are more important for short-term control than are biotic factors and the pathogens are affected by these factors similarly to chemical insecticides. In long-term control, all factors act upon host, pathogen, and their interaction in a more complex way. Environmental factors affect host susceptibility and density as well as the virulence and persistence of the pathogen or its dispersion, transmission, and infection processes. The same pathogen can affect target pest populations in the short or long term, depending on the behaviour of the host, the nature of its habitat, and the dosage of pathogen applied.

IV. Checking the Results of Microbial Control

Methods of evaluation depend on the nature of the habitat (crop), the behaviour of the host, and the action of the pathogen. In general, microbial preparations produced by industry and evaluated by economic entomologists or growers have to compete with chemical insecticides in terms of applicability and costs. With both short-term pathogens and chemicals, the rate of mortality is the effect to be measured, and the higher the mortality the better the insecticide is usually considered to be. Lack of specialists familiar with the special problems posed by the use of pathogenic organisms has caused serious difficulties during the course of obtaining registration. Authorities have rarely acknowledged the importance of the absence of residues toxic to warm-blooded animals or man or harmful to beneficial arthropods and bees (Hall, 1963).

There are some important features differentiating the methods of checking the effectiveness of long-term microbial control from those applied to chemical control. Unlike chemical control, immediate mortality is not the only criterion of measurement. Individuals sublethally infected by virus disease are sometimes needed to carry over the epizootic from one generation to the next e.g. *Neodiprion sertifer*, the European pine sawfly (Bird, 1953) and *N. swainei*, Swaine's jack-pine sawfly (Smirnoff, 1967). Here, local extinction is not desirable and medium mortality bringing the insect population below the economic threshold is superior to heavy mortality.

Another point is the selective removal of more females than males by pathogens. Female pine sawflies (*N. sertifer* and *Neodiprion pratti pratti*) have, for instance, one more larval instar than males of the same species. Hence, they are exposed longer to virus applications; males reach the resistant prepupal stage earlier (Bird, 1961; McIntyre and Dutky, 1961). The general aspects of a shift in the sex ratio through disease are discussed by Campbell (1963).

The relatively slow action of pathogens on hosts often makes it difficult to measure effectiveness by routine methods adapted to insecticide application. Sampling procedures are reviewed by Morris (1960). Sometimes, comparative counts of different instars have been combined in an effort to assess the complete effect of microbial control, e.g. against the gypsy moth, *Lymantria dispar* (Connola *et al.*, 1966). Some widely accepted corrections take account of the different intensities of pest outbreaks and make figures comparable. Before the complete effect of microbial control can be measured, natural limiting factors may influence the untreated check pest population so much that the usual correcting formulae, like those of Abbott (1925) or Schwerdtfeger (1932), become impracticable. Further, early application of pathogens to infect very young instars, because these are usually most susceptible, may prevent population counts before treatment. These and other reasons (p. 432, post-larval mortality) led to the conclusion (Franz, 1968) that, particularly after microbial control, the assessment of damage or leaf area preserved on the crop may often be a better method of measuring the effectiveness of control. The eventual conservation of cultivated plants above the economic threshold rather than quick kill of many pest individuals will be decisive for the evaluation of the method. This is true already for the short-term microbial control, but still more so for a permanent or semi-permanent effect in the long-term. In discussing the debilitating or sterilizing effect of pathogens, Neilson (1965) came to the same conclusion: "In forest entomological problems the effect any biological control agent may have in influencing the magnitude and direction of population fluctuations of the host over several generations is often much more important than the immediate insecticidal effect that might be achieved a few days after the first application."

V. Crop and Pest Management

After discussing trends in crop management and microbial control, it will be useful to clarify the relation of both to pest control or pest management. With the developing pattern of modern agriculture and forestry towards less diversity of plant cover, plant-feeding insects are encouraged to multiply and to become pests. Counter measures have long been predominantly concerned with killing these pests, rather than with preventing pest outbreaks by increasing the resistance of the ecosystem to them. Recent difficulties caused by the application of chemical pesticides as the only means of control led to more comprehensive methods of pest control–integrated control–which emphasize the need to acknowledge the entity of an ecosystem (Chapter 1).

One of the salient points of the integrated approach to pest control is not the total elimination, but only the reduction of the pest below the *economic threshold.* This threshold is easier to define than to determine. It is the level of pest abundance above which crop losses caused by, or to be expected from, the pest are higher than the minimum total cost of control measures. In assessing the cost of crop protection, deleterious indirect side-effects, like the triggering of outbreaks of facultative pests, have to be considered as costs. In order to cover such side-effects, as a rule of thumb, the cost of the insecticidal control of one pest which is approaching the tolerance level ("action threshold" of Stern *et al.*, 1959) can be doubled before it is used to determine the economic threshold (Steiner and Baggiolini, 1968). The prediction of population dynamics is required to assess the future of the pest population, to find a realistic value for the losses to be expected and the economic threshold. Then, population figures can be transformed into crop losses or expenses for control.

Usually, the higher the cash value of a crop, the lower the economic threshold of its pests. Cultural changes and population shifts influence this threshold. If the public has a high standard of living and, for instance, dislikes fruits showing minor defects of complexion, it is most difficult to set up an integrated control programme on the basis of a tolerance level of almost zero. However, threshold levels of pest populations are almost invariably higher than expected. This holds particularly for damage to parts of the plant that are not harvested or sold. Spectacular loss of leaf may not significantly alter the yield if it happens late in the season, e.g. with potatoes.

Crop losses plus control costs can be tolerated by the grower up to a certain limit, which may be called the *economy limit* (Fig. 2). This limit depends on the margin of profit on which the grower is operating. From this the amount afforded to losses due to the depradation of pests and to crop protection can be assessed. If no cheap control measures are available and control costs exceed the economy limit, it is economic to tolerate the crop loss. The range between the actual expenses for control plus crop losses and the economy limit, i.e. between

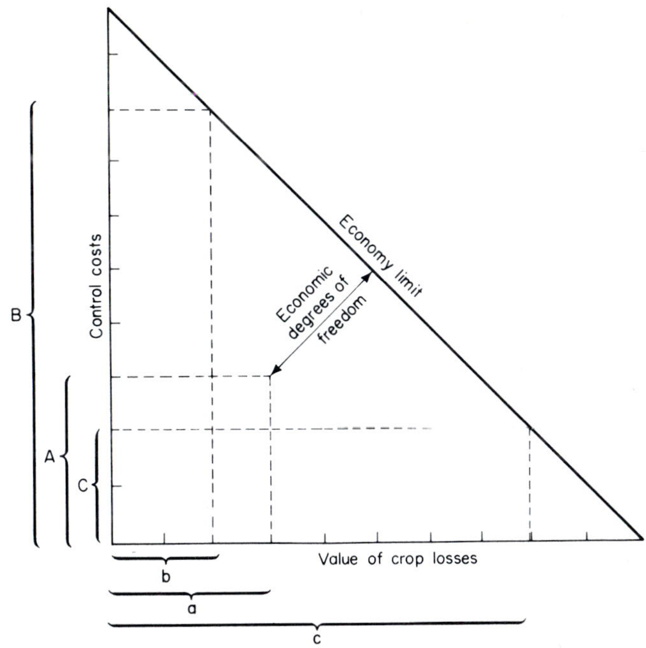

Fig. 2. Relationship between tolerable expenses for control and tolerable value of crop losses. The scale is such that one unit of expenses for control equals one unit of loss of crop value. The maximal control costs plus loss of crop value to be tolerated depends on economics: if expenses or losses exceed this limit (economy limit), there will be no economic justification any more for this crop to be grown under the specific conditions. Inside this frame, expenses for control and crop losses are interchangeable entities, but the tolerable total of these entities is constant. A = example for medium total control cost; a = corresponding economic threshold, expressed as crop loss to be tolerated. B = example for high control cost which allows only crop losses, b, if the economy limit is not to be exceeded. C = example for low control cost which allows high crop losses, c, before the economy limit is exceeded. In cases B and C, there are no economic degrees of freedom left. They can be regained if control costs, B, or crop losses, c, are reduced without altering the corresponding parameters, b, or C.

the lower and the upper limit for possible total losses, represents the economic degrees of freedom of Chant (1966) as indicated in Fig. 2.

Pest management procedures have their bearing on microbial control. The *permanence of a host population,* although at low levels, may insure long-term action of pathogens after occasional application (examples in Part X). Any prediction of population dynamics includes *assessment of losses to be expected from diseases.* This was shown for the nun moth, *(Lymantria monacha)* by precocious rearing from the egg by Janisch (1959) and is apparently now in regular use in some places in the U.S.S.R.; larvae of the potato beetle *(Leptinotarsa decemlineata),* or the brown-tail moth *(Nygmia phaeorrhoea =*

Euproctis chrysorrhoea) and of other caterpillars are classified according to their haemolymph condition (pathogens, haemocytes) to determine their state of health and outbreak potential (Lappa, 1967). Another parameter in the determination of the economic threshold is the *cost of control action.* Pathogens that permanently reduce the average host population level below the economic threshold, of course, economize so much that the tolerable level of the pest can be higher (example Cc in Fig. 2) than after costly single or repeated, short-term applications of control measures (example Bb in Fig. 2). Enough hosts may be conserved to maintain the disease in an enzootic state ready to react when insect density increases. This equation of pest numbers with degrees of economic damage and, in turn, with monetary losses is required for the stepwise development of pest management schemes in which biological measures are integrated appropriately, according to their merits and potentials.

Microbial control can be combined with other types of control. Pathogens of one type can be combined with *pathogens* of another type as well as with many chemical *pesticides.* Full efficiency of microbial control is frequently assured only if highly mobile *vectors* are present. Therefore, preservation of the floral and faunal diversity of an ecosystem can contribute to the dispersion of pathogens (Pimentel, 1961; Franz, 1964b; Rivers, 1967). The colonization of entomophages *(parasitic arthropods and predators)* before or together with pathogens has contributed to some outstanding successes, for instance with the European spruce sawfly *(Gilpinia (Diprion) hercyniae)* (p. 426). Microbial control can be combined with another method of biological control–*autocidal control*–during the preparatory stage, when the pest numbers have to be reduced before mass release of sterile or genetically inferior individuals is effective, and/or during the release phase so that artifical contamination or sublethal infection is combined with the genetic deterioration (Knipling, 1960; Lawson, 1966). *Resistant varieties* of cultivated plants may enhance the effect of pathogens. The effect of nuclear polyhedrosis virus (NPV) against the bollworm *(Heliothis zea)* and the tobacco budworm *(Heliothis virescens)* in Texas was, for instance, fully satisfactory if applied on a somewhat resistant variety of cotton (Fernandez *et al.,* 1969). Other examples of combinations with microbial control are given in Part X of this chapter.

There are already examples of complete success following the judicious integration (which is more than the simple addition) of various pest control methods. The spotted alfalfa aphid *(Therioaphis trifolii)* is being permanently suppressed in California and some neighbouring States by a combination of resistant alfalfa varieties, native and introduced parasites and predators, disease organisms where effects can be intensified by manipulating moisture conditions, and a particular pesticide at concentrations that permit natural enemies to survive and to be effective (Hagen and van den Bosch, 1968). Another example, still being developed, is the control of the tobacco hornworm *(Manduca quinquemaculata)* in North Carolina by a combination of: time of planting; insecticide applied rarely and only to the tops of the plants, because natural limitation factors often make control unnecessary; establishing artificial colonies of predatory *Polistes* wasps; destruction of post-harvest sucker growth to reduce the overwintering pest population, which depends on this food; application of *Bacillus thuringiensis* gradually replacing chemical insecticides (Rabb *et al.*, 1957; Lawson *et al.*, 1961). Also, *B. thuringiensis* is used in the integrated control schemes for apple orchards, e.g. in Canada (Jaques, 1965), in Germany (Steiner and Baggiolini, 1968) and against *Hyponomeuta* species at the blossom time in Germany.

The development of such pest management systems will continue to progress not because of their derivation from logical or ecological thinking, but because of fear of insecticide resistance and of toxic hazards in the human environment (Beirne, 1967). National and international (WHO sponsored) regulations and recommendations will also contribute to the shift away from the proximate remedy to the ultimate solution of plant protection by an integrated approach. Microbial control will become one element in the new direction. Its incorporation into crop and pest management systems should not be overlooked, although, in the rest of the chapter, it will be largely considered in isolation, from the viewpoint of its dependence on environmental factors.

VI. Stress and Outbreak Status of the Insect Population

Environmental influence on natural epizootics is similar to that on microbial control, particularly in the long-term. Therefore, observations on the effect of environment on natural diseases of insects will be used to supplement examples of applied microbial control. The influence of factors on the host, on the pathogen, and on their interrelation will be treated as in Fig. 1. Those factors will be selected which show a clear relation to diseases and to their application in biological control.

Before treating single factors, two complex effects of the environment on the host will be considered, stress and outbreak status. Weather, directly or indirectly, alters the general condition of the host in a way, termed *stress,* that predisposes it to infection and activates inapparent infections. This then disrupts the homeostasis of the insect (Steinhaus, 1960; Jaques, 1961, 1962). The effect of environmental factors as stressors depends greatly on their intensity. Numerous laboratory experiments have been reported on stressors and incitants of disease (Pimentel and Shapiro, 1962; Aruga, 1963; Tanada, 1965, 1967). Most of these papers deal with virus diseases, some also with protozoan diseases. Latent virus infections have been activated mainly by physical factors, food quality, application of various chemicals or other pathogens like insect viruses from other hosts or superinfection with species-specific virus. No universal stressor has yet been discovered, but temperature and humidity seem to act as stressors most commonly in nature (Bergold, 1958).

Dosages of *insecticides* sublethal to the target pest (host) have been used as stressors and incitants (Chapter 14). The ecological point of view is rarely considered in papers on this subject. Dosages of chemicals sublethal to the target host may well be detrimental to more susceptible insects, particularly to parasitic microhymenoptera. This is a real danger, because low dosages of broad spectrum and persistent insecticides (which have been used in many instances) may selectively kill the susceptible entomophagous arthropods and thereby endanger one of the great advantages of microbial control, its lack of harm to other members of the biocoenosis. Unpublished observations by the author after adding small amounts of DDT (12 g of pure DDT per hectare) to *B. thuringiensis* during experiments against the oak tortricid *(Tortrix viridana)* in 1968 point in this direction. The harmlessness to entomophages of insecticides used as stressors should be checked carefully before field application.

Other stressors are *pathogens* which induce activation of latent virus infections, e.g. granulosis of the fall webworm *(Hyphantria cunea)* activated by application of *B. thuringiensis* to late larval instars (Krieg and Schmidt, 1962). This is of practical importance because fall webworms live together in groups composed of different instars. Whereas young larvae are susceptible to *B. thuringiensis* older ones die only after induction of latent viruses.

Superinfection with viruses of the same kind has proved to be very effective in microbial control. The practical consequence is that control operations with many viruses are very likely to succeed if the untreated host population first shows signs of the disease. For instance, most successful virus (NPV) trials with the pine sawfly *(Neodiprion sertifer)* in Europe report slight incidence of the disease in the control plot and are therefore considered to be superinfections (Franz and Niklas, 1954; Kudler, 1965; Schönherr, 1965). Many other examples could be cited where natural mortality as an epizootic was either insufficient or too late. Application of the same pathogen, usually a virus, that had caused the incipient epizootic then resulted in drastic reduction of the host population, no doubt greatly supported by superinfection. So far, no observations have been published on the inhibition of virus diseases in the field by the occurrence of other diseases of the same or of a similar type (interference of viruses) (for inhibitions in the laboratory see Chapter 21).

Host populations of different *outbreak status* have shown different susceptibility to artificial (or natural) infection. Some observations indicate that some insect species, particularly those which undergo more or less cyclic gradations regularly terminated by epizootics (like the Lepidoptera: *Lymantria dispar; Lymantria monacha; Zeiraphera griseana; Dasychira pudibunda; Aporia crataegi*), become more tolerant of the pathogen involved (*Z. griseana*, Martignoni, 1957; *Phryganidia californica,* Martignoni and Schmid, 1961;

L. dispar, Vasiljević, 1961; *Malacosoma californicum (pluviale),* Wellington, 1962; general discussion of quality problems, Franz, 1965). Some experiments have investigated the problem of when to apply microbial control to achieve maximum effect and duration of control. Treatment of the pine processionary *(Thaumetopoea pityocampa)* with cytoplasmic polyhedrosis viruses (CPV) in France, the first field experiment of this type at the culmination of the gradation, although very successful (Biliotti *et al.*, 1959; Grison *et al.*, 1959) did not prevent the next outbreak from appearing simultaneously in treated and untreated regions about six years later (Grison, 1968). A French/Swiss joint application in 1967 against extremely low populations of the larch budmoth, *Z. griseana* and covering a whole valley of the Alps still awaits evaluation (Grison, 1968). Stairs (1965) has shown in Canada that artificial initiation of virus epizootics is possible at a very early stage of an outbreak of the forest tent caterpillar *(Malacosoma disstria).* Similarly in Japan, application of CPV of *Dendrolimus spectabilis* in pine forests caused high mortality during the early outbreak stages, but had less effect during culmination of the gradation (Koyama and Katagiri, 1968; Katagiri, 1969). It is quite natural that studies of this type which manipulate the pest and its epizootic by interference at an optimum moment were carried out in the forest where large and relatively undisturbed areas are available. The development of this transitional grade between short- and long-term microbial control will help to obtain maximum and lasting benefits from the use of endemic pathogens, fully exploiting their organismic nature.

VII. Physical Factors

A. TEMPERATURE

High temperatures sometimes increase the resistance of *host* insects to viruses (review, Tanada, 1965). These temperatures are within the range of normal summer air temperatures, e.g. 36° C, *Pieris rapae* with granulosis; 29.4° C, *Gilpinia (Diprion) hercyniae* infected by NPV; 39° C, *Trichoplusia ni* and *Heliothis zea* infected by NPV; 35° C, *Colias eurytheme* infected by CPV (Tanada and Chang, 1968). Exposure of GV of *P. brassicae* to slightly greater degrees of heat for a longer time (e.g. to 40° C for 20 days) destroyed most virus infectivity (David, 1967). Exposure of natural populations to extreme heat of summer may cause either failure of control operations or disappearance of latent infections. This (and radiation, p. 421) should be kept in mind when considering the use of viruses in hot climates. In contrast, Dikasova (1966) reports particularly good infection by GV of *Euxoa segetum* on cotton at 45° C.

Temperatures that inactivate the *pathogen* are usually too high to be encountered under natural conditions. *Bacillus thuringiensis* applied to beeswax foundation against *Galleria mellonella* is endangered by wax temperatures near

60° C (depending on exposure period) during processing (Kulikov, 1966; Burges and Bailey, 1968). Grinding must be carefully supervised during the formulation of germs to avoid detrimental heat.

Mostly, temperature influences the *host-pathogen relation* as a whole. In general, the optimum temperature range of the host also favours disease, apart from stress conditions mentioned above. Usually high temperatures accelerate disease and insects are killed more rapidly. This is of great practical importance when quick protection of crops is desired. As infection occurs *per os* with most pathogens (except fungi), it is due in part to an acceleration of feeding at high temperatures. The interrelation of the three-fold temperature regulated system plant, insect and pathogen during microbial control operations has been studied, for instance, with the oak tortricid, *T. viridana* controlled by *B. thuringiensis* (Franz *et al.*, 1967). Application of bacteria on oaks just showing the first small leaves gave satisfactory control as long as air temperatures of 15° C were reached daily for several hours. If temperatures remained low, at 8°-10° C, larvae ceased to feed. However, because of the lower thermal threshold of the plant, the leaves continued to grow, gradually decreasing the spore/crystal deposit per unit leaf area. An old rule from the era of stomach poison application becomes valid again–particularly on fast-growing leaves: apply the control agent when temperatures are likely to remain above the activity threshold of the host at least for some hours during the days following treatment. Higher doses can partially compensate the depressing effect of low temperature, e.g. an increase from 0.2% to 0.5% or 1.0% suspension when control of the ermine moth (*Hyponomeuta* sp.) is required at average day temperatures below 17° C (Rybina, 1966). As a general rule, an increase of *B. thuringiensis* dosages up to 10 times is recommended in the northern parts of the U.S.S.R. around Leningrad as compared to the South (Fedorintchik, 1964).

Similarly for viruses, GV of the red-banded leaf roller *(Argyrotaenia velutinana)* made a greater impact in southern U.S.A. than in the north (Glass, 1958). The European spruce sawfly, *Gilpinia (Diprion) hercyniae*, was controlled more rapidly in areas with three host generations per year compared to those with one or two generations (Bird, 1964). (Soil inhabiting insects see p. 422.) Thus, the geographical range for the use of some pathogens seems to be correlated to prevailing temperature conditions. As this seems to be a result of the thermal activity threshold of the host, the discovery of pathogen strains more active at low temperature, as reported for *B. thuringiensis* (Smirnoff, 1963), will probably be of no help. Obviously because entomophagous fungi usually invade the host through the integument, the temperature range of massive mortality caused by mycosis extends lower than usually observed with other diseases. Due to the overriding influence of humidity for fungi and the difficulty of separating influences predisposing the host and limiting the fungus, no clear-cut field experiences are available (Müller-Kögler, 1965).

The temperature influence in the soil has been compared in the laboratory for several pathogens attacking cockchafer larvae *(Melolontha melolontha)* at 17°, 20° and 25°C (Hurpin, 1968). Mycosis *(Beauveria tenella)* and bacteriosis *(B. popilliae* strain *"Melolontha")* had optima at 20°C, rickettsiosis *(Rickettsiella melolonthae)* at 17°C, nosematosis *(Nosema melolonthae)* at 20°C, coccidosis *(Adelina melolonthae)* was better the higher the temperature, and spindle-inclusion virosis *(Vagoiavirus melolonthae)* acted independently of temperature.

The "activator" role of temperature on the pathogen was important for the fungus, the "depressor" role on the host being equal in all experiments. The limitation of milky disease caused by *B. popilliae* strain *"melolonthae"* to third instar larvae during the summer of the year following cockchafer flights in France, and the presence of rickettsiosis in cold forest soils are examples of epizootic phenomena elucidated by these results, which agree with field results of Ferron (1967) on the same host using *B. tenella* and with American experience on the Japanese beetle *(Popillia japonica)* (Dutky, 1963). Limits for development and application of milky diseases are within the range of 15°-36°C soil temperature. The success of milky disease as a control factor is fairly dependent on the range of soil temperatures encountered and more particularly on the threshold temperatures of the various stages of the insect. The threshold for pupation is only about 1°C below that for disease development. This narrows considerably the area where the host can occur but the disease cannot. The pathogen is most effective where the soil temperature remains some time above 21°C (Tashiro, 1957).

B. HUMIDITY AND RAIN

Humidity may be an important environmental factor for the *host* as it can act as stress factor. In excess, it induces, for instance, epizootics of bacteria in the laboratory, particularly the potential pathogens (Bucher, 1963). Its impact on virus infections seems, in some cases, to be great, e.g. NPV of the gypsy moth *(L. dispar)* (Wallis, 1957), less so for *Galleria mellonella* and others (Pimentel and Shapiro, 1962). Its effect is probably connected with chain effects of metabolic disturbances of the host (Vago, 1963).

Humidity and rain may act favourably and prevent desiccation of *pathogens* unprotected by spore coats, membranes or inclusion bodies. Survival of rickettsiae or bacteria in carcasses, however, is secured more by the protective colloids surrounding them than by humidity. Of all protected pathogens, microsporidan spores seem to depend most on humidity but survive rarely for longer than a few months, except in diapausing hosts (Weiser, 1961). Conidia or spores of fungi depend on high humidity not for survival, but for infection (see below).

Dispersal of pathogens is sometimes assisted by rainfall, e.g. NPV for

N. sertifer in pine trees from high foci of diseased larvae to lower parts of the crown (Bird, 1961) and polyhedra in surface soil splashed on to the leaves of many plants (Jaques, 1967). Rain is also reported to assist the dispersal of disease after application of *B. thuringiensis* against *Dendrolimus sibiricus* in Russian forests (Kulagin and Lebedeva, 1965). Rain may be disadvantageous, however, during spraying or dusting with pathogens. The adhesiveness of modern commercial formulations properly dried on the leaf surface is so good that medium rainfall does not greatly reduce the residue (e.g. *B. thuringiensis*).

Survival and dispersion of the nematode *Neoaplectana carpocapsae* (DD 136) as vector of a bacterial disease depends on the availability of a surface film of water on the plant (Chapter 8). Addition of chemicals (originally developed for forest fire protection) can reduce evaporation and prolong survival of the nematodes (Webster and Bronskill, 1968). Further research in this direction may enlarge the present rather narrow ecological range for the utilization of these nematodes and broaden the field of microbial control which, at present, does not reach mining species.

Most authors consider the effect of humidity on the *host-pathogen relation* important mainly to fungal infections. Some differences in the results of spore germination at different relative humidities may reflect measurements made at the micro- and macroclimate levels. Müller-Kögler (1965) lists numerous examples showing how infections of different fungus species are influenced by the duration of high humidity, and by changes of humidity due to the microclimatic conditions on the insect or plant, climate and weather, site and type of crop. Sites having a relatively high air humidity have more fungus epizootics on insects than neighbouring dry sites and are predisposed to the use of fungi. Shade trees in coffee plantations facilitated fungal epizootics of *Coccus viridis* and *Saissetia coffeae* by *Cephalosporium.* Fungi caused mortality of *Euproctis chrysorrhoea (Nygmia phaeorrhoea)* in oak forests, of *Aradus cinnamomeus* in pine stands and of *Autographa gamma* in fields, that was proportional to the density of the plant cover. Although high air humidity does not seem to prevail in all fungal epizootics, particularly not in those caused by Entomophthoraceae, the intentional furthering of humid site conditions has frequently been tried for the stimulation of fungal pest control as will be discussed on p. 434.

C. LIGHT AND RADIATION

Light of a certain short wave length and intensity can have a stimulating effect on the germination, sporulation, and growth of *Beauveria bassiana* and some Entomophthorales (Müller-Kögler, 1965). Most germs, however, including sporeforming bacteria and occluded viruses are inactivated by sunlight, particularly by ultra-violet radiation. Special formulations of *B. thuringiensis* preparations were required to prolong the effectivity of spore and crystals exposed to sunlight. This problem is particularly relevant for regions having a sunny climate. Although heat transfered by long wave radiation can be destructive (see Section VII A), the main influence of sunlight on pathogens is exerted by its ultra-violet-component. Many experiments on viruses have shown that very short periods, even hours, suffice to inactivate NPV and GV exposed to sunshine. They are more susceptible in pure suspension than in haemolymph (e.g. NPV of *Bombyx mori,* Aizawa, 1955) or in tissue of dead larvae (e.g. GV of *Pieris brassicae,* David, 1967). Macerated larvae of *P. brassicae* retained GV infectivity after 43 hr of sunlight when smeared on the lower leaf surface, i.e. protected against ultra-violet. The better results of crude NPV suspensions, as compared with rather pure ones, during field experiments against gypsy moth *(L. dispar)* larvae in Sardegna (Magnoler, 1968) may also be interpreted as caused by better protection against sunlight. To avoid the highly destructive power of ultra-violet, application of NPV against *Heliothis* species in Texas has been carried out at night (Fernandez *et al.*, 1969).

D. OTHER PHYSICAL FACTORS

Wind is able to disseminate pathogens as shown experimentally using NPV of the alfalfa caterpillar *(Colias eurytheme)* over a distance of 2 m (Thompson and Steinhaus, 1950). Air transport of *B. thuringiensis* has been measured by suction traps in the forest (Grison and Bourguignon, 1965). Indirectly, wind contributes to desiccation of the substrate and the air, and may shorten longevity of unprotected pathogens.

Weather factors usually act together. Some may have great direct or indirect influences on host, pathogen, or their interplay. A typical consequence of a period of favourable weather is the increase of the *population density* of many pest insects. In addition to stressing the population by mutual disturbance (p 415), closer contact between individuals facilitates infection by diseases. Healthy insects may touch conidia of entomophagous fungi or feed on substrate contaminated with pathogens that infect *per os.* Special behaviour of diseased hosts like gregariousness or migration to the surface of the soil or to the tips of trees favours dispersion of pathogens. Mining and plant sucking species, on the other hand, are relatively well protected against this type of contamination. High population density and high incidence of disease may impair the health of the subsequent generation and increase the chance of infection from carcasses or other depots of pathogens densely distributed over the habitat. This concerns, for instance, diseases of soil inhabiting scarabaeids as listed on p. 419. Sufficient pest increase can be tolerated only in certain crops, like forests, with a high economic threshold. In other crops, man can increase the probability of infection by distributing pathogens instead of waiting until they increase as a result of high host population density.

As weather factors cannot be manipulated, their influence can be modified by special types of plantation, irrigation or by alterations like light in the greenhouse or water sprayed on fields and orchards, etc. This will be discussed in the last section of this contribution.

In contrast to weather favouring increase of insect populations, extreme weather like excessive humidity, heat or frost helps to limit insects. There is some evidence that latently or sublethally infected insects succumb more easily to extreme weather than healthy ones, e.g. microsporidan-infected European cornborers *(Ostrinia nubilalis)* in Illinois, U.S.A. (Zimmack and Brindley, 1957), silkworms, fall webworms (Veber and Jasić, 1961) and black blowflies *(Phormia regina)* (Kramer, 1968). This is an important long-lasting effect of disease. Research along this line is recommended particularly on introduced pests that have left their pathogens behind.

VIII. Habitat

A. TYPE OF HABITAT

The abode of insects contributes to their state of health. Plants, soil, and water are the main habitats. Most relevant points have already been mentioned. The habitat can protect the insect against destructive physical factors like heat and frost, or the pathogen against ultra-violet light and desiccation. Shadeless plantations, dry, sterile soils and water polluted by waste chemicals are enemical to the preservation of pathogens. The same number of insects in a unit area may be crowded or not, depending on the carrying capacity of the habitat, i.e. the availability of suitable places to live in. Habitats of some permanency are favourable for the persistence of regulatory biotic agents, even in man-made habitats (pp. 428-440).

B. SOIL

The soil may be considered as a special stratum of the habitat, with qualities important for both host and pathogen. Differences in the effect of fungus *(Beauveria)* infections observed in relation to soil type cannot be caused by the humidity of the interstitial air which is always near saturation while a soil is wet enough to support plant growth. Differences may be caused, however, by the different physical structure of soils, some of which retain spores on the soil particles by adhesive forces. Soil acidity also affects pathogens. A low pH may damage spores of *B. popilliae* (Beard, 1945). Numerous fungi are influenced by the acidity of the soil (Müller-Kögler, 1965). Chemical fertilizers or manuring with green plants affects the soil pH and thereby influences the type of fungi available to infect soil insects. Further possibilities of making soil more suitable for entomophagous fungi are given in Part X.

Pathogens have frequently been applied to soil and forest litter, because of its humid and stable nature. Spores of *B. popilliae* and *B. lentimorbus*, which cause milky disease, have been used extensively against Japanese beetle larvae in soil in the eastern U.S.A. Control has usually been good because the bacteria are able to persist for several years in the soil. Natural dispersal was extensive, but relatively slow. Therefore, it was necessary to apply the bacteria to disease-free populations in many places, particularly to recently infested areas and favourite breeding places like golf courses. Once established, the bacteria maintain themselves for many years, particularly when susceptible insects immigrate into the area. Because they kill the larvae before sporulation is completed, highly virulent strains are less persistent than strains of a lower virulence (Dutky, 1963). (Further details of the method are given in Chapter 3.) For long-term control, under conditions favourable for the persistence of the resting stages of the pathogen, and in a crop of high economic threshold, the use of highly virulent germs may endanger the persistence of the control. This is, of course, different for the control of surface-feeding insects on a very valuable crop, where quick kill (short-term control) may be more important than the production of new pathogens in the hosts. The problem is different for virus diseases of surface-feeding insects. After application of occluded viruses against lepidopterous larvae the pathogens are washed down and preserved relatively well in the soil. The drying of NPV of *Trichoplusia ni* on the soil before leaching appeared to influence the amount of virus detected at various depths in experimental columns (Jaques, 1969). This virus retained 25% of its original infectivity after five years in the soil under field conditions (Jaques, 1967). GV of *Pieris brassicae* and *P. rapae* also remain infective in the soil for several years (David and Gardiner, 1967; Harcourt and Cass, 1968).

Forest litter, where the pentatomid wheat bug *(Eurygaster integriceps)* hibernates in the Southern U.S.S.R., when enriched with the fungi *Aspergillus repens* or *Beauveria bassiana*, gave medium to high mortality (Evlakhova, 1954). Infected bugs were also released on hibernating sites in the litter (Tarasov, 1968). In other experiments, litter was piled up, mixed with bran or other milling offal and inoculated with the fungi. Growth and sporulation of fungi took place before the bugs arrived for hibernation (more examples and literature, Müller-Kögler, 1965). Although much labour is needed to use the soil for microbial control in this way, it is an interesting method for hibernating insects and for certain types of economy. In his study of the persistence of NPV of *T. ni* (see above), Jaques (1967) suggested application of the polyhedra suspension to the soil surface, not to the leaves. Polyhedra remain infective in the soil for years and are spread to the plant by rain splashing and cultivation of the soil. As the host feeds on several wild plants, neighbouring uncultivated soil may accumulate polyhedra from natural infections and preserve them as pathogen reservoirs.

IX. Biotic Factors

A. FOOD

Unfavourable food plants, usually accepted by insects under the influence of intraspecific competition, may predispose them to infection by diseases. Most observations concern virus diseases, e.g. *B. mori, L. dispar, Malacosoma neustria, H. cunea* (Tanada, 1967). The chemical composition of the diet, particularly high content of protein, may increase the susceptibility of insects to some viruses (e.g. *Galleria mellonella,* Shvetsova, 1950; Pimentel and Shapiro, 1962). *P. brassicae* is said to be influenced in its susceptibility by the pH of the cell contents–acid favoured fungus *(Beauveria bassiana),* alkaline *B. thuringiensis*; hence, the combination of both was recommended (Kalyuga, 1968).

The foliage of many plants, particularly conifers, contains bacteriostatic and bactericidal substances, which inhibit growth of *B. thuringiensis* (Kushner and Harvey, 1962). It is recommended that the effect of the natural leaf food on the infection should be examined before planned microbial control operations begin (Smirnoff, 1967). Plant varieties partially resistant to the pest insect may enhance the overall effect of control in combination with pathogens (p. 414). However, European cornborer *(Ostrinia nubilalis)* larvae, collected from corn varieties less susceptible to the borer, were also infected by microsporida less than others taken from the normal varieties (Chiang and Holdaway, 1960). The possibility of host plants resistant to a pest also influencing the susceptibility of the pest to pathogens, warrants further study. The most important influence of quality and quantity of food seems to be its stress effect mentioned earlier (p. 415).

B. PARASITES, PREDATORS AND OTHER GERM VECTORS

Entomophagous arthropods (Fig. 3) and other germ vectors, vertebrate and invertebrate, play an important three-fold role in microbial control. They transmit diseases, sometimes compete with pathogens for the insect host, and fulfil a compensatory role in the complex of natural factors limiting pests. These three functions should be understood when efforts are made to manipulate the environment. Many exhaustive reviews, e.g. Steinhaus (1954), Biliotti (1956), Franz (1961b, 1964b), DeBach, ed. (1964), Müller-Kögler (1965), Rivers (1967), Tanada (1963, 1967) should be consulted.

1. Vectors

Some pathogens are transmitted to new hosts only by vectors, e.g. *Neoaplectanid* nematodes (Chapter 8). Facultative vectors are found among parasites (parasitoids), predators (including birds and mammals), and scavengers. They transmit the germs mechanically, often passing them through the gut. Most carriers are non-susceptible although some parasitoids become infected, not

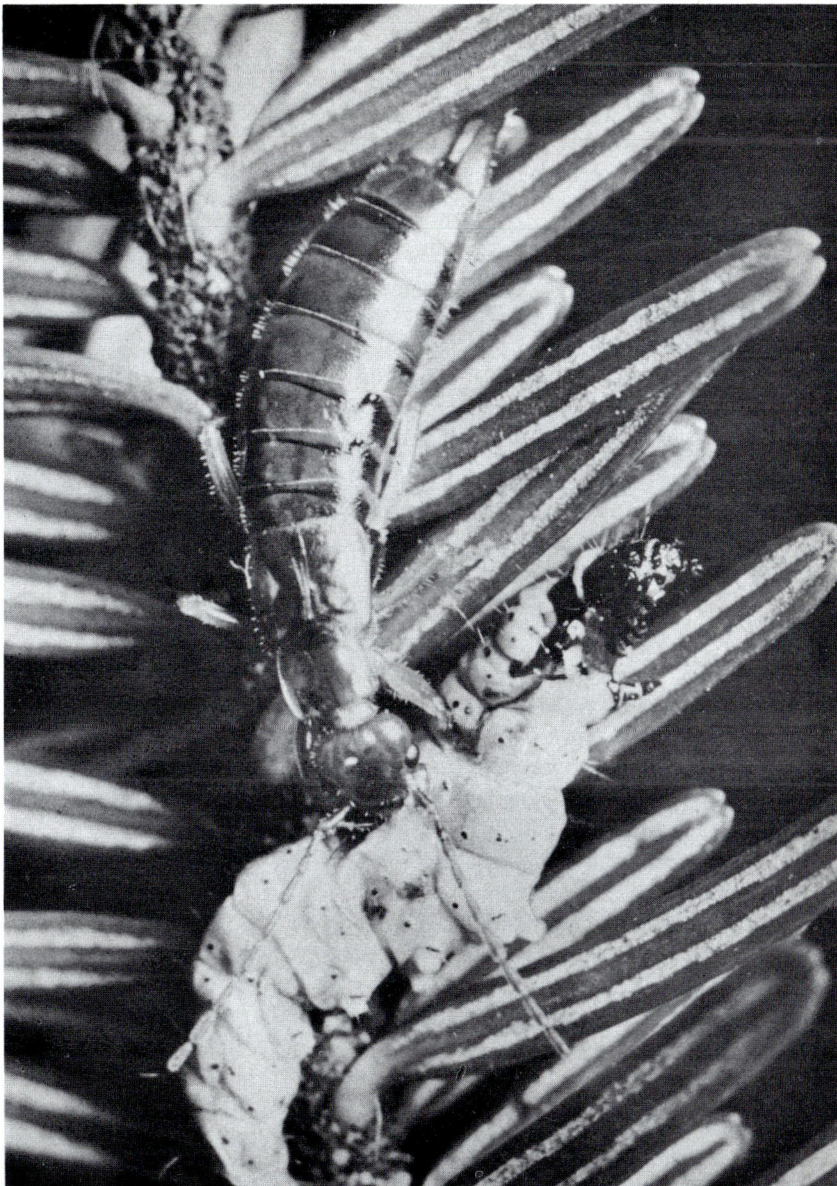

Fig. 3. Earwig, vector of virus diseases, feeding on larva of *Choristoneura murinana* killed by granulosis (photograph, J. M. Franz).

always to their own detriment. In addition, host insects themselves transfer diseases and contribute to the dispersion of epizootics. These vectors, proven as such by numerous experiments with all groups of pathogens, exert an effect in nature that is difficult to measure. It is a complex action, greatly influenced by physical factors and by the host's population density, and is a vital feature where long-term control is desired. Discussion of two general aspects show the far-reaching interrelationships between vectors and hosts.

a. Sawflies on coniferous trees. Studied particularly in Canada (Bird, 1961), these illustrate the importance of vectors for the dispersion and persistence of virus diseases. The NPV of the European spruce sawfly *Gilpinia (Diprion) hercyniae,* an insect introduced to eastern North America, probably came to the New World with imported parasites. The disease reached epizootic conditions in the early forties, without significant artificial dissemination by man. Together with parasites, it has kept the host's population below the economic threshold ever since. The persistence of the pathogen was assisted by (a) adult transmission of virus to the subsequent generation, probably more by contamination of the needles than by germinative transmission (Neilson and Elgee, 1968) and (b) by parasites, predators, and scavengers, some gifted with great searching capacity (e.g. low-density adapted Ichneumonidae of the genus *Exenterus*; Bird and Elgee, 1957). Female spruce sawflies move around after laying each egg, a behaviour more conducive to virus dispersion than laying clusters of eggs on a single twig as in the European pine sawfly *(N. sertifer).* This latter behaviour, and a smaller complex of introduced parasites, are considered to be responsible for more limited persistence and spread of the NPV of *N. sertifer. N. lecontei,* an endemic North American species, has an intermediate position for its specific virosis spreads more readily, apparently transmitted also by a larger parasite complex (Bird, 1961).

These three viroses illustrate persistence of a disease depending partly on host behaviour and partly on vector activity. They also illustrate transitions between long- and short-term microbial control and the duration of persistence, which, if the pathogen is applied at a medium dosage, can be longer than after high dosage application. Persistence caused by living organisms, both within and between generations, is called "biological persistence", in contrast to the "environmental persistence" of germs that endure extreme physical conditions (Franz, 1964a).

b. Practical utilization of disease vectors. This may take two forms: protection of vectors and their release. Protection requires the avoidance of any control action detrimental to organisms other than the target pest. Most insect pathogens used nowadays are more or less specific. Bacterial and virus diseases usually do not directly affect entomophagous insects (Franz, 1961a). Several fungi, like *Beauveria* sp. and some microsporida are exceptions (next section). The application of fungi to the soil or litter (p. 423) or in poor biocenoses (like potato fields) may be one way to avoid unnecessary destruction of other insects. The specificity of most insect pathogens, therefore, is a safeguard against impoverishment of the biocenosis. On the other hand, it is for crop management to assist in the conservation of refuge areas in cultivated landscapes where pesticides are used (Grison, 1968) (Part X). An indirect effect to entomophagous pathogens remains when populations of the host proper and possible alternate hosts are effectively suppressed by control action. It depends on the tolerance level for the pest whether or not sufficient numbers will survive to maintain the disease in enzootic conditions. Here again, many potential vector organisms are desirable, depending, as mentioned above, on the diversity of the ecosystem.

2. Competitors

Entomophages and pathogens compete for the host where too few hosts are available and when one organism prevents the development of the other. This becomes critical, mainly for parasites, if they have to complete their growth on an infected host. Usually, it is a problem of time coincidence (Biliotti, 1956). When the host has been parasitized before infection occurs, the parasite is usually able to complete its development, even if it does not reach its full size. This has been observed, for instance, with parasitic Diptera and Hymenoptera developing in virus-infected larvae of sawflies or Lepidoptera. Microsporidan infections of the host seem to affect parasitoids more than viroses or bacterioses. The host-pathogen-parasitoid interrelation is reviewed, for instance, by Kurstak (1966) in his study of *Ephestia küehniella,* attacked by *B. thuringiensis* and the ichneumonid, *Nemeritis canescens.* Well analysed field observations on the co-action and/or competition of entomophages and pathogens of Lepidoptera in Hawaii are given by Tamashiro (1968). A disease is very seldom incompatible with predaceous arthropods, although predators that prefer host larvae *(L. dispar, H. cunea)* diseased with microsporidoses, and remove them from the orchard, may decrease the infections inoculum in the habitat and thereby reduce the effectiveness of the disease (Weiser, 1956).

3. Supplementary Action

Pathogens and other natural enemies usually supplement each other. A rare chance to analyse this occurred with the European spruce sawfly *(G. hercyniae)* in Canada. Reactions of parasites to increased host populations came earlier than those of the virus (NPV), but the virosis alone was able to maintain the population at low levels. Both biotic agents together gave greater security and better suppression of the sawfly (Bird and Burk, 1961; Neilson and Morris, 1964).

The example of the complementary effects of introduced parasites, mycoses, endemic predators and a resistant variety of alfalfa, in the control of the spotted alfalfa aphid *(T. trifolii)* has already been mentioned (p. 414). It is remarkable in this context that a pathogenic fungus *(Entomophthora exitialis)* and parasites (Aphidiidae) operate at different times of the year the fungus being most effective in the desert areas of southern California during the winter months when the parasite, *Praon pallitans,* is in diapause; it disappears when the parasite becomes active in summer.

X. Crop Management

The principles outlined in Part V (pp. 412-415) will now be applied to particular types of crops, considering some examples from field tests, to assess future prospects of using microbial control in harmony with, and as part of, the requirements of crop management. It should be possible to overcome the widespread hesitancy of growers to accept this new method. This hesitancy is usually caused by the delay in control resulting from the incubation period and the relatively slow progress of the disease. Systematic effort by state agencies as well as by far-sighted industry (Franz, 1966) may be needed to educate growers to accept the ecological point of view and to give up the old ideal of quick eradication of a pest. In most instances the continued presence of insects on the crop can be tolerated as long as they are too few to cause economic damage. In other words, the economic threshold has to be established and used as guide line.

A. FOREST

Forests and shade trees are particularly suitable for microbial control (Franz, 1969). The relatively low value of the crop and its low annual gain in value permit only limited expenses for control. On the other hand, the economic threshold for most forest defoliators (sawflies and Lepidoptera) is higher than on any other crop. Finally, the ecological diversity of the forest and its freedom from annual upheavals are favourable to the development of stabilizing elements. Hence relatively high pest populations can be tolerated and relatively long-term degrees of control are desirable, with infrequent applications of the agents. Finally the selectivity of pathogens and their harmlessness for vertebrates greatly favour their use. Forests in many overpopulated countries are particularly esteemed as recreation areas and water reserves (p. 409). Pollution by toxic residues, even if they do not directly affect human food, should be avoided. This principle will become more widely recognized in the future, because pollution of the environment is one of the pressing ecological problems of the day. Ways to avoid it will be considered even if they involve expense.

Comparative costs of short-term forest insect control, using chemical insecticides or pathogens, are rarely available and depend on the economic situation of the country. In the U.S.S.R., *B. thuringiensis* is said to be 10 times (Gukasyan, 1963) or 4.5 times cheaper than DDT for control of *D. sibiricus* (Neudachin, 1965). The latter price was calculated for a huge operation using the so-called epizootiological method which consists of applying *B. thuringiensis* in strips 50-200 m apart. The effectiveness of this method is not undebated (Komyagin *et al.*, 1965), but the persistence and limited spread of the disease from spore reservoirs like webbed carcasses is well documented (e.g. Talalaev, 1959, 1965; Kulagin and Lebedeva, 1965). This seems to be one of the few examples of an effect of *B. thuringiensis* extending to the subsequent year and future generation of the pest (p. 420). The relatively low cost of "Dendrobacillin" (at least in the U.S.S.R.), one of the Russian *B. thuringiensis* preparations, may also depend on the price system of State-owned plants and cheap raw materials available for mass culturing the bacilli. In Germany, the cost of treatment (all expenses included) of oak forest against the tortricid, *T. viridana,* in a small helicopter operation covering 160 ha was 67 Deutschmarks (DM) per hectare (ha) for DDT (1.2 kg/40 l/ha) and 117 DM for the American *B. thuringiensis* preparation "Thuricide" (1 kg/75 l/ha) (1966). The price for the latter is not yet competitive, but may become so when several brands from other countries become available. In some European countries financial assistance is given to this type of experiment in order to acquaint foresters with preparations of limited competitive, but high safety value.

This point of view was important in the control of *T. viridana* in Germany which illustrates the economic considerations typical of *short-term application* in microbial control. Control was necessary because the quality of precious oaks used for veneer was threatened by an extended outbreak causing the formation of epicormic branches (Wasserreiser) after heavy defoliation. In addition, the valuable harvest of acorns was endangered. Because of financial restrictions, only the most valuable stands could be treated. The advantage of DDT was its more complete kill of the pest which also protected treated plots in the subsequent year, if they were somewhat isolated. The advantage of *B. thuringiensis* was its satisfactory control (around 80% of foliage and the oak-mast were saved) and its complete harmlessness (Franz, Krieg and Reisch, 1967). The plots (to be treated by helicopter) which were close to a city were, therefore, assigned to *B. thuringiensis* treatment, the others to DDT. As outbreaks of this tortricid are usually of limited duration in this part of Germany, the shorter effect of microbial control could be tolerated.

The general conclusion, valid at least in Europe, can be drawn that the advantage lies with microbial control, even in the short term, where highly valued forest crops are endangered (otherwise no control could be warranted), the outbreak does not last too long, and special circumstances emphasize the conservation and public health aspects.

Further *examples of short-term microbial control* in the forest concern mostly *B. thuringiensis.* Its use in Europe and the U.S.S.R. has recently been reviewed (Franz and Krieg, 1967), with satisfactory practical results against: *Dendrolimus sibiricus, Tortrix viridana, Selenephera (Selenophora) lunigera,*

Thaumetopoea pityocampa and *T. wilkinsoni, Zeiraphera griseana, Lymantria dispar* (in parts only moderate efficiency), *Panolis flammea* and *Archips crataegana.* In a pilot experiment the last species was also treated with an aerosol containing *Pseudomonas chlororaphis,* which caused 60-78% mortality after natural dispersion from a small focus to 60 ha, but this could not be repeated in a second experiment (Kudler *et al.,* 1959, 1965). Practically no natural spread has been observed with *B. thuringiensis* except to a limited extent on *D. sibiricus* (p. 429). The susceptibility to this pathogen differs greatly even among closely related species (Chapter 13). *Choristoneura murinana* is susceptible, but control was unsatisfactory because of the difficulty of completely covering quickly growing needles partially hidden in the tortricid's feeding web. In North America, satisfactory results with the gypsy moth *(L. dispar)* were obtained from eastern States, but the spruce budworm *(Choristoneura fumiferana)* proved to be as difficult to control by water or oil suspensions as its European relative mentioned above.

Several examples of *medium and long-term microbial control,* all concerning virus diseases, have already been quoted: *G. hercyniae* pp. 426-427; *N. sertifer* pp. 416, 426; *N. swainei* p. 411; *N. lecontei* p. 426; *N. pratti* p. 411; *D. spectabilis* p. 417; *T. pityocampa* p. 417; *M. disstria* p. 417; *M. californicum* p. 417.

This series is incomplete but is typical. The speed of action depends on the dosage used and the time of application. Where the tolerable level of damage is low, as in young pine plantations, treatment of sawfly *(N. sertifer)* eggs before eclosion gave control of second instar larvae. Where time was not pressing and the dosage used relatively low, the epizootic appeared as late as one to two years after application of NPV against *Malacosoma californicum* (Thompson, 1959).

Most of the virus diseases had already occurred in the area or even in the population treated. The biological persistence of virus infections for some years is a major advantage particularly in the forest where repeated applications can make the costs prohibitive. Although virus preparations are not yet available commercially for use against forest insects, it is safe to say that costs should be reasonable. The virus from 10 to 25 dead, fully grown larvae is usually considered sufficient to prepare a suspension for treatment of 1 ha of forest. Superinfection (p. 416) and treatment early in the course of a population increase (p. 417) may augment the efficiency and the long-term effect. The most outstanding success was the permanent suppression of the European spruce sawfly to subeconomic levels (p. 426). The risk of unintentional introduction of new pests is an unavoidable consequence of modern traffic; the aim should be to have effective pathogens available for introduction as soon as a new pest is established. This danger is particularly great for huge, newly planted forests of introduced tree species as in South America or New Zealand. Even-aged and uniform forests are frequently more susceptible to pest outbreaks than others more diverse in flora and age classes. Any diversity which modern forest management can afford, without sacrificing its economic aims, will contribute to better opportunities for natural or artificial epizootics among pest insects. These can develop at a tolerable pest density when, for instance, alternate hosts for and vectors of the pathogens are available and when the pest outbreak is damped by the co-action of several biotic factors.

B. ORCHARD

Crop management in orchards shows great variety. Some orchards are totally commercialized; others, like those producing fruit for juice only, are less intensively managed; some are managed without consideration of commercial aspects, like hobby gardens; or almost not managed at all, like apple trees along the streets. This variety causes great differences in the level of permissible damage. It is very low in fully commercialized orchards (p. 412); therefore, there is little chance for microbial control not fully competitive with insecticides. However, because of the well-known difficulties arising from total reliance on chemicals, there have been preliminary attempts to combine several techniques into an integrated system, particularly in apple orchards. Some microbial control preparations (mainly *B. thuringiensis*) have been incorporated into modified spray programmes against surface feeding (chewing) insects, predominantly lepidopterous larvae (Oatman, 1966; Steiner and Baggiolini, 1968). Less intensive management facilitates the acceptance of such preparations. Microbial pathogens have been particularly valued in orchards where the appearance of resistance against insecticides caused trouble with both the target pest and the accompanying species, like red spider mites. Also pathogens have been favoured by the need to control pests during the blossom period when pollinating insects must not be killed and most contact insecticides are prohibited (e.g. olive moth *Prays oleae,* Yamvrias, 1967) and *Hyponomeuta* sp. Finally, pathogens can be applied shortly before harvest, when chemical insecticides are undesirable.

Satisfactory control by Western European and North American standards has been obtained with *B. thuringiensis,* for instance, against the following Lepidoptera in orchards: fall cankerworm, *Alsophila pometaria*; grape leaf folder, *Desmia funeralis*; winter moth, *Operophtera brumata*; brown tail moth, *Euproctis chrysorrhoea (Nygmia phaeorrhoea)*; tent caterpillars, *Malacosoma* spp.; ermine moths, *Hyponomeuta* spp. (pp. 415, 418); fall webworm, *Hyphantria cunea* (reviews by Krieg, 1961, 1967a; Angus, 1968).

Viruses have been successfully used less frequently, for instance, the GV against the red-banded leaf roller, *Argyrotaenia velutinana* (p. 418) on apple, acting rather slowly, or recently with great promise, the specific GV against the codling moth, *Carpocapsa pomonella* (Falcon *et al.,* 1968). Application of microsporida *(Thelohania hyphantriae)* against the fall webworm and accompanying Lepidoptera in orchards, on a small scale in the C.S.S.R., is of ecological interest in that alternate hosts *(M. neustria, H. malinellus)* assisted in the dispersal of germs, served as pathogen reservoirs, and harboured the disease during winter *(E. chrysorrhoea)* (Weiser and Veber, 1955).

This series of examples shows that mainly insects chewing on open leaves are accessible to microbial control in orchards. As foliage pests they do not damage the crop directly. Difficulties arise with other species whose larvae bore into the buds (like several tortricids) and mine the leaves, twigs, or fruits. When weather conditions are favourable (p. 418), satisfactory control by *B. thuringiensis* can be obtained with some of them like *Hedya nubiferana (Argyroploce variegana)* and *Tmetocera ocellana* on opening apple buds (Herfs, 1965). The addition of effective phagostimulants would help to obtain better *per os* infection of this group of pests. The low amount of *B. thuringiensis* ingested by mining larvae also causes some *post-larval mortality* and reduction in fertility, e.g. with the eye-spotted budmoth *(Spilonota ocellana)* and the codling moth *(C. pomonella)* (Oatman and Legner, 1964; Angus, 1968). This is not only important when assessing the total mortality caused by the treatment, but also allows a gradual suppression of a tortricid population which cannot be controlled quickly by microbial methods. Long-term effects of repeated application should be thoroughly investigated when the use of microbial control in orchards is considered. The greater efficiency of GV than of *B. thuringiensis* against the codling moth may indicate the value of highly virulent pathogens where the pest ingests only traces of the treated plant cuticle.

Management of orchard crops can, in a limited way, contribute to improving environmental conditions for microbial control. Any reduction of regular pesticide sprays, adoption of integrated control programmes, and increase in the diversity of host plants (soil cover), even in commercial orchards, can improve the diversity and regulative potential of the biocoenosis (p. 414). Specific measures to increase air humidity may sometimes be advisable for entomophagous fungi. Subplanting melons into young citrus plantations has been recommended to favour appearance of *Entomophthora* on aphids (Tisdale, 1930; further examples, Müller-Kögler, 1965). The old technique of attracting egg-laying females of *Oryctes rhinoceros,* a pest of oil palms in the Pacific area, to heaps of rotten material treated with *Metarrhizium anisopliae* (Friederichs, 1919) is again being tested by the rhinoceros beetle project of the South Pacific Commission. A new virus proved to be more efficient (Marschall, 1970).

Any method that helps to reduce insecticide sprays should be particularly acceptable to hobby orchardists. These are inclined to overdose insecticides. Further, they do not sell their fruits and so, unlike commercial growers, are not compelled to obey exaggerated rules of aesthetic appearance of their product (p. 412). There is, however, a remarkable reaction of the public to the residue problem in some European countries. Special health shops sell unsprayed fruits recognizable by certain blemishes on the skin. Microbial control could be easier applied, if the existing very high standards of external perfection could be slightly reduced (which would not decrease the fruit quality), as it is normal for instance in some countries of eastern Europe. Juice producers are much better situated in this respect, because the tolerated level of chemical residues is very low for fruit juices. As a whole, while orchards are not unsuitable to microbial control the different degrees of management intensity influence their suitability. The development of integrated control methods which make more use of pathogens (like a combination of sterile male release and virus of the codling moth) may improve the situation in the near future.

C. PERENNIAL CROPS

Perennial crops other than forests and orchards share with these a quality beneficial to microbial control, i.e. the permanence of plant cover, allowing host and pathogen populations to persist in some degree of balance. Grasslands, lawns and fodder plants like alfalfa will be discussed as examples, among others such as some soft fruits and tropical cultures like sugar cane not discussed specifically. In most cases, the economic threshold is relatively high, allowing for some damage by pests before control becomes necessary economically. This is particularly true of grasslands not used permanently by grazing cattle, and of lawns. Aesthetic, more than production aspects, govern the damage that can be tolerated, for instance, on golf courses. Some cases of microbial control on perennial crops will exemplify the problems.

Bacteria have been used against grubs of the Japanese beetle with considerable success. This has already been mentioned in regard to the impact of weather factors (p. 419), pH of soil (p. 422), application to the soil (p. 423) and persistence of the pathogens *(B. popilliae* and *B. lentimorbus)* on the control achieved. Control has been widely accepted as satisfactory, which is reflected in the following figures: 244,000 lb of a standardized spore preparation were used from 1939 to 1953 in 14 eastern States of the U.S.A. (Fleming, 1961). The milky disease is now considered to be one of the potential weapons for regions newly invaded by the pest. Western North America is apparently now under invasion pressure, and great areas of southern and central Europe are both climatically suitable to the beetle and permanently endangered by aircraft transportation (Mayer, 1962). Thus, cheap mass production of the bacilli outside the living host would be an important achievement. Control can be economized by simultaneous application of spore dust and fertilizers (White, 1948). There are, however, thermal limits for the range of the disease (p. 419). In marginal regions, or when quick control on valuable lawns is desired, additional use of insecticides is warranted.

On grassland, *B. thuringiensis* plays an increasing role in the control of lepidopterous larvae like the fawn-coloured lawn moth *(Crambus bonifatellus)* and the salt-marsh caterpillar *(Estigmene acrea)* in the U.S.A., and the European skipper *(Thymelicus lineola)* in Canada (Arthur, 1968). It is still more important for control of the alfalfa caterpillar *(Colias eurytheme)* on alfalfa. Here, the low tolerance level of toxic insecticide residues (which become concentrated in products from the cattle), as well as exemption of *B. thuringiensis* from a tolerance limit by the Food and Drug Administration in the U.S.A., have paved the way for wider use of this bacillus. Although it is still rather expensive ($1.25-$1.90 for control of *T. lineola* per acre), it has the advantages of being commercially available and of acting rapidly. Farmers have learnt to accept the quick arrest of feeding as satisfactory relief although the caterpillars usually do not die until a few days later. As in most other cases, no persistent effect has been noted, perhaps because larvae do not stick firmly to the leaves.

As regards the persistence of effects, *virus* preparations are more satisfactory against the alfalfa caterpillar. Strip cutting of alfalfa, developed for integrated control in California (Schlinger and Dietrick, 1960), may also prolong the effect of virus after application. The tendency of virus-killed larvae to adhere to the plant is a disadvantage, which can be serious with a heavy larval population since cattle, for instance, reject alfalfa contaminated by large numbers of dead caterpillars. It might be advisable, as suggested by Cameron (1967), to get the disease established by using virus and accept the loss in crop value for one season (cutting period). As "supervised pest control" is accepted widely by alfalfa growers in the western U.S.A., a combined application of both pathogens could be further developed, geared to the actual outbreak situation, closely supervised as part of integrated control procedures.

Rickettsiae in scarabaeid larvae have only restricted applicability, at present, because they are not completely safe to warm-blooded animals (Krieg, 1963). It may be possible, however, for some foci to be established by microbial control experts in perennial crops or forests, with the intention of using the great biological persistence of the pathogen. Germinative transmission has been shown to occur (Krieg, 1967b; Niklas, 1969) with *Rickettsiella melolonthae* in the European chafers, *Melolontha* sp. and *Amphimallon solstitiale.* Spread is certainly enhanced by the remarkable environmental resistance of these pathogens (Hurpin, 1965; Niklas and Brammanis, 1969). The presence of an enzootic disease may increase the total mortality of some scarabaeids where their degree of damage is marginal (like *A. solstitiale, A. horticola* or *Maladera brunnea*) and thereby make other control measures superfluous (see also Chapter 7).

Fungi deserve mention here since agricultural practices have been reported to intensify their effect in perennial crops like alfalfa (p. 420). Irrigation can increase air humidity and provide the environment needed for sporulation of fungi like the Entomophthoraceae even at dry sites (Hall and Dunn, 1958). Even under improved conditions, aphid densities necessary to trigger epizootics may sometimes be higher than the economic injury level for the affected crop. The close density dependence of fungal epizootics has been demonstrated in experiments (Manglitz and Hill, 1964). Conservation of grass cover to keep the soil moist enough to allow fungal infection of grasshopper eggs in Siberia is an example of the use of agricultural techniques for the induction of epizootics (Rubtsov, 1939). Where humus is inadequate, green manuring and other means of improving the humus content have been reported to increase the effect of *B. tenella* and other fungi attacking white grubs of *Melolontha* (Schaerffenberg, 1952) (more examples, Müller-Kögler, 1965).

D. ANNUAL CROPS

The continuity of habitat typical of forests, orchards, and perennial crops is lacking in annual crops. This is a disadvantage in all cases of microbial control that depend on the continuing occurrence of hosts. It will be shown that, in spite of the frequent change of plant cover, some types of microbial control are feasible in annual crops, and also that the continuity of pathogens might be secured in other ways.

Annual crops comprise mainly vegetable crops, truck crops, cereals, cotton, and other plants that are totally removed after harvest. At harvest, pathogens adhering to the plants dissapear and so cannot influence subsequent attacks.

Rotation is a routine measure for many crops and in many, but not all, areas. It is meant to avoid exhaustion of particular soil components and the perpetuation of plant pests which profit from the permanent supply of susceptible hosts. Recent economic evolution in agriculture has favoured, however, the trend to grow permanently and in monoculture those crops which show optimum yield and maximum profit. This is sometimes advocated even in places where rotation has formerly been considered to be unavoidable and where damage by pest organisms increases with permanent culture, at least at the beginning. The simplification of management, along with high profit, seems to more than compensate for such losses. Two examples will show that microbial control can utilize such modern trends because it assists (unwillingly, no doubt) the coexistence of host and pathogen populations.

Sugar beets in Europe are frequently attacked by the beetle *Atomaria linearis* (Cryptophagidae). Where rotation was interrupted, natural mortality of the beetle due to a fungus disease *(Cephalosporium)* increased remarkably and made further control unnecessary, whereas rotation disrupted the incipient epizootic (Bombosch, 1963). A similar situation may occur with larvae of *Sitona lineata*, feeding on the roots of peas (Volk and Bombosch, 1968). Where the repeated culture of potatoes on the same field is permissible, the treatment of larvae of the Colorado potato beetle *(L. decemlineata)* with a microbial preparation (Beauverin) based on *B. bassiana* reduces the viability of the population, 29% of the surviving beetles having shown reduced fertility (Dyadechko and Sikura, 1963). Dead larvae and pupae augment and conserve the supply of conidia available in the soil. Müller-Kögler (1965) gives more examples concerning fungi, e.g. on *Cleonus punctiventris* and *Melolontha* sp. In Part VIII, the importance of the soil as a habitat for pathogens and the remarkable environmental persistence of NPV in the soil (Jaques, 1969) has been mentioned. The importance of uncultivated refuge areas harbouring a stock of biologically persistent pathogens should again be stressed (Grison, 1968). All these examples emphasize the possibility of retaining parts of the infectivity potential even for pests on annual crops, as long as they are grown on the same place.

In many other cases, typical short-term control remains the sole possibility because host plants including pests and pathogens are removed from the field at relatively short intervals and insufficient pathogens are left in the soil. Usually, the economic threshold of this type of crop is also rather low, e.g. for vegetables. Then, microbial control has to compete with chemical insecticides and it can satisfy growers only when at least one of two conditions can be met: (a) quick kill of the host; (b) no other insecticides are suitable because of either difficulties with toxic residues or with resistance. Microbial control has obtained full support by the growers where conditions (a) and (b) coincided and pathogens were available in the amount needed.

Availability of pathogens has restricted their large-scale use in annual crops so far to *B. thuringiensis* and *B. bassiana,* the latter was in the U.S.S.R. only. The acceptance of *B. thuringiensis* in the U.S.A. facilitated after it was exempted from residue tolerance on the following raw annual crops: artichokes, beans, broccoli, cabbage, cauliflower, celery, cottonseed, kale, lettuce, mustard greens, potatoes, spinach, sweet corn, tomatoes and turnip greens. Because residue tolerances for insecticides as well as the resistance of pest insects change with time and geographic area, the range of recommendations and hosts treated is not constant. In addition, the availability of certain formulations like dust preparations greatly influences the acceptance of preparations by growers (Hall, 1963). Species of *Pieris* and the diamond-back moth *(Plutella maculipennis)* are typical examples of highly susceptible pests on annual crops on which microbial control by *B. thuringiensis* alleviated trouble with toxic residues and/or insecticide resistance.

Difficulties arise when two or more pests, occurring simultaneously on the same plant, differ greatly in their susceptibility to the pathogen. This is the case, for instance, with the imported cabbage worm *(P. rapae)* and the cabbage looper *(T. ni)* in the U.S.A., the latter being about eight times less susceptible than the former (McEwen *et al.,* 1960). A worse situation is encountered in Europe, where *P. brassicae,* the susceptible species, is frequently accompanied by the non-susceptible noctuid *Mamestra brassicae.* In such cases, a combination of two pathogens will be necessary (p. 414), particularly where, to avoid residues or resistance, admixture with insecticides is undesirable. Such a mixture of insecticides and pathogens has been advocated, however, when the efficiency of both preparations alone was unsatisfactory, and their addition resulted in good control (Chapter 14). At present, the addition even of small amounts of chemicals to a microbial preparation would nullify the "no chemical residue" advantage of the pathogen (p. 416). A useful means of combination is sometimes an application of insecticides early in the growth period and their substitution by microbial preparations before harvest to avoid chemical residues (Hall, 1968).

Another difficulty in valuable annual crops is the relatively slow action of many pathogens (p. 411). Although feeding of the species most susceptible to *B. thuringiensis* stops very shortly after ingestion of sufficient toxic crystal, complete coverage of waxy leaves by sprays is difficult and feeding may continue long enough to cause some damage. Thorough supervision of the crop and early application of a well formulated pathogen preparation (sometimes dust is better than spray) against young larval instars is particularly important under such conditions.

Although many experiments on the use of *B. thuringiensis* have been reported, few records are available concerning its large-scale application in certain crops. Unsuccessful experiments, using poor preparations and sometimes premature publication, can create scepticism among growers that is difficult to overcome later. As usual, time should create a more balanced view and efficient preparations will be accepted, particularly if the difficulties connected with chemicals make them more prohibitive. At present, the wide-spread use of *B. thuringiensis* preparations in the U.S.A. seems to centre on regions where residue problems on annual crops are most critical, as on vegetables in California and Florida as well as on tobacco (mainly the sphingids of the genus *Manduca*) in the south-eastern States.

The development of *virus* preparations will increase the range of pests for which microbial preparations are available. Commercial virus preparations (NPV) against *Heliothis* and *Trichoplusia ni* are expected to be on the market in the U.S.A. soon, after long and thorough tests for efficiency and hygienic harmlessness (Allen, 1968). This will also alleviate the situation on crops where noctuids occur along with other Lepidoptera more susceptible to *B. thuringiensis* (vegetables, tobacco). It will be important to make follow-up studies on fields where the same crop is grown in successive years (like cotton) and a degree of transmission of the viral pathogens could be expected. Good kills, even during the second and third generations have been reported after the application of GV against the cutworm, *Agrotis segetum,* on cotton in the U.S.S.R. (Dikasova, 1966). The use of *fungi,* especially *Beauveria bassiana,* on annual crops has been developed mainly in Europe, predominantly the U.S.S.R. An experimental preparation based on *B. bassiana* is also being tested in the U.S.A. Its effect on young larvae of the Colorado potato beetle has been demonstrated in several European countries (Müller-Kögler, 1965). The non-specificity of the fungus and the difficulty of obtaining commercial preparations in most other countries has apparently limited its wider application to the U.S.S.R. (p. 435) where it is usually combined with low dosages of DDT (p. 416) (Sikura, 1967). It may also be used elsewhere if this beetle becomes more resistant to chemical insecticides. Experiments against the European corn borer, *O. nubilalis* have profited from the humid micro-environment in the leaf axil of corn. Favourable humid conditions have also been utilized for experiments to control the pentatomid, *Eurygaster integriceps,* during hibernation in the litter (p. 423). So far, no large-scale application against these two pests has been published. As mentioned earlier, the use of fungi requires special environmental conditions most likely to be found in the soil or in favourable micro-habitats.

E. PROTECTED CROPS

Glasshouses, mushroom houses, and similar places have one feature in common, close control of the environment by man. Some examples demonstrate the suitability of protected cropping for biological control, for instance the use of the predaceous mite, *Phytoseiulus persimilis* against phytophagous mites. Very little has, however, been done to develop the use of pathogens. Although the environmental conditions are man-made, it is seldom practicable to alter them merely to suit some beneficial organisms, becuase they are geared to the optimal culture of the crop. Only pathogens which can operate efficiently within these physical limits can be tried. Further, the value of protected crops is very high and, correspondingly, the economic threshold usually extremely low. The thresholds have been established for the major pests, but the real significance of less important species such as leafhoppers, thrips, capsids, leaf-eating caterpillars is still uncertain (Hussey, personal correspondence, 1968).

In mushroom houses, Diptera (Phoridae, Mycetophilidae, Cecidomyiidae) along with a tarsonemid mite are most important (Hussey, 1967). The possibility of enriching the soil with nematodes that attack the larvae of the first two Diptera families is, at present, being studied in England. Also strains of *B. thuringiensis* that produce exotoxin may be worthwhile trying. In glasshouses, Coccidae on various plants have been infected efficiently by *Cephalosporium* spp. in the C.S.S.R. (Neuzilova, 1957), but this example did not lead to practical usage. It may be, however, that the virus diseases of Tetranychidae, e.g. *Panonychus citri* (Gilmore and Tashiro, 1966), or exotoxin of *B. thuringiensis* (Krieg, 1968b) will become more important in future, owing to the marked resistance of many glasshouse mites to acaricides.

Most cases in glasshouses will require short-term control, whereas in mushroom culture, sterilized compost may harbour pests along with their inoculated antagonists in some sort of balance for a considerable period.

F. STORED PRODUCTS

Stored products are also usually kept under artificial conditions. Again, it will seldom be practicable to alter the conditions in order to suit pathogens. One has to chose pathogens that can survive and be efficient within the physical limits occurring in stores and factories.

The most advanced project is the protection of *beecomb* from wax moths *(Galleria mellonella* and *Achroia grisella)* with *B. thuringiensis.* Powdered preparations applied to the surface of empty comb protect it prophylactically from young larvae. Dipping and dusting of empty comb has the disadvantage that spores and crystals are partially removed from the comb by bees and by the crop of honey. Some spores would also enter the honey and possible spoilage of human food by eventual germination of spores cannot be excluded. This is avoided by incorporating the preparation into the foundation wax, where it largely remains, firmly embedded in the wax, which is spread by the bees throughout the comb. Experiments have shown that not all strains and formulations of *B. thuringiensis* are equally suitable, that *A. grisella* is less susceptible than the Greater Wax moth, and that the bacteria must not be heated above 60°C during manufacturing of the sheets of foundation wax (p. 417). New methods are now being tested and it cannot be doubted that beecomb protected by *B. thuringiensis* from wax moths will be commercially available in the near future, utilizing the harmlessness of the pathogen for honey-bees and man (Krieg and Franz, 1959; Johansen, 1962; Herfs, 1964; Burges and Bailey, 1968). Its safety when embedded in foundation wax has been approved and registered in Britain (Burges, personal communication, 1969).

In other types of stored products like grains, flour, or clothes, microbial control would also have to be applied as a prophylactic measure. For quick kill of established infestations, fumigation and other methods are better than relatively slow-acting microbial control. Since high dosages are required for prophylactic treatment, most discussion and experiments centre around *B. thuringiensis,* which controls only lepidopterous larvae. Several moths feeding on grain products, such as *Ephestia (Anagasta) kuehniella* and *Plodia interpunctella* are susceptible to the bacillus. An addition of 0.2-0.3% of the spore/crystal complex of *B. thuringiensis* to the flour results in 100% mortality of first instar larvae (Yamvrias, 1962; Krieg, 1964). Several authors have recommended practical use of this method in places where such moths are difficult to suppress in flour, but the admixture of such large quantities of live spores into flour might be unacceptable because they might cause saprophytic spoilage of some foods, such as soups, on occasions when the foods were not heated sufficiently to kill spores. Pure crystal preparations would not suffice against *E. kuehniella* as live spores are needed for lethal infection. Spores could persist long enough under dry conditions. Admixture into such products as grain, from which spores would be largely removed during processing, would probably be acceptable, but the commercial preparations still cost too much. For other pathogens such as protozoans like *Nosema* and viruses (e.g. of the *Tinea* species attacking clothes), the problems of usefulness of *in vivo* production, standardization, and storage (of microsporida) need much further research.

The occurrence of heavy epizootics in stored product insect populations suggests future possibilities of microbial control in this field (Burges, personal correspondence, 1968). In *developing countries* under warm climatic conditions, there is a need for a harmless food protectant that could be given to native farmers without fear or danger to human lives through misuse. Another prophylactic measure is to attack *residual insect populations* living in accumulations of debris in stores and factories, using pathogens as introductions. Diseased insects themselves would carry pathogens into the inaccessible parts of such accumulations.

The trends in storage and factory procedure are likely to have important effects on practices in insect control. Firstly, there is a trend towards mechanical handling of products. This would favour mechanically admixed powders of pathogens, but only if they were reliable and adequately standardized. The operational labour force is reduced by mechanization programmes. Less labour is available to remove debris. This parallels the second trend, that of increased mechanization of factories and mills, with the accompanying reduction in the stoppages of machinery for cleaning. Treatment of debris and static material with pathogens might be encouraged, where this could be done with minimal labour. For instance, after a periodic cleaning of a mill, the first run of grain could be heavily treated with pathogens to fill "dead spaces", like the boots of elevators, with food highly lethal to insects, and to allow some pathogenic material to fall in places where debris accumulates. Pathogens should be able to spread with the insect population. This is the case, as mentioned earlier, with the original host of *B. thuringiensis,* the Mediterranean flour moth *(E. kuehniella).* Food in storage is one step nearer to the consumer than the growing crop and degradation factors in stores are less likely to kill or remove pathogens than those outside. Consequently, higher standards of safety for man must be set (Krieg, 1968a).

References

Abbott, W. S. (1925). *J. econ. Ent.* **18,** 265-267.

Aizawa, K. (1955). *J. seric. Sci. Japan* **24,** 398-399. (In Japanese.)

Allen, G. E. (1968). Proc. U.S.-Japan Semin. Microbial Control Insect Pests, pp. 37-41. U.S.-Japan Committee Sci. Cooperation. Panel 8. Fukuoka.

Angus, T. A. (1968). *Wld Rev. Pest Control* **7,** 11-26.

Arthur, A. P. (1968). *J. Invertebrate Path.* **10,** 146-150.

Aruga, H. (1963). *In* "Insect Pathology. An Advanced Treatise" (E. A. Steinhaus, ed.), Vol. 1, pp. 499-530. Academic Press, New York.

Beard, R. L. (1945). *Connecticut Agric. exp. Stn. New Haven, Bull.* **491,** 503-583.

Beirne, B. P. (1967). "Pest Management", 123 pp. Hill, London.

Bergold, G. H. (1958). *In* "Handbuch der Virusforschung" (C. Hallauer and K. F. Meyer, eds), Vol. 4, pp. 60-142. Springer-Verlag, Vienna.

Biliotti, E. (1956). *Entomophaga* **1,** 45-53.

Biliotti, E., Grison, P., Maury, R. and Vago, C. (1959). *C.r. hebd. Séanc. Acad. Agric. Fr.* **45**, 407-409.

Bird, F. T. (1953). *Can. Ent.* **85**, 437-446.

Bird, F. T. (1961). *J. Insect Path.* **3**, 352-380.

Bird, F. T. (1964). Colloque international sur la pathologie des insectes et la lutte microbiologique. Paris 1962. *Entomophaga Mém. hors Sér.* No. 2, 465-473.

Bird, F. T. and Burk, J. M. (1961). *Can. Ent.* **93**, 228-238.

Bird, F. T. and Elgee, D. E. (1957). *Can. Ent.* **89**, 371-378.

Bombosch, S. (1963). *Z. Angew. Ent.* **52**, 313-342.

Bucher, G. E. (1963). *In* "Insect Pathology. An Advanced Treatise" (E. A. Steinhaus, ed.), Vol. 2, pp. 117-147. Academic Press, New York.

Burges, H. D. and Bailey, L. (1968). *J. Invertebrate Path.* **11**, 184-195.

Cameron, J. W. M. (1963). *Ann. Rev. Ent.* **8**, 265-286.

Cameron, J. W. M. (1967). *In* "Insect Pathology and Microbial Control" (P. A. van der Laan, ed.), pp. 182-196. North-Holland Publ. Co., Amsterdam.

Campbell, R. W. (1963). *Can. Ent.* **95**, 465-474.

Chant, D. A. (1966). *In* Symp. Scient. Aspects Pest Control (Washington, 1966) Natn. Acad. Sci., Natn. Res. Council, Publ. 1402, pp. 193-218.

Chiang, H. C. and Holdaway, F. G. (1960). *J. econ. Ent.* **53**, 918-924.

Connola, D. P., Lewis, F. B. and McDonough, J. L. (1966). *J. econ. Ent.* **59**, 284-287.

David, W. A. L. (1967). *In* "Insect Pathology and Microbial Control" (P. A. van der Laan, ed.), pp. 174-178. North-Holland Publ. Co., Amsterdam.

David, W. A. L. and Gardiner, B. O. C. (1967). *J. Invertebrate Path.* **9**, 342-347.

DeBach, P. (ed.) (1964). "Biological Control of Insect Pests and Weeds", 844 pp. Chapman and Hall, London.

Dikasova, E. T. (1966). *In* Biol. metod. bor'b. s vredit. sel'sk., lesn. khoz. i karant. sorn. (M. A. Rish, ed.), pp. 104-105. Izd. Fan, Tashkent. (In Russian.)

Dutky, S. R. (1963). *In* Insect Pathology. An Advanced Treatise" (E. A. Steinhaus, ed.), Vol. 2, pp. 75-115. Academic Press, New York.

Dyadechko, M. P. and Sikura, A. J. (1963). *Nauk. praci. Ukr. nauk.-dosl. inst. zakhistu roslin* **12**, 81-84. (In Ukrainian.)

Evlakhova, A. A. (1954). Sess. Sericult., Apicult., Plant Protect, Vet. Sci. Sections, Techn. Repts., Leningrad. (In Russian.)

Falcon, L. A., Kane, W. R. and Bethell, R. S. (1968). *J. econ. Ent.* **61**, 1208-1213.

Fedorintchik, N. S. (1964). *In* Colloque international sur la pathologie des insectes et la lutte microbiologique. Paris, 1962. *Entomophaga Mém. hors Sér.* No. 2, 51-61.

Fernandez, A. T., Graham, H. M., Lukefahr, M. J., Bullock, H. R. and Hernandez, N. S., Jr. (1969). *J. econ. Ent.* **62**, 173-177.

Ferron, P. (1967). *Entomophaga* **12**, 257-293.

Fleming, W. E. (1961). *U.S. Dep. Agric.* Leaflet No. 500, Washington, 6 pp.

Franz, J. M. (1961a). *In* "The Ecological Effects of Biological and Chemical Control of Undesirable Plants and Animals", pp. 93-105. Warsaw 1960. IUCN Symposium, Leiden.

Franz, J. M. (1961b). *In* "Handbuch der Pflanzenkrankheiten" (H. Richter, ed.), Vol. 6(3), 2nd edit., pp. 1-302. Verlag Parey, Berlin.

Franz, J. M. (1964a). *In* "Global Impacts of Applied Microbiology" (M. P. Starr, ed.), pp. 256-266. Almquist and Wiksell, Stockholm and John Wiley and Sons, New York.

Franz, J. M. (1964b). *Ann. appl. Biol.* **53**, 510-515.

Franz, J. M. (1965). *Z. Angew. Ent.* **55**, 319-325.

Franz, J. M. (1966). *Meded. Rijksfacult. Landbouwwetensch., Gent* **31**, 512-525.

Franz, J. M. (1969). 6. Congr. Forestal Mundial. Madrid 1966, **2**, 1915-1924.

Franz, J. M. (1968). *Anz. Schädl. kde.* **41**, 65-71.

Franz, J. M. and Krieg, A. (1967). *Gesunde Pfl.* **19**, 175-176, 178-180, 182.

Franz, J. and Niklas, O. F. (1954). *Nachrichtenbl. Deutsch. Pfl. schutzd., Braunschweig* **6**, 131-134.

Franz, J. M., Krieg, A. and Reisch, J. (1967). *Nachrichtenbl. Deutsch. Pfl. schutzd., Braunschweig* **19**, 36-44.

Friederichs, K. (1919). *Monogr. Angew. Ent. Berlin* (4), 116 pp.
Gilmore, J. E. and Tashiro, H. (1966). *J. Invertebrate Path.* **8,** 334-339.
Glass, E. H. (1958). *J. econ. Ent.* **51,** 454-457.
Grison, P. (1968) Symp. O.I.L.B. Darmstadt 1968, 31 pp. (mimeograph).
Grison, P. and Bourguignon, S. (1965). *C.r. hebd. Séanc. Acad. Agric. Fr.* **51,** 112-116.
Grison, P., Vago, C. and Maury, R. (1959). *Rev. Forest. Française* (5), 353-370.
Gukasyan, A. B. (1963). *Izv. Akad. Nauk SSSR, Ser. Biol.* **28,** 115-125. (In Russian.)
Hagen, K. S. and Bosch, R. van den (1968). *Ann. Rev. Ent.* **13,** 325-384.
Hall, I. M. (1961). *Adv. Pest Control Res.* **4,** 1-32.
Hall, I. M. (1963). *In* "Insect Pathology. An Advanced Treatise" (E. A. Steinhaus, ed.), Vol. 2, pp. 477-517. Academic Press, New York.
Hall, I. M. (1968). Proc. U.S.-Japan Semin. Microbial Control Insect Pests pp. 165-167. U.S.-Japan Committee Sci. Cooperation. Panel 8. Fukuoka.
Hall, I. M. and Dunn, P. H. (1958). *J. econ. Ent.* **51,** 341-344.
Harcourt, D. G. and Cass, L. M. (1968). *J. Invertebrate Path.* **11,** 142-143.
Herfs, W. (1964). *Z. Angew. Ent.* **54,** 233-237.
Herfs, W. (1965). *Z. Pfl. krankh.* **72,** 65-77.
Hurpin, B. (1965). *Proc. 12. Int. Congr. Ent. (London, 1964).* 727.
Hurpin, B. (1967). *In* "Insect Pathology and Microbial Control" (P. A. van der Laan, ed.), pp. 135-161. North-Holland Publ. Co., Amsterdam.
Hurpin, B. (1968). *J. Invertebrate Path.* **10,** 252-262.
Hussey, N. W. (1967). *Mushroom Indust. Conf., Torquay,* 1967. Leaflet 14 pp.
Janisch, E. (1959). *Z. Angew. Ent.* **43,** 371-386.
Jaques, R. P. (1961). *J. Insect Path.* **3,** 47-54.
Jaques, R. P. (1962). *J. Insect Path.* **4,** 1-22.
Jaques, R. P. (1965). *Can. Ent.* **97,** 795-802.
Jaques, R. P. (1967). *Can. Ent.* **99,** 820-829.
Jaques, R. P. (1969). *J. Invertebrate Path.* **13,** 256-263.
Johansen, C. (1962). *Glean. Bee Cult., Medina* **90,** 682-684.
Kalyuga, M. V. (1968). *Ent. Obozr., Moskva* **47,** 450-453. (In Russian.)
Katagiri, K. (1969). *Entomophaga* **14,** 203-214.
Knipling, E. F. (1960). *J. econ. Ent.* **53,** 415-420.
Komyagin, A. I., Poltev, V. I. and Lobanov, A. V. (1965). *In* Issled po biol. metod. bor'by s vredit. sel'skogo i lesn. khoz. (Dokl. k simp., 17-20. Nov. 1964) (A. I. Cherepanov, ed.), vyp. 2, pp. 14-18. Akad. Nauk SSSR, Sibirsk. Otd., Novosibirsk. (In Russian.)
Koyama, R. and Katagiri, K. (1968). Proc. U.S.-Japan Semin. Microbial Control Insect Pests, pp. 63-69. U.S.-Japan Committee Sci. Cooperation. Panel 8. Fukuoka.
Kramer, J. P. (1963). *Texas Rep. Biol. Med.* **26,** 199-204.
Krieg, A. (1961). *Mitt. Biol. BundAnst., Berlin-Dahlem* (103), 79 pp.
Krieg, A. (1963). *In* "Insect Pathology. An Advanced Treatise" (E. A. Steinhaus, ed.), Vol. 1, pp. 577-617. Academic Press, New York.
Krieg, A. (1964). *Z. Angew. Ent.* **51,** 13-23.
Krieg, A. (1967a). *Mitt. Biol. BundAnst., Berlin-Dahlem* (125), 106 pp.
Krieg, A. (1967b). *Umschau, Frankfurt/M.* **67,** 801-802.
Krieg, A. (1968a). *Zentralbl. Bakteriol. I. Abt. Ref.* **214,** 501-511.
Krieg, A. (1968b). *J. Invertebrate Path.* **12,** 478.
Krieg, A. and Franz, J. (1959). *Naturwissenschaften* **46,** 22-23.
Krieg, A. and Schmidt, L. (1962). *Nachr. bl. Beutsch. Pfl. Schutzd., Braunschweig* **14,** 177-182.
Kudler, J. (1965). *Lesnický časopis, Praha* **11,** 359-366. (In Czech.)
Kudler, J., Lysenko, O. and Hochmut, R. (1959). Trans. "First International Conference of Insect Pathology and Biological Control", pp. 73-80. Prague 1958.
Kudler, J., Lysenko, O. and Hochmut, R. (1965). Commun. Inst. Forest. Cechosl., pp. 219-226.
Kulagin, V. S. and Lebedeva, N. P. (1965). *In* Ispol. mikroorg. dl. bor'by s vred. nasekom.

les. vost. sibiri (E. V. Talalaev, ed.), **19**(1), pp. 29-34. Izv. biol.-geogr. nauchn. issled. Inst. pri Irkutsk gosudarst. Univ. im Zhdanova. (In Russian.)
Kulikov, N. S. (1966). *Pchelovodstvo* (10), 29. (In Russian.)
Kurstak, E. S. (1966). *Ann. Epiphyties, Paris* **17**, 335-383, 451-508.
Kushner, D. J. and Harvey, G. T. (1962). *J. Insect Path.* **4**, 155-184.
Laan, P. A. van der (ed.) (1967). "Insect Pathology and Microbial Control", 360 pp. North-Holland Publ. Co., Amsterdam.
Lappa, N. V. (1967). *In* "Insect Pathology and Microbial Control" (P. A. van der Laan, ed.), pp. 264-265. North-Holland Publ. Co., Amsterdam.
Lawson, F. R. (1966). Proc. FAO Symp. Integr. Pest Contr. Rome 1965 (3), pp. 27-45.
Lawson, F. R., Rabb, R. L., Guthrie, F. E. and Bowery, T. G. (1961). *J. econ. Ent.* **54**, 93-97.
Magnoler, A. (1968). *Entomophaga* **13**, 335-344.
Manglitz, G. R. and Hill, R. E. (1964). *Res. Bull. Neb. agric. Exp. Stn.* (217), 21 pp.
Marschall, K. J. (1970). *Nature, Lond.* **225**, 228-229.
Martignoni, M. E. (1957). *Mitt. Schweiz. Anst. Forstl. Versuchswesen* **32**, 371-418.
Martignoni, M. E. and Schmid, P. (1961). *J. Insect Path.* **3**, 62-74.
Mayer, K. (1962). *Nachr. bl. Deutsch. Pfl. schutzd., Braunschweig* **14**, 58-61.
McEwen, F. L., Glass, E. H., Davis, A. C. and Splittstoesser, C. M. (1960). *J. Insect Path.* **2**, 152-164.
McIntyre, T. and Dutky, S. R. (1961). *J. econ. Ent.* **54**, 809-810.
Morris, R. F. (1960). *Ann. Rev. Ent.* **5**, 243-264.
Müller-Kögler, E. (1965). "Pilzkrankheiten bei Insekten. Anwendung zur biologischen Schädlingsbekämpfung und Grundlagen der Insektenmykologie", 444 pp. Verlag Parey, Berlin.
Neilson, M. M. (1965). *J. Invertebrate Path.* **7**, 306-314.
Neilson, M. M. and Elgee, D. E. (1968). *J. Invertebrate Path.* **12**, 132-139.
Neilson, M. M. and Morris, R. F. (1964). *Can. Ent.* **96**, 773-784.
Neudachin, J. J. (1965). *In* "Use of Microorganisms for Controlling Forest Pests in East Siberia" (E. V. Talalaev, ed.), **19**(1), pp. 35-40. Izv. biol.-geogr. nauchn. issled. Inst. pri Irkutsk gosudarst. Univ. im Zhdanova. (In Russian.)
Neužilová, A. (1957). *Universitas Carolina, Biologica* **3**,(1), 7-29. (In Czech.)
Niklas, O. F. (1969). *Entomophaga* **14**, 225-228.
Niklas, O. F. and Brammanis, L. (1969). *Nachr. bl. Deutsch. Pfl. schutzd., Braunschweig* **21**, 11-12.
Oatman, E. R. (1966). *J. econ. Ent.* **58**, 1144-1147.
Oatman, E. R. and Legner, E. F. (1964). *J. econ. Ent.* **57**, 294.
Pimentel, D. (1961). *Ann. ent. Soc. Am.* **54**, 76-86.
Pimentel, D. and Shapiro, M. (1962). *J. Insect Path.* **4**, 77-87.
Rabb, R. L., Steinhaus, E. A. and Guthrie, F. E. (1957). *J. econ. Ent.* **50**, 259-262.
Rivers, C. F. (1967). *In* "Insect Pathology and Microbial Control" (P. A. van der Laan, ed.), pp. 252-263. North-Holland Publ. Co., Amsterdam.
Rubtsov, I. A. (1939). *Probl. Ecol. Biocenol., Leningrad* (4), 35-88. (In Russian.)
Rybina, L. M. (1966). *In* Biol. metod. bor'b. s vredit. sel'sk., lesn. khoz. i karant. sorn. (M. A. Rish, ed.), pp. 152-155. Izd. Fan, Tashkent. (In Russian.)
Schaerffenberg, B. (1952). *Anz. Schädl. kde.* **25**, 166-170.
Schlinger, E. I. and Dietrick, E. J. (1960). *Calif. Agric.* **14**(1), 8-9, 15.
Schönherr, J. (1965). *Z. Pfl. krankh.* **72**, 466-477.
Schwerdtfeger, F. (1932). *Z. Forst-, Jagdwes.* **64**, 146-167.
Shvetsova, O. I. (1950). *Mikrobiologija, Moskva* **19**, 532-542. (In Russian.)
Sikura, A. J. (1967). *Abstr. 6. Int. Pfl. schutz-Kongr. Wien 1967*, 655-656.
Smirnoff, W. A. (1963). *Can. Ent.* **95**, 127-133.
Smirnoff, W. A. (1967). *In* "Insect Pathology and Microbial Control" (P. A. van der Laan, ed.), pp. 179-180. North-Holland Publ. Co., Amsterdam.
Stairs, G. R. (1965). *Can. Ent.* **97**, 1059-1062.

Steiner, H. and Baggiolini, M. (1968). Landesanstalt für Pflanzenschutz, Stuttgart, 63 pp.
Steinhaus, E. A. (1949). "Principles of Insect Pathology", 757 pp. McGraw-Hill, New York.
Steinhaus, E. A. (1954). *Hilgardia* **23,** 197-261.
Steinhaus, E. A. (1960). *Bact. Rev.* **24,** 365-373.
Steinhaus, E. A. (ed.) (1963). "Insect Pathology. An Advanced Treatise", Vol. 1, 661 pp., Vol. 2, 689 pp. Academic Press, New York.
Stern, V. M., Smith, R. F., Bosch, R. van den and Hagen, K. S. (1959). *Hilgardia* **29,** 81-101.
Talalaev, E. V. (1959). Trans. "First International Conference of Insect Pathology and Biological Control", pp. 51-57. Prague 1958. (In Russian.)
Talalaev, E. V. (1965). *In* Ispol. mikroorg. dl. bor'by s vred. nasekom. les. vost. sibiri (E. V. Talalaev, ed.), **19**(1), pp. 71-77. Izv. biol.-geogr. nauchn. issled. Inst. pri Irkutsk gosudarst. Univ. im Zhdanova. (In Russian.)
Tamashiro, M. (1968). Proc. U.S.-Japan Semin. Microbial Control Insect Pests, pp. 147-153. U.S.-Japan Committee Sci. Cooperation. Panel 8. Fukuoka.
Tanada, Y. (1963). *In* "Insect Pathology. An Advanced Treatise" (E. A. Steinhaus, ed.), Vol. 2, pp. 423-475. Academic Press, New York.
Tanada, Y. (1965). *Entomophaga* **10,** 139-150.
Tanada, Y. (1967). *In* "Pest Control. Biological, Physical and Selected Chemical Methods" (W. W. Kilgore and R. L. Doutt, eds), pp. 31-88. Academic Press, New York.
Tanada, Y. and Chang, G. Y. (1968). *J. Invertebrate Path.* **10,** 79-83.
Tarasov, L. G. (1968). *Zashch. Rast., Moskva* **13**(8), 52-53. (In Russian.)
Tashiro, H. (1957). *J. econ. Ent.* **50,** 350-352.
Thompson, C. G. (1959). Trans. "First International Conference of Insect Pathology and Biological Control", pp. 201-204. Prague 1958.
Thompson, C. G. and Steinhaus, E. A. (1950). *Hilgardia* **19,** 411-445.
Tisdale, W. B. (1930). *Florida Agric. Exp. Stn. Rep.*, p. 96.
Vago, C. (1963). *In* "Insect Pathology. An Advanced Treatise" (E. A. Steinhaus, ed.), Vol. 1, pp. 339-379. Academic Press, New York.
Vasiljević, L. (1961). *Entomophaga* **6,** 269-276.
Veber, J. and Jasić, J. (1961). *J. Insect Path.* **3,** 103-111.
Volk, St. and Bombosch, S. (1968). *Anz. Schädl. kde.* **41,** 57-63.
Wallis, R. C. (1957). *J. econ. Ent.* **50,** 580-583.
Webster, J. M. and Bronskill, J. F. (1968). *J. econ. Ent.* **61,** 1370-1373.
Weiser, J. (1956). *Z. Pfl. krankh.* **63,** 625-638.
Weiser, J. (1961). "Die Mikrosporidien als Parasiten der Insekten" (W. Zwölfer, ed.), *Monogr. Angew. Ent.* (17) 149 pp. Verlag Parey, Hamburg.
Weiser, J. and Veber, J. (1955). *Československ. Parasitol.* **2,** 191-199. (In Czech.)
Wellington, W. G. (1962). *J. Insect Path.* **4,** 285-305.
White, R. T. (1948). *J. econ. Ent.* **41,** 113-114.
Yamvrias, C. (1962). *Entomophaga* **7,** 101-159.
Yamvrias, C. (1967). *In* "Insect Pathology and Microbial Control" (P. A. van der Laan, ed.), pp. 284-285. North-Holland Publ. Co., Amsterdam.
Zimmack, H. L. and Brindley, T. A. (1957). *J. econ. Ent.* **50,** 637-640.

CHAPTER 20

Possibilities of Pest Resistance to Microbial Control Agents

H. D. BURGES

Pest Infestation Control Laboratory, Slough, Buckinghamshire, England

I. Introduction

There can be great variation between closely related species of pests in their resistance to the same biological control agent. Often one is susceptible, whilst another is immune; others may be intermediate. It is inconceivable that these attributes remain static in a biological system, hence the capacity for the selective development of resistance to biological control agents must be considered. In this chapter the likelihood of this capacity causing troublesome resistance in microbial control programmes will be discussed, including comparisons with macrobial control agents and the resistance of mammals to disease. In contrast to mammals, very little is known about changes in resistance during the lifetime of individual insects, hence attention will be limited to the development of genetically transmissible resistance in populations.

II. Criteria for the Demonstration of Resistance

Resistance in an insect population is recognized by bioassay of a sample of the population in comparison with a known susceptible stock of insects, using for both the same preparations of lethal agent—the pathogen. Bioassay methods are described in Chapter 27. A shift of the probit line (the straight line of probit mortality graphed against log dosage; see Chapter 27, Fig. 1) caused by resistance is expressed by the resistance factor (RF). This is the ratio of the LD_{50} values for the resistant and susceptible populations and can be regarded as a comparison of average resistance values.

A look at probit lines shows that their slopes (b) are very important too (Dyte and Blackman, 1967). Sometimes the slope for the resistant stock (Fig. 1,

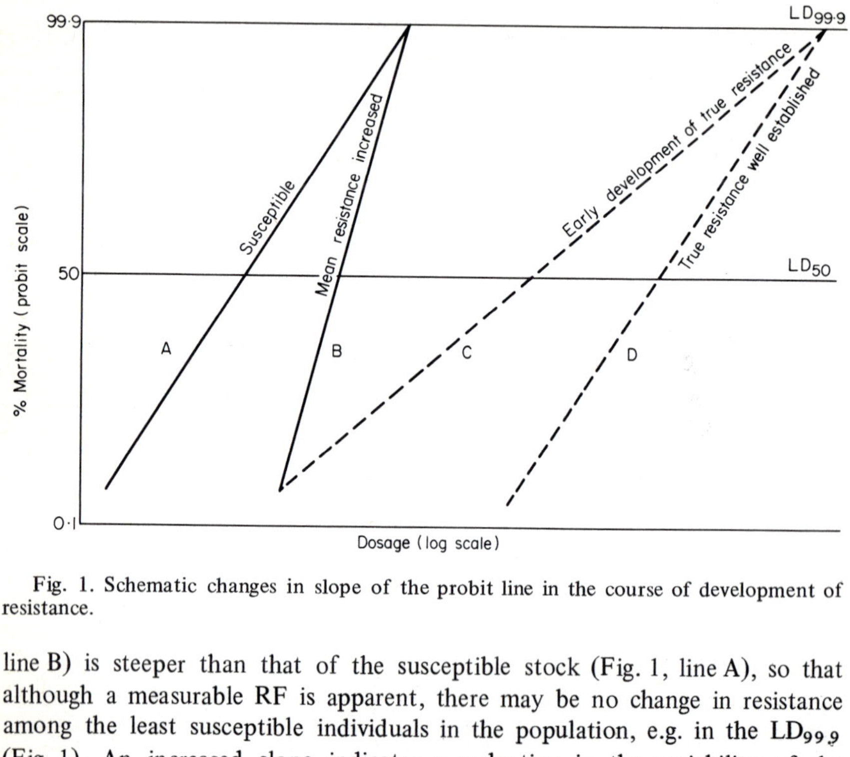

Fig. 1. Schematic changes in slope of the probit line in the course of development of resistance.

line B) is steeper than that of the susceptible stock (Fig. 1, line A), so that although a measurable RF is apparent, there may be no change in resistance among the least susceptible individuals in the population, e.g. in the $LD_{99.9}$ (Fig. 1). An increased slope indicates a reduction in the variability of the population (Chapter 27). In this case selection pressure of the pathogen that produced the increase in average resistance (i.e. at the LD_{50} level) may have done no more than weeded out the more susceptible individuals from the breeding population. True resistance involves a shift in the $LD_{99.9}$ (Fig. 1, lines C and D).

The appearance of true resistance is often accompanied by a lowering of the slope (Fig. 1, line C), indicating increased variability. This may be caused by a semi-dominant resistance gene (or genes) being present most frequently in the heterozygous state in a gene complex not fully adapted to its presence or by a mixture of susceptible and resistant insects in the population. Later, under continued selection pressure by the lethal agent, the slope may increase as insects homozygous for the resistance gene may be favoured and as the gene complex becomes better adapted to the presence of the resistance gene (Fig. 1, line D). However, homozygosity does not necessarily produce a slope parallel to that of the susceptible strain. Thus bioassays should be sufficiently detailed to show the slope of probit lines if the real significance of RF values is to be demonstrated.

Reliance on bioassay at only one dosage level can be entirely misleading. For instance, Sidor (1959) quoted mortalities shown on the left of Fig. 2 for three stocks of insect at a single dosage. The application of assumed slopes in the figure shows how the resistant stock could have appeared the most susceptible at a higher dosage level.

Unfortunately, much of the information about resistance to insect pathogens does not include slopes and so its value must be critically considered. Slopes so far encountered in bioassays of insect pathogens fall into two bands, one between $b = 0.8$ and 2.1 for pathogens not producing known toxins, and the other between $b = 1.7$ and 8 for *Bacillus thuringiensis*, which produces toxins

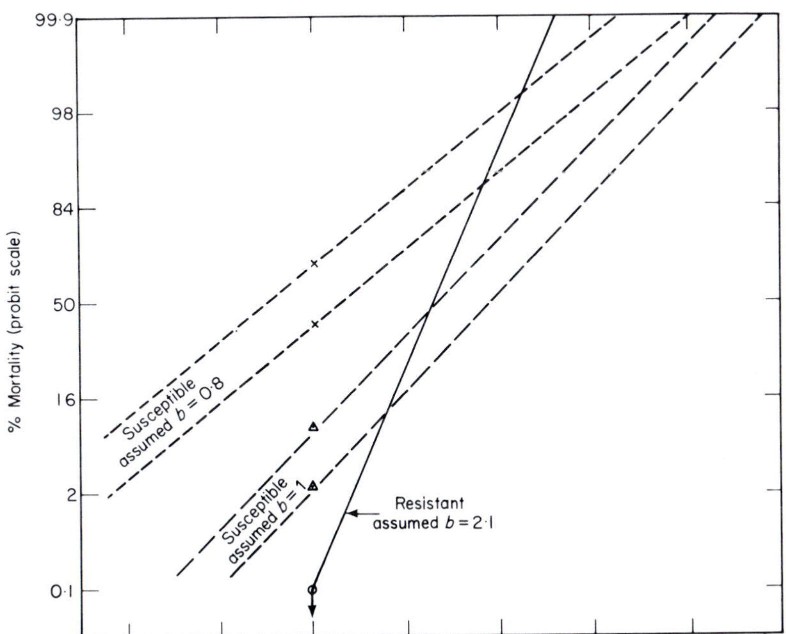

Fig. 2. Assumed slopes (b) drawn through mortality values of Sidor (1959) at a single dosage level of granulosis virus for three stocks of *Pieris brassicae*, each stock shown by o, Δ and x respectively. The slopes approach the extremes to be expected for assays of insect viruses.

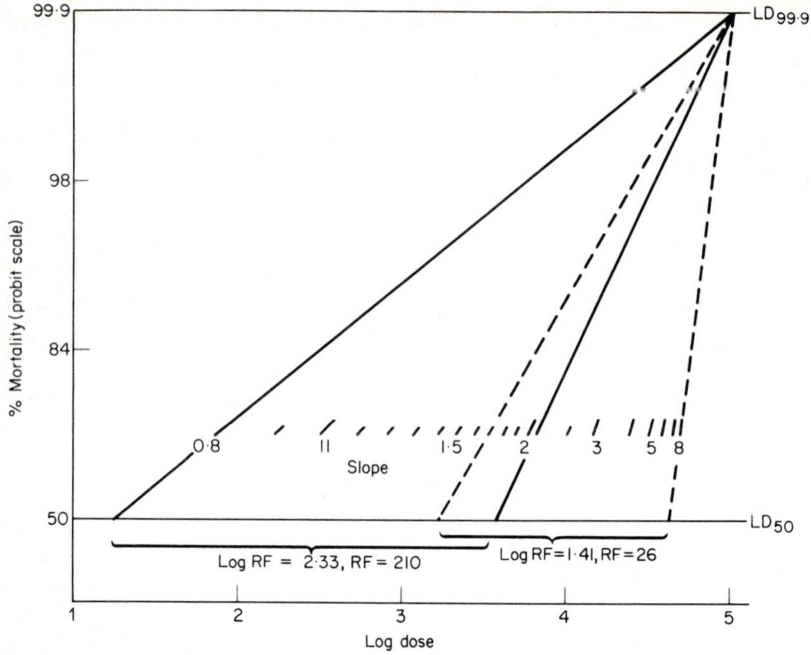

Fig. 3. Change in the resistance factor (RF) when probit lines of different slope (b) are drawn through one $LD_{99.9}$ point. The RF is antilog (log $LD50_1$-log $LD50_2$).

(Table IV in Chapter 27). Probit lines with these slopes drawn through a single $LD_{99.9}$ dosage in Fig. 3 show that alteration of slope across the extremes of each band produced apparent RF values of x210 and x26 respectively. Thus, if slopes are unknown, true resistance altering the $LD_{99.9}$ value is certain to be involved only when these RF values are exceeded. Values for other ranges can be read from Fig. 3.

III. Resistance of Insects to Microbial Control Agents

I have found no records of indisputable resistance of insects to microbial agents in field trials or control programmes. However, few such agents have been used for long and it is doubtful whether anything less than high levels of resistance would have been detected.

Some studies have been made on naturally occurring disease epizootics. Bird and Elgee (1957) speculated that, after a population crash due to polyhedrosis virus disease, the recovery of the European spruce sawfly, *Gilpinia (Diprion) hercyniae,* might have been due to the development of resistance, but they offered no evidence that the insects were in fact more resistant during the recovery. During a granulosis epizootic in the larch bud moth, *Eucosoma griseana,* LD_{50} values in assays with larvae from two consecutive generations changed from 0.0067 μg/larva to 0.254 and 0.291, indicating an increase in average resistance to the virus (Martignoni, 1957). However, the slopes also changed from 0.5 to 1.2 and 1.3 respectively, with the result that the LD_{99} values in the second generation were *lower* than in the first, indicating no change in the resistance of the least susceptible larvae. Since the second generation followed peak mortality in the epizootic, this example appears to be a case of the epizootic weeding out the more susceptible insects.

A species-specific disease of unexpectedly low virulence in comparison with similar diseases in other insect species suggests the possibility of genetically acquired resistance, a possibility which cannot be ignored, as for instance with the polyhedrosis disease of the spruce budworm, *Choristoneura fumiferana,* which is about $\times 4000^{-1}$ as active (w/w) as the polyhedrosis disease of the silkworm (Bergold, 1948, 1951), and with some strains of *Bacillus thuringiensis,* which are 100 times more active in some hosts than in others (Burgerjon and Biache, 1967). Even without the slopes of probit lines, such large differences indicate true differences in resistance at the $LD_{99.9}$ level (section II) and in these examples the techniques used for testing the different hosts are sufficiently similar to ensure that the recorded differences in activity of the pathogens were not due to technique. Absolute comparability of technique can, however, rarely be attained. Thus techniques that provide optimal growing conditions for the different hosts can be regarded as comparable, but if the food plant is different, inhibitors may be involved or the thickness and surface texture of leaf may alter the dosage of a sprayed suspension where the deposit is expressed in terms of weight of pathogen per unit weight of leaf, although W. A. L. David was unable to demonstrate an effect of leaf thickness (personal communication). Ignoffo and Garcia (1969) achieved virtual comparability by using the same artificial medium for different hosts and so demonstrated similar activities for different viruses that appeared very different in virulence in their respective hosts in field tests.

Variation in the resistance of different wild stocks of the same pest suggests more convincingly that resistance might have been developed in some stocks, but is not proof. Without knowing the slopes of probit lines, Sidor (1959) claimed a granulosis-resistant stock of the large white butterfly, *Pieris brassicae,* to be cross-resistant to a cytoplasmic polyhedrosis virus. Mortalities due to polyhedrosis are shown in Fig. 2 for the granulosis-resistant stock and two susceptible ones. The imaginary slopes in Fig. 2 show that true resistance at the $LD_{99.9}$ level is not demonstrated if the slope for the resistant stock had been much greater than those for the susceptible stocks, but otherwise Sidor's claim is valid. Maléki-Milani (1969) produced evidence of similar calibre that larvae of the cabbage moth, *Mamestra brassicae,* collected from a field population, and also larvae from a laboratory population, were more susceptible to cytoplasmic polyhedrosis than larvae of another strain which had been bred at La Minière for many years, and which had suffered attacks of polyhedrosis that might have led to the selection of resistant insects (A. Burgerjon, personal communication). Kartman (1953) found differences in resistance to the canine heartworm, a filaroid nematode *Dirofilaria immitis,* in two pairs of interfertile intermediate-host species, i.e. *Aedes aegypti* compared with *A. albopictus* (difference of x20), and *Culex pipiens* compared with *C. quinquefasciatus* (x2.5). Study of hybrids revealed that genetic factors influenced the resistance. Also geographical strains of *A. aegypti* varied in susceptibility. Differences occurred not only in the susceptibility of the mosquitoes to infection, but also in the degree of development of the parasite permitted in the mosquito, ranging from complete inhibition to normal formation of the infective larval stage capable of infecting the primary vertebrate host. Kartman (1953) reviewed many instances of such variation involving this and other vertebrate pathogens, and Kartman (1950) reviewed evidence of over 30 workers indicating variation in susceptibility of *A. aegypti* to the filarial nematode, *Wuchereria bancrofti.* Ossowski (1958, 1960a, b) found that nuclear polyhedrosis virus collected from distant plantations was more effective against the wattle bagworm, *Kotochalia junodi,* than virus collected from the local plantation in which tests were performed. Resistance might have been acquired by the local insects to the local virus as suggested by Ossowski, but loss of virulence of the local stock of virus also seems a possible explanation. Finally, Ayuzawa *et al.* (1969) reported differences in the resistance of different laboratory races of the silkworm, *Bombyx mori,* to the cytoplasmic polyhedrosis virus of another moth, *Dendrolimus spectabilis.*

The production of resistant stocks of insects in the laboratory proves that resistance to microbial agents can be obtained experimentally. Pasteur reared a stock of silkworms resistant to the microsporidan responsible for pebrine. He did this by careful selection of individual silkworms immune to the disease, subsequently rearing them in pure strains. This discovery, as much as any other, saved the silkworm industry of France (Steinhaus, 1949). Selective methods have also produced a stock of silkworm resistant by 16-fold to the cytoplasmic-polyhedrosis virus (Watanabe, 1967), a stock resistant to the flacherie virus (Uzigawa and Aruga, 1966) and another to the muscardine fungus (Koidsumi and Wade, 1955). Rothenbuhler and Thompson (1956) obtained large differences between a genetical line of honey-bee selected for susceptibility and other lines selected for resistance to *Bacillus larvae,* which causes American foulbrood disease (see also Park, 1936; Park *et al.*, 1937; Bamrick and Rothenbuhler, 1961; Thompson and Rothenbuhler, 1957). Similarly, laboratory strains of the mosquito *A. aegypti* (but not of a *Culex* hybrid) susceptible and resistant to infection with *Dirofilaria immitis* have been obtained by selection for eight generations (Kartman, 1953), and also a stock of *P. brassicae* resistant to granulosis disease (Rivers, 1959; Sidor, 1959; David and Gardiner, 1960,

1965a). Although the assays with *P. brassicae* were not designed to measure the degree of difference in susceptibility, inspection of the data suggests that a virus-free stock was in the order of x100 more resistant than a very susceptible stock, and very roughly x10 less resistant than a resistant stock, giving an overall difference in the order of x1000 between the resistant and the very susceptible stocks (David and Gardiner, 1965a). Thus a degree of resistance as high as some of those obtained against chemicals (e.g. x800 in houseflies against dieldrin; Crow, 1957) has been recorded against an insect pathogen.

Latent diseases are often activated by a number of well-known factors that stress the host insect. Aizawa *et al.* (1961) obtained a strain of silkworm resistant to activation of virus by cold conditions, independent of resistance to infection with virus. In experiments in which the virus was not fed to the larvae, unfamiliar food increased the incidence of granulosis in a susceptible stock of *P. brassicae* but not in a resistant one (David and Gardiner, 1965b).

Little is known about the number of generations in which resistance to microbial agents develops. Among the examples quoted above, Aizawa *et al.* (1961) selected their silkworms for 13 generations, and Watanabe (1967) and Kartman (1953) selected for eight. Ignoffo (1967) states: "Fragmentary evidence indicates that it takes 30-40 generations of exposure to microbial insecticides to induce some level of resistance equivalent to that of chemical insecticides."

Variation of resistance to insect pathogens in an insect population and variation of the infective dose picked up by the insect are commonly large, as shown by the very low slopes of probit lines (Table IV in Chapter 27), which gives scope for natural selection of survivors.

Resistance has been reported to a microbial toxin. The housefly, *Musca domestica,* developed eight-fold resistance to the exotoxin of *Bacillus thuringiensis* in 27 generations of selection and 14-fold in 50 generations, a knowledge of slopes of the probit lines showing the resistance to be about 10-fold at the LD_{99} level (Harvey and Howell, 1965), but no resistance was obtained after 27 generations at a low selection pressure by Feigin (1963). One strain (but not a second strain) of *Drosophila melanogaster* developed 2.5-fold resistance in 30 generations at an unspecified intensity of selection (Herrewege, 1969).

This positive evidence is counterbalanced by negative evidence in the form of many reports of lack of development of resistance to microbial agents, some of which are listed by Ignoffo (1967) and by Martignoni and Schmid (1961).

IV. Resistance of Mammals to Microbial Control Agents

Study of the microbial control of the rabbit with myxomatosis in Australia has proved the development of inherited resistance in the rabbit and also a reduction in the virulence of the virus in a microbial control programme. In

Australia the European rabbit, *Oryctolagus cuniculus,* developed distinct resistance to the introduced Brazilian myxoma virus in seven years. Parallel with this, virus strains of moderate virulence replaced the virulent strain as dominant forms, because the reduction of virulence lengthened the survival of diseased rabbits and hence the time that less virulent virus was available for transmission by the insect vectors to healthy rabbits (Fenner, 1965; Pimentel, 1968). As one of two possible terminal associations between the rabbit and its disease, Fenner suggests that the virus will still cause moderately severe disease with an appreciable mortality, much as smallpox does in human communities. However, the reproductive power of the rabbit is such that this sort of disease need not seriously interfere with its population size. In the field of human epidemiology, the ravages of tuberculosis and measles introduced for the first time are notorious and suggest that resistance has been acquired in populations where these diseases are endemic, although the resistance problem in mammals is complicated by the acquisition of resistance during the lifetime of an individual.

V. Resistance of Insects to Macrobial Control Agents

I have found only one reference to the development of resistance in a macrobial control programme. The larch sawfly, *Pristiphora erichsonii,* developed an immunity to the introduced ichneumonid *Mesoleius tenthredinis* in about 27 years, the parasite being rendered harmless in the host's body by encapsulation (Muldrew, 1953). Simmonds (1967) stated: "There has been no development of resistance by a pest to any insect parasites or predators, except possibly with one ichneumonid parasite of the larch sawfly [see above] and this only in certain populations."

I have found one reference to the development of resistance to a macrobial agent in the laboratory. In a system in which the housefly, *Musca domestica,* was allowed to evolve under pressure from a parasitic wasp, *Nasonia vitripennis,* fly numbers at the start of each wasp generation being kept constant, Pimentel (1968) found that resistance developed in the fly and some avirulence in the wasp. He considered that the resistance was more important than the avirulence. In another experiment, the host numbers were allowed to fluctuate with the result that some degree of balance and stability evolved—the host numbers remaining at a relatively high level and those of the parasite at a low level, in comparison with violent fluctuations in the numbers of both species in the control, which was so arranged that evolution of the host was prevented.

VI. Interaction in the Evolution of Host and Pathogen

Biological control agents are alive, a unique advantage over chemicals. They are subject to variation, which may lead to the natural development of more effective strains, to the conquest of newly-acquired host resistance, or a capacity to infect new species. Pimentel (1968) believes that the evolution of resistance tends to stabilize populations of host and controlling agent by a process of genetical feedback. In this process pathogen density influences selective pressure on the host; this pressure influences the genetic constitution of the host and, in turn, the effects of the host's genetic constitution alter pathogen abundance, which may then alter the genetical make-up of the pathogen. A tendency towards the evolution of avirulence or of virulence of the agent would probably be determined by where selection pressure is exerted. Thus transmission of disease by the eating of dead bodies might lead towards an increase in virulence, whereas transovarial transmission might lead towards chronic disease of moderate severity with survival up to the point at which the adult reproduces. In the laboratory, instances of increased or reduced virulence have been frequently reported after repeated passage of the pathogen through the same, or another, host species (Chapter 30). Examples of differences in virulence between strains of pathogens are common. These are particularly numerous among pathogens of mammals, for instance, distinct strains of the influenza virus of different virulence have caused successive epidemics of disease in man. However, among insects convincing variations in virulence of virus strains have yet to be shown (David and Gardiner, 1965a), although other types of pathogens exist as strains of different virulence, e.g. 12 strains of *Bacillus thuringiensis* show different activities against many host species (e.g. Burgerjon and Biache, 1967). Also pathogens produce toxins, which may vary in toxicity as much as strains of pathogens vary in virulence, e.g. Pendleton (1969) found large differences in the crystalline toxins of different strains of *B. thuringiensis.*

VII. Consideration of Relevant Facts About Resistance to Chemicals

The discussion of the expression of resistance in section II was developed from a knowledge of resistance to chemicals: further discussion of this subject yields ideas that must be considered in relation to pathogens.

In the development of resistance to chemicals, a small degree of polyfactorial vigour tolerance generally appears first, without much change in the slopes of the probit lines (Brown, 1967). Possibly, since it applies to chemical insecticides in general, such vigour tolerance developed against chemicals would also extend to pathogens, and vigour tolerance to one pathogen might extend to others.

With chemicals, after the development of vigour tolerance, there usually follows a variable number of generations with little change, then large increases in resistance appear rapidly, usually monofactorial (Crow, 1957; Brown, 1967). Information about changes in the resistance of wild insect populations to pathogens is limited to suggestions that endemic pathogens have weeded out the more susceptible individuals of *Eucosoma griseana* and *Phryganidia californica*

(Martignoni, 1957; Martignoni and Schmid, 1961). Since the pathogens were endemic it is possible that one or more resistance genes were already common in the population. In the event of resistance developing to an exotic pathogen introduced into a population that had never experienced that pathogen before, the pattern might follow that outlined for chemicals.

Resistance to chemicals develops only in populations containing resistance genes. The same can be expected with pathogens, so attempts to demonstrate resistance experimentally in the laboratory should involve insect populations based on many individuals, preferably gleaned from the survivors of field populations exposed to the pathogen over as wide as possible an area. Also fresh insects from widely scattered field populations and from different countries could be interpolated continually into the experimental stock.

Reversion of resistant stocks is rarely complete and resistance to chemicals is redeveloped rapidly. This is because neither the resistance gene, nor the complex of supporting genes evolved with the main resistance gene, slip back to their former state of extreme rarity. If a pathogen is enzootic, particularly if it causes periodic epizootics, moderate numbers of the resistance and supporting genes may be present in the insect population, and there would almost certainly be periodic ebb and flow of resistance build-up and reversion.

The higher the selection pressure, the faster is the development of resistance to chemicals. This seems a good reason for the use of minimal dosages of pathogens to allow the survival of sub-economic insect populations—a case argued for other reasons elsewhere (Chapter 19).

Resistance to chemicals has been greatest amongst those most persistent. Thus, if selection pressure is maintained, the persistence of pathogens, such as viruses, in a population would favour the development of resistance in contrast to others, like *B. thuringiensis,* that do not persist.

With monofactorial resistance to chemicals, homozygous resistant insects often suffer troubles, such as low fecundity, until a supporting gene complex has been evolved. Thus in experiments on the development of resistance to pathogens, all factors except the dosage of pathogen should be kept optimal for breeding of the insects. Sometimes results advantageous to the insect, e.g. longer adult life and consequent greater egg production, eventually accompany the development of resistance to chemicals.

VIII. Conclusions and Research Requirements

On grounds of fundamental biological principle, the existence of a capacity of insects to develop resistance to microbial control agents is undeniable. The production of resistance in the laboratory offers proof of this capacity. However, there is scant evidence on which to predict whether resistance will become of widespread importance in practice. It shows no signs of doing so at present in such well-known microbial control successes as the use of the *Bacillus popilliae* group against the Japanese beetle and the virus of the spruce sawfly *Gilpinia (Diprion) hercyniae.* However, most attempts at microbial control are in their infancy and are not studied in sufficient detail to reveal resistance. No more can be suggested than a possibility that some wild insect populations are already to some degree resistant to enzootic pathogens and that this resistance might be increased if selection pressure on the host was increased by a microbial control programme. Much would depend on the degree of selection pressure, on the scale of the programme and whether it becomes as intense as the use of some chemicals today. More pronounced resistance might develop to an exotic pathogen, but this suggestion is made mainly by analogy to chemicals, although it receives a little support from the development of resistance to a single virus used extensively to control a mammal, the rabbit. One factor not present in chemicals is the ability of at least some pathogens to change and counter resistance. This may prove important, particularly in pathogens that persist. Furthermore, by genetic manipulation of microbial control agents in the laboratory, any natural tendency to defeat resistance by the evolution of more effective strains can probably be supplemented, and possibly developed at a greater rate than would occur naturally.

The available evidence suggests that resistant insects are less likely to appear in macrobial than in microbial control.

Reduction of virulence of biological agents may also occur. This has no equivalent with chemicals. Together with resistance, it may lead towards balance and stability in populations after the introduction of an agent, although population levels at which balance is achieved would be bound to vary and may be above levels that can be tolerated economically.

The need for research is obvious. At this stage, when the development of resistance has been demonstrated in the laboratory without answering the question of whether resistance will develop in biological control programmes, more emphasis should be given to field studies in which samples of insects are taken into the laboratory for accurate bioassay to test for resistance. The bioassays should be sufficiently detailed to show the slopes of probit lines, which indicate whether RF values demonstrate real resistance at the $LD_{99.9}$ level. At the beginning of a programme, assays are required to obtain base line data for comparison with future wild generations of agents and pests. Many microbial agents can be preserved in their original state of virulence by a variety of methods, such as deep freezing. For future reference, *these agents should be preserved from the time of their initial discovery.* Laboratory stocks of insects, derived from wild populations before the start of a programme are more difficult to maintain unchanged for reference purposes, because they may change in resistance, both if bred free from pathogens, and in their presence. Nevertheless reference stocks of insects would be very useful. Microbial control programmes should be studied in sufficient detail to reveal any resistance that may develop and also every opportunity should be taken of studying changes in the susceptibility of insects after a pathogen appears in a new area, naturally or by introduction. For instance, a granulosis virus of *Hyphantria cunea* appeared in Europe in 1957 and reduced this major pest to a minor role (Vasiljević, in press): recently the pest has started to increase again (Vasiljević, personal communication).

References

Aizawa, K., Furuta, Y. and Nakamura, K. (1961). *J. seric. Sci. Japan* **30**, 405-412. (In Japanese with English summary.) Cited in Aizawa, K. (1963). *In* "Insect Pathology. An Advanced Treatise" (E. A. Steinhaus, ed.), Vol. 1, pp. 381-412. Academic Press, New York.

Ayuzawa, C., Yushinobu, A. and Kurata, K. (1969). *Bull. seric. exp. Stn Japan* **23**, 469-497.

Bamrick, J. F. and Rothenbuhler, W. C. (1961). *J. Insect Path.* **3**, 381-390.

Bergold, G. (1948). *Z. Naturf.* **3B**, 25-26.

Bergold, G. H. (1951). *Can. J. Zool.* **29**, 17-23.

Bird, F. T. and Elgee, D. E. (1957). *Can. Ent.* **89**, 371-378.

Brown, A. W. A. (1967). *Wld Rev. Pest Control* **6**, 104-114.

Burgerjon, A. and Biache, G. (1967). *Entomologia exp. appl.* **10**, 211-230.

Crow, J. F. (1957). *A. Rev. Ent.* **2**, 227-246.

David, W. A. L. and Gardiner, B. O. C. (1960). *J. Insect Path.* **2**, 106-114.

David, W. A. L. and Gardiner, B. O. C. (1965a). *J. Invertebrate Path.* **7**, 285-290.

David, W. A. L. and Gardiner, B. O. C. (1965b). *J. Invertebrate Path.* **7**, 347-355.

Dyte, C. E. and Blackman, D. G. (1967). *J. stored Prod. Res.* **2**, 211-228.

Feigin, J. M. (1963). *Ann. Ent. Soc. Am.* **56**, 878-879.

Fenner, F. (1965). *In* "The Genetics of Colonising Species" (H. G. Baker and G. L. Stebbins, eds), pp. 485-499. Academic Press, New York.

Herrewege, J., van (1969). Ph.D. Thesis, Univ. Lyon, 90 pp.

Harvey, T. L. and Howell, D. E. (1965). *J. Invertebrate Path.* **7**, 92-100.

Ignoffo, C. M. (1967). *In* "Insect Pathology and Microbial Control" (P. A. van der Laan, ed.), pp. 91-117. North-Holland Publ. Co., Amsterdam.

Ignoffo, C. M. and Garcia, C. (1969). *J. Invertebrate Path.* **14**, 282-283.

Kartman, L. (1950). Ph.D. Thesis, Johns Hopkins Univ. Baltimore. Cited in Kartman (1953).

Kartman, L. (1953) *Expl Parasit.* **2**, 27-78.

Koidsumi, K. and Wade, Y. (1955). *Jap. J. appl. Zool.* **20**, 184-190.

Maléki-Milani, H. (1969). Ph.D. Thesis, Univ. Paris, 117 pp.

Martignoni, M. E. (1957). *Mitt. schweiz. Anstalt forstl. Versuchswesen* **32**, 371-418.

Martignoni, M. E. and Schmid, P. (1961). *J. Insect Path.* **3**, 62-74.

Muldrew, J. A. (1953). *Can. J. Zool.* **31**, 313-332.

Ossowski, L. L. J. (1958). *Nature, Lond.* **181**, 648.

Ossowski, L. L. J. (1960a). *Ann. appl. Biol.* **48**, 299-313.

Ossowski, L. L. J. (1960b). *J. Insect Path.* **2**, 35-43.

Park, O. W. (1936). *Am. Bee J.* **76**, 12-15.

Park, O. W., Pellett, F. C. and Paddock, F. B. (1937). *Am. Bee J.* **77**, 20-25 and 34.

Pendleton, I. R. (1969). *J. Invertebrate Path.* **13**, 423-428.

Pimentel, D. (1968). *Science* **159**, 1432-1437.

Rivers, C. F. (1959). *Trans. 1st Int. Conf. Insect Path. Biol. Control, Prague,* 1958, pp. 205-210.

Rothenbuhler, W. C. and Thompson, V. C. (1956). *J. econ. Ent.* **49**, 470-475.

Sidor, C. (1959). *Ann. appl. Biol.* **47**, 109-113.
Simmonds, F. J. (1967). *J. R. Soc. Arts* **115**, 880-898.
Steinhaus, E. A. (1949). "Principles of Insect Pathology", 757 pp. McGraw-Hill, New York.
Thompson, V. C. and Rothenbuhler, W. C. (1957). *J. econ. Ent.* **50**, 731-737.
Uzigawa, K. and Aruga, H. (1966). *J. seric. Sci. Japan* **35**, 23-26. (In Japanese.)
Vasiljević, L. In press. *Entomophaga*.
Watanabe, H. (1967). *J. Invertebrate Path.* **9**, 474-479.

CHAPTER 21

Interactions Between Pathogens

ALOYSIUS KRIEG

Biologische Bundesanstalf für Land- und Forstwirtschaft, Institut für biologische Schädlingsbekämpfung, Darmstadt, Germany

After inoculation of culture media or of susceptible hosts with several pathogens, interactions between micro-organisms may result in co-existence, synergism, or antagonism. All these types of interaction have been observed with insect pathogens. Antagonism is equivalent to a reduction in virulence, whereas synergism enhances virulence as a result of the interaction. In principle, synergism and antagonism are possible between different micro-organisms as well as between strains of one and the same pathogen.

Owing to the restricted space available to this topic, reference is made only to the most important papers dealing with such interactions. Results which could not be adequately analysed, as well as reports based on insignificant effects, have not been considered.

I. Bacteria

A special kind of interaction is that between different pathogenic factors connected with one and the same micro-organism. In whole cultures of *Bacillus thuringiensis,* for example, three factors may act together: spores, endotoxin crystals and exotoxin. Angus and Heimpel (1959) found endotoxin crystals to be highly effective against some lepidopterous larvae such as *Bombyx mori.* However, according to the same authors and to Burgerjon and Yamvrias (1959), living spores are necessary in addition to endotoxin crystals to induce significant mortality in moths like *Ephestia (Anagasta) kuehniella.* Finally, in *Mamestra (Barathra) brassicae,* high mortality of the larvae may be induced only by a combination of all three pathogenic factors (Burgerjon and de Barjac, 1962).

Zurabova (1968) mechanically mixed separately fermented cultures of different strains (serotypes) of *B. thuringiensis* after sporulation. The mixture was more potent than the equivalent quantity of any one culture, indicating synergism between the different strains. In contrast, she obtained no such increase in potency when the different strains were grown together in the same culture, so that possibly the different strains were antagonistic during their growth in culture. The dominance of one strain in infections in larvae of *Philosamia cynthia,* fed a mixture of different strains, was caused by antagonism rather than pathogenicity (Pendleton, 1969). Krieg (1970) showed that antagonism between *B. thuringiensis* strains is caused by bacteriocins. Bacteriocins of another type are well-known from some gram-negative potential pathogens such as *Pseudomonas aeruginosa* (Paterson, 1965) and *Serratia marcescens* (Prinsloo, 1966).

A possible consequence of mixed infections of pathogens *in vivo* or *in vitro* are recombinations of genetic factors, which may give rise to new types. Especially, the origin of strains of increased virulence from moderately virulent ones could be expected. In this connection, some attention should be paid to the work of Reeves (1966), who succeeded in establishing *in vitro* artificial genetic transformation of "pathogenicity" from a virulent variety of *B. thuringiensis* to an apathogenic one.

Bacteriophages also may cause genetic conversion or transduction. This is possible because the genetic material of phages and that of their host bacteria are derived from common ancestors of lysogenic bacteria. Bacteriophages have been reported from *P. aeruginosa* (Paterson, 1965) and from *S. marcescens* (Prinsloo, 1966) as well as from *B. thuringiensis* (reviewed by Krieg, 1961, 1967). Commercial preparations of *B. thuringiensis* often contain lysogenic bacteria or are contaminated by phages. It is therefore possible that, in some cases of reduced efficiency, the activity of bacteriophages during the vegetative phase of the fermentation process cause incomplete sporulation and scanty production of parasporal crystals.

It has not been established whether bacteriophages have any significance in disease therapy. According to experience in other branches of applied microbiology, the selection of resistant clones of bacteria minimizes the therapeutic effect of the phages within a very short time after bacteriophage infection. Furthermore, negative results have been obtained with specific phages on *B. thuringiensis* infections of *B. mori* (Afrikian, 1960). It has also been reported that infections of *S. marcescens* by phages did not significantly influence the pathogenic efficiency of the host-bacterium against the armyworm, *Pseudaletia unipuncta* (Goodwin, 1968).

Mixed infections of insects with different types of pathogenic bacteria are rare in nature. In most bacterioses, only one type or species is involved as causative agent. An antagonism between different bacteria, due to antibiotics, may prevent mixed infections. For example, Vaňková (1957, 1965) demonstrated *in vitro* production of an antibiotic-like substance, effective against other gram-positive bacteria, by several varieties of *B. thuringiensis.* Beard (1946) recorded that *Bacillus popilliae* inhibits the development of *Bacillus lentimorbus* in grubs of the scarabaeid beele, *Popillia japonica,* inoculated with both bacteria. In cases of antagonism *in vivo* immunity factors may be involved, for example bactericides produced by host insects (Stephens-Chadwick, 1967; Kawarabata and Aizawa, 1967; Mohrig and Messner, 1968).

The effect of combinations of different bacteria *in vivo* was studied by Stephens (1959) on the grasshopper, *Melanoplus bivittatus.* She found no synergistic effect in combinations of *P. aeruginosa* with *S. marcescens.* Comparable results have been obtained by Steinhaus (1959) on the wax moth *Galleria mellonella*: while *B. thuringiensis* helped *S. marcescens* to act as a secondary invader, *S. marcescens* actually reduced the efficiency of *B. thuringiensis.* These observations of Steinhaus may be elucidated by the results of Isakova (1964). She found that at doses not high enough to kill larvae rapidly by toxicosis due to the crystal toxin, larvae died more slowly due to septicaemia. In a species such as *G. mellonella* with a poor gut microflora, the septicaemia was caused predominantly by vegetative cells of *B. thuringiensis,* but in *Pieris brassicae,* which has a rich gut flora, the body cavity was invaded by mutualistic gut bacteria, mostly Enterobacteriaceae. In the latter case, the crystal is evidently acting as a pace-maker to the secondary invaders by interfering with the normal functioning and possibly the defence mechanisms of the gut. White (1968) obtained similar results.

Another problem concerns the possible protection of insects from bacterial infection by competing microflora in the gut. White (1968) found that erythromycin controlled *Streptococcus faecalis/faecium* in *P. brassicae,* but its use for extended periods usually led to the development of a species of *Aeromonas* that could give rise to a fatal septicaemia. Without the antibiotic, the *Streptococcus* probably prevented the development of the *Aeromonas.* Infection experiments with *Pseudaletia unipuncta* by Goodwin (1968) showed that *Pseudomonas aeruginosa* induces a very high mortality only in larvae fed on an axenic diet. In larvae fed with corn-leaf under xenic conditions, this bacterium did not commonly produce lethal septicaemia. Probably, *P. aeruginosa* was inhibited by the gut microflora and/or by antibiotic plant fractions. Similar results, however, were not obtained with *S. marcescens,* which induced a constant mortality (of about 30%) in both xenic-corn-fed and axenic-diet-fed caterpillars. When *P. aeruginosa* and *S. marcescens* were applied simultaneously to axenic-diet-fed larvae, the induced mortality was about 50%, intermediate between the mortalities caused by either bacterium alone. This confirmed the results of Stephens (1959) who found that these two facultative pathogens do not act synergistically. Combinations of *S. marcescens* or *P. aeruginosa* with *Streptococcus faecalis* var. *liquefaciens* induce significant mortality in axenic-reared larvae of *P. unipuncta* (Goodwin, 1968). No mortality, however, could be induced in this host either by combinations of *Enterobacter cloacae* and *Enterobacter aerogenes* with *S. faecalis* var. *liquefaciens* or by application of either species alone.

Combinations of different bacteria have also been tested by Kudler and Lysenko (1964) against some lepidopterous larvae. The mortality induced by a mixture of *B. thuringiensis* with gram-negative bacteria like *Pseudomonas, Serratia, Enterobacter,* and *Flavobacterium* was never higher than that caused by the most effective component, *B. thuringiensis.*

Some attention should also be paid to interactions between obligate pathogenic (bacteria-like) rickettsiae and potentially pathogenic bacteria. Although Hurpin and Robert (1968) observed inhibition of *Rickettsiella melolonthae* by a well-established *Bacillus popilliae* infection in cockchafer larvae *(Melolontha melolontha),* also double infections with both pathogens occasionally occurred. Simultaneous application of both pathogens induced no increase in mortality compared with that caused by the more virulent rickettsia alone. It is of some interest that Wille (1959) found a bacterial septicaemia in *Melolontha* larvae as a result of a preceding infection with *R. melolonthae.*

II. Viruses

Mixed virus infections are not uncommon in nature. They have been observed in many Lepidoptera, for example, with nuclear and cytoplasmic polyhedroses in *Mamestra (Barathra) brassicae, Bombyx mori, Thaumetopoea pityocampa,* with nuclear polyhedrosis and granulosis in *Choristoneura fumiferana, C. murinana, Agrotis (Euxoa) segetum, Spodoptera (Laphygma) frugiperda, Nephelodes emmedonia, Pieris rapae, Pseudaletia unipuncta, Trichoplusia ni,* and with cytoplasmic polyhedroses and granuloses in *A. segetum* and *Pieris brassicae.*

After infection of the larvae of *Antheraea pernyi* or *B. mori* with two types of nuclear polyhedrosis virus, sensitive cells became infected with only a single virus type (Gershenson, 1956). This phenomenon may be due to interference at cellular level. In some rare cases, however, cell nuclei have been found to be infected by both types of the virus, which may presuppose recombination of insect viruses. Delayed mortality due to interference between two strains of a nuclear polyhedrosis virus in *Hyphantria cunea* has been reported by Aruga *et al.* (1961b) and between two cytoplasmic polyhedrosis viruses in *B. mori* by Aruga *et al.* (1961a, 1963). Later, Tanada and Chang (1964) studied interactions of two cytoplasmic polyhedrosis viruses in *B. mori* and *Colias eurydice.* In

C. eurydice a remarkable antagonism occurred. The degree of interference varied with the sequence in time of feeding, with the relative doses applied, and with the age of larvae used. Again, nearly all infected cells contained only one type of virus. Double infections of cells occurred very rarely. According to recent investigations (Aruga, 1967), there is no interference between the nuclear polyhedrosis of fat body cells and the cytoplasmic polyhedrosis of gut cells in *B. mori,* but a remarkable interference was found between a cytoplasmic polyhedrosis and a nuclear polyhedrosis virus both of the gut epithelium. Interference also occurred between the gut cytoplasmic polyhedrosis and the so-called flacherie virus. Attempts to elucidate virus inhibition by postulation of an immune inhibition factor and presence of interferon have been made by Kawarabata and Aizawa (1967). In this connection, it should also be mentioned that development of resistance or cross-resistance may occur as a result of a long association between the host population and the same or another pathogen.

Increased effectiveness of viruses following double infection is known from other branches of virology. In insect virology, Tanada (1959) suggested synergism on the basis of quantitative response by a test population of *P. unipuncta.* He observed increased efficiency of a nuclear polyhedrosis virus after stimulation with a granulosis virus in the same host. Bird (1959), however, found no evidence for a synergistic action with double infections of *C. fumiferana* with granulosis and nuclear polyhedrosis. He mentioned that the prior infection interfered with the second. Single cells were found to be infected by only one of the two viruses and double infection of cells was again rare. It should be mentioned that virus synergism (Tanada, 1959) as well as antagonism (interference) (Aruga, 1967) may also be induced if one of the virus partners is inactivated by heat or ultra-violet irradiation. But this statement could not be confirmed generally. Lowe and Paschke (1968), for example, mentioned that synergism after simultaneous infection of *T. ni* with nuclear polyhedrosis and granulosis viruses was produced only by combinations of two infectious inocula. No synergism or interference occurred, however, when an infectious and thermally inactivated agent were combined.

A latent virus infection of an insect may be activated, not only by viruses which are pathogenic for the host in question, but also by foreign viruses. Bergold (1951) found stimulation of nuclear polyhedrosis of *C. fumiferana* by the granulosis virus of *C. murinana.* Krieg (1957b) reported activation of an inapparent nuclear polyhedrosis of the gut epithelium of the sawfly, *Neodiprion sertifer,* by two different viruses to which this host is not sensitive: cytoplasmic polyhedra from the moth *Dasychira pudibunda* and nuclear polyhedra from the butterfly, *Aporia crataegi.* Recently, similar results have been obtained by Longworth and Cunningham (1968). These authors induced cytoplasmic polyhedrosis in larvae of the butterfly, *Aglais urticae,* by feeding of nuclear polyhedra from the gypsy moth, *Lymantria dispar.*

It is suggested that the polyhedral protein, and not active virions, played a significant role in the activation of latent virus infections by foreign viruses with inclusion bodies. Unfortunately activation of latent viruses following inoculation by foreign viruses hampers work on the host range of insect viruses (Smith, 1963).

III. Viruses with Bacteria or Rickettsiae

Latent viroses may also be activated by non-viral pathogens such as *B. thuringiensis.* For example, Vasiljević (1957) reported that up to 90% of larvae of *Hyphantria cunea,* which had ingested *B. thuringiensis,* died of a nuclear polyhedrosis instead of bacteriosis. Only 10-15% of untreated caterpillars, however, died of polyhedrosis. Krieg and Schmidt (1962) observed that only young caterpillars of *H. cunea* died with symptoms of bacteriosis after feeding on *B. thuringiensis,* whereas, after the same treatment the older larvae died with symptoms and signs of an activated granulosis. Other bacteria also may be suitable activators. Food treated with *Serratia marcescens* induced an outbreak of nuclear polyhedrosis causing 100% mortality in a latently infected population of *Neodiprion sertifer* (Krieg, unpublished). Similar results with this host have been obtained by Kudler and Lysenko (1964) after use of *S. marcescens* (52% mortality) and *Pseudomonas chlororaphis* (20-100% mortality). It is apparent, therefore, that artificial infection with bacteria may have a greater effect in populations having latent infection of virus than in healthy ones.

However, a remarkable inverse effect has also been reported. In laboratory experiments, Sicker *et al.* (1965) fed *B. thuringiensis* to caterpillars of *Malacosoma neustria* from a population suffering from a latent nuclear polyhedrosis. Surprisingly, a lower mortality of the treated larvae occurred compared with untreated larvae from the same population.

Viruses may also induce secondary bacterioses. Bacterial septicaemia has been observed after application of specific nuclear polyhedra in *B. mori* (Vago, 1956a) and *Aporia crataegi* (Krieg, 1957a). It is well known that unpurified virus suspensions usually have a greater effect than purified ones. For example, Magnoler (1968) reported this effect in the nuclear polyhedrosis of *Lymantria dispar.* It is suggested that such increase in efficiency is due to bacterial contamination of the impure virus suspensions with potential pathogens.

Some field trials have also been carried out with intentionally combined suspensions of viruses and bacteria. For example, Semel (1961) combined *B. thuringiensis* with nuclear polyhedra for the control of *Trichoplusia ni.* However, no increase in mortality, compared with that caused by the virus alone, was observed. Combinations of *B. thuringiensis* with polyhedrosis viruses induced no enhanced efficiency in *Malacosoma fragile* (Stelzer, 1965) and *Mamestra (Barathra) brassicae* (Krieg, 1967). Shekhurina (1966), however, reported positive results with similar combinations in the field. She used granulosis virus of the moth *Agrotis (Euxoa) segetum* and *B. thuringiensis* simultaneously against *Agrotis (Euxoa) exclamationis. B. thuringiensis* alone induced 60% and the virus alone 75% mortality, while a combination of both pathogens achieved 92%.

Combinations of rickettsiae and viruses have been used by Hurpin and Robert (1968). They obtained an efficiency intermediate between that of each pathogen alone (rickettsiosis about 58%, and virosis about 78% morbidity) within a temperature range of 17°-25° C. The lower the temperature the greater was the percentage of rickettsiosis, but higher temperatures increased the percentage of virosis following simultaneous infections. Each pathogen-host relationship appears to have its own temperature optimum, and the effect of double infections may be different at different temperatures.

IV. Other Pathogens

Double infections of insects by different protozoans are well known. For example, Wiser (1956) reported mixed infections with several microsporida in *Euproctis chrysorrhoea* and *Lymantria dispar.*

Vago (1956b) studied synergism between microsporidosis and granulosis in *Sesamia cretica.* Later, Atger and Vago (1960) also found synergism between microsporida and nuclear polyhedrosis in *Samia cynthia* and *B. mori.* A similar synergistic effect between microsporidosis and granulosis as well as with cytoplasmic polyhedrosis was observed by Huger (1960) in *Agrotis (Euxoa) segetum,* and between microsporidosis and cytoplasmic polyhedrosis by Tanada (1962) in *Colias eurytheme.* Lipa (1968) mentioned a synergistic effect of simultaneous infections with a microsporidon, a cytoplasmic and a nuclear polyhedrosis in *Heliothis zea.*

Weakening of insect hosts by toxins may also favour bacterial infection. For example, Lepesme (1938) obtained no striking mycosis after application of *Aspergillus flavus* to the locusts *Schistocerca gregaria* and *Locusta migratoria,* but instead a secondary infection by potential pathogens such as *Pseudomonas aeruginosa* and *Serratia marcescens.* Similar observations have been reported by Vago (1963) with *Aspergillus, Rhizopus* and *Fusarium* as pace-makers for secondary bacterioses. Combinations of *Beauveria bassiana* and *B. thuringiensis* have been tested against Orthoptera (Brinkman and Tonkonoshenko, 1967), Mallophaga (Hoffman and Gingrich, 1967) and Coleoptera (Sandner and Cichy, 1967) though without any significant synergistic effect. However, Kalyuga (1968) used a combination of *B. bassiana* and *B. thuringiensis* with some success against the lepidopteran, *Pieris brassicae.* Combinations of both pathogens induced 93-98% mortality. Each pathogen, alone, however, induced 88% *(B. bassiana)* and from 58 to 86% *(B. thuringiensis)* mortality, respectively.

Masera (1934) reported an antagonistic effect by *S. marcescens* on the insect pathogen *B. bassiana*: the mortality induced in the beetle, *Tenebrio molitor,* by the fungus was markedly reduced by the bacterium.

A probable synergistic effect occurred in larvae of *Melolontha melolontha* infected with *Rickettsiella melolonthae* in which mixed infections with fungi were found also (Wille, 1959), beside the specific infection.

Recently, Koyama and Katagiri (1967) described populations of *Dendrolimus spectabilis,* attacked by the fungus, *Isaria farinosa,* which showed a remarkably high incidence of virosis after feeding on cytoplasmic polyhedra, probably as a result of synergism between the two pathogens. Interactions between fungi and viruses have also been found by Telenga (1958) and by Evlakhova and Shvetsova (1961). In both cases *B. bassiana* activated a latent polyhedrosis virus disease of the host larvae *(Malacosoma neustria* and *Plusia gamma,* respectively).

A simultaneous infection of the geometrid moth, *Eulype hastata,* by a protozoan (*Nosema* sp.) and a fungus (*Entomophthora* sp.) have been reported by Steinhaus (1959). Hurpin (1965) described an interesting linkage phenomenon between *Beauveria tenella* and *Nosema melolonthae.* After a combined application to the grubs of *N. melolonthae,* the microsporidan survived the fungal epizootic, and in spite of a temporary disappearance of the host, the microsporidan finally suppressed the development of a new host population.

Natural infections of insects with several fungi are rare. According to Müller-Kögler (1965) antibiotic antagonism may prevent such mixed infections *in vivo. In vitro,* however, *Beauveras, Paecilomyces* and *Cephalosporium* showed no antagonism in mixed cultures (Fassatiova, 1964).

V. Conclusions

From observations on simultaneous infections it is concluded that they may or may not have synergistic or antagonistic effects as expressed by changes in mortality of insect hosts. The effect depends not only on the nature of the micro-organisms participating in the process, but also on other parameters such as their virulence, the relative doses applied, and the sequence in time of infection. In addition, predisposing factors such as the influence of climate (especially temperature) and the effect of stress conditions, are involved. Finally, unforeseen results may be produced by interactions between applied pathogens and pathogens already existing in the population.

Therefore results concerning interrelationships between pathogens obtained under restricted experimental conditions, should not be generalized.

References

Afrikian, E. G. (1960). *J. Insect Path.* **2**, 299-304.

Angus, T. A. and Heimpel, A. M. (1959). *Can. Ent.* **91**, 352-358.

Aruga, H. (1967). Abstr. Proc. Joint U.S.-Japan Semin. Microbial Control Insect Pests, pp. 17-18. U.S.-Japan Committee Sci. Cooperation. Panel 8. Fukuoka.

Aruga, H., Hukuhara, T., Fukuda, S. and Hashimoto, Y. (1963). *J. Insect Path.* **5**, 415-421.

Aruga, H., Hukuhara, T., Yoshitake, N. and Ayudhya, I. N. (1961a). *J. Insect Path.* **3**, 81-92.

Aruga, H., Yoshitake, N., Watanabe, H., Hukuhara, T., Nagashima, E. and Kawai, T. (1961b). *Jap. J. appl. Ent., Zool.* **5**, 141-144. (In Japanese.)

Atger, P. and Vago, C. (1960). *Revue. Path. vég., Ent. agric. Fr.* **39**, 205-209.

Beard, R. L. (1946). *Science* **103**, 371-372.

Bergold, G. H. (1951). *Can. J. Zool.* **29**, 17-23.

Bird, F. T. (1959). *J. Insect Path.* **1**, 406-430.

Brinkman, L. I. and Tonkonoshenko, A. P. (1967). *Probl. vet. san.* (Kuibischev) **28**, 325-331. (In Russian.)

Burgerjon, A. and de Barjac, H. (1962). *Verhandlung. 11. int. Kongr. Ent., Wien 1960,* **2**, 835-839.

Burgerjon, A. and Yamvrias, C. (1959). *C.r. hebd. Séanc. Acad. Sci. Paris* **249**, 2871-2872.

Evlakhova, A. A. and Shvetsova, O. I. (1961). *Zashch. Rast. Moskva* **7**, 43-44. (In Russian.)

Fassatiova, O. (1964). *Entomophaga Mém. hors Sér.* **2**, 159-161.

Gershenson, S. M. (1956). *Dokl. Akad. Nauk S.S.S.R.* **110**, 1199-1201.

Goodwin, R. H. (1968). *J. Invertebrate Path.* **11**, 358-370.

Hoffman, R. A. and Gingrich, R. E. (1967). *J. econ. Ent.* **61**, 85-88.

Huger, A. (1960). *Ztschr. Pfl. Krankh.* **67**, 65-77.

Hurpin, B. (1965). *J. Invertebrate Path.* **7**, 39-44.

Hurpin, B. and Robert, P. (1968). *J. Invertebrate Path.* **11**, 203-213.

Isakova, N. P. (1964). *Entomophaga Mém. hors. Sér.* No. 2, 175-178.

Kalyuga, M. V. (1968). *Ent. Obozr.* **47**, 450-453.

Kawarabata, T. and Aizawa, K. (1967). Abstr. Proc. Joint U.S.-Japan Semin. Microbial Control Insect Pests, pp. 53-54. U.S.-Japan Committee Sci. Cooperation. Panel 8. Fukuoka.

Koyama, R. and Katagiri, K. (1967). Abstr. Proc. Joint U.S.-Japan Semin. Microbial Control Insect Pests, pp. 24-26. U.S.-Japan Committee Sci. Cooperation. Panel 8. Fukuoka.

Krieg, A. (1957a). *Z. Pfl. Krankh.* **64**, 657-662.

Krieg, A. (1957b). *Archiv ges. Virusforschg.* **7**, 212-219.

Krieg, A. (1961). "*Bacillus thuringiensis* Berliner". *Mitt. Biol. Bundesanstalt Land-u Forstwirtsch., Berlin-Dahlem* **103**, 79 pp.

Krieg, A. (1967). "Neues über *Bacillus thuringiensis* und seine Anwendung". *Mitt. Biol. Bundesanstalt Land-u. Forstwirtsch., Berlin-Dahlem* **125**, 106 pp.

Krieg, A. (1970). *J. Invertebrate Path.* **15**, 291.

Krieg, A. and Schmidt, L. (1962). *Nachrichtenbl. dtsch. Pflanzenschutzd. (Braunschweig)* **14**, 177-182.

Kudler, J. and Lysenko, O. (1964). FAO/IUFRO Symp. "Int. Dangerous Forest Diseases and Insects", **2**, IX, 8 pp. Oxford 1964.

Lepesme, P. (1938). *Bull. Soc. Hist. nat. Afr. Nord* **29**, 372-384.

Lipa, J. J. (1968). *Bull. ent. Pologne* **38**, 611-616.

Longworth, J. F. and Cunningham, J. C. (1968). *J. Invertebrate Path.* **10**, 361-367.

Lowe, R. E. and Paschke, J. D. (1968). *J. Invertebrate Path.* **12**, 86-92.

Magnoler, A. (1968). *J. Invertebrate Path.* **11**, 326-328.

Masera, E. (1934). *Annali Sper. agr.* **15**, 117-150.

Mohrig, W. and Messner, B. (1968). *Biol. Zentralbl.* **87**, 439-470.

Müller-Kögler, E. (1965). "Pilzkrankheiten bei Insekten. Anwendung zur biologischen Schädlingsbekämpfung und Grundlagen der Insektenmykologie", 444 pp. Verlag Parey, Berlin.

Paterson, A. C. (1965). *J. gen. Microbiol.* **39,** 295-303.
Pendleton, I. R. (1969). *J. Invertebrate Path.* **13,** 235-240.
Prinsloo, H. E. (1966). *J. gen. Microbiol.* **45,** 205-212.
Reeves, E. L. (1966). *Diss. Ohio State Univ.* 52 pp.
Sandner, H. and Cichy, D. (1967). *Ekologia Polska* Ser. A. **15,** 325-333.
Semel, M. (1961). *J. econ. Ent.* **54,** 698-701.
Shekhurina, T. A. (1966). *In* Biol. metod. borb. s vredit. sel'sk lesn. choz. karant. sorn. Tashkent 1966, pp. 194-197. (In Russian.)
Sicker, W., Magnoler, A. and Huger, A. (1965). *Z. Pfl. Krankh.* **72,** 599-605.
Smith, K. M. (1963). *In* "Insect Pathology. An Advanced Treatise" (E. A. Steinhaus, ed.), pp. 457-497. Academic Press, New York.
Steinhaus, E. A. (1959). *Hilgardia* **28,** 351-380.
Stelzer, M. J. (1965). *J. Invertebrate Path.* **7,** 122-125.
Stephens, J. M. (1959). *Can. J. Microbiol.* **5,** 313-315.
Stephens-Chadwick, J. (1967). *Fedn. Proc. Fedn. Am. Socs exp. Biol.* **26,** 1675-1679.
Tanada, Y. (1959). *J. Insect Path.* **1,** 215-231.
Tanada, Y. (1962). *J. Insect Path.* **4,** 495-497.
Tanada, Y. and Chang, G. Y. (1964). *J. Insect Path.* **6,** 500-516.
Telenga, N. A. (1958). Cit. after Müller-Kögler (1965).
Vago, C. (1956a). *J. Silkworm* **8,** 39-47.
Vago, C. (1956b). *Entomophaga* **1,** 82-87.
Vago, C. (1963). *In* "Insect Pathology. An Advanced Treatise" (E. A. Steinhaus, ed.), pp. 339-379. Academic Press, New York.
Vaňková, J. (1957). *Fol. Biol. Praha* **3,** 175-182.
Vaňková, J. (1965). *Proc. 12th Int. Congr. Ent. London 1964,* p. 739.
Vasiljević, L. A. (1957). *Mem. Inst. Plant Prot. Beograd* **7,** 79 pp. (Serbo-Croat.).
Weiser, J. (1956). *Ztschr. Pfl. Krankh.* **63,** 625-638.
Weiser, J. (1963). *In* "Insect Pathology. An Advanced Treatise" (E. A. Steinhaus, ed.), pp. 291-334. Academic Press, New York.
White, A. G. (1968). "The histopathological effects and the site of action of *Bacillus thuringiensis* in the larva of *Pieris brassicae* and its bioassay against the larva of *Galleria mellonella",* 185 pp. Ph.D. Thesis, Univ. Leeds.
Wille, H. (1959). Trans. "First International Conference of Insect Pathology and Biological Control", pp. 127-141. Prague 1958.
Zurabova, E. (1968). *In* "XIII Int. Congr. Ent., Abstr. Paper", 311 pp. Moscow 1968.

CHAPTER 22

Safety of Insect Pathogens for Man and Vertebrates

A. M. HEIMPEL

United States Department of Agriculture, Agricultural Research Service, Entomology Research Division, Beltsville, Maryland, U.S.A.

I. Introduction

The idea of using pathogens of insects as control agents is not new. According to Martignoni (1964) the production of these pathogens started some time after 1880 and continued over the years. However, in many cases, these attempts never got past the experimental stage because many of the most promising bacterial and viral pathogens were found to be fastidious and grow only in living insect tissue. Consequently, these pathogens could be produced only on living insects artificially reared, at great expense, on natural plant foliage during a limited season of each year. Of course, naturally infected insects in the field were often collected to provide sources of these micro-organisms, though these collections provided "filthy" preparations of indefinite or varied composition.

From these early developments in microbial control there are no records of safety tests. Perhaps such tests were carried out though no publications are available. Scientists, working with these micro-organisms, observed their extreme specificity and came to the conclusion, perhaps widely valid, that insect pathogens were, for the greater part, innocuous to other life forms.

For the last three decades the trend in selection of pesticides has been towards the highly toxic chemical and it became obvious to the legislators in various countries that something must be done to protect the public consuming foodstuffs treated by insecticidal sprays.

II. Registration of Microbial Insecticides

A. UNITED STATES OF AMERICA

The U.S.A. has been the greatest user of insecticides and it was this country that first created a law requiring registration of any materials used to treat food crops. So it was that Congress prepared the Federal Insecticide, Fungicide and Rodenticide Act which became law on 25 June 1947.

The Pesticide Regulation Division (PRD) of the United States Department of Agriculture (USDA) was established to carry out the dictates of this legislation. Upon receipt of an application for registration and labeling of a pesticide, fungicide or rodenticide product, the PRD is responsible for approving proof of the efficacy and safety of said product when it is to be used on food crops or otherwise. This action is always coordinated with the establishment of a level of tolerance or an exemption from tolerance provided by the Food and Drug Administration (FDA), United States Department of Health, Education and Welfare.

The type of tolerance level permissible on crops, at market time, is based on toxicological data. In the case of some highly toxic compounds, the foodstuff must have no detectable insecticide left, whereas certain chemicals may have a prescribed amount of residue on the marketed crop; this is defined as a prescribed level of tolerance.

In the case of microbial agents to control insects the regulatory agencies have made it clear that they required proof of safety sufficient to allow the granting of an exemption of tolerance. Since these agents are living entities capable of propagating in nature, they must be proved safe for all other life forms.

Consequently, when a petition for registration and labeling of a microbial agent is filed with the PRD, the petitioner must supply the following information.

1. A method of production of the microbial agent with demonstration of adequate techniques for production of a uniform product and for its standardization.

2. A method to provide evidence that extraneous biotypes have been eliminated or controlled to an acceptable level.
3. Efficacy of the product must be demonstrated by data from thorough field testing in various parts of the country, on all of the insects' host plants proposed for treatment in the petition.
4. Safety of the product for vertebrates, plants and beneficial insects must be established by applying a protocol of tests that has the approval of the PRD.
5. There must be an exemption from tolerance requirements issued by the FDA. These exemptions from tolerance must cover all food or feed crops that are to be treated or that may be contaminated.

For several years now intensive discussions on the proper protocol of tests for establishing exemption of tolerance for insect viruses have been carried out between the USDA and the FDA. The latter organization has appointed a panel of distinguished scientists to consult on the development of such a protocol. As this publication goes to press, this panel has not yet reported their conclusions to the FDA. However, from past experience it is possible to give a tentative and possibly incomplete statement of the general requirements for establishing exemption of tolerance.

In very general terms, the microbial agent must be shown harmless for other life forms from the plant and animal kingdoms. It must be demonstrated that the agent fails to multiply in small farm animals, rodents, and man. In these cases multiplication of the insect pathogen can be established only by the detection of concentrations of the micro-organism above that to be expected after dilution during serial passage. This should be demonstrated in the host animal as well as in tissue culture lines taken from various animals.

Test animals should be committed to acute toxicity tests using the micro-organism, e.g. intravenous injection, intraperitoneal injection, and oral feeding accompanied by pathological examinations of tissues from representative test and control animals from at least two species. Inhalation and dermal exposure data should be included using at least two animal species.

Chronic toxicity tests involving 90-day feeding tests with two species of animals fed varying doses of the micro-organism must be conducted. The carcinogenicity of the micro-organism should be tested, usually in small rodents.

The safety of the micro-organism must be established for game birds, game and commercial fish, shellfish and Crustacea (e.g. shrimp). Any materials used in formulation of the pathogen preparation must be demonstrated to be innocuous and evidence of techniques for production-batch-control by acute toxicity tests must be provided (usually by intraperitoneal injection of a rodent).

B. COUNTRIES OTHER THAN THE U.S.A.

There is very little difference between the regulations and procedures in force in the U.S.A. and most of the other countries throughout the world that use considerable amounts of insecticides.

For example, in Sweden, the Pesticide Act (1964) is administered by the National Poisons and Pesticide Board and the requirements to register a pesticide with this organization are essentially the same as those listed above for the U.S.A.

Similarly in West Germany, recent legislation in the form of the Plant Protection Law (1967) is administered by the Federal Biological Institute for Agriculture and Forestry. The Federal Health Service is also involved in a somewhat similar fashion to the FDA in the United States of America. Germany is one of the few countries, along with France, Russia and the U.S.A. that have manufactured microbial agents (specifically, products based on varieties of *Bacillus thuringiensis*).

In Holland the Pesticide Act of 1962 is administered by the Committee of Phytopharmacy and this Committee reports to two Ministries, the Ministry of Social Affairs and Public Health and the Ministry of Agriculture and Fisheries.

In New Zealand the registration and use of pesticides including microbial agents is covered by the Agricultural Chemicals Act, 1959, and is administered by the Agricultural Chemicals Board comprised of representatives from the Department of Agriculture, the Health Department and from farming, industrial, and merchant organizations. Non-voting technical experts from government and industry are consulted. The Board makes recommendations to Parliament who set the law, on usable pesticides, by publication in the Parliamentary Gazette.

In Canada a pesticide must be registered under the Pest Control Products Act (Canada) administered by the Canada Department of Agriculture, Plant Products Division, Production and Marketing Branch, Ottawa. The Food and Drug Directorate of the Department of National Health and Welfare judge the safety and set the tolerances of the various pesticides. In addition each Province has its statutes governing the use of pesticides (e.g. Ontario–The Pesticides Act, 1967, which includes reference to microbial agents).

A rather novel approach is used in Great Britain (England, Wales and Scotland). In 1957, a voluntary scheme (formerly known as the "Notification of Pesticides Scheme" and now called "Pesticides Safety Precautions Scheme") was negotiated and drawn up by the Ministry of Agriculture, Fisheries and Food, the Ministry of Health, with corresponding Scottish Departments, and Industrial Associations. Under this scheme industry must notify the government of the introduction of a new pesticide or new ingredient and also provides the safety and toxicological data to the appropriate advisory committee to the government agencies. The material must be withdrawn from the market if considered unsafe. If approved under the above-mentioned scheme then an application is made to another advisory committee under the Agricultural Chemicals Approval Scheme and data supporting the efficacy of the new material must be tendered for approval before final clearance for sale and use.

Microbial agents are authorized for use in France by an Anti-Parasite Committee that views reports tendered by the Laboratoire de Phytopharmacide de l'Institut National de la Recherche Agronomique, in collaboration with the Service de la Protection des Vegetaux (Paris).

The Japanese do not have a law governing the registration of pesticides including microbial agents. However, all such materials must be approved by the Ministry of Agriculture.

The following is a list of countries and the agencies in their respective governments responsible for authorizing the distribution and use of pesticides. This information was drawn in part from a report by Hurpin and Müller-Kögler entitled "Enquete sur les conditions d'homologation des préparations á base de *Bacillus thuringiensis*" for the 1964 Work Group on Insect Pathology and Microbial Control, sponsored by the International Commission on Biological Control. Belgium: Conseil Supérieur d'Hygiène Publigue et Institut d'Hygiéne et d'Epidémiologie. Czechoslovakia: Central Inspection and Testing Institute of Agriculture (at Brno) and the Ministry of Health. Iran: Research Institute of Plant Protection and Quarantine (Evin-Teheran) and the Bureau of Control of Chemical Products (Bongake-Chimiai). Italy: Ministry of Health. Poland: Institute of Plant Protection (Poznan). Spain: Station of Agricultural Phytopathology of the National Institute of Agricultural Investigations. Switzerland: Federal Agricultural Experimental Stations at Lansamme, Oerlikon and Wadenswil in collaboration with the Interfederal Commission of Toxicology.

So much for the requirements of registration. Now let us examine what we know of safety of the insect pathogens for other life forms. To avoid confusion we will discuss the various types of pathogens separately.

III. Bacteria

A. SPOREFORMING BACTERIA

1. Bacillus popilliae

One of the first organisms to be used extensively in the field was the milky disease organism, *Bacillus popilliae,* isolated and described by Dutky (1937, 1940). Dutky (1941) obtained a U.S. Patent for a method for control of the Japanese beetle, *Popillia japonica,* using this bacterium and later a second patent for a process for propagating the bacterium (Dutky, 1942). The States on the Eastern seaboard of the U.S.A. were plagued by the Japanese beetle and as a consequence when Dutky proposed cooperative programs between the Bureau of Entomology (Federal) and the States to distribute the milky disease, his proposal was met with considerable enthusiasm from several future collaborators.

Dutky then petitioned the Bureau of Entomology and Plant Quarantine, Public Health Service, Bureau of Animal Industry and Bureau of Plant Industry and the Apiculture Division for permission to distribute the organism in nature.

In his proposal he reported that he had fed spores to starlings and to chickens without adverse effects, the bacterium having remained viable without germinating during the trip through the birds' guts. He also pointed out that the bacterium requires highly specific conditions to germinate, and perhaps more significant, it does not grow at the temperature of the vertebrate body. These arguments proved sufficient, at that time, for permission to carry out the program. During the next few years 184,000 lb of the Dutky milky-disease preparation was distributed over approximately 194,000 sites in 14 States and in the District of Columbia.

No harmful effects were ever detected following this broadcast of milky disease. However, one very amusing episode marked this process in Maryland. A lady who owned a farm in an area treated with milky disease lost some chickens; this resulted in a magistrate's hearing in an endeavour to collect her loss from the county commissioners. After testimony from Dr. C. R. Davis of the Maryland Livestock Sanitary Commission that the product had been thoroughly tested and found non-toxic to chickens, Dr. George Langford of the University of Maryland who was in charge of the work for the State was called to the stand. He stated that he believed the bacterium to be harmless to vertebrates and then, asking for some of the spore preparation and a spoon, he promptly ate a heaping spoonful of the spore dust, washing it down with a glass of water. The magistrate immediately suspended the case pending further observation of Dr. Langford. This excellent gentleman is alive and healthy today and is the Maryland State Entomologist.

The above-mentioned experiments are to my knowledge the only reported tests for safety that have been carried out with any of the milky disease organisms, although plans for test are now being contemplated by the Agriculture Research Service of the USDA.

2. Bacillus thuringiensis

In October 1956 Dr. E. A. Steinhaus met with Dr. R. A. Fisher and Mr. J. M. Sudarsky of the Pacific Yeast Products (later to become Bioferm Corporation) to arrange the experimental work on submerged fermentation of *Bacillus thuringiensis* var. *thuringiensis* that led to the product Thuricide. Several other companies including Rohm and Haas, Merck, Sharpe and Dohme, Grain Processing Company and Nutrilite Products Incorporated began producing competitive products shortly thereafter; all but Bioferm and Nutrilite gave up production after a few years.

Initial field work and safety studies, including human volunteer tests, were necessary and occupied the period from 1956 to 1958 when the FDA granted a temporary exemption from tolerance and the PRD issued an experimental permit, allowing the use of *B. thuringiensis* on vegetables and forage crops. On 14 April 1960, the FDA granted full exemption from tolerance, allowing commercial application of *B. thuringiensis* based preparations to food and forage crops.

Let us examine the experimental work necessary to permit registration. In 1959 Steinhaus reported that Brown *et al.* (1958) had tested *B. thuringiensis* var. *thuringiensis* and the varieties, *alesti, sotto, entomocidus* and *subtoxicus* in an attempt to select pathogenic strains for mice. The method used was the same used by Brown and his colleagues with *Bacillus cereus* strains. To quote Steinhaus: "Except for two deaths occurring immediately after inoculation, and judged not to be caused by the bacillus, none of these strains [of *B. thuringiensis*], after cultivation on blood-dextrose medium showed any toxicity or pathogenicity for mice. Dr. Brown concludes that these strains cannot be converted to a pathogenic state for mice, under the conditions quoted in the paper by him and his colleagues."

There has always been the fear in regulatory and scientific circles that insect pathogens might be induced or selected in such a way that they would convert to vertebrate pathogens; this is often as a result of misinformation or a lack of understanding of the genetics of such a process. In the previously described work by Brown *et al.* (1958), they worked with *B. cereus* strains and by selection on suitable media obtained virulent strains from populations that were, to all intents and purposes, avirulent. In such a case the change is a one-step process involving pathogenicity. Since Brown tested this possibility in *B. thuringiensis* without finding the capacity to become pathogenic for vertebrates in the populations tested, we can dispense with this aspect for the present.

What are the possibilities of virulent strains of *B. thuringiensis* pathogenic for vertebrates developing? This is best answered by Steinhaus (1959) and since I doubt that his comments can be improved upon, I shall quote him. "It is generally considered that naturally occurring pathogens are relatively stable in the genetic sense; which means that their specific value within a given environment may reflect the gradual accumulation of a series of genetic determinants making the strain concerned specifically fit to multiply in its particular natural environment. To obtain a variant with high fitness to an entirely different environment it would now be necessary that there occur appropriate changes in several determinants rather than just one genetic alteration in order to change the avirulent type into a type pathogenic for vertebrates. Since it is known that genetic determinants change at relatively low rates the probability of the occurrence of a series of the changes required to make potential variants fit for another environment would be exceedingly low."

From the knowledge we have about insect pathogens, I believe that Steinhaus' remarks apply particularly well to insect viruses; they also appear to fit the situation regarding the crystal-forming bacteria. However, they may not apply to all of the entomogenous fungi, protozoa and rickettsiae; this will be fully discussed in the ensuing sections.

Most of the experimental work on safety carried out with *B. thuringiensis* is given in the paper by Fisher and Rosner (1959). A summary of this data is in order. The *B. thuringiensis* strain tested in this work was the NRS 996, isolated by Mattès in 1927. Spores were formulated with a diatomaceous earth filler. The filler alone was implicated in some toxic effects on plants during the tests, particularly when massive doses were used. This product, named Thuricide, was used in most tests at about 9×10^9 viable spores/g, determined by plate counts. In tests on man 3×10^9 viable spores/g were used.

a. Virulence of Thuricide following serial passage through mice. Mice were injected intraperitoneally and 6 hr later blood was drawn by cardiac puncture and was injected intraperitoneally into a second group of mice. This serial passage was repeated with five more groups of mice and none of the terminal group showed abnormal symptoms. Since one death occurred in the first test group, the bacterium, by itself and the carrier alone were tested by intraperitoneal injection. None of the bacteria-injected mice died but the carrier injections caused toxic symptoms with severe irritation of the peritoneum.

b. Persistence of B. thuringiensis *in the blood of mice.* White mice were injected intraperitoneally with *B. thuringiensis* and *B. cereus.* Cardiac punctures were made at preselected intervals and blood was plated on trypline glucose extract agar. Both *B. thuringiensis* and *B. cereus* were still in the blood at 48 hr but had disappeared by 72 hr.

c. Pathogenicity of B. thuringiensis *by parenteral administration into guinea pigs.* Guinea pigs were injected intraperitoneally with vegetative cells of *B. thuringiensis, B. cereus* and *Bacillus subtilis.* Table I shows that the guinea pig withstood large doses of bacteria from broth culture, but a number of animals succumbed to the massive doses from slant cultures.

TABLE I

Tests of guinea pigs treated with vegetative rods of sporeforming bacteria (Fisher and Rosner, 1959)

Organism	Broth culture		Slant culture	
	No. injected	No. deaths	No. injected	No. deaths
B. thuringiensis	10	0	10	7
B. cereus	5	0	5	5
B. subtilis	–	–	5	0

d. Inhalation toxicity of B. thuringiensis *in mice.* Mice were exposed four distinct times to gram quantities of Thuricide, each exposure, while confined in a 30 cm square chamber fitted with a powder blower. No untoward symptoms or change in feeding or weight were detected and gross pathological examinations were negative.

e. Allergenicity of Thuricide in guinea pigs. Sensitizing doses were given in two ways to guinea pigs: (1) by intracutaneous injection, (2) by the abrasion-patch technique. Topical application on the intact skin was also made. A slight erythema was noticeable in the injected and abraded animals indicating local irritation. No effect was observed from challenging doses given two weeks after the last sensitizing treatments. Topical applications had no effect.

f. Inhalation and ingestion of Thuricide by human volunteers. Eighteen volunteers received physical and laboratory examinations and then commenced a five-day course of ingestion of 1 g each of Thuricide each day. In addition, five of the test subjects inhaled 100 mg of the powder daily for five days. All subjects were then thoroughly reexamined and again 4-5 weeks later. All people tested remained healthy and all the extensive laboratory tests were negative.

The data on man also included records of eight employees exposed to the bacterial preparation during the course of manufacturing the product. These exposure periods totalled 25 hr in some cases. All the exposed personnel were in good health and showed no harm from the exposure.

g. Acute oral toxicity of Thuricide. Suspensions (33%) of Thuricide were placed directly into the stomachs of rats. Doses up to 24 g of Thuricide (2×10^{12} spores/kg body wt) were used. There were no deaths or symptoms of toxicity after one week and gross pathology examinations were negative.

In addition, Fisher and Rosner (1959) reported that tests carried out by other collaborators showed, through acute and chronic feeding tests, that no toxicity was apparent in chicks, laying hens, young swine and hogs, fish, adult honey-bees, and honey-bee larvae. Tests on honey-bees are described in Chapter 23, in which it is concluded that honey-bees are harmed only by high concentrations of exotoxin such as are never likely to be acquired in practice.

Thus it was that, based on the Bioferm Corporation's petition, which is part of the foregoing description of experiments, the Food and Drug Administration granted full exemption from tolerance on 14 April 1960, and the product was registered under the trade name Thuricide by the Pesticide Regulation Division, USDA.

B. NON-SPOREFORMING BACTERIA

There are two non-sporeformers that have been seriously considered from time to time as potentially useful microbial control agents. Unfortunately, such a proposal should not be seriously contemplated on the grounds of safety since both organisms have an extensive record of pathogenicity to man and/or other animals. It is not possible to give a complete bibliography of their involvement with vertebrates; a brief citation of some of the latest literature must suffice.

1. Pseudomonas aeruginosa

Pseudomonas aeruginosa has been implicated in cases of mastitis in cows (Brown, 1956), of atrophic rhinitis in service personnel (Shuman *et al.*, 1956), infections in newly-bred mares (Doll, 1956) and of pneumonia in mink (Gorham, 1956). This organism has also been reported from man as a hazard in intensive surgery cases (Tinne *et al.*, 1967); in respiratory infections (Phillips, 1967; Fierer *et al.*, 1969); an urinary infection (Moore and Forman, 1966) and a case of nephritis (Weiser, personal communication).

2. Serratia marcescens

Serratia marcescens has been reported to cause septicemia in man (Black *et al.*, 1967; Dodson, 1968); intestinal infections (McCormack and Kunin, 1966) and infections in man (Magnuson and Elston, 1966).

IV. Viruses

The above synopsis of the work carried out by the Bioferm Corporation to prove the safety, and incidentally the efficacy, of *B. thuringiensis* makes one point abundantly clear. Before anyone approaches a regulatory agency, in any country, with an application to register a microbial agent (or any control agent) you must have a product; it is not possible to register a bacterium or a virus.

As late as 1960, this was not properly understood in the U.S.A., witness the approach made to the FDA by Dr. F. L. McEwen. As an associate Professor of Entomology, Dr. McEwen sent a clear, concise presentation entitled, "The use of the polyhedrosis virus of the cabbage looper to control the cabbage looper on food crops," to the FDA requesting information regarding requirements for proving the virus efficacious and safe. The reply included the basic requirements for registering a prouduct given previously in this presentation. McEwen's reply thanking the FDA terminated this contact.

In 1962, the Agriculture Research Service of the USDA made a similar request, concerning the cabbage looper nuclear polyhedrosis virus (NPV), to the PRD and the FDA. As contacts began and conferences occurred between these agencies, it became abundantly clear that a product must be manufactured and tested. For several years, Dr. C. M. Ignoffo had been working in Brownsville, Texas, for the USDA, developing methods for growing the cabbage looper *Trichoplusia ni* and the corn earworm (cotton bollworm) *Heliothis zea,* on semi-artificial media, in order to produce the NPV's specific for these insects. It was decided that production of the viruses was now feasible, and sufficient virus formulation was on hand to carry out initial field studies for efficacy and for safety tests.

A. TESTS WITH OCCLUDED VIRUSES ON ANIMALS

1. Tests in the U.S.A. by the FDA

Ignoffo and Heimpel (1965) tested the NPV of *H. zea,* using white mice and guinea pigs, to determine the toxicology and pathogenicity of the virus for vertebrates. Virus preparations used were tested against *H. zea* larvae to establish the level of virulence in the insect. Careful bacterial counts were also made by the plating method.

Mice and guinea pigs were exposed to virus powder (500 mg/mouse and 100 mg/guinea pig) in closed containers for 2 hr and then observed for two months. Controls were treated with wheat flour. One guinea pig became ill and recovered after 24 hr, another died in this experiment and histopathological examination showed it had succumbed to an acute pneumonia. No signs of virus infected were detected. The experiment was repeated with no further deaths. All other guinea pigs in these experiments were healthy and made normal weight gains during the observation period. None of the white mice became unhealthy and all made normal weight gains over the two-month test period.

Shaved guinea pigs were injected intradermally on the back with three antigens, (1) polyhedra, (2) insect debris plus washed polyhedra and (3) insect debris from which the polyhedra had been removed. Mild oedema occurred immediately after injection but lasted only 15 min. All guinea pigs remained healthy and made normal weight gains. Challenging doses were given after 25 days. In all animals in groups 2 and 3, the skin became whealed around the site of the injection over an area of skin approximately $250 \times 500\ mm^2$; this reaction soon faded. However, the guinea pigs in group 1 (washed polyhedra) did not react to the challenging dose, indicating that polyhedra as *per se* did not act as an antigen (possibly they were not available as antigens due to the inertness of the polyhedral protein in the vertebrate body).

Guinea pigs were injected intraperitoneally with protein dissolved from polyhedra and with freed virus rods. During two months' observation all animals remained healthy, their temperatures and weight gains were normal.

White mice were force-fed polyhedra suspended in water. All animals remained healthy, temperatures and weight were normal for two months.

Newly-weaned, white mice were injected intracerebrally with large doses of freed virus rods. All animals survived for two months; temperature and weight gains were normal.

Heimpel (1966) carried out very similar tests to those reported by Ignoffo and Heimpel (1965), using the NPV of *Trichoplusia ni.* Again, there was no evidence of toxicity or pathogenicity for the animals tested.

Heimpel and West (unpublished; under a contract issued to the Rosner-Hixson Laboratories by the USDA) tested four NPV's and a granulosis virus (Table II). In each test all animal groups were made up of equal numbers of males and females. There was no evidence of toxicity or pathogenicity in either sex (Table II).

2. Tests in the U.S.A. by Industry

Two companies have made many tests of pathogenicity and toxicity using their respective products based on the NPV of *H. zea.* The animals involved in

TABLE II

Tests of white mice and guinea pigs treated with insect viruses

Virus	Test animal	Number of animals: Treated	Deaths	Control	Deaths	Type of test	Status of virus	Dose ($\times 10^9$)
Granulosis	Mice	30	4	30	4	Peritoneal	Granules	24
virus	Mice	20	0	20	3[b]	Venous	Freed	30
Estigmene	G. pig	30	4[b]	30	4[b]	Peritoneal	Granules	24
acrea	G. pig	20	0	0[d]		Cutaneous	Freed	30
NPV[a] of	Mice	20	2[b]	20	3[b]	Venous	Freed	35.0
Trichoplusia	G. pig	20	0	0[d]		Cutaneous	Freed	1.75
ni								
NPV[a] of	Mice	20	1[b]	20	3[b]	Venous	Freed	35.0
Heliothis	G. pig	20	0	0[d]		Cutaneous	Freed	1.75
zea								
NPV[a] of	Mice	20	0	20	0	Venous	Polyhedra	0.1
Spodoptera	Mice	30	3[c]	30	4[c]	Peritoneal	Polyhedra	1.0
exigua	Mice	20	2[c]	20	3[c]		Polyhedra	1.0
	Mice	20	2[c]	20	3[c]	Venous	Freed	35.0
	G. pig	30	5[c]	30	4[c]	Peritoneal	Polyhedra	1.0
	G. pig	20	0	0[d]		Cutaneous	Freed	1.75
NPV[a] of	Mice	30[c]	0	30	0	Venous	Polyhedra	0.1
Spodoptera	Mice	30	3[b]	30	4[b]	Peritoneal	Polyhedra	1.0
frugiperda	Mice	20	3[b]	20	3[b]	Oral	Polyhedra	1.0
	Mice	20	0	20	3[b]	Venous	Freed	35.0
	G. pig	30	2[b]	30	4[b]	Peritoneal	Polyhedra	1.0
	G. pig	10	0	0[d]		Cutaneous	Polyhedra	1.0
	G. pig	10	0	0[d]		Cutaneous	Freed	1.75

[a] NPV = Nuclear polyhedrosis virus.
[b] Cause of death, broncho-pneumonia.
[c] Cause of death, broncho-pneumonia complicated by kidney infections.
[d] No control animals. Control sites selected on test animals.

most of the tests were white mice, rats, guinea pigs, and dogs. Other animals tested will be mentioned separately.

Intravenous, intraperitoneal and subcutaneous injections in rodents caused no harm to the test animals.

Acute toxicity feeding tests (usually 21 days) and subacute feeding tests (90 days) were conducted separately on rodents. Again no harmful effects were detected in the test animals. The progeny of some of the animals were observed for abnormal effects; however, none were detected.

Two-year feeding studies of rats, and repeated subcutaneous injections of mice over an 18-month period, were made to assess the carcinogenic potential of the virus, without detecting any increase in the incidence of cancer.

Inhalation studies on guinea pigs revealed no undue effects. Guinea pigs were exposed dermally without irritation. Challenging doses of viral products injected subcutaneously did not elicit any detectable response (Meinecke *et al.*, 1970).

NPV of the *H. zea* was introduced into the culture system of several established lines of mammalian tissue culture. None of the cell cultures showed any cytological changes or any evidence of viral replication. Other attempts to infect mammalian tissue culture lines with live insect viruses also failed (Ignoffo, 1968). Juvenile oysters, *Crassostrea virginica,* adult brown shrimps, *Penacus aztecus,* the longnose killifish *Fundulus similis,* spot, *Leiostomus xanthurus,* mature grass shrimps, *Palaemonetes pugio,* sheepshead minnows, *Cyprinodon variegatus,* the white sucker, *Catastomas commersoni,* the black bull head, *Ictalurus melas* and the rainbow trout, *Salmo gairdneri* were tested with viral preparation, by feeding and in the case of the sheepshead minnow by intraperitoneal injection. No effect was detected in any of these animals at dosages approximating the normal level of application for insect control. The rainbow trout were sensitive to dosage at 25 times the normal level of application, probably due to the resulting turbidity in the water.

Feeding tests were conducted using the English sparrow, valley quail and the mallard duck without harming any of them. Extensive insect tests on polyhedra collected from the feces of the mallard duck indicated that the virus remained unharmed and unchanged after passage through the bird's gut.

B. TESTS WITH OCCLUDED VIRUSES ON MAN AND HUMAN PRODUCTS

Statements by the two companies regarding the health of several individuals constantly exposed to the virus from *H. zea* during its production and processing were tendered as part of the petitions to the regulatory agencies. Full records and medical examinations of all individuals were made and the examining physicians declared that there were no changes in the health of the subjects under exposure.

Polyhedra of the *H. zea* NPV were incubated in human gastric juice (at pH 2.1 and neutralized to pH 7.0) and samples taken at six intervals from 10 min up to 2 hr. At pH 2.1, about half of the virus was non-pathogenic for *H. zea* larvae after 40 min incubation and most or all of the virus was killed in 2 hr. The virus incubated at pH 7.0 was unharmed (Chautani *et al.*, 1968).

Heimpel and Buchanan (1967) carried out human feeding tests using volunteers from the Entomology Research Division, Agricultural Research Service, USDA. Ten men and women were each fed 5.82 billion polyhedra over the course of five days after a thorough physical and laboratory examination and were then observed for a month. Intensive examinations were given each of the test group 10 and 30 days after the start of the experiment. A group of six men and women served as controls and consumed insect protein separated from the same virus preparation. The controls were examined at the same times as the test group. No significant change in the condition of any individual in the test or control groups was detected, nor were any differences noted between the two groups. All of the individuals from both groups are alive and healthy at the time of this writing, two years from the time of the experiment. The authors concluded that the virus had no harmful effects on the test subjects.

C. TESTS WITH NON-OCCLUDED VIRUS

Giran (1966) tested, against mammals, the non-inclusion virus that develops in the nuclei of cells of the greater wax moth larvae, *Galleria mellonella* (densonucleosis virus, described in Chapter 2, p. 35). The disease organism is small (21-23 mμ). Virus particles in physiological saline solution were injected intraperitoneally in adult mice, rabbits and newborn mice; subcutaneously in rabbits; and intracerebrally in newborn mice. Adult mice and rabbits also were fed the live virus. None of the treated animals died and no pathological symptoms were detected.

D. CONCLUSIONS ABOUT VIRUSES

These data, collectively, indicate that the insect viruses are the safest of all the microbial agents proposed for insect control and are infinitely safer for other life forms than chemical agents.

V. Protozoa

The Microsporida are the most common protozoans found in insects and have been frequently tested as microbial control agents for insects. Unfortunately, members of the order Microsporida are found infecting vertebrates and crustacea as well. The following is by no means a complete bibliography of microsporidan diseases of animals other than insects; however, it will suffice to emphasize the need for extensive safety tests with these organisms before use in the field.

Nosema spp. have been detected associated with tumors, in the brain and in infections of rodents (Arison and Cassaro, 1966; Canning, 1965; Nelson, 1962; Petri, 1966; Petri and Schmidt, 1966; Weiser, 1964, 1965). A species of *Thelohania* has also been detected in rodents (Doby *et al.*, 1963).

Plistophora nyotrophica caused high mortality in the common toad, *Bufo bufo* (Canning *et al.*, 1964).

Microsporida are common parasites of fresh and salt water fish (Cope, 1959; Dechtiar, 1965; Haley, 1954a, b; Hoffman, 1967; Jakowska, 1964; Kabata, 1959; Schäperclaus, 1954; Sinderman, 1961; Stunkard and Lux, 1965; Summerfelt, 1964; Wales and Wolf, 1955; Weissenberg, 1968). The genera involved are *Nosema, Glugea* and *Plistophora.*

Several reports of Microsporida in Crustacea have also been published; some of the hosts are of commercial importance. Hutton (1959) and Iverson and Manning (1959) reported microsporidal diseases in the salt water and the pink shrimp respectively. Sprague (1965, 1966) isolated two species of *Plistophora* from the blue crab and other decapods.

There does not appear to have been any cross-infection tests made to mammals using the above-mentioned isolates. It is highly doubtful whether species identification is sufficiently reliable to forego thorough testing of insect microsporidal pathogens before exposing vertebrates to these organisms.

Finally there have been reports and discussions of microsporidal infections in man (Matsubayashi *et al.*, 1959; Viting, 1965; Weiser, 1966; Werner, 1965).

Protozoan pathogens frequently occur in insect infestations of stored food (Burges, personal communication), but none of these pathogens has caused disease in man and domestic animals. This is an indication that these particular protozoans are not pathogenic in vertebrates.

VI. Fungi

A. ENTOMOGENOUS FUNGI ASSOCIATED WITH VERTEBRATES

There are only a few groups of fungi or separate species that have, in the past, been seriously considered and worked with in the field for insect control. Concomitantly these fungi kill tons of insects, the world over, every year. They are listed in Table I of Chapter 5 and include some like the Entomophthoraceae and the Laboulbeniales which have fastidious culture requirements. The Entomophthoraceae, *Beauveria bassiana* and *Metarrhizium anisopliae,* are the entomopathogenic fungi most frequently studied, and their relations to other living animals are also better known. Indeed, these are the only fungi associated with insects that have been identified in the literature causing aberrant conditions in mammals.

The Entomophthoraceae have been implicated in horse and human disease since the organism *Entomophthora coronata* has been identified as the causal agent of phycomycosis in horses and man, although it is the only species of this genus involved to date (Emmel, 1958; Emmons and Bridges, 1961; Bridges and Emmons, 1961; Bridges *et al.*, 1962; Emmons, 1964; Bras *et al.*, 1965; Restrepo *et al.*, 1967; Andrade *et al.*, 1967; Zilton *et al.*, 1967; Martinson and Clark, 1967; Lowe *et al.*, 1968). An isolate from horses, provided by C. W. Emmons, proved pathogenic for wax moth larvae (Roberts, personal communication).

On the other hand D. M. Macleod (personal communication) made it clear that he believes the animals and individuals reported above may have been in poor condition and thus more susceptible to infection.

Macleod (1954) reported several cases of isolation of *Beauveria* sp. from tissues of vertebrates and Georg *et al.* (1962) demonstrated *Beauveria bassiana* as the causal agent of pulmonary mycosis in the giant tortoises, *Testudo elephantopus* and *T. gigantea elephantina,* that had been stressed by chilling. *Beauveria (Tritirachium) shiotae* was isolated from an abscess in the bile duct of a man.

B. TOXICITY AND PATHOGENICITY TESTS

The genus *Aspergillus* has some species that are insect pathogens and also several members which are pathogenic to vertebrates (e.g. Ford and Friedman, 1967; Papavassiliou and Stylianea, 1969). Schaerffenberg (1968) reported on animal tests with the fungi, *B. bassiana* and *M. anisopliae.*

Subcutaneous and intravenous injections of 0.5 ml of 2% spore suspensions of these fungi were made in two groups of rats for each fungus. No morbid changes were detected in the test rats and investigation of tissues showed the absence of fungal mycelium in the blood and organs, after a two-month observation period.

In inhalation experiments, rats were exposed to 4 mg of pure spore dust/m^3 in a sealed tin box. Two groups of 10 rats were treated for each fungus. No pathogenic or toxic effects, or allergic manifestations, were noted over two months.

"Fungal Bran" containing *B. bassiana* and *M. anisopliae* were each fed to three groups of 10 rats with the following variations.

1. One group of rats received 6 g of fungal bran mixed 1 : 1 with sugar and rolled oats/animal. Afterwards supplement of bread, fruit and vegetable refuse was fed (water *ad libitum*). All of these animals survived, were normal, exhibited no loss in weight and had unreduced appetites.
2. The second group was fed fungal bran, rolled oats and sugar (water *ad libitum*). These animals exhibited loss of appetite, low consumption of food and weight losses averaging 30%.
3. The third group received only 10 g of fungal bran/day/animal (water *ad libitum*). Three animals died after three weeks; the others suffered an average weight loss of 40%, contracted diarrhea and stopped feeding. Their appetites returned after placing them on a normal diet; weight losses were regained in three weeks. Ten control rats fed on bran and water suffered weight losses up to 30% in three weeks, an obvious state of stress, but exhibited none of the other symptoms.

This experiment tends to support Macleod's opinion that physically stressed animals may be susceptible to some action by these fungi.

Müller-Kögler (1965) reports that injection of *Paecilomyces (Spicaria) farinosus* spores into rabbits did not adversely affect the animals.

3. Human Allergic Reactions

There have been several reports from scientists working with *B. bassiana* of moderate to severe allergic reactions to spore preparations (Müller-Kögler, 1967). In most cases the symptoms were tiredness or weakness, neck or head pains and giddiness. In most cases, the symptoms disappeared in a relatively short time. It is possible that these reactions could be avoided by wearing masks and protective clothing (see also Chapter 5).

In view of the literature available on these fungi it is highly probable that regulatory agencies would require extensive experimental data on toxicity and pathogenicity as well as data on their mutability (see also Chapter 5).

VII. Rickettsiae

The rickettsiae affecting insects have been studied to a limited extent (Dutky and Gooden, 1952; Krieg, 1962a), but very few toxicity and pathogenicity tests have been carried out. *Rickettsiella melolonthae* and *R. grylli* are able to infect mammals lethally, especially mice by the nasal and intraperitoneal route (Krieg, 1955; Giroud *et al.,* 1958; Mandin *et al.,* 1967). For instance, Krieg (1962b) injected more than 5×10^8 *R. melolonthae* particles intraperitoneally and intranasally into white mice. One of the eight mice injected intraperitoneally and three of the eight mice injected intranasally died with typical symptoms of rickettsiosis. In addition, higher doses of *R. melolonthae* injected intravenously may induce a severe rickettsiosis in rabbits. From the lungs of a rabbit, suffering from an artificial infection of *R. melolonthae,* the pathogen could be reisolated in a form virulent for *Melolontha* sp. (Krieg, personal communication). Suitor (1964) was able to cultivate *R. melolonthae* and *R. popilliae in vitro* in both entodermal cells of chicken and McCoy cells.

It is almost certain that this display of pathogenicity by the insect rickettsiae eliminates them as candidates for microbial control of insects.

VIII. Discussion, Conclusions and Research Requirements

It seems incredible that so many good scientists have worked so long with insect pathogens without testing them for safety, yet this is, until very recently, the case. Experience with these organisms apparently convinced the research workers that the organisms were harmless. To a great extent, recent findings bear out their assumptions.

Insect viruses of the *Borrelinavirus* (NPV), *Smithiavirus* (cytoplasmic polyhedrosis), *Bergoldiavirus* (granulosis) and *Moratorvirus* (densonucleosis) types (Chapter 2) are apparently harmless for other life forms. Indeed, they are likely the safest of all organisms associated with insects. In addition to the data already given in this presentation, reports from more than two dozen scientists from all over the world have established that representatives of all the above virus types have been injected, during the course of serological investigations, into more than 1500 vertebrates (mostly guinea pigs, rabbits, mice, chickens and frogs) without deaths due to virus infection. In these investigations all of the conventional routes of injection were employed including intraperitoneal, intravenous, subdermal and intradermal routes.

In my experience, the regulatory agencies in the U.S.A. have been correct, cautious, but extremely fair in their handling of the petitions for clearance and labeling of microbial pathogens of insects. I believe their comportment, in the realization that precedents were being made, was highly laudable; serving the best public interest.

The requirements for clearance of *Bacillus thuringiensis* and of the nuclear polyhedrosis virus from *H. zea* were extensive and expensive, but the proof finally procured was convincing, final and imminently worthwhile. It is my opinion that some relaxation of the requirements concerning the viruses might now be tolerated as subsequent viruses are presented for labeling and registration; a much less extensive protocol of tests might be envisaged in view of the high level of specificity of the insect viruses and due to the high cost of development of these very useful organisms.

There is little doubt left that the crystalliferous bacteria related to *Bacillus thuringiensis* are safe for use as microbial insecticides. The extensive use given products based on these bacteria, over the last eight years, fully justifies the decision to grant exemption of tolerance by the regulatory agencies in the U.S.A. and by similar organizations in other countries. There is a Russian product that contains not only a variety of *Bacillus thuringiensis*, but also strains of *Bacillus cereus*. To my knowledge these *B. cereus* strains have not been adequately tested for safety. In view of the work done by Brown *et al.* (1958) on "masked mammalian pathogens" in *B. cereus* populations, this type of preparation cannot be considered safe until proper tests have been conducted on the contained *B. cereus* strains.

The non-sporeforming bacteria should be examined with great care. Many show potential as pathogens or secondary invaders in man and in other animals. Their variability and, in some cases, their high mutation rate commands attention.

For the same reason, the fungi and protozoans, particularly the Microsporida, will require extensive testing and a more definitive means of identification before they can be considered for general use as microbial control agents.

The rickettsiae, that are now available for consideration, should, in my opinion, be excluded from the micro-organisms proposed for microbial control of insects.

So it would appear that the insect viruses and the crystalliferous bacteria are the most likely candidates for microbial control at the present time. Since we are barely becoming familiar with the variety and numbers of these micro-organisms, it is hardly appropriate to predict their future potential. However, enough are now available to occupy the full attention of all interested scientists for the next decade or two at least.

The reliability of any microbial control product, both as to its activity and to its microbial content, is clearly the responsibility of the manufacturer. Granted, the regulatory agencies share this burden. However, it has been my experience that the manufacturers in the U.S.A. have always taken this responsibility very seriously. So it was that a practice, of testing each batch of *B. thuringiensis* produced, was instituted routinely during the exploratory phases of the work on production of this organism by Bioferm Corporation. This excellent practice has been continued in all plants producing microbial agents in this country.

Briefly, each microbial batch produced is injected intraperitoneally into rodents to detect any harmful, extraneous biotypes in the product. Concurrently, the product is plated out on a variety of bacteriological media to identify any extraneous micro-organisms present. Such a practice eliminates the possibility of the inclusion of harmful biotypes with the manufactured bacteria or virus. This safety check should be considered essential to any production of commercial microbial agents.

Apparently, workers exposed continually to the crystalliferous bacteria and the insect viruses have shown no ill effects after several years of exposure. However, should the production of entomogenous fungi ever be contemplated, it would be wise to provide masks and protective clothing to exposed personnel, in view of the previous reports of allergenic reactions in man.

We appear to have reached the threshold of a new era in the field of insect control. This is not to say that insect pathogens will, ultimately, completely replace the use of chemical insecticides; but with our growing knowledge of the side-effects of some chemical pesticides and after the decided development of resistance to chemicals in some of our most important insect pests, it is obvious that these microbial agents have a role to play. Safety of use is one of the mainstays of the proposal for microbial control. When some chemicals are sprayed in a field, it is analogous to shooting a shotgun, loaded with buck-shot, into a crowd to kill an individual; conversely, the microbial agent can be compared to the use of a rifle to eliminate that one undesirable from the crowd without harm to any other. We no longer, in some cases, need to create invertebrate deserts in our fields and forests.

References

Andrade, Z. A., Paula, L. A., Sherlock, I. A. and Cheever, A. W. (1967). *Am. J. trop. Med. Hyg.* **16**, 31-33.

Arison, R. N. and Cassaro, J. A. (1966). *Cancer Res.* **26**, 1915-1920.

Black, W. A., Pollock, A. and Bachelor, E. L. (1967). *J. clin. Pathol.* **20**, 883-886.

Bras, G., Gordon, C. C., Emmons, C. W., Prendegast, K. M. and Sugar, M. (1965). *Am. J. trop. Med. Hyg.* **14,** 141-145.
Bridges, C. H. and Emmons, C. W. (1961). *J. Am. vet. med. Ass.* **138,** 579-589.
Bridges, C. H., Romane, W. M. and Emmons, C. W. (1962). *J. Am. vet. med. Assoc.* **140,** 673-677.
Brown, E. R., Moody, M. D., Treece, E. L. and Smith, C. W. (1958). *J. Bacteriol.* **75,** 499-509.
Brown, R. W. (1956). *In* "The Year Book of Agriculture 1956. Animal Diseases" (A. Stefferud, ed.), p. 245. U.S. Government Printing Office, Washington.
Canning, E. U. (1965). *Trans. R. Soc. trop. Med. Hyg.* **59,** 371.
Canning, E. U., Elkan, E. and Trigg, P. I. (1964). *J. Protozool.* **11,** 157-166.
Chauthani, A. R., Murphy, D., Claussen, D. and Rehnborg, C. S. (1968). *J. Invertebrate Path.* **12,** 145-147.
Cope, O. B. (1959). *Trans. Am. microscop. Soc.* **78,** 157-162.
Dechtiar, A. O. (1965). *Can. Fish Culturist* **34,** 35-38.
Doby, J. M., Jeannes, A. and Rault, B. (1963). *C.r. hebd. Séanc. Acad. Sci. Paris* **257,** 248-251.
Dodson, W. H. (1968). *Archs intern. Med.* **121,** 145-150.
Doll, E. R. (1956). *In* "The Year Book of Agriculture 1956. Animal Diseases" (A. Stefferud, ed.), p. 539. U.S. Government Printing Office, Washington.
Dutky, S. R. (1937). Ph.D. Thesis, 113 pp. Rutgers Univ., New Brunswick, New Jersey.
Dutky, S. R. (1940). *J. agric. Res.* **61,** 57-68.
Dutky, S. R. (1941). U.S. Patent 2,258,319.
Dutky, S. R. (1942). U.S. Patent 2,293,890.
Dutky, S. R. and Gooden, E. L. (1952). *J. Bacteriol.* **63,** 743-750.
Emmel, M. W. (1958). *Proc. 1st Ann. Florida Conf. for Veterinarians* **1,** 18-19.
Emmons, C. W. (1964). *Riv. Patol. veg.* **4** (Ser. III), 329-337.
Emmons, C. W. and Bridges, C. H. (1961). *Mycologia* **53,** 307-312.
Fierer, J., Traylor, P. M. and Gezon, H. M. (1969). *New Eng. J. Med.* **276,** 991-996.
Fisher, R. A. and Rosner, L. (1959). *J. agric. Fd Chem.* **7,** 686-688.
Ford, S. and Friedman, L. (1967). *J. Bacteriol.* **94,** 928-933.
Georg, L. K., Williamson, W. M., Tilden, E. B. and Getty, R. E. (1962). *Sabouradia, J. Intl. Soc. hum. anim. Mycol.* **2,** 80-86.
Giran, F. (1966). *Entomophaga* **11,** 405-407.
Giroud, P., Dumas, N. and Hurpin, B. (1958). *C.r. hebd. Séanc. Acad. Sci. Paris* **247,** 2499-2501.
Gorham, J. R. (1956). *In* "The Year Book of Agriculture 1956. Animal Diseases" (A. Stefferud, ed.), p. 568. U.S. Government Printing Office, Washington.
Haley, A. J. (1954a). *Trans. Am. Fish. Soc.* **83,** 84-90.
Haley, A. J. (1954b). *J. Parasitol.* **40,** 482-483.
Heimpel, A. M. (1966). *J. Invertebrate Path.* **8,** 98-102.
Heimpel, A. M. and Buchanan, L. K. (1967). *J. Invertebrate Path.* **9,** 55-57.
Hoffman, G. L. (1967). *In* "Parasites of North American Freshwater Fish", pp. 65-78. University of California Press, Berkeley and Los Angeles.
Hutton, R. F. (1959). Fla. St. Board of Conservat., Tallahassee Tech. Serv. Bull. No. **26,** 36 pp.
Ignoffo, C. M. (1968). *Bull. ent. Soc. Am.* **14,** 265-276.
Ignoffo, C. M. and Heimpel, A. M. (1965). *J. Invertebrate Path.* **7,** 329-340.
Iverson, E. S. and Manning, R. B. (1959). *Trans. Am. Fish. Soc.* **88,** 130-132.
Jakowska, S. (1964). *Ann. Cong. Latino-Am. Zool.* **1,** 265-273.
Kabata, Z. (1959). *Parasitol.* **49,** 309-315.
Kreig, A. (1955). *Naturwissenschaften* **42,** 609-610.
Kreig, A. (1962a). *Deutsche Ent. Z.* **9,** 31.
Krieg, A. (1962b). *Z. F. Parasiteu.* **21,** 309-320.
Lowe, R. E., Rumbaugh, R. G. and Patterson, R. S. (1968). *J. Invertebrate Path.* **11,** 506-507.

Macleod, D. M. (1954). *Can. J. Bot.* **32,** 818-890.
McCormack, R. C. and Kunin, C. M. (1966). *Pediatrics* **37,** 750-755.
Mandin, J., Giran, F. and Vago, C. (1967). *Entomophaga* **12,** 295-301.
Martignoni, M. E. (1964). *In* "Biological Control of Insect Pests and Weeds" (P. De Bach and E. I. Schlinger, eds), pp. 579-609. Rheinhold Publ. Corp., New York.
Martinson, F. D. and Clark, B. H. (1967). *Am. J. trop. Med. Hyg.* **16,** 40-47.
Matsubayashi, H., Koike, T., Mikata, I., Takei, H. and Hagiwara, S. (1959). *Arch. Path.* **67,** 181-187.
Magnuson, C. W. and Elston, H. R. (1966). *Ann. intern. Med.* **65,** 409-418.
Meinecke, C. F., McLane, W. C. and Rehnborg, C. S. (1970). *J. Invertebrate Path.* **15,** 207-210.
Moore, B. and Forman, A. (1966). *Lancet* **2,** 929-931.
Müller-Kögler, E. (1965). *In* "Pilzkrankheiten bei Insekten", p. 130. Verlag Paul Parey, Hamburg and Berlin.
Müller-Kögler, E. (1967). *In* "Insect Pathology and Microbial Control" (P. A. van der Laan, ed.), pp. 339-353. North-Holland Publ. Co., Amsterdam.
Nelson, J. B. (1962). *Proc. Soc. Exp. Biol. Med.* **109,** 714-717.
Papavassiliou, J. and Stylianea, A. (1969). *Zentr. Bakteriol. Parasitenk. Abt I. Orig.* **209,** 412-414.
Petri, M. (1966). *Acta path. microbiol. scand.* **66,** 13-30.
Petri, M. and Schmidt, P. (1966). *Acta. path. microbiol. scand.* **66,** 437-446.
Phillips, I. (1967). *S. Hyg.* **65,** 229-235.
Restrepo, A., Greer, D. L., Robledo, M., Diaz, C., Lopez, R. and Bravo, C. (1967). *Am. J. trop. Med. Hyg.* **16,** 34-39.
Schaerffenberg, B. (1968). *Entomophaga* **13,** 175-182.
Schäperclaus, W. (1954). *In* "Fischkran Kheiten", pp. 355-358. Academie-Verlag, Berlin.
Shuman, R. D., Andrews, J. S. and Earl, R. L. (1956). *In* "The Year Book of Agriculture 1956. Animal Diseases" (A. Stefferud, ed.), p. 351. U.S. Government Printing Office, Washington.
Sinderman, C. J. (1961). *J. Parasitol.* **47** (Suppl.), p. 34.
Sprague, V. (1965). *J. Protozool.* **12,** 66-70.
Sprague, V. (1966). *J. Protozool.* **13,** 196-199.
Steinhaus, E. A. (1959). *J. econ. Ent.* **52,** 506-508.
Stunkard, H. W. and Lux, F. E. (1965). *Biol. Bull.* **129,** 371-387.
Suitor, E. C., Jr. (1964). *J. Insect Path.* **6,** 31-40.
Summerfelt, R. C. (1964). *Trans. Am. Fish. Soc.* **93,** 6-10.
Tinne, J. E., Gordon, A. M., Bain, W. H. and Mackey, W. A. (1967). *Brit. Med. J.* **2,** 313-315.
Viting, A. I. (1965). *Zhur. Neu. Psi. S.S. Korsakova* **65,** 1641-1645.
Wales, J. H. and Wolf, H. (1955). *Calif. Fish Game* **41,** 183-187.
Weiser, J. (1964). *Parasitol.* **54,** 749-751.
Weiser, J. (1965). *J. Protozool.* **12,** 78-83.
Weiser, J. (1966). *Proc. 1st Congr. Parasitol.* **1,** 445-446.
Weissenberg, R. (1968). *J. Protozool.* **15,** 44-57.
Werner, H. (1965). *Zentral. Bakteriol. Parasit. Infection. Krankh. Hyg.* **197,** 558-565.
Zilton, A., Paula, L. A., Sherlock, I. and Cheever, A. (1967). *Am. J. trop. Med. Hyg.* **16,** 31-33.

CHAPTER 23

The Safety of Pest-insect Pathogens for Beneficial Insects

L. BAILEY

Rothamsted Experimental Station, Harpenden, Herts, England

I. Introduction

One of the most important reasons for the current interest in pathogens of pest insects lies in the hope that they will be sufficiently specific, in contrast to many insecticides, not to harm beneficial insects. In nature at least, pathogens do not infect at random. Because of this fact it has, perhaps, been more a belief than a hope that insect pathogens are, for all practical purposes, host-specific. In spite of trouble resulting from a similar attitude to modern synthetic insecticides (Smith and van den Bosch, 1967), little heed was at first paid to the possibility that pest-insect pathogens would also affect beneficial insects in the field. Recently there has been more caution and tests are becoming usual. Most of these tests have been done with honey-bees.

II. Effects of Pest-insect Pathogens on Beneficial Insects

A. HONEY-BEES

Many experiments have been made with *Bacillus thuringiensis* on honey-bees *(Apis mellifera)* and some of the most significant have been selected for

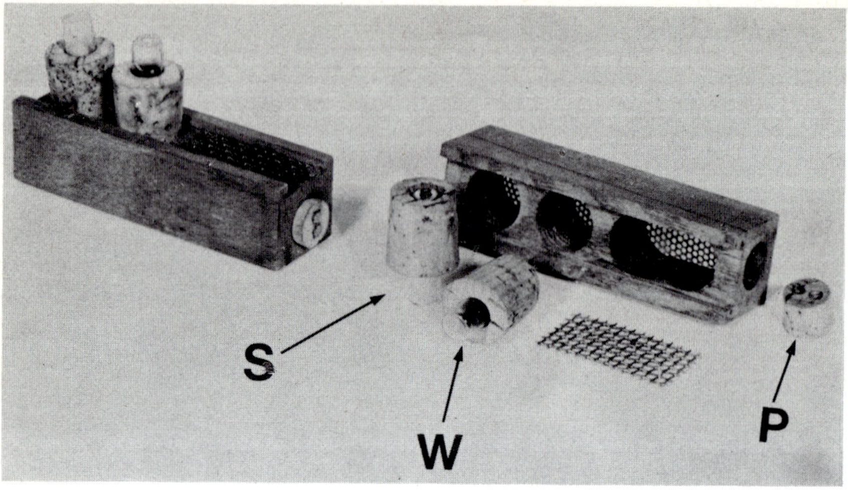

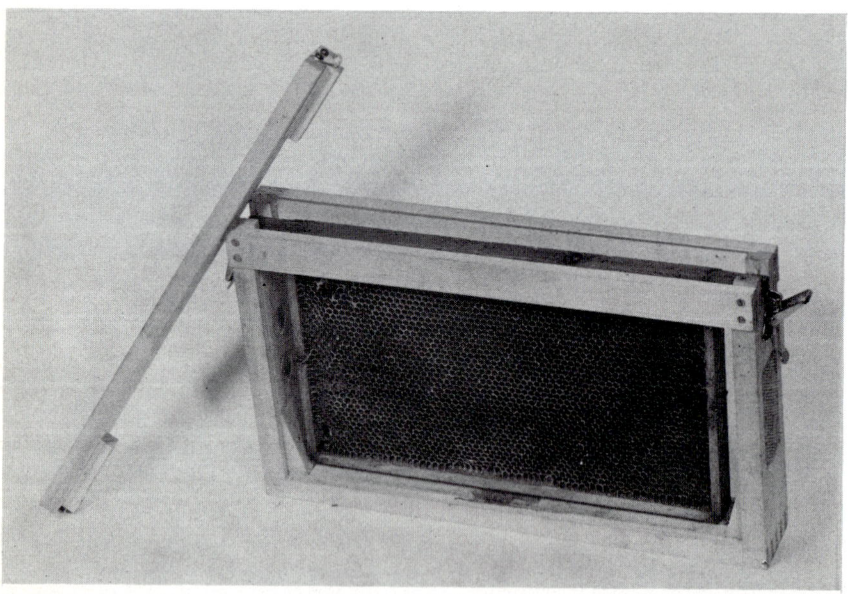

Fig. 1. Simple equipment for laboratory work with bees. (a) Cage (13 cm long) for about 20 adult bees. The feeder vials contain strong sucrose solution, S, and water, W. Holes (5 mm diameter) in the cork, P, contain pollen taken from bee combs. Newly-emerged bees live eight or more weeks at 30° or 35°C. (b) Box for incubating pupae in bee combs to obtain newly-emerged bees. Such bees neither fly nor sting for about 24 hr and so are easily handled. (c) Cages are incubated conveniently in shallow trays. (d) Frame for identifying individual larvae in their comb (scale is in inches).

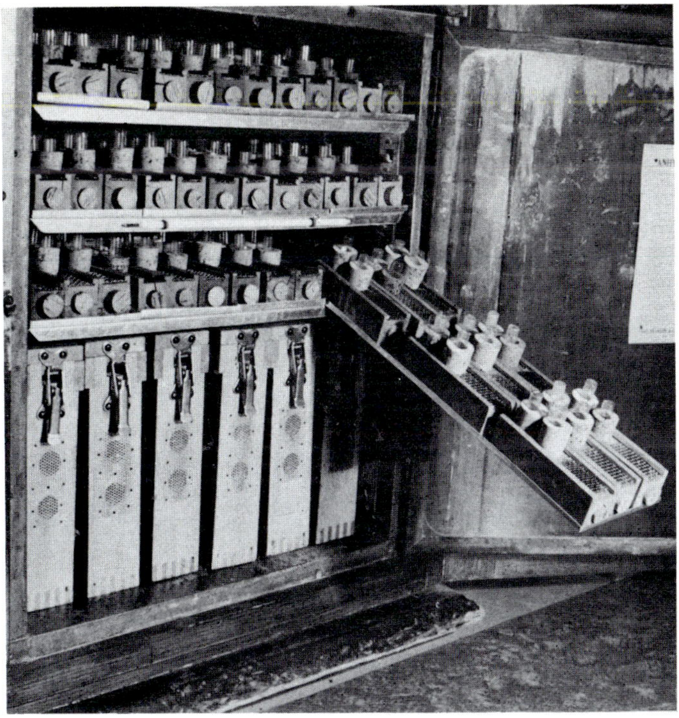

(c)

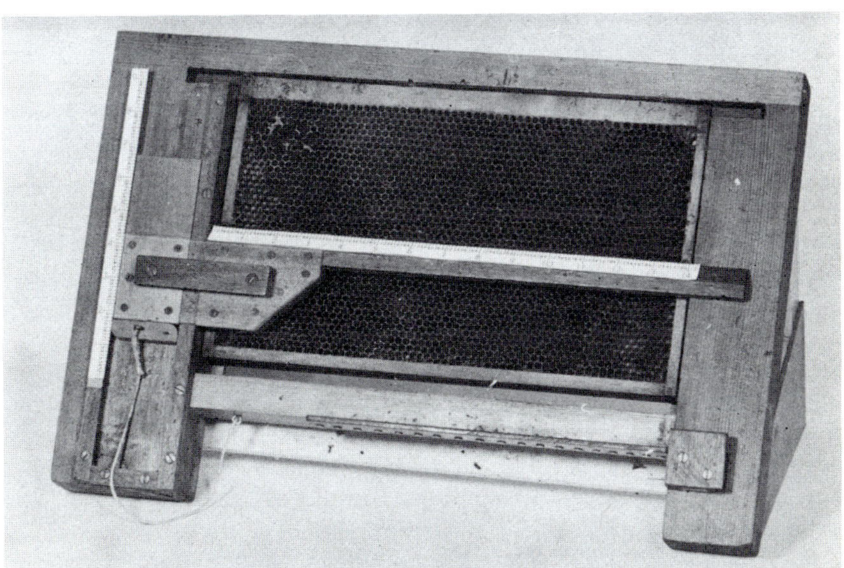

(d)

discussion here. Wilson (1962) dusted 5 g of a commercial preparation of *B. thuringiensis* into bee colonies six times at 11-day intervals without causing obvious effects. Lecomte and Martouret (1959) sprayed rape in greenhouses with preparations of *B. thuringiensis* var. *alesti* containing seven-fold the concentration of bacteria needed to control *Pieris brassicae* caterpillars, but free from exotoxin, which is poisonous for bees and produced by some other strains (Cantwell *et al.*, 1966, and below), without harming bee colonies that were foraging on the crop. Franz *et al.* (1967) noticed no harmful effects on non-lepidopterous insects, including bees, when they controlled the oak tortricid *(Tortrix viridana)* by spraying *B. thuringiensis* over forests from aircraft, whereas previous sprays with DDT had greatly decreased the arthropod fauna. Burges and Bailey (1968) caused no obvious harm to bees they supplied with wax impregnated with *B. thuringiensis* of two serotypes, or to the larvae the bees reared in the combs they built of the wax. The combs stayed proof against wax moths *(Galleria mellonella)* for several years. Several other workers have made observations similar to these field tests and the results have been substantiated by laboratory experiments, although these have shown that concentrated preparations of *B. thuringiensis* are harmful when adult bees consume much. Krieg and Herfs (1962, 1963) made some of the most detailed experiments. They found that, although 10^7 vegetative cells of *B. thuringiensis* per ml of sucrose syrup fed *ad lib.* to caged bees were harmless; the same concentration of spores together with the associated crystals killed all the bees. The heat-stable exotoxin, also produced by cultures of some strains of *B. thuringiensis,* was poisonous for bees too. That of var. *thuringiensis* (serotype 1) was the most toxic of five strains tested on bees, but 3×10^5 spores + associated toxins/bee/day were harmless. Martouret and Euverte (1964) found that 0.2 mg of spores + crystals, or of spores + crystals + exotoxin, of serotype 1 per bee/day killed all the bees in 14 and 7 days respectively. Haragsin and Vaňková (1968) tested spores + crystals of 12 strains of *B. thuringiensis*: at 10^8 spores/ml of food, variety *alesti* was the most toxic, killing about 40%, and var. *galleriae* the least toxic, killing 0.5%, for adult bees; at 10^8 spores/dm^2 of brood-comb, var. *bombycis* was most toxic, killing about 0.5%, and var. *galleriae* the least toxic, killing none, for young larvae. Cantwell *et al.* (1966) found that the crystal alone did not kill bees, but the exotoxin did, and so did large concentrations of spores alone, although there is no evidence that the spores germinate or multiply in bees. Cantwell *et al.* (1964) found, as did Krieg and Herfs (1963), that about 0.3 mg of heat-sterilized exotoxin/ml of sucrose syrup fed to bees was harmful, but they considered bees were likely to ingest such amounts in the field only when between 20 and 700 lb of *B. thuringiensis* preparations were applied per acre of crops. They thought it improbable that this very large amount would be used in agricultural practice.

Sekariah and Seth (1959) found *B. thuringiensis* of an undefined strain in dead pupae in bee colonies that seemed to have foulbrood, and Krieg and Herfs

(1963) found *B. thuringiensis* in the haemocoele of adult bees that had died after eating very many of the bacteria. However, as there is no evidence that spores germinate or multiply in living bees, *B. thuringiensis* might well act saprophytically as does *Bacillus alvei* and other bacilli that multiply in the remains of larvae killed by European foulbrood and other causes (Bailey, 1963). Shimanuki and Hartman (1963) observed that up to 30% of larvae, that each had 1700 spores of *B. thuringiensis* placed in their food when they were 16 hr old, were removed from the colony within four days by nurse bees. Larvae treated when 32 hr old suffered less. However, Heimpel (unpublished), who observed similar effects, noted that the ejected larvae were alive and did not die of infection with *B. thuringiensis* when they were incubated in the laboratory. I have noticed that many larvae, especially the youngest, are frequently ejected when more than about 1 mg of foreign material of various kinds, including non-infective matter, is placed in their food. Such contamination is unlikely in nature when *B. thuringiensis* is used to control pests.

It can be concluded that there is no evidence that bees will be harmed by *B. thuringiensis* in practice.

Few attempts have been made to infect bees with insect pathogens other than *B. thuringiensis.* Cantwell *et al.* (1966) fed small bee colonies each with more than 10^{10} polyhedra of the polyhedrosis viruses of the cabbage looper, *Trichoplusia ni,* and the corn earworm, *Heliothis zea*, and with similar numbers of capsules of the granulosis virus of the red-banded leaf roller, *Argyrotaenia velutinana,* and saw no harmful effects. They also report others who saw no ill effects when honey-bees were fed the polyhedrosis virus that attacks the greater wax moth, *Galleria mellonella.* I have injected adult honey-bees with suspensions of virus particles released with dilute alkali from the polyhedra of this virus and caused no apparent harm, whereas *G. mellonella* larvae injected with similar preparations died of polyhedrosis. Similarly, bees appeared unharmed when I injected them with *Tipula* iridescent virus that was infective for *G. mellonella,* and with densonucleosis virus of *G. mellonella* (Chapter 2; Meynadier *et al.* 1964).

Pest-insect pathogens that have multiplied in bees in laboratory tests are the fungus, *Beauveria bassiana*, (U.S.D.A., 1965) and the nematode, *Neoaplectana carpocapsae* ("DD-136"), (Cantwell *et al.*, 1966). *B. bassiana*, which needs a humid atmosphere to penetrate insect cuticle, and *N. carpocapsae* which infects bee larvae kept on moist filter paper, could conceivably attack larvae in their cells, where they are constantly wet with liquid food. In spite of the widespread occurrence of *B. bassiana*, however, it has never been found attacking bees in nature.

B. OTHER BENEFICIAL FIELD INSECTS

Few examples are recorded of other beneficial insects becoming infected with pest-insect pathogens. Bracken and Bucher (1966) found the bacterium, *Serratia marcescens,* present in laboratory cultures of wax moth larvae, causing a fatal septicaemia in emerged adults of an ichneumonid, *Exeristes comstockii,* that had been reared on the larvae. Issi and Maslennikova (1964, 1966) found the microsporidan, *Nosema polyvora*, of *Pieris brassicae* infecting and killing adults of the Braconid parasite *Apantales glomeratus*, although the infected parasitic insects lived long enough to transmit *N. polyvora* to healthy individuals of *P. brassicae.* Weiser (1963) also states that "parasitic insects, such as Hymenoptera" are susceptible to infection by Microsporida infecting their hosts, although Steinhaus (1954) reports others finding that *P. brassicae* infected with Microsporida were not parasitized by *Apanteles* spp.

Pathogens of pest insects may well affect useful parasites of the same host in an indirect way much more severely than by infecting them. For example, Harcourt (1966) observed that a granulosis virus of *Pieris rapae* in Canada killed the caterpillars before Tachinid parasites, *Phryxae vulgaris,* in them could complete their development. Steinhaus (1954) refers to Tachinid parasites in Europe that did not attack one of their hosts, the nun-moth caterpillar, *Lymantria monacha,* when this was already infected with polyhedrosis viruses, and to the polyhedrosis virus that killed alfalfa caterpillars in California before their Braconid parasite, *Apantales medicaginis,* completed its development. Thus, artificially distributed pathogens, like insecticides, might well diminish the population of beneficial parasitic insects by killing their hosts. Even spontaneous epizootics can cause similar effects. Ullyett and Schonken (1940) and Ullyett (1947) observed that the fungus, *Entomophthora sphaerosperma,* sometimes spread to so many caterpillars of *Plutella maculipennis* on crucifers that too few arthropod parasites of the moth survived to control severe outbreaks of the pest the next season. Similarly, Jaques *et al.* (1968) observed that populations of insects parasitizing the apple leaf-roller, *Pseudexentera mali,* and the winter moth, *Operophtera brumata,* decreased when the pests were sprayed with the entomogenous fungi, *Metarrhizium anisopliae* and *Beauveria bassiana.*

By contrast, a few observations have suggested that pathogens do not necessarily seriously affect parasitic insects. Evlakhova and Voronina (1967) observed that Braconid parasites, *Aphidius* spp., completed their normal life-cycle in pea aphids, *Acyrthosiphon pisum,* infected with entomophthorous fungi. Shaw *et al.* (1967) noted that three species of predatory mite seemed unharmed by feeding on virus-infected *Panonychus citri,* and laid only slightly fewer eggs than mites fed on virus-free individuals. Zondag (1965, 1967) observed that a nematode parasitizing the wood-wasp, *Sirex noctilio,* in New Zealand did not attack insect parasites of the wasp. However, there are reports of parasites of *Sirex* spp. in Europe being attacked by a similar nematode.

C. THE SILKWORM

The silkworm, *Bombyx mori,* is special in being a domesticated insect; it can be reared in isolation from pathogens used against pest insects in the field.

Nevertheless, it is illegal to disseminate foreign preparations of any pathogen in Japan for fear they may endanger silkworms. Some strains of *B. thuringiensis*, notably var. *thuringiensis*, which are effective against pest insects, are relatively harmless to silkworms (Angus, 1968; Angus and Norris, 1968). They may be similar to the enzootic types reported to be widespread in Japan and that have been recovered from the dust in silkworm farms (Aizawa, 1967). However, what is harmless for silkworms is not necessarily harmless for beneficial field insects. For example, *B. thuringiensis* var. *thuringiensis* is more harmful than *B. thuringiensis* var. *sotto* to honey-bees (Krieg and Herfs, 1962), but var. *sotto* is one of the most harmful to silkworms (Angus and Norris, 1968).

Other pest-insect pathogens that attack silkworms include *Beauveria bassiana, Metarrhizium anisopliae* and other fungi (Madelin, 1966), *Tipula* iridescent virus (Smith, 1967) and the cytoplasmic polyhedrosis virus of the pine caterpillar, *Dendrolimus spectabilis* (Aruga *et al.*, 1963).

Pest-insect pathogens that have failed to infect silkworms in laboratory tests include *Bacillus popilliae* and *Bacillus lentimorbus* (Aizawa, 1967), which cause the "milky diseases" of Japanese beetle larvae, *Popillia japonica*, and the nuclear polyhedrosis virus of *Galleria mellonella* (Gershenson, 1957; Aizawa, 1967). However, Aizawa found that the infectivity of *G. mellonella* polyhedrosis virus for wax moth larvae was neutralized by antiserum prepared against silkworm polyhedrosis virus, which shows some relationship between the viruses, further suggested by the fact that injecting the silkworm virus kills *G. mellonella* larvae (Aizawa, 1962; see also Chapter 30).

III. Specificity of Pathogens

Although major effects by pest-insect pathogens on beneficial field insects may be improbable, the observations discussed so far indicate that wide host ranges are not uncommon. Experiments with beneficial insects are too few, however, to give a good idea of the potential host ranges of insect pathogens. For this purpose the specificity of insect pathogens for all kinds of insects should be considered.

A. CROSS-INFECTIVITY TESTS

Many attempts to infect species widely different from that of the original host have failed, e.g. with *B. thuringiensis* (Heimpel and Angus, 1963; Kreitz, 1966), *B. popilliae* (Dutky, 1963) and several kinds of virus (Gershenson, 1957; Neilson, 1964; Bailey and Gibbs, 1964; Bailey, 1965; Weiser and Vago, 1966; Hurpin and Robert, 1967; Ignoffo, 1968a). However, many others have succeeded. The best known pathogens with wide host ranges are some of the fungi. *Metarrhizium anisopliae* is known to attack more than 50 insect species in seven insect orders (Roberts, 1968). *Beauveria bassiana* may have an even wider host range, knowledge of which continues to expand rapidly. *Entomophthora sphaerosperma* attacks species in most if not all of the large orders of insects in nature (Gustafsson, 1965). Several workers have transmitted other *Entomophthora* spp. between widely different hosts in the laboratory (Thaxter, 1888; Yendol and Paschke, 1966; Prasertphon, 1963). Wilding (1969) transmitted various species of *Entomophthora* from one species of aphid to others and then easily returned them to their original host species, which suggests that mutants were not being selected by passaging the fungi in "foreign" species.

The very wide host ranges attributed to some species of Microsporida, especially *Nosema apis,* by early workers (see Thomson, 1960) were probably mistaken. Adequately controlled experiments (e.g. Kramer, 1964) have not confirmed their results. Nevertheless, Smirnoff (1968) showed that the microsporidan *Thelohania pristiphorae* from the larch sawfly larva, *Pristiphora erichsonii,* would infect the completely unrelated tent caterpillars, *Malacosoma disstria* and *M. americanum*, when fed to them (see also Chapter 30, p. 668).

The viruses were at one time considered to be very host-specific (Smith, 1967) but there are now several records of cross-infection between species (Stairs, 1960; Smith, 1967; Ignoffo, 1968a) and between genera (e.g. Gershenson, 1957; Neilson, 1964; Ignoffo, 1968b; Smith, 1967). In fact nuclear polyhedrosis virus for controlling *Adoxophyes orana (reticulana)* is best cultured in the much larger *Mamestra brassicae* (Ponsen, 1966). Gershenson (1964) reported that all of many species of Nymphalidae tested are susceptible to all of several kinds of nuclear polyhedroses of Lepidoptera that have been tested. He also stated that the cytoplasmic polyhedrosis viruses were even less specific than the nuclear ones and thought it possible that all Lepidoptera spp. are susceptible to every such virus. Neilson (1964) imported a cytoplasmic polyhedrosis virus of *Vanessa cardui* from England to Canada, where it seemingly did not occur, not even in an occult form, and successfully infected 11 species in 10 genera of Lepidoptera out of 18 species tested. Recent serological tests have supported the results of these cross-infectivity tests. Cunningham (1968) showed that the virus particles from nuclear polyhedra of four Nymphalidae of different, although closely related, genera were serologically indistinguishable as were those of two *Lymantria* spp. and those from granulosis capsules of three *Pieris* spp. Moreover, Cunningham and Longworth (1968) showed that viruses from cytoplasmic polyhedra in seven unrelated species of the Nymphalidae, Arctiidae, Notodontidae, Lymantridae and Hepialidae, were very closely related serologically or were indistinguishable. At least some polyhedrosis viruses, therefore, have a very wide host range within the Lepidoptera. Smith (1967) considers there is evidence of nuclear and cytoplasmic polyhedra being successfully transmitted to Neuroptera, and there is no doubt that *Tipula* iridescent virus (TIV) and the very similar *Sericesthis* iridescent virus have very wide host ranges. TIV has been transmitted by injection and by mouth to species of several insect orders (Smith *et al.*, 1961; Smith, 1967). Bailey and Gibbs (1964) transmitted acute bee-paralysis virus to several *Bombus* spp. Admittedly many examples of the non-specificity of insect viruses have been shown by injecting them into foreign hosts. This method might well by-pass almost insurmountable barriers to infection, such as gut enzymes and lack of appropriate cell-wall receptors in the gut epithelium. For example, the infective dose of acute or chronic bee-paralysis virus by injection is about 10^2 particles, whereas by mouth the dose is 10^{10} or more (Bailey, 1965; Bailey and Gibbs, 1964). By contrast, Gershenson (1964) observed that the cytoplasmic polyhedrosis viruses were less infective by injection than by mouth, possibly because the appropriate receptors for these viruses are in the gut, which is the only organ infected by them. Mitsuhashi (1967) infected the green rice leaf-hopper, *Nephotettix cincticeps,* with *Chilo* iridescent virus (which is very similar to TIV) from the rice stem borer, *Chilo suppressalis*, by allowing the hopper to ingest a suspension of the virus through a thin membrane. These insects presumably have similar virus receptors on their gut epithelium, which perhaps reflects their common food.

B. FACTORS INFLUENCING INFECTION

1. Age

Many failures to infect "foreign" hosts by mouth may have occurred because the insects were not treated when they were susceptible. Susceptibility to infection in some insects is brief and most usual when the insect is young. Aruga *et al.* (1963) infected young silkworms by feeding them cytoplasmic polyhedra of the pine caterpillar *(Dendrolimus spectabilis),* whereas previous workers had failed to infect older larvae. Gershenson (1964) and others (see Stairs, 1968) noted that young larvae of Lepidoptera were more easily infected with nuclear polyhedra than old ones. Age affects the susceptibility of a host to other pathogens as well as viruses. Smirnoff (1968) who transmitted a microsporidan from the larch sawfly to tent caterpillars found that, whereas many first instar tent caterpillars became infected, very few second and no third instars did. Baird (1957), who transmitted *Entomophthora muscae* between several species of Diptera, noticed that the youngest individuals of *Musca domestica* were the most susceptible. The first, and also the sixth, instars of *G. mellonella* are most susceptible to *B. thuringiensis* (Morrison and Perron, 1963). In addition to insect pathogens known to have alternative hosts, others that are most infective for the youngest hosts are *Bacillus larvae* of larval bees (Bailey, 1963), the fungus *Ascosphaera apis* of larval bees (Bailey, 1967), sacbrood virus of bees (Bailey, 1969), Sigma virus of *Drosophila melanogaster* (Seecoff, 1968) and also the parasitic mite *Acarapis woodi* of adult honey-bees. Various insect and mite species also usually acquire "circulative" viruses from their plant hosts most rapidly when they are immature (Swenson, 1967). Clearly, the age of the host must be taken into account when testing the host ranges of pathogens.

2. Ecology

Ecological factors, in addition to the intrinsic changes with age of insects, profoundly affect susceptibility. They probably limit the possible host ranges of pathogens and so increase their effective specificity in nature.

Many *Entomophthora* spp. that grow readily as saprophytes nevertheless infect only a few groups of insects. Gustafsson (1965) could see no clear physiological reason for this and surmised that the explanation was "probably of an ecological nature". The apparent specificity of some *Entomophthora* spp. for some insect species in mixed populations in the field, noted for example by Hall and Dietrich (1958), Bohart (1949), MacLeod *et al.* (1966), may depend on micro-ecological factors that affect infection of different species differently. Giard (1888) observed that, in nature, *Entomophthora telaria* occurred in *Ragonycha melanura* only when this beetle was with an infected bug, probably *Phygadicus urticae*, on the same plant, *Galiopsis tetrahit*. This suggests that the insects were susceptible to the same infection because they were sharing the same habitat.

Nearly all entomopathogenic fungi infect insects by penetrating the integument. Environmental factors, especially humidity, radiant energy and ambient temperature, may, therefore, play a great part in determining their host ranges. These factors will affect the interior of insects less than the body surface. Accordingly, pathogens that multiply, germinate or are released only in conditions specific to the gut of some species may be less likely than fungi to infect foreign hosts. For example, the obligate bacterial pathogens–*Bacillus popilliae, B. larvae, Clostridium brevifaciens, Streptococcus pluton*–which seem to have very narrow host ranges, all need narrow ranges of oxidation potentials and other essential factors to start their infective cycles (Dutky, 1963; Bailey and Lee, 1962; Bucher, 1961; Bailey and Gibbs, 1962); and also the polyhedrosis viruses may be limited to insects with a gut lumen alkaline enough to dissolve the silicon-bound polyhedral protein (Estes and Faust, 1966; Faust and Adams, 1966). Nevertheless, slight differences in temperature can spell the difference between success and failure for some of these pathogens. The fungus *Ascosphaera apis,* for example, commonly attacks honey-bees in Britain and some parts of Europe in spring, when the weather is very changeable and the bee larvae are sometimes chilled (Bailey, 1967), but it has never been shown to attack honey-bees in N. America. Yet it has been found attacking solitary bees *(Megachile inermis* and *Anthophora prufica)* in Utah (Baker and Torcheo, 1968). Presumably honey-bees in N. America are less likely to be chilled than in some European countries. The Microsporida seem a highly specialized group; they multiply intracellularly and, though the conditions they require are unknown, some specific mid-gut factors may be needed to release the polar filaments. Yet *Nosema bombycis* spores will infect vertebrate embryo cells when these are maintained at 28° C (Ishihara, 1968). Their inability to infect similar tissues at 37° resembles the inability of *Nosema apis* to multiply in bees at 37° (Lotmar, 1943), whereas the parasite multiplies rapidly when the bees are kept at 35° or colder. Similarly *Tipula* and *Sericesthis* iridescent viruses do not multiply in *Galleria mellonella* when this insect is kept above 30° (Day and Mercer, 1964; Tanada and Tanabe, 1965). Temperature is important for the success of other pathogens, in addition to those with known alternative hosts. *B. popilliae* of the Japanese beetle (Dutky, 1963), Sigma virus of *D. melanogaster* (see Seecoff, 1968) and acute bee-paralysis virus (Bailey and Milne, 1969) for example, multiply or cause symptoms only within narrow temperature ranges. Temperature is important, therefore, in the study of potential new hosts for pathogens but its effect has rarely been systematically investigated.

IV. Outlook

There is no evidence that any of the pest-insect pathogens currently favoured for biological control, notably *B. thuringiensis, B. popilliae* and some polyhedrosis viruses, would harm beneficial field insects. This fact, together with the many failures to transmit pathogens to hosts that are very different from the insect in which they were found, has characteristically led pest-insect pathologists to be optimistic. They might well continue safely to hold this attitude. However, the many articles written about pest-insect pathogens invariably extol their specificity and rarely discuss the possible width of their host ranges. This neglect may foster complacency.

Cameron (1967) said "there is no known case where a microbial pathogen of an insect has caused infection or other serious injurious effects in higher animals". This statement depends on a limited definition of an insect pathogen. Many viruses, rickettsiae and protozoa that multiply in vertebrates, and viruses that multiply in plants, also multiply and sometimes cause symptoms in insects (Kramer, 1967; Chamberlain, 1968; Maramorosch, 1968), some of which are unrelated to the usual vectors (Hurlbut and Thomas, 1960). Rabies, vesicular stomatitis and Sindbis viruses, which resemble the "insect pathogen", Sigma virus, multiply in *Drosophila melanogaster* (Plus and Atanasiu, 1966; Périès *et al.,* 1966; Berkaloff *et al.,* 1967) and the flies infected with rabies virus lay fewer eggs and die sooner than uninfected individuals. Strains of *Salmonella typhimurium,* a common cause of food poisoning in man, multiply in and kill larvae of *Galleria mellonella* that ingest them (Kurstak and Vega, 1967). Other facts that make dubious any forecast of the specificity of an insect pathogen are that *B. thuringiensis* infects and kills earthworms (Smirnoff and Heimpel, 1961), and that nucleic acid of silkworm polyhedrosis virus will infect and multiply in cultured mammalian cells, producing polyhedra and virus particles, indistinguishable from those that form in the silkworm (Himeno *et al.*, 1967). Many different kinds of pathogen clearly infect several very different hosts with little respect to our present systems of biological classification. Their ability to spread to novel hosts within the Insecta should hardly be surprising. The wonder seems rather that host specificity is so evident than that some insect pathogens have wide host ranges. Admittedly these host ranges are limited compared with the broad spectra of insecticides and, as infectivity—especially in nature—is probably a multifactorial quality, a change in the several factors that might enable a pathogen to infect a novel host may be improbable. However, there is no certainty that such changes do not occur and that pathogens will stay restricted to the pests against which they are directed, especially when they are disseminated artificially thereby giving mutants increased opportunities.

In spite of the desirability of insect pathogens that affect only pest insects, it is remarkable how much interest is aroused by those that are the least specific. Dutky (1959) refers to *Beauveria bassiana* with its wide, undefined host range, as a "magnificent pathogen". Stairs (1968) referring to adapting polyhedrosis viruses to "foreign" hosts by initially infecting these with very many nuclear polyhedra, says "it may be possible to adapt viruses to economically important species that are not presently susceptible to a virus". This could well apply to useful insects exposed to viruses applied artificially in the field to control pest insects. Cunningham and Longworth (1968), when referring to the apparent identity of many cytoplasmic polyhedrosis viruses, say the biological control of Lepidoptera will be "considerably increased if many species are infected with the same virus". In addition to the silkworm, useful Lepidoptera such as *Cactoblastis cactorum,* that control weeds, may be vulnerable to these viruses. *C. cactorum* is probably susceptible to *B. thuringiensis* too, although there is little evidence that this pathogen spreads readily when accidentally introduced into populations of susceptible insects in field conditions, whereas it can in food stores and warehouses. Commercial interests find specific pathogens unattractive because they are usually difficult to culture, and the demand for them would be much less than for broad spectrum pathogens. Equally important, they obviously do not usually severely decrease populations of their hosts in nature. These enzootic pathogens would be ideally employed when encouraged to multiply and spread by cultural practices that knowledge of their ecology might help to devise.

All beneficial insects, except the silkworm, are wild, and they will inevitably encounter pathogens that are artificially distributed in the field. Pathogens intended for use this way should be tested at least against honey-bees. Honey-bees are self-supporting in rural areas, plentiful and readily available and so are more convenient for tests than many other kinds of field insects.

Newly-emerged adults should be fed and sprayed with the pathogens and incubated at 30° and 35° (Fig. 1): small colonies in the field should similarly be fed and sprayed and their larvae frequently examined for disease during the next few weeks. However, failure to harm bees or any other test insect in experiments such as these does not prove they are insusceptible. The uninitiated experimenter could easily miss the well-known honey-bee pathogens themselves when the often very precise circumstances needed for them to multiply and spread are absent (Bailey, 1968).

To sum up, present evidence with beneficial insects is not discouraging for the continued tests of pest-insect pathogens or for their use in agricultural practice. However, pathogens are not free from hazards as they are mutable and many of all kinds already span very wide host ranges.

References

Aizawa, K. (1962). *J. Insect Path.* **4**, 122-127.

Aizawa, K. (1967). *Mushi* **39**, 97-102.

Angus, T. A. (1968). *Wld. Rev. Pest Control* **7**, 11-26.

Angus, T. A. and Norris, J. R. (1968). *J. Invertebrate Path.* **11**, 289-295.

Aruga, H., Hukuhara, T., Fukuda, S. and Hashimoto, Y. (1963). *J. Insect Path.* **5**, 415-421.

Bailey, L. (1963). "Infectious Diseases of the Honey Bee." 175 pp. Hutchinson, London.

Bailey, L. (1965). *J. Invertebrate Path.* **7**, 132-140.

Bailey, L. (1967). *In* "Insect Pathology and Microbial Control" (P. A. van der Laan, ed.), pp. 162-167. North-Holland Publ. Co., Amsterdam.

Bailey, L. (1968). *A. Rev. Ent.* **13**, 191-212.

Bailey, L. (1969). *Ann. appl. Biol.* **63**, 483-491.

Bailey, L. and Gibbs, A. J. (1962). *J. gen. Microbiol.* **28**, 385-391.

Bailey, L. and Gibbs, A. J. (1964). *J. Insect Path.* **6**, 395-407.

Bailey, L. and Lee, D. C. (1962). *J. gen. Microbiol.* **29**, 711-717.

Bailey, L. and Milne, R. G. (1969). *J. gen. Virology* **4**, 9-14.

Baird, R. B. (1957). *Can. Ent.* **89**, 432-435.

Baker, G. M. and Torcheo, P. F. (1968). *Mycologia* **60**, 189-190.

Berkaloff, A., Berreur, P. and Cals, P. (1967). *C.r. hebd. Séanc. Acad. Sci. Paris* **264**, 1545-1548.

Bohart, G. E. (1949). *Pan-Pacif. Ent.* **25**, 82 only.

Bracken, G. K. and Bucher, G. E. (1966). *J. Invertebrate Path.* **9**, 130-132.

Bucher, G. E. (1961). *Can. J. Microbiol.* **7**, 641-655.

Burges, H. D. and Bailey, L. (1968). *J. Invertebrate Path.* **11**, 184-195.

Cameron, J. W. (1967). *In* "Insect Pathology and Microbial Control" (P. A. van der Laan, ed.), pp. 182-196. North-Holland Publ. Co., Amsterdam.

Cantwell, G. E. Knox, D. A. and Michael, A. S. (1964). *J. Insect Path.* **6**, 532-536.

Cantwell, G. E., Knox, D. A., Lehnert, T. and Michael, A. S. (1966). *J. Invertebrate Path.* **8**, 228-233.

Chamberlain, R. W. (1968). *In* "Insect Viruses" (K. Maramorosch, ed.), pp. 38-58. Springer-Verlag, Berlin.

Cunningham, J. C. (1968). *J. Invertebrate Path.* **11**, 132-141.

Cunningham, J. C. and Longworth, J. F. (1968). *J. Invertebrate Path.* **11**, 196-202.

Day, M. F. and Mercer, E. H. (1964). *Aust. J. biol. Sci.* **17**, 892-902.

Dutky, S. R. (1959). *Adv. appl. Microbiol.* **1**, 175-200.

Dutky, S. R. (1963). *In* "Insect Pathology" (E. A. Steinhaus, ed.), Vol. 2, pp. 75-115. Academic Press, London.

Estes, Z. E. and Faust, R. M. (1966). *J. Invertebrate Path.* **8,** 145-149.
Evlakhova, A. A. and Voronina, E. G. (1967). *In* "Insect Pathology and Microbial Control" (P. A. van der Laan, ed.), pp. 280-281. North-Holland Publ. Co., Amsterdam.
Faust, R. M. and Adams, J. R. (1966). *J. Invertebrate Path.* **8,** 526-530.
Franz, J. M., Krieg, A. and Reisch, J. (1967). *NachrBl. dt. PflSchutzdienst. Stuttg.* **19,** 36-44.
Gershenson, S. (1957). *Rep. Acad. Sci. USSR* **113,** 1161-1162.
Gershenson, S. (1964). *Entomophaga, Mém. hors. Sér.* **2,** 361-372.
Giard, A. (1888). *Bull. Scient. Fr. Belg.* **3,** 298-309.
Gustafsson, M. (1965). *Lantbr Högsk. Annlr* **31,** 103-212.
Hall, I. M. and Dietrich, E. J. (1958). *Calif. Agric.* **9,** 5-16.
Haragsin, O. and Vaňková, J. (1968). *Annls Abeille* **11,** 31-40.
Harcourt, D. G. (1966). *Can. Ent.* **98,** 653-662.
Heimpel, A. M. and Angus, T. A. (1963). *In* "Insect Pathology" (E. A. Steinhaus, ed.), Vol. 2, pp. 21-73. Academic Press, London.
Himeno, M., Sakai, F., Onodera, K., Nakai, H., Fukuda, T. and Kawade, Y. (1967). *Virology* **33,** 507-512.
Hurlbut, H. S. and Thomas, J. I. (1960). *Virology* **12,** 391-407.
Hurpin, B. and Robert, P. (1967). *Entomophaga* **12,** 175-180.
Ignoffo, C. M. (1968a). *In* "Insect Viruses" (K. Maramorosch, ed.), pp. 129-167. Springer-Verlag, Berlin.
Ignoffo, C. M. (1968b). *Bull. ent. Soc. Am.* **14,** 265-276.
Ishihara, R. (1968). *J. Invertebrate Path.* **11,** 328 only.
Issi, I. V. and Maslennikova, V. A. (1964). *Ent. Rev., Wash.* **43,** 56-58.
Issi, I. V. and Maslennikova, V. A. (1966). *Ent. Rev., Wash.* **45,** 275-277.
Jaques, R. P., Stultz, H. T. and Huston, F. (1968). *Can. Ent.* **100,** 813-818.
Kramer, J. P. (1964). *Entomophaga, Mém. hors. Sér.* No. 2, 95-99.
Kramer, J. P. (1967). *In* "Insect Pathology" (E. A. Steinhaus, ed.), Vol. 1, pp. 251-272. Academic Press, London.
Kreitz, G. (1966). *Waldhygiene* **6,** 183-187.
Krieg, A. and Herfs, W. (1962). *Entomophaga, Mém. hors Sér.* No. 2, 193-195.
Krieg, A. and Herfs, W. (1963). *Entomologia exp. appl.* **6,** 1-9.
Kurstak, E. and Vega, C. E. (1967). *Can. J. Microbiol.* **14,** 233-237.
Lecomte, J. and Martouret, D. (1959). *Annls Abeille* **2,** 171-175.
Lotmar, R. (1943). *Beih. Schweiz. Bienenztg.* **1,** 261-284.
MacLeod, D. M., Cameron, J. W. M. and Soper, R. S. (1966). *Revue roum. Biol. Ser. Bot.* **11,** 125-134.
Madelin, M. F. (1966). *A. Rev. Ent.* **11,** 423-448.
Maramorosch, K. (1968). *In* "Current Topics in Microbiology and Immunology" (K. Maramorosch, ed.), Vol. 42, pp. 94-107. Springer-Verlag, Berlin.
Martouret, D. and Euverte, G. (1964). *J. Insect Path.* **6,** 198-203.
Meynadier, G., Vago, C., Plantevin, G. and Atger, P. (1964). *Revue Zool. agric. appl.* **63,** 207-208.
Mitsuhashi, J. (1967). *J. Invertebrate Path.* **9,** 432-434.
Morrison, F. O. and Perron, J. M. (1963). *Phytoprotection* **44,** 106-115.
Neilson, M. M. (1964). *J. Insect Path.* **6,** 41-52.
Périès, J., Printz, P., Canivet, M. (1966). *C.r. hebd. Séanc. Acad. Sci. Paris* **262,** 2106-2107.
Plus, N. and Atanasiu, P. (1966). *C.r. hebd. Séanc. Acad. Sci. Paris* **263,** 89-92.
Ponsen, M. B. (1966). *Meded. Rijksfac. LandbWet. Gent* **31,** 553-557.
Prasertphon, S. (1963). *J. Insect Path.* **5,** 318-335.
Roberts, D. W. (1968). *In* "Insect Pathology and Microbial Control" (P. A. van der Laan, ed.), pp. 243-246. North-Holland Publ. Co., Amsterdam.
Seecoff, R. (1968). *In* "Current Topics in Microbiology and Immunology" (K. Maramorosch, ed.), Vol. 42, pp. 60-93. Springer-Verlag, Berlin.
Sekariah, P. C. and Seth, R. N. (1959). *Indian Vet. J.* **36,** 19-23.
Shaw, J. G., Moffitt, C. and Scriven, G. T. (1967). *J. econ. Ent.* **60,** 1751-1752.

Shimanuki, H. and Hartman, P. A. (1963). *Bact. Proc.* **63,** p. 10.
Smirnoff, W. A. (1968). *J. Invertebrate Path.* **11,** 321-325.
Smirnoff, W. A. and Heimpel, A. M. (1961). *J. Insect Path.* **3,** 403-408.
Smith, K. M. (1967). "Insect Virology". Academic Press, London.
Smith, K. M., Hills, G. J. and Rivers, C. F. (1961). *Virology* **13,** 233-241.
Smith, R. F. and van den Bosch, R. (1967). *In* "Pest Control" (W. W. Kilgore and R. L. Doutt, eds), pp. 295-340. Academic Press, London.
Stairs, G. R. (1960). *Can. Ent.* **92,** 906-908.
Stairs, G. R. (1968). *In* "Insect Viruses" (K. Maramorosch, ed.), pp. 1-23. Springer-Verlag, Berlin.
Steinhaus, E. A. (1954). *Hilgardia* **23,** 197-261.
Swenson, K. G. (1967). *In* "Methods in Virology" (K. Maramorosch and H. Koprowski, eds), Vol. 1, pp. 267-307. Academic Press, London.
Tanada, Y. and Tanabe, A. M. (1965). *J. Invertebrate Path.* **7,** 184-188.
Thaxter, R. (1888). *Mem. Boston Soc. Nat. Hist.* **4,** 133-201.
Thomson, H. M. (1960). *J. Insect Path.* **2,** 346-385.
Ullyett, G. C. (1947). *Ent. Mem. Dep. Agric. Un. S. Afr.* **2,** 74-202.
Ullyett, G. C. and Schonken, D. B. (1940). *Un. S. Afr. Sci. Bull. Dep. Agr. Forestry,* No. 218, 24pp.
U.S.D.A. (1965). *Agric. Res., Wash.* **14,** 8-9.
Weiser, J. (1963). *In* "Insect Pathology" (E. A. Steinhaus, ed.), Vol. 2, pp. 291-334. Academic Press, London.
Weiser, J. and Vago, C. (1966). *J. Invertebrate Path.* **8,** 314-319.
Wilding, N. (1969). *Rep. Rothamsted exp. Stn. for 1968,* pp. 230-231.
Wilson, W. T. (1962). *J. Insect Path.* **4,** 269-270.
Yendol, W. G. and Paschke, J. D. (1966). *J. Invertebrate Path.* **7,** 414-422.
Zondag, R. (1965). *Rep. Forest Res. Inst. N.Z.* 1964, pp. 53-62.
Zondag, R. (1967). *Rep. Forest Res. Inst. N.Z.* 1966, pp. 57-64. Wellington, N.Z.

CHAPTER 24

Production of Pathogens in Artificial Media

H. T. DULMAGE and R. A. RHODES

Entomology Research Division, Agricultural Research Service
Brownsville, Texas, U.S.A.
and
U.S. Department of Agriculture,
Northern Utilization Research and Development Division,
Peoria, Illinois, U.S.A.

I. Introduction

While many organisms are pathogenic to insects or produce chemicals toxic to them, only three are at present being produced or studied to any degree in large-scale fermentations. One, *Bacillus thuringiensis,* is grown primarily for its toxins; the other two, *Bacillus popilliae* and *Beauveria bassiana*, are used as invasive insect pathogens. Two fungi, *Metarrhizium anisopliae* and *Acrostalagmus aphidum*, have been grown in pilot plant. In this chapter, we examine general fermentation technology, discuss the production of *B. thuringiensis* and *B. popilliae* in detail, and review some of the problems associated with the production of the fungal pathogens.

II. Microbial Technology

A. BASIC PRINCIPLES

The parasitic nature of infectious organisms does not necessarily exclude saprophytic growth, although the selectivity of pathogens for certain hosts indicates that highly specific conditions may be required for propagation *in vitro.* Formation of insecticidal products of cells also requires the initial or concomitant proliferation of the organism, and the production of maximum yields of such products may demand specific distortions of normal cell growth or metabolism. However, because the metabolic processes of the microbial cell are ordered and because it must maintain this organization to survive, the cell itself restricts the amount of distortion which can be imposed to enhance one aspect of metabolism. Productivity is mediated by the inherent potential of the cell and by the mechanisms that control cell functions. The consistency of cellular properties, together with predictable alterations produced by modification of growth conditions, imply the presence of both metabolic and genetic control mechanisms. All fermentative processes, including the production of microbial control agents, ultimately depend on these mechanisms (Rhodes, 1966).

B. MODIFICATION OF MICROBIAL CHARACTERISTICS

Commercial production of micro-organisms or microbial products invariably requires selection of a specific strain best suited to the process and, furthermore, it is often necessary to seek modification of the characteristics of the organism involved. These changes may be needed to permit growth under economic fermentation conditions or to increase production of a desired product. Such changes may be brought about by mutation—i.e. alteration of the genetic material of the cell by mutagenic agents—or by transfer of genetic material into the cell. Mutations are rare events and detection may be difficult unless some means of selecting for a particular mutant is available. When the selection procedure is time-consuming, for example, when bioassays are required, it may not be practical to examine the required number of isolates to detect a desired variant. The conditions under which desoxyribonucleic acid transfer occurs are specific, and the spontaneous occurrence of transfer probably is negligible. However, where operative, transfer offers means for introducing a new, desirable characteristic in cells, but detection is under the same constraints as described for mutation.

C. MAINTENANCE OF CULTURES

Repeated transfer of cultures on artificial media can cause undesirable changes in the organism, such as a decrease in its capacity to sporulate. Among insect pathogens, diminished virulence has been reported from repeated growth outside the host (Müller-Kögler, 1965; Seman, 1964). Pathogenicity or sporogenesis can often be restored by passage through an appropriate host insect (Müller-Kögler, 1965; Kawakami, 1960). Modification of the pathogenicity of *B. thuringiensis* by insect passage has been reported (Aizawa and Fujiyoshi, 1967).

The most accepted form of culture maintenance has been lyophilization where spores or vegetative cells suspended in sterile serum are rapidly frozen in tubes in a dry ice bath and dried under vacuum; the tubes are sealed while evacuated. Other methods include: storage under refrigeration, storage frozen under liquid nitrogen, and storage of spores in sterile dry soil.

D. MEDIA

Microbial cells require water, carbon for biosynthesis and energy, nitrogen, mineral elements and growth factors. The levels and forms of these substances depend on the fermentation process used. Thus a carbon source suitable for a semi-solid fermentation might not be suitable for a deep-tank fermentation. In addition, precise requirements for specific processes are set by the organism involved and by the physiological state desired in the cells. In some cases, optimum growth or yield of product may occur only within very narrow limits of medium composition; in other cases, an organism may accept wide variations in media without apparent effect on the fermentation.

1. Sources of Carbon

Carbon is the prime raw material for synthesis of new cell material or cell products. Usually, carbohydrates are the most available and economic carbon sources. Polysaccharides cannot enter the cell, and organisms that utilize them form extracellular hydrolytic enzymes. Starch, for example, can be used in *B. thuringiensis* fermentations because this organism is usually an active amylase producer. Economic considerations largely exclude the use of pure sugars. Most often, molasses, raw grain mashes, grain processing by-products, or enzyme-hydrolyzed grain starches provide needed carbohydrates.

Cells are the major carbonaceous product in fermentations. About 3-5 g of fungal cells, 1-3 g of bacterial cells, and 1-5 g of yeast cells are produced per 100 ml of fermentation liquor (Aiba *et al.*, 1965).

2. Sources of Nitrogen

The nitrogen required by micro-organisms can sometimes be supplied by ammonium salts. More often, organic nitrogen must be supplied in the form either of single amino acids or of complex materials–including specific peptides, nucleic acids and vitamins. As a group, parasitic organisms have more extensive requirements than do saprophytes. Most organisms grow faster when organic nitrogen is supplied, even though it is not essential. The cheapest forms of organic nitrogen are protein-rich materials of plant and animal origin. These include soybean meals, distillers' solubles, corn steep liquor, oil-free cottonseed endosperm flour, yeast extracts, and whey or casein hydrolysates. The level of carbon sources in a medium frequently dictates the level of nitrogen compounds required. The complex needs, characteristic of some pathogens, may require the use of animal sera or insect hemolymph.

3. Mineral Elements

Inorganic salts are essential for growth of micro-organisms. These include potassium, magnesium, phosphorus, sulfur and lesser quantities of calcium, zinc, iron, cobalt, copper, molybdenum, manganese, or other minerals. Particular activities may involve requirements beyond those for growth. For example, manganese is required for sporulation and calcium for heat stability in spores. Ordinarily, elements needed in trace quantities are coincidentally supplied in water and crude fermentation substrates. Some natural waters may contain harmful amounts of certain trace minerals; in such cases, deionized or distilled water may be required.

4. Growth Factors

The vitamins essential as components of enzyme systems are needed by all microbial cells; they must be supplied if the cell cannot synthesize them. A deficient capacity to biosynthesize almost any essential cell component will result in a specific requirement. The unique demands of so-called fastidious organisms often turn out to be an unsuspected need for relatively common components such as oleic acid. Requirements for specific natural products often reflect imbalance of nutrients in the medium.

E. CONDITIONS FOR MICROBIAL GROWTH

The cultural conditions essential for maximum cell mass usually are not those that afford maximum yield of a metabolic product. In addition, the most robust cells frequently are produced under conditions which afford less than maximum cell yield. The latter is particularly important when it is realized that insect pathogens must manifest appropriate levels of virulence.

1. pH

Optimum growth of most bacteria occurs near pH 7; yeasts and molds tolerate greater acidity, but do not necessarily prefer it. During growth, products of microbial metabolism often cause major shifts in pH, and still further changes may occur when growth is culminated by subsequent metabolism of the primary products. Frequently, but not always, utilization of carbohydrates lowers the pH of a medium, while utilization of proteins raises it. In such cases, the pH range desired during the fermentation may influence the choice and level of these nutrients. The pH of fermentation media is most frequently controlled by buffers or by the automatic addition of sterile alkali or acid.

2. Oxygen

Micro-organisms differ in their need for oxygen and vary in their requirements during different phases of growth. It is difficult to supply sufficient oxygen to rapidly growing cultures. This problem will be discussed in the section on large-scale fermentations.

3. Temperature

Almost all micro-organisms have a fairly wide range of temperature at which some proliferation occurs. The optimum for producing either cells or cell products must be determined empirically. Usually, it will be somewhat below the maximum temperature at which growth occurs, and the best temperature for product formation often is not the same as that for maximum growth. Optimum growth of most insect pathogens would be expected to be close to those temperatures normally encountered in the insect (25-32° C). These vary according to the climatic zone. Since temperature-adapted strains of insect pathogens have been detected in the field (Evlakhova and Švecova, 1965), it may be desirable to grow insect pathogens at temperatures closely compatible with the area in which they are to be disseminated.

F. LARGE-SCALE FERMENTATIONS

The requirements of any aerobic fermentation demand an intimate association between micro-organism, nutrients, and air. While this is not difficult to obtain in the laboratory, the maintenance of good aeration becomes increasingly difficult when fermentations are scaled up. Furthermore, the economics of large-scale production demand that the fermentation occupies as little space as possible. The semi-solid fermentation is designed to meet these requirements for micro-organisms in surface culture. The deep-tank fermentation is used when a liquid or submerged culture is preferred.

1. Semi-solid Fermentations

In the semi-solid fermentation, the organism is grown in a liquid nutrient which has been absorbed on the surface of small particles of a carrier. This achieves a high ratio of surface area to volume and furnishes, in a relatively small space, a large liquid-gas interface. Usually, wheat bran is used as the carrier in these fermentations, although ground corn, peanut meal, oat or rice hulls, cottonseed meal, and alfalfa meal have been used. Inorganic carriers such as expanded volcanic glass, diatomaceous earth, vermiculite, and pumice are sometimes used. Since moist bran has a tendency to clump and reduce aeration efficiency, a mixture of bran and inorganic carrier is frequently used. Organic carriers often furnish nutrients to the fermentation as well as serving as an absorption base. Bran, an excellent source of starch and protein, has been used for many years in amylase and proteinase fermentations.

In a typical semi-solid fermentation, bran, water, and a suitable nutrient solution are mixed and sterilized by flowing steam; the medium then is inoculated with a spore suspension, a fermented bran culture, or a submerged culture seed. The moisture content of the final mixture is adjusted with water to between 50 and 70%. During the early part of the fermentation, air between 80 and 100% R.H. is passed over the bran to aerate the fermentation without drying the bran. The temperature of the air is carefully controlled, since the air also regulates the temperature of the fermentation. After an appropriate fermentation period, the moist air is replaced by dry air to gradually dry the bran and terminate the fermentation. When the moisture content of the bran has dropped to about 4%, the bran is harvested.

The semi-solid fermentation is an inexpensive process. The equipment used is comparatively simple and unsophisticated. Absolute sterility is not maintained. However, the same factors that make a semi-solid process inexpensive also limit the control that can be maintained over the fermentation. For maximum yields of cells or products, careful regulation of the various stages of the fermentative process is usually required. Consequently, most modern fermentations use the deep-tank procedures described below.

Recovery of the product from semi-solid fermentations is simple only when the product is soluble in a suitable solvent and therefore easy to extract from the final bran cake. However, in some applications, purified materials are not required so long as the activity produced is available for use. In this case, the final bran need only be dried and ground. Total production costs for such materials are very low.

Underköfler and Hickey (1954) and Prescott and Dunn (1959) should be consulted for a more detailed review of the semi-solid fermentation process.

2. Submerged Fermentations

Modern fermentations use pure cultures growing dispersed in liquid media. In laboratory studies flasks are agitated on a shaking machine, which splashes the liquid to increase the liquid-gas interface for gas exchange and so improve aeration. Pilot plant studies and large-scale production use deep-tank fermentors. These range in size from 5 liters in a laboratory model up to 200,000 liters in production vessels. Air is introduced at the bottom of the tank. Submerged turbine impellers intimately mix air, media and organisms. Water jackets or cooling coils control temperature. Foaming can be a problem in fermentors and is controlled by the addition of such insoluble liquids as oils, polyglycols, and silicones, which must be closely regulated by automatic devices because antifoams reduce oxygen absorption rates (Bungay *et al.*, 1960).

Maintenance of sterility during fermentation is extremely important in the deep-tank process. Air must be filtered to prevent entry of contaminant organisms. Devices for agitation, pH control, and antifoam addition are designed for sterilization *in situ* and for operation without introducing contaminants. Media and other ingredients must be sterilized, usually by heating. Everything, except inocula added after sterilization, must be sterile, and samples must be taken only through valves kept sterile by flowing steam.

A deep-tank fermentation is inoculated with a seed culture produced in increasing volumes of media in shake flasks and small fermentors. Transfers are timed when the organism is in a vigorous stage of growth and made aseptically. The production fermentor is then inoculated with 0.1-10% by volume of the final seed, depending on the requirements of the organism. Rigorous control of temperature, aeration, pH, and foaming are maintained throughout the fermentation. Occasionally, to obtain maximum yields, fermentation conditions must be changed during the production run.

Recovery of product from submerged fermentations is often difficult, since there is only a small amount of the desired material in a large amount of fermentation liquor. If the product is insoluble, as when recovering the organism itself, filtration or centrifugation can be employed. Otherwise, solvent extraction, precipitation, or absorption on resins, charcoal, or other similar materials must be used. Both fermentation and recovery costs are higher than those in a semi-solid fermentation. However, yields are usually greater in the deep-tank process and the product can be concentrated; these more than compensate for the increased costs.

III. *Bacillus thuringiensis* Fermentation

A. INTRODUCTION

Since all *B. thuringiensis* formulations are sold primarily for control of lepidopterous pests, industry is primarily interested in the crystalline toxin (= crystal or δ-endotoxin). However, spores may play a secondary role in the insecticidal activity, and the heat-stable exotoxin (= β-exotoxin or fly-factor) has practical potential. All three components are produced both in semi-solid and in submerged fermentations, both of which are used commercially.

There are advantages and disadvantages in each type of fermentation. The semi-solid process yields a wettable powder or dust formulation containing spores, crystals, and exotoxin simply by drying and grinding the final bran cake. The product, being dry, is inherently stable. However, bran is a major constituent of the final formulation. Bran is difficult to wet and tends to swell when wetted, characteristics that make it an unsatisfactory component of a wettable powder. Thus, although the semi-solid product has been a satisfactory dust base, it has been difficult to use as a wettable powder.

Submerged fermentations have mainly been used to produce flowable formulations–suspensions of the spore-crystal complex. These can be used as sprays, but, of course, are not available as dusts. In the past, liquid formulations of the complex tended to deteriorate and require refrigerated storage, but now they have been stabilized and can be stored at room temperature. Originally, flowables did not contain the exotoxin. However, it can be precipitated from the beer and recovered along with the spores and crystals, which is sometimes done today. Dulmage *et al.* (1970) have developed a recovery procedure to produce a dry preparation of the spores and crystals for use as a wettable powder or a dust. This process will be used commercially in 1970.

B. MEASUREMENT OF ACTIVITY

While standardization of *B. thuringiensis* preparations will be discussed at length in another chapter, it would be useful to review some of the methods of reporting the insecticidal activity of these materials.

1. Viable Spore Count

Spores of *B. thuringiensis* are resistant to pasteurization. Most viable spore counts are made on suspensions of spores that have been exposed to a temperature of 65°C for 10 or 15 min. In some cases it may be necessary to expose the spores to a temperature of around 80°C for a brief period–i.e. to "heat-shock" them–to induce germination.

2. Spore-crystal Complex

a. Diet dilution unit (DDU_{50}). The diet dilution unit is the reciprocal of the LD_{50} determined in terms of the concentration of a sample in artificial diet. In the absence of a standard, the diet dilution unit is a useful tool, since the unit varies directly with potency and since it permits the direct comparison of total activities in liquids and solids. However, the diet dilution unit, like the LD_{50}, has the disadvantage of varying with the species and age of insect used, and it is not reliable for comparing independent observations from unrelated assays (Dulmage *et al.*, 1970).

b. International unit (IU). In 1966, at Wageningen, The Netherlands, a working party proposed that potencies of the crystal of *B. thuringiensis* be determined through bioassays in which LD_{50}'s of unknown *B. thuringiensis* samples were compared with those of a standard. They recommended as a primary reference standard, E-61, a material prepared at the Institut Pasteur, Paris, France, and assigned it a potency of 1000 IU/mg. Thus, potencies of *B. thuringiensis* materials would be expressed in international units/mg relative to this standard. The use of the standard prevents the interference of the variables inherent in the diet dilution assay, and, when a standard is available, the international unit should be preferred (Burges, 1967).

3. Heat-stable Exotoxin

The exotoxin prevents the metamorphosis of fly larvae into the adult form and the toxin is generally measured in bioassays against this insect. Activity of the test sample can be expressed as the LC_{50} based on weight of pure toxin, because pure toxin has now been isolated and reference samples are available (Chapter 12).

C. SEMI-SOLID FERMENTATION

A process patented by Mechalas (1963) for the large-scale production of *B. thuringiensis* toxins on bran-based semi-solid media is presented in Fig. 1. The diagram shows two passages in shake flasks, the usual procedure, although the Mechalas patent shows only one. In a typical fermentation, the seed for the semi-solid fermentation was produced by passing *B. thuringiensis* through shake flasks and then into a seed fermentor. Tne medium in the flasks was composed of 15 g dextrose, 5.0 g corn steep liquor, 5.0 g yeast autolysate, and 4.0 g K_2HPO_4/liter of water, adjusted to pH 7.0-7.2 with NaOH. The flasks were incubated 8 hr at 30° C. The fermentor medium contained 10 g dextrose, 4.5 g corn steep, 6.0 g yeast autolysate, 3.5 g K_2HPO_4, 0.43 g NaOH, and 0.1 g $CaCl_2$/liter of water. The fermentor was inoculated with 0.1% by volume of the shake flask seed and incubated 16 hr at 30° C. Approximately 400 ml of this fermentor seed was used to inoculate each kilogram of the semi-solid production medium.

Production of the spores and toxins was carried out on a semi-solid medium composed of 545 g wheat bran, 380 g expanded perlite, 62 g soybean meal, 36 g dextrose, 3.6 g lime, 0.9 g NaCl, 0.29 g $CaCl_2$, and 160 ml water. After partial sterilization with flowing steam for 60 min, the mixture weighed about 1 kg. This was inoculated with 400 ml of fermentor seed yielding a final mixture with moisture content 60% by weight and pH 6.9. In an actual fermentation, about 250 kg of the inoculated bran was placed in bins with perforated bottoms through which air at 30-34° C and 95-100% R.H. was passed at about 0.4-0.6 vol air/vol inoculated medium/min for the first 3 hr and 1.0-1.2 vol thereafter. The

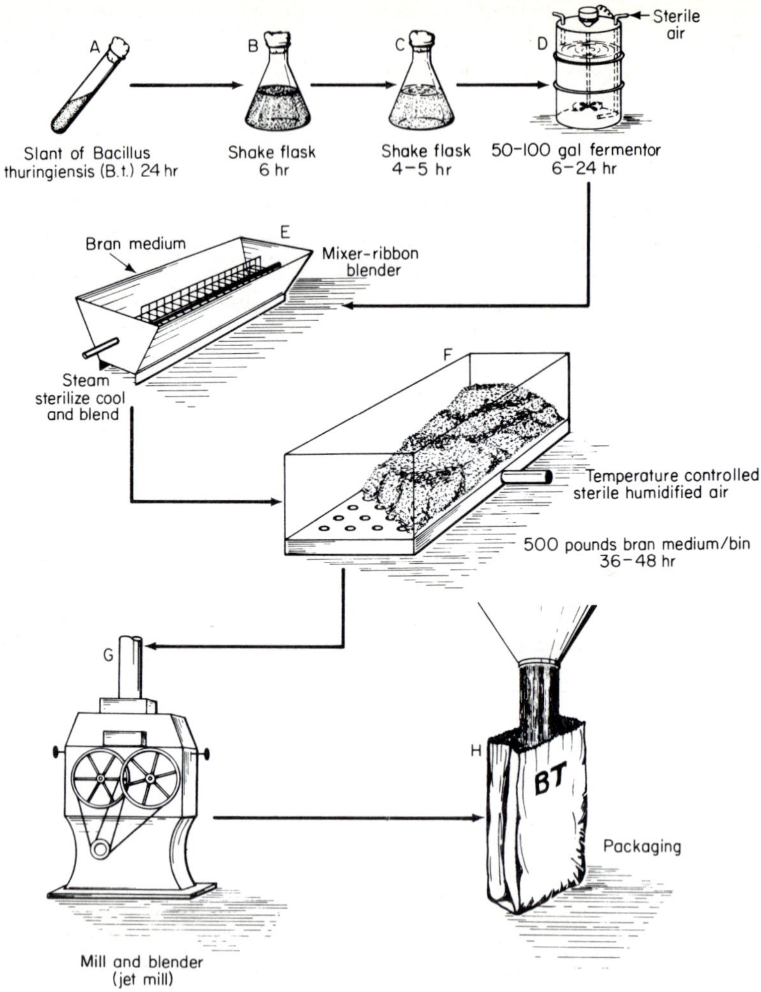

Fig. 1. Semi-solid fermentation of *B. thuringiensis.* Drawing by E. Cantu and H. Dulmage (unpublished).

bins were incubated for about 36 hr, during which time the pH rose to 7.5 and the moisture content dropped to about 53%. At this time dry air at 50-55° C was passed through the bran for another 36 hr. The bran medium was then harvested and ground through 80 mesh screens. The final product had a moisture content of 4% and a pH of 7.0. The product was active against a typical lepidopteran, the salt-marsh caterpillar *(Estigmene acrea)* and a typical dipteran, the housefly *(Musca domestica).* The amount of activity was not reported.

The process just described is a typical semi-solid fermentation. While it can be very closely controlled through the seed fermentor, many problems arise in the bin fermentation. The bran itself is not sterilized during the heating process, although the level of micro-organisms is usually reduced so much that they do not interfere with the fermentation. The introduced air is clean, but not sterile. The lower layers of bran effectively filter contaminants from the air and prevent their spread throughout the mixture; as a result, these layers often become heavily contaminated. This in itself would not be a problem, aside from reducing the yield of good product. However, the air tends to develop channels as it passes through the bran, resulting in poor aeration and temperature control in parts of the bran mass (Underköfler *et al.*, 1947). This can be overcome only by thoroughly mixing the bran one or more times during the fermentation. This mixing may spread the contaminants from the bottom layer through the bin with a loss in quality of the final product. Both problems can be overcome by sterile-filtering the air and replacing the bin containers with tumbling perforated drums (Takamine, 1913, 1914). Such procedures, however, are costly and decrease the economic advantages of the semi-solid process.

The strain of *B. thuringiensis* used and the fermentation conditions greatly influence the production of crystals in semi-solid media. Dulmage, in a Symposium on the Identification and Assay of Viruses and *B. thuringiensis* used for Insect Control, held in London, England, in July, 1964, described work on this aspect of the fermentation at Nutrilite Products, Inc. Table I shows a comparison of six strains of *B. thuringiensis* var. *thuringiensis* in semi-solid fermentation. All strains produced approximately the same level of spores in the bran medium. Yet, a very wide spread in insecticidal activity was found—from 1 : 10 to 1 : 20,000—a 2000-fold range. The influence of fermentation conditions on crystal production is shown in Table II. When one strain was

TABLE I

Production of insecticidal activity by six strains of Bacillus thuringiensis *var.* thuringiensis *in a semi-solid bran medium*

Strain No.	Lowest active dilution[a]
B-1	1 : 20,000
B-2	1 : 10,000
B-3	1 : 10,000
B-4	1 : 3,000
B-5	1 : 500
B-6	1 : 10

[a] Lowest dilution of 10% suspension of bran at which significant kill (10% or greater) of *Estigmene acrea* was observed on each of three consecutive assays. There were virtually no deaths in the controls.

TABLE II

Production of insecticidal activity by a single strain of Bacillus thuringiensis *var.* thuringiensis *in six semi-solid fermentation runs*[a]

	Assays on harvested bran		
Run No.	Spore count x 10^9/g dry wt	IU/mg[b] dry wt	IU/10^6 spores ratio
1	6	240	40
2	17	1400	82
3	7	940	130
4	3	840	280
5	11	840	76
6	5	650	130

[a]Media for all runs were identical.
[b]Assay insect: *Estigmene acrea.*

grown in six separate fermentations on the same semi-solid medium, spore production varied from 3 x 10^9 to 17 x 10^9 spores/g. Potencies of these products varied from 240 to 1400 IU/mg. Ratios of international unit to spore count in different fermentations ranged from 40 to 280 IU/10^6 spores. Thus the potencies produced did not depend solely on the extent that the organism grew, but was also influenced by fermentation conditions.

Since the quantity of crystal produced can be altered by strain selection and by modification of fermentation procedures, it is probable that the potency of materials produced from bran can be increased. However, to attain significant gains from such changes, close control of the fermentation will be required. In view of the drawbacks associated with the semi-solid fermentation, this control will be difficult to achieve. Consequently, the submerged process is likely to supplant the semi-solid procedure in future production of *B. thuringiensis* toxins.

D. SUBMERGED FERMENTATION

Ignoffo (1967) presented a diagram of the fermentative procedures used by the International Mineral and Chemical Corporation (IMC) to produce their flowable formulation of the *B. thuringiensis* spores and toxins. A slightly modified version of this diagram is reproduced in Fig. 2. Ignoffo did not specify the media or fermentation procedures used, but it is assumed that the fermentation was based on the Megna patent (1963) and proceeded as follows: inoculum for a production fermentor was prepared by passing *B. thuringiensis* sequentially through two media in shake flasks and then to a seed fermentor. Nutrient broth was used for the initial shake flask, and a medium composed of 1% beet molasses, 0.85% corn steep solids, and 0.1% $CaCO_3$ was used for the

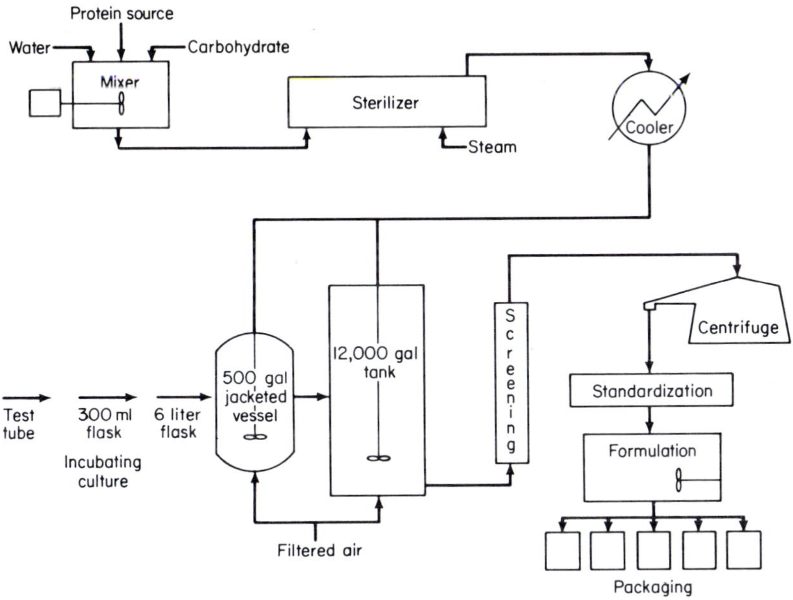

Fig. 2. Submerged fermentation of *B. thuringiensis.* Drawing by E. Cantu from C. Ignoffo (1967).

second shake flask and for the seed fermentor. Each shake flask seed was incubated 24 hr. The seed fermentor was allowed to incubate until vigorous vegetative growth was attained, it was then used to inoculate the production tank. The composition of the medium in the production tank could vary, but was limited to 3-4% solids and was so designed that the "fermentable carbohydrate and nitrogen available for growth present in said fermentation medium were exhausted at approximately the same time after the commencement of sporulation". A typical medium contained 1.86% beet molasses, 1.4% cottonseed flour (Pharmamedia), 1.7% corn steep liquor solids, and 0.1% $CaCO_3$. When sporulation was complete, the beer was passed through a fine screen to remove any coarse particles, centrifuged, diluted with various stabilizing agents, and packaged as a flowable formulation. In the Megna patent, it was specified that the final product had insecticidal activity and that the final fermentation beer contained 2-5 x 10^9 viable spores/ml. There was no statement as to how much insecticidal activity such a fermentation produced.

In the patent just described, Megna claimed a recovery process based on the filtration of the fermentation liquor with the assistance of a filteraid such as Celite 512. He stated that any imbalance in the supply of nitrogen and carbohydrate would result in incomplete sporulation, fracturing of intact cells, germination of spores, and/or autolysis, which would make the recovery of the product by filtration more difficult. In the present International Mineral and Chemical Corporation process (Ignoffo, 1967), recovery is accomplished by centrifugation, thus avoiding filtration problems.

A process patented by Drake and Smythe (1963) has also been used in the industrial production of *B. thuringiensis* in the U.S.A. They disagreed with the requirements of Megna that limited the level of nutrients in the fermentation medium to 3-4% and preferred 6-10% total nutrients. Furthermore, they did not believe that it was critical to exhaust the carbohydrate and nitrogen sources near the onset of sporulation as Megna suggested. A typical medium contained 6.8% corn starch, 0.64% sucrose, 1.94% casein, 4.7% corn steep, 0.6% yeast and 0.6% phosphate buffer. Since some of the ingredients were liquids, the actual total solid content was 12.3%. The final liquor before harvest contained 14×10^9 viable spores/ml; other trials yielded counts greater than 15×10^9 spores/ml. This patent claimed production of activity against the southern armyworm, the salt-marsh caterpillar, and housefly larvae. Unfortunately, yields of product were not specified nor bioassays standardized, so it is impossible to know how much activity was produced.

The Drake and Smythe patent is notable for two important observations besides the fermentation: (1) the exotoxin was precipitated from fermentation liquors with $CaCl_2$ or $BaCl_2$, and (2) a mixture of inclusion bodies and water-soluble toxins from which the spores had been removed retained its activity against the salt-marsh caterpillar, the southern armyworm and the housefly larvae. In an interesting experiment, a water-soluble product with activity against armyworms was isolated from a filtered beer presumably free from spores and crystals.

Other patents on the submerged fermentation of *B. thuringiensis* exist. Bonnefoi (1960) patented the production of spores and toxins in an aerated liquid medium containing 0.6-1.0% N (amino acids), 1-2% sugar, and traces of calcium, zinc, manganese, and magnesium. The product was dried and mixed with appropriate carriers to make a powder. Shell Internationale Research (1969) patented a medium consisting of 2.3% casein, 1.0% molasses, and 2.3% Scotaferm (a by-product of the fermentation of alcoholic beverages). This patent stated that fermentations could be carried out with any of several strains of *B. thuringiensis*, blending the products of the different fermentations, but claimed that at least one of the components of the mixture had to be from a fermentation of serotype IX. This requirement for serotype IX is surprising and does not conform to the authors' experience.

In a recent paper, Majumber (1968) stated that the virulence of *B. thuringiensis* was entirely dependent upon the production of "viable spores with attached parasporal rhomboidal crystals" and added that this sporulation depended upon the presence of D-xylose in the medium at levels of less than 0.025%. This did not take into account the separate activity of the crystal.

Majumber also suggested assay by injection of spores into the hemocoele of the cockroach. Again, while the spores should initiate a septicemia, the vital gut wall barrier has been bypassed and activity of the crystal toxin is not demonstrated.

The paper and patents referred to above have been primarily concerned with the production of *B. thuringiensis* spores. Yet several workers have reported differences in insecticidal activity between various serotypes and preparations of *B. thuringiensis* (Angus, 1956, 1965, 1967; Menn, 1960; Heimpel and Angus, 1960, 1963; Vaňková, 1964; Burgerjon, 1965; Burgerjon and Biache, 1967; Broersma and Buxton, 1967; Angus and Norris, 1968; Dulmage, 1970a). The isolate of *B. thuringiensis* used and the fermentation conditions employed in the semi-solid fermentation influenced the production of the crystal, and the

TABLE III

Characteristics of the insecticidal activities of powders recovered from fermentation beers of different variants of Bacillus thuringiensis *grown on tryptone-based and Proflo-based media*

Variant	Medium[a]	Characteristics of powder			
		Spore count x 10^9/g	DDU_{50}/g	$DDU_{50}/10^9$ spores[b]	DDU_{50} recovered/ liter beer[b]
aizawai	Tryptone	76	76,000	1,000	150,000
	Proflo	120	34,000	280	230,000
alesti	Tryptone	53	<3,700	<70	<5,000
	Proflo	22	<2,200	<100	<5,800
dendrolimus	Tryptone	95	43,000	450	86,000
	Proflo	250	<2,500	<10	<15,000
entomocidus	Tryptone	36	26,000	720	61,000
	Proflo	110	240,000	2,200	1,000,000
finitimus	Tryptone	42	<2,900	<70	<5,800
	Proflo	41	4,100	100	29,000
galleriae	Tryptone	46	17,000	370	33,000
	Proflo	120	44,000	370	240,000
kenyae	Tryptone	9	63,000	7,000	180,000
	Proflo	60	100,000	1,700	650,000
morrisoni	Tryptone	69	83,000	1,200	250,000
	Proflo	70	98,000	1,400	600,000
sotto	Tryptone		Poor growth		
	Proflo	7	<280	<40	<1,600
subtoxicus	Tryptone	31	220,000	7,100	620,000
	Proflo	85	53,000	620	340,000
thuringiensis	Tryptone	22	230,000	10,500	420,000
	Proflo	160	180,000	1,100	1,100,000
tolworthi	Tryptone	14	810,000	58,000	3,000,000
	Proflo	130	100,000	770	580,000

[a]For formulae of media, see Table IV.
[b]Assay species *Pectinophora gossypiella*.

TABLE IV

Media for the fermentation of Bacillus thuringiensis

Ingredient	Level (g/liter)		
	Tryptone medium	Proflo medium	Soybean meal medium
Tryptone	10.0		
Proflo		10.0	
Soybean meal			15.0
Bacto-peptone®		2.0	
Dextrose	5.0	15.0[a]	5.0
Corn starch	5.0		5.0
Yeast extract	2.0	2.0	
K_2HPO_4	1.0		
KH_2PO_4	1.0		
$MgSO_4.7H_2O$		0.3	0.3
$FeSO_4.7H_2O$		0.02	0.02
$ZnSO_4.7H_2O$		0.02	0.02
$CaCO_3$		1.0	1.0
All media diluted to volume with distilled H_2O			

[a]In later experiments, level reduced to 10.0 g.

amount produced did not depend solely on the growth of the organism. Dulmage (1970b) studied crystal production by different strains of *B. thuringiensis* in submerged culture. Table III lists the results. The production of the insecticidal activity (due mainly to toxin) was dependent both on the strain and on the medium. No one strain–and no one medium–was necessarily superior. Yields (DDU_{50}/liter) were greater with most cultures on the Proflo medium, but *dendrolimus* and *tolworthi* produced more toxin on the tryptone medium. If the cultures are judged on the basis of the tryptone medium, *tolworthi* is best, but on the Proflo medium, *thuringiensis* is superior. Efficiency of production, measured as $DDU_{50}/10^9$ spores, also varied from culture to culture and, with each culture, from medium to medium. Since there was no correlation between spore production and insecticidal activity, these results point out the danger of evaluating fermentations by spore count.

The most recent advance in the commercial production of the crystal toxin has been the use of a newly isolated strain of *B. thuringiensis* var. *kurstaki,* HD-1, reported by Dulmage (1970a), and the recovery of spores and crystals by a process developed by Dulmage *et al.* (1970). Media used by Dulmage in his studies with HD-1 are presented in Table IV. They were not selected as the best media for toxin production, but are representative of media that support the growth of *B. thuringiensis* isolates. The Proflo and the soybean meal media would be economical for commercial production; the tryptone medium would not. A flow sheet for the recovery process is presented in Table V and can be summarized as follows: the whole beer was centrifuged to recover spores and crystals. The cream from the centrifugation was suspended in 4-6% lactose solution and precipitated with 4 vol. of acetone. Lactose, precipitated along with the crystals and the spores, helped to prevent clumping and to make the final product easier to resuspend. The precipitate was recovered by filtration with suction in a Buchner funnel using Whatman No. 1 paper. Filteraid was not needed. The precipitate was washed with acetone and dried.

TABLE V

Flow sheet: Process for recovery of spore-crystal complex of Bacillus thuringiensis

	Whole beer, pH 8.4-8.7
	Adjust to pH 7.0 with HCl
	Centrifuge
Supernatant	Residue
(Discard)	Suspend in 0.1-0.05 vol (Based on original beer) 4-6% lactose
	Stir 30 min
	Add slowly while stirring 4 vol acetone
	Stir 30 min
	Let stand 10 min
	Filter with suction
Filtrate	Residue
(Discard)	Stir with small volume acetone
	Filter with suction
Filtrate	Residue
(Discard)	Stir with small volume acetone
	Filter with suction
Filtrate	Residue
(Discard)	Dry overnight, room temperature

The product recovered from the above fermentation has been named the HD-1 formulation. Dulmage (1970a) investigated the level of crystal toxin production relative to spore count and compared it with two commercial experimental formulations and with the French standard, E-61. While the four materials had similar spore counts, the level of toxin in the HD-1 formulation was unusually high (Table VI). HD-1 has now been produced on a commercial

TABLE VI

Comparison of spore counts and international units of spore-crystal preparations of Bacillus thuringiensis[a]

Preparation	Spores x 10^9/g	IU/mg
E-61	18	1,000[b]
HD-1-PL-1	18	16,000
Commercial "A"	17	75
Commercial "B"	18	900

[a] Bioassay insect: *Heliothis virescens.*

[b] E-61, the proposed international standard, has 1000 IU/mg by definition.

scale by Abbott Laboratories, North Chicago, Illinois and by International Minerals and Chemical Corporation, Skokie, Illinois. Comparative bioassays between the commercial HD-1 and two commercially-marketed materials are shown in Table VII. The improved potency of this formulation measured in these bioassays has been confirmed in field trials (McGarr *et al.*, 1970; Kenney, unpublished; Dulmage *et al.*, 1971).

TABLE VII

Average potencies of formulations of the spore-crystal complex of Bacillus thuringiensis, *expressed on weight or application basis*

Formulation	Potency in *Heliothis virescens*	
	Weight basis	Application basis
HD-1 powder	12,000 IU/mg	5.40 x 10^9 IU/lb
Thuricide 90TS flowable	860 IU/mg	0.81 x 10^9 IU/qt
Biotrol 25W 183 powder	530 IU/mg	0.24 x 10^9 IU/lb

Yields of crystal have thus been increased in submerged fermentation. Since the production of the toxin responds to strain selection and alteration in fermentation conditions, it may be expected that yields will be improved markedly in the future. This should lead to formulations more active at lower cost and broaden the use of this valuable microbial insecticide.

IV. Production of *Bacillus popilliae in vitro*

A. INTRODUCTION

The pioneering work of Dutky showed that milky disease is an effective means for the biological control of the Japanese beetle, *Popillia japonica*; closely related beetles of the family Scarabaeidae also are infected (Dutky, 1963; Tashiro and Steinkraus, 1966). In nature, the causative bacteria, *B. popilliae* and *B. lentimorbus*, are obligate pathogens because they grow as vegetative and sporulating cells only within infected larvae. Spores survive outside the host but vegetative cells die rapidly in any menstruum except hemolymph or complex growth media (St. Julian *et al.*, 1963). Although techniques now have been devised that permit extensive vegetative growth in fermentors, effective sporulation has not been achieved. Use of milky disease for control is limited by the inability to produce large quantities of infective spores in artificial culture (Rhodes, 1965, 1967).

Fermentative production of a specific product usually requires an "unnatural" physiology induced by mutation and specific environment for maximum yield. In a sense, the opposite is true in developing means for production of an insect pathogen. Here, genetic and physiological bases for the complex interrelationships that characterize a specific host-parasite relationship must be retained while the pathogen is grown in an artificial environment. The problems encountered in attempts to devise techniques for large-scale production of milky disease spores indicate the inherent difficulties.

A process for production of the milky disease bacteria has several requirements that must be consistently met: (1) large populations should be produced per unit fermentation volume, (2) a high proportion of the vegetative cells should sporulate, (3) growth and sporulation should occur under fermentation conditions amenable to large-scale processing, (4) the resultant spores should be stable and infective under field conditions, (5) virulence and propagative characteristics of the disease induced in host populations by *in vitro* spores should be equivalent to those caused by the native pathogen.

Research with *B. popilliae* has been emphasized because this organism is superior to *B. lentimorbus* as a control agent and is less fastidious in artificial culture.

B. SELECTION OF STRAINS

B. popilliae can be isolated in pure culture by plating spores obtained from diseased larvae. Massive accumulation of spores in the hemolymph gives diseased larvae a milky appearance. These spores retain viability indefinitely in the dry state. Even when diseased hemolymph is obtained under rigorously aseptic conditions, the dried spores cannot be considered a pure culture in the microbiological sense. The nutritive medium required for growth of *B. popilliae* is also almost invariably suitable for contaminant organisms, which grow rapidly and interfere with growth of *B. popilliae.* In addition, spores from hemolymph germinate poorly.

The bacteria are isolated by germinating spores on solid media so that separated clones of vegetative cells develop; vegetative cells can be preserved by lyophilization after further plating (Haynes *et al.*, 1961; Lingg *et al.*, 1967). These cells contain the unaltered genome of the original spore because they produce authentic milky disease when injected into larvae (Pridham *et al.*, 1964). However, the genetic complement of all spores is not identical and strains of varied properties can be isolated. Dutky (1963) has reported variation in pathogenicity among naturally occurring strains studied in larvae.

A strain of *B. popilliae,* NRRL B-2309, was selected for current research because it grows rapidly in artificial media and because both vegetative cells and spores are infective by injection; spores of this strain produced in larvae are also infective by feeding. Additional strains have been selected from spontaneous variants of the parent in artificial culture. These include strains which differ in rate of growth, metabolic capacity, colonial characteristics, infectivity, and extent of sporogenesis *in vitro. B. popilliae* is variable and care must be taken to stabilize characteristics during propagation. Variation in artificial culture represents the selective pressure applied to the population by nonparasitic existence. The disparity between conditions in larvae and in artificial culture is a continuing problem in efforts to obtain strains with characteristics appropriate to control use.

C. VEGETATIVE GROWTH OF *BACILLUS POPILLIAE*

Because only one spore is formed by each progenitor cell, it is necessary to establish conditions for maximum production of vegetative cells in fermentations. Under optimum conditions, about 2×10^9/ml viable vegetative cells of *B. popilliae* are achieved in growth periods of 16-18 hr in aerated fermentors. The pattern of growth is shown in Fig. 3. Somewhat smaller populations develop in shaken flasks (Rhodes *et al.*, 1966; Sharpe, 1966).

B. popilliae requires oxygen both for metabolism of carbohydrates and for maximum growth (Costilow *et al.*, 1966). Although vegetative growth occurs under reduced oxygen tension, and possibly even anaerobically in adapted cultures, the yield of cells is less. Larval hemolymph contains dissolved oxygen, which diminishes, during proliferation of the pathogen, to about one-half that of normal larvae or of diseased larvae which contain mainly spores (Weiner *et al.*, 1966).

The minimal growth requirements of *B. popilliae* in a synthetic medium include 11 amino acids, thiamine, and barbiturate (Sylvester and Costilow, 1964). However, growth is very limited in synthetic media and serial transfer is often not successful. Highest cell yields are obtained in media containing

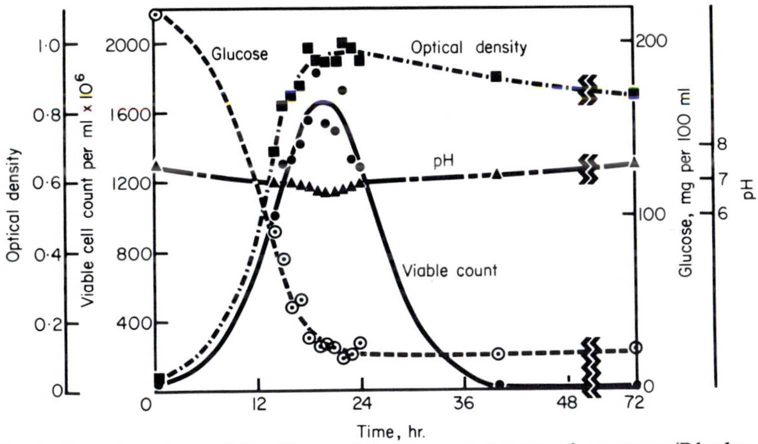

Fig. 3. Growth pattern of *Bacillus popilliae* in aerated 2-liter fermentors (Rhodes *et al.*, 1966).

complex nitrogen sources. *B. popilliae* appears to require unknown growth factors or a balance of nutrients which is best satisfied by specific yeast extracts (Rhodes *et al.*, 1966). The standard growth medium (designated MD) contains 1.5% yeast extract, 0.3% K_2HPO_4, and 0.2% glucose (autoclaved separately and added aseptically); part of the yeast extract can be replaced by other organic nitrogen sources, such as enzymatically hydrolyzed casein. Tryptone is sometimes included in MD medium because it enhances viability, and filter-sterilized media afford significantly better growth (Sharpe, 1966). The cooking periods required for heat sterilization of large volumes render media unsuitable for growth, and filter-sterilization is required. Although growth equivalent to that in MD medium occurs on less expensive formulations based on corn steep liquor or some other nitrogen sources, such media do not support growth through serial transfer. Commercially, inocula could be prepared on the MD medium and production then done on an alternative medium.

The logarithmic phase of bacterial growth is generally followed by a stationary phase during which there is little net change in cell numbers. The stationary phase may last for hours before viability appreciably declines, especially if deleterious products formed during the logarithmic growth phase are neutralized. Sporogenesis occurs during the post-logarithmic phase in sporeforming bacteria. However, cells in cultures of *B. popilliae* die without sporulating. Characteristically, fewer than 0.1% of cells remain viable 24 hr after the point of maximum population (Fig. 3). Cultures that reach less than maximum populations survive proportionally longer. Accordingly, longevity can be increased by modifications of growth conditions which tend to restrict growth: suboptimal temperature, minimal inocula, limited nutrient, or reduced oxygen supply. Viability is also extended by inclusion of particulate carbon in the medium or by dialysis during growth. At best, cultural techniques achieve limited survival. Cells do not lyse although, upon continued incubation, bizarre shapes occur among survivors. Residual viability is not the result of sporulation by a fraction of the population or of emergence of uniquely resistant cells; cultures isolated from the surviving cells behave identically to the original. Costilow *et al.* (1966) have suggested that accumulation of peroxide is the cause of death (Pepper and Costilow, 1965). Rhodes (1965) has proposed that death occurs because cells are committed to sporogenesis, which they cannot accomplish under existent conditions. Whatever the reason, rapid death of cultures is apparently the symptom not the cause of asporogeny.

Vegetative cells from flask culture or small fermentors infect Japanese beetle larvae when injected, and spores are formed normally during the ensuing disease (Pridham *et al.*, 1964). The number of vegetative cells required to induce disease varies with their physiological state. About 10^3 logarithmic phase cells per larva are optimal. Greater dosages are required if cells are taken from the decline phase of the growth curve or from poor growth conditions. It appears unlikely that the host is somehow repeatedly selecting sporulating strains during proliferation in larvae and that asporogenic variants invariably are selected during growth in laboratory media. Milky disease has been induced in larvae by injection of vegetative cells of strains exhibiting a unique property and the same strain then has been reisolated from spores produced in the insect.

Injection of excessive numbers of vegetative cells causes an overwhelming infection which kills larvae before spores are formed. Possibly, the metabolic activities of large vegetative populations overwhelms the nutritive balance in the hemolymph or toxic amounts of foreign cell material may be liberated during growth and death of many invading cells. We have found that injection of large numbers of dead vegetative cells is lethal, and Dutky (1963) has stated that toxic material is produced by *B. popilliae* grown in artificial culture. Therefore, death associated with massive infection of hemolymph may involve toxin formation *in vivo*.

D. SPORULATION OF *BACILLUS POPILLIAE* IN LARVAE

Spores are the stable infective form by which milky disease is disseminated in nature. About 5 x 10^9 spores/larva (ca. 5 x 10^{10}/ml hemolymph) accumulate in the hemolymph during the 7- to 21-day developmental period of the disease. The appearance of *B. popilliae* spores is shown in Fig. 4. The structure of spores

Fig. 4. *Bacillus popilliae.* (a) Sporangia, *sp*, each with a refractile spore, *s*, and a smaller refractile parasporal body, *p*, from a milky diseased *Popillia japonica* larva. Phase contrast x4500. (b) Surface view of spore freed from sporangium x64,000, scanning electron microscopy by G. St. Julian and L. D. Bulla. (c) Live vegetative cells, *v*, dead granular vegetative cells, *dv*, pre-spores, *ps*, and spores, *s*, in hemolymph from larva in intermediate stage of infection. Phase contrast x4500. (d) Same stages from colonies on agar plates.

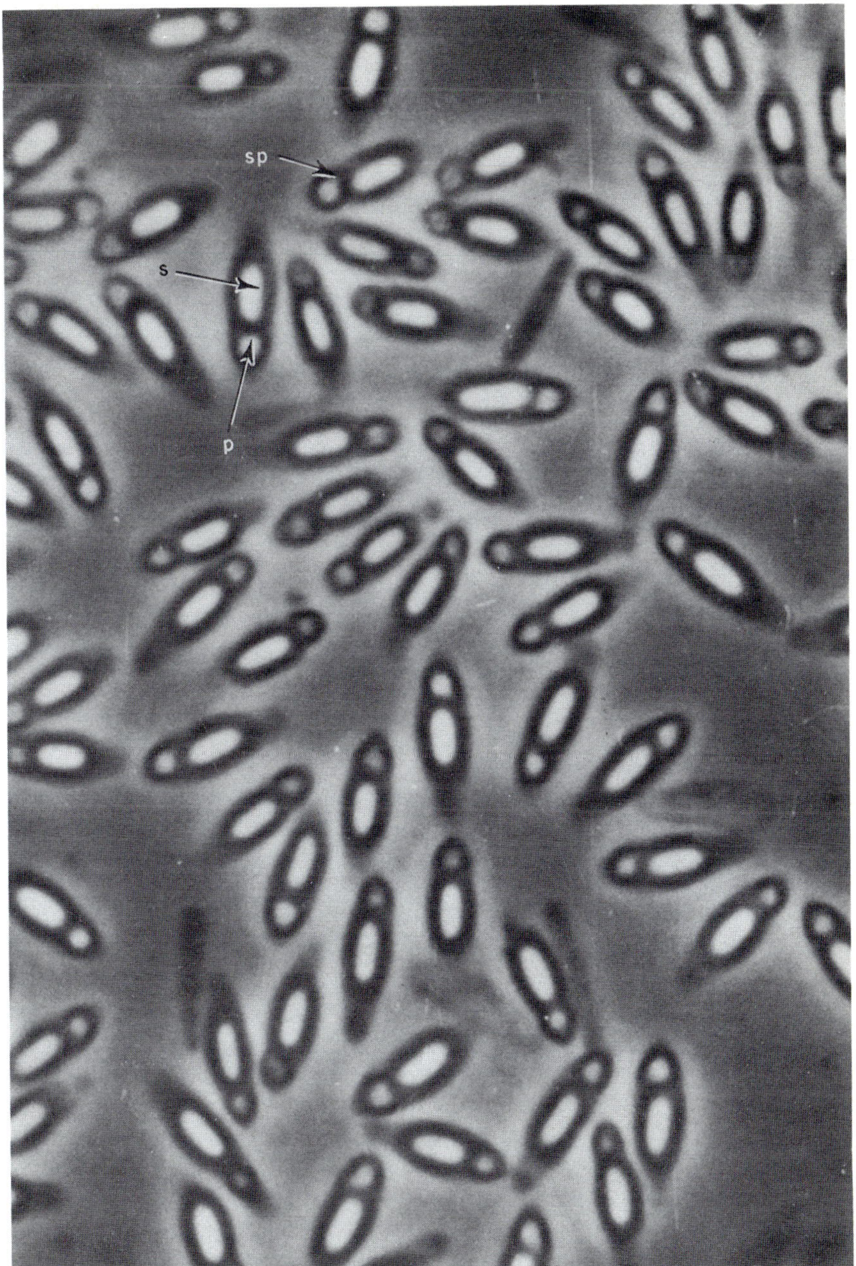

Fig. 4(a).

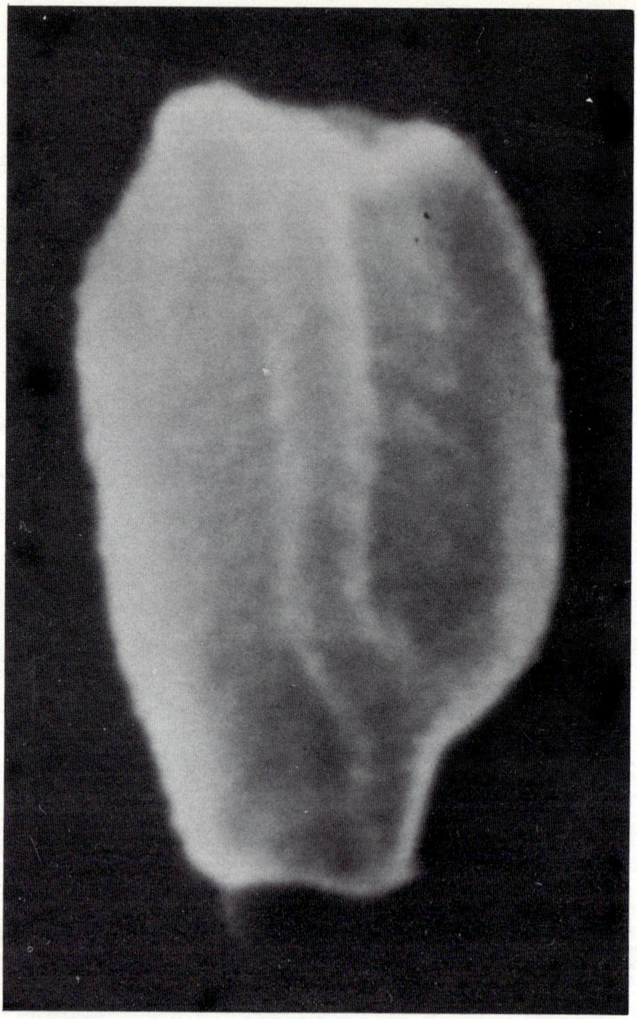

Fig. 4(b).

and the stages of sporogenesis in hemolymph have been established by electron microscopy (Black, 1968a). Figure 4(b) shows the characteristic, heavily ridged surface structure and Fig. 5 a longitudinal section of a spore. The cytology of sporogenesis in *B. popilliae* is similar to that recorded for other bacteria (Murrell, 1967). Spores of both *B. popilliae* and *B. lentimorbus* invariably are encased in a sporangium derived without drastic change from the vegetative cell wall (Hrubant and Rhodes, 1968; Bulla *et al.*, 1970b). Spores of *B. popilliae* germinate by protrusion through the spore and sporangium of a germ tube which

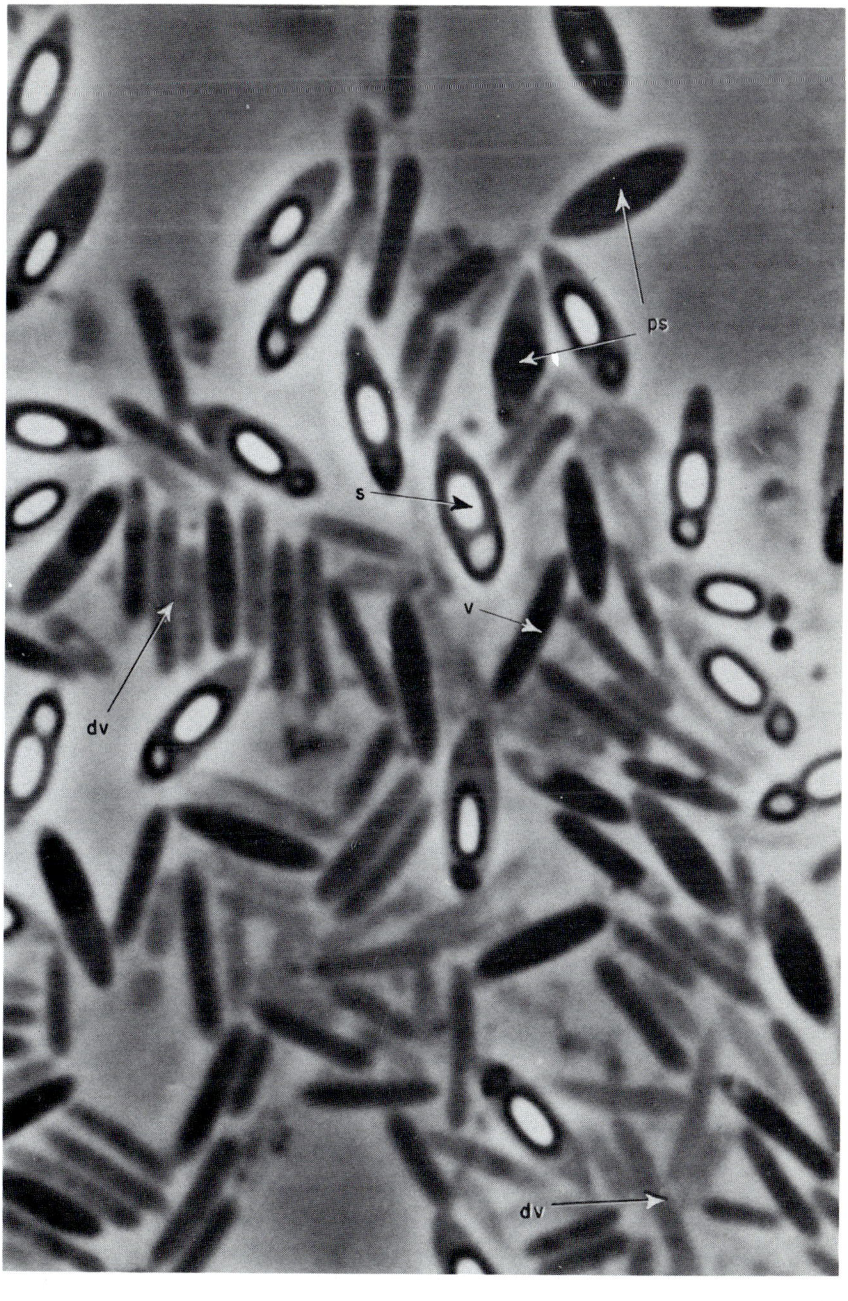

Fig. 4(c).

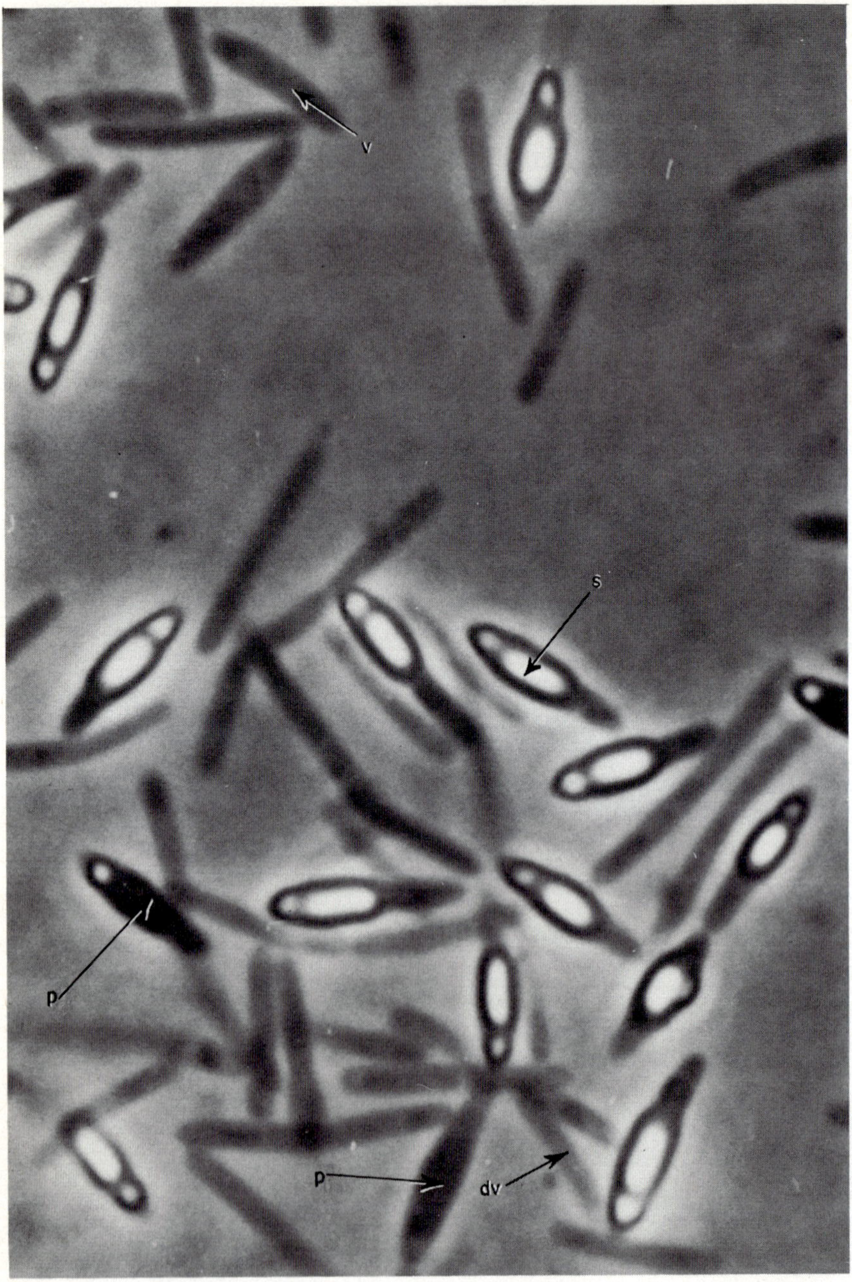

Fig. 4(d).

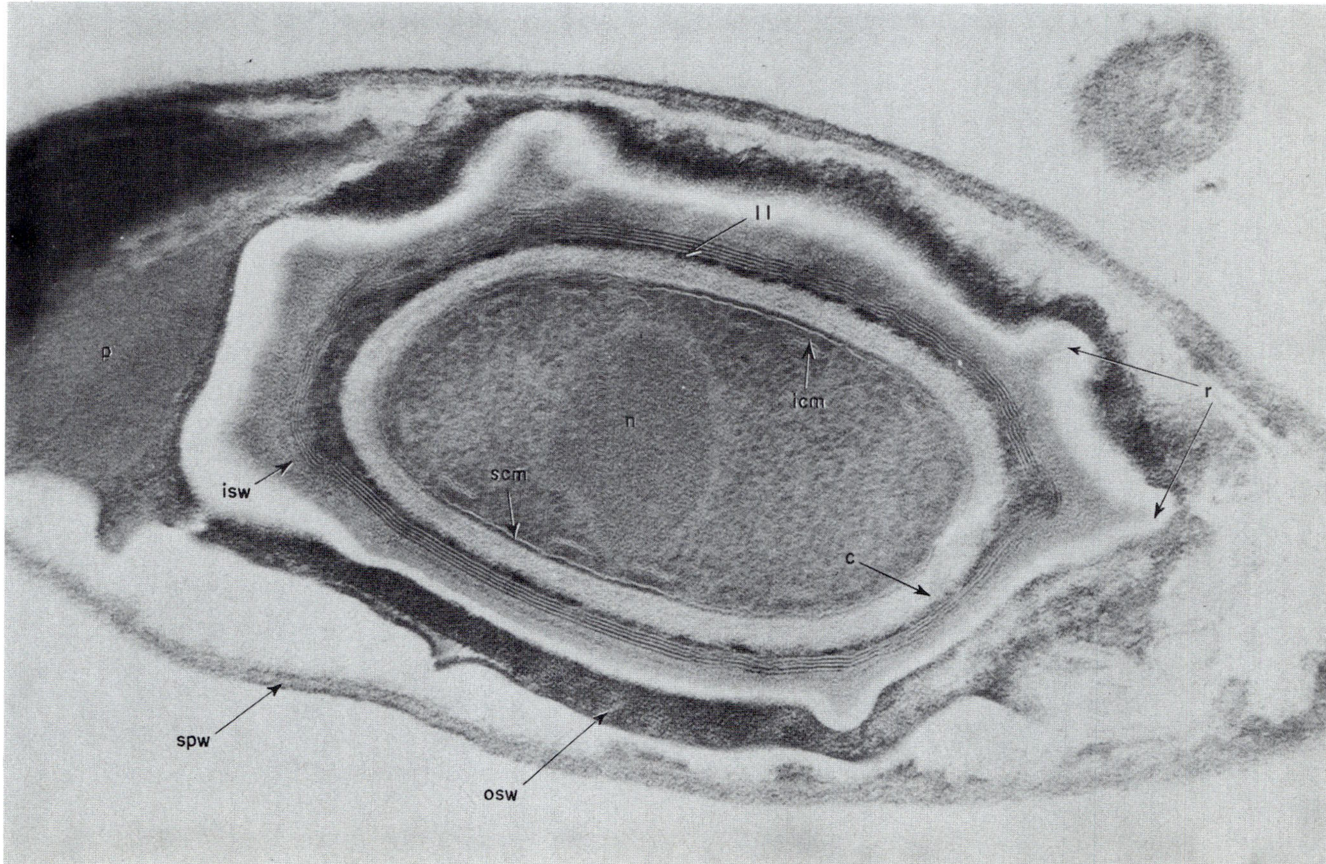

Fig. 5. Longitudinal section of spore of *Bacillus popilliae* from hemolymph; sporangial wall, *spw*; outer spore wall, *osw*; intermediate spore wall *isw*; laminated layer, *ll*; cortex, *c*; spore core membrane, *scm*; intracore membrane, *icm*; nucleoplasm, *n*; spore wall ridges, *r*; paraspore, *p*. Transmission electron microscopy ×125,000 by S. H. Black,

then divides to form the initial vegetative cell. Ordinarily, protrusion occurs at the end of the spore opposite the paraspore; the paraspore becomes phase dark and disappears after germination is complete.

There is mounting evidence that vegetative growth in hemolymph includes a large proportion of cells which never sporulate. Hemolymph contains only vegetative cells during the initial three to four days of infection. Intermediate stages are characterized by the simultaneous occurrence of vegetative cells, prespores, and spores (Fig. 4(c)). Vegetative cells never exceed 1-3 x 10^9/ml of hemolymph and decline in number as prespores and spores replace them. A large proportion, perhaps most, vegetative cells appear granular and nearly devoid of cytoplasm throughout the disease process; presumably, such cells are dead. Most cells in stages of overt sporulation remain phase dark and apparently viable, although death occurs at any stage prior to formation of the fully mature spore. Dead vegetative cells are destroyed or removed from the hemolymph, presumably by phagocytosis or lytic processes. Consequently, more than 90% of the cells in "milky" larvae are spores. Accumulation of spores in hemolymph depends upon slow and continued proliferation and sporulation by strains of moderate virulence rather than a prolonged phase of exclusively vegetative growth followed by synchronous sporulation throughout the population (St. Julian *et al.*, 1970).

Three considerations crucial to developing a technique for spore production arise from observations on sporulation in larvae:

(1) Larval hemolymph may be a relatively poor environment for sporulation of milky disease bacteria.

(2) Strains of *B. popilliae* best suited for *in vitro* production because of their rapidity of growth and sporulation might be relatively unsuited for control use because they would kill larvae prematurely without forming sufficient spores to spread disease in the field.

(3) The ultimate method for *in vitro* production of spores may involve continuous culture with separate environments for growth and sporulation phases, or a dialysis technique that continuously removes metabolic products and replenishes nutrients, so simulating the living processes of the host.

E. SPORULATION OF *BACILLUS POPILLIAE* IN ARTIFICIAL CULTURE

As yet, there is no technique for inducing extensive sporulation *in vitro.* Nevertheless, milky disease bacteria are sporogenic in laboratory culture. First, several strains form significant numbers of spores *in vitro* under specific cultural conditions. Second, changes in cell structure and composition that are interpreted as the consequence of aborted sporulation regularly occur in a large proportion of cells of many strains. Third, changes in enzyme activity have been found in *B. popilliae* cells which are reminiscent of sporulation processes in other bacteria and which are related to enzymes contained in spores.

Authentic spores are formed in colonies by 15-20% of the cells of selected strains. Sporulation occurs only under highly specific conditions of medium and inoculum (Rhodes *et al.*, 1965; Sharpe *et al.*, 1970), and predominantly in a ring near the periphery of colonies in cells on or near the surface. Vegetative growth occurs exclusively for the first four days; prespores and refractile spores appear immediately thereafter; subsequently, the refractile spores develop resistance to heat and desiccation, and sporulation ends in about 10-15 days. Most cells do not sporulate and the center of colonies becomes filled with dead cells and cellular debris. Vegetative growth often continues for a short period after sporulation and extends the colony beyond the zone of sporulation. The cytology of sporogenesis by cells in colonies is analogous to that recorded in cells from larval hemolymph (Black, 1968b). Spores are shown in Fig. 4. There are differences between spores from larvae and those from artificial culture. Mature spores formed in larvae are uniform and compact with a dense sporangium; the shape of the paraspore is indefinite (Fig. 4(a)). In general, spores from artificial culture have a less dense sporangium and the paraspore is rhomboid and separated from the spore (Fig. 4(d)). These differences apparently reflect relative maturity of the spores because those from larvae during intermediate stages of infection (Fig. 4(c)) strongly resemble *in vitro* spores. Usually, the paraspore develops refractility after the spore *in vivo* (Fig. 4(c)); the converse is true in artificial culture (Fig. 4(d)). Conditions within colonies can be considered similar to those in a chemostat because of continuous diffusion within the colony and the solid medium.

Growth in a liquid medium containing particulate carbon also results in spore formation (Haynes and Rhodes, 1966, 1969). Unlike sporulation on solid media, which is restricted to specific variants, many strains exhibit limited sporulation (ca. 0.1-1%) in liquid media containing carbon. It has been theorized that carbon promotes sporulation by absorption of deleterious materials originally present in the medium or formed during growth.

Cultures which sporulate in either system become asporogenic when transferred repeatedly as vegetative cultures. Maximum sporulation occurs with inocula only one or two vegetative transfers from spores previously engendered *in vitro*. Spores from artificial culture germinate more readily than do those from larvae and they can be readily used to initiate vegetative cultures.

Selected strains form a spore analog when growing in diphasic culture (solid agar base overlaid with liquid nutrient medium in a shaken flask). These cells are swollen and contain a spore primordium separated from the sporangium by a membrane; further development does not occur (Black, 1968b).

The formation of an intracellular refractile body lacking the cytological characteristics of spores is an apparent alternative to sporulation in many strains of *B. popilliae.* As many as 80% of cells develop this structure under conditions often proximate to those which cause sporulation. Refractile bodies also have been detected in limited quantity during proliferation in larvae. Refractile bodies may represent abortive or unbalanced development after commitment to sporulation and probably include unorganized spore or parasporal material. Vegetative cells, spores, and refractile bodies differ in composition and enzyme content. Spores contain less protein, desoxyribonucleic acid, and ribonucleic acid than do vegetative cells; like all bacterial spores, they contain a small, but definite, amount of dipicolinic acid. Refractile bodies differ from spores by the occurrence of a large amount of poly-B-hydroxybutyrate and by the absence of dipicolinic acid (Mitruka *et al.*, 1967). Spores from hemolymph or from colonies contain heat-stable catalase; vegetative cells do not. Catalase is formed by cells of sporogenic strains at the time sporulation is initiated. Although refractile bodies also contain catalase, it is not heat stable. Most probably, the energy yielding processes needed for biosynthesis in sporulation are impaired in artificial culture (Bulla *et al.*, 1970a); the resultant imbalanced metabolism gives rise to both uncoupled enzyme reactions and disorganized cell structures.

Sporogenic strains appear to arise by selection from the population of a small percentage of cells capable of forming spores under a particular cultural condition. Conversely, sporogenic capacity is lost if these strains are grown repeatedly as vegetative cells. Both emergence of sporogenic strains and loss of sporeforming ability reflect the variability of *B. popilliae.*

Conditions for emergence of sporogenic strains involve complex media based on yeast extract and other natural products. The need for complex ingredients prevents identification of exact nutritive requirements. However, study of these strains may allow identification of the metabolic differences between sporogenic and asporogenic strains as well as between vegetative growth and sporulation in sporogenic strains; this information could provide the clue to conditions which promote spore formation.

Strains sporogenic on solid media form limited numbers of spores in liquid media during extended incubation without agitation following an initial period of shaken aerobic growth. Selection of a sporogenic strain from liquid culture is difficult because, unlike development on solid media, sporulating cells are not isolated as clones from those not sporulating.

F. SUITABILITY OF SPORES FROM ARTIFICIAL CULTURE

Spores produced in colonies are infective when injected into Japanese beetle larvae but they are not infective when fed (Schwartz and Sharpe, 1970). Strains most sporogenic *in vitro* form fewer than the normal number of spores in larvae; this characteristic could retard spread of the disease. However, the large number of inexpensive spores made available by fermentation could make this characteristic of relatively minor consequence. In addition, selective pressure in the insect should subsequently cause emergence of strains with appropriate pathogenic characteristics in diseased larvae.

Spores of *B. popilliae* must survive for years in soil in order to perpetuate the disease and to provide continuous control. However, it is presumed that spores must germinate before infection can occur, although neither route nor mechanism of invasion from gut into hemocoel is known. If spores germinate prematurely, i.e. away from the site of invasion in a susceptible host, the organism will die because vegetative cells cannot survive or sporulate again except in the hemolymph. Therefore, germination only in specific circumstances is a necessary characteristic of infective *B. popilliae* spores. Usually, less than 1% of spores from diseased larvae germinate in artificial culture (St. Julian and Hall, 1968; Splittstoesser and Steinkraus, 1962). Limited germination also occurs in larvae because injection of at least 1000-fold more spores than vegetative cells are required to induce comparable rates of infection (Pridham *et al.*, 1964). Thus, large numbers of spores must be used in soil to achieve significant control. At this time, tests indicate that between 10^7 and 10^9 spores/g of soil are required to achieve 50%, or greater, infection of larvae.

Spores produced in artificial culture germinate more readily than do spores from hemolymph. The requirement for inocula prepared from spores automatically tends to select strains which germinate best. It is probable that premature germination in the larval gut or in wet soil by spores produced *in vitro* is the reason why they are not infective when fed. Thus, loss of infectivity may be attributed to changes in characteristics other than those usually associated with invasiveness by pathogens, and infectivity can be lost because some characteristic necessary for artificial culture is contrary to those needed for infection.

Because of the inherent variability of *B. popilliae*, selection of specific strains that embody the desired attributes of sporogenesis, stability, and infectivity appears to be a fruitful approach to devising methods for large-scale production. Current methods and existent strains are not entirely suitable, but characterization of these strains may provide the information necessary to devise techniques for large-scale production of spores.

V. Production of Fungal Pathogens *in vitro*

A. SEMI-SOLID FERMENTATION

Beauveria bassiana, *Metarrhizium anisopliae*, and *Acrostalagmus aphidum* can all be grown in semi-solid fermentation. The media and procedures are similar to those employed in the *B. thuringiensis* semi-solid fermentation, and the reader is referred to pp. 515-518. A liquid inoculum is used to inoculate the bran, and many of the media developed for submerged fermentation are useful for its production. Many fungi prefer corn meal in the medium and, in the authors' experience, *A. aphidum* required it. A useful seed medium has been: soybean meal, 10.0 g; corn meal, 10.0 g; glucose, 15.0 g; NaCl, 5.0 g; $CaCO_3$, 2.0 g/liter distilled water. Semi-solid media similar to those used for *B. thuringiensis* are often satisfactory, but it may be preferable, and with *A. aphidum* essential, to replace about half the bran in the formulations with corn meal. Since the developing mycelium binds the bran medium tightly, it is usually necessary for maximum yields to mix the fermenting bran once or twice before sporulation begins. To obtain sporulation after the mycelium is well grown, drying of cultures should be as fast as possible. Müller-Kögler (1960) reports a decrease in the germination capacity of the conidia if this is not done.

The semi-solid fermentation is preferable for many of these fungi, since the conidia do not need to be recovered from the bran base. The dry conidia-bran mixture is relatively stable, but cannot be stored for prolonged periods of time.

B. SUBMERGED FERMENTATION

In submerged culture, many entomopathogenic fungi do not produce true conidia. Instead, dimorphic fungi with blastospores are obtained; these are considered to be in the "yeast phase" instead of the "mycelium phase" (Müller-Kögler, 1967). Samšiňáková (1966) has reported the production of blastospores by *B. bassiana.* She obtained a yield of 10-15 g dry blastospores/liter beer. Adámek (1965) obtained approximately 18 g dry blastospores of *M. anisopliae*/liter beer. Blastospores have been observed by Dulmage in submerged cultures of *A. aphidum.*

Vezina *et al.* (1965) have reported the production of true conidia by *Aspergillus ochraceus,* an insect pathogen. Several other members of the Fungi imperfecti also are known to do so. Blastospores obtained in submerged culture are difficult to preserve and easily lose their viability. The submerged cultivation of the fungal insect pathogens would be more useful if true conidia could be obtained. Much work needs to be done in this area.

References

Adámek, L. (1965). *Folia Microbiol Praha* **10,** 255-257.

Aiba, S., Humphrey, A. E. and Millis, N. F. (1965). "Biochemical Engineering". Academic Press, New York.

Aizawa, K. and Fujiyoshi, N. (1967). Proc. Joint U.S.-Japan Semin. Microbial Control Insect Pests, pp. 79-83. U.S.-Japan Committee Sci. Cooporation. Panel 8. Fukuoka, Japan.

Angus, T. A. (1956). *Can. J. Microbiol.* **2,** 111-121.

Angus, T. A. (1965). *Bact. Rev.* **29,** 364-372.

Angus, T. A. (1967). *J. Invertebrate Path.* **9,** 256-260.

Angus, T. A. and Norris, J. R. (1968). *J. Invertebrate Path.* **11,** 289-295.

Black, S. H. (1968a). *J. Invertebrate Path.* **12,** 148-157.

Black, S. H. (1968b). *J. Invertebrate Path.* **12,** 158-167.

Bonnefoi, A. (1960). French Patent 1,225,179.
Broersma, D. B. and Buxton, J. A. (1967). *J. Invertebrate Path.* **9**, 58-69.
Bulla, L. A., St. Julian, G., Rhodes, R. A. and Hesseltine, C. W. (1970a). *Can. J. Microbiol.* **16**, 243-248.
Bulla, L. A., St. Julian, G., Rhodes, R. A. and Hesseltine, C. W. (1970b). *Appl. Microbiol.* **18**, 490-495.
Bungay, H. R., Simons, C. F. and Hosler, P. (1960). *J. Biochem. Microbiol. Technol. Eng.* **2**, 143-155.
Burgerjon, A. (1965). *Entomophaga* **10**, 21-26.
Burgerjon, A. and Biache, G. (1967). *In* "Insect Pathology and Microbial Control" (P. A. van der Laan, ed.), pp. 294-296. North-Holland Publ. Co., Amsterdam.
Burges, H. D. (1967). *In* "Insect Pathology and Microbial Control (P. A. van der Laan, ed.), pp. 306-338. North-Holland Publ. Co., Amsterdam.
Costilow, R. N., Sylvester, C. J. and Pepper, R. E. (1966). *Appl. Microbiol.* **14**, 161-169.
Drake, B. B. and Smythe, C. V. (1963). U.S. Patent 3,087,865.
Dulmage, H. T. (1970a). *J. Invertebrate Path.* **15**, 232-239.
Dulmage, H. T. (1970b). *J. Invertebrate Path.* **16**. (In press.)
Dulmage, H. T., Correa, J. A. and Martinez, A. J. (1970). *J. Invertebrate Path.* **15**, 15-20.
Dulmage, H. T., Wolfenbarger, D. A., Lukefahr, M. J. and Correa, J. A. (1971). *J. econ. Ent.* (In press.)
Dutky, S. R. (1963). *In* "Insect Pathology" (E. A. Steinhaus, ed.), Vol. 2, pp. 75-115. Academic Press, New York.
Evlakhova, A. A. and Švecova, O. I. (1965). *Ent. Obozr.* **44**, 721-726.
Haynes, W. C. and Rhodes, L. J. (1966). *J. Bacteriol.* **91**, 2270-2274.
Haynes, W. C. and Rhodes, L. J. (1969). *J. Invertebrate Path.* **13**, 250-255.
Haynes, W. C., St. Julian, G., Shekleton, M. C., Hall, H. H. and Tashiro, H. (1961). *J. Insect Path.* **3**, 55-61.
Heimpel, A. M. and Angus, T. A. (1960). *J. Insect Path.* **2**, 311-319.
Heimpel, A. M. and Angus, T. A. (1963). *In* "Insect Pathology, an Advanced Treatise" (E. A. Steinhaus, ed.), Vol. 2, pp. 21-73. Academic Press, New York.
Hrubant, G. R. and Rhodes, R. A. (1968). *J. Invertebrate Path.* **11**, 371-376.
Ignoffo, C. M. (1967). *In* "Insect Pathology and Microbial Control" (P. A. van der Laan, ed.), pp. 91-117. North-Holland Publ. Co., Amsterdam.
Kawakami, K. (1960). *Bull. Sericult. exp. Sta.* (Tokyo) **16**, 83-99.
Lingg, A. J., McMahon, K. J. and Herzmann, C. (1967). *Appl. Microbiol.* **15**, 163-165.
Majumber, S. K. (1968). *In* "Pesticides Symposium 1964" (S. K. Majumber, ed.), pp. 167-174. Acad. Pest Contr. Sci., Mysore, India.
McGarr, R. L., Dulmage, H. T. and Wolfenbarger, D. A. (1970). *J. Econ. Ent.* **63**, 1357-1358.
Mechalas, B. J. (1963). U.S. Patent 3,076,922.
Megna, J. C. (1963). U.S. Patent 3,073,749.
Menn, J. J. (1960). *J. Insect Path.* **2**, 134-138.
Mitruka, B. M., Costilow, R. N., Black, S. H. and Pepper, R. E. (1967). *J. Bacteriol.* **94**, 759-765.
Müller-Kögler, E. (1960). *Ztschr. Pflan. Krankh.* **67**, 663-668.
Müller-Kögler, E. (1965). *In* "Pilzkrankheiten bei Insekten" (Anwendung Biologischen Schadlingbekampfung und Grundlagen der Insektenmykologie), pp. 86-89. Parey, Berlin and Hamburg.
Müller-Kögler, E. (1967). *In* "Insect Pathology and Microbial Control" (P. A. van der Laan, ed.), pp. 339-353. North-Holland Publ. Co., Amsterdam.
Murrell, W. C. (1967). *In* "Advances in Microbial Physiology" (A. H. Rose and J. F. Wilkinson, eds), Vol. 1, pp. 133-251. Academic Press, New York.
Pepper, R. E. and Costilow, R. N. (1965). *J. Bacteriol.* **89**, 271-276.
Prescott, S. C. and Dunn, C. G. (1959). *In* "Industry Microbiology", pp. 666-682; 844-858. McGraw-Hill Book Co., New York.
Pridham, T. G., St. Julian, G., Adams, G. L., Hall, H. H. and Jackson, R. W. (1964). *J. Insect Path.* **6**, 204-213.

Rhodes, R. A. (1965). *Bacteriol. Rev.* **29**, 373-381.
Rhodes, R. A. (1966). *In* "Bioengineering and Food Processing" (M. R. Sfat, ed.), Vol. 62, pp. 21-29. American Institute of Chemical Engineers.
Rhodes, R. A. (1967). Proc. Joint U.S.-Japan Semin. Microbial Control Insect Pests, pp. 85-92. U.S.-Japan Committee Sci. Cooporation. Panel 8. Fukuoka, Japan.
Rhodes, R. A., Roth, M. S. and Hrubant, G. R. (1965). *Can. J. Microbiol.* **11**, 779-783.
Rhodes, R. A., Sharpe, E. S., Hall, H. H. and Jackson, R. W. (1966). *Appl. Microbiol.* **14**, 189-195.
St. Julian, G. and Hall, H. H. (1968). *J. Invertebrate Path.* **10**, 48-53.
St. Julian, G., Pridham, T. G. and Hall, H. H. (1963). *J. Insect Path.* **5**, 440-445.
St. Julian, G., Sharpe, E. S. and Rhodes, R. A. (1970). *J. Invertebrate Path.* **15**, 240-246.
Samšiňáková, A. (1966). *J. Invertebrate Path.* **8**, 395-400.
Schwartz, P. H. and Sharpe, E. S. (1970). *J. Invertebrate Path.* **15**, 126-128.
Seman, E. O. (1964). *Bot. Z. S.S.S.R.* **49**, 1473-1477.
Sharpe, E. S. (1966). *Biotechnol. Bioeng.* **8**, 247-258.
Sharpe, E. S., St. Julian, G. and Crowell, C. (1970). *Appl. Microbiol.* **19**, 681-688.
Shell Internationale Research Maatschappij, N.V. (1969). Netherlands Patent 68 16,397.
Splittstoesser, D. F. and Steinkraus, K. H. (1962). *J. Bacteriol.* **84**, 278-282.
Sylvester, C. J. and Costilow, R. N. (1964). *J. Bacteriol.* **87**, 114-119.
Takamine, J. (1913). U.S. Patent 1,054,324.
Takamine, J. (1914). *Ind. Engn. Chem.* **6**, 824-828.
Tashiro, H. and Steinkraus, K. H. (1966). *J. Invertebrate Path.* **8**, 382-389.
Underkofler, L. A., Severson, G. M., Goering, K. J. and Christensen, L. M. (1947). *Cereal Chem.* **24**, 1-22.
Underkofler, L. A. and Hickey, R. J. (1954). "Industrial Fermentations", Vol. II. Chemical Publishing Co., New York.
Vaňková, J. (1964). *Mém. hors. Sér. Entomophaga, No. 2,* 271-291.
Vezina, C., Singh, K. and Sehgal, S. N. (1965). *Mycologia* **57**, 722-736.
Weiner, B. A., Kwolck, W. F., St. Julian, G., Hall, H. H. and Jackson, R. W. (1966). *J. Invertebrate Path.* **8**, 308-313.

CHAPTER 25

Propagation of Arthropod Pathogens in Living Systems

CARLO M. IGNOFFO and W. FRED HINK

International Minerals and Chemical Corporation, Libertyville, Illinois, U.S.A.
and
Faculty of Entomology, Ohio State University, Columbus, Ohio, U.S.A.

I. Introduction

The annual sales of chemical insecticides are expected to reach 0.5 billion dollars during 1970 (Neumayer *et al.*, 1969). Microbial insecticides probably account for less than 0.5% of all insecticides sold. This, despite the fact that the use of entomopathogens is historically older than the use of chemical insecticides. One major reason why microbial insecticides have not been exploited, in spite of numerous examples of successful uses, is their need of complex production techniques. Natural, living, microbial insecticides, in general, require more specialized production technology than that required for synthetic chemical insecticides. The available systems for mass production of microbial insecticides were categorized and described earlier (Briggs, 1963; Martignoni, 1964; Ignoffo, 1967). To summarize, these systems depend on the available substrates: (1) living whole organisms; (2) embryonated eggs or cultures of organs, tissue, dispersed cells or established cell lines; (3) fermentation media; (4) completely defined chemical substrates or various combinations of the above such as replication of animal viruses in bacteria hosts, which are in turn produced by fermentation (Abel and Trautner, 1964; Bayreuther and Romig, 1964). Propagation using non-living substrates, methods 3 and 4 above, are covered in Chapter 24. Our chapter is restricted to mass propagation of fungi, protozoans, bacteria, rickettsiae and viruses in living systems, both whole and excised.

II. Propagation in Whole Organisms

A. FUNGI PROPAGATION

Most entomogenous fungi are not obligate pathogens. Of more than 500 species, less than 2% were propagated in living hosts for subsequent use to control insects (Table I). Most were produced using either surface or submerged fermentation techniques (Ignoffo, 1967; Anderson and Ignoffo, 1967) and include many species of Moniliaceae, a few Zythiaceae and Entomophthoraceae but no Coelomomycetaceae species. Propagation techniques, similar to those described for other obligate pathogens, have never been fully developed or applied to obligate fungi (Table II). Detailed accounts of host-rearing, inoculation, incubation, recovery and yields, etc. are for the most part nonexistent. Available information is usually restricted to the period prior to 1940. Insecticidal use of such obligate fungi as were propagated relied mostly on introduction or colonization with dead or living diseased insects. This technique with slight variation was successfully used to control the spotted alfalfa aphid, *Therioaphis maculata*, with *Entomophthora exitialis, E. virulenta, E. coronata*

TABLE I

Estimated number of described pathogens and those propagated using whole organisms or tissue-cell technology[a]

Insect pathogen	Described	Propagated[b]	Propagation technique: Whole organism	Propagation technique: Tissue-cell
Fungi	530	30	8	0
Viruses	298	49	49	15
Protozoans	210	26	24	2
Bacteria	90	7	4	0
Rickettsiae	6	2	2	2

[a] Compiled from Steinhaus, 1949; Kreig, 1961, 1963; Müller-Kögler, 1965; Weiser, 1961, 1963.

[b] Includes estimated numbers propagated using both living and non-living technology.

TABLE II

Taxons of arthropod pathogens propagated in living hosts for use in insect control

Class	Order	Family	Genus	Species
		Fungi		
Phycomycete	Blastocladiales	Coelomomycetaceae	*Coelomomyces*	*stegomyiae*
	Entomophthorales	Entomophthoraceae	*Entomophthora* (*=Empusa*)	*aulicae, erupta, grylli, sphaerosperma*
Fungi Imperfecti (Deuteromycete)	Sphaeropsidales	Zythiaceae	*Aschersonia*	*aleyrodis*
	Moniliales	Moniliaceae	*Acrostalagmus*	*aphidum*
			Beauveria	*bassiana*
		Protozoa		
Rhizopodea	Amoebida	Endamoebidae	*Melamoeba* (*Malpighamoeba*)	*locustae*
Telosporea	Eucoccida	Adeleidae	*Adelina*	*tribolii*
	Neogregarinida	Schizocystidae	*Mattesia*	*dispora, grandis*
Microsporidea	Microsporida	Nosematidae	*Nosema*	*bombycis, carpocapsae, culisetae, curvidentis, infesta, lotmaris, lymantriae, mesnili, muscularis, otiorrhynchi, plodiae, phylotreta, serbica, whitei*
			Glugea	*gasti*
			Plistophora	*schubergi, scolyti*
			Perezia	*pyraustae*
			Thelohania	*hyphantriae, pristiphorae, similis, weiseri*
		Bacteria		
Schizomycetes	Eubacteriales	Bacillaceae	*Bacillus*	*popilliae, lentimorbus*
			Clostridium	*brevifaciens, malacosomae*
		Rickettsiae		
Microtatobiotes	Rickettsiales	Wolbachieae	*Enterella*	*culicis, stethorae*
			Rickettsiella	*grylli, melolonthae, popilliae, tipulae*

(Hall and Dunn, 1958); green apple bug with *E. erupta* (Dustan, 1924a, b); brown-tail caterpillar with *E. aulicae* (Speare and Colley, 1912); mosquitoes with *Coelomomyces stegomyiae* (Laird, 1960, 1966); European apple sucker with *E. sphaerosperma* (Dustan, 1923); grasshopppers with *E. grylli* (Edington, 1899; Howard, 1902); chinch bugs with *Beauveria bassiana* (Snow, 1895; Forbes, 1895); whitefly with *Aschersonia aleyrodis* (Berger, 1910); a zygaenid caterpillar with *B. bassiana* (Burkill, 1914) and potato aphid with *Acrostalagmus aphidum* (Shands *et al.*, 1958, 1963). A comprehensive review of other insect-fungus associations is presented by Müller-Kögler (1965).

1. Blastocladiales

Recent field trials (Laird, 1969, personal communications; Couch, 1968) demonstrated that a *Blastocladiales*, i.e. *Coelomomyces* spp., could be a promising microbial insecticide. Laird showed that *Coelomomyces* could be established in new areas and its incidence increased in areas where it already occurred. Propagation techniques, however, using either artificial media or living host are not available. Attempts to transmit the disease under laboratory conditions, an obvious prerequisite for an obligate pathogen being considered as a microbial insecticide, were, with one or two notable exceptions, generally unsuccessful. Laird (1959), after several failures, infected *Aedes aegypti* larvae using sporangia of *C. stegomyiae* collected from *A. albopictus*. Diseased larvae, debris and bottom-sediment from habitats known to harbor *Coelomomyces*-diseased larvae, and filter paper containing dried remains of diseased larvae were used as inoculum. Laboratory infections occurred after larvae were exposed for 13-24 days to inoculum placed in distilled water, buffered at pH 6.6. Development of infected larvae was severely retarded. Couch (1968) has continually maintained laboratory infection in the malaria mosquito, *Anopheles quadrimaculatus,* for about two years. Yields generally were $2\text{-}5 \times 10^3$ sporangia/mosquito larva ($2\text{-}5 \times 10^6$ sporangia/g larva), with a maximum yield of 63,000 sporangia/larva or 6.3×10^7 sporangia/g larva (Couch, 1968). Assuming 100 zoospores/sporangia, a maximum of 6.3×10^6 zoospores/larva or 6.3×10^9 zoospores/g larva was possible (Table III).

The aquatic habitat of *Coelomomyces* spp., its natural persistence, and the susceptibility of aquatic insect pests, which are normally difficult to control using pathogens, make it an attractive candidate for consideration as a microbial insecticide. Species of two families of aquatic Diptera (Simulidae–blackflies and Culicidae–mosquitoes), which are serious pests of man, and a species of backswimmer *Notonecta* sp. (Hemiptera: Notonectidae) are susceptible to *Coelomomyces* (Bogoyavlensky, 1922; Couch and Umphlett, 1963). Further consideration of *Coelomomyces* as a microbial insecticide must await the accumulation of more data. Initial efforts should center on factors responsible

TABLE III

Estimated yields of fungi, protozoans, bacteria, and rickettsiae obtained from insect hosts reared on either natural or synthetic diets

Pathogen species	Host species	Host substrate	Yield x 10^6 per Host	Yield x 10^6 per Gram-host	Reference
		Fungi[a]			
Coelomomyces stegomyiae	mosquito	dog food	6	6300	Couch, 1968
		Protozoans[b]			
Glugea gasti	boll weevil	synthetic	68-250	4600	McLaughlin, 1969, personal communication
Malamoeba locustae	grasshopper	foliage	3	3-4	Taylor and King, 1937
Mattesia grandis	boll weevil	synthetic	2-4	100	McLaughlin, 1969, personal communication
Nosema infesta	potato tuberworm	potato	10	400	Hall, 1954
Nosema lymantriae	gypsy moth	leaves	30-50	300-500	Weiser, 1969, personal communication
Thelohania hyphantriae	fall webworm	leaves	10	100	Weiser, 1969, personal communication
		Bacteria[b]			
Bacillus popilliae	Japanese beetle	seeds	1100	4900	Dutky, 1942
Clostridium malacosomae	eastern tent caterpillar	leaves	20	100	Bucher, 1969, personal communication
		Rickettsiae[c]			
Rickettsiella popilliae	Japanese beetle	seeds	3×10^5	75×10^6	Dutky and Gooden, 1952

[a]Zoospores.
[b]Spores or cysts.
[c]Rickettsiae.

for infection of susceptible or potentially susceptible hosts capable of being mass produced.

2. Entomophthorales

As early as 1912 Speare and Colley described propagation of *Entomophthora aulicae* in field-collected caterpillars of the brown-tail moth, *Nygmia phaeorrhoea.* The procedure was successfully used for four years (1908-1911 inclusive) to produce 10^5 diseased caterpillars/season. Results were less promising when a Japanese species of *Entomophthora* was propagated on gypsy moth, *Lymantria (Porthetria) dispar,* caterpillars. The following is a synopsis of the propagating procedure described by Speare and Colley (1912). Young brown-tail caterpillars were used as the primary host, although at least 16 other caterpillar species could be used as alternate hosts. Webs, containing larvae, were collected from natural infestations and stored at 2-3°C until needed. Propagation began 1-2 months before the intended spring or fall use of the fungus. Separate wooden boxes (11 x 27 x 27 in) were used for either rearing or infecting larvae. The bottom of the box was covered with a thin layer of soil or gravel and the inner-opening of the top rimmed with tanglefoot. About 200 webs with larvae were placed in each box and the larvae fed field-collected raspberry, oak, willow or cherry leaves. Greenhouse-grown raspberry or lettuce was used during winter and early spring. Rearing was done at 27°C. Living, diseased larvae, introduced into boxes containing healthy larvae, served as the inoculum. Viability of the inoculum, during seasons when host larvae were not available, was maintained by serial passage using larvae stored at low temperature. A "high humidity" was maintained in the infecting-boxes to insure spore discharge and host infection. Spore discharge from the introduced diseased larvae was sufficient to infect 50-85% of the larvae within 10 days. Dead and dying caterpillars were removed daily and replaced with healthy larvae. This process was repeated until the required number of diseased larvae were produced. Yields of "hundreds of thousands" of spores/mature caterpillar were obtained. An estimated annual capacity of 2×10^{11} spores (2×10^5 caterpillars/year; 10^6 spores/larva) was achieved.

Dustan (1923, 1924, 1927) also used disease introduction to propagate *E. sphaerosperma* or *E. erupta* on the apple sucker, *Psylla mali,* and green apple bug, *Lygus communis,* respectively. Resting spores of *Entomophthora* were used as inoculum. After a number of infecting techniques were tried Dustan decided that transferring leaves bearing diseased insects, netted diseased flying adults, or infected nursery trees were the best techniques for propagating and using *Entomophthora.* Resting-spore inoculum, preserved over-winter in ground-cages, was transferred to small cages containing apple seedlings infested with *P. mali* or *L. communis.* The initial inoculum was propagated in small cages, then transferred to larger cages (20 ft tall) built over apple trees. A high humidity was maintained by frequent watering and spraying. Diseased insects from these cages were then introduced into orchards.

3. Sphaeropsidales

Berger (1910, 1921, 1932) used citrus trees to "propagate" the red *Aschersonia (Aschersonia aleyrodis)* on the common whitefly *(Dialeurodes citri)* and the winged whitefly *(D. citrifolii)*. The above technique, however, was abandoned when Fawcett (1908) successfully propagated *Aschersonia* spp. on artificial media. Berger (1910) used the following technique to propagate *A. aleyrodis* on natural infestations of whiteflies. Citrus leaves bearing pustules containing spores and mycelia of *A. aleyrodis* were agitated in water and the contents filtered through cheesecloth. Approximately 40 pustules/pint of water was used as inoculum for propagation as well as for field control of whiteflies. This amounts to 10^4-10^5 spores/ml if one assumes a pustule sphere (diameter 1000 μ) packed with spores (diameter 20-30 μ) or 0.4-4 x 10^9 spores/mature orange tree. Initial infection of the whitefly population was observed within 10 days with maximum infection occurring within three weeks. Fungus spores are "produced in enormous quantities as red elevations or pustules" emanating from dead larvae. The calculated increase in yield over the inoculum using the above procedure (based upon yield of 17 x 10^4 leaves/mature orange tree; 1 pustule/leaf; 10^6 spores/pustule: inoculum of 4 x 10^8 spores/tree) was less than 500-fold. In light of modern developments *Aschersonia* spp. should be reconsidered as a potential microbial insecticide especially since artificial culturing techniques are possible.

B. PROTOZOA PROPAGATION

Of about 210 protozoans only two dozen or so have been propagated in living systems for possible use as microbial insecticides (Table I). All but one belong to the classes Telosporea and Microsporidea (Table II). Most are microsporida of the family Nosematidae. Species of the orders Eucoccida and Haplosporida are potential microbial insecticides for control of stored products, pasture and bark beetles (Weiser, 1963); however, none have actually been propagated for this use. Lepidoptera, Orthoptera, Coleoptera and Hymenoptera served as hosts for mass propagation of protozoan pathogens. Readers are referred to Weiser (1961, 1963, 1966) and Lipa (1963) for additional reports of protozoans associated with insects. Grasshoppers *(Melanoplus, Locusta)* or cockroaches were used by Taylor and King (1937), and Weiser (1969, personal communication) to propagate species of Endamoebidae or Nosematidae. Zimmack *et al.* (1954), Weiser (1957, 1969, personal communication), McLaughlin and Bell (1969, personal communication) and Smirnoff (1966) used caterpillars *(Antheraea, Aporia, Cydia (Carpocapsa), Crambus, Ephestia, Euproctis, Hyphantria, Lymantria, Malacosoma, Ostrinia, Pieris, Plodia, Tineola)*, beetles *(Anthonomus,*

Otiorrhynchus, Phyllotreta, Pityokteines, Scolytus, Tribolium) or a sawfly *Pristiphora* to propagate species of Schizocystidae or Nosematidae. Diptera *(Culex, Anopheles, Culiseta)* also were used to propagate species of Nosematidae (Weiser, 1969, personal communication). Yields of protozoans have varied from 3-4600 x 10^6 spores/g host (Table III).

1. Rhizopodea: Endamoebidae

As early as 1936, Taylor and King (1937) propagated *Malameba (Malpighamoeba) locustae* in grasshoppers. Although *Melanoplus differentialis* was primarily used, *M. mexicanus, M. femur rubrum* as well as 37 other species of Acrididae were also susceptible. In the procedure used by Taylor and King (1937) for propagating *M. locustae*, naturally infected male and female *M. differentialis* were caged separately and fed plant foliage. Fecal pellets containing *Malameba* cysts, collected at 24-hr intervals, were blended in 500 ml of water. Coarse particles were removed by passing the suspension through a sieve. The suspension was standardized by number of cysts/ml. The average yield/day for two days of production was 3 x 10^6 cysts/female and 2 x 10^6 cysts/male or an average of ~3.8 x 10^6 cysts/g grasshopper/day.

2. Telosporea: Schizocystidae; Nosematidae

a. Propagation of Mattesia *and* Glugea. McLaughlin and Bell (1969, personal communication) produced two sporozoans, *Mattesia grandis* and *Glugea gasti,* in boll weevil larvae. Adults, although susceptible, were not used because larvae were easier and less expensive to rear. Alternative hosts also could be used. *Mattesia* infections in insects span a wide variety of hosts, i.e. 12 Lepidoptera, 3 Coleoptera, 1 Siphonaptera, 1 Hymenoptera. Since cabbage loopers *(Trichoplusia ni),* bollworms *(Heliothis zea),* budworms *(H. virescens),* and pink bollworms *(Pectinophora gossypiella)* are susceptible (Ignoffo and Garcia, 1965) and can be mass produced (Ignoffo, 1964a, 1965a; Richmond and Ignoffo, 1964), they are potential hosts for propagating *Mattesia.*

The following procedure, based on the boll weevil rearing procedure and diet developed by Vanderzant and Davich (1958), Earle *et al.* (1959) and Gast and Davich (1966), was successfully used by McLaughlin and Bell (1969, personal communication) to produce *M. grandis* and *G. gasti* spores. Boll weevil eggs, implanted in an agar-base, semisynthetic-diet solidified in a Petri dish, were incubated at 30°C and 50-60% R.H. Gast and Davich (1966) found this humidity necessary to minimize microbial contamination and to prevent desiccation of the diet. From about 100 to 150 eggs/dish, yields ranged from 40 to 90 adults/dish (Gast and Davich, 1966). Two to four days (instar II) or 4-6 days (instar III) later, larvae and media were sprayed with a water suspension of either *G. gasti* or *M. grandis* spores. A chromographic sprayer delivered 1 ml of 10^6 spores/ml to each dish or about 150 spores/mm^2 of diet surface. Treated dishes were placed at 30°C until weevils emerged, 10-13 or 6-10 days later with either *G. gasti* or *M. grandis* spores respectively. Adults were caged and fed for 2-4 days *(G. gasti)* or 5-6 days *(M. grandis)* to permit further development of the protozoan infection and to optimize sporulation.

Diseased weevils, mostly dead, were blended in water to release the spores from infected tissue. The spore-weevil suspension was next filtered through a four-ply cheesecloth pad, differentially centrifuged, filtered, washed and centrifuged again to concentrate the spores. Spores were stored at 4°C in water for no longer than two weeks *(G. gasti)* or two months *(M. grandis)* prior to use in field experiments. Longer storage proportionally decreased spore viability, i.e. percentage infection of weevils.

After several months of production the yield of *G. gasti* and *M. grandis* spores averaged 68×10^6 and 17×10^5 spores/weevil respectively. The maximum yield was 25×10^7 *G. gasti* and 4×10^6 *M. grandis* spores/larva. The average yield, based upon a 15-mg weevil, was 46×10^8 *G. gasti* and 10^8 *M. grandis* spores/g weevil. Assuming a yield of one gram of weevils/dish (average 67 weevils/dish) the increase in production over that used for inoculation was 100- and 5000-fold for *M. grandis* and *G. gasti* respectively. Cost of producing weevils, excluding overheads, was 0.342 cents/weevil.

b. Propagation of Thelohania *and* Nosema *spp.* Weiser (1969, personal communication) propagated 13 species of *Nosema*, four species of *Thelohania*, and two species of *Plistophora* in immature stages of laboratory-, field- or insectary-reared Diptera, Coleoptera, Orthoptera or Lepidoptera. Larvae of *Hyphantria cunea* were the primary host for propagation of *Thelohania hyphantriae*; however, *Euproctis chrysorrhoea* and *Malacosoma neustria* also were used. *Nosema lymantriae, N. serbica* and *N. muscularis* were propagated in *Lymantria dispar* larvae.

The caterpillars for propagating *Thelohania* or *Nosema* were reared to instar II-IV on mulberry, oak or willow leaves. Selected trees, and/or egg masses or caged caterpillars on foliage were sprayed with a suspension of $1\text{-}5 \times 10^5$ spores/ml.

Larvae were produced in batches of 500-1000 individuals. About 10-20 days later, depending upon the protozoan species and environmental conditions, diseased larvae and/or pupae were collected and refrigerated for further processing. Accumulated larvae were blended in water, and spores were purified and concentrated by differential sedimentation and/or centrifugation. Spores stored in water, with or without antibiotics, at 4-8°C lived for at least 12 months. The average yield of *T. hyphantriae* or *N. lymantriae* spores was 10^7 or $3\text{-}5 \times 10^7$ spores/larva respectively. The average increase of *Thelohania* and *Nosema* production over inoculation was x1000 and x5000 respectively.

Larvae of the sod webworm, *Crambus bonifatellus* were initially used by Hall (1954) to propagate *Nosema infesta*. When rearing difficulties were encountered with *Crambus*, Hall tried buckeye caterpillars, *Junonia coenia*, and finally settled on potato tuberworms, *Gnorimoschema operculella*. Finney *et al.* (1947) developed a tuberworm mass-rearing technique which Hall used with slight modifications to propagate *N. infesta*. Egg-sized potatoes dipped in a suspension of *Nosema* spores (5×10^6 spores/ml) were infested with neonates and incubated at 28°C until tuberworms matured. After 10 days mature, infected larvae were collected and blended in water to release *Nosema* spores, filtered through cheesecloth, standardized as to number of spores/ml, and stored at 5° or –30°C. Infectivity was lost within 6-12 months at 5°C but was still present after 12 months' storage at –30°C.

Yields were not reported by Hall (1954); however, if one assumes an average yield of 1×10^7 spores/larva and a larval weight of 25 mg/larva, then an average of 4×10^8 spores/g larva was probably achieved. Spore yields steadily decreased with repeated passage through tuberworms and propagation was eventually terminated because yield became less than inoculum. The increase in yield over that used for the inoculum, based on an average of 50 larvae/potato, was ~100-fold. Host propagation cost was less than 0.1 cent/tuberworm (Finney *et al.*, 1947).

C. BACTERIA PROPAGATION

Bacteria are generally propagated by fermentation and it is only when this system cannot be used that living systems are considered. Of 90 bacterial species described from insects, only four were propagated in living hosts (Table I). All four are spore formers, *Bacillus* or *Clostridium*, classified as in Table II. Species of *Bacillus* are aerobes or facultative anaerobes, while those of *Clostridium* are anaerobes or aerotolerant.

Larvae of the Japanese beetle, *Popillia japonica* (Scarabaeidae), were used by Dutky (1942) to propagate *Bacillus popilliae* and *B. lentimorbus*, and tent caterpillars, *Malacosoma* spp. (Lasiocampidae), by Bucher (1969, personal communication) for *Clostridium brevifaciens* and *C. malacosomae*. Production yields ranged from 1 to 49×10^8 spores/g host (Table III). It was Dutky's pioneering studies with the milky-disease bacterium which demonstrated that a production protocol could be developed and successfully used to propagate an obligate insect pathogen. Products, using Dutky's procedure, are still available and sold for Japanese beetle control under the trade names Doom and Japidemic.

1. Clostridium *Species*

Laboratory propagation of *C. brevifaciens* and *C. malacosomae* for use as bacterial insecticides was accomplished by Bucher (1957, 1959, 1961a, b, 1969, personal communication) using field-collected eastern tent caterpillars, *Malacosoma americanum*. Two other species *M. pluviale* and *M. disstria* could be used; however, *M. americanum* was preferred because field-collected eastern tent caterpillars were relatively free of virus and were not known to be naturally infected with *Clostridia.* Host susceptibility of *Clostridium* is restricted to *Malacosoma.* Bucher used the following procedure to propagate either *C. brevifaciens* or *C. malacosomae* in *M. americanum.* Larvae, collected from tents on naturally infested trees and separated by size into lots of 20-25, were placed into pint-size ice cream cartons or quart-size plastic boxes. Instar IV larvae were fed a bouquet of leaves (chokecherry, apple or other Rosaceae), dipped in a suspension containing 10^3-10^4 spores/ml. Fresh leaves were provided daily. All larvae were dead after 6-10 days of incubation at 20-26°C.

After death the entire contents of the incubating containers were collected. Spores were released during the disease but most spores were excreted in diarrhetic feces shortly before death. Plant parts, dead larvae and frass were washed separately with gentle agitation to release spores. After repeated washings, supernatants were pooled, sieved through cheesecloth and centrifuged at 2000 g. The spore-debris-sediment was standardized (number of spores/ml) in water and stored at 4-6°C, where spores lived for several years. Laboratory production capacities, assuming continuous availability of larvae of 2-4 million diseased larvae/year were possible using the above procedures. Bucher obtained maximum yields of 2×10^7 spores/larva or $\sim 10^8$ spores/g larva. A calculated 50,000-fold increase in spore yield over inoculum was obtained.

2. Bacillus *Species*

Although Japanese beetle grubs were the primary host for propagating *B. popilliae,* at least 50 other Scarabaeidae are also susceptible (Dutky, 1963). Other milky disease organisms, *B. lentimorbus* and *B. euloomarahae,* can also be propagated in scarabaeid grubs.

The procedure and technology for propagating *B. popilliae* in *Popillia japonica,* as presented herein, was condensed from studies of Dutky (1941a, b, c, 1942a, b, 1963), White and Dutky (1940, 1942) and White and McCabe (1943). Mature grubs ($\sim$225 mg/grub), collected from naturally infested soil, were injected with 10^6 spores/grub in a volume of 30 μl (4.4×10^6 spores/g grub). Mature grubs were preferred; however, smaller instar II or III grubs also could be used. Injected larvae were each placed in 1-in cubicles and covered with soil containing 0.5-1 lb of seeds (Dutch clover : Red top grass; 1 : 1) per 100 lb soil. Moisture level of the soil is prepared to 60% of its balling point. Germinating seeds provided food during incubation. Propagation was in batches of 500 grubs/incubator-box, five layers of 100 grubs/layer, at 30°C for 10-12 days.

After incubation, diseased grubs were recovered by screening, dropped in an ice-water-bath and washed to remove adhering soil. The ice-water prevented cannibalism and minimized spore loss. Collected larvae were packed in ice and refrigerated at 0-2°C until sufficient numbers were obtained for further processing. Diseased grubs were processed into a spore-grub tissue suspension using a meat chopper. This suspension, standardized to number of spores/ml, was mixed with precipitated calcium carbonate. A high-speed impeller-type-blower and heated-air were used to produce a fine, dry, dust concentrate containing 10^9 spores/g. An average yield of 1.1×10^9 spores/grub (range $0.4\text{-}1.6 \times 10^9$) was attained at an estimated plant-scale production of 0.5-5 million diseased grubs/year. The minimum-average yield (under starvation conditions) was 2×10^9 spores/g grub as contrasted to a maximum-average yield of 7.1×10^9 spores/g grub. The average increase in yield over that used to inoculate grubs was ~1100-fold. The retail price of Doom or Japidemic is 1.3-1.4 cents/g, which calculates to a cost of ~15 cents/grub.

D. RICKETTSIAE PROPAGATION

1. Arthropod Associations

Rickettsiae associated with insects are grouped into Rickettsieae, Ehrlichieae and Wolbachieae. Species of Rickettsieae and Ehrlichieae, although pathogenic for lice, fleas, mites and ticks in varying degrees, are also pathogenic to man or other vertebrates. Species of Wolbachieae are specifically associated with arthropods; however, none were ever produced for wide-scale use as microbial insecticides (Tables I, II). Two genera, *Rickettsoides,* which grow on the surface of gut epithelium, and *Wolbachia,* which grow intracellularly, are relatively harmless for their arthropod hosts (Krieg, 1961). Two other genera *Enterella* and *Rickettsiella* are true entomopathogens and are potential candidates for consideration as microbial insecticides, especially since their host range includes some very important insect pests.

Several mosquito species *Culex quinquefasciatus* (Brumpt, 1938), *C. fatigans, C. molestus, Anopheles quadrimaculatus* and *Aedes aegypti* (Micks *et al.*, 1961) are susceptible to *Enterella culicis* or a closely related species of *Enterella.* Several species of a coccinellid beetle *Stethorus* are highly susceptible to *E. stethorae* (Hall and Badgley, 1957). Close to a dozen species of scarabaeids or closely related beetles are susceptible to *Rickettsiella melolonthae* (Krieg, 1958a, b; Hurpin, 1960; Niklas, 1960) originally isolated from *Melolontha melolontha* (Wille and Martignoni, 1952). The scarabaeids *Popillia japonica, Phyllophaga anxia, P. ephilida* and *Amphimallon majalis* are susceptible to *R. popilliae* originally isolated from the Japanese beetle (Dutky and Gooden, 1952). Other pest species, a dipteran *Tipula paludosa* and orthopterans *(Gryllus bimaculatus, Acheta domesticus)* are susceptible either to *R. tipulae* (Huger, 1958) or *R. grylli* (Vago and Martaja, 1963) respectively.

2. Rickettsiella *Species*

Cultivation of *Rickettsiella* in Diptera (Huger, 1958) and stored-product beetles (Krieg, 1955) suggest the possible substitution of continuously available, easily reared hosts for scarabaeid grubs. The host-rearing techniques used to propagate *B. popilliae* (Dutky, 1942) and recovery techniques of *R. popilliae* (Dutky, 1959) were used to develop the following protocol. Field-collected grubs, injected with ~25 rickettsiae/larva, were incubated at 27°C using the procedure developed for *B. popilliae* propagation. Aureomycin or penicillin (20 μg/larva) was used to inhibit development of injected bacteria without seriously affecting virulence of *R. popilliae*. *Rickettsiella*, however, were sensitive to dihydrostreptomycin and sodium sulfadiazine. Much higher doses (~7 x 10^8 rickettsiae/g soil) were required for soil inoculation. After 35 days of incubation diseased grubs were harvested, washed in water, blended and centrifugally-filtered through a Celite filter-cake. The Celite-filter containing rickettsiae was slurried with water and filtered through filter paper. Rickettsia particles were counted using dark-field microscopy and refrigerated. No loss in activity was detected after one year's storage at 4°C or three years' storage at −79°C. About 10^{-5} of original activity was still present after three years' storage at 4°C. Yields of 3.3 x 10^{11} rickettsiae/larva or 75 x 10^{12} rickettsiae/g grub were obtained. The increase in yield for the injection or soil inoculation technique was 13 x 10^9 or x 29 respectively.

Further consideration of *Enterella* and *Rickettsiella* for mass propagation as microbial insecticides must await future demonstration of effective field control of pest species, propagation-feasibility and vertebrate-safety (Mandin *et al.*, 1967).

E. VIRUS PROPAGATION

Many persons feel that viruses are potentially excellent insecticides due to their specificity and activity against economically important arthropods (Steinhaus, 1949; Bird, 1950; Martignoni, 1964; Heimpel, 1965; Anderson and Ignoffo, 1967; Ignoffo, 1966, 1967, 1968a). About 300 virus "species", representing five natural groups, are described (Table I). Four of the groups, i.e. nuclear polyhedrosis (NPV), cytoplasmic polyhedrosis (CPV), granulosis (GV) and non-inclusion virus (NIV), were propagated and used as viral insecticides (Table IV). From a recently described new group of pox-like insect viruses, ~15 have been isolated, and are at present being considered as another potential group of viral insecticides (Roberts, 1969, personal communication). Although ~20% were "mass" propagated, only five, all NPV, were industrially produced, mostly for experimental field use (Appendix 6, Section IV). Viruses were propagated mostly in caterpillars; however, sawflies and mites were also used. Immature stages, although the predominant choice of most investigators, were not exclusively used. Pupae (Vago and Atger, 1961) or adults (Martignoni, 1964) also were used. Hosts were either collected from natural and/or induced field infestations or continuously reared on natural and/or artificial diets. Artificial

TABLE IV

Arthropod species used as hosts for propagation of arthropod viruses

	Nuclear polyhedrosis	
Adoxophyes orana (reticulana)	*Hibernia defoliaria*	*Peridroma margaritosa*
Aporia crataegi	*Kotochalia junodi*	*Plusia gamma*
Choristoneura fumiferana	*Lymantria (Porthetria) dispar*	*Prodenia eridania*
Colias philodice eurytheme	*Lymantria fumida*	*Prodenia ornithogalli*
Dendrolimus spectabilis	*Malacosoma fragile*	*Prodenia praefica*
Gilpinia (Diprion) hercyniae	*Malacosoma neustria*	*Spodoptera (Prodenia) litura*
Heliothis virescens	*Mamestra (Barathra) brassicae*	*Spodoptera (Laphygma) exigua*
Heliothis zea	*Neodiprion sertifer*	*Spodoptera (Laphygma) frugiperda*
Hemerocampa pseudotsugata	*Neodiprion swainei*	*Trichoplusia ni*
	Cytoplasmic polyhedrosis	
Adoxophyes orana (reticulana)	*Hemerocampa pseudotsugata*	*Pectinophora gossypiella*
Dasychira pudibunda	*Lymantria fumida*	*Thaumetopoea pityocampa*
Dendrolimus spectabilis	*Mamestra (Barathra) brassicae*	*Trichoplusia ni*
	Granulosis	
Argyrotaenia velutinana	*Eucosma griseana*	*Spodoptera (Laphygma) exigua*
Choristoneura fumiferana	*Hyphantria cunea*	*Spodoptera (Laphygma) frugiperda*
Choristoneura (Cacoecia) murinana	*Pieris brassicae*	*Trichoplusia ni*
Cydia (Carpocapsa) pomonella	*Pieris rapae*	
	Non-inclusion virus	
Panonychus citri		

diets and continuously reared hosts are at present the best approach to systematic, mass propagation of viral insecticides. This combination relieves dependence on seasonal availability of hosts or their food and permits development of controlled production protocols. Other factors which may influence production, recovery and standardization of viral insecticides were summarized previously (Ignoffo, 1965b).

1. Nuclear Polyhedrosis Virus (NPV)

There are about 125 described NPV associated with four major insect orders, Lepidoptera, Hymenoptera, Diptera, Orthoptera. Associations with Lepidoptera account for ~90% of all NPV. About 25% of described NPV were mass propagated in either caterpillars or sawfly larvae (Table IV). The following sawfly larvae were used to propagate NPV: European spruce sawfly, *Gilpinia (Diprion) hercyniae* (Balch and Bird, 1944); European pine sawfly, *Neodiprion sertifer* (Breny, 1951); and the Swaine jack-pine sawfly, *N. swainei* (Smirnoff, 1961). Caterpillars used for NPV propagation were the alfalfa caterpillar, *Colias philodice eurytheme* (Steinhaus and Thompson, 1949); tent caterpillar, *Malacosoma fragile, M. neustria* (Clark and Thompson, 1954; Franz, 1969, personal communication); armyworm-leafworm complex, *Spodoptera litura, Prodenia eridania, P. praefica, P. ornithogalli* (Abul Nasr, 1959); *Spodoptera exigua, S. frugiperda* (Ignoffo, 1969, personal communication); bollworm-budworm complex, *Heliothis zea, H. virescens* (Ignoffo, 1965c, 1966); cabbage moth, *Mamestra brassicae* (Ponsen, 1966); cabbage looper, *Trichoplusia ni* (McEwen and Hervey, 1958, 1959; Ignoffo, 1964a, b, 1966); gamma noctuid, *Plusia gamma* (Vago and Cayrol, 1955); gypsy moth complex, *Lymantria dispar* (Rollinson *et al.*, 1965), *L. fumida* (Koyama and Katagiri, 1967); spruce budworm, *Choristoneura fumiferana* (Stairs and Bird, 1966); wattle bag worm, *Kotochalia junodi* (Ossowski, 1957); variegated cutworm, *Peridroma margaritosa* (Ignoffo, 1969, personal communication); Douglas-fir tussock moth, *Hemerocampa pseudotsugata* (Thompson, 1969, personal communication); *Hibernia defoliaria* (Franz, 1969, personal communication); pine caterpillar, *Dendrolimus spectabilis* (Koyama *et al.*, 1966); apple leafroller, *Adoxophyes orana (reticulana)* (Ponsen, 1966); black-veined white moth, *Aporia crataegi* (Franz, 1969, personal communication). Yields of NPV ranged from 2 to 50×10^8 polyhedral inclusion bodies (PIB)/g larva for sawfly larvae to 6-43 $\times 10^9$ PIB/g larva for caterpillars (Table V). Additional associations of NPV and caterpillars are cited in Ignoffo (1966a, 1968a).

a. NPV of Heliothis: *Noctuidae.* A series of papers described in detail the host-rearing protocol, virus infecting procedure, bioassay, safety, and field-effectiveness (Ignoffo, 1965a, c, d, e: Ignoffo and Heimpel, 1965; Ignoffo *et al.*, 1965) of the NPV of the cotton bollworm, *Heliothis zea.* This virus is at present being considered for registration as the first commercial U.S.A. viral insecticide.

TABLE V

Estimated yield of arthropod viruses from hosts grown on natural and/or synthetic diets

Pathogen species	Host substrate	Yield × 10^8 per Host	Yield × 10^8 per Gram-host	Reference
		Nuclear polyhedrosis[a]		
Gilpinia hercyniae	Pine	2	50	Bird and Burk, 1961
Heliothis zea	Synthetic	150	300	Ignoffo, 1965
Lymantria dispar	Leaves: synthetic	10-25	100	Lewis, 1969, personal communication
Mamestra brassicae	Cabbage: synthetic	40	60	Ponsen, 1966
Neodiprion sertifer	Pine	1	25	Lewis, 1969, personal communication
Neodiprion swainei	Pine	0.1	2	Smirnoff, 1964
Trichoplusia ni	Broccoli, cotton	60-80	200-260	McEwen and Hervey, 1959; Ignoffo, 1966
	Synthetic	130	430	Ignoffo, 1966
		Cytoplasmic polyhedrosis[a]		
Dendrolimus spectabilis	Pine: synthetic	5	20-30	Koyama and Katagiri, 1968
Thaumetopoea pityocampa	Pine	15	46	Martouret and Dusaussoy, 1959
		Granulosis[b]		
Cydia pomonella	Synthetic	10	200	Falcon, 1969, personal communication
		Non-inclusion virus[c]		
Panonychus citri	Lemons	0.0003	10	Shaw, 1969, personal communication; Gilmore and Munger, 1963

[a]Polyhedral inclusion bodies.
[b]Granule inclusion bodies.
[c]Minimum infective dose (MID)/host or gram host based upon 1 nanogram diseased mites/ml = 1 MID and 1 mite = 30 μg.

The primary host for propagation of *Heliothis* NPV was *H. zea*. The same stock of *H. zea* used for virus propagation in 1962 (Ignoffo, 1965a, c) is still in use. Over 100 generations, ~13/year, were reared. Other *Heliothis* species *(H. virescens, H. armigera, H. paradoxa, H. phloxophaga)* were also used for NPV propagation. The procedure (Fig. 1), used to rear *Heliothis*, generally applies to many NPV propagation techniques. Cotton bollworm larvae were individually reared in plastic 2-oz cups from neonates or eggs on an artificial diet at 30°C. In later modifications clear, orientated, polystyrene trays containing 50 (0.5 oz) cubicles/tray and covered with a heat-sealable Mylar film were used to rear larvae individually, both for continuity of the bollworm culture and for virus propagation (Ignoffo and Boening, 1970). Large 1.5-oz cubicles, 30/tray, worked better for rearing larvae to pupation. After six days (average body wt ≃179 ± 12 mg/larva) the surface of the medium in each cup was sprayed with 0.2 ml of a virus suspension containing 1.8×10^7 PIB/ml. This was a dose of 3.6×10^6 PIB/cup; ~2500 PIB/mm^2 or ~2×10^4 PIB/g larva. Sprayed cups containing larvae were incubated at 24° C. More than 99% of the larvae, weighing 500-600 mg/larva, were dead after 10 days' incubation. Living infected larvae, when desired, were collected after 5-7 days. Larvae, frozen to facilitate manual collection, were stored in ice cream cartons at –20° C.

Inclusion bodies were recovered, purified and concentrated from diseased larvae by blending with water, filtering through sieves and differential centrifugation. Viruses processed to a freeze-dried powder or water suspensions of PIB were stored at 5 or –20°C prior to field use. Preparations were standardized as to number of LD 50 units, number of PIB and number of secondary biotypes/mg or ml (Ignoffo, 1965b, 1966b; Ignoffo and Heimpel, 1965; Martignoni, 1967). A total of 215,000 bollworms and budworms (bollworms, 200,000; budworms, 15,000) were produced in 17 weeks of pilot production for an estimated production of 660,000 larvae/year. Six persons were employed in the NPV program, four to rear *Heliothis* and two to propagate the NPV. Estimated production cost was 7 cents/*H. zea* larva and 2.8 cents/*H. virescens* larva. Labor accounted for approximately 60% of total cost. Yields averaged 15×10^9 PIB/larva (3×10^{10} PIB/g larva) with a range of 6-36 x 10^9 PIB/larva (1.2-7.2 x 10^{10} PIB/g larva). The increase in PIB, based upon the actual amount of inoculum used, was >4000. The increase in PIB based on a known *per os* LD 99 dose was $>10^6$.

b. NPV of Trichoplusia: *Noctuidae.* Briggs (1963) described a technique which Flood used to propagate the NPV of cabbage loopers, *Trichoplusia ni*. Flood relied on heavy looper populations in field-grown crops as a source of loopers. Selective insecticides were used to control egg and larval parasites. The inoculum was applied using field sprayers, and diseased larvae were hand-harvested 4-8 days later. Virus diseased larvae were blended in water, filtered and quick-frozen in 1-pint volumes.

Diet-formula, rearing equipment and procedures used to propagate the cabbage looper NPV on an artificial diet were described by Ignoffo (1966a). In general, the diet and technique were similar to those used for propagation of *Heliothis* NPV. After 6-7 days' feeding on artificial diet at 30° C the looper's medium was sprayed with 0.2 ml of a suspension of 5×10^6 PIB/ml. This is a calculated dose of $\sim 1 \times 10^5$ PIB/larva or $\sim 5 \times 10^5$ PIB/g larva (210 mg/larva). Larvae on treated diet in 8-oz capped jars were placed at 23° C. Diseased larvae were harvested 4-5 days later and stored at −20° C. Suspensions (8×10^9 PIB/ml) stored frozen in water at −20° C were viable for at least 15-18 months (McEwen and Hervey, 1959). Processing to obtain PIB was identical to that described for *Heliothis* NPV.

A total of 20,520 larvae (2904 8-oz jars) were processed by two workers during a six-week pilot program for an estimated annual production of 168,000 larvae. Yields averaged 13×10^9 PIB/larva (43×10^9 PIB/g larva) or an estimated 10^4 increase in PIB over that used for inoculum (Ignoffo, 1966a). McEwen and Hervey (1959) obtained yields of 8×10^9 PIB/larva or 26×10^9 PIB/g larva when larvae were reared on cole-crop foliage. Field-collected diseased larvae averaged 6×10^9 PIB/larva or 20×10^9 PIB/g larva (Ignoffo, 1966).

c. NPV of Adoxophyes: *Tortricidae.* Ponsen (1966) used cabbage moth larvae, *Mamestra brassicae,* as an alternative host for propagation of NPV and CPV of the apple leafroller, *Adoxophyes orana,* after earlier studies (Ponsen and DeJong, 1964) demonstrated that cabbage worms were susceptible. Cabbage worms were used because they were larger, easier to rear, and an artificial diet modified from Adkisson *et al.* (1960) was available (Ponsen, 1966). Neonate larvae were fed cabbage leaves for three days, then transferred to artificial diet treated with NPV virus. Yields of 4×10^9 PIB/larva or $\sim 16 \times 10^9$ PIB/g larva were obtained. Cost of production using *A. orana* as the host was estimated at 0.5 cents/larva with a laboratory-production capacity of $\sim 11 \times 10^3$ larvae/year.

d. NPV of Lymantria: (Porthetria): *Lymantriidae.* Lewis (1969, personal communication) propagated gypsy moth NPV using a laboratory strain of gypsy moths reared on an artificial diet (Odell and Rollinson, 1966). This diet and a similar procedure also were used to propagate the NPV of the eastern tent caterpillar. Earlier propagation relied on field-collected larvae (Rollinson and Lewis, 1962). Instar IV larvae (average 69 mg/larva), were fed in groups of 10-1000 on leaf-bouquets or diet surface sprayed with a dose of 10^5-10^7 PIB/larva or 10^6-10^8 PIB/g larva. Rearing and incubation were at 25° C. The PIB recovery technique was described by Rollinson and Lewis (1962). After 12-20 days the dead, diseased larvae were collected, blended with water, filtered through a fine plastic screen and differentially centrifuged (750, 2000, 5000 r.p.m.) to concentrate PIB. Final PIB suspensions were counted and stored in buffer (pH 7) at 4° C. Lypholized, flash-evaporated or air-dried PIB were prepared when long-term storage was planned. Yields of 1-2.5×10^9 PIB/larva or

$\sim 10^{10}$ PIB/g larva were obtained, which was an increase of 10^2-10^4-fold over the inoculum used. Laboratory-production capacity of a million diseased larvae/year ($\sim 10^{15}$ PIB/year) was achieved. Vago and Atger (1961) produced 30 g of "pure" PIB ($\sim 3 \times 10^{13}$ PIB or ~ 12.5-30.0×10^3 diseased larvae) by administering 1-3 x 10^3 PIB/mature larva. PIB were recovered from pupae.

e. NPV of Neodiprion: *Diprionidae.* Smirnoff (1964, 1969, personal communication) used large wooden racks (9 x 3 x 1 ft) indoors and an outdoor carousel to rear field-collected larvae of the jack pine sawfly, *Neodiprion swainei.* Three million instar II larvae on 35 racks at 25-30° C, were fed on pine foliage sprayed with 5-25 x 10^7 PIB/rack (50 ml/rack, 1-5 x 10^6 PIB/ml). About 5 x 10^5 larvae were handled at one time using the outdoor carousel. The inoculum dose was 3-18 x 10^3 PIB/larva or 1-6 x 10^5 PIB/g larva. Fresh foliage, treated with virus, was provided twice-daily for the first three days and fresh untreated foliage for another 10-18 days.

During 2-3 weeks of incubation diseased, dead and dying larvae were collected and stored at 4°C. Inclusion bodies were concentrated by centrifugation after blending with water and filtering through cheesecloth and nylon. PIB suspensions were stored in polyethylene containers at 4° C. Yields from three million larvae averaged 10^7 PIB/larva or 2 x 10^8 PIB/g larva (Smirnoff, 1969, personal communication). An average of 6-13 x 10^6 PIB/larva was obtained from 10^5 larvae (Smirnoff, 1964). Yield was 3-4 x 10^3 times the inoculum. Production costs, including salary and supplies but excluding overheads, were 0.04-0.09 cents/larva, based upon an average of 10^7 PIB/larva (Smirnoff, 1964). PIB were stored dried or in dilute mixtures of water and virus. Shorter periods of storage in benzene or fuel oil were also possible (Smirnoff *et al.*, 1962).

European pine sawfly *(N. sertifer)* NPV also was propagated on field-collected instar III-IV larvae (Lewis, 1969, personal communication; Rollinson *et al.*, in press. Larvae on red pine foliage were sprayed with 4 ml of 10^6 PIB/ml for every 1000-2000 larvae (2-4 x 10^3 PIB/larva $\simeq$7-13 x 10^4 PIB/g larva). The treated larvae, and foliage, placed in ventilated cardboard boxes (1000-2000 larvae/box), were incubated in an outdoor insectary ($\sim$21° C). Diseased larvae were manually collected and processed using the method of Lewis (1960).

An average yield of 10^8 PIB/larva or 25 x 10^8 PIB/g larva was obtained, which was an increase of $\sim 10^4$-fold over that used for inoculum. Production capacities of 1-2 million larvae/year, during a three-month spring production period, were achieved at an estimated cost of 1-2 cents/larva.

2. Cytoplasmic Polyhedrosis Virus CPV

There are $\sim$100 described CPV associated with Lepidoptera, Diptera and Neuroptera. Lepidopteran hosts account for $\sim$95% of the described CPV. Less than a dozen caterpillar species (Table IV) were hosts for propagation of CPV, i.e. cabbage moth, *Mamestra brassicae,* and apple leafroller, *Adoxophyes orana* (Ponsen, 1966); pine caterpillar, *Dendrolimus spectabilis* (Koyama *et al.*, 1966); Japanese larch lymantrid, *Lymantria fumida* (Koyama and Katagiri, 1967, 1968); pine processionary caterpillar, *Thaumetopoea pityocampa* (Martouret and Dusaussoy, 1959); Douglas-fir tussock moth, *Hemerocampa pseudotsugata* (Thompson, 1969, personal communication); tussock moth, *Dasychira pudibunda* (Franz, 1969, personal communication); cabbage looper, *Trichoplusia ni,* and pink bollworm, *Pectinophora gossypiella* (Ignoffo, 1969, personal communication). The CPV of the pine processionary caterpillar was one of the first insect viruses produced in large quantities and used as a viral insecticide. Yields of CPV ranged from 20-46 x 10^8 PIB/g larva (Table V).

a. CPV of Thaumetopoea: *Thaumetopoeidae.* Martouret and Dusaussoy (1959) used 175 pine trees, in three locations, to rear pine processionary caterpillars for CPV propagation. Rows of trees were infected with 1335 colonies of field-collected larvae. When required, additional food was given as "garlands" of pine branches draped over defoliated branches of the young trees. Each of 132 garlands was made from 10 pine branches. Rearing and virus propagation conditions were 16-20°C and 65-80% R.H.

Trees bearing instar V larvae were sprayed twice (five-day interval) with ~3 x 10^9 PIB/tree. Dead and moribund larvae, observed two weeks after the first spraying, were collected over a three- to five-week period. A total of 170,779 larvae were produced during a two-month period for an estimated capacity of 10^6 larvae/year. Inoculum for this level of production was ~10^{12} PIB (160 g of 7 x 10^9 PIB/g). Yields from mature larvae (~330 mg/larva) ranged from 1.2-2.7 x 10^9 PIB/larva or 3.6-8.4 x 10^9 PIB/g larva. The average yield was 1.5 x 10^9 PIB/larva or 4.6 x 10^9 PIB/g larva. Yields from instar III or IV larvae were of the same order, based on body weight, as that of mature instar V larvae. Counts from instar III or IV larvae averaged 3-5 x 10^7 PIB/larva (3-5 x 10^9 PIB/g larva) or 5-6 x 10^8 PIB/larva (5-6 x 10^9 PIB/g larva) respectively. The increase of yield over inoculum was 227-fold.

PIB were recovered as follows. Diseased larvae were pulped (Latapie crusher-pulper), fermented for 15 days, then filtered under vacuum through a filter-press and nylon cloth (100 μ diameter). Activity was estimated using PIB counts. The purified filtrate was spray dried on bentonite. Nine tons of dust (2.2 x 10^7 PIB/g) containing 0.72% PIB and 225 kg of 3.5% PIB were produced for the 1968 field trials and 15.4 tons (2 x 10^7 PIB/g) were produced for 1969 field trials (Grison, 1960).

b. CPV of Dendrolimus: *Lasiocampidae.* Koyama and Katagiri (1968) used both artificial diet and pine needles to propagate CPV of the pine caterpillar, *Dendrolimus spectabilis.* A dose of 10^6 PIB/ml was used to spray instar VII larvae feeding on pine branches. Diseased larvae, collected 20 days after inoculation, were stored at 0-5°C. Yields of 5×10^8 PIB/larva (~2-3 x 10^9 PIB/g larva) were attained.

3. Granulosis Virus (GV)

About a dozen caterpillar species were used as hosts for propagation of GV (Table IV). Techniques varied from using field-collected larch budmoth larvae, *Eucosma griseana* (Martignoni and Auer, 1957) to using a continuously-reared laboratory stock of codling moth larvae, *Cydia (Carpocapsa) pomonella* (Falcon, 1969, personal communication; Falcon *et al.*, 1968). Other caterpillar hosts used to propagate GV were cabbageworms, *Pieris rapae* and *P. brassicae* (Biliotti *et al.*, 1956; Tanada, 1956; McEwen and Hervey, 1959); red banded leafroller, *Argyrotaenia velutinana* (Glass, 1958); spruce budworm, *Choristoneura fumiferana* (Stairs and Bird, 1966); fir-shoot roller, *Choristoneura (Cacoecia) murinana*, and fall webworm, *Hyphantria cunea* (Franz, 1969, personal communication; Franz, 1961); armyworm, *Spodoptera exigua, S. frugiperda*, and cabbage looper (Ignoffo, 1969, personal communication).

The described protocol was developed by Falcon (1969, personal communication). Codling moth larvae were continuously reared using a modification of Dickson *et al.*'s (1952) procedure. Neonate larvae were individually reared in 0.5-oz jelly-cubicles (Ignoffo and Boening, 1970) on a semisynthetic diet modified after Ignoffo (1963) by J. F. Howell. The oriental fruit moth, *Grapholitha molesta*, is also susceptible to the codling moth granulosis and might serve as an alternative host. Larvae were reared in complete darkness to prevent their tunneling into the diet for 10 days at 20-26°C, then each was fed a drop of water containing 1×10^7 capsules, i.e. ~2×10^8 capsules/g larva. Larvae at this stage are in instars IV-V and average 46 mg/larva (range 40-58). Capsules (1.1×10^8 capsules/ml) were administered *per os* using a syringe equipped with a 1-in, 25-27 gauge needle. Treated larvae were incubated at 20-26°C for 2-3 days. To facilitate handling and to minimize virus loss, living larvae were collected and stored at 4-6°C until needed.

Capsules were recovered from diseased larvae by trituration (sterile tissue grinder) and differential centrifugation. Approximately 500 larvae were processed at one time. Low speed centrifugation (<500 r.p.m.; 2 min) eliminated the insect debris, and high speed centrifugation (>10,000 r.p.m.; 30 min) concentrated the capsules from the supernatant. Capsule suspensions were standardized using electron microscopy (Williams and Backus, 1949). Counts were based upon addition of a known number of polystyrene-latex particles to a known volume of capsule suspension. The average yield was ~10^9 capsules/larva or ~2×10^{10} capsules/g larva. Yields of virus produced in 1966 and 1967, on a smaller scale, were 6.6×10^9 and 1.9×10^9 capsules/larva respectively. Increase in capsule yield over inoculum was 100- to 660-fold.

Production capacity, based upon seven months of laboratory production in 1968, was estimated at 140,000 larvae/year and cost, excluding labor and overheads, was 0.3 cents/larva.

4. Non-Inclusion Virus (NIV)

There are ~2 dozen described NIV of arthropods. All but three are associated with insects. The NIV have the most extensive variety of hosts. Five orders of insects (Lepidoptera, Hymenoptera, Diptera, Coleoptera, Orthoptera) and one order of an arachnid (Acarina) harbor NIV. One NIV isolated from a dipteran *(Tipula paludosa)* infects three species of Coleoptera, seven of Diptera and 12 of Lepidoptera (Smith *et al.*, 1961). To our knowledge only one, i.e. citrus red mite, *Panonychus citri,* NIV was propagated for insecticidal use (Table IV). The citrus red mite is the only known susceptible acarine host (Shaw *et al.*, 1967); however, this may be a reflection of no attempted transmission to other arthropods. Certainly the evidence from other NIV (35 of 39 attempts to cross-transmit NIV to alien hosts were successful) indicates a possibly wider host range (Ignoffo, 1968b).

The following procedure was used by Gilmore and Munger (1963) to propagate the NIV of citrus red mite. The virus propagation procedure was an extension of techniques developed earlier to continuously rear citrus red mites for toxicological and biological studies (Munger and Gilmore, 1960; Chamber and Moffitt, 1967). Green lemons (2-in diameter) racked in wire frames (18 x 18 in), 32 lemons/rack, were the mite food. Adult mites (250/lemon) were allowed to oviposit (~1800 eggs/lemon/24 hr) on lemons for 72-96 hr. Afterwards adult mites were transferred to fresh lemons and the process repeated. A specially constructed tower and air-jet were used to transfer adults (Munger and Gilmore, 1960). Egg-infested lemons were incubated at 27°C and 60-70% R.H. in incubators containing 10 racks. Mites in the protonymph stage (nine days after oviposition) were used for virus propagation. Each rack of 32 lemons was finely sprayed with 8 ml of a suspension containing 100 μg triturated diseased mites/ml. The minimum dose necessary to produce infections was 2 μg diseased mites/ml or the virus extracted from 0.05 to 0.1 mite (Gilmore and Munger, 1963). In more recent tests a dose of 1 ng diseased mites/ml infected some mites fed sugar + water through an inert membrane (Shaw, 1969, personal communication). Virus-treated mites and lemons were incubated at 21-35°C. At peak infection (9-12 days after inoculation) each lemon supported 300-500 diseased mites. Diseased dead mites, living mites, cast skins, webbing and other debris were brushed from the lemon surface, placed in a vial, weighed and stored at –20°C. Virus diseased mites could be stored as a frozen-glycerin suspension, or vacuum-dried, freeze-dried or chemically-dried preparations at –25°C for >46 weeks. Infectivity was completely lost within 10 weeks when aqueous suspensions were stored at 7 or 25°C. After evaluating several storage conditions diseased mites were routinely stored at −25°C in loosely stoppered vials over anhydrous calcium chloride. No appreciable loss of infectivity was detected after 66 weeks of storage.

The average yield from each rack of 32 lemons was 100 mg of diseased mites. Yields as high as 250 mg/rack were obtained. The increase in virus over inoculum was 125- to 312-fold. A propagation capacity of 50-100 g of diseased mites/year (2-5 x 10^6 diseased mites/year) was obtained at a labor and material cost of ~0.2-0.4 cents/mite ($80-100/g mite).

F. CONCLUSIONS AND RESEARCH

More than a thousand arthropod pathogens are described and yet only about 10% have been mass propagated regardless of the technology employed (Table I). Surprisingly, in spite of its inherent difficulty, whole organism technology accounted for ~80% of the total propagated. Viruses, probably because of their potential as insecticides, their specificity and availability, accounted for ~45% of the total propagated in living systems. Living systems are only considered when the pathogen is highly desirable as a microbial insecticide and no other system is available. Development of systems for continuous mass-rearing arthropods (Knipling, 1955, 1959; Baumhover *et al.,* 1955; Steiner *et al.,* 1965; Gast and Vardell, 1963; Ignoffo, 1966a) has made propagation of obligate insect pathogens technically feasible. Commercial feasibility for the most part must still be proven.

Any development which will result in lower production costs, i.e. media simplification, flexible production system, automated production, will greatly stimulate further consideration of obligate pathogens as microbial insecticides. Media simplification, for example, has reduced costs of producing a cannibalistic host ~10-fold. The same production system used to produce a non-cannibalistic host may further reduce costs 1/2 to 1/10. Automation would reduce the number of production personnel, which accounts for approximately 60-70% of total production costs. The single greatest expenditure is construction of a production plant. Because of this, research and development should obtain information that would permit a basic plant design capable of rearing many different arthropod hosts. Attainment of these objectives would insure production, eventual use and wide acceptance of microbial insecticides formulated from obligate pathogens.

III. Propagation in Avian Embryos

Attempts to culture insect viruses in fertilized eggs failed and attempts with other arthropod pathogens, with the exception of rickettsiae, are few. Arthropod rickettsiae *(Wolbachia, Rickettsiella)* were cultivated in embryonated eggs (Steinhaus, 1942) or mammalian host (Krieg, 1955; Giroud *et al.*, 1958). Of the two genera *Rickettsiella* is a true entomopathogen. Since it is pathogenic to mammals, its development into a microbial insecticide is most unlikely. The granulosis virus of *Peridroma margaritosa* and *Junonia coenia* and the NPV of *Colias philodice eurytheme, Spodoptera exigua, Bombyx mori, Phryganidia californica* and *Heliothis zea,* both crude and purified, were inoculated into embryonated chick eggs (Steinhaus, 1951; Hink and Ignoffo, 1969, personal communication). Presence of virus could not be demonstrated in chicken tissue or egg-fluids. *B. mori* NPV also would not grow in embryonated eggs (Aizawa, 1961). In Aizawa's studies there was some interaction between host and virus. Embryos died and PIB morphology was changed by alternate passage through eggs and insects. Future corroboration of Aizawa's study is required. In a more recent study turkey eggs could not be infected with viral rods or purified inclusion bodies of *B. mori* CPV (Cantwell *et al.,* 1968).

IV. Propagation in Tissue-cell Systems

The concept of propagating arthropod pathogens in insect tissue culture was demonstrated for all major pathogen groups being considered as potential insecticides. Available information, however, on yields and technology is from laboratory propagation of milligram- to gram-quantities. Application of laboratory technology to commercial systems has yet to be demonstrated and judging from our present rate of development will not be realized for some time. The technology is available! The necessity for its use, at least at present, is not! The need must be coupled with major developments in insect-tissue technology, namely (1) development of prolific, high yield per volume cell lines; (2) simplification of culture media; (3) propagation of high pathogen titers in selected cell lines; and (4) design and development of plant-scale equipment and routine production procedures. Pathogen propagation in tissue cultures offers distinct advantages over *in vivo* propagation. Tissue cultures are relatively free of secondary biotypes, can be stored, easily regulated, and may cost less than *in vivo* systems.

A. GENERAL PROCEDURES

Aseptic conditions are used in culturing insect organs, tissues, and cells. All glassware, media, and equipment must be sterilized. Insect cells, like many cultured cells, are sensitive to growth inhibitors; therefore, glassware must be chemically clean and purified water used to formulate media.

Primary explants were grown in hanging or standing drops, roller tubes, shaking flasks, spinner flasks, T-flasks, or polystyrene disposable flasks. The optimum temperature for cell growth was 26-30°C. Insects must be surface sterilized before dissection and removal of explant tissues. Ethyl alcohol (70%) was used to sterilize the exterior of fruit fly, *Drosophila melanogaster,* larvae and silkworm, *Bombyx mori,* pupae (Burdette *et al.,* 1968; Grace, 1958a). Ovaries from adult *Heliothis zea* were aseptically removed and surface sterilized with 0.5% sodium hypochlorite (Hink and Ignoffo, 1970). Sodium hypochlorite was considered an ideal disinfectant because of its excellent microbiocidal activity, stability, solubility, low mammalian toxicity, detectability (acid KI-colorimetric reaction) and ease of neutralization with thiosulfate (Ignoffo and Dutky, 1963). Hyamine solution (0.1-0.4%) sterilized the exterior of nymphal leafhopper, *Agallia constricta,* and variegated cutworm larvae, *Peridroma saucia* (Hirumi and Maramorosch, 1963; Martignoni and Scallion, 1961). Eggs of *A. constricta* were treated with 75% EtOH followed by 0.1% $HgCl_2$ (Chiu *et al.,* 1966) and *D. melanogaster* eggs subjected to 3% sodium hypochlorite and then 0.05% $HgCl_2$ in 70% EtOH (Horikawa and Fox, 1964). After surface sterilization, care must be taken to prevent introducing the disinfectant into the primary culture.

Various agents were used to dissociate tissue. Trypsin and Versene damaged the integument of *P. saucia* (Martignoni *et al.,* 1958). Undamaged cells were obtained using a hepatopancreas extract of the snail, *Helix aspersa.* Trypsin, Versene, hyaluronidase, and the hepatopancreas extract were tried on epidermal, intestinal, and gonadal tissues of four lepidopteran species (Aizawa and Vago, 1959a). Trypsin, hyaluronidase, and Versene destroyed cells at concentrations used in vertebrate tissue culture; however weaker concentrations were not detrimental and dispersed cells formed monolayers. The embryonic tissues of *D. melanogaster* dissociated in Ca- and Mg-free saline containing 0.12% Versene and 0.15% crude trypsin (Lesseps, 1965). Embryos up to 11 hr old yielded uniform suspensions of single cells and older embryos produced large undissociated groups of cells. Ovaries of *Heliothis zea* were dissociated using 0.25% trypsin in a balanced salt solution after trituration and agitation (Hink and Ignoffo, 1970). Treatment of *A. constricta* embryos with 0.25% trypsin did not separate cells but improved cell outgrowth from primary explants (Chiu *et al.,* 1966). Apparently insect cells are more sensitive to dissociating agents than vertebrate cells. Cell separation by mincing or trituration may be as effective as enzyme treatment.

B. EXPLANTS OR CELL LINES

Our discussion on tissues will focus on those capable of long-term maintenance or development into cell lines. None of the established cell lines (Table VI) were commercially used; however, all are potential substrates for propagation of obligate insect pathogens.

Embryonic tissue is often selected to start cultures because it is generally assumed to be in a state of active growth and thus to contain all the necessary hormones and growth factors (Horikawa and Fox, 1964; Horikawa *et al.,* 1966). Growth potential of cells is often related to embryo age. Two-hour embryo transplants did not grow. In contrast 8-hr embryo cells grew logarithmically.

TABLE VI

Available long-term cultures or established insect cell lines

Insect	Primary explant	Time in culture or number of subcultures[a]	Reference
Lepidoptera			
Antheraea eucalypti	pupal ovaries	44 subcultures	Grace, 1962a
Bombyx mori	larval ovaries	12 subcultures	Vao and Chastang, 1958
Bombyx mori	larval gonads	22 subcultures	Gaw, Liu and Zia, 1959
Bombyx mori	larval ovaries	3 years	Grace, 1967
Chilo suppressalis	larval hemocytes	32 months	Mitsuhashi, 1967a
Cydia (Carpocapsa) pomonella	embryo	22 subcultures	Hink, 1969, personal communication
Heliothis zea	adult ovaries	98 subcultures	Hink and Ignoffo, 1970
Spodoptera frugiperda	pupal ovaries	15 subcultures	Vaughn, 1969, personal communication
Trichoplusia ni	adult ovaries	96 subcultures	Hink, 1970
Diptera			
Aedes aegypti	macerated larvae	3 years	Grace, 1966
Aedes aegypti	minced larvae	115 subcultures	Singh, 1967
Aedes aegypti	embryo	22 subcultures	Peleg, 1968
Aedes albopictus	minced larvae	115 subcultures	Singh, 1967
Aedes vexans	minced pupae	18 subcultures	Sweet and Dupree, 1968
Aedes vittatus	minced larvae	8 subcultures	Singh and Bhat, 1969, personal communication
Anopheles stephensi	minced larvae	38 subcultures	Schneider, 1969
Culiseta inornata	minced adult	7 subcultures	Sweet and Dupree, 1968
Drosophila melanogaster	embryo	520 days	Horikawa, Ling and Fox, 1966
Drosophila melanogaster	embryo	14 months	Echalier and Ohannessian, 1969
Homoptera			
Agallia constricta	embryo	20 months	Chiu and Black, 1967
Agallia quadripunctata	embryo	20 months	Chiu and Black, 1967
Orthoptera			
Blaberus craniifer (fuscus)	embryo	2 years	Landureau, 1968
Leucophaea maderae	heart	18 months	Vago, 1969, personal communication
Periplaneta americana	embryo	2 years	Landureau, 1968

[a]At time of publication or communication.

Seecof and Unanue (1968) observed development of nerve- and muscle-like cells from morphologically similar cells of a 3-7 hr embryo of *D. melanogaster.* The cultures were not maintained for more than 30 days. Leafhopper embryonic tissue was successfully cultivated as a primary culture (Hirumi and Maramorosch, 1964a) and developed into a cell line (Chiu and Black, 1967). Primary explants from trypsinized cockroach embryos, *Periplaneta americana* and *Blaberus craniifer (fusca),* were subcultured and established as cell lines (Landureau, 1966, 1968). Honey-bee, *Apis mellifera,* mosquito, *Aedes aegypti,* and spruce budworm, *Choristoneura fumiferana* embryonic tissues were also successfully cultured as primary explants (Giauffret *et al.,* 1967; Peleg, 1966; Sohi 1968).

The gonadal tissues of caterpillars were successfully cultured many times. Wyatt's pioneering work (1956) demonstrated that cells of *B. mori* ovary exhibited rapid mitosis in medium formulated to simulate hemolymph. Wyatt's formulation (1956) was the basis for subsequent insect tissue culture media (Gaw *et al.,* 1959; Grace, 1967; Vago and Chastang, 1958). Ovarian tissues from other lepidopteran species also were cultured (Grace, 1958a; Jones and Cunningham, 1960; Lender and Duveau-Hagege, 1963; Sen Gupta, 1961; Stanley and Vaughn, 1968). Mosquito cell lines were established from primary cultures of macerated insects (Grace, 1966; Singh, 1967; Sweet and Dupree, 1968). Until recently, all established insect cell lines were started from immature tissue. Sweet and Dupree (1968) first successfully subcultured cells from adult tissue, i.e. a mosquito, *Culiseta inornata.* Hink and Ignoffo (1970) and Hink (1970) first established a cell line from adult lepidopteran ovaries *(H. zea* and *T. ni).*

Hemocytes, which seem suitable for culture because no treatment is necessary to disperse cells, do not proliferate as well as embryonic and ovarian tissues. Hemocytes *(P. saucia)* will attach to the culture vessel and develop monolayers (Martignoni and Scallion, 1961). Monolayers survive for 10-15 days; however subculturing was not attempted. The first hemocyte cell line was established from larval hemocytes of the rice stem borer, *Chilo suppressalis* (Mitsuhashi, 1967a).

Imaginal discs provided mitotically active cells which differentiated *in vitro* for several weeks (Schneider, 1964; Oberlander and Fulco, 1967). These cells are embryologically determined and consequently long-term growth was not achieved.

Explants of intestinal tissue (Sen Gupta, 1961), cephalic ganglia and lymph glands (Raimondi and Ghini, 1963), neuroblasts, circulatory organs, and Malpighian tubules (Hirumi and Maramorosch, 1964b), trachea (Martin and Junko, 1967) and epidermis (Miciarelli *et al.,* 1967) produced cellular outgrowths and mitotically active cells. However, no cell lines were established from these explants.

C. CULTURE MEDIA AND GROWTH FACTORS

The hydrogen ion concentration, osmotic pressure, oxygen tension, ion balance, and nutrients are some important factors considered when formulating media. The composition of insect tissue-culture media was reviewed by Smith (1967) and Vago (1967) and will not be discussed here except as it pertains to increase of cell growth, longevity and media simplification.

Cell migration, mitosis, and longevity of silkworm ovarian tissues increased after addition of ring or prothoracic gland extracts (Grace, 1958b). Brain, prothoracic gland, and corpus allatum extracts increased vesicle formation, tissue bud formation, and cell migration in leg explants of the cockroach, *Leucophaea maderae* (Marks and Reinecke, 1965). Addition of ecdysone to imaginal discs of the greater wax moth, *Galleria mellonella,* increased growth and percentage of cultures showing *in vitro* metamorphosis (Oberlander and Fulco, 1967). Ecdysone supplement was also beneficial to cultures of ocular imaginal discs of *D. melanogaster* (Burdette *et al.,* 1968).

Vertebrate sera and chick-embryo extracts are also beneficial to insect cells and tissues cultured *in vitro.* A simple medium containing salts, trehalose, oestradiol, and a growth-stimulating chick-embryo extract was used to culture heart, gonadal, and imaginal tissues of the blowfly, *Calliphora erythrocephala,* and salivary glands of *D. melanogaster* (Demal and Leloup, 1963). Kitamura (1965) demonstrated that calf serum stimulated cellular migration and maintained healthy cell sheets in primary explants of the mosquito, *Culex pipiens.* Calf serum was better than chicken plasma or bovine serum. Martignoni and Scallion (1961) found that fetal bovine serum provided better growth conditions for *P. saucia* hemocytes than human, lamb, or horse sera. A hemolymph-independent (HI) line of *Heliothis* cells grew better in fetal bovine serum than in sera from man, cattle, rabbit, guinea pig, rat, or chicken (Shapiro and Ignoffo, 1969, personal communication). Fetal bovine sera also enhanced growth of Grace's *Antheraea eucalypti, Aedes aegypti,* and *B. mori* cell lines (Sohi and Smith, 1970). Compounds which stimulate vertebrate cell growth may be useful for insect cell lines. Methyl and propyl parabens stimulated growth of organ cultures (White, 1967). Trace metals were required for maximum growth of L-cells (Thomas and Johnson, 1967). Fetuin promoted growth of several different mammalian cells (Puck *et al.,* 1968). Insulin stimulated cell proliferation of rat mammary carcinoma (Heuson *et al.,* 1967), and dimethylnitrosamine increased growth and longevity of embryo hamster cells (Huberman *et al.,* 1968).

Prior to 1960 insect tissue culture media were supplemented with either heterologous or homologous insect hemolymph. An advance of major technical importance was the replacement of hemolymph with vertebrate sera or extracts (Vago and Chastang, 1962a, b). Vertebrate serum or chick embryo extracts supported growth of hemocytes and gonads without the need for insect hemolymph. However, cultures in HI medium did not survive as long as those with hemolymph. Ovarian *B. mori* tissue produced cellular outgrowths in HI medium containing salts, sugars, lactalbumin hydrolysate, and yeast extract (Aizawa and Sato, 1963). Long-term culture of cells in HI medium was first achieved by Horikawa *et al.* (1966). Many insect cell lines are now grown in HI media (Table VII). Cell lines of *A. eucalypti* and *A. aegypti,* originally established by Grace (1962a, 1966) in media with hemolymph, were adapted to proliferate in HI media (Nagle *et al.,* 1967; Sohi, 1969; Yunker *et al.,* 1967). Cells from ~10 insect species were subcultured and established in HI media since 1966. Another major advancement in insect tissue culturing was the replacement of individual amino acids and vitamins with protein hydrolysates and yeast extracts (Chiu and Black, 1967; Horikawa *et al.,* 1966; Landureau, 1968; Mitsuhashi, 1967; Singh, 1967).

Metabolic studies of cultured insect cells should be employed to optimize and simplify arthropod tissue culture media. Trehalose, a sugar of insect hemolymph, appears necessary for *in vivo* insect cell growth; however, an *A. eucalypti* cell line utilizes glucose as easily as trehalose (Clements and Grace, 1967). Cholesterol, important for *in vivo* growth, is not required for *in vitro* cell growth. Histidine, threonine, and tryptophan are not synthesized by insects but insect cell cultures synthesize them in signficant amounts (Grace and Brzostowski, 1966). Insect hemolymph contains high amino acid concentrations yet leafhopper tissues required lower amino acid concentrations than are normally present in hemolymph (Mitsuhashi and Maramorosch, 1964).

D. PATHOGEN PROPAGATION

1. Virus Propagation

The first successful infection of insect cells with an obligate insect pathogen was by Trager (1935). Little was reported for 23 years until Grace (1958c) observed NPV in cultured ovarian tissues of tussock moths, *Hemerocampa leucostigma.* These cells carried a *latent* infection and PIB formation occurred after changing the composition of the growth medium. *In vitro* NPV infection of *B. mori* tissues was reported by Aizawa and Vago (1959b), Gaw *et al.* (1959), and Medvedeva, 1959). After 1959, 20 successful infections of insect tissue or cell culture with virus were reported.

Viral inoculum must be free of contaminants or obtained aseptically from diseased insects. Primary explants are usually inoculated when subcultured or 2-3 days after subculturing. Diseased hemolymph is most often used as inoculum. If properly timed, hemolymph may contain infectious nucleic acid, naked virus rods, and/or PIB. Purified nucleic acid, purified virions, infected cell cultures, tissue explants, and triturated whole diseased insects were also used as viral inoculum (Table VII). Use of *B. mori* NPV in *B. mori* ovarian tissue was the most investigated virus-cell-culture system. Infectivity of various inocula are somewhat contradictory. Vaughn and Faulkner (1963) and Miloserdova (1965) obtained infection using diseased insect hemolymph and purified virions

TABLE VII

Explants, tissue and/or cell lines reported susceptible to arthropod viruses

Host tissue	Virus species[a]	Inoculum[b]	Reference
Bombyx mori			
gonads	*B. mori* NPV	hemolymph, tissue culture	Trager, 1935; Aizawa and Vago, 1959; Vaughn and Faulkner, 1963; Faulkner and Vaughn, 1965, Vago and Chastang, 1960; Medvedeva, 1959; Gaw *et al.*, 1959; Miloserdova, 1965.
gonads	*B. mori* NPV	virions	Faulkner and Vaughn, 1965; Krywienczyk and Sohi, 1967; Vago and Chastang, 1960.
hemocytes	*B. mori* NPV	hemolymph	Miloserdova, 1965
cell culture	*B. mori* NPV	hemolymph	Vago and Croissant, 1963
gonads	Densonucleosis	virion	Vago *et al.*, 1966
Galleria mellonella			
ovary, fat tissue, hemocytes	*G. mellonella* NPV	hemolymph	Sen Gupta, 1963; Heitor, 1963
larval ovary	Densonucleosis	hemolymph	Vago and Luciani, 1965
Antheraea eucalypti			
pupal ovaries	CPV	latent infection	Grace, 1962b
cell line	*B. mori* NPV	virions	Grace, 1968, personal communication
cell line	SIV	virions	Bellett and Mercer, 1964

larval ovaries	NPV	latent infection	Grace, 1958c
Peridroma saucia			
larval hemocytes	*P. saucia* NPV	triturated tissue	Martignoni and Scallion, 1961
Lymantria dispar			
larval and pupal ovaries	*L. dispar* NPV and CPV *B. mori* NPV *Antheraea pernyi* NPV *Pieris brassicae* granulosis	hemolymph, virions, explant	Vago and Bergoin, 1963
Drosophila melanogaster			
embryo	sigma	triturated tissue	Ohanessian and Echalier, 1967
Chilo suppressalis			
cell line	CIV	accidental infection	Mitsuhashi, 1967a
Nephotettix cincticeps and *Laodelphax striatella*			
embryo	CIV	virions	Mitsuhashi, 1967b
Antheraea pernyi			
larval testicular cysts	*A. pernyi* NPV	hemolymph	Medvedeva, 1959

[a] NPV, nuclear polyhedrosis virus; CPV, cytoplasmic polyhedrosis virus; SIV, *Sericesthis* iridescent virus; TIV, *Tipula* iridescent virus; CIV, *Chilo* iridescent virus.

[b] Hemolymph–hemolymph from larvae infected with virus: tissue culture–virus infected tissue culture; explant–explants from virus infected larvae, virions–purified virions; triturated tissue–triturated virus infected insects; accidental infection–accidently virus infected.

combined with dissolved PIB protein but could not obtain infection when using purified virions alone. PIB protein may play some, as yet unknown, role in the infective process. Diseased adipose tissue and infected tissue fragments initiated viral infection of cultured *Lymantria dispar* ovaries (Vago and Bergoin, 1963). Purified virions seldom were infectious. Other studies showed that purified virions will infect *B. mori* ovarian cultures (Krywienczyk and Sohi, 1967). However, susceptibility to purified virions was extremely variable and high virus titers sometimes failed to infect while lower titers were infectious (Faulkner and Vaughn, 1965). This variability could be due to treatments used to release virions from PIB or low sensitivity of the assay (Shapiro and Ignoffo, 1969).

Infection of established cell lines with pathogenic insect viruses will give impetus to consideration of insect cell lines as substrates for production of viral insecticides. Established cell lines, for the most part, were susceptible to NIV. Grace's *A. eucalypti* cells support growth of *Sericesthis* iridescent virus (SIV) (Bellet and Mercer, 1964), *Tipula* iridescent virus (TIV) and *Chilo* iridescent virus (CIV) (Hukuhara and Hashimoto, 1967). Purified virions were used in SIV studies and hemolymph from infected *G. mellonella* larvae in TIV and CIV studies. Inoculation of cell lines with occluded viruses (NPV, CPV, GV) usually failed. Grace (1969, personal communication) infected an *A. eucalypti* cell line with purified virions from *B. mori* NPV. About 20% of the cells were infected and NPV formed 2.5 days after inoculation. Our tests indicated that nucleic acid, isolated from diseased insect tissue, can provide inoculum for infecting cell cultures. Infectious DNA was isolated from *B. mori* NPV (Onodera *et al.*, 1965) and tissues of infected *B. mori* larvae (Dobrovol's'ka *et al.*, 1965). Infectious RNA was isolated from *B. mori* CPV and midgut epithelium of infected larvae (Kawase and Miyajima, 1968). Himeno *et al.* (1967) reported that viral DNA from *B. mori* NPV initiated inclusion body formation in a cell line derived from human amnionic tissue; however, similar tests with *Heliothis* virus in four primate lines (one monkey, three man) were unsuccessful (Ignoffo, 1968b).

Incubation periods of 1-14 days were reported following viral inoculation of insect cells. Inclusion bodies of *B. mori* NPV formed in *B. mori* ovarian tissue 1-4 days after inoculation. Only 1-4 PIB/nucleus (seven maximum) were formed. This is the lowest of any virus-cell system studied to date (Gaw *et al.*, 1959; Vago and Chastang, 1960; Vaughn and Faulkner, 1963). Cultured hemocytes of *P. saucia*, infected with *P. saucia* NPV, produce 50 PIB/cell five days after infection (Martigoni and Scallion, 1961). Cultured tussock moth ovaries produced 10-20 PIB/cell seven days postinfection (Grace, 1958c). Ovarian tissue of *A. eucalypti* produced CPV again, presumably a latent CPV, after subjecting the cultures to *B. mori* NPV. Based upon PIB counts in published photographs the cytoplasm of infected cells contained 300-500 PIB/cell (Grace, 1962b). Generally, cultured cells produce fewer PIB/infected cell than than cells in living insects (Vago and Bergoin, 1963). In our experience less than 10% of the cell populations of a given culture is ever infected. Mammalian cell lines generally yield 1-30 x 10^3 virions (DNA or RNA)/cell (Sharp and Kim, 1966; Levy *et al.*, 1966; Spendlove *et al.*, 1966). This yield is an estimated 33-100 PIB/cell based on a mean of 30 DNA or 300 RNA virions/PIB. Progression of NPV infections in primary cell cultures is similar to that observed in whole organisms (Vago and Croissant, 1963). Cytological changes *in vitro* follow those observed in tissues of living insects (Krywienczyk and Sohi, 1967; Martignoni and Scallion, 1961).

SIV multiplication in the *A. eucalypti* cell line was investigated both qualitatively and quantitatively by Bellett and Mercer (1964) and Bellett (1965a, b). Virus antigen appeared in cytoplasm 2-3 days after inoculation when ~90% of the cells were infected. Infectious material was demonstrated in the medium 4.5 days after inoculation. Maximum production of infectious units was reached seven days postinoculation. A yield of 495 infectious units/cell was attained. Grace (1962) reported a CPV increase of 300-fold in *A. eucalypti* ovarian tissues. Trager (1935) obtained a 10,000-fold increase of *B. mori* NPV in ovarian tissue culture, which was comparable to that obtained in whole larvae (Aizawa, 1959). The larval increase, however, occurred within 2-3 days as compared to nine days of tissue culture. Viruses reported propagated in insect explants, tissue or cells are listed in Table VIII.

TABLE VIII

Insect pathogens propagated on insect explants, tissue or dispersed cell substrates

Inclusion viruses	Non-inclusion viruses
Antheraea eucalypti	*Chilo suppressalis*
Antheraea pernyi	*Drosophila melanogaster*
Bombyx mori	*Sericesthis* iridescent
Galleria mellonella	*Tipula* iridescent
Heliothis zea	**Protozoans**
Hemerocampa leucostigma	*Nosema bombycis*
Lymantria dispar	*Nosema mesnili*
Peridroma margaritosa	**Rickettsiae**
Peridroma saucia	*Rickettsiella melolonthae*
Pieris brassicae	*Rickettsiella popilliae*
Samia cynthia walkeri	

2. Protozoa and Rickettsiae Propagation

A protozoan, *Nosema mesnili,* which is a *Pieris brassicae* pathogen, developed in cultured tissues of *P. brassicae* (Sen Gupta, 1964). Larval tissue infected with *N. mesnili* sporozoites and trophozoites, when placed in culture medium, developed spores seven days later. Morphologically, spores produced *in vitro* resembled those developed *in vivo.* Pathogenicity and spore yield were not assessed. A *Nosema* of *B. mori (N. bombycis)* developed in *B. mori* ovarian primary explants, Grace's *A. eucalypti* and *A. aegypti* cell lines, and primary cell cultures of rat, mouse, rabbit and chick embryo (Ishihara, 1968; Ishihara and Sohi, 1966; Kawarabata and Ishihara, 1968; Trager, 1937). Sporulation occurred in all cells except mouse, rabbit, and chick embryo cells. Spores formed in insect cell lines, *B. mori* primary explants and rat embryo primary culture.

Rickettsiae, like sporozoans, are obligate parasites. *Rickettsiella* of beetles, *Melolontha melolontha,* grow in KB, Hep_2, chicken embryo, and rabbit kidney cells. Elements appear in cytoplasm three days after inoculation, accumulate in cytoplasmic vacuoles, but do not form the characteristic crystalloid inclusion bodies observed in living insects. Tissue incubated 10 days produced rickettsiosis when injected into *M. melolontha* larvae. Pathogenicity was retained during three *in vitro* serial passages (Pourquier *et al.,* 1963). *Rickettsiella popilliae,* which replicates in Grace's *A. eucalypti* cell line, morphologically resembles that obtained *in vivo* (Suitor and Paul, 1968).

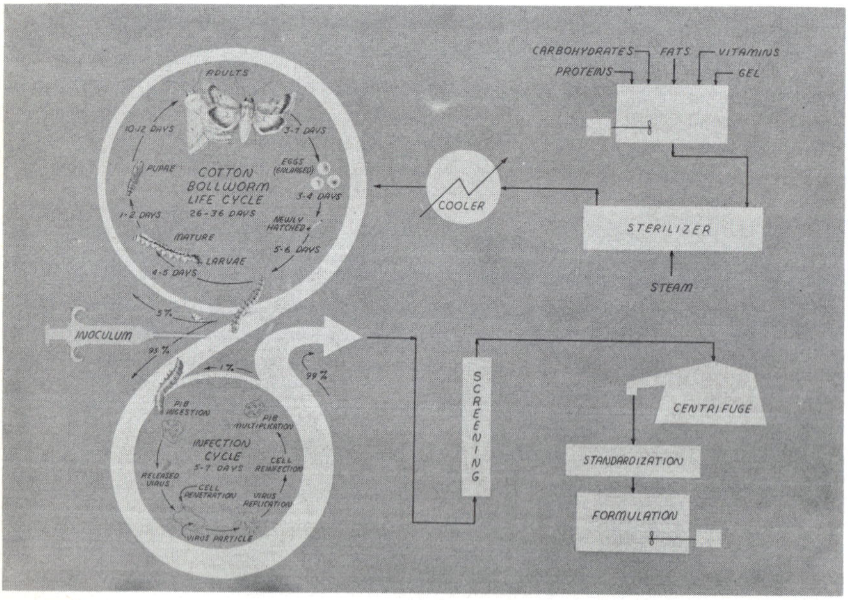

Fig. 1. Schematic representation of the propagation of a nucleopolyhedrosis virus in a living host system.

E. CONCLUSIONS AND RESEARCH

Four goals must be achieved before commercial use of either tissue explants or cell lines can be seriously considered. First, we must develop a prolific tissue or cell line capable of producing large numbers of infectious units quickly. This logically, although not necessarily, presupposes developing a prolific cell line which produces a large number of cells/unit volume. Second, and really concurrently, the cells must be susceptible. Although this appears obvious, it in fact rarely was achieved on a continuous basis even under "pampered" laboratory conditions. Third, the culture media must be simplified either by reducing the number of ingredients to those actually required for growth or through substitution of less expensive natural ingredients for expensive purified chemicals now being used. Fourth, development of a propagation technology and production-plant equipment which permits systematic, continuous, clean and safe propagation.

At present we have barely achieved the first objective, establishment of potential cell lines, and are many years away from developing a propagation technology. We say this not in despair but to challenge others to explore propagation of obligate insect pathogens in tissue or cell culture systems.

References

Abel, P. and Trautner, T. A. (1964). *Z. Verbindungsl.* **95,** 66-72.
Abul-Nasr, S. (1959). *J. Insect Path.* **1,** 112-120.
Adkisson, P. L., Vanderzant, E. S., Bull, D. L. and Allison, W. E. (1960). *J. econ. Ent.* **53,** 759-762.
Aizawa, K. (1959). *J. Insect Path.* **1,** 67-74.
Aizawa, K. (1961). *Entomophaga* **6,** 197-201.
Aizawa, K. and Vago, C. (1959a). *C.r. hebd. Séanc. Acad. Sci., Paris* **249,** 928-930.
Aizawa, K. and Vago, C. (1959b). *Annls Inst. Pasteur, Paris* **96,** 455-460.
Aizawa, K. and Sato, F. (1963). *Annls Épiphyt.* **14,** 125-126.
Anderson, R. F. and Ignoffo, C. M. (1967). "Microbial Technology". Reinhold Publ. Co., New York.
Balch, R. E. and Bird, F. T. (1944). *Scient. Agric. Ottawa* **25,** 65-80.
Baumhover, A. H., Graham, A. J., Hopkins, D. E., Dudley, F. H., New, W. D. and Bushland, R. C. (1955). *J. econ. Ent.* **48,** 462-466.
Bayreuther, K. E. and Romig, W. R. (1964). *Science* **146,** 778-779.
Bellett, A. J. D. (1965a). *Virology* **26,** 127-131.
Bellett, A. J. D. (1965b). *Virology* **26,** 132-141.
Bellett, A. J. D. and Mercer, E. H. (1964). *Virology* **24,** 645-653.
Berger, E. W. (1910). Report of Entomologist, pp. xxxv-xliv. Florida Agric. Expt. Stn.
Berger, E. W. (1921). *Quart. Bull. State Plant Board Florida* **5,** 141-154.
Berger, E. W. (1932). *Proc. Florida State Hort. Soc.* **45,** 131-136.
Biliotti, E., Grison, P. and Martouret, D. (1956). *Entomophaga* **1,** 35-44.
Bird, F. T. (1950). Can. Dom. Dep. Agric. Forest Insect Invest. Bi-Monthly Prog. Rep., Vol. 6, pp. 2-3, Sept.-Oct.
Bird, F. T. and Burk, J. M. (1961). *Can. Ent.* **93,** 228-238.
Bogoyavlensky, C. V. (1922). *Arkh. Russ. Protist Obshch.* **1,** 113-119.
Breny, R. (1951). *Parasitica (Gembloux)* **7,** 118-124.
Briggs, J. D. (1963). *In* "Insect Pathology. An Advanced Treatise" (E. A. Steinhaus, ed.), Vol. 2, pp. 519-548. Academic Press, New York.
Brumpt, E. (1938). *Annls Parasit. hum. comp.* **16,** 153-158.
Bucher, G. E. (1957). *Can. J. Microbiol.* **3,** 695-709.
Bucher, G. E. (1959). *Can. Ent.* **91,** 411-416.

Bucher, G. E. (1961a). *J. Insect Path.* **3,** 439-445.
Bucher, G. E. (1961b). *Can. J. Microbiol.* 7, 641-655.
Burdette, W. J., Hanley, E. W. and Grosch, J. (1968). *Tex. Rep. Biol. Med.* **26,** 173-180.
Burkill, I. H. (1914). *Gardens' Bull. (Singapore)* **1,** 207-208.
Cantwell, G. E., Faust, R. M. and Poole, H. K. (1968). *J. Invertebrate Path.* **10,** 161-162.
Chamber, D. L. and Moffitt, C. (1967). *J. econ. Ent.* **60,** 1748-1749.
Chiu, R. and Black, L. M. (1967). *Nature, Lond.* **215,** 1076-1078.
Chiu, R., Reddy, D. V. R. and Black, L. M. (1966). *Virology* **30,** 562-566.
Clark, E. C. and Thompson, C. G. (1954). *J. econ. Ent.* **47,** 268-272.
Clements, A. N. and Grace, T. D. C. (1967). *J. Insect Physiol.* **13,** 1327-1332.
Couch, J. N. (1968). Proc. Joint U.S.-Japan Semin. Microbial Control Insect Pests, pp. 93-101. U.S.-Japan Committee Sci. Cooperation. Panel 8. Fukuoka.
Couch, J. N. and Umphlett, C. J. (1963). *In* "Insect Pathology. An Advanced Treatise" (E. A. Steinhaus, ed.), Vol. 2, pp. 150-188. Academic Press, New York.
Demal, J. and Leloup, A. M. (1963). *Annls Epiphyt.* **14,** 91-93.
Dickson, R. C., Barnes, M. M. and Turzan, C. L. (1952). *J. econ. Ent.* **45,** 66-68.
Dobrovol's'ka, H. M., Kok, I. P., Smirnova, I. A. and Chistyakova, A. V. (1965). *Mykrobiol Zh.* **27,** 73-75.
Dustan, A. G. (1923). *Agric. Gaz. Can.* **10,** 16-19.
Dustan, A. G. (1924a). *Ann. Rep. ent. Soc. Ontario* **54,** 63-67.
Dustan, A. G. (1924b). *Proc. Acad. ent. Soc.* **9,** 14-36.
Dustan, A. G. (1924c). *Can. Dep. Agric. Pamph.* **45,** 1-13.
Dustan, A. G. (1927). *J. econ. Ent.* **20,** 68-75.
Dutky, S. R. (1941a). U.S. Patent 2,258,319.
Dutky, S. R. (1941b). *J. econ. Ent.* **34,** 215-216.
Dutky, S. R. (1941c). *J. econ. Ent.* **34,** 217-218.
Dutky, S. R. (1942a). *Bur. Ent. Plant Quarantine* ET-192.
Dutky, S. R. (1942b). U.S. Patent 2,293,890.
Dutky, S. R. (1959). *Adv. appl. Microbiol.* **1,** 175-200.
Dutky, S. R. (1963). *In* "Insect Pathology. An Advanced Treatise" (E. A. Steinhaus, ed.), Vol. 2, pp. 75-115. Academic Press, New York.
Dutky, S. R. and Gooden, E. L. (1952). *J. Bacteriol.* **63,** 743-750.
Earle, N. W., Gaines, R. C. and Roussel, J. S. (1959). *J. econ. Ent.* **52,** 710-712.
Echalier, G. and Ohannessian, A. (1969). *C.r. hebd. Séanc. Acad. Sci., Paris* **268,** 1771-1773.
Edington, D. (1899). *Cape of Good Hope Bacteriological Institute Ann. Rep., 1898,* pp. 9-10, 84-90. Grahamstown, Cape of Good Hope.
Falcon, L. A., Kane, W. R. and Bethell, R. S. (1968). *J. econ. Ent.* **61,** 1208-1213.
Faulkner, P. and Vaughn, J. L. (1965). Proc. XII Int. Congr. Ent., pp. 717-720.
Fawcett, H. S. (1908). Special Study 1, Univ. State Florida.
Finney, G. L., Flanders, S. E. and Smith, H. S. (1947). *Hilgardia* **17,** 437-483.
Forbes, S. A. (1895). *Illinois State Ent. 19th Rep.,* pp. 16-176.
Franz, J. M. (1961). *Ann. Rev. Ent.* **6,** 183-200.
Gast, R. T. and Davich, T. B. (1966). "Insect Colonization and Mass Production". Academic Press, New York and London.
Gast, R. T. and Vardell, H. (1963). *U.S. Dep. Agric., Agric. Research Service,* ARS 33-89.
Gaw, Z., Liu, N. T. and Zia, T. U. (1959). *Acta virol.* **3,** Suppl. 55-60.
Giauffret, A., Quiot, J., Vago, C. and Poutier, F. (1967). *C.r. hebd. Séanc. Acad. Sci., Paris* **265,** 800-803.
Gilmore, J. E. and Munger, F. (1963). *J. Insect Path.* **5,** 141-151.
Giroud, P., Dumas, N. and Hurpin, B. (1958). *C.r. hebd. Séanc. Acad. Sci., Paris* **247,** 2499-2501.
Glass, E. H. (1958). *J. econ. Ent.* **51,** 454-457.
Grace, T. D. C. (1958a). *J. gen. Physiol.* **41,** 1027-1034.
Grace, T. D. C. (1958b). *Aust. J. biol. Sci.* **11,** 407-417.
Grace, T. D. C. (1958c). *Science* **128,** 249-250.
Grace, T. D. C. (1962a). *Nature, Lond.* **195,** 788-789.
Grace, T. D. C. (1962b). *Virology* **18,** 33-42.

Grace, T. D. C. (1966). *Nature, Lond.* **211,** 366-367.
Grace, T. D. C. (1967). *Nature, Lond.* **216,** 613.
Grace, T. D. C. and Brzostowski, H. W. (1966). *J. Insect Physiol.* **12,** 625-633.
Grison, P. (1960). *Z. angew Ent.* 47, 24-31.
Hall, I. M. (1954). *Hilgardia* **22,** 535-565.
Hall, I. M. and Badgley, M. E. (1957). *J. Bacteriol.* **74,** 452-455.
Hall, I. M. and Dunn, P. H. (1958). *J. econ. Ent.* **51,** 296-298.
Heimpel, A. M. (1965). *Wld Rev. Pest. Control* **4,** 150-159.
Heitor, F. (1963). *Annls Épiphyt.* **14,** 213-215.
Heuson, J. C., Coune, A. and Heimann, R. (1967). *Expl Cell Res.* **45,** 351-360.
Himeno, M., Sakai, F., Onodera, K., Nakai, H., Fukada, T. and Kawade, Y. (1967). *Virology* **33,** 507-512.
Hink, W. F. (1970). *Nature, Lond.* **226,** 466-467.
Hink, W. F. and Ignoffo, C. M. (1970). *Expl Cell Res.* **60,** 307-309.
Hirumi, H. and Maramorosch, K. (1963). *Annls Epiphyt.* **14,** 77-79.
Hirumi, H. and Maramorosch, K. (1964a). *Expl Cell Res.* **36,** 625-631.
Hirumi, H. and Maramorosch, K. (1964b). *Contr. Boyce Thompson Inst. Pl. Res.* **22,** 259-268.
Horikawa, M. and Fox, A. S. (1964). *Science* **145,** 1437-1439.
Horikawa, M., Ling, L. and Fox, A. S. (1966). *Nature; Lond.* **210,** 183-185.
Howard, L. O. (1902). U.S.D.A. Yearbook 1901, pp. 459-470.
Huberman, E., Saltzberg, S. and Sachs, L. (1968). *Proc. natn. Acad. Sci. U.S.A.* **59,** 77-82.
Huger, A. (1958). Koll. Arbgr. Insektenpathol. u. mikrobiol. Bekampfung, Paris, France.
Hukuhara, T. and Hashimoto, Y. (1967). *J. Invertebrate Path.* **9,** 278-281.
Hurpin, B. (1960). Abstr. 11th Int. Ent. Kongr. Wien. Austria, 875-880.
Ignoffo, C. M. (1963). *Ann. ent. Soc. Am.* **56,** 178-182.
Ignoffo, C. M. (1964a). *J. Insect Path.* **6,** 318-326.
Ignoffo, C. M. (1964b). *J. Insect Path.* **6,** 237-245.
Ignoffo, C. M. (1965a). *J. Invertebrate Path.* **7,** 217-226.
Ignoffo, C. M. (1965b). *Entomophaga* **10,** 29-40.
Ignoffo, C. M. (1965c). *J. Invertebrate Path.* **7,** 209-216.
Ignoffo, C. M. (1965d). *J. Invertebrate Path.* **7,** 315-319.
Ignoffo, C. M. (1965e). Proc. 1965 Beltwide Cotton Production Mechanization Conf., pp. 26.
Ignoffo, C. M. (1966a). *In* "Insect Colonization and Mass Production" (Carroll N. Smith, ed.), pp. 501-530. Academic Press, New York.
Ignoffo, C. M. (1966b). *J. Invertebrate Path.* **8,** 547-548.
Ignoffo, C. M. (1967). *In* "Insect Pathology and Microbial Control" (P. A. van der Laan, ed.), pp. 91-117. North-Holland Publ. Co., Amsterdam.
Ignoffo, C. M. (1968a). *In* "Current Topics in Microbiology and Immunology" (K. Maramorosch, ed.), Vol. 42, pp. 129-167. Springer-Verlag, Berlin, Heidelberg, New York.
Ignoffo, C. M. (1968b). *Bull. ent. Soc. Am.* **14,** 265-276.
Ignoffo, C. M. and Boening, O. P. (1970). *J. econ. Ent.* **63,** 1696-1697.
Ignoffo, C. M., Chapman, A. J. and Martin, D. F. (1965). *J. Invertebrate Path.* 7 227-235.
Ignoffo, C. M. and Dutky, S. R. (1963). *J. Insect Path.* **5,** 422-426.
Ignoffo, C. M. and Garcia, C. (1965). *J. Invertebrate Path.* **7,** 260-262.
Ignoffo, C. M. and Heimpel, A. M. (1965). *J. Invertebrate Path.* **7,** 329-340.
Ishihara, R. (1968). *J. Invertebrate Path.* **11,** 328.
Ishihara, R. and Sohi, S. S. (1966). *J. Invertebrate Path.* **8,** 538-540.
Jones, B. M. and Cunningham, I. (1960). *Nature, Lond.* **187,** 1072-1074.
Kawarabata, T. and Ishihara, R. (1968). Abstract, Proc. Soc. Invertebrate Path., Coloumbus.
Kawase, S. and Miyajima, S. (1968). *J. Invertebrate Path.* **11,** 63-69.
Kitamura, S. (1965). *Kobe J. med. Sci.* **11,** 23-30.
Knipling, E. F. (1955). *J. econ. Ent.* **48,** 459-462.
Knipling, E. F. (1959). *Science* **130,** 902-904.

Koyama, R. and Katagiri, K. (1967). *Bull. Govt. Forest exp. Stn.* **207,** 1-10.
Koyama, R. and Katagiri, K. (1968). Proc. Joint U.S.-Japan Semin. Microbial Control Insect Pests, pp. 63-69. U.S.-Japan Committee Sci. Cooperation. Panel 8. Fukuoka.
Koyama, R., Katagiri, K., Iwata, Z., Kushida, T., Kimura, S., Yanbe, T., Kondo, H., Kaminaga, S., Ibata, K. and Matsueda, A. (1966). *Trans. 77th Japanese Forest Soc.,* 359-374. (In Japanese.)
Krieg, A. (1955). *Naturwissenschaften* **42,** 609-610.
Krieg, A. (1958a). *Z. Naturforsch.* **13,** 374-379.
Krieg, A. (1958b). *Z. Naturforsch.* **13,** 555-557.
Krieg, A. (1961). "Grundlagen der Insektenpathologie. Viren-, Rickettsien- und Bakterien-Infektionen". Steinkopff, Darmstadt, Germany.
Krieg, A. (1963). *In* "Insect Pathology. An Advanced Treatise" (E. A. Steinhaus, ed.), Vol. 1, pp. 577-617. Academic Press, New York.
Krywienczyk, J. and Sohi, S. S. (1967). *J. Invertebrate Path.* **9,** 568-570.
Laird, M. (1959). *Ecology* **40,** 218.
Laird, M. (1960). *Am. Inst. Biol. Sci., Tech. Report* 84-92.
Laird, M. (1966). *World Health Organization Chronicle* **21,** 18-26.
Landureau, J. C. (1966). *Expl Cell Res.* **41,** 545-556.
Landureau, J. C. (1968). *Expl Cell Res.* **50,** 323-337.
Lender, T. and Duveau-Hagege, J. (1963). *Annls Épiphyt.* **14,** 81-89.
Lesseps, R. J. (1965). *Science* **148,** 502-503.
Levy, J. P., Silvestre, D., Leclerc, J. C. and Boiron, M. (1966). *Virology* **29,** 681-683.
Lewis, F. B. (1960). Northeastern Forest Exp. Stn. Forest Research Note 109, pp. 1-8.
Lipa, J. J. (1963). *In* "Insect Pathology. An Advanced Treatise" (E. A. Steinhaus, ed.), Vol. 2, pp. 335-361. Academic Press, New York.
Mandin, J., Giran, F. and Vago, C. (1967). *Entomophaga* **12,** 295-301.
Marks, E. P. and Reinecke, J. P. (1965). *Gen. comp. Endocr.* **5,** 241-247.
Martignoni, M. E. (1964). *In* "Biological Control of Insect Pests and Weeds" (P. H. DeBach, ed.), pp. 579-609. Reinhold Publ. Co., New York.
Martignoni, M. E. (1967). Pacific Northwest Forest and Range Experiment Station Rep. U.S.D.A. Forest Service, February, 1967. Corvallis, Oregon, U.S.A.
Martignoni, M. E. and Auer, C. (1957). *Mitt. Schweiz. Zentanst. Forstl. Versuchsw.* **33,** 73-93.
Martignoni, M. E. and Scallion, R. J. (1961). *Nature, Lond.* **190,** 1133-1134.
Martignoni, M. E., Zitcer, E. M. and Wagner, R. P. (1958). *Nature, Lond.* **128,** 360-361.
Martin, B. and Junko, N. (1967). *Biochem. Z.* **346,** 491-495.
Martouret, D. and Dusaussoy, G. (1959). *Entomophaga* **4,** 253-259.
McEwen, F. L. and Hervey, G. E. R. (1958). *J. econ. Ent.* **51,** 626-631.
McEwen, F. L. and Hervey, G. E. R. (1959). *J. Insect Path.* **1,** 86-94.
Medvedeva, N. B. (1959). (Transl. from Russian.) *Probl. Virol.* **4,** 64-71.
Miciarelli, A., Sbrenna, G. and Colombo, G. (1967). *Experientia* **23,** 64-66.
Micks, D. W., Julian, S. R., Jr., Ferguson, M. J. and Duncan, D. (1961). *J. Insect Path.* **3,** 120-128.
Miloserdova, V. D. (1965). (In Russian, English summary.) *Vop. Virus* **10,** 417-420.
Mitsuhashi, J. (1967a). *Nature, Lond.* **215,** 863-864.
Mitsuhashi, J. (1967b). *J. Invertebrate Path.* **9,** 432-434.
Mitsuhashi, J. and Maramorosch, K. (1964). *Contr. Boyce Thompson Inst. Pl. Res.* **22,** 435-460.
Müller-Kögler, E. (1965). "Pilzkrankheiten bei Insekten". Paul Parey, Berlin.
Munger, F. and Gilmore, J. E. (1960). *J. econ. Ent.* **53,** 964-966.
Nagle, S. C., Crothers, W. C. and Hall, N. L. (1967). *Appl. Microbiol.* **15,** 1497-1498.
Neumayer, J., Gibbons, D. and Trask, H. (1969). Chemical Week Report, April 12, 1969.
Niklas, O. F. (1960). Mitt. biol. Bundesanstalt Land-u Fortwirtsch., No. 101, 60 pp. Berlin-Dahlem.
Oberlander, H. and Fulco, L. (1967). *Nature, Lond.* **216,** 1140-1141.
Odell, T. M. and Rollinson, W. D. (1966). *J. econ. Ent.* **59,** 741-742.
Ohanessian, A. and Echalier, G. (1967). *Nature, Lond.* **213,** 1049-1050.

Onodera, K., Komano, T., Himeno, M. and Sakai, F. (1965). *J. molec. Biol.* **13,** 532-539.
Ossowski, L. L. J. (1957). *Ann. appl. Biol.* **45,** 81-89.
Peleg, J. (1966). *Experientia* **22,** 555-558.
Peleg, J. (1968). *Virology* **35,** 617-619.
Ponsen, M. B. (1966). *Meded. Rijksfaculteit Land. Wetenschappen Gent,* **31,** 553-557.
Ponsen, M. B. and DeJong, D. J. (1964). *Entomophaga* **9,** 253-255.
Pourquier, M., Mandin, J. and Vago, C. (1963). *Annls Épiphyt.* **14,** 193-197.
Puck, T. T., Waldren, C. A. and Jones, C. (1968). *Proc. natn. Acad. Sci. U.S.A.* **59,** 192-199.
Raimondi, G. R. and Ghini, C. (1963). *Annls Épiphyt.* **14,** 153-159.
Richmond, C. A. and Ignoffo, C. M. (1964). *J. econ. Ent.* **57,** 503-505.
Rollinson, W. D., Hubbard, H. B. and Lewis, F. B. *J. econ. Ent.* **62.** (In press.)
Rollinson, W. D. and Lewis, F. B. (1962). Northeastern Forest Expt. Stat. Forest Research Note 130, pp. 1-6.
Rollinson, W. D., Lewis, F. B. and Waters, W. E. (1965). *J. Invertebrate Path.* **7,** 515-517.
Schneider, I. (1964). *J. exp. Zool.* **156,** 91-104.
Schneider, I. (1969). *J. Cell Biol.* **42,** 603.
Seecof, R. L. and Unanue, R. L. (1968). *Expl Cell Res.* **50,** 654-660.
Sen Gupta, K. (1961). *Folia biol.* **7,** 400-408.
Sen Gupta, K. (1963). *Indian J. exp. Biol.* **1,** 222-224.
Sen Gupta, K. (1964). *Curr. Sci.* **33,** 407-408.
Shands, W. A., Simpson, G. W. and Hall, I. M. (1963). Maine Agricultural Expt. Bull. Tech. Series F6.
Shands, W. A., Thompson, C. G., Simpson, G. W. and Wave, H. E. (1958). *J. econ. Ent.* **51,** 184-186.
Shapiro, M. and Ignoffo, C. M. (1969). *J. Invertebrate Path.* **14,** 130-134.
Sharp, D. G. and Kim, K. S. (1966). *Virology* **29,** 359-366.
Shaw, J. G., Moffitt, C. and Scriven, G. T. (1967). *J. econ. Ent.* **60,** 1751-1752.
Singh, K. R. P. (1967). *Curr. Sci.* **36,** 506-508.
Smirnoff, W. A. (1961). *J. Insect Path.* **3,** 29-46.
Smirnoff, W. A. (1964). Forestry Chronicle **40,** 187-194.
Smirnoff, W. A. (1966). *J. Invertebrate Path.* **8,** 360-364.
Smirnoff, W A., Fettes, J. J. and Haliburton, W. (1962). *Can. Ent.* **94,** 477-486.
Smith, K. M. (1967). "Insect Virology". Academic Press, New York.
Smith, K. M., Hills, G. H. and Rivers, C. F. (1961). *Virology* **13,** 233-241.
Snow, F. H. (1895). 4th Ann. Rep. Dir. Univ. Kansas, 1894, 46 pp.
Sohi S. S. (1968a). *Can. J. Zool.* **46,** 11-13.
Sohi, S. S. (1969). *Can. J. Microbiol.* **15,** 1197-1200.
Sohi, S. S. and Smith, C. (1970). *Can. J. Zool.* 48, 427-432.
Speare, A. T. and Colley, R. H. (1912). "The Artificial Use of the Brown-tail Fungus in Massachusetts, with Practical Suggestions for Private Experiment, and a Brief Note on a Fungous Disease of the Gypsy Caterpillar", 29 pp. Wright & Potter, Boston.
Spendlove, R. S., Leunette, E. H., Knight, C. O. and Chin, J. N. (1966). *J. Bacteriol.* **92,** 1036-1040.
Stairs, G. R. and Bird, F. T. (1966). *Can. Ent.* **97,** 411-416.
Stanley, M. S. M. and Vaughn, J. L. (1968). *Ann. ent. Soc. Am.* **61,** 1067-1072.
Steiner, L. F., Harris, E. J., Mitchell, W. C., Fujimoto, M. S. and Christenson, L. D. (1965). *J. econ. Ent.* **58,** 519-522.
Steinhaus, E. A. (1942). *Public Hlth Rep.* (U.S.) **57,** 1375-1377.
Steinhaus, E. A. (1949). "Principles of Insect Pathology", 757 pp. McGraw-Hill, New York.
Steinhaus, E. A. (1951). *Hilgardia* **20,** 629-678.
Steinhaus, E. A. and Thompson, C. G. (1949). *J. econ. Ent.* **42,** 301-305.
Suitor, E. C. and Paul, F. (1968). *Abstract, Proc. Soc. Invertebrate Path., Columbus.*
Sweet, B. H. and Dupree, L. T. (1968). *Mosquito News* **28,** 368-373.
Tanada, Y. (1956). *Hawaii Farm Sci.* **4,** 6-7.
Taylor, A. B. and King, R. L. (1937). *Trans. Am. microscop. Soc.* **56,** 172.
Thomas, J. A. and Johnson, M. J. (1967). *J. natn. Cancer Inst.* **39,** 337-345.
Trager, W. (1935). *J. exp. Med.* **61,** 501-513.

Trager, W. (1937). *J. Parasit.* **23,** 226.
Vago, C. (1957). *C.r. hebd. Séanc. Acad. Sci., Paris* **245,** 2115-2117.
Vago, C. (1967). *In* "Methods in Virology" (K. Maramorosch and H. Koprowski, eds), Vol. 1, pp. 567-602. Academic Press, New York.
Vago, C. and Atger, P. (1961). *Entomophaga* **6,** 53-56.
Vago, C. and Bergoin, M. (1963). *Entomophaga* **8,** 253-261.
Vago, C. and Cayrol, R. (1955). *Annls Inst. natl. Rech. Agron. Ser. C. Annls Épiphyt.* **6,** 421-432.
Vago, C. and Chastang, S. (1958). *Experientia* **14,** 110-111.
Vago, C. and Chastang, S. (1960). *C.r. hebd. Séanc. Acad. Sci., Paris* **251,** 903-905.
Vago, C. and Chastang, S. (1962a). *Entomophaga* **7,** 175-179.
Vago, C. and Chastang, S. (1962b). *C.r. hebd. Séanc. Acad. Sci., Paris* **255,** 3226-3228.
Vago, C. and Croissant, O. (1963). *Annls Épiphyt.* **14,** 43-51.
Vago, C. and Luciani, J. (1965). *Experientia* **21,** 393-394.
Vago, C. and Martaja, R. (1963). *C.r. hebd. Séanc. Acad. Sci., Paris* **256,** 1045-1047.
Vago, C., Quiot, J. and Luciani, J. (1966). *C.r. hebd. Séanc. Acad. Sci., Paris* **263,** 799-800.
Vanderzant, E. S. and Davich, T. B. (1958). *J. econ. Ent.* **51,** 288-291.
Vaughn, J. L. and Faulkner, P. (1963). *Virology* **20,** 484-489.
Weiser, J. (1957). *Ceskoslov. parasitol.* **4,** 359-367.
Weiser, J. (1961). Monograph. *Angew. Ent.* **17,** 1-149.
Weiser, J. (1963). *In* "Insect Pathology. An Advanced Treatise" (E. A. Steinhaus, ed.), Vol. 2, pp. 291-334. Academic Press, New York.
Weiser, J. (1966). "Nemoci Hmyzu" (Diseases of Insects), 554 pp. Academia, Praha.
White, A. A. (1967). *Proc. Soc. exp. Biol. Med.* **126,** 588-591.
White, R. T. and Dutky, S. R. (1940). *J. econ. Ent.* **33,** 306.
White, R. T. and Dutky, S. R. (1942). *J. econ. Ent.* **35,** 679-682.
White, R. T. and McCabe, P. J. (1943). U.S. Dep. Agric. Bur. Ent. Plant Quarantine E-605, pp. 1-7.
Williams, R. C. and Backus, R. C. (1949). *J. Am. chem. Soc.* **71,** 4052-4057.
Willie, H. and Martignoni, M. E. (1952). *Z. Allgem. Pathol. u. Bakteriol.* **15,** 470-474.
Wyatt, S. S. (1956). *J. gen. Physiol.* **39,** 841-852.
Yunker, C. E., Vaughn, J. L. and Coryy, J. (1967). *Science* **155,** 1565-1566.
Zimmack, H. L., Arbuthnot, K. D. and Brindley, T. A. (1954). *J. econ. Ent.* **47,** 641-645.

CHAPTER 26

Economics of Microbial Control

H. T. DULMAGE

Entomology Research Division, Agricultural Research Service, U.S. Department of Agriculture, Brownsville, Texas, U.S.A.

I. Introduction

About 2000 insect pathogens have now been isolated, and we have learned that some of them can supplement or replace chemicals in the control of insects. Researchers are meanwhile searching for other pathogens that might be used in insect control. However, except for a few private and confidential studies by industry, the costs of the production and application of these organisms have not been investigated. Consequently, we still do not have sufficient knowledge of the economic potential of microbial insect control. It is elementary to state, yet easy to forget, that the most effective microbial agent will find little use if it is too expensive to apply, i.e. if the returns from its use are not commensurate with the investment necessary for its development.

This is not to say that because of insufficient knowledge about the economics of microbial insect control the prospects are discouraging. They are not. Indeed, what we do know about the production of microbial control agents and the control they achieve should make us optimistic about the future, though most of them at present are still too expensive for widespread application. I do not think this situation will continue; I believe we can have real hope that the use of pathogens will offer an economic means of controlling insects. In this chapter, I shall attempt to discuss the current costs of microbial pathogens and to make some predictions about the future of this method of control.

II. Economics of the Development of a Microbial Insecticide

A. CONTRIBUTIONS OF UNIVERSITY AND GOVERNMENT AGENCIES

The financial risks involved in the complete development of a microbial insecticide would be too high for a private company to undertake if much of the essential basic research were not being done by university and government agencies throughout the world, particularly in Canada, England, France, Germany, The Netherlands, Russia, and the U.S.A. Table I shows the expenditures of the United States Government in 1967 for basic research on pests and pest controls including the pathogens (Anonymous, 1968). Although pathogens are grouped with predators and parasites in the table, it would be

TABLE I

U.S. government-financed research on pests, pesticides, and pest control, 1967 (Anonymous, 1968)

Area of research	Scientific man-years, GS-11 and above[a]	Funding (in thousands of dollars)
Population dynamics	1,038	33,205
Pesticide kinetics	621	11,778
Development of analytical methods	91	3,200
Miscellaneous research other than control	103	1,774
Toxicology, physiology, and behavior of nontarget organisms	144	6,412
Total expenditure on research other than control methods	1,997	56,369
Control methods:		
Discovery and synthesis of chemicals	130	5,483
Field evaluation and methods of application	279	9,385
Mode of action, including resistance in target organisms	59	2,023
Sterilization and physiological alteration	80	3,029
Cultural control, management practices, and physical protection	117	4,323
Chemical attractants, repellents, and other stimulants	74	2,351
Integrated control	35	1,994
Development of resistant host species	275	9,173
Parasites, predators, and pathogens	116	4,749
Total expenditures, all control methods	1,165	42,510
Total, all expenditures	3,162	98,880

[a] GS-11 scientists are considered able to plan and carry out independent research and are the equivalent of a Ph.D. either by training or experience.

reasonable to assume that pathogen research accounted for about one-third to one-half of that joint budget. Thus the U.S. Government spent about $2 million studying insect pathogens and assigned 40-60 senior scientists to these projects. This money was spent primarily in searching for new pathogens and in developing means of producing and utilizing them. This contrasts to the amounts spent by the government for research on chemical pesticides which were largely devoted to evaluating compounds previously synthesized and screened by industry. Thus, the overall expenditures for research were markedly higher for chemical insecticides than for microbial agents, but the expenditures for the development of new products were probably greater for the microbial agents. I would expect this to be true in any country where private industry exists since the study of pathogens is a new and, to a manufacturer, a high risk field which he is reluctant to enter. Governments, therefore, have had to do much of this work.

B. ECONOMICS OF INDUSTRIAL RESEARCH

1. Comparison of Development Costs of Chemical and Microbial Agents

Chemical Week (Anonymous, 1969) estimated that a company must spend between $3 and $6 million to bring a new chemical insecticide to market. These expenditures, of course, include the research on products that for one reason or another fail in the laboratory, in field tests, or on the market: the successful product must pay for them. Table II shows the chances of success and the total cost of research and development for a typical chemical pesticide in 1964. The odds were 1000 : 1 that the new chemical would fail to survive the initial

TABLE II

Cost of research and development (R & D) of a successful chemical pesticide (Anonymous, 1969)

Step	Average cost/ compound	Chance of reaching next step	Cumulative odds	Total R & D cost
	$			$
Synthesis and initial screening	4,000	1 : 100	1 : 100	400,000
Toxicity testing	100,000	1 : 10	1 : 1,000	1,000,000
Field evaluation	400,000	1 : 4	1 : 4,000	1,600,000
Product development	200,000	1 : 2	1 : 8,000	400,000
Process development and pilot plant	200,000	1 : 1.5	1 : 12,000	300,000
Test marketing	200,000	1 : 1.5	1 : 18,000	300,000
Commercialization	1,000,000[a]	1 : 2	1 : 36,000	2,000,000
Totals	2,104,000			6,000,000

[a] This assumes no marketing organization has been established. Otherwise the commercialization step would be reduced to $200,000.

screening and testing for toxicity, and 36 : 1 that it would fail to reach the market even if it survived the preliminary steps.

A company has better odds that a microbial insecticide will survive initial screening and testing for toxicity. Firstly, a considerable amount of prescreening and selection has been done by government agencies; secondly, there is some hope that most microbial insecticides will be harmless to other living things. Thus, the early odds against a pathogen may be as low as 4 : 1; while the remaining odds against reaching the market will again be 36 : 1. These are the odds against the success of a particular *manufacturer*—not a particular *pathogen.* One manufacturer's attempts to develop a pathogen may fail; another may succeed with the same organism. Still, if we take the two estimates, each manufacturer must consider that for every microbial agent he attempts to develop, the odds are 144 : 1 against its successful marketing.

There are three areas in which the costs of research and development of an insect pathogen may be considerably higher than those of a chemical agent: (1) the initial studies which require expensive and time-consuming bioassays; (2) the testing for toxicity which must be very exacting—and expensive—to meet the demands of government agencies who are concerned lest insect pathogens which might persist and multiply in the environment, should be infectious to man; and (3) the field trials which will often have to be extended beyond the normal range due to the specialized requirements of some pathogens. The other research and development costs will be about the same for the two types of agents. Thus, it is more expensive to develop a microbial agent. So, despite better chances of success, the overall costs of the research and development required to put these pathogens on the market may be about the same as those for marketing a chemical.

A similar conclusion was reached by Grison (1967) in a tabulation of the same costs (Table III). The three years that have passed since this table was prepared have shown that the estimated costs for the field trials and toxicological studies were too low. If they are adjusted to the actual cost, the total costs of development of microbial and chemical agents become about equal. This similarity is not at all discouraging.

2. Expenditures for Industrial Research

Manufacturers keep information on their expenditures for research on microbial pathogens confidential. However, it is possible to make reasonable estimates. In the U.S.A., two companies are producing and selling preparations of *Bacillus thuringiensis.* They also do most of the industrial research on insect pathogens. The sizes of their staffs indicate that their expenditures run to no more than $400,000 per year. Research by other companies, both inside the U.S.A. and throughout the world, is limited and probably does not exceed $200,000 per year. Thus, the worldwide total for industrial investigation of

TABLE III

Comparison of the costs of research and development of a chemical or a microbiological insect control agent[a]

Step	Chemical control agent	Microbiological control agent
	$	$
Synthesis and selection	500,000	80,000
Laboratory testing	200,000	480,000
Field trials	300,000	250,000
Toxicological studies	350,000	250,000
License	25,000	25,000
Formulation	80,000	100,000
Product depreciation	450,000	355,000
Equipment and plant depreciation	350,000	270,000
Market studies and demonstration trials	250,000	200,000
Totals	2,505,000	2,010,000

[a] Grison (1967). Data provided by C. M. Ignoffo, International Minerals & Chemicals Corporation, Libertyville, Ill. 60048.

insect control with microbial pathogens probably totals no more than $600,000 per year. This contrasts with the $100 million per year spent by industry in investigating chemical pesticides (Simmonds, 1967).

3. *Validity of Patents*

Firstly any company planning to begin research on insect control with microbial pathogens must consider whether it will have to share its developments with competitors. There is no positive answer, but so much of the preliminary screening of microbial agents is done by public agencies that there is certainly some doubt whether a pathogen itself could be patented. However, companies engaged in antibiotic fermentations often protect themselves by patenting, not the producing organism, but the processes of production and recovery that lead to more economical production of the antibiotic. There is no reason why this type of patent could not be applied to the production of insect pathogens. Thus, patent procedures are probably available by which a company should be able to protect the fruits of its endeavors.

4. *Market Size*

Before a manufacturer can commit any sizeable amount of money to research, he must consider whether the potential sales justify the investment. Obviously, intensive investigation is justified with an agent like *B. thuringiensis* which has the potential of controlling many insects of major economic importance; the available market is large. Similarly, viruses active against major pests have the potential of quantity sales and warrant considerable study. However, a private company cannot justify spending much money experimenting with the production of pathogens that are active only against insects of limited distribution; the return from sales will be too small. As a result such research will probably become the responsibility of governments. However, the means of producing one pathogen will often also apply to others so it may be economically practical for a manufacturer to produce microbial agents with limited market potential once the manufacturing procedures have been established.

III. Cost of Production of Microbial Insecticides

A. BACTERIA AND FUNGI

1. Semi-solid Fermentations

Semi-solid fermentations (Chapter 24) have the advantage of being inexpensive if little or no purification of the end-product is required. Ideally, the final bran-pathogen complex is simply dried, ground, and packaged with a minimum of formulation. Therefore, since the bran base provides a very large proportion of the weight of the final product, the cost of different pathogens will vary little on a *weight* basis. However, the quantity of the product needed per application will vary with the pathogen so the cost of treatments can vary considerably. A common rule of thumb is that the production costs of a dried ground bran material will average 50 cents/lb. Packaging, distribution, and reasonable profits will raise the retail price of such a material to about $2/lb.

2. Deep-tank Fermentations

Although a fermentation in deep tanks is much more expensive than a semi-solid fermentation, it can be controlled much more closely, and its yield potentials are higher, so it is usually necessary to turn to a deep-tank process to improve the potency of a product. Since the product must be recovered from the fermentation beer and formulated, costs vary considerably, depending on the yield of pathogen and the complexity of the recovery.

Actual costs and production figures for deep-tank production of microbial pathogens are not available, though Tables IV and V show the estimated costs for the fermentation and recovery of *B. thuringiensis* by an acetone precipitation process developed by Dulmage *et al.* (1970). The figures are derived from an analysis prepared by Sohns *et al.* (1966) for the recovery of a microbial polymer by methanol precipitation from a deep-tank fermentation; though they are hypothetical and extrapolated from a different fermentation, they are reasonable and illustrate the type of analysis necessary for any deep-tank production of a microbial pathogen. This hypothetical plant would produce base material at a cost of $1.69/lb so the retail price of undiluted base would be

TABLE IV

Hypothetical fixed capital investment for plant producing 800,000 lb B. thuringiensis *base per year by acetone precipitation*[a] *(Sohns* et al., *1966).*

Item		Investment
		$
Land and improvements		25,000
Buildings		210,000
Fermentors (10-15,000 gal; 3-800 gal; 2-90 gal)	341,600	
Accessory fermentation equipment	74,200	
Recovery equipment	193,000	
Other plant equipment	124,600	
Subtotal	733,400	733,400
Installation of equipment		256,000
Piping, wiring, instruments		347,000
Engineering and contracting fees		243,000
Contingencies		200,000
Total hypothetical fixed capital investment		2,015,000

[a]Yield: 10 g base/liter of beer. Operations: 300 days/yr; 24 hr/day.

TABLE V

Hypothetical "cost to make" of B. thuringiensis *base by acetone precipitation (Sohns* et al., *1966)*[a]

Cost item	Cost/lb
	$
Raw materials	0.211
Acetone	0.200
Utilities:	
Steam	0.162
Water	0.032
Electricity	0.138
Labor and supervision	0.300
Maintenance	0.113
Fixed charges	0.294
Miscellaneous factory supplies and expenses	0.017
Charge on working capital	0.018
General plant overhead	0.206
Total "cost to make"	1.691

[a]Yield: 10 g base/liter of beer. Operations: 300 days/yr; 24 hr/day.

about \$7/lb. Since *B. thuringiensis* products currently retail at slightly over \$2/lb and assay about 800 International Units (IU) per mg, the base produced in this fermentation must be active enough to be diluted at least 3.5 times–i.e. it must have a potency in excess of 2800 IU/mg. Thus the potency of the fermentation product will determine the economic feasibility of the process.

B. VIRUSES

1. Production Methods

Viruses are produced only in living tissue. It is tantalizing to speculate about their production in tissue culture, but such a procedure would be prohibitively expensive in the present state of our technology. We must therefore produce virus in living insects, and the cost of producing such insect viruses is closely tied to the rearing cost of the host insect.

2. Costs of Insect Rearing

Although much depends on the yield of virus per larva and the amount of virus needed per application in the field, it is reasonable to assume that total rearing costs of the host must not exceed 0.5-2.0 cents/larva if the production of the virus is to be economically sound. These expenses are highly variable and depend on the cost of the diet, the rearing containers, and the labor involved. Artificial diets generally cost between 25 and 75 cents/liter, and support between 100 and 3500 larvae/liter. Thus diet contributes between 0.02 and 0.75 cent/larva to the rearing cost. Noncannibalistic insects can be grown in simple trays, and the container cost per larva may be as low as 0.01 cent, but cannibalistic insects must be kept separate, and this requirement can raise the cost of the container to 0.75 cent/larva or more. Fortunately, the use of honeycomb-like materials (Roberson and Noble, 1968) promises to reduce the cost of rearing cannibalistic insects to between 0.05 and 0.2 cent/larva. Labor costs depend on the amount of time required for handling the eggs and larvae and also on the size of the egg-producing stock needed. The manpower involved in maintaining a stock culture for the supply of eggs can be considerable if the yield of fertile eggs per adult female is low. Labor costs vary too much to be reported accurately, but they usually fall between 0.3 and 1.0 cent/larva. Mechanization should reduce this cost in the future.

3. Recovery and Formulation Costs

The cost of recovering and formulating viral materials is relatively low because the materials are so highly concentrated that only small amounts of reagents and accessory materials are needed. As long as no great degree of purification is required, these costs should remain under 0.05 cent/larva.

IV. Economics of the Use of Microbial Insect Control Agents

Burges (1964), Heimpel (1965), Franz (1966), and Dulmage (1967) discussed the practical aspects of the use of pathogens for insect control. If the pathogen does not have the capacity to persist in the environment,. the economics are simple because it must then be applied like a chemical. If the use of the pathogen results in satisfactory control and helps to avoid restrictions on insecticidal residues (and if it is cheap enough), it is an economic agent. Sometimes the specificity of the pathogen will still preclude its use—for example, when there is a multivalent infestation with one of the pests insensitive to the control agent. Such a condition might be handled by way of combinations of pathogens, but these would have to be cheap enough to be economically feasible.

Some pathogens have the power of persisting and spreading in the environment. With such agents, even if costs of application are high, the treatment may be a bargain. For example, J. M. Cameron (personal communication) stated that the cost of introducing the virus of the European spruce sawfly, *Gilpinia (Diprion) hercyniae,* probably did not exceed $50,000, but introducing this virus over 15 years ago in an area near Sault Ste. Marie, Canada, appears to have contributed to the control of the pest ever since. Also, Simmonds (1967), who analyzed the economics of the introduction of specific insects as control agents (and these can illustrate the potential of introduced pathogens) reported that the introduction of a lady beetle, *Cryptognatha nodiceps,* on to the island of Principe had controlled the coconut scale, *Aspidiotus destructor,* over the past 10 years; the average benefit in increased crop yields was $169,000/year compared with the $9400 it cost to introduce this predator. Such returns on investment are spectacular and can be expected only with agents that give long-term control; therefore, industry probably cannot be expected to investigate the use of introduced viruses because sales would be low even though the economic benefits would be high. However, the potential value of introduced viruses warrants considerable research on the part of public agencies.

V. The Future

As government regulations on the use of chemical insecticides increase and as insects develop resistance to these chemicals, the need for biological control agents will increase. There is no reason to doubt that the cost of producing insect pathogens will decrease as our technology improves, and there is every reason to hope that these pathogens will come into their own as practical, economical, insect control agents.

References

Anonymous (1968). "A Study of Federally Financed Research on Pests, Pesticides and Pest Control by the Federal Committee on Pest Control". U.S. Government Printing Office, 1968-0-362-075.

Anonymous (1969). *Chemical Week,* **104,** April **26,** 36-38.

Burges, H. D. (1964). *World Crops* 1-8 (Sept.).

Dulmage, H. T. (1967). *In* "Insect Pathology and Microbial Control" (P. A. van der Laan, ed.), pp. 120-124. North-Holland Publ. Co., Amsterdam.

Dulmage, H. T., Correa, J. A. and Martinez, A. J. (1970). *J. Invertebrate Path.* **15**, 15-20.
Franz, J. M. (1966). *Mededelingen Rijksfaculteit Landbouwwetenschappen Gent* **31**, 512-525.
Grison, P. (1967). *Phytiat.-Phytopharm.* **16**, 63-74.
Heimpel, A. M. (1965). *World Rev. Pest Control* **4**, 150-161.
Roberson, J. L. and Noble, L. W. (1968). *J. econ. Ent.* **61**, 331-332.
Simmonds, F. J. (1967). *Jl. R. Soc. Arts* (October) 880-898.
Sohns, V. E., Rogovin, S. P. and Grifin, E. L., Jr. (1966). *U.S. Dep. Agric.* ARS-71-33.

CHAPTER 27

Standardization and Assay of Microbial Insecticides

H. D. BURGES and E. M. THOMSON

Pest Infestation Control Laboratory, Agricultural Research Council, Slough, Bucks, England

I. Introduction

In early attempts to control insects by microbial means, little importance was attached to the measurement of the quantities of pathogen applied because the pathogens were expected to spread naturally. The species, strain or biotype of the organism (Chapter 2) was considered the vital factor. This is still largely true of organisms used as introductions, but when organisms incapable of effective spread are applied as microbial insecticides, measurement of concentration and viability become important. Consequently only microbial insecticides will be considered in this chapter.

The amount of a microbial insecticide that will achieve control depends on the susceptibility of the pest population and the potency of the microbial product. As for chemical insecticides, susceptibility is measured by laboratory and field trials and need not concern us here. Measurement of potency is equivalent to the assessment of the amount of active ingredient in a chemical insecticide. However, microbial insecticides can rarely be measured chemically: other methods are required and will form the subject of this chapter.

Although methods and units suitable for microbial insecticides must be designed primarily to achieve standardization, they should also be agreeable internationally and easy to understand in practice. Standardization can, therefore, be defined as "the adoption of the most appropriate units for the measurement of the insecticidal potency of a pathogenic preparation". It enables a manufacturer to reproduce a product of constant potency and compare its potency with that of other products.

In the early stages of the development of microbial insecticides, it was hoped that counts of viable organisms would suffice, assuming, when toxins were involved, that each organism always produced a constant amount of toxin. However, this proved inadequate, as was clearly demonstrated for the microbial insecticide, *Bacillus thuringiensis* (Krieg, 1965a; Burgerjon, 1965; Vago and Burges, 1964; Burges *et al.*, 1967; Heimpel, 1967). The potency of a preparation can be predicted to a limited extent by carefully controlling the production processes. Some aspects of the potency can be measured by seroassay and maybe eventually by chemical estimation. However, all aspects of potency can be measured together only by bioassay with the insect species to be controlled. But bioassay too has its problems. In the present chapter, all these methods are examined carefully and critically to select the best means of standardization. Due attention will be paid to small technical details because these are likely to govern success or failure in standardization techniques.

II. Prediction of Yield : Quality Control

Careful control of inocula and the production process often enables the yield of a pathogen to be predicted within certain limits. Frequently this is a good first approximation, but it cannot be trusted as the final standardization, because variations may occur at many stages in production.

With *in vitro* production, e.g. that of *B. thuringiensis*, contaminants similar in appearance to the pathogen may dilute the yield, phages may strike in varying degree, or the virulence of the strain may alter. If mild, these abnormalities remain undetected by microscopic checks and counts during the course of production. Different strains may vary in behaviour in the same medium (Burgerjon and Biache, 1967; Conner and Hansen, 1967; Chapter 24). The same strain may behave differently in different media (Rogoff *et al.*, 1969).

With *in vivo* production, at present restricted to insects, host specimens of even size, health, physiology and genetical constitution can be mass-produced by carefully controlled breeding techniques. A predictable disease condition can be obtained by accurate inoculation and so the potency of a pathogenic preparation can be expressed in terms of the number of cadavers it contains. Despite every control, variations arise because neither insect nor pathogen is entirely stable and other diseases may intervene.

It can be concluded that, when quality control is good, yield gives a useful first approximation to the activity of a pathogen preparation, but must be checked by other means.

III. Counts of Pathogenic Organisms and Particles

The basic component in a pathogen preparation is the organism, a count of which gives a measure of the potency of the preparation. This situation may be complicated by the death of some of the organisms, by the aggregation in bundles (e.g. virus polyhedra) or clumps (e.g. spores) of varying size, by crystals of toxin and by water-soluble toxins. Particle counts distinguish toxin crystals, but not live from dead organisms or numbers of organisms in bundles.

In all counts, the first task is to suspend the organisms in buffer, separate them one from another and dilute to a suitable level. A known volume of the suspension is examined microscopically for a particle count or applied to a nutrient medium for a count of viable organisms. A number of counts are averaged and the precision of this estimate is obtained with the help of simple statistics.

A. PREPARATION OF A DILUTE HOMOGENEOUS SUSPENSION

When the preparation is in the form of a dried powder, the first task is to wet and suspend a weighed sample. This is aided by the addition of an anionic detergent as wetting agent (not cationic ones; Norris and Powell, 1961). With both a suspended powder or a preparation already in suspension, the particles or organisms rapidly sink and so thorough stirring is vital between each step.

The next task is to separate the particles or organisms both one from another and from solid impurities. Powders should first be soaked for 30 min. Separation can be accomplished in a blender, homogenizer, sonifier or by shaking with glass beads. With a blender, the efficiency of separation depends largely on the speed of the machine and the duration of treatment. However, besides splitting clumps, the treatment also damages organisms or particles; as a result, there is an optimum duration for the attainment of maximal counts. For instance, Heimpel (in Burges *et al.*, 1967) obtained increasing viable spore counts on blending or sonifying suspensions of powders containing *B. thuringiensis* for up to 5.5 min, after which the counts fell. The count at 5.5 min was 6.7 times the value at 0.5 min. Comparative counts after 1 min blending at different laboratories have been extremely variable (Section III D). Different blenders have different characteristics and also the actual speed of the blades in any one bowl of the bottom drive type varies greatly according to the state of lubrication of the bearings. In the authors' opinion, homogenizing 0.5 g of powder in a ground glass, long-stemmed homogenizer ("Griffith's tube", Baird and Tatlock, Chadwell Heath, England), with 10 slow up and 10 down strokes while rotating the plunger through a half circle 20 times per stroke, gives results most likely to be replicated by different people in different laboratories. These homogenizers are common laboratory equipment, easily obtained. Equivalent treatment in other apparatus is about 5 min in a well-lubricated Waring blender and 1-2 hr shaking with glass beads. Shorter periods should be used for preparations supplied as suspensions or those containing structures more delicate than bacterial spores.

Foam produced by homogenization tends to trap spores and this should be prevented by an antifoam. Neutral buffer should be included in the solution to prevent aggregation of the separated organisms. The wetting agent, and the keeping of suspensions in a compact shape, minimize the retention of organisms by glass surfaces. Since we are considering resistant stages able to withstand physical extremes, none of these ingredients will harm them.

The following solution is widely used and strongly recommended as suspending and diluting liquid: 0.0425 g KH_2PO_4/litre distilled water, adjusted to pH 7.2 with NaOH, with 0.2 ml Triton X-100 wetting agent (Rhom and Haas, Philadelphia) and 0.4 ml Dow Corning Anti-foam A. For plate counts of viable organisms this should be autoclaved at 15 p.s.i. for 25 min in volumes of no more than 250 ml to ensure penetration of heat. Alternatively, for particle counts 0.5% V/V saturated solution of formalin should be added to deter contaminants and immobilize active organisms (Norris and Powell, 1961).

B. COUNTS OF PARTICLES

Particles can be counted microscopically and electronically but, by these methods, it is impossible to count spores and crystals of *B. thuringiensis* in powders which contain a high proportion of debris.

1. Counting Chambers

Of the microscopic methods, a counting chamber is best used when an oil immersion objective is not required. A known volume of suspension is trapped between a thick, precision made, coverglass and a precision ground, square ruled, sunken platform on a slide (dust free!). A concentration of about 10^8 particles/ml is convenient. If excess liquid drains into a well which surrounds the platform, the chamber must be reloaded. The slide is slightly moistened and the coverglass worked down on to it until coloured rings appear, but, despite this, poor adhesion of slip to slide often causes 10-50% extra liquid to be trapped. This is the principal source of error but can be minimized by measuring the real depth at each filling by interferometry (Norris and Powell, 1961). After allowing the particles to settle for 2 min, the average number per small square is found, all particles lying across the top and left lines of each square being included to avoid counting the same particle twice. The number of particles/ml of suspension is calculated from this value. At least 400 particles should be counted, in four lots of 100, setting up the chamber four times to reduce the error due to the imperfect fit of the coverglass. Before each use, the apparatus should be examined microscopically to detect any particles left from previous counts.

Phase contrast and dark field microscopy enable unstained particles to be counted. The former is simpler, but some cells may be invisible. Very high standards of cleanliness are required with the latter. Both are excellent for recognizing refractile bodies, such as bacterial spores and inclusion bodies of viruses, and for distinguishing germinated from dormant bacterial or *Nosema* spores. Live dormant spores cannot be distinguished in this way from spores that have recently died. Unstained refractile particles can often be counted by transmitted light, or particles can be stained by dilute stain (e.g. methylene blue) in the suspending liquid.

Chambers 0.1 mm deep in a thick slide give more accurate results than those, like the Helber, 0.02 mm deep on a thin slide (Cook and Lund, 1962). The short focal length of high power objectives such as x60 may dictate the use of the latter.

2. Counts of Particles in Agar Films

If an oil immersion objective need be used, particles can be counted in an agar film. Equal volumes of suspension and agar solution containing a little indian ink are mixed at 45°C, and about 0.005 ml of the mixture placed on an ordinary slide warmed to 45°C. A cover slip is put on and the agar sets as a film 10-20 μ thick. The average number of particles per field is obtained with the aid of a graticule previously measured against a calibrated slide, or more precisely with an image-splitting eyepiece (Powell and Errington, 1963). The depth of the agar is measured directly with the vernier of the fine adjustment on the microscope by focusing on indian ink particles just above the slide and others just below the cover slip (Weibull, 1960).

3. Counts of Particles in Stained Films

A fixed film can be used when staining is necessary to distinguish the particles, particularly if more than one type of particle is present, and if the oil immersion objective is required. A drop of known volume (e.g. 0.01 ml), from a calibrated pipette (Cook and Yousef, 1956) or a microsyringe, is spread evenly over an area of 1 sq cm on a slide. Particles must not be allowed to settle in a syringe between delivery of drops. The smear is fixed and stained. The average number of particles per field is obtained as with agar films above, care being taken to traverse the width of the smear because the particles are not randomly distributed (Hanks and James, 1940). Other sources of error are the failure of some organisms to stain and the loss of some organisms during fixation and staining. By this method one can also obtain ratios of different organisms or particles, such as spores and crystals of *B. thuringiensis.* An excellent stain combination for the latter is naphthol blue black and carbol fuchsin (Smirnoff, 1962).

4. Electronic Counts

A Coulter counter is expensive, but counts many samples very rapidly, although the samples must be purer than would normally be obtained in industrial microbial insecticides (p. 601). Particles down to 1 μ in diameter are counted and a size distribution can be obtained by counting different size ranges. A convenient sample size is 0.05 ml, containing for instance about 20,000 virus polyhedra, which are counted in 14 sec as they pass at high speed through an aperture. Martignoni and Iwai (1968) give full operational details of 10 repeat counts made in pairs of alternating polarity for each sample.

5. Counts Under the Electron Microscope

Granulosis capsules can be counted under the electron microscope by adding a known number of polystyrene-latex granules and taking a ratio (Williams and Backus, 1949).

C. COUNTS OF VIABLE ORGANISMS

A dilute suspension of viable organisms is applied to a suitable nutrient medium and colonies are allowed to grow; these are counted on the assumption that every viable organism produces a single colony. At present, this method can be used only for bacteria and fungi able to grow *in vitro* on agar-based media. Cell culture monolayers may be used for viruses when monolayers sufficiently continuous to produce readily visible plaques are developed. Live protozoan spores, e.g. those of *Nosema,* could be counted microscopically if an efficient chemical or physical method of germinating all the spores of a sample *in vitro* could be found.

1. Preparation of Suspensions

Before applying a suspension of bacteria or fungi to the medium, it must be diluted to a level that will allow distinct colonies to grow. Suitable steps are 1 : 100, with 1 : 10 for the last two dilutions. Generally the last three dilutions should be plated in quadruplicate. A fresh pipette *must* be used for each dilution. Suspensions must be shaken at least 30 times immediately before pipetting. After filling the pipette the tip should be touched on the side of the flask to remove the liquid on the outside. On delivering the sample the tip should be held about 1 cm above, but never touching, the liquid. With a blow out pipette a second blow, about 3 sec after the first, removes liquid draining to the tip.

Suspensions of bacterial spores should be heat shocked to break dormancy, e.g. 15 min at 65° C. Fungal spores sometimes take a variable time to germinate. Plating on microscope slides enables detection of spores that germinate slowly (Müller-Kögler, 1967). For conidiospores and blastospores of *Beauveria bassiana,* Müller-Kögler and Samšiňáková (1969) recommend the percentage germination after 24 or 36 hr as a standard.

2. Plating

Of a variety of plating procedures, the pour plate is the best for spores of all organisms that form distinct colonies below the surface of a transparent agar medium. One ml of the suspension is pipetted into each petri dish then, before it has begun to dry, about 12 ml of medium at 45° C is added and mixed immediately with six circular, clockwise movements, six anticlockwise, six backwards and forwards, and finally six sideways. The plates are allowed to set and dry, then incubated inverted (overnight at 30° C for *B. thuringiensis*). Colonies on plates bearing between 30 and 300 colonies are counted. Various mechanical counting aids are available (Meynell and Meynell, 1965).

Alternatively, for many fungi, and for bacteria that form suitable colonies best on the agar surface, 0.5 ml of suspension can be spread over well dried plates. Müller-Kögler (1967) describes methods for fungi.

D. PRECISION OF COUNTS OF PARTICLES AND VIABLE ORGANISMS

In counting procedures, there are two types of errors, those inherent in random sampling of a suspension and operational errors. The most important errors are cumulative systematic ones and any that greatly outweigh all others.

In Table I, estimates of precision of 19 examples have been classified: examples mainly involving errors inevitable in random sampling with a reasonable amount of labour (column 2), and those with various systematic or large errors (column 3), e.g. errors caused by differences in equipment and technique used by different operators, or difficulties created by the impurities in commercial microbial insecticides.

Since random sampling is used in all methods of standardization, its effects will be considered first. The numbers of particles, organisms or colonies counted follow the Poisson distribution and, therefore, the standard error (s) due to random sampling is the square root of the total number counted. Seen as a proportion of this total, s decreases rapidly as more are counted, until after about 400 the rate of decrease diminishes to a very low level (Meynell and Meynell, 1965). Thus one should aim to count at least 400. The confidence limits that encompass 95% of replicate counts are ±1.96 s about the observed

TABLE I

Precision and labour involved in different methods of standardizing microbial insecticides. Examples are numbered 1 to 23

Method	95% Confidence limits (as % about the mean)		Man-hours of labour
	Attainable by one operator with a usual amount of labour	Results of several operators or poor single-operator results that could often be improved	
Colony count	(1)90-110 (2)68-138	(12) 76-132 (13) 11-288	(20)1
Particle count in counting chamber	(3)85-115 (4)62-138 (5)77-123	(14) 88-140 (15)133-164 (16) 7-193 (17) 8-295	(21)1.5
Particle count in Coulter counter	(6)99-101 (pure) (7)90-110	(18) 68-132 (range, not limit)	(22)0.5
Bioassay (potency ratios)	(8)84-119 (9)83-120 (10)74-135 (11)66-151	(19) 23-177	(23)5

(1) Based on random (Poisson) error on a count of 400 colonies (p. 599) (Eisenhart and Wilson, 1943).

(2) Limits of mean of four viable spore count plates (Burges *et al.*, 1967) based on *s* within the four replicate plates by one operator on any one day, calculated by analysis of variance (see also p. 600) on 248 plates (Mather, 1964). Average total colonies on the four plates was 819.

(3) Obtained by increasing the random error of a count of 400, i.e. (1) above, by 50% assuming "thc standard error of a [particle] count under the best conditions need be no more than 50% greater than the error due to random sampling" (Norris and Powell, 1961).

(4) Calculated limits of a single count based on variation (analysis of variance) within triplicate microscopic counts of seven nematode cultures (p. 600) (Nash and Fox, 1969).

(5) Using the standard deviation from Table II, last line, as the error value *s* (limits are $\pm t_{14}s$) in finding the limits of one count.

(6) Based on a Coulter count of 75,000 particles of 92.1-98.5% purity (Martignoni and Iwai, 1968).

(7) As (4) from Coulter counts: 1238-18,632 nematodes counted in each replicate.

(8) *B. thuringiensis* assayed with *Trichoplusia ni* on artificial medium, $b = 5$, five doses, 25 larvae/dose. Precision good because of steep slope.

(9) *B. thuringiensis* assayed with *Ephestia kuehniella* (Cavard method; Burges *et al.*, 1967); $b = 2.3$, 100 larvae/dose, five doses. Precision good despite low slope, because large numbers of larvae can be used.

(10) Virus polyhedra assayed with *Heliothis zea* on artificial medium, $b = 1.1$, 200 larvae/dose, five doses. Low slope necessitates the use of many larvae and so a very efficient assay system with artificial media must be used.

(11) Limits of the ED_{50} (not potency ratio, see p. 611) of *Pseudomonas aeruginosa* assayed by injection into grasshoppers, $b = 2.0$, 20 larvae/dose, five doses. Precision poor because of low slope and great variation between assays.

(12) Limits of the mean of two plates (200-400 colonies), surface-inoculated with drops of bacterial suspension (p. 599).

count, e.g. 400 ± 39 or, expressed as a percentage, 100 ± 10% (Table I, example 1). The limits for viable organism counts often agree well with these theoretical values (Eisenhart and Wilson, 1943), although Bucher and Morse (1963) obtained wider limits with *Pseudomonas aeruginosa* due to frequently obtaining less than 400 colonies/count and unaccountable variation between plates (Table I, example 12).

All methods of estimating pathogens involve measurements of the volume of liquid in which the organisms are suspended. The accuracy of pipetting and similar operations depends largely on the individual, whose performance varies from day to day. The most important errors are systematic ones. A systematic 1% error in six decimal dilutions would cause a 6% error in the count in the final dilution. Combining this with a 5% random error on a count of 400 colonies would amount to $\sqrt{5^2 + 6^2} = 7.8\%$. This would increase the corresponding limits from 100 ± 10 (Table I, example 1) to 100 ± 15. However, Snyder (1947) considered that pipetting errors were unlikely to be significant in colony counts, and it seems unlikely that they are important in other types of counts.

It is important to keep a check on variation. Eisenhart and Wilson (1943) give a quick method of testing for deviations from chance variation between replicate plates in routine viable spore counts and this method can also be used with particle counts.

---

(13) As (2) but basing the limits on an *s* that includes variation between operators (p. 600).

(14) and (15) Based on the best and the worst of five series of 5-16 counts, each series with a different operator (p. 600) (Table I in Norris and Powell, 1961, no transformation used). The limits, based on the true volume of suspension in the chamber, are expressed as % of the expected volume to show the systematic error.

(16) Polyhedra counts by 13 operators, Table II, mean limits of lines 1-3.

(17) Limits of an individual count calculated by including the variation between two operators in the error *s* of an analysis of variance using a square root transformation (p 600) (Martignoni and Iwai, 1968).

(18) See p. 601.

(19) Limits of individual potency ratios of three *B. thuringiensis* powders assayed with four assay species (Table III in Burges *et al.*, 1967). Each species involved its own assay technique used at two different laboratories. Small variations in technical details for the same technique at different laboratories combined to give different results and so variation between laboratories was included in the *s* obtained by analysis of variance.

(20) The estimate assumes a supply of clean equipment and undiluted stock solutions on the shelf, used items cleared away but not cleaned, and includes calculation of result. One bacterial preparation measured using four replicate plates (Ignoffo, personal communication).

(21) Assumptions as (20) but includes cleaning the counting chamber. The chamber is loaded four times from the same suspensions, totalling 400 particles counted (Ignoffo, personal communication).

(22) Assumptions as (20). Four pairs of counts are made on the same sample (Martignoni and Iwai, 1968).

(23) Assumptions as (20). Includes breeding stock insects, making media, setting up, reading and calculating results for one series of five concentrations for the standard preparation and a similar series for the test preparation (Ignoffo, personal communication).

With *B. thuringiensis* powders, variation in viable spore counts often considerably exceeded chance variation (Table I, example 2; Burges *et al.*, 1967). However, examination revealed a far more serious effect resulting from the difficulty of distintegrating clumps of spores and fermentation solids (p. 593). Mean counts varied from 8.3×10^9 to 545×10^9 with three *B. thuringiensis* powders plated by 13 different workers in seven different countries, following a standard technique using blenders (Burges *et al.* 1967). By far the greatest variation was that between operators, due probably to the use of different blenders (p. 593). Limits of the mean of four replicate plates were impossibly wide when variation between operators was included in the error (Table I, example 13). This can be improved (p. 594).

With particle counts in counting chambers, the actual volume of a suspension in a chamber is greatly affected by variability in fitting the coverglass (p. 594). Norris and Powell (1961) concluded that, under the best conditions (pp. 593-597), the increase in actual error due to all causes need be no more than 50% of the random error (Table I, example 3). However, they found that, if undetected, it could cause a large, systematic over-estimate (Table I, examples 14 and 15).

With particle counts in chambers, variability may be due to both impurities and operators–including variable fitting of the coverglass. Counts by one individual with nematodes (Table I, example 4, count in an open dish) produced wider limits than those obtained by Norris and Powell (1961) with bacteria under ideal conditions (Table I, example 1), as did 15 counts of virus polyhedra by one operator (Table II; Table I, example 5, count in a chamber). The latter were part of interlaboratory comparisons, organized by Ignoffo, with three dried preparations of a nucleopolyhedrosis virus containing about 85-95% host particulate material and about 5-15% inclusion bodies. Although an attempt was made to standardize the equipment and procedures, individuals for the most part used their own routine procedure. The preparations used were not typical commercial preparations, but laboratory batches where host particulate material was not eliminated. Variation between operators and between laboratories (Table II), produced impossibly wide limits for an individual count (Table I, example 16). In another series of tests, two skilled operators at different laboratories counting the same six impure preparations of virus polyhedra obtained mean counts of 54×10^8 and 23×10^8. In a statistical analysis, using the error term due only to operators, confidence limits for a single count were extremely wide (Table I, example 17). Clearly operator error is demonstrably great and little reliance can be placed on counts until operator performance has been synchronized and steps taken to allow for variable fit of coverglasses etc. (pp. 593-599). Spores, but not crystals, of *B. thuringiensis* in commercial liquid formulations can be counted in chambers using phase contrast microscopy, more accurately than in stained smears, but less accurately than by viable spore count.

TABLE II

Variation in counts of inclusion bodies from dried preparations of a nucleopolyhedrosis virus containing particulate host tissue (Ignoffo, personal communication)

Number of: Operators	Laboratories	Counts (n)	Sample	Mean polyhedra per mg x10^7	Standard deviation	95% confidence limits of an individual count expressed as % of mean[a]
13	many	17	A	8.2	3.6	8 to 192
13	many	17	B	5.5	3.0	−15 to 215
13	many	17	C	8.4	2.9	28 to 172
4	1	5	A	6.9	1.6	35 to 165
4	1	5	B	5.1	1.7	7 to 192
4	1	5	C	8.8	1.2	62 to 138
3	1	3	A	6.1	0.7	50 to 149
3	1	3	B	3.4	1.1	−39 to 239
3	1	3	C	5.2	1.3	−7 to 208
1	1	15	D	2.8	0.3	77 to 123

[a] $\frac{100\,(\text{mean} \pm t_{n-1}\,(\text{standard deviation})}{\text{mean}}$, data not transformed

Crystals in these liquids can be counted only in stained smears, but precision is low. It is impossible to count spores and crystals in powder formulations microscopically.

Large numbers of pure particles, e.g. 75,000, can be counted rapidly and easily with a Coulter counter, thus greatly reducing the limits. Martignoni and Iwai (1968) obtained good results with purified virus polyhedra containing no more than 7.9% of particulate impurities in the same size range as polyhedra (Table I, example 6). With 17.1% of impurities, microscopic counts averaged only 51.4% of corresponding Coulter counts. Expressing 51.4% and the value for the Coulter counts (100%) as percentages of their mean (75.7%) produces an unsatisfactory range of 68-132%, example 18 in Table I, which compares unfavourably with limits down column 2 of the table. However, good results were obtained with immature stages of the nematode, *Neoaplectana carpocapsae* (DD-136), Coulter counts (Table I, example 7) being consistently less variable than visual ones (example 4).

Viewing the subject of precision as a whole, Table I, column 2, shows what can be attained in well controlled systems. Column 3 shows the effect of some important sources of error, which are particularly likely to occur when more than one operator or laboratory are involved.

IV. Seroassay

The amount of crystal in a spore-crystal preparation of *B. thuringiensis* can be determined quantitatively by its reaction with specific antiserum in a gel diffusion test. A full account of this technique, which was developed by H. M. Chapman, W. H. Kingham and J. R. Norris (personal communication), has not been published so will be described here.

A. TECHNIQUE

The test is set up in trays. Each tray contains six rows of seven cups formed by cementing a sheet of perspex (1/8 in thick) to another sheet of perspex (1/16 in thick), perforated with holes 5/8 in in diameter.

The antigen is prepared by suspending a known weight of the spore-crystal preparation in universal buffer. Stock buffer is made by mixing, in order, 125 ml each of 0.4 *M* aqueous solutions of Na_2CO_3, 2-amino-2-methyl-propanol, $NaH_2PO_4 2H_2O$ and citric acid, then 3.4 ml of the reducing agent 2-mercapto-ethanol is added before adjusting the final pH to 10 with 1 *M* NaOH and bringing the volume to 1 litre with distilled water. This stock solution is used at a 1 : 8 dilution. It is important to re-adjust the pH of the buffer after the bacteria are added before shaking overnight to dissolve all the crystal. The antigen is the supernate obtained after centrifuging, and it can be stored frozen.

The antiserum is obtained by injecting rabbits with either suspensions of spores and crystals or alkaline solutions of crystal (Cooksey, 1968).

Antiserum is incorporated into pure agar, e.g. Ion agar No. 2 (Oxoid Ltd.). Equal volumes of 2% (*W/V*) agar in water and double strength universal buffer, pH 10, are mixed at 50°C then 5% (*V/V*) antiserum added with constant stirring. Using a warmed pipette the mixture is then dispensed into the cups in the perspex tray. After cooling, wells 1/8 in in diameter are cut in the centre of the agar discs using a sharp stainless steel tube. The antigen is diluted in an arithmetic series with universal buffer and the wells filled in duplicate by means of a Hamilton syringe, beginning with the most dilute antigen. A standard is run simultaneously. Should the antigen solution overspill any well this must be discarded and another well filled. The tray is incubated for 48 hr in a saturated atmosphere, after which the diameter of the outermost precipitin rings can be measured. If different numbers of rings are formed in standard and test material, a homology test should be set up. To do this, wells are cut in agar in a small petri plate, then a central well is filled with antiserum and peripheral wells with the antigens. Rings that link, and these may not always be the outermost ones, are the rings to be measured.

The rings are most easily measured with a micrometer eyepiece in a dissecting microscope. The diameter plotted against the log of the concentration gives a straight line between diameters of 5.7 and 9.6 mm. The antigen concentration of the unknown can be compared with that of the standard by the ratio of the reciprocals of the slopes (Cooksey, 1968). Alternatively, the square of the diameter can be plotted against antigen concentration. This is also a proportional relationship.

B. SIGNIFICANCE OF THE METHOD

The accuracy and reproducibility are very good with pure spore-crystal preparations, but decrease with impurities. We have found the method unsuccessful with a commercial preparation containing a substance to protect the crystal against ultra-violet light, possibly due to a masking effect of this additive. The successful seroassay measures the quantity of crystal in a spore-crystal mixture in arbitrary units of one of its antigenic components. The units can be calibrated in terms of weight of intact crystal by testing against an antigen solution containing a known weight of pure crystal. Successive batches of antiserum must be recalibrated.

The seroassay can also give an indirect measurement of pathogenicity in special cases. The serounits can be calibrated against bioassay data where the same strain of bacterium is used against an insect sensitive to the crystal alone, e.g. *Pieris brassicae* and *Bombyx mori.* The relationship is strictly limited to such cases. If the spore plays any role in pathogenicity, seroassay and bioassay cannot be correlated in this way. Where comparison is to be made, care should be taken to breed the insects for bioassay under carefully controlled conditions because some gut bacteria prevalent in sub-optimal breeding conditions may kill larvae stressed by eating doses of crystal normally sub-lethal (Rogers, 1967; White, 1968).

V. Bioassay

The potency of a microbial insecticide depends on an ensemble of factors, the combined effect of which can be measured comprehensively by only one sensitive instrument, the insect. However, the insect is live, hence variable and complex. Its use to measure the activity of a pathogen–another live, variable, complex entity–inevitably calls for a procedure designed to contend with variation. This is achieved by allowing known numbers of the pathogen to act on suitable numbers of insects. The result is easily distilled to tangible values with the help of graphs and statistics. In practice, variation is minimized by careful control of techniques and conditions: statistics are simplified by approximation until they reach the level of a graph supplemented by a little elementary calculation.

A. THEORY OF BIOASSAY

Basically a number of insects are dosed with the microbial insecticide and an effect is measured. The desired effect in the field is death of the insect, so this is commonly selected in bioassay. It is an all or nothing effect, each insect being classified as alive or dead and the results expressed as percentages of dead insects. Meynell and Meynell (1965), Krieg (1965a, b) and Wiegand (1962, 1968) discuss the use of this effect, and of other effects, such as the time taken to die, which is sometimes more accurate, but more difficult to interpret.

Most information is gained by using a range of doses. Graphing mortality against dose gives an S-shaped curve, which is approximated to a simple straight line by converting mortality to a probit scale and dose to logs. The straight line that fits the points best is a form of average of the results. It can be regarded as an estimate of the true performance of the population of which the insects used were a sample.

The reliability of this estimate is shown by the limits within which the true values are likely to lie with a selected degree of certainty, usually 95%. These are the fiducial limits. Since the range of these limits (Fig. 1) is least at the dose giving 50% mortality, the 50% effective dose or ED_{50} is the most useful value to consider when comparing the activities of different preparations. Since low ED_{50}'s indicate high potencies, some people find it easier to express results as the reciprocal of the ED_{50}, which varies directly with potency. When the ED_{50}

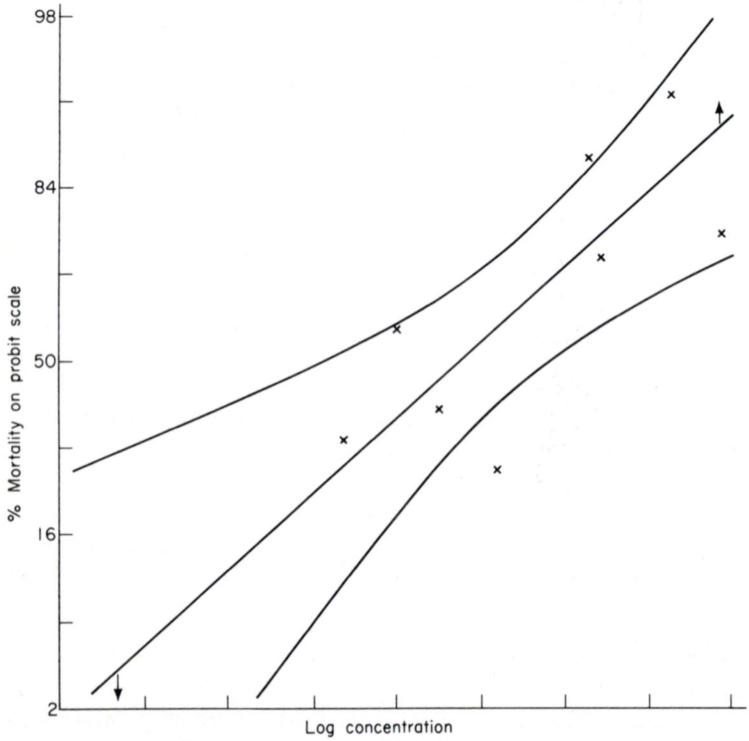

Fig. 1. The fiducial limits (outer lines) of a probit line (adapted from Finney, 1952).

dosage is expressed as concentration of the pathogenic preparation in an artificial insect diet, Dulmage *et al.* (1970) term the reciprocal the "diet dilution unit" (DDU).

Results (ED_{50} or DDU) with the same sample of microbial insecticide may differ with different populations of insects, e.g. those available on successive days. The populations may differ in susceptibility, i.e. position of the line along the dosage axis, and in variability, i.e. slope of the line. Table III shows how these differences largely cancel out when potency ratios are obtained from the ED_{50}'s of a test material and of one particular lot of microbial insecticide designated as a standard and included in the same assay. Thus potency ratios vary much less than the ED_{50}'s from which they are obtained (Sun, 1950; Mechalas and Anderson, 1964; Table III of Chapter 12). By adopting an arbitrary number of potency units for the standard, the potency of the test sample can be expressed in these units (Table III). When the stock of the standard is almost exhausted, a new stock can be calibrated against the original.

TABLE III

Measurement of the potency of two preparations of Bacillus thuringiensis *by bioassay with* Ephestia kuehniella *(Burges, unpublished)*

Assay	ED_{50}[a] standard preparation A	ED_{50}[a] test preparation B	Potency ratio A/B	Potency units[b] (*E. kuehniella*: standard A)	95% fiducial limits
1	31.6	46.8	0.676	676	490 to 934
2	100.5	832.0	0.126	126	37 to 427
3	23.4	100.0	0.234	234	154 to 356
4	38.0	85.2	0.447	447	339 to 589
			Weighted mean	345	170 to 701

[a] ED_{50} = dose causing 50% mortality.
[b] Adopting an arbitrary number of potency units for the standard = 1000.

The lines and their slopes for standard and test preparations vary proportionately in different batches of insects only if the modes of action of the preparations are identical, i.e. the standard must be homologous. Thus a chemical insecticide would be a poor standard for comparison with a pathogen. A strain of pathogen in the test preparation different from that in the standard–partial homology–is less satisfactory than the same strains in both–true homology (Burges, 1967; Fig. 1 in Chapter 13).

Only organisms which store well, without loss of viability, and formulations offering the best storage properties should be used as standards. With *B. thuringiensis*, a powder, stored dry (no more than 8% moisture) at a low humidity and about 5°C in the dark, should have an almost indefinite life. This pioneer among microbial insecticides was the first to have an agreed international standard, E61, as a result of co-operative work between 21 laboratories (Burges *et al.*, 1967; Dulmage, 1970).

B. PRACTICAL ASPECTS OF BIOASSAY TECHNIQUE

Recent experience in the bioassay of pathogens has indicated some ways of obtaining less variable results more easily.

A key factor in the reduction of variation is careful control of the physiological state of the insects, by controlling both the conditions in which they are bred and those during exposure to the pathogen. Food, temperature, humidity, population density and sometimes day length are important during breeding. The size of larvae is usually standardized by choosing those of the same age in precisely controlled breeding conditions. The larvae of some species, e.g. the wax moth, *Galleria mellonella,* grow at very different rates–even the offspring of one mother–despite rigidly controlled conditions. With such species, equal sized larvae of known age must be selected either visually or by weight. The labour involved in weighing is sometimes worth while, because it shows the dose of pathogen/g insect body weight.

The route of infection by the pathogen in the assay should be the same as that in the field. Injection of pathogens into the insect body cavity is useless for standardization of microbial insecticides.

The developmental stage most severely attacked by the pathogen is usually best for assay purposes. With larvae, the youngest that can be handled with low natural mortality should be chosen. Eggs are often easily handled, e.g. approximate numbers of newly-laid eggs of *Ephestia (Anagasta) kuehniella* are placed on a layer of dried flour paste containing the pathogen, so that larvae are exposed to the pathogen from hatching and, later, survivors and dead bodies are easily and accurately counted (Burgerjon and Yamvrias, 1959; Cavard in Burges *et al.*, 1967).

A number of criteria give measures of potency very similar, but more consistent than, those obtained using mortality. For instance, in the assay of *B. thuringiensis*, one may use paralysis of silkworms (Angus, 1967; Angus and Norris, 1968) and photometric measurement of the food eaten by *Pieris brassicae* caterpillars (Burgerjon, 1962).

With the peroral route of infection, the dose acquired by each insect depends on the amount of food eaten. Appetite at different times in the instar varies enormously (Burges, 1960). Ideally larvae should be used at the same time after moulting, but as this is usually impracticable, at least those in recognizable pre- and post-moult conditions should be discarded. Pendleton (1969) found that instar III larvae of *Philosamia cynthia* var. *ricini* changed in colour from green to white 2-3 days after the moult at a very constant weight (58-62 mg each). The appetite of larvae of *P. brassicae* varied even when measured at a constant time following a moult, variability in the proportions of leaf discs eaten by individual larvae in eight batches ranging from 40 ± 10 to 11 ± 10 (mean % ± S.E.).

A period of starvation before exposure is incorporated in some techniques, but opinion of the value of this practice varies. Starvation increases susceptibility to *B. thuringiensis* (Angus, 1956; Rogers, 1967) and it ensures that all larvae feed, but it does not reduce variation in appetites (Rogers, 1967).

The condition of the food affects the amount that insects eat. Leaves should always be fresh and of even thickness (Burgerjon, 1962). Golebiowska (in Burges *et al.*, 1967) obtained very different ED_{50}'s for newly-hatched *E. kuehniella* larvae on *B. thuringiensis* powders mixed directly into dry flour, and on the same powders mixed into an aqueous slurry of flour, dried and reground, although these differences largely disappeared in the potency ratios. Artificial media have the advantage of being more easily reproducible than foliage, but the stability of the pathogen in the medium must be checked carefully (Rogers, 1967) and antibiotics or preservatives omitted if they affect the pathogen. These media can be used in highly efficient automated systems where large numbers of larvae must be kept singly, e.g. *Heliothis zea.*

It is essential to apply the microbial insecticide evenly to the insect's food. The same precautions as when preparing suspensions of pathogens for counting are needed (Section III A). When a syringe is used to dispense drops, settling of particles must be avoided, e.g. by magnetic stirring in the syringe (Angus 1967). After application to foliage, or other surfaces like beeswax, suspensions should be dried rapidly to avoid deterioration such as might be caused by the germination of spores during tardy drying. Dipping gives good distribution of properly formulated suspensions (Section III A) over finely pubescent foliage if the leaves are shaken after dipping and allowed to dry, petiole downwards, to avoid a drip drying on the tip of each leaf. Fine, non-drenching sprays should be used on smooth waxy leaves, preferably dispensing known volumes in oil in a spray tower (Potter, 1952) or in water in a chamber (Burgerjon, 1956; Rosický and Weiser, 1951). Directional spraying of known volume, for instance with a scent spray, is less satisfactory due to variable bounce of spray droplets hitting the leaves and to a variable amount missing the leaves. Pendleton (1969) found that a small amount of pure agar (0.25%) added to a suspension of pure *B. thuringiensis* crystals enabled the suspension to be spread on leaves and to dry evenly in air at 30°C. Suspensions can be mixed very evenly in an artificial medium that gels on cooling (Splittstoesser and McEwen, 1961) or in the sticky liquid portion of *Galleria* medium, which is then used to coat flakes of baby cereal very evenly (Hoopingarner and Materu, 1964; Burges and Bailey, 1968). The acidicity (pH 4) of the honey in the medium prevents premature germination of *B. thuringiensis* spores. Powders can be mixed evenly into a meal or powdery medium by a combination of pounding in a mortar and mixing in a rotary mixer (Burges, 1964). Suspensions can be sprayed on to a meal while it is being actively stirred, followed by further mixing as described above for powders. Intimate mixing can be obtained in liquids or slurries which may subsequently be dried in thin layers (Burgerjon and Yamvrias, 1959), but some separation or settling may occur during drying.

The problem of the amount of food plus pathogen eaten by the insect is aggravated with *B. thuringiensis* by the crystal causing early paralysis of the buccal region and gut, which prevents further feeding. Rogers (1967) greatly reduced the scatter of his points about a straight line, without altering the slope, by grouping data according to the amount of pathogen actually eaten by each insect, compared with the same data graphed against concentration of pathogen suspension applied to the food. With *Galleria mellonella,* White (1968) found this practice unsuccessful because it greatly lowered the slope.

The amount of pathogen ingested can be measured in various ways. Laan and Geest (personal communication) applied a known quantity of pathogen suspension to small discs of leaf. One disc was given to each larva and those not quickly eating all the food were discarded. In a very good modification of this technique, N. H. E. Gibson and M. Galowalia (personal communication) applied the bacteria, diluted in cabbage juice, to the blunt tips (3 x 4 mm) of small triangles of cabbage leaf. Each dried tip was inserted through a slit in the base of a small plastic dish and was eaten within 5 min by a larva. Larvae will drink a drop of suspension placed by syringe on their mouthparts (Angus, 1967) or larvae can be force-fed by inserting the needle into the buccal cavity (Martouret, 1962; Heimpel, personal communication) or anus (Norris, personal communication). The fact that larvae receive all the dose in one concentrated gulp does not matter for standardization assay. Forced feeding involves a variable degree of shock and any larva that regurgitates the suspension must be discarded. Silkworms physically damaged during forced feeding with bacterial suspensions are readily recognized by rapid discoloration due to septicaemia, or 4000 spores of *Bacillus cereus* per larva added to the inocula of control larvae cause the same effect (Heimpel, personal communication). Rogers *et al.* (1966) added a radioisotope (^{32}P as orthophosphate in dilute HCl) to a suspension applied to discs of leaf. The amount of suspension eaten was estimated from the residual radioactivity on the uneaten leaf. However, Rogers (1967) found that, on drying, the distribution of the dissolved ^{32}P salt on the leaf was different from that of suspended particles. He overcame this by adding 3% polyethylene glycol (Carbowax "6000") to the ^{32}P solution. This substance promotes evenness of drying. White (1968) used a radioisotope in broodcomb for *G. mellonella.* Chauthani (1968) ensured that the whole dose was eaten by covering an artificial medium with a thick layer of molten paraffin wax through which was inserted, before cooling, a glass rod about the diameter of a larva. Later the rod was removed, leaving a hole in the wax, into which was inserted the dose of pathogen. The larva had to eat all the treated part of the medium as it burrowed downwards in the hole.

Some general precautions should be noted. Larvae of some species are cannibalistic, or eat dead bodies, and must be kept singly in cartons, e.g. *Heliothis zea* (Chauthani, 1968) or gelatin capsules 8 mm in diameter and 24 mm long, e.g. *G. mellonella* (Burges and Thomson, unpublished). The exposure period should be minimal to allow the effect to show in most of the insects, since variation tends to increase with time. Systems that allow the insects to walk away from, or fall off, treated food should be avoided. Observation of the effect should be easy. In doubtful cases, death is assumed if the insect fails to respond to touch or, in insects that sham death, to *gentle* warming. Some insects, e.g. *E. kuehniella,* are difficult to find because they burrow, which can be avoided by using a very thin layer of medium (Burgerjon and Yamvrias, 1959). The addition of 10% glycerol makes a mixture of flour and yeast powder suitable for other storage moths and produces better adhesion of the food to glass (Burges, unpublished).

Up to this point, the discussion applies more or less to viruses that form inclusions and bacteria and protozoans that form spores, because these can be transmitted *per os.* The use of fungi has not reached a point where standardization is necessary and, for bioassay, the uncertainty of the relative importance of infection *per os,* through the cuticle and through the spiracles presents problems. Bioassay of fungi is discussed in Chapter 5. At present the best approach is probably to apply spores to the environment of the test insects–food for storage insects, soil for soil-dwelling insects and air for leaf-feeding insects–in conditions (particularly humidity) believed to be optimal for the fungus. Vacuum dusting should be avoided in case release of the vacuum draws spores abnormally into the spiracles. Assays for the exotoxin of *B. thuringiensis* are discussed in Chapter 12.

In designing an assay the number of concentrations, the interval between them and the number of insects must be decided. Initially these decisions depend on how far the activity of the test preparation and the susceptibility of the insects can be predicted. It may be best to conduct a small preliminary assay with widely spaced concentrations, or, alternatively, a large number of concentrations may suffice. In the definitive assay, points nearest to the ED_{50} carry most weight and there should always be at least one point above or below the ED_{50}. Ideally the points should be spaced between 15 and 85% mortality: one must aim at this without undue risk of missing the activity range. A common combination is five concentrations at intervals of x2: insect numbers will be discussed further in Section V D.

For routine purposes, assay results can be assessed in a few minutes by plotting percentage mortality against dosage on logarithmic probability paper for test and standard, and obtaining the potency ratios of the ED_{50}'s. In our experience, the lines in some assays tend to curve at low mortalities, so less weight should be given to these mortalities. Litchfield and Wilcoxon (1949) give a quick approximate method of obtaining the confidence limits of the ED_{50}, potency ratio and slope (including those for heterogeneous data) accurate enough for most purposes (Bucher and Morse, 1963). Limits should always be given in published work.

C. PRECISION OF BIOASSAY

There are no absolute measurements against which the precision of a bioassay can be judged, the only yardstick being the reproducibility of results in a series of identical experiments.

Reproducibility of results expressed as potency ratios hinges on the reproducibility of the ED_{50}'s comprising the ratios. The factors influencing this are revealed by the components in the calculation of the approximate standard error, s, of the log ED_{50}:

$$s = \frac{1}{b\sqrt{n\Sigma w}}$$

where b is the slope of the graph line of probit mortality on log dose, n is the number of larvae at each dose, and Σw is the sum of the weighting coefficients.

The size of Σw depends on the mortalities obtained and is lowest when these are symmetrical about the ED_{50}. In assays with good symmetry, the precision is governed mainly by b and n.

In assays with insect pathogens, b is typically low (Table IV), thus tending towards low precision. The effect of b on the confidence limits of a potency ratio obtained by simultaneous assays with two preparations giving the same slope is given in Fig. 2. From which the precision to be expected by the use of different numbers of insects (n) can also be seen. In Table I, example 8, limits of 84-119 are obtained at a slope of 5, and only 25 larvae/dose. In example 9, 100 larvae/dose must be used to obtain similar precision because the slope is only 2.3. In example 10 with a much lower slope of 1.1, the use of 200 larvae/dose gives much less precision (limits 74-135) and the assay must be replicated three times to increase precision to limits of 85.3-117.1, i.e. near those in examples 8 and 9.

The values in Fig. 2 apply when the mortalities in the assay fit the graph line well. If the mortalities are heterogeneous about the line for either the standard or the test preparation, the confidence limits are widened by the use of a heterogeneity factor in their calculation. This factor is greatest when the number of doses (k) in the assay is least. It is t_{2k-2}: tables of t appear in most statistics books. For example, when $k = 5$, $t_8 = 2.31$, which is used instead of $t_\infty = 1.96$ for homogeneous data as in Fig. 2. The span of the confidence limits of the log potency ratio is thus increased by a factor of 2 (2.31/1.96).

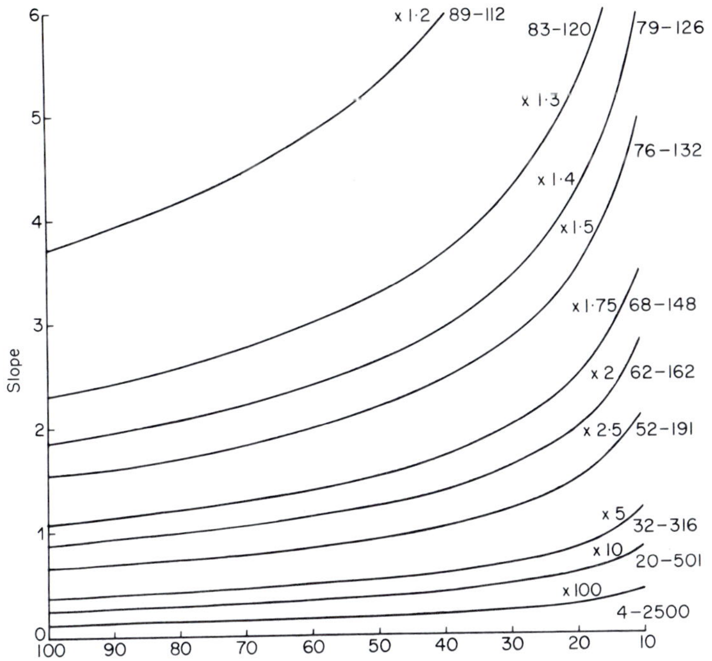

Fig. 2. The effect of slope, and the number of insects used at each of five doses of microbial insecticide, on the confidence limits (right-hand values) of potency ratios and the differences (left-hand values) needed between two potency ratios for significance at the 95% level.

The values in Fig. 2 were intended for results in which the potency ratios of repeated assays do not differ significantly, so that the variation between them can be ignored (Bliss, 1952). The confidence limits of the mean of the successive potency ratios are then much narrower than those for the potency ratio of any one assay. If, however, the differences are significant, the between-assay variation must be incorporated in the calculation of the limits of the mean ratio (Bliss, 1952), which may result in little narrowing of the limits of the mean compared with those calculated for individual ratios. Should this be so, it is of course vital to do more than one assay, because the precision of a single assay might give an exaggerated view of the precision of the system. For instance, Bucher and Morse (1963) obtained unavoidable heterogeneity between eight assays of *Pseudomonas aeruginosa* with grasshoppers, resulting in limits of the mean potency of 66-151% of the ED_{50} for the whole series (Table I, example 11). These limits would have been 71-140% if the assays had been homogeneous. In this example limits of the ED_{50} are quoted instead of those for a potency ratio because a *Pseudomonas* preparation cannot be stored as a standard. In an extensive series of assays with *B. thuringiensis*, heterogeneity between assays

TABLE IV

Slope, b, *in assays with insect pathogens*

Pathogen	*b*		No. of assays or strains	Host species	Reference
	Mean	Range			
Polyhedrosis virus	1.1	1.1-1.2	3 assays	*Heliothis zea*	Chauthani, 1968
Polyhedrosis virus	1.2	1.0-1.2	2 assays	*Heliothis zea*	Ignoffo, 1965, 1966
Polyhedrosis virus	1.4	–	1 assay	*Heliothis virescens*	Ignoffo, 1966
Polyhedrosis virus	2.1	–	1 assay	*Trichoplusia ni*	Ignoffo, 1964
Polyhedrosis virus	1.1	–	1 assay	*Spodoptera exigua*	Ignoffo, personal communication
Polyhedrosis virus	0.8	–	–	*Bombyx mori*	Bergold, in Bucher, 1958
Polyhedrosis virus	0.9	–	1 assay	*Choristoneura fumiferana*	Bergold, in Bucher, 1958
Polyhedrosis virus	1.0	0.8-1.2	2 assays	*Phryganidia californica*	Martignoni and Schmid, 1961
Granulosis virus	1.0	1.0-1.0	2 assays	*Pieris rapae*	Martignoni and Schmid, 1961
Granulosis virus	1.0	0.5-1.3	3 assays	*Eucosoma griseana*	Martignoni, 1957
Lymphotropha tribolii	1.5	–	3 assays	*Tribolium castaneum*	Ashford, 1967
Nosema locustae	0.8	–	–	*Melanoplus bivittatus*	Bucher, 1958
Nosema oryzaephili	1.3	–	1 assay	*Oryzaephilus surinamensis*	Burges *et al.*, in press
Nosema whitei	1.1	0.8-1.3	5 assays	*Tribolium castaneum*	R. J. Milner, personal communication
Pseudomonas aeruginosa	1.9	1.1-2.7	8 assays	*Melanoplus bivittatus*	Bucher and Morse, 1963
Bacillus popilliae	1.6	–	12 assays	*Popillia japonica*	Beard, in Bucher, 1958
Bacillus larvae	0.8	–	1 assay	*Apis mellifera* larvae	Woodrow, in Bucher, 1958
Bacillus thuringiensis	1.8	1.7-1.8	2 assays	*Trichoplusia ni*	Ignoffo *et al.*, 1968
Bacillus thuringiensis	4.9	–	14 assays	*Trichoplusia ni*	Splittstoesser and McEwen, 1961

Bacillus thuringiensis	2.0	1.4-2.6	8 assays	*Trichoplusia ni*	Hall, in Burges *et al.*, 1967
Bacillus thuringiensis	2.7	1.9-4.2	6 assays	*Trichoplusia ni*	Ignoffo, in Burges *et al.*, 1967
Bacillus thuringiensis	2.0	–	8 assays	*Estigmene acrea*	Mechalas and Anderson, 1964
Bacillus thuringiensis	1.8	1.3-2.2	9 assays	*Estigmene acrea*	Dulmage, in Burges *et al.*, 1967
Bacillus thuringiensis	1.2	0.9-1.4	24 assays	*Ephestia kuehniella*	Golebiowska, in Burges *et al.*, 1967
Bacillus thuringiensis	2.3	1.6-2.8	12 assays	*Ephestia kuehniella*	Cavard, in Burges *et al.*, 1967
Bacillus thuringiensis	3.6	1.8-5.5	11 assays	*Bombyx mori*	Aizawa, in Burges *et al.*, 1967
Bacillus thuringiensis	4.5	3.2-7.9	10 strains	*Bombyx mori*	Angus, personal communication
Bacillus thuringiensis	3.4	–	1 assay	*Bombyx mori*	N. H. E. Gibson and M. Galowalia, personal communication
Bacillus thuringiensis	2.3	1.1-4.8	15 assays	*Galleria mellonella*	Burges, in Burges *et al.*, 1967
Bacillus thuringiensis	2.4	1.9-3.0	3 assays	*Ostrinia nubilalis*	Raun, in Burges *et al.*, 1967
Bacillus thuringiensis	1.7	1.1-2.7	11 assays	*Pieris brassicae*	Burgerjon, in Burges *et al.*, 1967
Bacillus thuringiensis	3.8	3.4-4.4	3 assays	*Pieris brassicae*	N. H. E. Gibson and M. Galowalia, personal communication
Bacillus thuringiensis crystal	2.0	0.7-2.6	10 assays	*Pieris brassicae*	Rogers, 1967
Bacillus thuringiensis crystal	5.5	–	1 assay	*Bombyx mori*	Angus, in Bucher, 1958
Bacillus thuringiensis crystal	3.3	1.4-6.9	11 strains	*Philosamia cynthia*	Pendleton, 1969
Bacillus thuringiensis exotoxin	3.4	3.3-3.6	2 assays	*Musca autumnalis*	Yendol and Miller, 1967
Bacillus thuringiensis exotoxin	1.9	–	–	*Musca domestica*	Table I of Chapter 12
Bacillus thuringiensis exotoxin	4.7	–	–	*Galleria mellonella*	Table I of Chapter 12
Bacillus thuringiensis exotoxin	7.8[a]	–	1 assay	*Drosophila melanogaster*	Benz and Perron, 1967
Bacillus thuringiensis exotoxin	4.3[b]	4.3, 4.3	2 assays	*Drosophila melanogaster*	Benz and Perron, 1967
Bacillus thuringiensis exotoxin	2.0	–	1 assay	*Drosophila melanogaster*	Krieg, 1966

[a]Without yeast.
[b]With yeast.

resulted in widely spaced confidence limits in a number of systems (Burges *et al.*, 1967). Variation in the results from different laboratories caused even wider limits (Table I, example 19).

D. DEVELOPMENT OF A BIOASSAY SYSTEM AND IMPROVING ITS PRECISION

The above considerations show three logical steps in the development of a bioassay system, the trial of technique, establishment of its reproducibility and finally deciding how to make the best use of the system.

Figure 2 has been constructed for easy reference to precision at each step and the rapid methods of Litchfield and Wilcoxon (1949) are recommended for the simple calculation of the essential values (ED_{50} and b). Some people envisage precision most easily in terms of confidence limits and others in terms of sensitivity, i.e. the size of difference between two products that the assay will detect. For the latter, the smallest differences between potency ratios that would be significant at the 5% level have been included in Fig. 2.

1. *Initial Technique*

Reference to Section V B should enable a technique to be selected that will give minimum variation for a reasonable outlay of labour and materials. Initially the technique can be tried with five or more dosages of a single product. As soon as a trial with mortalities reasonably symmetrical about the ED_{50} is obtained, the goodness of fit of points about the graph line can be assessed (Litchfield and Wilcoxon, 1949). If there is heterogeneity, attempts should be made to improve the technique (pp. 606-610), examining such factors as the precision with which the dose reaches individual insects and the possibility of bias–maybe in size or activity–of insects allocated between doses (ideally this allocation should be at random).

At this stage reference to Fig. 2 will show whether enough insects have been used to give the target precision with the value of b obtained in the initial trial. If the slope is low and the amount of work is to be kept within reason, it may be necessary to try to increase the slope by a modification of technique, e.g. change in temperature, age of insect, food, or exposure period. In addition, an examination of factors affecting insect appetite or the evenness of application of the pathogen to the food may be rewarding.

2. *Reproducibility*

The next step is to compare a test sample of the pathogen preparation with another sample designated as standard and to repeat the comparison several times. The slopes (b) for the standard and for the test materials in an assay may differ. The lines for each material should, therefore, be fitted independently of each other, until experience with the system tells whether b varies significantly.

If it does not, parallel lines can be fitted (e.g. Mechalas and Anderson, 1964). Slopes are more likely to vary from one assay to the next, because the batches of insects are different, so lines for successive assays should also be fitted independently until experience has been gained.

If differences between the replicate potency ratios are large, such technical aspects as the reproducibility of assay conditions, physiological state of the insects, possibility of deterioration of the pathogen before it reaches the insect, pH of pathogen suspensions, etc. need examination.

These differences are large enough to warrant such an examination if the standard error of the mean log potency ratio,

$$s_{\overline{M}} = \frac{\sqrt{\Sigma M^2 - (\Sigma M)^2/k}}{k(k-1)}$$

substantially exceeds an estimate of $s_{\overline{M}}$ obtained from the error within the assay,

$$s_{\overline{M}} = \frac{\Sigma(s_M)}{k\sqrt{k}}$$

where M is a log potency ratio, $\overline{M}$ is the mean log potency ratio, Σ indicates summation, and k is the number of potency ratios (Bliss, 1952). Litchfield and Wilcoxon's quick methods do not give the standard errors of log potency ratios (s_M), but these are easily calculated from the fiducial limits of the potency ratios as

$$s_M = \frac{1}{1.96} \log \frac{\text{(upper limit)}}{\text{(potency ratio)}}$$

3. Final Form of the Assay

When the reproducibility of the assay has been found, reference to Fig. 2 will establish the best combination of number of insects and number of replicate assays to use for the standardization of a test microbial insecticide to the required degree of precision.

Since the slope b plays such a key role, it is worth considering how much it can be increased. Of the pathogens in Table IV, all those which are believed to attack by infectivity without producing toxins (i.e. all except *B. thuringiensis*), produced slopes predominantly below 2. Meynell and Meynell (1965) state that b with such pathogens is not likely to exceed 2 because it is believed that the micro-organisms act independently of each other. Thus it is worth expending considerable effort to raise b to 2, but above this level there may be little to gain from major undertakings such as genetically based insect breeding systems. According to Martignoni and Schmid (1961), in those insect species that show cycles of population abundance terminated by virus epizootics, insect populations collected just before an epizootic are likely to give lower slopes than those collected afterwards when the population has become scarce (e.g. slope ranges of

Eucosoma griseana and *Phryganidia californica*, Table IV). Meynell and Meynell (1965) and Bucher (1958) point out that *b* is often high in assays of chemical poisons ($b \simeq 20$), so that values exceeding 2 might be expected in pathogens that produce toxins. In Table IV, the slope for *B. thuringiensis* is predominantly near 2 with two instances about 5; one of the latter, that with *Bombyx mori*, varying considerably with strain of bacterium. However, Rogers (1967) obtained a value near 2 (Table IV) with almost spore-free crystal fed to *P. brassicae*, even though an accurate measurement of dose per insect was employed. Also, with crystal similar to that of Rogers from 11 different bacterial strains, Pendleton (1969, personal communication) obtained slopes varying between 1.4 and 6.9 (mean 3.3) with larvae of *Philosamia cynthia*. Pendleton has limited evidence that this variation in slope was due to the bacterial strain rather than to variation between batches of insects. Thus although the crystal toxin of *B. thuringiensis* may sometimes produce slopes considerably in excess of 2 this has not always been the experience to date. Slopes with the exotoxin of *B. thuringiensis* were mainly well above 2 (Table IV).

Precisionwise, the assay of *B. thuringiensis* in an artificial medium with *T. ni* (Table IV, Splittstoesser and McEwen, 1961) is excellent because of the steep slope. That used by Cavard (in Burges *et al.*, 1967) with *E. kuehniella* is even better, because large numbers of larvae can be used with little labour, with a slope slightly exceeding 2 at 25°C (Table IV) and steeper at 30°C, a temperature near the maximum at which larvae complete development. This effect of high temperature could be a result of faster metabolism and feeding of the insect or faster multiplication of the bacterium (Smirnoff, 1967).

VI. Discussion, Conclusions and Research Requirements

The important achievements, to date, in the standardization of microbial insecticides are the realization of the significance of the available alternatives and the advance of some methods towards the limit of technical development. Only *B. thuringiensis* is at present sufficiently used commercially to require an international system of standardization. It is important to anticipate the requirements of other organisms in order to introduce well based systems when the time comes.

In general, the methods available for standardization fall into two broad groups: one time-consuming, involving bioassay; the other relatively quick, including all methods except bioassay (Table I). Since a quick, easy method is obviously desirable, the merits of the quick methods for different types of pathogen will be considered first.

Pure toxins, or preparations in which a toxin is the only active component, constitute the simplest type of pathogen. The exotoxin of *B. thuringiensis* falls into this category, also the crystal toxin when used against those few host species in which it is effective alone. When specific chemical methods become available, they will be the best. Seroassay for the crystal toxin is valuable, particularly for research on unformulated, relatively pure, preparations; but impurities and formulation ingredients in some commercial preparations upset the method. To obtain the relationship of seroassay units to potency, the method must be calibrated initially by bioassay. This does not apply to chemical measurements, because the unit involved is weight of active ingredient just as with chemical insecticides.

The next group comprises those pathogens which will not readily germinate to form colonies on agar plates and which can be estimated by particle counts. Virus polyhedra, the *Bacillus popilliae* group, protozoans, many fungi and nematodes fall into this group. The limitations of the particle count are that it takes no account of whether the particles have died or deteriorated and it cannot be used after particulate formulation ingredients have been added. The speedy Coulter counter can be used only for microbial preparations far purer than likely to be produced on an industrial scale and, in combination with microscopic examination for viability, for nematodes. Except for some nematodes, this group of pathogens is mainly produced *in vivo* and is unlikely to be troubled by attenuation of the stock.

The next group grow *in vitro* without producing toxins. It comprises some bacteria and fungi. Either a viable spore count or particle count can be used. The viable spore count detects death of non-dormant spores, but neither method measures attenuation, attack by phages and variable dormancy.

The final group consists of fungi and crystalliferous bacteria, toxigenic *in vitro*. Again, viable spore or particle counts can be used, subject to the limitations mentioned above and that these methods are unable to measure variable toxin production.

In a well tried and well understood industrial process, with carefully controlled substrate and conditions, these quick methods can give quite reliable estimates of potency, depending largely on the experience and acumen of the staff in charge. However, this proviso and the factors outlined above introduce elements of unreliability intolerable in a product offered for sale. Thus a method free from these limitations is required and the only one available is the more time-consuming bioassay (Table I). Good assay procedures have not been developed for nematodes and, in this group, reliance must at present be placed on particle counts. Assay procedures for fungi need study.

Bioassay values must be expressed in arbitrary units related to a particular batch of material designated as a standard. This is a reliable and simple system with a host-species-specific pathogen, such as a virus, or with a broad-spectrum pathogen used against the insect species involved in the assay.

Thus the various methods of standardization each have their uses. In general, the first step is control of production conditions to give predictable yields, then the quality check of each batch by one of the quick methods, finally the check by bioassay of potency of large bulks assembled for sale. This bioassay check gives the definitive information that allows the formulator to adjust the product to the advertised level of potency by the addition of the correct amount of inert ingredient. The whole process is illustrated for *B. thuringiensis* in Fig. 3.

PRODUCTION STEP	*STANDARDIZATION METHOD*
Batch production process	*Rigid control of conditions: yield*
↓	
Harvested batch	*Quality check by quick method (viable spore count). Safety tests in mice etc.*
↓	
Blending batches into bulks	*Bioassay of bulks with* Trichoplusia ni
↓	
Formulation to standard potency	*Use bioassay results*
↓	
Sale	*Recommended treatment rates for* T. ni *and like species based on* T. ni *assay. Rates for other groups of species based on assay results with subsidiary assay species*
↓	
Statutory checks	T. ni *assay in government laboratories*

Fig. 3. Proposed role of different standardization methods in the production and marketing of *Bacillus thuringiensis.*

Future trends in the standardization of microbial insecticides depend on how much their use increases. At present, standardization rests with the few active commercial firms who maintain a level of potency adequate to meet their individually recommended application levels. Extensive increase in use would necessitate agreed methods to provide a basis of comparison between different products. This goal is readily attainable with species-specific pathogens, but it presents difficulties with broad-spectrum pathogens, such as *B. thuringiensis,* which at present is the most advanced in commercial development.

These difficulties arise because bioassay results, expressed in standard units obtained with one host species, often do not apply to another host species. This may happen if the test preparation is formulated in a different way to the standard preparation (Dulmage, 1970), or most likely if the strains should differ in the two preparations and one strain is intrinsically more potent in one host species than in the other (Burges, 1967; Burges *et al.,* 1967). This is not surprising, because one would expect different strains of pathogen to become adapted in nature to particular species of hosts. Also an analogy can be drawn with chemical insecticides: the relative potency of two chemicals is frequently reversed in different insect species.

This poses the question of which species to choose as assay species. The obvious answer is to choose the pest against which the pathogen is used most, providing it is a convenient species from the point of view of assay technique. If it is not, a species similar in its reaction to the pathogen should be chosen. Gradually, comparative information on other pests could be assembled and such subsidiary assay species adopted as are found necessary to provide information for those pests that differ substantially from the main assay species. This is already done at the level of the individual commercial company. If the use of the microbial insecticide expands vastly, it could be extended between companies. Since *Trichoplusia ni* is one of the pests attracting the most use of this pathogen and since it is also one of the best assay species, easy to breed, free from quarantine restrictions in all countries, and adapted to a standard artificial assay medium, it seems a good universal test species. *Ephestia kuehniella* is a strong candidate for a secondary assay role, because it is cosmopolitan and even more suitable from the technical bioassay point of view than *T. ni.* Both species measure the spore-crystal complex. Another species is necessary to measure the exotoxin, which attacks a much greater range of insects. However, the situation is a dynamic one, because strains with improved activity are adopted from time to time by the manufacturers (Dulmage, 1970). The degree of improvement differs for different host species and may even involve reduced activity against some hosts. Furthermore, the desirable characters from several recognized strains may be combined by genetical manipulation into one artificial strain and the new strain so fabricated will neither be recognizable to anyone but its architect, nor alignable to any known host spectrum. The practical outcome of this situation may well be a greater consumer-reliance on the know-how of the manufacturer of the broad-spectrum microbial insecticide than is at present expected with chemicals.

Be this as it may, it is the function of research to provide the tools for use when required by practice. At present research can be most profitably applied to the study of precision.

The precision *obtainable,* as opposed to *obtained,* in practice with a reasonable amount of labour is between examples (1) and (2) in Table I for colony counts, between (3) and (4) or (5) for particles counted in a counting chamber, and between (8) and (10) for bioassay. Industrial samples contain too many inactive particles for the Coulter counter to be used. However, particle counts, viable spore counts and bioassay have one point in common–the pronounced disagreement between recent results from different laboratories (Table I, column 3; Table II; Burges *et al.,* 1967). If comparative tests are to be used in practice, consistent results must be obtainable at different laboratories. Luckily the difficulties can be easily remedied.

The main reasons for inconsistency of particle counts with counting chambers are variation in the *actual* depth of the liquid in the chamber and in the ability of different operators to recognize the correct particles. These difficulties can be overcome by the measurement of depth with an interferometer each time a chamber is used, and by the development of a chamber usable with an oil immersion objective. The problems with the latter are the thickness of the coverglass and the pull exerted by the immersion oil, which moves the coverglass. These problems could probably be overcome by the development of a long, but narrow, chamber with a thin fixed coverglass. Each chamber would have to be calibrated by interferometry, and if there were significant variations in depth along the length of the chamber, an average value could be taken and counts always made to follow a traverse lengthwise along the platform. Inconsistency in viable spore counts mainly originates from the use of different blenders, which could probably be overcome by using cheap, standard glass homogenizers (p. 594).

Differences in bioassay results are caused by the cumulative differences of many points in technique. The answer is technical standardization down to the last detail, e.g. samples of the same batch of food and of the same stock of insects could be distributed between laboratories; temperatures, humidities, day lengths, containers, apparatus (particularly homogenizers), insect size etc., could be standardized.

One of the advantages of using an artificial medium is that several insect species may grow on it, thus enabling different specific pathogens to be compared on their particular host insect in identical conditions. In this way, Ignoffo and Garcia (1969) compared the pathogenicity of five nuclear polyhedrosis viruses in their respective hosts.

Research centres around the development of new methods and improvement of existing ones. The following suggestions particularly need attention:

1. Development of a counting chamber for use with an oil immersion objective (see above).
2. Further exploration of mechanical electronic counting methods.
3. Search for an *in vitro* viability test for *Nosema* spores.
4. Development of a chemical assay for the exotoxin of *B. thuringiensis.*
5. Investigation of seroassay for some viruses.
6. Assessment of how far standardization of the spore-crystal complex of *B. thuringiensis* by a selected host species is valid for other pest species.
7. Interlaboratory reproducibility tests for (a) particle counts as described on pp. 593-601, (b) viable spore counts (pp. 592-594 and 596-601), (c) bioassay of *B. thuringiensis* with a single host species by a single, precisely-controlled technique.
8. Development of a quick significance test between potency ratios extending the methods of Litchfield and Wilcoxon (1949).
9. Development of specialist assays, e.g. one that would measure the suitability of a *B. thuringiensis* preparation for use in the special conditions of the honey-bee hive.

10. Development of quick assays to measure the potency of individual bacterial colonies in work on mutations.

References

Angus, T. A. (1956). *Can. J. Microbiol.* **2,** 416-426.
Angus, T. A. (1967). *J. Invertebrate Path.* **9,** 256-260.
Angus, T. A. and Norris, J. R. (1968). *J. Invertebrate Path.* **11,** 289-295.
Ashford, R. W. (1967). Ph.D. Thesis Univ. Lond., 146 pp.
Benz, G. and Perron, J.-M. (1967). *Experientia* **23,** 871-873.
Bliss, C. I. (1952). "The Statistics of Bioassay". Academic Press, New York.
Bucher, G. E. (1958). *Proc. Xth int. Congr. Ent., Montreal, 1956* **4,** 695-701.
Bucher, G. E. and Morse, P. M. (1963). *J. Insect Path.* **5,** 289-308.
Burgerjon, A. (1956). *Annls Épiphyt.* **7,** 675-684.
Burgerjon, A. (1962). *Annls Épiphyt.* **13,** 59-72.
Burgerjon, A. (1965). *Entomophaga* **10,** 21-25.
Burgerjon, A. and Biache, G. (1967). *Entomologia exp. appl.* **10,** 211-230.
Burgerjon, A. and Yamvrias, C. (1959). *C.r. hebd. Séanc. Acad. Sci. Paris* **249,** 2871-2872.
Burges, H. D. (1960). *J. Insect Physiol.* **5,** 317-334.
Burges, H. D. (1964). *Mém. hors Sér. Entomophaga* No. 2, 323-327.
Burges, H. D. (1967). *Nature, Lond.* **215,** 664-665.
Burges, H. D. *et al.* (1967). *In* "Insect Pathology and Microbial Control" (P. A. van der Laan, ed.), pp. 314-337. North-Holland Publ. Co., Amsterdam.
Burges, H. D. and Bailey, L. (1968). *J. Invertebrate Path.* **11,** 184-195.
Burges, H. D., Canning, E. U. and Hurst, J. A. *J. Invertebrate Path.* (In press.)
Chauthani, A. R. (1968). *J. Invertebrate Path.* **11,** 242-245.
Conner, R. M. and Arne Hansen, P. (1967). *J. Invertebrate Path.* **9,** 12-18.
Cook, A. M. and Lund, B. M. (1962). *J. gen. Microbiol.* **29,** 97-104.
Cook, A. M. and Yousef, R. T. (1953). *J. Pharm. Pharmac.* **5,** 141-144.
Cooksey, K. E. (1968). *Biochem. J.* **106,** 445-454.
Dulmage, H. T. (1970). *J. Invertebrate Path.* **15,** 232-239.
Dulmage, H. T., Correa, J. A. and Martinez, A. J. (1970). *J. Invertebrate Path.* **15,** 15-20.
Eisenhart, C. and Wilson, P. W. (1943). *Bact. Rev.* **7,** 57-137.
Finney, D. J. (1952). "Probit Analysis". Cambridge Univ. Press. Cambridge.
Hanks, J. H. and James, D. F. (1940). *J. Bact.* **39,** 297-305.
Heimpel, A. M. (1967). *In* "Insect Pathology and Microbial Control" (P. A. van der Laan, ed.), pp. 355-359. North-Holland Publ. Co., Amsterdam.
Hoopingarner, R. and Materu, M. E. A. (1964). *J. Insect Path.* **6,** 26-30.
Ignoffo, C. M. (1964). *J. Insect Path.* **6,** 237-245.
Ignoffo, C. M. (1965). *J. Invertebrate Path.* **7,** 315-319.
Ignoffo, C. M. (1966). *J. Invertebrate Path.* **8,** 531-536.
Ignoffo, C. M., Clemente, G. and Gasparotto, V. A. (1968). *J. Invertebrate Path.* **11,** 97-103.
Ignoffo, C. M. and Garcia, C. (1969). *J. Invertebrate Path.* **14,** 282-283.
Krieg, A. (1965a). *Entomophaga* **10,** 3-20.
Krieg, A. (1965b). *Entomophaga* **10,** 49-54.
Krieg, A. (1966). *Entomologia exp. appl.* **9,** 185-190.
Litchfield, J. T., Jr. and Wilcoxon, F. (1949). *J. Pharmac. exp. Ther.* **96,** 99-113.
Martignoni, M. E. (1957). *Mitt. schweiz. Anst. forstl. VersWes.* **32,** 371-418.
Martignoni, M. E. and Iwai, P. J. (1968). Pacif. N.W. Forest and Range Expl. Station. U.S. Forest Service Res. Note, PNW-85, 14 pp.
Martignoni, M. E. and Schmid, P. (1961). *J. Insect Path.* **3,** 62-74.
Martouret, D. (1962). *XIth int. Congr. Ent. Vienna, 1960* **2,** 849-855.
Mather, K. (1964). "Statistical Analysis in Biology". Methuen, London.
Mechalas, B. J. and Anderson, N. B. (1964). *J. Insect Path.* **6,** 218-224.

Meynell, G. G. and Meynell, E. (1965). "Theory and Practice in Experimental Bacteriology". Cambridge Univ. Press, Cambridge.
Müller-Kögler, E. (1967). *In* "Insect Pathology and Microbial Control" (P. A. van der Laan, ed.), pp. 339-353. North-Holland Publ. Co., Amsterdam.
Müller-Kögler, E. and Samšiňáková, A. (1969). *Entomophaga* **14**, 369-382.
Nash, R. F. and Fox, R. C. (1969). *J. Invertebrate Path.* **13**, 153-154.
Norris, K. P. and Powell, E. O. (1961). *Jl R. microsc. Soc. Part 2* **80**, 107-119.
Pendleton, I. R. (1969). *J. Invertebrate Path.* **13**, 423-428.
Potter, C. (1952). *Ann. appl. Biol.* **39**, 1-28.
Powell, E. O. and Errington, F. P. (1963). *Jl R. microsc. Soc.* **82**, 39-49.
Rogers, A. H. (1967). Ph.D. Thesis, Univ. Leeds, 145 pp.
Rogers, A. H., White, A. G. and Gibson, N. H. E. (1966). *Lab. Pract.* **15**, 426-430 and 434.
Rogoff, M. H., Ignoffo, C. M., Singer, S., Gard, I. and Prieto, A. P. (1969). *J. Invertebrate Path.* **14**, 122-129.
Rosický, B. and Weiser, J. (1951). "Moderni Insekticidy" (Modern Insecticides). Přirodověd. Vydavatelstvi, Praha. (In Czechoslovakian.)
Smirnoff, W. A. (1962). *J. Insect Path.* **4**, 384-386.
Smirnoff, W. A. (1967). *In* "Insect Pathology and Microbial Control" (P. A. van der Laan, ed.), pp. 125-130. North-Holland Publ. Co., Amsterdam.
Synder, T. C. (1947). *J. Bact.* **54**, 641-654.
Splittstoesser, C. M. and McEwen, F. L. (1961). *J. Insect Path.* **3**, 391-398.
Sun, Y. P. (1950). *J. econ. Ent.* **43**, 45-53.
Vago, C. and Burges, H. D. (1964). *J. Insect Path.* **6**, 544-547.
Weibull, C. (1960). *J. Bact.* **79**, 155.
White, A. G. (1968). Ph.D. Thesis Univ. Leeds, 185 pp.
Wiegand, H. (1962). *NachBl. dt. Pflanzenschutzdienst, Berl.* **12**, 241-250.
Wiegand, H. (1968). *Archiv Pflanzenschutz* **4**, 53-74.
Williams, R. C. and Backus, R. C. (1949). *J. Am. Chem. Soc.* **71**, 4052-4057.
Yendol, W. G. and Miller, E. M. (1967). *J. econ. Ent.* **60**, 860-864.

CHAPTER 28

Formulation of Microbial Insecticides[1]

T. A. ANGUS and P. LUTHY

Insect Pathology Research Institute, Canada,
Department of Fisheries and Forestry,
Sault Ste. Marie, Ontario, Canada

I. Introduction

It is our purpose in this chapter to discuss the form in which pathogenic micro-organisms can best be brought into contact with insects following production in the laboratory or factory. We are, as government employees, of necessity only observers of the commercial scene and so lack direct knowledge of specific innovations whose adoption ensures some economic advantage for a particular product or manufacturer. Ideally the accumulated experience of all groups, commercial and non-commercial, should be brought to bear but understandably this is not always possible in view of the confidential nature of some industrial research.

For economic and technical reasons, microbial insecticides have developed along similar lines to conventional chemical preparations. Important specific differences, of course, do exist because microbial insecticides do not directly

[1] Contribution No. 136.

depend on the effect of a poisonous chemical but exploit the activity of living (or self-replicating) entities. An exception is the enterotoxinosis caused by *Bacillus thuringiensis* (see Chapter 13) wherein a pre-formed toxic protein is essential for infection to occur. Generally, however, it is the multiplication of a micro-organism in the host tissues that leads to disease and death. The aim of the formulator then is to avoid practices that might inhibit or harm the pathogen and wherever possible to enhance the possibility of infection. Thus, not only must one avoid agents in any way antimicrobial but also, with *B. thuringiensis,* any compounds capable of denaturing the protein comprising the toxic crystal. Any attempt to utilize a particular species of micro-organism in an insecticide formulation should be based on an intimate knowledge of the host-parasite relationship.

The widespread use in agriculture, forestry and public health programmes of an ever-increasing array of biocides such as chemical insecticides, herbicides and fungicides has led to many technical articles about application equipment and methods, with characteristics of formulations, and with additives that assist toxic action in a variety of ways. Happily it is unnecessary to refer in detail to such matters since they are more than adequately covered in easily available reviews and standard texts (Bailey and Smith, 1951; Brown, 1951; Metcalf *et al.*, 1951; Potts, 1958; Martin, 1959). However, it might be helpful to review very briefly some characteristics of insecticides so that the meaning of some technical terms, as used by us, will be clear.

II. Attributes of Insecticides

By strict definition, an insecticide is simply a compound that kills insects and conceivably could include mineral acids, corrosive compounds and so on. In practice the term generally refers to a compound developed for, or usually used for, that purpose (the active chemical); or it refers to a biocide diluted and applied in such a way as to enhance its insecticidal activity (the formulated material). Modern chemical insecticides are based on a very wide range of organic and inorganic compounds of differing solubilities. Usually the active principle is diluted with a solid or liquid *carrier* or *extender.* The liquids include water, oil, volatile solvents and mixtures or emulsions of these. Often the insecticidal compound is a solid and if the carrier is a *solvent* as well as a diluent, it enables uniform and widespread application as a *spray.*

If a liquid insecticide is undesirable, a dry one may be used as a *dust.* Here the active compound may be diluted by blending it with *extenders* such as fine clays, diatomaceous earth and so on; these are sometimes referred to as *fillers.* In some cases the active compound may be adsorbed on an inert solid, which is often referred to as a *carrier.* If the extender or carrier is attractive to the target insect as a food, oviposition site or the like it is sometimes referred to as a *bait* preparation.

Chemical insecticides may act as either *contact* or *stomach poisons.* The latter must be ingested, although they do not necessarily act only in the gut area. Contact poisons may impinge on the target insect at the time of application or, as it moves about, the insect may later come into contact with the poison. Because of its nature (waxy, smooth, oily, etc.) the sprayed surface may not easily wet. This is frequently true for many kinds of foliage and may be counteracted by *spreaders,* which are usually *wetting-agents* that reduce the surface tension of the spray droplet. Wetting agents may also be added to dry formulations to produce *"wettable-powders"* which can then be more easily suspended in water.

Unfortunately the compounds that ensure spreading or wetting may also accelerate the washing-off of coatings by rain or dew. To increase adhesion, *stickers* or *adhesives* of various types are included in insecticide formulations. These are compounds that form a layer or discrete spots which, when dry, resist weathering. In the case of volatile active compounds the sticker may also slow up loss of activity due to evaporation. Some of the finely particulate extenders and carriers help bind chemicals to the foliage surface because of surface effects.

If the liquid carrier is a mixture of water and oil (or some other water-immiscible solvent), emulsifiers are added to stabilize emulsions. In some dust formulations, *anti-caking agents* are included to prevent the formation of lumps. Finally the action of some chemicals is potentiated or enhanced by other compounds that are not insecticidal themselves; they are sometimes referred to as synergists (Brown *et al.*, 1967). Not all the ingredients of a formulation can be neatly catalogued for some are multipurpose. For instance, in long-acting insecticidal paints the oil-solvent mixture functions as diluent, solvent, spreader and finally as sticker. There are also some commercial additives that function both as spreader and sticker.

The terms cited above embrace an extensive list of proprietary compounds that reflect the numerous ways and circumstances in which chemicals are used as insecticides. Some of the terms used are directly applicable to microbial insecticides, and others are less apt or appropriate.

The desirable attributes in a microbial pathogen to be used for insect control have been discussed by several authors (Bucher, 1956; Cameron, 1963; Hall, 1963; Angus, 1965; Dulmage, 1967; Rivers, 1967) (see also Chapter 1). Few, if any, insect pathogens completely meet these criteria so that it is important that whatever potential they possess should not be diminished by inappropriate processing. Although many micro-organisms pathogenic for insects have been studied, only some have been seriously considered for use as microbial insecticides; they have been discussed in several reviews and include viruses, bacteria, fungi and protozoans (Dutky, 1959; Briggs, 1963; Bucher, 1964; De

Bach, 1964; Vaňková, 1964; Angus, 1965; Heimpel, 1965; Rogoff, 1966; Heimpel, 1967; Ignoffo, 1967; Angus, 1968).

Choice of formulation may be vitally important in practical application. For instance, if heavy rainfall is expected, a dust would be unsuitable and a spray containing a good sticker would be required. A dust may be best on some low plants, such as lettuce, because better treatment may be given to undersides of leaves. In sunny climates the inclusion of a protectant against sunlight is important.

III. Liquid Formulations

A. WATER

Microbial insecticides used as sprays are suspensions of unicellular entities whose ability to infect disappears if the cell is disrupted physically or chemically. In this they differ from the chemical insecticides which are usually applied in solution. Dissolving the pathogens would of course destroy them. As a result water is frequently used as a diluent for many microbial insecticides and is generally the liquid of choice.

The inclusion bodies found in some insect virus diseases are made up of virions occluded in a crystalline protein matrix. The bodies are very stable in water; aqueous suspensions have been stored at 3°C for years without any serious decrease in virulence. The endospores of many *Bacillus* species are also relatively stable in water but it should be noted that the presence of certain compounds may trigger premature germination; the specific requirements differ from species to species (Ignoffo, 1964; Sussman and Halvorson, 1966). The spores of many fungal pathogens, on the other hand, will germinate when a threshold humidity is reached (Sussman and Halvorson, 1966; Hedlund and Pass, 1968; Yendol, 1968). Some kinds of fungal resting spores must undergo a ripening or maturation process before they will germinate but fungal conidiospores germinate readily in water (Clark *et al.*, 1968; Krejová, 1968). Therefore, the storage of fungus spores in water or at high humidity should be avoided. The spores of certain protozoans will germinate in water if the pH is appropriate and if certain ions are present; in this they resemble *Bacillus* spores. Unlike bacterial and fungal spores, protozoan spores are very sensitive to desiccation (Kellen and Lindegren, 1968; Steinhaus, 1960).

The above remarks about the suitability of water as a diluent are true for relatively resistant forms such as polyhedra and spores. The so-called vegetative phases of bacteria, fungi and protozoans are sometimes adversely affected by storage in conditions that are markedly hypertonic or hypotonic. For prolonged storage then, water purity (in terms of pH, ion content, and organic content) is a factor in the retention of virulence of certain kinds of pathogens (Chambers,

1968; Magnoler, 1968). Purity is not so critical if the water is to be added just before the spray is applied.

Water, of course, is the diluent most often used when preparing wettable powders for use. The wettable powder types of microbial insecticides are essentially dried cells extended with suitable fillers, wetting agents and spreaders.

B. OILS

Oils of various kinds have long been used in insecticide preparations. Fuel oil has been widely favoured as a vehicle in forest spraying because it dissolves many chlorinated hydrocarbon insecticides. Equally important are its cheapness and many desirable spraying characteristics, including good sticking and spreading qualities. Use of oil as a carrier for microbial insecticides came about, in part, from the need to fit such products into established procedures and to utilize existing equipment (Angus *et al.*, 1961; Clark and Reiner, 1956).

Oil suspensions of *B. thuringiensis* have been used experimentally. Initially some difficulty was experienced in preparing uniform suspensions but this was met by preliminary wetting of the dry microbial insecticide with an emulsifer-water mixture before final dispersion in the oil carrier.

In view of the tendency of fungal spores to germinate prematurely or abortively in water, and the sensitivity of the vegetative phases of some micro-organisms, it would seem desirable to study further the use of oil carriers. The storage of micro-organisms under oil is a long-established laboratory procedure. Lewis and Connola (1966) found that diesel oil killed bacterial spores, although it is not known whether the presence of the oil during heat shock treatment prior to plating caused spore mortality.

The use of oils is sometimes limited by possible phytotoxicity. In some circumstances foliage damage can be tolerated but where the foliage is used as a food (lettuce, cole crops, etc.) the oil residue might be unacceptable.

C. EMULSIONS

The use of emulsion preparations for microbial insecticides stemmed in part from the need to adapt them to oil spraying equipment in forestry operations (Angus *et al.*, 1961). There is, however, another reason that arises out of production techniques. Some manufacturers of *B. thuringiensis* preparations produce the pathogen by the aerated broth method and, when the fermentation is complete, the spores and crystals are harvested as a thick creamy paste by centrifugation. It is obviously more direct (and conceivably less harmful to the spores) to omit drying and suspend the pathogen in a concentrated emulsion that can be later diluted in water.

The composition of any particular emulsion will of course depend on a number of factors including the amount and kind of pathogen but basically would include: an emulsifier to marry the oil and water phases, a salt additive to achieve isotonicity (where required), possible wetting agents and/or stickers (Lewis and Connola, 1966). A wide range of emulsifiers is available; those of the type permitted in foods and cosmetics have been used with success (Angus *et al.*, 1961; Smirnoff, 1967; Frear, 1968; Jaques *et al.*, 1968).

The type of emulsion (oil-in-water, water-in-oil) and its stability varies with the components and the kind of generating equipment used. If a permanent emulsion cannot be achieved, it is desirable that the emulsion should be such that it can be re-established by simple mixing or back-pumping (Winchester, 1967). The emulsion preparation of *B. thuringiensis* marketed as "Thuricide 90TS" (International Minerals and Chemical Corp., Skokie, Illinois) is stable over long periods of time providing freezing is avoided. Settling does occur, but the sediment is easily dispersed.

IV. Dusts

The earliest microbial insecticides were formulated in dry form and were used as dusts or wettable powders. The fillers or carriers used included such compounds as attapulgite, Fuller's earth, pyrophyllite, talc, kaolin, bentonite and other inert materials. Many of these are still used as they are in chemical insecticides (Watkins and Norton, 1955). It has been reported that the abrasive action of some kinds of dusts increases the susceptibility of some insects to fungal infection (Chapter 5). In such cases, the dust functions not only as a carrier or diluent but also as a synergist.

A dry formulation is sometimes indicated because of product history. For instance, the insect viruses are obligate pathogens and can be produced only in the living tissues of the particular host (or to a limited degree in cell cultures). In laboratory studies the inclusion bodies can be freed of host tissue residues but this is laborious and time-consuming. In commercial production, the moribund host containing the pathogen is macerated and diluted with inert carrier. A liguid formulation may putrify because of the tissue residues and perhaps be less stable (aesthetically less acceptable) than a dry powder. This is also true for the commercial formulation of *Bacillus popilliae,* the causative agent of Japanese beetle milky-disease. In the case of one *B. thuringiensis* formulation, the pathogen is cultured on a semi-solid medium (Rogoff, 1966) so that it is preferable to process it as a dust or wettable powder rather than attempt to separate the spores and crystals from the medium solids. When grinding and mixing materials containing the pathogens to obtain a sufficiently fine powder, care should be taken to avoid increase in temperature or physical damage that would harm the pathogen.

The choice of the inert filler for use in a dust formulation is subject to the general proviso that it be non-toxic to the pathogen being used. Further, after application, water in the form of rain or dew should not yield a solution hostile to the pathogen (unfavourable pH, high salt concentration, etc.).

The decision as to the most desirable form (spray or dust) varies with the crop being protected, the target insect, climatic conditions and, of course, the particular pathogen being utilized. Such comparative tests as have been made are limited and do not indicate any consistent superiority of one form over another for field use.

V. Additives

A. SPREADERS

Spreaders or wetting agents are added to the water diluent to ensure "wetting" of the surface to be sprayed (Furmidge, 1959a, b; Hartley, 1960; Frear, 1968). For a complete explanation of the factors involved reference should be made to standard physical chemistry texts. Briefly, a spreader enables a stable liquid/solid interface to be formed. Many materials have been used including dried milk, powdered casein, dried blood, gelatin, saponins, soaps, etc. Many of these were used empirically at first, but latterly emphasis has been on the use of highly specific compounds of known performance (Hartley, 1960). In so far as microbial insecticides are concerned, it is essential that the compound used should not encourage premature growth or germination and that it should not inhibit successful establishment of the pathogen. Some factors are likely to be rather subtle, e.g. although detergents such as sodium dodecyl sulphate do not inactivate the crystal toxin of *B. thuringiensis,* they open up the structure of the crystal and make it more sensitive to destruction by other means (Cooksey, personal communication). In Table I is a list of some spreaders or wetting agents that have been used or recommended for use in microbial insecticides.

B. STICKERS

Some of the spreaders noted above (i.e. soap, saponin, and some modern synthetic compounds) are cleansing agents so that although their use aids wetting and film formation, it also hastens removal by rain or dew. To counteract this (and in some cases where no special spreaders have been added) it is necessary to add adhesives or stickers to ensure the formation of a weather-resistant film on foliage (Geering and Lloyd, 1962; Frear, 1968). This is especially important where the pathogen is like a "stomach poison", i.e. must be ingested with the foliage.

As with the spreaders, the stickers added should not decrease pathogenicity. A number of compounds such as flour, dextrines and gums have been used (Martin, 1959). Modern stickers include many proprietary compounds such as Lovo (amine-stearate solutions), and synthetic lattices, such as polyvinyl chloride, which form water-dispersible suspensions that dry and cure to

TABLE I

Additives that have been added to preparations of microbial insecticides

Kind of additive[a]	Type of pathogen[b]	Reference	Compatibility[c]
Diluent (dust)			
Pyrophylite	Bt.	Commercial literature	Rec.
Talc	Bt.	Commercial literature	Rec.
Celite	Bt.	Commercial literature	Rec.
Chalk	Bt.	Commercial literature	Rec.
Starch	Bt.	Commercial literature	Rec.
Synthetic silicates	Bt.	Commercial literature	Rec.
Kaolin	Bt.	Commercial literature	Rec.
Bentonite	Bt.	Commercial literature	Rec.
Attapulgite	Bt.	Commercial literature	Rec.
Lactose	Bt.	Ignoffo and Graham (1967)	Lab.
Lactose	V	Ignoffo (1965)	Lab.
Magmabentonite	V	Smirnoff (1967)	Field
Wetting Agents and Spreaders			
Alkyl phenols	Bt.	Herfs (1965), Heimpel (1967)	Field
Vatsol OT	Bt.	Herfs (1965), Heimpel (1967)	Lab.
Sandovit	Bt.	Herfs (1965), Heimpel (1967)	Lab.
Novémol	Bt.	Herfs (1965), Heimpel (1967)	Field
Petro AG	Bt.	Herfs (1965), Heimpel (1967)	Field
Colloidal X77	Bt.	Tanada and Reiner (1962)	Field
Colloidal X77	V	Elmore (1961), Tanada and Reiner (1962)	Field
Triton X45	V	McEwen and Hervey (1958)	Lab.
Triton X100	V	Clark and Reiner (1956)	Lab.
Triton X100	V	Ignoffo *et al.* (1965)	Field
Triton X114	Bt.	Jaques and Fox (1960)	Field
Triton X155	Bt.	Herfs (1965), Heimpel (1967)	Lab.
Laters surfactant	Bt.	Morris (1969)	Lab.
Igepal CO-630	Bt.	Morris (1969)	Lab.
Arlacel "C"	V	Clark and Reiner (1956)	Lab.
Tween 20	f	Jaques *et al.* (1968)	Lab.
Adhesives and Stickers			
Tung oil	Bt.	Lewis and Connola (1966)	Field
Arabol E77L	Bt.	Commercial literature	Rec.
Molasses	Bt.	Commercial literature	Rec.
Powdered skim milk	Bt.	Commercial literature	Rec.
Powdered skim milk	V	Commercial literature	Rec.
Glutolin	Bt.	Herfs (1965), Heimpel (1967)	Field
Methocel	V	Clark and Reiner (1956)	Lab.
Methocel	Bt.	Angus (1959), Herfs (1965), Heimpel (1967)	Lab.
Polyvinyl chloride latexes	Bt.	Angus (1959), Herfs (1965), Heimpel (1967)	Field
Dried blood	V	Smirnoff (1967)	Field
Corn syrup	Bt.	Stelzer (1967)	Field

TABLE I–*cont.*

Kind of additive[a]	Type of pathogen[b]	Reference	Compatibility[c]
Adhesives and Stickers–*cont.*			
Corn syrup	V	Stelzer (1967)	Field
Latex D	Bt.	Herfs (1965), Heimpel (1967)	Rec.
Geon latex 652	Bt.	Angus (1959)	Lab.
Geon latex 652	V	Smirnoff (1967)	Field
Plyac	Bt.	Morris (1969)	Lab.
Casein	Bt.	Morris (1969)	Lab.
Folicote	Bt.	Morris (1969)	Lab.
Lovo 190	Bt.	Geering and Lloyd (1962)	Lab.
Lovo 192	Bt.	Geering and Lloyd (1962), Morris (1969)	Lab.
Emulsifiers			
9D 207	Bt.	Lewis and Connola (1966)	Field
9D 207	V	Wolfenbarger (1965)	Field
Pinolene 1882	Bt.	Morris (1969)	Lab.
Tween 80	Bt.	Angus *et al.* (1961)	Field
Tween 80	V	Clark and Reiner (1956)	Lab.
Span 80	Bt.	Angus *et al.* (1961)	Field
Span 80	V	Clark and Reiner (1956)	Lab.
Triton B 1956	Bt.	Tanada (1956), McEwen and Hervey (1959), Fox and Jaques (1961)	Field
Triton B 1956	V	McEwen and Hervey (1959)	Field
Triton B 1956	V	Clark and Reiner (1956)	Lab.
Bait Constituents			
Ground corn meal	Bt.	Commercial literature	Rec.
Cottonseed oil	p	McLaughlin *et al.* (1968)	Field
Honey	p	McLaughlin *et al.* (1968)	Field
Hydroxy ethyl cellulose	p	McLaughlin *et al.* (1968)	Field
Miscellaneous			
Sodium chloride	Bt.	Lewis and Connola (1966)	Field
Propionic acid	Bt.	Lewis and Connola (1966)	Field
Xylene	Bt.	Lewis and Connola (1966)	Field
Lactose	V	Ignoffo and Graham (1967)	Lab.
Benzene	V	Smirnoff (1961)	Field
Boric acid	Bt.	Doane and Wallis (1964)	Lab.

[a] In some cases, the function is assumed since it is not stated in original reference.
[b] Bt., *B. thuringiensis;* f, fungus; V, Virus; p, protozoan.
[c] Lab.: In laboratory tests no indication that the additive was harmful to the pathogen.
Field: Good results obtained in field trials implying that under the conditions stated the additive did not significantly reduce effectiveness.
Rec.: Use of additive noted or recommended without supporting evidence about effect on pathogen; presumably harmless.

water-insoluble films. In Table I is a list of some stickers that have been used or recommended for use in microbial insecticides.

C. PROTECTANTS

Some insect pathogens are highly susceptible to damage by desiccation, and by exposure to sunlight, or to ultra-violet radiation (Stephens, 1957; Cantwell and Franklin, 1966; Cantwell, 1967; David, 1967; David *et al.*, 1968; Gudauskas and Canerday, 1968; Jaques, 1968). The pathogens include bacteria (both spore and vegetative phase), virus (free virions and polyhedra), fungi, and by inference, protozoans which are usually short-lived outside of their hosts. To counter this, formulations have been modified to minimize such effects.

Of the protection systems that have been suggested, one is referred to as encapsulation. Spores and crystals of *B. thuringiensis* encapsulated (presumably) by a method similar to that used in producing smudge-proof carbon paper, proved to be less sensitive to sunlight while toxicity was unaffected (Raun and Jackson, 1966; Raun *et al.*, 1966; Anon., 1967; Greaves *et al.*, 1968).

It has also been suggested that clumping of spores and crystals, induced by addition of precipitants, would produce granules or "clusters" of spores and crystals in which the centremost spores would be protected from sunlight. Depending on the clump size achieved, this might necessitate an additional grinding stage to achieve uniformity.

One well-known commercial formulation of *B. thuringiensis* ("Thuricide 90TS") has been treated to increase its resistance to damage by sunlight. Another formulation ("Thuricide SS" and "Super Thuricide") with increased resistance to ultra-violet light and heat has been developed. It contains 50% solids, the spore count per gram is one-half that of "Thuricide 90TS" and the specific gravity is higher. No information has been given on the nature of the additives used. It has been reported that *Pseudomonas aeruginosa*, a bacterial pathogen of grasshoppers, can be made more resistant to desiccation by a coating of a mixture of mucin, sucrose and casein (Stephens, 1957).

VI. Compatibility with Other Pesticides

From time to time, it has been suggested that microbial insecticides might be combined with chemical pesticides used in agriculture and forestry. Once again the important point is that the additive should not interfere with the action of the microbial pathogen. *A priori*, one would not recommend adding fungicidal chemicals to suspensions of fungal spores and experimental data indicate that some fungal pathogens of insects are sensitive to fungicides used against plant pathogens (Hall and Dunn, 1958; Jaques and Patterson, 1962; Yendol, 1968).

Bacterial and viral pathogens seem to be less sensitive to chemical pesticides, and in Table II data from several sources are summarized indicating that microbial insecticides of this type are compatible with a wide range of chemical pesticides. Here, as in Table I, the use of a wide range of experimental procedures makes meaningful comparison difficult. The data though informative should not be regarded as definitive.

When low dosages of pathogens and microbial insecticides are applied together, a synergistic effect sometimes results and sometimes an inhibition of the pathogen. A combination may show both effects depending on the concentration of the chemical. The highest concentrations inhibit the pathogen, either by direct damage before it is eaten by the insect, or by depressing its multiplication in the insect (Chapter 14; reviews by Pristavko, 1967a, b; Franz, 1961; Cameron, 1963). There is need for much more intensive investigation of such mixtures.

Some manufacturers stress in their literature that, although many of the commonly used pesticides seem to be compatible with virus and bacterial formulations, "contact time" should not exceed 12 hr. This would seem to be especially important when using fungicides with microbial insecticides. McEwen *et al.* (1960) found reduced viability of spores after 3 hr exposure to five insecticides and two fungicides.

VII. Future Research

It is traditional (and probably wise) that prophetic utterances should be both cryptic and brief. As we see it, it appears that much more study should be devoted to the development of multi-component mixtures that include different kinds of pathogens and insecticides. Enough work, albeit preliminary, has been done to indicate that with some combinations the total effect can be greater than the sum of the parts.

The increasing emphasis on "integrated control" will make it desirable to give additional study to compatibility, not only in complex mixtures but also in circumstances where chemical and microbial insecticides are used sequentially (Fox and Jaques, 1961). Prolonged or sustained use of chemicals at increasing dosages has led to emergence of resistant insect populations. It would be of interest to determine if a pest species could as effectively respond when under simultaneous (or sequential) attack from a chemical poison and a variety of pathogens each relying on differing modes of action.

Little or no study has been given to the question of possible synergists for microbial insecticides (apart from sub-lethal dosages of chemical insecticides). One or two clues have been provided, e.g. Doane and Wallis (1964) found that borax synergized *B. thuringiensis,* but the subject is well-nigh untouched (Chapter 14). Search should be particularly along the lines of furthering the process of infection, possibly for instance an abrasive material could combine the function of diluent and agent to damage the gut.

TABLE II

Chemical pesticides that have been used with microbial insecticides

Pesticide	Type of pathogen[a]	Reference	Compatibility[b]
Insecticides			
Azinphosmethyl	Bt.	Herfs (1965), Heimpel (1967)	Rec.
Azinphosmethyl	V	Commercial literature	Rec.
Bidrin	Bt.	Commercial literature	Rec.
Carbaryl	Bt.	McEwen *et al.* (1960), Herfs (1965), Heimpel (1967)	Field
Carbophenothion	Bt.	McEwen *et al.* (1960), Herfs (1965), Heimpel (1967)	Field
DDD	Bt.	Commercial literature	Rec.
DDT	Bt.	Herfs (1965), Heimpel (1967)	Field
DDT	V	Wolfenbarger (1965)	Field
Demeton	Bt.	McEwen *et al.* (1960)	Field
Diazinon	Bt.	Commercial literature	Rec.
Dieldrin	Bt.	Commercial literature	Rec.
Dinitrocresol	Bt.	Herfs (1965), Heimpel (1967)	Field
Endosulfan	Bt.	Herfs (1965), Heimpel (1967)	Field
Endrin	Bt.	Herfs (1965), Heimpel (1967), Commercial literature	Rec.
Endrin	V	Hofmaster and Ditman (1961), Wolfenbarger (1965), Girardeau and Mitchell (1968)	Field
Malathion	Bt.	Commercial literature	Rec.
Malathion	Bt.	Herfs (1965), Heimpel (1967)	Unc.
Malathion	V	Hofmaster and Ditman (1961)	Field
Methyl parathion	Bt.	Herfs (1965), Heimpel (1967), Commercial literature	Field
Methyl parathion	V	Ignoffo *et al.* (1965)	Unc.
Methyl trithion	Bt.	Commercial literature	Rec.
Mevinphos	Bt.	Commercial literature	Rec.
Mevinphos	V	Hofmaster and Ditman (1961), Wolfenbarger (1965)	Field
Naled	Bt.	Creighton *et al.* (1964), Herfs (1965), Heimpel (1967)	Field
Naled	V	Hofmaster and Ditman (1961)	Field
Parathion	Bt.	McEwen *et al.* (1960)	Field
Parathion	V	Hofmaster and Ditman (1961), Getzin (1962), Wolfenbarger (1965)	Field
Perthane	V	Hofmaster and Ditman (1961)	Field
Phosphamidon	Bt.	Commercial literature	Rec.
Pyrethrins	Bt.	Commercial literature	Rec.
Rotenone	Bt.	Commercial literature	Rec.
Ryania	Bt.	Oatman (1966), Commercial literature	Field
Strobane	Bt.	Commercial literature	Rec.
TDE	Bt.	Commercial literature	Rec.
Tepp	Bt.	McEwen *et al.* (1960), Commercial literature	Unc.

TABLE II–*cont.*

Pesticide	Type of pathogen[a]	Reference	Compatibility[b]
Insecticides–*cont.*			
Tepp	V	McEwen and Hervey (1958)	Field
Toxaphene	Bt.	Herfs (1965), Heimpel (1967)	Field
Toxaphene	V	Hofmaster and Ditman (1961), Getzin (1962), Wolfenbarger (1965)	Field
Trichlorfon	Bt.	Herfs (1965), Heimpel (1967)	Field
Fungicides			
Captan	Bt.	McEwen *et al.* (1960)	Field
Chloranil	Bt.	McEwen *et al.* (1960)	Field
COCS	Bt.	McEwen *et al.* (1960)	Field
Copper oxychloride	Bt.	Herfs (1965), Heimpel (1967)	Field
Daconil	Bt.	Commercial literature	Rec.
Difolatan	Bt.	Commercial literature	Rec.
Dichlone	Bt.	Herfs (1965), Heimpel (1967)	Field
Dimethoate	Bt.	Commercial literature	Rec.
Dithane M22, M45, Z78	Bt.	Commercial literature	Rec.
Dyrene	Bt.	Commercial literature	Rec.
Dodine	Bt.	McEwen *et al.* (1960), Jaques (1963), Oatman (1968)	Field
Ferbam	Bt.	McEwen *et al.* (1960)	Field
Folpet	Bt.	Commercial literature	Rec.
Glyodin	Bt.	McEwen *et al.* (1960), Jaques (1963)	Unc.
Maneb	Bt.	McEwen *et al.* (1960), Jaques (1963)	Field
Phenyl mercuric acetate	Bt.	McEwen *et al.* (1960)	Field
Sulphur	Bt.	McEwen *et al.* (1960)	Field
Thiocarbamates	Bt.	Herfs (1965), Heimpel (1967)	Field
Zineb	Bt.	Herfs (1965), Heimpel (1967)	Field
Ziram	Bt.	Herfs (1965), Heimpel (1967)	Field
Acaricides			
Aramite	Bt.	Commercial literature	Rec.
Difocol	Bt.	Herfs (1965), Heimpel (1967), Commercial literature	Field
Tetradifon	Bt.	Commercial literature	Rec.
Miscellaneous			
Maleic hydrazide	Bt.	Commercial literature	Rec.

[a] Bt., *B. thuringiensis*; V, Virus.

[b] Lab.: In laboratory tests no indication that the additive was harmful to the pathogen.
Field: Good results obtained in field trials implying that, under the conditions stated, the additive did not significantly reduce effectiveness.
Rec.: Use of additive noted or recommended without supporting evidence about effect on pathogen; presumably harmless.
Unc.: On the basis of the reported data, or because of the unavailability of the original reference, the effect of the additive on the pathogen is uncertain.

Most study has been devoted to formulating microbial insecticides against phytophagous and soil-inhabiting insects. This should continue along existing lines. The discovery of effective protectants against solar radiation is an urgent necessity. Only one or two attempts have been made to utilize pathogens against water-inhabiting species of insects (Laird, 1960; Sikorowski and Madison, 1968). In view of the public health importance of some species this would seem to merit further attention.

References

Angus, T. A. (1959). *Can. Ent.* **91,** 254-255.

Angus, T. A. (1965). *Bact. Rev.* **29,** 364-372.

Angus, T. A. (1968). *Wld Rev. Pest Control* 7, 11-26.

Angus, T. A., Heimpel, A. M. and Fisher, R. A. (1961). *Bi-Monthly Prog. Rep. Can. Dep. Forestry* **17,** 1-2.

Anon. (1967). *Int. Pest Control* 8, 8.

Bailey, S. F. and Smith, L. M. (1951). "Handbook of Agricultural Pest Control". Industry Publications Inc., New York.

Briggs, J. D. (1963). *In* "Insect Pathology. An Advanced Treatise" (E. A. Steinhaus, ed.), Vol. 2, pp. 519-548. Academic Press, New York.

Brown, A. W. A. (1951). "Insect Control by Chemicals". John Wiley and Sons, Inc., New York.

Brown, N. C., Chadwick, P. R. amd Wickham, J. C. (1967). *Int. Pest Control* **6,** 10-13.

Bucher, G. E. (1956). *Proc. Int. Cong. Ent.* 10th Montreal **4,** 695-701.

Bucher, G. E. (1964). *Ann. ent. Soc. Que.* **9,** 30-42.

Cameron, J. W. M. (1963). *Ann. Rev. Ent.* **8,** 265-286.

Cantwell, G. E. (1967). *J. Invertebrate Path.* **9,** 138-140.

Cantwell, G. E. and Franklin, B. A. (1966). *J. Invertebrate Path.* **8,** 256-258.

Chambers, D. L. (1968). *J. Invertebrate Path.* **10,** 245-251.

Clark, E. C. and Reiner, C. E. (1956). *J. econ. Ent.* **49,** 703-704.

Clark, T. B., Kellen, W. R., Fukuda, T. and Lindegren, J. E. (1968). *J. Invertebrate Path.* **11,** 1-7.

Creighton, C. S., Cuthbert, F. P., Jr. and Reid, W. J., Jr. (1964). *J. Insect Path.* **6,** 102-110.

David, W. A. L. (1967). *In* "Insect Pathology and Microbial Control" (P. A. van der Laan, ed.), pp. 174-178. North-Holland Publ. Co., Amsterdam.

David, W. A. L., Gardiner, B. O. C. and Woolner, M. (1968). *J. Invertebrate Path.* **11,** 496-501.

De Bach, P. ed. (1964). "Biological Control of Insect Pests and Weeds". Chapman and Hall Ltd., London.

Doane, C. C. and Wallis, R. C. (1964). *J. Insect Path.* **6,** 423-429.

Dulmage, H. T. (1967). *In* "Insect Pathology and Microbial Control" (P. A. van der Laan, ed.), pp. 120-124. North-Holland Publ. Co., Amsterdam.

Dutky, S. R. (1959). *In* "Advances In Applied Microbiology" (W. W. Umbreit, ed.), Vol. 1, pp. 175-200. Academic Press, New York.

Elmore, J. C. (1961). *J. econ. Ent.* **54,** 47-50.

Fox, C. J. S. and Jaques, R. P. (1961). *Can. J. Plant Sci.* **41,** 428-430.

Franz, J. M. (1961). *Ann. Rev. Ent.* **6,** 183-200.

Frear, D. E. H. (ed.) (1968). "Pesticide Handbook-Entoma 20th Edition". College Science Publishers, State College, Pennsylvania.

Furmidge, C. G. L. (1959a). *J. Sci. Fd Agric.* **5,** 267-273.

Furmidge, C. G. L. (1959b). *J. Sci. Fd Agric.* **5,** 274-282.

Geering, Q. A. and Lloyd, J. H. (1962). *J. econ. Ent.* **55**, 786-790.
Getzin, L. W. (1962). *J. econ. Ent.* **55**, 442-445.
Girardeau, J. H., Jr. and Mitchell, E. R. (1968). *J. econ. Ent.* **61**, 312-313.
Greaves, J. H., Rowe, F. P., Redfern, R. and Ayres, P. (1968). *Nature, Lond.* **219**, 402-403.
Gudauskas, R. T. and Canerday, D. (1968). *J. Invertebrate Path.* **12**, 405-411.
Hall, I. M. (1963). *In* "Insect Pathology. An Advanced Treatise" (E. A. Steinhaus, ed.), Vol. 2, pp. 477-517. Academic Press, New York.
Hall, I. M. and Dunn, P. H. (1958). *J. econ. Ent.* **51**, 341-344.
Hartley, G. S. (1960). *Chem. Ind.* 448-452.
Hedlund, R. C. and Pass, B. C. (1968). *J. Invertebrate Path.* **11**, 25-34.
Heimpel, A. M. (1965). *Wld Rev. Pest Control* **4**, 150-161.
Heimpel, A. M. (1967). *Ann. Rev. Ent.* **12**, 287-322.
Herfs, W. (1965). *Z. Pflkrankh.* **72**, 584-599.
Hofmaster, R. W. and Ditman, L. D. (1961). *J. econ. Ent.* **54**, 921-923.
Ignoffo, C. M. (1964). *Entomophaga* **2**, 293-298.
Ignoffo, C. M. (1965). *J. Invertebrate Path.* **7**, 209-235.
Ignoffo, C. M. (1967). *In* "Insect Pathology and Microbial Control" (P. A. van der Laan, ed.), pp. 91-117. North-Holland Publ. Co., Amsterdam.
Ignoffo, C. M., Chapman, A. J. and Martin, D. F. (1965). *J. Invertebrate Path.* **7**, 227-235.
Ignoffo, C. M. and Graham, H. M. (1967). *J. Invertebrate Path.* **9**, 390-393.
Jaques, R. P. (1963). *Can. J. Plant Sci.* **43**, 301-306.
Jaques, R. P. (1968). *Can. J. Microbiol.* **14**, 1161-1163.
Jaques, R. P. and Fox, C. J. S. (1960). *J. Insect Path.* **2**, 17-23.
Jaques, R. P. and Patterson, N. A. (1962). *Can. Ent.* **94**, 818-825.
Jaques, R. P., Stultz, H. T. and Huston, F. (1968). *Can. Ent.* **100**, 813-818.
Kellen, W. R. and Lindegren, J. E. (1968). *J. Invertebrate Path.* **11**, 104-111.
Krejzovà, R. (1968). *J. Invertebrate Path.* **12**, 460.
Laird, M. (1960). *Am. Inst. Biol. Sci. Tech. Rep.* (unnumbered).
Lewis, F. B. and Connola, D. P. (1966). *U.S. Forest Service Research Paper* NE-50.
Magnoler, A. (1968). *J. Invertebrate Path.* **11**, 326-328.
Martin, H. (1959). "The Scientific Principles of Crop Protection". Edward Arnold (Publishers) Ltd., London.
McEwen, F. L. and Hervey, G. E. R. (1958). *J. econ. Ent.* **51**, 626-631.
McEwen, F. L. and Hervey, G. E. R. (1959). *J. Insect Path.* **1**, 86-94.
McEwen, F. L., Glass, E. H., Davis, A. C. and Splittstoesser, C. M. (1960). *J. Insect Path.* **2**, 152-164.
McLaughlin, R. E., Daum, R. J. and Bell, M. R. (1968). *J. Invertebrate Path.* **12**, 168-174.
Metcalf, C. L., Flint, W. P. and Metcalf, R. L. (1951). *In* "Destructive and Useful Insects". Third Edition, pp. 255-386. McGraw-Hill Book Co., Inc., New York.
Morris, O. N. (1969). *J. Invertebrate Path.* **13**, 134-146.
Oatman, E. R. (1966). *J. econ. Ent.* **59**, 368-373.
Oatman, E. R. (1968). *J. econ. Ent.* **61**, 62-64.
Potts, S. F. (1958). "Concentrated Spray Equipment, Mixtures and Application Methods". Dorland Books, Caldwell, New Jersey.
Pristavko, V. P. (1967a). *Ent. Rev.* **46**, 443-446.
Pristavko, V. P. (1967b). *In* "Insect Pathology and Microbial Control" (P. A. van der Laan, ed.), pp. 212-214. North-Holland Publ. Co., Amsterdam.
Raun, E. S. and Jackson, R. D. (1966). *J. econ. Ent.* **59**, 620-622.
Raun, E. S., Sutter, G. R. and Revelo, M. A. (1966). *J. Invertebrate Path.* **8**, 365-375.
Rivers, C. F. (1967). *In* "Insect Pathology and Microbial Control" (P. A. van der Laan, ed.), pp. 252-263. North-Holland Publ. Co., Amsterdam.
Rogoff, M. H. (1966). *In* "Advances in Applied Microbiology" (W. W. Umbreit, ed.), Vol. 8, pp. 291-313. Academic Press, New York.
Sikorowski, P. P. and Madison, C. H. (1968). *J. Invertebrate Path.* **11**, 390-397.
Smirnoff, W. A. (1961). *J. Insect Path.* **3**, 29-46.

Smirnoff, W. A. (1967). *Can. Dep. Forestry and Rural Development Bi-Monthly Research Notes* **23,** 35-36.
Steinhaus, E. A. (1960). *J. Invertebrate Path.* **2,** 225-229.
Stelzer, M. J. (1967). *J. econ. Ent.* **60,** 38-41.
Stephens, J. M. (1957). *Can. J. Microbiol.* **3,** 995-1000.
Sussman, A. and Halvorson, H. O. (1966). "Spores, Their Dormancy and Germination". Harper and Row, New York.
Tanada, Y. (1956). *J. econ. Ent.* **49,** 320-329.
Tanada, Y. and Reiner, C. (1962). *J. Insect Path.* **4,** 139-154.
Vaňková, J. (1964). *Entomophaga Mém. hors Sér.* No. 2, 273-291.
Watkins, T. C. and Norton, L. B. (1955). "Handbook of Insecticide Dust Diluents and Carriers". Dorland Books, Caldwell, New Jersey.
Winchester, J. M. (1967). *Int. Pest Control* **5,** 23-25.
Wolfenbarger, D. A. (1965). *J. Invertebrate Path.* **7,** 33-85.
Yendol, W. G. (1968). *J. Invertebrate Path.* **10,** 116-121.

CHAPTER 29

Perennial Laboratory Culture of Disease-Free Insects

THOMAS J. HELMS and EARLE S. RAUN

Department of Entomology, University of Nebraska, Lincoln, Nebraska, U.S.A.

I. Introduction

The rearing of insects in the laboratory has become a necessary part of entomological research. When gross biological function, life-history and ecology were the order of the day, continual laboratory rearing was unnecessary for most insect species. As entomologists began to investigate the biochemical aspects of insect life, field observation and collection were no longer sufficient. Consequently, entomological research units began to rear their particular insect(s) under artificial conditions. In some cases these attempts were met with immediate success–in others continual failure hampered efforts. Each failure, however, was educational, providing additional insight into the insect and its requirements. Today many insect species are continually being reared under laboratory conditions (Appendix 6).

Disease is one of the major obstacles to breeding insects. The scientist requires insects that are as near normal as possible. Normal insects can be regarded as healthy insects bred in typical, favorable field conditions with a gene complex typical of a field population. Insects bred in the laboratory are abnormal to some extent, maybe only in as far as they have not experienced typical field conditions. Disease is a more severe form of abnormality.

This chapter deals primarily with methods by which microbial disease can be eliminated, reduced, or confined in laboratory colonies of insects. However, some nutritional considerations are included. Experiences found successful through trial and error by many entomologists have been compiled, without attempting to cite all possible methods. The goal? To provide scientists with some suggestions for rearing normal insects.

II. Rearing and Handling Facilities

The prevention or suppression of disease in insect laboratory colonies is multifaceted. Whether the maladies are infectious or non-infectious, optimum rearing conditions must be provided. Frequently, the exact conditions best suited to a given insect species are not fully known and conditions used in initial rearing attempts are selected by an "educated guess".

Often accommodation originally planned for another purpose must be renovated and modified, each facility with its own design, so no blue-print will fit all situations. The researcher must use his own ingenuity to satisfy the necessary requirements.

Spatial isolation from possible sources of contamination is desirable. Contamination might take the form of parasitic arthropods, insect pathogens, stray or wild arthropods, or chemicals in water or air. The greatest hazards are from areas where insect pathogens are being produced or studied. The insect breeding facility itself could be a source of contamination to other programs of work. If there is insufficient space to rely on isolation alone, disease spread should be prevented by special equipment such as disease-handling cabinets and rooms equipped with air filtration.

Proper humidity, temperature and light conditions are essential. Smith (1966) edited a book which dealt with the colonization and mass-rearing of various groups and species of insects. Each has its own requirements which must be met in order to produce healthy insects. Humidity too high or too low may cause abnormality or even colony elimination. As examples, some epizootics occur under conditions of high humidity, while low humidity may prevent normal emergence of the adult from the pupa and subsequent wing expansion.

Suitable temperatures are likewise limited for healthy insect rearing. Controlled fluctuations in temperature may be required to trigger the mating response, as in several Lepidoptera, including the European corn borer, *Ostrinia nubilalis* (Sparks, 1963). Constant-temperature rooms should be designed so that the temperature can be altered, because it is sometimes desirable to speed up or slow down breeding, or to eliminate disease by altering the temperature. Steinhaus (1945) eliminated a non-sporeforming bacterial infection from a colony of the potato tuberworm, *Phthorimaea operculella,* by reducing the rearing temperature. Tanada and Chang (1968) demonstrated resistance to a cytoplasmic-polyhedrosis virus in the alfalfa caterpillar, *Colias eurytheme,* when reared at 35° C. Similar studies have demonstrated resistance to nuclear-polyhedrosis and granulosis viruses in other insects.

The importance of the quality and quantity of light, as well as day-length, must be considered. Photoperiod and temperature in the control of diapause is extensively discussed in a book by Lees (1955) and many papers have since been published on this subject. Quality of light may affect such functions as mating, since infrared irradiations appear to be involved in attracting one sex to another in some species (Callahan, 1965).

The above factors which influence non-infectious disease also indirectly affect infectious diseases, because insects are predisposed to them if they are not growing well. Infectious maladies can be largely avoided by preventing the causative organism from reaching the insect. This requires continuous sanitation. Walls and laboratory furniture should be of a non-porous material which will withstand periodic cleaning and disinfection. Surfaces that catch and accumulate dust should be avoided as far as possible. Working surfaces should be porcelain, enamel or of an epoxy-type. Although many laboratories employ stainless steel for bench-tops, recent studies have shown that it is too porous to provide the best sanitizable surface (Chaturvedi and Maxcy, 1969). Bench-tops should be cleaned frequently and, just prior to use, treated with antimicrobial agents. Simply working above a moistened surface, such as wet paper towels laid on the bench, prevents much contamination by fungi, and many antimicrobial solutions can be used.

Various means such as air filtration have been used to reduce air borne contamination in rearing rooms. In the cotton boll weevil laboratory at State College, Mississippi air passes into the room through a wall built of filter material as in aero-space "clean rooms" (McLaughlin, personal communication). Miskimen (1965) used a 2-in-thick fiberglass filter, impregnated with hexachlorophene, on the air-conditioning system. Charcoal filters can be used to extract fumes and smells. Rooms or equipment can be decontaminated with fumigants such as triethylene and propylene glycols (McLaughlin, personal communication), ethylene oxide and others (Kelsey, 1967; Winge-Heden, 1963). Fumigation must be followed by a period of airing, during which ingress of contamination must be prevented.

Some laboratories employ a positive pressure in rearing rooms. In such facilities fans force air through filters, and maintain a positive pressure in the rearing rooms to prevent the entry of contaminated air from other parts of the building, or from the outside. To make this system feasible, windows must be thoroughly sealed or blocked. Additionally, a double-door entrance to the laboratory, with a 30-W germicidal lamp operating continuously in the space between the doors (atrium), may be of value (Miskimen, 1965). Miskimen also used additional lamps for 14 hr daily, one lamp per 1000 sq ft of floor area. In similar rooms for handling pathogens, the maintenance of a negative pressure by extracting air through an absolute filter prevents the escape of pathogens from the room.

In addition to air flow into the rearing area, we must consider the flow of personnel. Too frequently an insect rearing unit takes great pains to sanitize, sterilize, disinfect and filter everything except people working and moving from one area to another, so leading to trouble. Ideally, personnel should specialize so that those working in the rearing area would remain there throughout the working day. If this is not possible, however, the worker and his clothing must be disinfected before return to the rearing area. In veterinary and medical research where sanitation is necessary, personnel take showers and change clothing each time they move from one area to another. This regimen may not be entirely necessary in insect pathology, but it should be considered. David and Gardiner (1966) have outlined less stringent procedures for the maintenance of virus-free insect stock. A minimal requirement should be thorough scrubbing of hands with a change of laboratory coat, for which a locker area is desirable.

Various cages and containers have been developed for insect rearing. Screen wire, glass, various plastics, metal and wood have been used. Wood should be avoided because it can provide a substrate on which contaminating fungi can grow. Whether metal or plastic cages and containers are employed depends on the type and stage of insect, and the available sterilizing facilities. Many disinfectants corrode metals, and heat sterilization deforms many plastics. Autoclaving has been a standard practice in many laboratories. Others wash with soap and water, then sanitize with alcohol, chlorocresol, cresol, mercuric chloride, phenol, sodium hypochlorite, or fumigate with methyl bromide or formaldehyde. Sodium hypochlorite is particularly good for dipping. Formalin solutions have a long-standing reputation as efficient and relatively inexpensive antimicrobial agents. Ignoffo and Dutky (1963) recommended sodium hypochlorite for general laboratory disinfection after viability and infectivity tests with *Bacillus* and *Beauveria* spores and a nuclear-polyhedrosis virus. Yendol (1968) demonstrated that commercial fungicides (maneb, zineb, ferbam, dodine, and captan) affect conidia of several of the *Entomophthora*. General laboratory (food industry) disinfectants were discussed by Goldenberg and Relf (1967). Other papers by Bean (1967), Hugo (1967), and Walters (1967) may be of general interest. Sterilization facilities should be adequate to sterilize equipment after every use.

Disposable plastic and waxed card containers are available in many sizes and shapes, and frequently cost no more, in the long run, than the labor involved in washing and sterilizing non-disposable types. These are frequently used directly from the shipping containers without sanitizing, or they may be rinsed with disinfectant solutions and allowed to dry before use. (When trying a new type of plastic rearing container remember that your insect may be susceptible to that particular plastic.) Matsuda and Matsuura (1967) utilized flexible plastic bags (isolators) for rearing silkworms. They sterilized the inner side of the isolators with a spray of 2% peracetic acid.

Adequate arrangements must usually be made to prevent the escape of arthropods, particularly those capable of transmitting infectious diseases of man or animals. The simplest procedure is to stand insect cultures on traps of oil. A filter paper sealed across the mouth of a culture jar by molten paraffin wax not only keeps in the occupants, but also keeps out unwanted mites and psocids, and, to a large extent, pathogens. For sealing cracks, crevices and other unneeded openings from the rearing area, tanglefoot or other trapping material, and moats around some areas, may be necessary. Kohls (1937) recommends the provision of locker rooms, mirrors and other "deticking" facilities.

III. Colony Acquisition and Elimination of Disease

The success of a rearing program largely depends on obtaining a disease-free and genetically sound initial stock. These insects may be obtained from another laboratory or collected from the field; there are points for and against both methods.

Acquisition of a new colony from another laboratory has the advantage that the history of the parental stock is known. Disease transferrence is thus reduced, and the likelihood of the presence of disease in the colony is known, although many diseases can remain undetected unless specifically sought. However, this colony may not be genetically identical to wild populations. Generation after generation in the laboratory, each with a correspondingly reduced gene pool, will, in all likelihood, have selected a strain specifically adapted to laboratory rearing. If the investigator is willing to accept this restriction, acquisition from an established colony is the easiest approach. The same rearing procedures and sanitation regime should then be followed in the new location.

Some laboratories have found that introducing wild stock revitalizes the laboratory colony (Maddox, personal communication). However, precautions against disease must be taken as described below or the entire colony may become infected.

Field acquisition of the initial insects is probably the commonest method and assures a good genetic base from which to start. For a few generations, the colony will usually be genetically typical of the field population so that experimental results should more nearly reflect what might be expected in the field.

The main drawback of starting the colony from field collections is the danger of bringing an insect pathogen into the rearing facility. This danger is least when ecological conditions are ideal for the insect, because, at this time, a feral population usually contains mostly healthy insects.

The egg is usually the best stage to start a colony because it is least likely to carry, and most easy to free from, disease. Many pathogens, particularly bacteria and fungi, are not transmitted within the egg and can easily be eliminated by surface sterilization. If difficult to collect in the field, the first eggs laid in the laboratory may be surface sterilized. If the eggs are inaccessible, immature or adult stages must be used to start the colony and the isolation approach discussed later must be adopted.

Eggs and other stages are surface sterilized by immersion in germicidal solutions. Martignoni and Milstead (1960) recommend two quaternary ammonium compounds (QAC), Hyamine® 10-X (Rohm & Haas Company, Philadelphia, Pa.) and Zephiran® chloride (Winthrop Laboratories, New York, N.Y.), for surface sterilization of insects. Formalin and sodium hypochlorite are the most common materials used on eggs (Bucher and Williams, 1967; Getzin, 1962; Golanski, 1961; Grisdale, 1968; Vail *et al.,* 1968). Trichloracetic acid (Bergold, 1942) and sodium hydroxide-potassium permanganate (Tarasevich, 1953) have also been used. Sometimes pathogens are trapped in the outer coats of the egg and can be removed by dissolving the proteinaceous protective egg coat with trypsin (Zimmack and Brindley, 1957) and then washing in a mixture of 2% sodium hydroxide and 2% formaldehyde.

Surface sterilization, however, does not reduce many viral and protozoan pathogens which are transmitted within the ovum. Few techniques show promise of eliminating such viral contaminants though some Microsporida have been eliminated by exposing eggs to temperatures just below the upper limit for survival, as shown by Allen and Brunson (1947) with the potato tuberworm, *P. operculella,* Astaurov (1956) with the silkworm, *Bombyx mori,* and Raun (1961) with the European corn borer, *Ostrinia nubilalis.*

Others have found that eggs can be collected from isolated females and kept separate. After the oviposition period, females are dissected and the various tissues examined microscopically for Microsporida. Only eggs from uninfected females are retained.

A program not unlike the "specific pathogen free" (SPF) approach for ridding an organism of pathogens has been accomplished with the cotton boll weevil, *Anthonomus grandis,* by McLaughlin (1966). Two disease organisms, *Glugea gasti* (*Nosema* sp.), a microsporidan, and *Mattesia grandis,* a neogregarine, were eliminated by two methods: the "Family Unit" and "Quarantine" methods.

A. FAMILY UNIT METHOD

The microsporidan may be acquired *per os* as well as being passed to progeny transovum. The disease may be acute or chronic and adults may not show disease symptoms. For these reasons maintenance of the integrity of family units through the F_2 generation was required. With a known incidence of 20% (based on examination of 50 stock colony adults), McLaughlin set up 30 family units each containing three adult females. Therefore, about 18 units (20% of 3 x 30) were likely to contain infected adults. When all F_1 adults and immature progeny (larvae and pupae) were killed and examined for the pathogen after 30 days, this proved to be a slight under-estimate (Fig. 1). The F_2 adults not sacrificed were allowed to breed, maintaining the integrity of units, until F_6 without the reappearance of disease. The units were then considered disease-free.

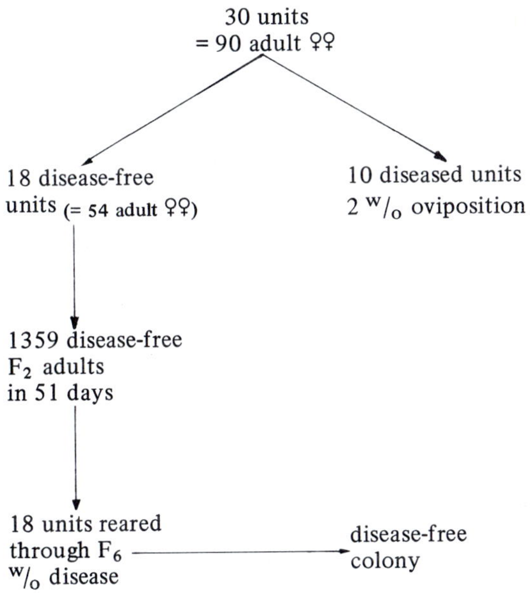

Fig. 1. Flow diagram of a Family Unit method of eliminating pathogens from insect stocks (McLaughlin, 1966).

B. QUARANTINE METHOD

M. grandis infected adults are easily detected because symptoms always appear within 10 days after infection. The disease is rarely passed transovum and healthy adults generally emerge earlier than those infected. Because of the advantages of a larger parental stock the quarantine method was devised. It takes advantage of mechanical rearing techniques instead of the small numbers per unit used in the family unit method, which involved excessive man-days to bring to completion.

The gregarine was introduced into the F_3 generation, of the microsporidosis-free adults (from the family unit experiment described above), by association with infected weevils. Cages of F_4 and F_5 generation adults were selected for the test: disease-free colonies were established by the F_5 and F_6 generations, respectively. Figure 2 is a flow diagram of the F_4 parental stock. Because healthy adults usually emerge before the infected ones, F_5 adults were collected for a period of only four days, the remaining larvae and pupae being destroyed. Emerging adults were placed in subunits of 30 or less each.

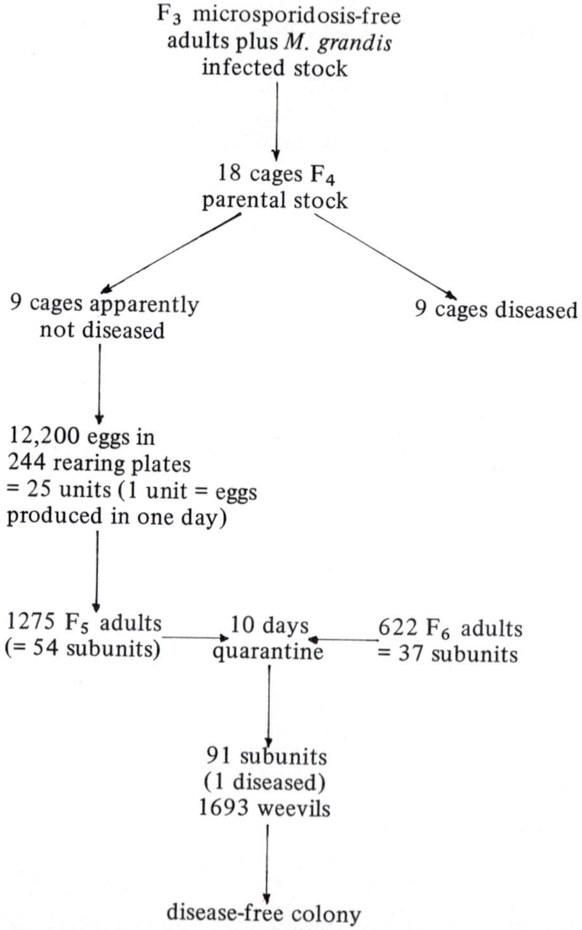

Fig. 2. Flow diagram of Quarantine method of eliminating pathogens from insect stocks, modified from an original diagram by McLaughlin (1966).

Selective breeding has removed other kinds of insect pathogens. Of particular interest is David and Gardiner's (1966) attempt to remove a granulosis virus from the European cabbageworm, *Pieris brassicae.* Their result, after many years of hard work, is a stock "apparently free of virus". One of the main reasons for the difficulty was that the virus is passed transovum and may still be present in an occult state. Yet, Getzin (1962) was able to rid cabbage loopers, *Trichoplusia ni,* of a nuclear-polyhedrosis virus by surface sterilization of eggs and rearing the larvae on an artificial diet.

In acquiring a new colony one can never be certain that a latent virus is not being carried by the insect. Under adverse conditions it could appear and wipe out the colony. Various workers have advocated that the insects be placed under stress conditions while in quarantine in order to induce the latent malady to appear. The stress condition most frequently advocated is crowding, others are higher or lower than normal temperatures, reduced food supply, and even chemicals. Diseased insects can then be removed from the colony, and only the apparently healthy retained, followed by surface sterilization of eggs.

IV. Colony Maintenance

Once freed from disease, insect colonies require constant vigilance and care to keep them so. As soon as the disease-free condition is established the breeding area should be sterilized by more thorough than usual cleaning or, ideally, by fumigation with formalin vapor. Sanitation, air filtration and the maintenance of a disease-free supply of food are the main defenses against the re-introduction of disease (Sections II and III) but, in addition, periodic microscopical checks for chronic, inapparent disease are necessary. A routine prophylactic treatment is useful, such as a period at high temperature in each generation where a heat-sensitive pathogen is known to be a major disease hazard. A routine period of stress may also be usefully interpolated to reveal disease. Finally the general breeding performance should be watched in case genetical weakness appears or symbionts suffer damage. Genetical troubles may necessitate a cross-breeding system, as with the rice stem borer, *Chilo suppressalis* (Iwata, 1965).

V. Diet Considerations

A thorough discussion of diets for the mass-production of insects would be unnecessarily repetitive because of the recent work edited by Smith (1966). This is, without doubt, a vade-mecum for those desiring to rear one or a great variety of insects. The purpose of this section, therefore, is to give the investigator some general principles to establish his particular insect's diet.

The terminology used to describe artificial foods substituted for natural foods is confusing. The culture environment is also artificial in the sense of being different to the species' natural habitat, even if a natural food is used. The terms "medium" and "diet" are synonymous as far as insect culture is concerned. "Medium" would be best reserved for reference to the culture of micro-organisms, leaving "diet" for insect culture. "Synthetic diet" means the use of basic ingredients, such as the sugars, together with supplements, such as yeast extract. Other terms that refer to the chemical composition of insect diets are: oligidic, without chemical identity; "meridic", with partial chemical identity; and, holidic, complete chemical identity (except for pure, inert materials) or chemically defined. One often encounters the terms axenic and xenic in titles of papers on insect cultivation. According to Steinhaus and Martignoni (1967), axenic cultivation refers to the rearing of one or more individuals of a single species in, or on, a non-living medium, e.g. an insect free from micro-organisms; xenic cultivation refers to the rearing of one or more individuals of one species in association with an unknown number of species of other organisms.

Practically every investigator who attempts to artificially culture an insect develops techniques that specifically fit his immediate situation and particular insect. As a consequence of the artificial situation, the investigator is challenged by a host of biological problems (i.e. ecology, physiology, behavior, etc.). Conversely, however, it is interesting to note the wide variety of artificial situations to which many insects can adapt themselves. In sum, the investigator's objective in any mass-rearing program is the production of healthy animals, as near normal as he requires, with minimal expense for materials and handling time.

Every insect diet, whether natural or artificial, provides carbohydrate, fat and protein, or the raw materials for their synthesis. Cholesterol and the B vitamins are essential organic components in all insect diets. Many insect species harbor internal symbionts that synthesize all or part of the required vitamins. Many insects can synthesize enough vitamin C to satisfy their needs, but unlike vertebrates they cannot synthesize cholesterol from acetic acid. Essential inorganic dietary requirements are principally water and salts (minerals).

Until recently, most artificial diets, particularly those for phytophagous insects, have contained some part of the insect's natural food. The so-called "corn leaf factor" of the European corn borer, for example, was ultimately

TABLE I

Diet for the European corn borer, Ostrinia nubilalis, *used successfully for 32 generations (Lewis, personal communication)*

Ingredients	Amount	Ingredients	Amount	Ingredients	Amount
Agar	280 g	Ascorbic acid[a]	120 g	Dextrose (D-glucose)	400 g
Casein	440 g	Cholesterol	32 g	Fumidil-B (Fumagillin acid)[d]	1500 p.p.m.
Wheat germ	32 g	Salt mixture No. 2[b]	144 g		
Water	12,000 ml	Sorbic acid[c]	32 g	Vitamin supplement[b]	92 g

[a] Merck and Co., Inc., Rahway, New Jersey, U.S.A.
[b] Nutritional Biochemicals Corp., Cleveland, Ohio, U.S.A.
[c] Dissolved in 160 ml 95% ethyl alcohol.
[d] Lewis and Lynch (1969).

determined to be ascorbic acid (Chippendale and Beck, 1964). When sufficient ascorbic acid is added to diets without natural food plant components, many insects that require the vitamin molt and reproduce normally (Vanderzant *et al.*, 1962; Vanderzant and Richardson, 1963; and many others). Suitable substitutes for other dietary plant factors have been found. For example: casein, wheat germ, and egg albumin (Tables I and V) provide principally amino acids; vegetable oils (Tables IV and V) provide fatty acids; sugars and starches of various kinds (Tables I, IV, V and VI) provide simple sugars. Yeasts are dietary supplements rich in B vitamins and protein (Tables II-V). Amino acids, vitamins,

TABLE II

Diets for storage insects (Burges, personal communication)

Wheat, wheatfeed (finely ground wheat bran), and glycerol on a damp pad of cotton (7 : 3 : 1)	Hairy grain beetle, *Typhaea stercorea*
Wheat and wheatfeed on a damp pad (7 : 3)	Meal moth, *Pyralis farinalis*
Wheatfeed and yeast (10 : 1)	Cigarette beetle, *Lasioderma serricorne*; biscuit beetle, *Stegobium paniceum*; slender horned flour beetle, *Gnathocerus maxillosus*; long headed flour beetle, *Latheticus oryzae*; small-eyed flour beetle, *Palorus ratzeburgii*
Wheatfeed and yeast on a damp pad (10 : 1)	Lesser mealworm and black fungus beetle, *Alphitobius diaperinus* and *A. laevigatus*; depressed flour beetle, *Palorus subdepressus*
Wheatfeed, yeast, and glycerol (10 : 1 : 3)	Mediterranean flour moth, *Ephestia (Anagasta) kuehniella*[a]; tropical warehouse moth, *E. (Cadra) cautella*[a]; warehouse moth, *E. elutella*[a]; Indian-meal moth, *Plodia interpunctella*[a]; corn moth, *Nemapogon granellus*[a]
Wheatfeed, rolled oats, and yeast (5 : 5 : 1)	Rust-red grain beetle, flat grain beetle, and other cucujid beetles, *Cryptolestes capensis, C. pusillus,* etc.; larger cabinet beetle, *Trogoderma inclusum, Trogoderma* spp.; merchant grain beetle and saw-toothed grain beetle, *Oryzaephilus mercator* and *O. surinamensis*; yellow and dark mealworms, *Tenebrio molitor*[a] and *T. obscurus*[a]
Baby cereal, yeast, glycerine, and honey (50 : 5 : 22 : 23)	Lesser and greater wax moths, *Achroia grisella*[a], *Galleria mellonella*
Wheatfeed, fishmeal, and yeast (8 : 4 : 1)	Ptinid beetles; dark and black flour beetles, *Tribolium destructor* and *T. madens*
Wholemeal flour and yeast (12 : 1)	Rust-red and confused flour beetles, *T. castaneum* and *T. confusum*
Wheatfeed, rolled oats, fishmeal, and yeast (5 : 5 : 2 : 1)	Oriental, German, American and Australian cockroaches, *Blatta orientalis*[a], *Blatella germanica*[a], *Periplaneta americana*[a] and *P. australasiae*[a]
Fishmeal, yeast, and (16 : 1) flannel	Case bearing and common clothes moths, *Tinea columberiella* and *T. bisselliella*; furniture and varied carpet beetles, *Anthrenus flavipes* and *A. verbasci*; black carpet beetle and fur beetle, *A. megatoma* and *A. pellio*
Fishmeal, yeast, and (16 : 1) bacon ends	Hide, bacon, leather, etc. beetles, *Dermestes* spp.[a]

[a] Drinking water provided in the culture either on damp filter paper or in a corked tube with a wick of filter paper or cotton.

TABLE III

Diet for several noctuid larvae: cabbage looper, Trichoplusia ni*; alfalfa looper,* Autographa californica*; yellow-striped armyworm,* Prodenia ornithogalli*; beet armyworm,* Spodoptera exigua*; tobacco budworm,* Heliothis virescens*; cotton bollworm (corn earworm),* H. zea*; armyworm,* Pseudaletia unipuncta*; and, variegated cutworm,* Peridroma saucia *(Shorey and Hale, 1965)*

Ingredients	Amount	Ingredients	Amount	Ingredients	Amount
Agar	128 g	Ascorbic acid	32 g	Dried brewer's yeast	320 g
Sorbic acid	10 g	Formaldehyde (40%)	20 g	Methyl *p*-hydroxy-benzoate	20 g
Water	6400 g	Soaked pinto beans	2133 g		

TABLE IV

Diet for the olive fruit fly, Dacus oleae *(Tzanakakis and Economopoulos, 1967). Heat is not required during preparation*

Ingredients	Amount	Ingredients	Amount
Brewer's yeast	7.5 g	Cellulose powder for column chromatography	26.0 g
Olive oil[a]	2.0 g		
Potassium sorbate	0.05 g	Methyl *p*-hydroxybenzoate	0.2 g
2N HCl	3.0 ml	Roasted peanuts (as purchased on the market)	6.0 g
Sucrose	2.0 g	Soya hydrolysate, enzymatic[b]	3.0 g
Tap water	55.0 ml	Tween-80 (polyoxyethylene sorbitan monooleate)	0.75 ml

[a] Minerva® Olive Oil.
[b] Nutritional Biochemicals Corp., Cleveland, Ohio, U.S.A.

TABLE V

Diet for both larvae and adults of the cotton boll weevil, Anthonomus grandis. *Glasshouse cultures of the host plant are not needed for oviposition (Sterling and Adkisson, 1966)*

Ingredients	Amount	Ingredients	Amount	Ingredients	Amount
Agar	1.3 g	Cholesterol	0.01 g	Alphacel (cellulose powder)	1.3 g
KOH (1%)	2.4 ml	Egg albumen	0.8 g	Brewer's yeast	1.3 g
Sucrose	1.7 g	Inhibitor[b]	1.7 ml	Cottonseed meal	13.8 g
Water	70.8 ml	Polyotic®[a]	0.7 g	Vitamin mixture[c]	2.6 ml
		Wesson oil	0.9 ml	Wheat germ oil	0.4 ml

[a] Tetracycline hydrochloride (A.I., 25 g/lb), American Cyanamid Company.
[b] Contained 10 g sorbic acid and 10 g methyl *p*-hydroxybenzoate per 100 ml 96% ethanol.
[c] Contained more ascorbic acid, alpha tocopherol and choline chloride than the diets used by Vanderzant (1957) and Vanderzant, Richardson and Davich (1959) which also contained the vitamins niacinamide, calcium pantothenate, thiamin (HCl), riboflavin, pyridoxin (HCl), folic acid, biotin, and vitamin B_{12}.

cholesterol, mixtures of the required salts, etc. may be substituted easily, particularly in a liquid diet (Table VI), and are sold commercially in pure or semi-pure forms. Agar is an ingredient common to many artificial diets because of its water-holding capacity and its holding qualities for other ingredients as well. Bulk or roughage is an important ingredient for insects with chewing mouthparts particularly those that normally feed on coarse or abrasive substances including fresh plant material. This is easily provided in unpurified foods such as those fed to stored products insects (Table II), in the form of pure cellulose (Tables IV and V), or the agar itself may be sufficient. In most artificial diets to which lipids are added (e.g. olive oil, Wesson oil, etc., Tables IV and V), an emulsifier or wetting agent (e.g. Tween-80) is necessary for proper mixing.

The physical nature of the rearing medium is an important aspect of artificial rearing that may be easily overlooked. It must be as acceptable to the insect as the natural medium. For example, Mittler and Dadd (1964) and Kieckhefer and Derr (1967) prepared "sachets" of liquid diet for aphids from two Parafilm® membranes which may have also provided a substitute for waxy plant surfaces. With tunneling insects, such as the European corn borer, strips of cardboard with

TABLE VI

Chemically defined diet for the pea aphid, Acyrthosiphon pisum, *successful for three generations (Auclair, 1965)*

Ingredients	Amount	Ingredients	Amount	Ingredients	Amount
1-amino acids and amides (mg)				Vitamins (mg)	
Alanine	100	DL-Homoserine	800	Ascorbic acid	10.0
Arginine	400	Isoleucine	200	Biotin	0.1
Asparagine	300	Leucine	200	Calcium pantothenate	5.0
Aspartic acid	100	Lysine mono-HCl	200	Choline chloride	50.0
Cysteine	50	Methionine	100	Folic acid	1.0
Cystine	5	Phenylalanine	100	*i*-Inositol	50.0
Gamma-amino butyric acid	20	Proline	100	Nicotinic acid	10.0
		Serine	100	*p*-Aminobenzoic acid	10.0
Glutamic acid	200	Threonine	200	Pyridoxine HCl	2.5
Glutamine	600	Tryptophan	100	Riboflavin	5.0
Glycine	20	Tyrosine	20	Thiamine HCl	2.5
Histidine	200	Valine	200	Other	
				Cholesterol benzoate	2.5 mg
				K_3PO_4	500.0 mg
				$MgCl_2 \cdot 6H_2O$	200.0 mg
				Salt mixture No. 2[a]	5.0 mg
				Sucrose	35.0 g
				Water to make	100.0 ml

[a] Nutritional Biochemicals Corp., Cleveland, Ohio, U.S.A.

large corrugations may be placed above the medium. These examples provide some evidence that normal behavioral responses may be elicited by substitute factors in the artificial environment. Some insects, however, are successfully cultured on diets in simple containers without such factors.

The following references, although not a comprehensive list, describe other insect diets and rearing techniques: human bot fly, *Dermatobia hominis,* Banegas *et al.* (1967); a dolicopodid fly, *Medetera aldrichii,* McGhehey and Nagel (1966); horn fly, *Haematobia irritans,* Schmidt *et al.* (1967); muscoid flies, *Musca* spp., *Fannia* spp. and *Stomoxys calcitrans,* Schoof (1964); an acridid, *Aulocara elliotti,* Anderson and Hastings (1966); house cricket, *Acheta domesticus,* Patton (1967); termites, Becker (1965); California five-spined ips, *Ips confusus,* Bedard (1966); cereal leaf beetle, *Oulema melanopus,* Connin *et al.* (1968); cotton boll weevil, *A. grandis,* Earle *et al.* (1966), Moore *et al.* (1967), and Vanderzant (1967b); foreign grain beetle, *Ahasverus advena,* Hill (1965); false wireworm, *Eleodes suturalis,* Matteson (1966); European corn borer, *O. nubilalis,* Beck *et al.* (1968); European pine shoot moth, *Rhyacionia buoliana,* Chawla and Harwood (1968); greater wax moth, *Galleria mellonella,* Dutky *et al.* (1962); cabbage looper, *Trichoplusia ni,* Ignoffo (1963a); gypsy moth, *Lymantria dispar,* Leonard and Doane (1966); Douglas-fir tussock moth, *Hemerocampa pseudotsugata,* Lyon and Flake (1966); pink bollworm, *Pectinophora gossypiella,* Richmond and Ignoffo (1964); red-banded leaf roller, *Argyrotaenia velutinana,* Rock *et al.* (1964); peach tree and lesser peach tree borers, *Sanninoidea exitiosa* and *Synanthedon pictipes,* Russell (1968); salt-marsh caterpillar, *Estigmene acrea,* Vail *et al.* (1967) and Vanderzant (1967b); corn earworm (also bollworm or tomato fruitworm), *Heliothis zea,* Vanderzant (1968); corn leaf aphid, *Rhopalosiphum maidis,* Kieckhefer and Derr (1967); green peach aphid, *Myzus persicae,* Mittler and Dadd (1964); lygus bug, *Lygus hesperus,* Strong and Kruitwagen (1969) and Vanderzant (1967a).

Many antimicrobial agents that inhibit fungi and bacteria, and to a lesser extent protozoans and viruses, are incorporated into artificial diets for insects. Relatively low concentrations of such compounds as formaldehyde, methyl *p*-hydroxybenzoate, potassium sorbate and sorbic acid are regularly added singly or in combination as preservatives, inhibitors or antiseptics (e.g. Table III). Some investigators have successfully controlled or prevented certain diseases by adding antibiotics such as benzylpenicillinic acid, erythromycin, fumagillin, tetracycline, and others. However, these are not used universally. It is imperative that essential symbiotic micro-organisms are not killed: for example, in the dermestid beetles, *Attagenus megatoma* and *Trogoderma parabile* (Boush *et al.*, 1968); the cigarette beetle, *Lasioderma serricorne* (Milne, 1963); aphids (Mittler, personal communication); termites; certain cockroaches; and many others. In addition to the references cited on artificial diets, some information on application of, and micro-organisms affected by, various antimicrobial agents may be gained from: Afrikian (1960), Bailey (1953), Chawla *et al.* (1967), Dunkel and Boush (1968), Gochnauer and Furgula (1962), Golanski (1961), Henry (1968), Hitchcock (1964), Ignoffo (1963b), Ignoffo and Garcia (1968), Lewis and Lynch (1969), McLaughlin and Keller (1964), Ouye (1962), Riddiford (1967), and Vail *et al.* (1968).

References

Afrikian, E. G. (1960). *J. Insect Path.* **2,** 299-304.
Allen, H. W. and Brunson, M. H. (1947). *Science* **105,** 394.
Anderson, N. L. and Hastings, E. (1966). *Ann. ent. Soc. Am.* **59,** 718-719.
Astaurov, B. L. (1956). *In* "Infectious and Protozoan Diseases of Beneficial and Harmful Insects" (V. I. Poltev and M. C. Paveleva, eds), pp. 63-93. Office of Agricultural Literature, Moscow.
Auclair, J. L. (1965). *Ann. ent. Soc. Am.* **58,** 855-875.
Bailey, F. (1953). *Bee World* **37,** 136-137.
Banegas, A. D., Mourier, H. and Graham, O. H. (1967). *Ann. ent. Soc. Am.* **60,** 511-514.
Bean, H. S. (1967). *J. appl. Bacteriol.* **30,** 6-16.
Beck, S. D., Chippendale, G. M. and Swinton, D. E. (1968). *Ann. ent. Soc. Am.* **61,** 459-462.
Becker, G. (1965). *Zeit. angew. Zool.* **52,** 385-398.
Bedard, W. D. (1966). *Ann. ent. Soc. Am.* **59,** 931-938.
Bergold, G. (1942). *Sonderdruck Naturwissenschaften* **30,** 422-423.
Boush, G. M., Dunkel, F. V. and Burkholder, W. (1968). *J. econ. Ent.* **61,** 644-646.
Bucher, G. E. and Williams, R. (1967). *J. Invertebrate Path.* **9,** 467-473.
Callahan, P. S. (1965). *Ann. ent. Soc. Am.* **58,** 727-745.
Chaturvedi, S. K. and Maxcy, R. B. (1969). *Fd Technol.* **23,** 67-70.
Chawla, S. S. and Harwood, R. F. (1968). *Wash. Agric. exp. Stn., Tech. Bull.* No. 59.
Chawla, S. S., Howell, J. F. and Harwood, R. F. (1967). *J. econ. Ent.* **60,** 307-308.
Chippendale, G. M. and Beck, S. D. (1964). *Ent. exp. Appl.* **7,** 241-248.
Connin, R. V., Cobb, D. L., Arnsman, J. C. and Lawson, G. (1968). USDA-ARS Report 33-125.
David, W. A. L. and Gardiner, B. O. C. (1966). *J. Invertebrate Path.* **8,** 325-333.
Dunkel, F. V. and Boush, G. M. (1968). *J. Invertebrate Path.* **11,** 281-288.
Dutky, S. R., Thompson, J. V. and Cantwell, G. E. (1962). *Proc. ent. Soc. Wash.* **64,** 56-58.
Earle, N. W., Walker, A. B. and Burks, M. L. (1966). *Ann. ent. Soc. Am.* **59,** 664-669.
Getzin, L. W. (1962). *J. Insect Path.* **4,** 486-488.
Gochnauer, T. A. and Furgala, B. (1962). *J. Insect Path.* **4,** 489-491.
Golanski, K. (1961). *J. Insect Path.* **3,** 11-14.
Goldenberg, N. and Relf, C. J. (1967). *J. appl. Bact.* **30,** 141-147.
Grisdale, D. B. (1968). *J. Invertebrate Path.* **10,** 425.
Henry, J. E. (1968). *J. Invertebrate Path.* **11,** 224-233.
Hill, S. T. (1965). *Bull. ent. Res.* **55,** 681-690.
Hitchcock, J. D. (1964). *J. Insect Path.* **6,** 408-410.
Hugo, W. B. (1967). *J. appl. Bact.* **30,** 17-50.
Ignoffo, C. M. (1963a). *Ann. ent. Soc. Am.* **56,** 178-182.
Ignoffo, C. M. (1963b). *J. Insect Path.* **5,** 395-397.
Ignoffo, C. M. and Dutky, S. R. (1963). *J. Insect Path.* **5,** 422-426.
Ignoffo, C. M. and Garcia, C. (1968). *J. Invertebrate Path.* **10,** 430-432.
Iwata, Y. (1965). *Wld. Rev. Pest Control* **4,** 162-173.
Kelsey, J. C. (1967). *J. appl. Bact.* **30,** 92-100.
Kieckhefer, R. W. and Derr, R. F. (1967). *J. econ. Ent.* **60,** 663-665.

Kohls, G. M. (1937). *In* "Culture Methods for Invertebrate Animals" (P. S. Galtsoff, F. E. Lutz, P. S. Welch and J. G. Needham, eds), pp. 246-256. Comstock Publishing Co., Ithaca, New York.
Lees, A. D. (1955). "The Physiology of Diapause in Arthropods". Cambridge University Press, New York.
Leonard, D. E. and Doane, C. C. (1966). *Ann. ent. Soc. Am.* **59,** 462-464.
Lewis, L. C. and Lynch, R. E. (1969). USDA-ARS Special Report V-409.
Lyon, R. L. and Flake, H. W., Jr. (1966). *J. econ. Ent.* **59,** 696-698.
Martignoni, M. E. and Milstead, J. E. (1960). *J. Insect Path.* **2,** 124-133.
Matsuda, M. and Matsuura, Y. (1967). *J. Seric. Sci., Tokyo* **36,** 403-408.
Matteson, J. W. (1966). *J. econ. Ent.* **59,** 26-27.
McGhehey, J. H. and Nagel, W. P. (1966). *Ann. ent. Soc. Am.* **59,** 290-292.
McLaughlin, R. E. (1966). *J. econ. Ent.* **59,** 401-404.
McLaughlin, R. E. and Keller, J. C. (1964). *J. Insect Path.* **6,** 481-485.
Milne, D. L. (1963). *J. ent. Soc. S. Africa* **26,** 43-63.
Miskimen, G. W. (1965). *Ann. ent. Soc. Am.* **58,** 820-823.
Mittler, T. E. and Dadd, R. H. (1964). *Ann. ent. Soc. Am.* **57,** 139-140.
Moore, R. F., Jr., Whisnant, F. F. and Taft, H. M. (1967). *J. econ. Ent.* **60,** 237-241.
Ouye, M. T. (1962). *J. econ. Ent.* **55,** 854-857.
Patton, R. L. (1967). *Ann. ent. Soc. Am.* **60,** 1238-1242.
Raun, E. S. (1961). *J. Insect Path.* **3,** 446-448.
Richmond, C. A. and Ignoffo, C. (1964). *J. econ. Ent.* **57,** 503-505.
Riddiford, L. M. (1967). *Science* **157,** 1451-1452.
Rock, G. C., Glass, E. H. and Patton, R. L. (1964). *Ann. ent. Soc. Am.* **57,** 617-621.
Russell, W. G. (1968). *J. econ. Ent.* **61,** 1450-1451.
Schmidt, C. D., Harris, R. L. and Hoffman, R. A. (1967). *Ann. ent. Soc. Am.* **60,** 508-510.
Schoof, H. F. (1964). *Bull. Wld Hlth Org.* **31,** 539-544.
Shorey, H. H. and Hale, R. L. (1965). *J. econ. Ent.* **58,** 522-524.
Smith, C. N. (ed.) (1966). "Insect Colonization and Mass Production". Academic Press, New York.
Sparks, A. N. (1963). *Proc. N. Centr. Br., ent. Soc. Am.* **18,** 95.
Steinhaus, E. A. (1945). *J. econ. Ent.* **38,** 718-719.
Steinhaus, E. A. and Martignoni, M. E. (1967). "An Abridged Glossary of Terms Used in Invertebrate Pathology". Pacific Northwest Forest and Range Experiment Station, USDA, Forest Service.
Sterling, W. L. and Adkisson, P. L. (1966). *J. econ. Ent.* **59,** 1074-1077.
Strong, F. E. and Kruitwagen, E. (1969). *Ann. ent. Soc. Am.* **62,** 148-155.
Tanada, Y. and Chang, G. Y. (1968). *J. Invertebrate Path.* **10,** 79-83.
Tarasevich, L. M. (1953). *Mikrobiologiya* **22,** 311-315.
Tzanakakis, M. E. and Economopoulos, A. P. (1967). *J. econ. Ent.* **60,** 660-663.
Vail, P. V., Henneberry, T. J., Kishaba, A. N. and Arakawa, K. Y. (1968). *J. Invertebrate Path.* **10,** 84-93.
Vail, P. V., Henneberry, T. J. and Pengalden, R. (1967). *Ann. ent. Soc. Am.* **60,** 134-138.
Vanderzant, E. S. (1957). *J. econ. Ent.* **50,** 219-221.
Vanderzant, E. S. (1967a). *J. econ. Ent.* **60,** 813-816.
Vanderzant, E. S. (1967b). *Ann. ent. Soc. Am.* **60,** 1062-1066.
Vanderzant, E. S. (1968). *Ann. ent. Soc. Am.* **61,** 120-125.
Vanderzant, E. S., Pool, M. C. and Richardson, C. D. (1962). *J. Insect Physiol.* **8,** 287-297.
Vanderzant, E. S. and Richardson, C. D. (1963). *Science* **140,** 989-991.
Vanderzant, E. S., Richardson, C. D. and Davich, T. B. (1959). *J. econ. Ent.* **52,** 1138-1143.
Walters, A. H. (1967). *J. appl. Bacteriol.* **30,** 56-65.
Winge-Heden, K. (1963). *Acta path. microbiol. scand.* **58,** 225-244.
Yendol, W. G. (1968). *J. Invertebrate Path.* **10,** 116-121.
Zimmack, H. L. and Brindley, T. A. (1957). *J. econ. Ent.* **50,** 637-640.

CHAPTER 30

Strain Improvement and Preservation of Virulence of Pathogens

KEIO AIZAWA

Institute of Biological Control, Faculty of Agriculture, Kyushu University, Fukuoka, Japan

I. Introduction

Knowledge about the characteristics of various kinds of insect pathogens and about their host-parasite relationships are accumulating. Many successful applications of insect pathogens have been reported, stimulated on the one hand by progress in insect microbiology, and on the other by the importance and value of microbial control as one of the selective methods of insect pest control.

Problems of pathogenicity, virulence, and strain selection are important in applied insect microbiology and have been discussed frequently (Steinhaus, 1949; MacLeod, 1954a; Tanada, 1959, 1963; Krieg, 1961, 1967; Briggs, 1963; Cameron, 1963; Aizawa, 1963; Martignoni, 1964; Smirnoff, 1964; Hall, 1964; Bucher, 1964; Müller-Kögler, 1965, 1967; Vago and Bergoin, 1968; Stairs, 1968; Angus, 1968) and reviewed by Tanada (1964, 1967b). Although many trials have been conducted, the systematic screening and breeding of insect pathogens are still primitive when compared, for example, with those in the production of antibiotics.

As Dutky (1959) mentioned, there are no general rules applicable to the selection of strains and no simple procedures for screening out the most promising. However, attempts to change the virulence and to select strains of insect pathogens will be collated and the results reviewed in this chapter, so that the present status of our knowledge can be assessed for the benefit of applied insect microbiology.

II. Pathogenicity and Virulence

A. DEFINITIONS AND CONTROLLING FACTORS

Steinhaus and Martignoni (1962) give comprehensive definitions of the term "pathogenicity" and "virulence", but in this review, pathogenicity will be used simply in the qualitative sense as the ability of a strain or species of micro-organism to produce disease in various hosts. Virulence will be used in the simple quantitative sense as the degree of pathogenicity against a specific host in controlled conditions within a group or species of micro-organism. Virulence varies in different physical conditions, such as temperature and humidity. These factors control the extent to which the virulence can be expressed. The innate virulence of a pathogen can be measured only in conditions that allow its full expression.

B. METHOD OF ESTIMATION OF VIRULENCE

Virulence is estimated by bioassay (see Chapter 27), which has been frequently discussed, particularly in relation to the standardization of *Bacillus thuringiensis* (Burgerjon, 1959, 1964, 1965; Krieg, 1965a, b; Burges, 1967a, b; Burges *et al.*, 1967), viruses (Ignoffo, 1964, 1965a, b, c, 1966a, b, 1967, 1968; Heimpel, 1967), and fungi (Müller-Kögler, 1965, 1967). Bioassay results are expressed as the LD_{50}, ED_{50} (Wittig, 1963), ID_{50}, or LC_{50} (in terms of the number of polyhedra, dilution of free virus suspension, weight of *B. thuringiensis* product, or number of spores or crystals per larva or unit of body weight, that affects half the insects). In bioassay, measured quantities of a pathogen are applied to a homogeneous host strain selecting insects which are comparable in age and body weight (Tanada, 1967b).

III. Strain Improvement and Preservation of Virulence

A. VIRUSES

Ossowski (1958, 1960, 1962) suggested the existence of virus strains with different virulence because equal concentrations of nuclear polyhedra from different localities did not produce the same degree of mortality in the wattle bagworm, *Kotochalia junodi.* Nuclear-polyhedrosis viruses of the tent caterpillars, *Malacosoma americanum, M. pluviale* and *M. disstria* are equally infectious for *M. disstria.* Nuclear-polyhedrosis virus from a European species, *M. alpicola,* acted much more slowly than the other native viruses (Stairs, 1964b). Batches of granular inclusions derived from two races of the butterfly, *Pieris brassicae,* were equal in virulence, but different stocks of the host varied in susceptibility (David and Gardiner, 1965).

According to Bergold (1958), "ineffective" viruses, like the granulosis virus of the moth, *Choristoneura fumiferana,* are possible mutants of low infectivity. In some insect viruses, strains forming polyhedra of different shapes are known. A strain of the nuclear-polyhedrosis of *Hyphantria cunea* with polyhedra in the form of tetrahedrons, which appear triangular in optical section, was more virulent than a "hexahedron" strain which appears tetragonal (Aruga *et al.,* 1961). Hukuhara and Hashimoto (1966) and Hukuhara (1968) found that a "tetragonal" strain was more virulent and, in addition, multiplied more rapidly than a "hexagonal" one although there was no serological difference. Stairs (1964a) selected a strain of granulosis virus producing only cuboidal inclusion bodies in *C. fumiferana,* but did not mention virulence.

The problem of virus strains should be considered in the standardization of virus products. Ignoffo (1965c) states that variations in bioassay results may be attributed to the existence of virus strains in the sample. He collected samples of virus from different areas and was able to pass them through insects continuously over a period of several years (Ignoffo, 1966b). Cameron (1962) suggested that an automatic selection of virus strains in an insect in the field might account for great variations in mortality. Allen (1968) obtained a strain of nuclear-polyhedrosis virus of *Heliothis* with two-fold increase in virulence, although his recently developed methods are not described in detail.

These papers indicate that virus strains with different virulence exist in natural insect populations and will be selected for microbial control by insect pathologists, but in laboratory conditions, the characteristics of a virus strain seem to be consistently preserved.

1. Change in Virulence

a. Passages through insects. With the nuclear-polyhedrosis virus of the sawfly, *Neodiprion sertifer,* Smirnoff (1961) selected a strain of increased virulence from the first larvae to die after inoculation at a concentration of 2×10^4 polyhedra/ml. In successive passages of the nuclear-polyhedrosis virus of *Galleria mellonella,* the virility increased gradually over the 1st to the 8th generations and reached 88% mortality, but during the 9th to the 12th generations, it remained unchanged at 75-80% mortality (Veber, 1964). The virulence of the nuclear-polyhedrosis virus of the gypsy moth, *Lymantria dispar,* increased five times above that of the original strain by serial passages through a new insect host (Fedorintchik, 1964). Further investigation is needed to decide whether or not an increase in the number of virus bundles (per polyhedron) after serial passages (Machay and Lovas, 1957) is a rather general phenomenon.

Aizawa (1962) reported successive passages of the nuclear-polyhedrosis virus of the silkworm, *Bombyx mori,* through *G. mellonella.* The virus titre of the infected *Galleria* haemolymph (bioassayed in *Galleria*) increased gradually and, after the 8th passage, reached 4.0-5.0 (–log LD_{50}, i.e. 0.003 ml diluted haemolymph was injected into each larva and the dilution at the LD_{50} level was 10^{-4}-10^{-5}). The infected haemolymph of *Galleria* was also infectious for the silkworm, and its titre (when assayed in the silkworm) was nearly the same as that of silkworm haemolymph typically infected with silkworm nuclear-polyhedrosis. The *Galleria*-adapted virus was neutralized by an antiserum formed in the rabbit against silkworm virus produced in the silkworm. The sectional shape of the polyhedra in the original silkworm polyhedrosis and in the early passages of virus through *Galleria* was nearly hexagonal. After successive passages through *Galleria,* tetragonal polyhedra were formed and sometimes a few triangular ones were observed.

Smirnoff (1963a) adapted the nuclear-polyhedrosis virus of the sawfly, *Trichiocampus viminalis,* to *Trichiocampus irregularis* and the adapted virus showed a pronounced increase of virulence.

The cultivation of the nuclear-polyhedrosis viruses of the alfalfa caterpillar, the beet armyworm, and the silkworm in chick embryos was unsuccessful (Steinhaus, 1951; Aizawa, 1961). However, after passages of the silkworm virus through silkworm pupae and chick embryos alternately, a variant virus which formed tetragonal polyhedra in the silkworm pupae and larvae was obtained. In further successive passages, the number of polyhedra decreased and sometimes triangular polyhedra were observed. The symptoms in the infected larvae entirely changed and became very similar to those of the so-called "clear head" disease. However, the infectivity of the haemolymph was 6.5-7.0 (LD_{50}, –log dilution, 0.005 ml injected/larva) and the virus was still neutralized with antiserum against the original nuclear-polyhedrosis virus of the silkworm (Aizawa, 1961). In this experiment, inasmuch as the virus was selected from the point of view of polyhedron formation, the virulence was not modified.

b. Attenuated virus. After *Galleria*-adapted silkworm nuclear-polyhedrosis virus (BG virus) (Aizawa, 1962) had been passed through *Galleria* for more than 80 generations, its virulence against the silkworm decreased. Table I shows the decrease in the virulence of BG virus when the polyhedron suspension was administered perorally to newly-hatched silkworm larvae. If the supernatant from homogenized, infected *Galleria* larvae (i.e. free virus) is injected into silkworm pupae, virulence was different among silkworm strains (Table II). In certain silkworm strains, virulence of BG virus was low either by injection of free virus or by feeding of polyhedra. In this connection the following should be noted. The nuclear-polyhedrosis virus native of *G. mellonella* is highly infectious

TABLE I

Virulence of the attenuated BG strain of the silkworm nuclear-polyhedrosis virus, assayed by feeding of polyhedra in different strains of silkworm larvae[a]

Expt. No.	Silkworm strain	LD_{50} (No. of polyhedra/ml)	
		Bombyx mori virus	*Galleria*-adapted *Bombyx mori* virus (BG-7801)
1	J 124 x C 122 (Futo)	$10^{4.5}$	$10^{8.0}$
	Fuji x Sakura	$10^{5.5}$	$10^{8.8}$
2	J 124	$10^{5.0}$	$10^{6.8}$
	C 124	$10^{3.8}$	$10^{5.8}$
	J 124 x C 124	$10^{5.8}$	$10^{8.0}$

[a] Aizawa *et al.*, unpublished.

TABLE II

Virulence of strains of the silkworm nuclear-polyhedrosis virus assayed by injection of free virus[a]

Virus strains	LD_{50} (-log dilution, 0.005 ml injected/larva)			
	Galleria mellonella (larvae)	Silkworm strains (pupae)		
		C 124 x J 124	Ryuhaku x Shuko	Shuko x Ryuhaku
B	2.65	6.30	–	–
	–	6.83	–	6.67
BG-87	3.83	5.16	5.37	–
BGC-27	3.33	≦2.62	<2.50	–
Gm-8	3.75	4.16	<2.50	–
GmC-6	>4.50	4.36	<2.50	–

B: Nuclear-polyhedrosis virus of *Bombyx mori.*
BG: *Galleria*-adapted B virus.
BGC: *Chilo suppressalis*-adapted BG virus.
Gm: Nuclear-polyhedrosis virus of *Galleria mellonella* (supplied by Dr. Y. Tanada, University of California).
GmC: *Chilo suppressalis*-adapted Gm virus.

[a] Aizawa *et al.*, unpublished.

for the greater wax moth, but it shows very low infectivity against some silkworm strains by injection. If the virus is injected into silkworm pupae, adults emerge and remain healthy. However, a few polyhedra were observed in silkworm adults when external symptoms were not discernible in the moths. The nuclear-polyhedrosis virus of *G. mellonella* is neutralized by antiserum against silkworm nuclear-polyhedrosis virus. The shape and size of polyhedra of the *Bombyx* and the *Galleria* viruses are different (Gershenson, 1957), but the viruses are serologically related (Aizawa, 1967). Furthermore, when a sublethal dose of BG polyhedra was administered to newly-hatched silkworm larvae, followed in a later instar by a challenge with the silkworm nuclear polyhedra, the larvae overcame the challenge.

The rice stem borer, *Chilo suppressalis,* has been found to be susceptible to the BG virus. This virus was successively passed through borers (BGC virus), as a result of which it was found to have become attenuated when free virus was bioassayed by injection in the silkworm (Table II).

When an insect virus is successively passed through another insect host, one should consider the change of virulence. Increased virulence should be available for microbial control, and the attenuated virus might be used for the control of the virus diseases of beneficial insects, particularly in the silkworm.

B. BACTERIA

1. Bacillus thuringiensis *and Related Bacteria*

a. Pathogenicity and susceptibility. According to the strain of bacterium and the species of host insect in question, the pathogenicity and virulence of *B. thuringiensis* may depend only on the toxicity of the crystal, or on a combination of this toxicity with the pathogenicity of the spore, or possibly mainly on the latter. For instance, the difference in virulence of the *alesti (anduze)* and *berliner* varieties against *P. brassicae* is accounted for by the structure of the crystals and their digestion by the chyle (Lecadet and Martouret, 1964). Thus the basis of the virulence of *B. thuringiensis* is complicated, and no attempt will be made in the following discussion to distinguish between the different causes of virulence.

The virulences of *B. thuringiensis* strains have been compared in many different hosts with varying degrees of accuracy (Herfs, 1962, 1963; Vaňková, 1964, 1965; Ridet, 1966; Burgerjon and Biache, 1967; Broersma and Buxton, 1967; Burges *et al.,* 1967; Angus, 1967; Angus and Norris, 1968).

The addition of 1% boric acid to a *B. thuringiensis* suspension resulted in a distinctly higher mortality than in larvae treated with either alone (Doane, 1965; Doane and Wallis, 1964). Mucin is an agent promoting infection by *Pseudomonas aeruginosa* in grasshoppers (Stephens, 1959). These agents probably alter the susceptibility of the insect host and not the virulence of the pathogen.

In the bioassay of pathogens, Tanada (1967b) claims to use a homogeneous host strain. Table III shows our results on the virulences of two strains of *B. thuringiensis* which were measured with six silkworm strains. The virulence of *B. thuringiensis* strain B varied considerably among silkworm strains when compared with that of *B. thuringiensis* strain A. The LD_{50} values for bacterial

TABLE III

Virulence of two strains of Bacillus thuringiensis *against the silkworm,* Bombyx mori[a]

B. thuringiensis strains	Expt. No.	Larval instar[b]	Silkworm strains: LD_{50} (Spores/g body wt perorally)					
			Daizo	C 115	Okusa	C 124	Shungetsu	J 124
A	684	IV_4-V_4	3.7×10^4	2.9×10^4	–	5.2×10^4	–	–
	685	IV_3-IV_4	3.9×10^4	1.4×10^4	4.2×10^4	5.7×10^4	2.6×10^4	9.8×10^3
	686	IV_2-IV_5	2.2×10^4	6.7×10^4	8.7×10^4	2.8×10^4	3.4×10^4	–
B	684	IV_4-V_4	1.9×10^7	2.9×10^7	–	4.2×10^6	–	–
	685	IV_3-IV_4	$>3.9 \times 10^7$	$>2.0 \times 10^7$	4.9×10^7	8.6×10^6	2.1×10^6	2.1×10^6
	686	IV_2-IV_5	$>4.2 \times 10^7$	$>4.3 \times 10^7$	5.1×10^7	4.7×10^6	4.4×10^6	4.7×10^6

[a] Aizawa *et al.*, unpublished.

[b] IV_4 indicates the fourth day of the fourth instar.

strain A probably do not differ significantly from each other. With bacterial strain B, the LD_{50} values of silkworm strains Shungetsu and J 124 appear to be clearly less than those for Daizo, C 115 and Okusa.

b. Change in virulence.

(i) Variants, Steinhaus and Jerrel (1954) sometimes found two crystals and one spore in a sporangium of *B. thuringiensis.* This has been also observed by Krieg (1963), Surany (1967), and Norris (personal communication). As mentioned by Toumanoff (1955), Vaňková (1957), Fitz-James and Young (1959), and Somerville *et al.* (1968), sporulating acrystalliferous mutant strains (sp^+ cr^-) with loss of virulence are commonly obtained, for example, by repeated cultivation in alkaline media (pH 9; Toumanoff and Vago, 1952), formaldehyde treatment (Fitz-James and Young, 1959), and repeated transfer at 48-hr intervals (Lemoigne *et al.,* 1956). Also, according to Somerville *et al.* (1968), sp^- cr^+ strains which show abortive sporulation exist, but are extremely rare. Evlakhova and Chvetzova (1964) selected virulent strains and based their selection on the types of crystal, pathogenicity, and serological characteristics.

(ii) Change in virulence by subculturing. Unfavourable physical conditions and the presence of inhibitors in the *in vitro* culture medium of *B. thuringiensis* may depress the growth of the bacteria or the production of spores or crystals, and so lower the virulence of the bacterial yield of that culture. Such a loss of virulence is, however, likely to be restored if the bacterium is recultured in an optimal medium in the absence of the inhibitory factor. Smirnoff (1963b) reported that *B. thuringiensis (cereus)* var. *dendrolimus* sporulated and formed crystals in a normal way in a medium containing 1 *M* urea, unlike the other varieties and species studied. This indicates that urea inhibits the crystal formation of most varieties. Smirnoff (1967a) observed the influence of temperature on the growth *in vitro* of crystalliferous bacteria and reasoned that this might explain the difference in the expression of virulence in insects at different temperatures. He suggested that it is desirable to select bacterial strains more active at the low temperatures common in the natural environment of the host insects.

Antibacterial substances are contained in plant leaves (Gukasian, 1958; Kushner and Harvey, 1962; Smirnoff, 1967b) which inhibit the formation of crystals. The effect of valine, leucine, and isoleucine on the production of exotoxin by *B. thuringiensis* and related bacteria was examined by Conner and Hansen (1967). Valine enhanced the growth of var. *thuringiensis* and stimulated the production of exotoxin.

(iii) Change in virulence by passages through insects. Toumanoff (1956, 1958) passed *Bacillus cereus* through *G. mellonella* and *P. brassicae* and obtained a crystalliferous strain. The same result was obtained by Le Corroller (1958) by means of successive passages of *B. cereus* through *G. mellonella.* According to Krieg (1967) there is some doubt about this result since crystalliferous bacteria have been isolated from *G. mellonella* larvae which were not treated with crystalliferous bacteria. Schvetsova and Zurabova (1967) passed *Bacillus subtilis* through various insects without the appearance of a crystal former. When they passed *B. thuringiensis* through the moths, *Mamestra (Barathra) brassicae* and *Hadena sordida,* a decrease of virulence was found. Stephens (1957) passed *B. cereus* spores through hibernating codling moth larvae eight times, and found the virulence increased 50 times. *B. cereus* isolated from insects showed a higher degree of virulence for the codling moth than strains isolated from apples (Stephens, 1952).

c. Strain improvement and preservation of virulence.

(i) Screening. Cosenza and Lewis (1966) isolated four strains of "wild" type *B. thuringiensis,* belonging to serotype 1, from gypsy moth larvae and found significant differences in their mortality and rate of action. For example, the LC_{50} of two isolates, 34 and 1A, was 2.65×10^6 and 1.75×10^7 viable spores/ml, respectively; the LC_{50} in crystals/ml was 2.0×10^6 and 5.0×10^7/ml, respectively.

Kushner and Lisson (1959) selected strains of *B. cereus* that could grow at a pH of 10.3 instead of the normal 7.5. These strains produced lecithinase and the resistance to the alkaline pH was not lost after several transfers on a neutral medium. Chislett and Kushner (1961) observed that the spores of these strains germinated at a higher pH than spores of an alkali-sensitive strain. Regrettably, there was no test of pathogenicity. Isakova and Stroeva (1968) isolated virulent strains of *B. thuringiensis (cereus)* var. *galleriae* not only from *G. mellonella* but also from the moths, *Cydia (Carpocapsa) pomonella, Agrotis segetum* and *H. sordida* and the sawfly, *Neodiprion sertifer.* Strains selected from these were used for industrial production of Entobacterin-3 in 1964-1965. Freeze-dried preparations maintained their original virulence after storage for one year.

(ii) Induced change, improvement, and preservation of virulence. Smirnoff and Cantin (1967) observed the occurrence of deformed cells in crystalliferous bacteria by the irradiation of ^{60}Co γ-rays at 456,560 rads. After four successive transfers the number of deformed cells did not exceed 20% and the period of lysis became normal. Nasedkina and Zotkina (1968) obtained highly virulent and phage-resistant strains of *B. thuringiensis (cereus)* var. *galleriae* by the combined treatment of phage and ethylenimine.

Gukasian and Mashanov (1966) obtained a more virulent strain of *Bacillus tuviensis* (for characteristics of this species, see Gukasian, 1967) by X-ray (5000-400,000 rads) or ^{60}Co γ-ray (5000-200,000 rads). After growth in cultures overnight, bacteria were irradiated and then subcultured on broth agar or potato agar media. Strains of greater virulence were obtained by irradiation with ^{60}Co γ-rays and culture on potato agar. For example, strains of low virulence (mortality: 16-28%) were improved to strains showing 76% mortality (20,000 rads), and 64% mortality (5000 rads). Similar results were obtained by ultra-violet irradiation (Mashanov, 1967a,b). Strains of *Bacillus insectus* (characteristics of this species, see Gukasian, 1967) of increased virulence killed larvae of *Dendrolimus sibericus* both in the laboratory and in the field (Mashanov, 1966).

Norris (personal communication, 1968) increased the virulence of a strain of *B. thuringiensis* against *P. brassicae* by selection of mutants caused by ultra-violet irradiation. The virulence was upgraded seven-fold. It is quite interesting to note that, even before the treatment and selection, this strain had a tendency to produce more than one crystal per cell, but afterwards multiple crystal formation was the rule. Although Norris mentioned that there were also changes in the growth media used during the experiments, the increase in virulence cannot be explained by only the change of culture media.

In the sericultural countries, it has been hoped to select and breed a *B. thuringiensis* strain of low toxicity for the silkworm while remaining highly toxic to injurious insects. Aizawa (1967) and Aizawa and Fujiyoshi (1968) obtained some variants of *B. thuringiensis* both by ultra-violet irradiation and by possible bacteriophage conversion. The LD_{50} (spores/larva) for the silkworm with these strains is 10^6-10^7, but 10^4 in the common cabbageworm, *Pieris rapae crucivora,* and 10^4-10^5 in the fall webworm, *H. cunea.* The diamond-back moth, *Plutella maculipennis,* is also highly susceptible to these crystal formers. Using artificial diets, the LD_{50} in *C. suppressalis* was shown to be less than 10^5. The pine caterpillar, *Dendrolimus spectabilis,* and the small oraesia, *Oraesia emarginata,* however, are relatively resistant.

2. Bacillus popilliae *and* Bacillus lentimorbus

a. Change in virulence by passages through insects. B. popilliae strain *Melolontha* is the most virulent strain for larvae of the cockchafer, *Melolontha melolontha.* Three strains were passed through the host insect for three or four generations, but the virulence was not modified (Hurpin, 1959). In other scarabaeid beetles, the New Zealand strain of *B. popilliae* infecting *Odontria zealandica* showed a low pathogenicity to *Amphimallon majalis.* The spores propagated in *Popillia japonica* had about the same pathogenicity to both species, but after successive passages through *Amphimallon* they became more potent against that species and lost their potency against *Popillia* (Fleming, 1958). Dutky (1963) mentioned that selected strains from *Popillia* are frequently much more virulent for another insect than its indigenous strain and passages through the new host generally show an increase in virulence.

b. Change in virulence on artificial media and screening of strains. Steinkraus and Provvidenti (1958) obtained a few, but consistent, sporeforming strains of *B. popilliae* on artificial media. Some strains which lost the ability to form spores on artificial media recovered the ability to form typical spores when injected into the larval host, even after 100 transfers on artificial media. Pridham *et al.* (1964) observed considerable variation in infectivity among different strains of milky disease bacteria. With *B. lentimorbus*, "low-phosphate" (K_2HPO_4, 0.3%) and "high-phosphate" (K_2HPO_4, 0.6%) propagation media resulted in cells of different physiological state, which played an important role in infectivity, although the numbers of viable cells injected also influenced the infectivity. According to Rhodes (1965), the most severe disease caused by bacterial cells grown in the high-phosphate medium was nearly twice as severe as that caused by cells grown in the low-phosphate medium. One strain, avirulent when grown in low-phosphate medium, exhibited slight infectivity if grown in high-phosphate medium.

From the "wild-type" of *B. popilliae*, Rhodes *et al.* (1965) isolated a strain which was sporogenic when plated on acetate agar. Neither the parent strain nor other strains of *B. popilliae* produced spores when tested on acetate agar. Spores produced on acetate agar resembled those produced in the haemolymph of diseased Japanese beetle larvae and caused milky disease. Growth characteristics of *B. popilliae* in flask cultures were studied by Rhodes *et al.* (1966), and they obtained a large number of vegetative cells without loss of virulence. According to Rhodes (1968), the milky disease bacteria are variable and the development by selection and mutation of strains sporogenic *in vitro* is under investigation. However, in a selected strain under specific conditions, authentic spores are formed rapidly in colonies by as many as 20% of the cells. Unlike sporulation on solid media, which is restricted to a few variants, many of the available strains form spores in liquid media containing carbon. Some of the newer variants which sporulate efficiently in artificial medium grow vigorously in haemolymph and larvae die before the formation of the maximum numbers of spores.

A satisfactory cell suspending fluid is 0.1% trypton (Difco) solution for *B. popilliae* and *B. lentimorbus* in infection experiments with Japanese beetle larvae (Julian *et al.*, 1963). *B. popilliae* and *B. lentimorbus* were preserved by lyophilization and remained viable during subsequent storage in lyophil for at least 12-20 months (Haynes *et al.*, 1961).

3. *Non-sporulating Bacterial Pathogens*

The existence of strains and varieties of non-sporulating bacteria with different virulence has been reviewed by Tanada (1967b).

The enhancement of virulence by passages through insects seems to be unsuccessful. For example, Bucher (1963) failed to select invasive strains of *P. aeruginosa.* Bucher (1963) and Heimpel (1964) mentioned the role of bacterial enzymes but strains of *P. aeruginosa,* which exhibit identical ability to digest gelatin, showed different virulence (Lysenko, 1965).

Steinhaus (1959) could not enhance the virulence of *Serratia marcescens* by repeated passages through *G. mellonella* or the beetle *Tenebrio molitor.* Bucher (1963) pointed out that selection of invasive bacteria by host passages should be conducted by feeding insects, not by injection, particularly with those non-sporulating bacterial pathogens which are regarded as potential pathogens (Bucher, 1960, 1963).

C. FUNGI

1. Variation in Virulence

According to MacLeod (1954a, b), some variations in morphological and cultural characteristics were observed in entomogenous fungi such as *Beauveria, Isaria, Spicaria, Hirsutella, Metarrhizium, Cephalosporium* and *Syngliocladium (Sorosporella).* Sometimes a decrease of virulence or growth rate has been observed (Müller-Kögler, 1965, 1967; Seman, 1964).

Arkhipova (1965) tested *Beauveria bassiana, B. globulifera, Metarrhizium anisopliae, Paecilomyces farinosus (Spicaria farinosa), Hirsutella subulata, Verticillium, Fusarium* and *Mucor racemosus* against the codling moth, *Cydia (Carpocapsa) pomonella,* under laboratory conditions and found the most pathogenic to be *Beauveria globulifera* and *M. anisopliae. B. globulifera* remained virulent over a wide temperature range, but *M. anisopliae* was less virulent at low temperatures and the ability of fungi to attack insects was altered by humidity.

2. Change in Virulence by Subculturing and Passages through Insects

Virulence was reduced in a strain of *Entomophthora (Empusa) aphidis* that had been grown *in vitro* for only one year, but not in *Metarrhizium, Beauveria,* and *Spicaria rileyi* (Rockwood, 1950).

Kerner (1958) observed an increase of virulence of *P. farinosus (S. farinosa)* (estimated by LT_{50}) after passages through insect hosts. After successive subculturings, Fox and Jaques (1958) reported a decline in the virulence of *M. anisopliae* against the wireworm, *Agriotes obscurus.* They frequently used fresh isolates of the pathogen from naturally infected wireworms.

Schaerffenberg (1959, 1964) reported a decrease of virulence during successive subculturings. *B. bassiana* from the Colorado potato beetle, *Leptinotarsa decemlineata,* was subcultured for 30 generations. Fifty larvae of instar IV were dusted with 200 mg of spores of each fungal generation. Mortality within 15 days in the first two generations was 75-100% and subsequently 100% up to the 16th generation, then it decreased in the following generations to only 50% at the 30th. Schaerffenberg emphasizes that *B. bassiana* must be passed through the insect in order to preserve its full virulence.

Kawakami (1960) described changes in seven entomogenous fungi, *B. bassiana, Spicaria prasina, P. farinosus (S. farinosa), Isaria fumosorosea, M. anisopliae, Aspergillus oryzae* and *Aspergillus flavus,* cultured successively for 5-19 generations at intervals of 30 or 180 days. In most of the species the rate of growth, formation of aerial mycelium, corenia, and spores decreased during successive transfers. The trends were marked when the intervals were shortened thus increasing the number of transfers. However, *B. bassiana* did not show these changes and in *A. flavus* spore formation increased. After these repeated transfers on culture media, the characteristics were restored by passage through the host insect. The virulence decreased progressively with successive transfers and recovered after passage through the insect. The degree of decrease of virulence varied on different culture media.

Velitskaya (1968) mentioned that the strains of *B. bassiana* most virulent for insects were also the most damaging for paramecia and corn seeds, and in some instances paramecia will be used as a marker for the estimation of virulence against insects.

3. Strain Improvement and Preservation of Virulence

Induced variation of fungi by physical and chemical mutagens from the point of view of physiological characteristics and strain improvement have been reported, particularly by Russian workers (Evlakhova, 1958, 1959, 1960, 1964; Evlakhova and Chvetzova, 1964; Evlakhova and Martens, 1961; Evlakhova and Shvetzova, 1965; Ewlachowa, 1962; Kirsanova, 1968).

Evlakhova and Martens (1961) and Ewlachowa (1962) obtained virulent strains by irradiation with X-rays and ^{60}Co γ-rays. *B. bassiana* isolated from the moths, *Zeuzera pyrina* and *Cossus cossus,* and *A. flavus* from *Locusta migratoria* were assayed in *Eurygaster integriceps* and *Cydia (Carpocapsa) pomonella.* X-Ray irradiation at 1200-4000 rads, and even at 40 rads, was effective. The effect depended on the species, the dose, and the developmental stage of the fungus. The best results were obtained with young cultures bearing mycelium and at early sporulation. With these variants the mortality caused by *B. bassiana* increased by 30-40% but there was no increase with *A. flavus.* In *B. bassiana,* the virulence was preserved for 7-10 generations. Treatment with ultrasonic vibration and ultra-violet light did not effect the occurrence of virulent strains.

The virulence of a strain of *B. bassiana* obtained by ^{60}Co γ-ray irradiation was superior by 50% to that of the original one for the control of *E. integriceps* (Fedorintchik, 1964). Evlakhova and Chvetzova (1964) obtained virulent strains of *B. bassiana* by treatment with DDT, Lindane, γ-rays, and X-rays. For example, the mortality caused by the original strain in larval instar IV of *E. integriceps* was 65% but 94-100% with the selected strain. Evlakhova and Shvetzova (1965) treated *B. bassiana* with DDT, Lindane, X-rays and γ-rays, and obtained virulent strains which persisted for 7-10, or 15 generations.

Roberts (1968) recommended the use of genetic manipulation to increase the virulence of insect pathogenic fungi before beginning field work, in preference to the use of strains found in nature. He suggested new approaches and possibilities, such as the growth of mutants on media containing short chain fatty acids, selection of spores which germinate quickly in the presence of compounds from the exocuticle, increase of the capability to produce toxins, genetic recombination, and use of markers.

D. RICKETTSIAE AND PROTOZOANS

Very little information is available about the change in virulence of rickettsiae and protozoans. Hurpin (1965) examined the effect of pH, temperature, antibiotics, and disinfectants on the virulence of *Rickettsiella melolonthae* but these results illustrate the stability rather than the virulence of the pathogens.

Passages of *Nosema infesta* through a host other than its natural host, the moth, *Crambus bonifatellus,* reduced its virulence against the latter (Hall, 1954). *Thelohania pristiphorae,* a microsporidan pathogen of the larch sawfly, *Pristiphora erichsonni,* was adapted to the tent caterpillars, *M. disstria* and *M. americanum,* by Smirnoff (1968). The virulence of the native strain assayed in the larch sawfly remained unchanged during six passages through the tent caterpillars. The mortality caused by the original and adapted strains of *T. pristiphorae* remained around 15%.

IV. Concluding Remarks and Future Research

The change in virulence, selection and improvement of strains, as well as the preservation of virulence in insect pathogens have been reviewed. Although many trials have been conducted, particularly by Russian workers, our knowledge is still rudimentary when compared, for example, with that relating to the production of antibiotics.

Certain projects can be chosen as being of prime importance in research. The first is the simplification of methods for bioassay of virulence or the discovery of markers representing virulence. In recent years, the standardization of *B. thuringiensis* and virus preparations has improved and this will contribute to the selection of pathogens of increased virulence. Another project concerns the study of the genetics of insect pathogens, because this plays an important role not only in insect microbiology but also in the selection and breeding of suitable strains.

Following these, when a potent pathogen is found, aspects of the mechanisms of infection such as the synergistic association of two or more micro-organisms (Tanada, 1967b) and the environmental factors (Tanada, 1967a) should be considered.

References

Aizawa, K. (1961). *Entomophaga* **6,** 197-201.

Aizawa, K. (1962). *J. Insect Path.* **4,** 122-127.

Aizawa, K. (1963). *In* "Insect Pathology. An Advanced Treatise" (E. A. Steinhaus, ed.), Vol. 1, pp. 381-412. Academic Press, New York and London.

Aizawa, K. (1967). *Mushi* **39**, *Suppl.*, 97-102.
Aizawa, K. and Fujiyoshi, N. (1968). Proc. Joint U.S.-Japan Semin. Microbial Control Insect Pests, pp. 79-83. U.S.-Japan Committee Sci. Cooperation. Panel 8. Fukuoka.
Allen, G. E. (1968). Proc. Joint U.S.-Japan Semin. Microbial Control Insect Pests, pp. 37-41. U.S.-Japan Committee Sci. Cooperation. Panel 8. Fukuoka.
Angus, T. A. (1967). *J. Invertebrate Path.* **9**, 256-260.
Angus, T. A. (1968). *Wld Rev. Pest Control* 7, 11-26.
Angus, T. A. and Norris, J. R. (1968). *J. Invertebrate Path.* **11**, 289-295.
Arkhipova, V. C. (1965). *Ent. Obozr.* **44**, 89-99. (In Russian with English summary.)
Aruga, H., Yoshitake, N., Watanabe, H., Hukuhara, T., Nagashima, E. and Kawai, T. (1961). *Jap. J. appl. Ent. Zool.* **5**, 141-144. (In Japanese with English summary.)
Bergold, G. H. (1958). *In* "Handbuch der Virusforschung" (C. Hallauer and K. F. Meyer, eds), Vol. 4, pp. 60-142. Springer-Verlag, Vienna.
Briggs, J. D. (1963). *In* "Insect Pathology. An Advanced Treatise" (E. A. Steinhaus, ed.), Vol. 2, pp. 519-548. Academic Press, New York and London.
Broersma, D. B. and Buxton, J. A. (1967). *J. Invertebrate Path.* **9**, 58-69.
Bucher, G. E. (1960). *J. Invertebrate Path.* **2**, 172-195.
Bucher, G. E. (1963). *In* "Insect Pathology. An Advanced Treatise" (E. A. Steinhaus, ed.), Vol. 2, pp. 117-147. Academic Press, New York and London.
Bucher, G. E. (1964). *Ann. ent. Soc. Québec* **9**, 30-42.
Burgerjon, A. (1959). *Entomophaga* **4**, 201-206.
Burgerjon, A. (1964). *Entomophaga Mém. hors Sér.* No. 2, 255-262.
Burgerjon, A. (1965). *Entomophaga* **10**, 21-25.
Burgerjon, A. and Biache, G. (1967). *Ent. exp. app.* **10**, 211-230.
Burges, H. D. (1967a). *In* "Insect Pathology and Microbial Control" (P. A. van der Laan, ed.), pp. 306-314. North-Holland Publ. Co., Amsterdam.
Burges, H. D. (1967b). *Nature, Lond.* **215**, 664-665.
Burges, H. D. *et al.* (1967). *In* "Insect Pathology and Microbial Control" (P. A. van der Laan, ed.), pp. 314-338. North-Holland Publ. Co., Amsterdam.
Cameron, J. W. M. (1962). *Verhand. XI Int. Kongr. Ent. (Wien, 1960)* **2**, 769-776.
Cameron, J. W. MacBain (1963). *Ann. Rev. Ent.* **8**, 265-286.
Chislett, M. E. and Kushner, D. J. (1961). *J. gen. Microbiol.* **25**, 151-156.
Conner, R. M. and Hansen, P. A. (1967). *J. Invertebrate Path.* **9**, 114-125.
Cosenza, B. J. and Lewis, F. B. (1966). *J. Invertebrate Path.* **8**, 520-525.
David, W. A. L. and Gardiner, B. O. C. (1965). *J. Invertebrate Path.* **7**, 285-290.
Doane, C. C. (1965). *Proc. XIIth Int. Congr. Ent. (London, 1964)*, p. 735.
Doane, C. C. and Wallis, R. C. (1964). *J. Insect Path.* **6**, 423-429.
Dutky, S. R. (1959). *Adv. Appl. Microbiol.* **1**, 175-200.
Dutky, S. R. (1963). *In* "Insect Pathology. An Advanced Treatise" (E. A. Steinhaus, ed.), Vol. 2, pp. 75-115. Academic Press, New York and London.
Evlakhova, A. A. (1958). *In* "Biologičeskij Metod Bor'by s Vrediteljami sel'skochozjajstvennych Kul'tur i lesnych nasaždenij" (V. P. Vassilijev, N. A. Telenga and N. P. Djadečko, eds), pp. 16-17. Izdanie Ministerstva sel'skogo Chozjajstva Moldavskoj SSR, Kišinev.
Evlakhova, A. A. (1959). *In* "Biologičeskij Metod Bor'by s Vrediteljami Rastenij" (N. A. Telenga, N. S. Sčerbinovskij and N. P. Djadečko, eds), pp. 42-52. Izdatel'stvo Ukrainskoi Akademii Sel'skochozjajstvennych Nauk, Kiev.
Evlakhova, A. A. (1960). *In* "Méthodes chimiques de lutte contre les ravageurs, les maladies et les mauvaises herbes" (V. P. Vassilijev, ed.), pp. 15-16. Izdatel'stvo Ukrainskoi Akademii Sel'skochozjajstvennych Nauk, Kiev. (In Russian.)
Evlakhova, A. A. (1964). *Trudy Vsesojuznogo Instit. Zashtity Rastenij* **21**, 95-100.
Evlakhova, A. A. and Chvetzova, O. I. (1964). *Entomophaga Mém. hors Sér.* No. 2, 521-529.
Evlakhova, A. A. and Martens, B. K. (1961). *In* "Materialy simpoziuma po primeneniyu biofiziki v oblasti zashchity rastenii", pp. 20-21. Leningrad. (In Russian.) *(Rev. appl. Ent.* 51, *Ser. A)*, 522-523.

Evlakhova, A. A. and Shvetsova, O. I. (1965). *Ent. Obozr.* **44**, 721-726.
Ewlachowa, A. A. (1962). *Verh. XI Int. Kongr. Ent. (Wien, 1960)* **2**, 861-862.
Fedorintchik, N. S. (1964). *Entomophaga Mém. hors Sér.* No. 2, 51-61.
Fitz-James, P. C. and Young, I. E. (1959). *J. Bacteriol.* **78**, 743-754.
Fleming, W. E. (1958). *Proc. Xth Int. Congr. Ent. (Montreal, 1956)* **3**, 115-125.
Fox, C. J. S. and Jaques, R. P. (1958). *Can. Ent.* **90**, 314-315.
Gershenson, S. M. (1957). *Dok. Akad. Nauk S.S.S.R.* **113**, 1161-1162.
Gukasian, A. B. (1958). *Rap. Ecole des Sciences de Sibérie U.R.S.S.* 7, 85-101. (In Russian.) (After Smirnoff, 1967b.)
Gukasian, A. B. (1967). *In* "Kristallonosnye mikroorganizmy i perspektivy ikh ispoljzovanija v lesnom khozjajstve" (Akademija Nauk S.S.S.R., Sibirskoe otdelenie institut lesa i drevesiny, A. B. Gukasian, ed.), pp. 5-20. Nauka, Moscow.
Gukasian, A. B. and Mashanov, A. I. (1966). *In* "Mikroorganizmy v borbe s vrediteljami lesnogo khozjajstva" (Akademija Nauk S.S.S.R., Sibirskoe otdelenie institut lesa i drevesiny, A. B. Gukasian, ed.), pp. 233-244. Nauka, Moscow.
Hall, I. M. (1954). *Hilgardia* **22**, 535-565.
Hall, I. M. (1964). *In* "Biological Control of Insect Pests and Weeds" (P. DeBach, ed.), pp. 610-628. Chapman and Hall, London.
Haynes, W. C., Julian, G., St., Jr., Shekleton, M. C., Hall, H. H. and Tashiro, H. (1961). *J. Insect Path.* **3**, 55-61.
Heimpel, A. M. (1964). *Entomophaga Mém. hors Sér.* No. 2, 23-33.
Heimpel, A. M. (1967). *In* "Insect Pathology and Microbial Control" (P. A. van der Laan, ed.), pp. 355-359. North-Holland Publ. Co., Amsterdam.
Herfs, W. (1962). *Deut. Ent. Zeitsch.* **9**, 466-470.
Herfs, W. (1963). *Entomophaga* **8**, 163-181.
Hukuhara, T. (1968). Proc. Joint U.S.-Japan Semin. Microbial Control Insect Pests, pp. 7-11. U.S.-Japan Committee Sci. Cooperation. Panel 8. Fukuoka.
Hukuhara, T. and Hashimoto, Y. (1966). *Jap. J. appl. Ent. Zool.* **10**, 149-155. (In Japanese with English summary.)
Hurpin, B. (1959). *Entomophaga* **4**, 233-248.
Hurpin, B. (1965). *Proc. XIIth Int. Congr. Ent. (London, 1964)*, p. 727.
Ignoffo, C. M. (1964). *J. Insect Path.* **6**, 318-326.
Ignoffo, C. M. (1965a). *J. Invertebrate Path.* **7**, 209-216.
Ignoffo, C. M. (1965b). *J. Invertebrate Path.* **7**, 315-319.
Ignoffo, C. M. (1965c). *Entomophaga* **10**, 29-40.
Ignoffo, C. M. (1966a). *In* "Insect Colonization and Mass Production" (C. N. Smith, ed.), pp. 501-530. Academic Press, New York.
Ignoffo, C. M. (1966b). *J. Invertebrate Path.* **8**, 547-548.
Ignoffo, C. M. (1967). *In* "Insect Pathology and Microbial Control" (P. A. van der Laan, ed.), pp. 91-117. North-Holland Publ. Co., Amsterdam.
Ignoffo, C. M. (1968). *In* "Insect Viruses" (Current Topics in Microbiology and Immunology, Vol. 42) (K. Maramorosch, ed.), pp. 129-167. Springer-Verlag, Berlin, Heidelberg, and New York.
Isakova, N. P. and Stroeva, I. A. (1968). *In* "Proceedings All-Union Scientific Research Institute for Plant Protection, Vol. 31 (Biological Methods of Plant Protection)" (L. S. Zimin, ed.), pp. 371-379. All-Union Lenin Academy of Agr. Sci., Leningrad. (In Russian with English summary.)
Julian, G., St., Jr., Pridham, T. G. and Hall, H. H. (1963). *J. Insect Path.* **5**, 440-450.
Kawakami, K. (1960). *Bull. Sericult. exp. Stn.* **16**, 83-99. (In Japanese with English summary.)
Kerner, G. (1958). *Trans. 1st Int. Conf. Insect Path. Biol. Control (Praha, 1958)*, pp. 169-176.
Kirsanova, R. V. (1968). *Mycologia and Phytopathologia (Leningrad)* **2**, 183-193. (In Russian.)
Krieg, A. (1961). "*Bacillus thuringiensis* Berliner. Über seine Biologie, Pathologie und

Anwendung in der biologischen Schädlingsbekämpfung", 79 pp. Paul Parey, Berlin and Hamburg.

Krieg, A. (1963). *In* "Recent Progress in Microbiology" (N. E. Gibbons, ed.), Vol. 8, pp. 134-140.

Krieg, A. (1965a). *Entomophaga* **10**, 3-20.

Krieg, A. (1965b). *Entomophaga* **10**, 49-54.

Krieg, A. (1967). "Neues über *Bacillus thuringiensis* und seine Anwendung", 106 pp. Paul Parey, Berlin and Hamburg.

Kushner, D. J. and Harvey, G. T. (1962). *J. Insect Path.* **4**, 155-184.

Kushner, D. J. and Lisson, T. A. (1959). *J. gen. Microbiol.* **21**, 96-108.

Lecadet, M.-M. and Martouret, D. (1964). *Entomophaga Mém. hors Sér.* No. 2, 205-212.

Le Corroller, Y. (1958). *Annls Inst. Pasteur, Paris* **94**, 670-673.

Lemoigne, M., Bonnefoi, A., Beguin, S., Grison, P., Martouret, D., Schenk, A. and Vago, C. (1956). *Entomophaga* **1**, 19-34.

Lysenko, O. (1965). *Proc. XIIth Int. Congr. Ent. (London, 1964)*, p. 717.

Machay, L. and Lovas, B. (1957). *Biol. Közlemények* **5**, 7-18.

MacLeod, D. M. (1954a). *Can. J. Bot.* **32**, 818-890.

MacLeod, D. M. (1954b). *Ann. N.Y. Acad. Sci.* **60**, 58-70.

Martignoni, M. E. (1964). *In* "Biological Control of Insect Pests and Weeds" (P. DeBach, ed.), pp. 579-609. Chapman and Hall, London.

Mashanov, A. I. (1966). *In* "Mikroorganizmy v borbe s vrediteljami lesnogo khozjajstva" (Akademija Nauk S.S.S.R., Sibirskoe otdelenie institut lesa i drevesiny, A. B. Gukasian, ed.), pp. 223-232. Nauka, Moscow. (In Russian.)

Mashanov, A. I. (1967a). *In* "Kristallonosnye mikroorganizmy i perspektivy ikh ispoljzovanija v lesnom khozjajstve" (Akademija Nauk S.S.S.R., Sibirskoe otdelenie institut lesa i drevesiny, A. B. Gukasian, ed.), pp. 129-131. Nauka, Moscow. (In Russian.)

Mashanov, A. I. (1967b). *In* "Kristallonosnye mikroorganizmy i perspektivy ikh ispoljzovanija v lesnom khozjajstve" (Akademija Nauk S.S.S.R., Sibirskoe otdelenie institut lesa i drevesiny, A. B. Gukasian, ed.), pp. 132-135. Nauka, Moscow. (In Russian.)

Müller-Kögler, E. (1965). "Pilzkrankheiten bei Insekten", xvi + 444 pp. Paul Parey, Berlin and Hamburg.

Müller-Kögler, E. (1967). *In* "Insect Pathology and Microbial Control" (P. A. van der Laan, ed.), pp. 339-353. North-Holland Publ. Co., Amsterdam.

Nasedkina, G. A. and Zotkina, N. Z. (1968). *In* "Proceedings of All-Union Scientific Research Institute for Plant Protection. Vol. 31 (Biological Methods of Plant Protection)" (L. S. Zimin, ed.), pp. 380-384. All-Union Lenin Academy of Agric. Sci., Leningrad. (In Russian with English summary.)

Ossowski, L. L. J. (1958). *Nature, Lond.* **181**, 648.

Ossowski, L. L. J. (1960). *J. Insect Path.* **2**, 35-43.

Ossowski, L. L. J. (1962). *Verh. XI Int. Kongr. Ent. (Wien, 1960)* **2**, 810-814.

Pridham, T. G., Julian, G., St., Jr., Adams, G. L., Hall, H. H. and Jackson, R. W. (1964). *J. Insect Path.* **6**, 204-213.

Ridet, J.-M. (1966). *Entomophaga* **11**, 355-364.

Rhodes, R. A. (1965). *Bact. Rev.* **29**, 373-381.

Rhodes, R. A. (1968). Proc. Joint U.S.-Japan Semin. Microbial Control Insect Pests, pp. 85-92. U.S.-Japan Committee Sci. Cooperation. Panel 8. Fukuoka.

Rhodes, R. A., Roth, M. S. and Hrubant, G. R. (1965). *Can. J. Microbiol.* **11**, 779-783.

Rhodes, R. A., Sharpe, E. S., Hall, H. H. and Jackson, R. W. (1966). *Appl. Microbiol.* **14**, 189-195.

Roberts, D. W. (1968). Proc. Joint U.S.-Japan Semin. Microbial Control Insect Pests, pp. 129-134. U.S.-Japan Committee Sci. Cooperation. Panel 8. Fukuoka.

Rockwood, L. P. (1950). *J. econ. Ent.* **43**, 704-707.

Schaerffenberg, B. (1959). *Anz. Schädlingskunde* **32**, 87-90.

Schaerffenberg, B. (1964). *J. Insect Path.* **6**, 8-20.

Schvetsova, O. I. and Zurabova, E. R. (1967). *Mikrobiologija* **36**, 614-620. (In Russian with English summary.)
Seman, E. O. (1964). *Botan. Žur.* **49**, 1473-1477. (In Russian.)
Smirnoff, W. A. (1961). *J. Insect Path.* **3**, 29-46.
Smirnoff, W. A. (1963a). *J. Insect Path.* **5**, 104-110.
Smirnoff, W. A. (1963b). *J. Insect Path.* **5**, 389-392.
Smirnoff, W. A. (1964). *Ann. ent. Soc. Queb.* 9, 43-53.
Smirnoff, W. A. (1967a). *In* "Insect Pathology and Microbial Control" (P. A. van der Laan, ed.), pp. 125-130. North-Holland Publ. Co., Amsterdam.
Smirnoff, W. A. (1967b). *Phytoprotection* **48**, 119-127.
Smirnoff, W. A. (1968). *J. Invertebrate Path.* **11**, 321-325.
Smirnoff, W. A. and Cantin, M. (1967). *J. Invertebrate Path.* **9**, 357-363.
Somerville, H. J., Delafield, F. P. and Rittenberg, S. C. (1968). *J. Bacteriol.* **96**, 721-726.
Stairs, G. R. (1964a). *Virology* **24**, 520-521.
Stairs, G. R. (1964b). *J. Insect Path.* **6**, 164-169.
Stairs, G. R. (1968). *In* "Insect Viruses" (Current Topics in Microbiology and Immunology, Vol. 42) (K. Maramorosch, ed.), pp. 1-23. Springer-Verlag, Berlin, Heidelberg and New York.
Steinhaus, E. A. (1949). "Principles of Insect Pathology", xi + 757 pp. McGraw-Hill, New York, Toronto and London.
Steinhaus, E. A. (1951). *Hilgardia* **20**, 629-678.
Steinhaus, E. A. (1959). *Hilgardia* **28**, 351-380.
Steinhaus, E. A. and Jerrel, E. A. (1954). *Hilgardia* **23**, 1-21.
Steinhaus, E. A. and Martignoni, M. E. (1962). "An Abridged Glossary of Terms Used in Insect Pathology", 20 pp. Mimeographed Series No. 6. Department of Insect Pathology, University of California, Berkeley.
Steinkraus, K. H. and Provvidenti, M. L. (1958). *J. Bacteriol.* **75**, 38-42.
Stephens, J. M. (1952). *Can. J. Zool.* **30**, 30-40.
Stephens, J. M. (1957). *Can. Ent.* **89**, 94-96.
Stephens, J. M. (1959). *Can. J. Microbiol.* **5**, 73-77.
Surany, P. (1967). *In* "Insect Pathology and Microbial Control" (P. A. van der Laan, ed.), pp. 247-248. North-Holland Publ. Co., Amsterdam.
Tanada, Y. (1959). *Ann. Rev. Ent.* **4**, 277-302.
Tanada, Y. (1963). *In* "Insect Pathology. An Advanced Treatise" (E. A. Steinhaus, ed.), Vol. 2, pp. 423-475. Academic Press, New York and London.
Tanada, Y. (1964). *In* "Biological Control of Insect Pests and Weeds" (P. DeBach, ed.), pp. 548-578. Chapman and Hall, London.
Tanada, Y. (1967a). *J. Sericult. Sci. Japan* **36**, 333-339.
Tanada, Y. (1967b). *In* "Pest Control" (W. W. Kilgore and R. L. Doutt, eds), pp. 31-88. Academic Press, New York and London.
Toumanoff, C. (1955). *Annls Inst. Pasteur, Paris* **89**, 644-653.
Toumanoff, C. (1956). *Annls Inst. Pasteur, Paris* **90**, 660-664.
Toumanoff, C. (1958). *Trans, 1st Int. Conf. Insect Path. Biol. Control (Praha, 1958)*, pp. 65-71.
Toumanoff, C. and Vago, C. (1952). *C.r. hebd. Séanc. Acad. Sci. Paris* **235**, 1715-1717.
Vago, C. and Bergoin, M. (1968). *Adv. Virus Res.* **13**, 247-303.
Vaňková, J. (1957). *Folia Biologica* **3**, 175-182.
Vaňková, J. (1964). *Entomophaga Mém. hors Sér.* No. 2, 271-291.
Vaňková, J. (1965). *Proc. XIIth Int. Congr. Ent. (London, 1964)*, p. 739.
Veber, J. (1964). *Entomophaga Mém. hors Sér.* No. 2, 403-405.
Velitskaya, I. S. (1968). *In* "Proc. All-Union Scientific Research Institute for Plant Protection, Vol. 31 (Biological Methods of Plant Protection)" (L. S. Zimin, ed.), pp. 407-414. All-Union Lenin Academy of Agric. Sci., Leningrad. (In Russian with English summary.)
Wittig, G. (1963). *In* "Insect Pathology. An Advanced Treatise" (E. A. Steinhaus, ed.), Vol. 2, pp. 591-636. Academic Press, New York and London.

CHAPTER 31

Aposymbiosis, A Possible Method for Antimicrobial Control of Arthropods

ALOYSIUS KRIEG

Biologische Bundesanstalt für Land- und Forstwirtschaft, Institut für biologische Schädlingsbekämpfung, Darmstadt, Germany

1. Symbiotic Associations and Aposymbiosis

Micro-organisms may be associated not only with diseased but also with healthy insects. The micro-organisms of healthy insects—commensals or symbiotes—are localized mostly in the alimentary canal or in special mycetomes. Although these microbes reproduce themselves within their host, no remarkable disturbances have been found. Therefore, it is concluded that an equilibrium has been developed during co-evolution of commensals and their hosts. With obligate symbiosis even a form of "negative parasitism" may exist between macro- and micro-organism.

Symbiosis, in a wider sense, also includes the normal microflora of the intestine. In some insects, a special flora is necessary for their normal growth and development. There are many transitional stages between an autochthonous gut microflora and a facultative microsymbiosis, e.g. in Muscidae, Pyrrhocoridae and Coptosomidae. A specific symbiosis with micro-organisms is known from well defined physiological groups of arthropods whose food is nutritionally incomplete, for example blood (Anoplura; some Heteroptera), or plant juices (Trypetidae; some Heteroptera and Homoptera). Other groups of such insects with microsymbiotes feed on hairs and feathers, e.g. Mallophaga, or on wood and stored products, e.g. Coleoptera such as Curculionidae and Blattidae.

The physiological significance of symbiotes for their host has been analysed in only a few cases. In blood-sucking insects microsymbiotes may synthesize the B-vitamin complex, and in insects feeding on plant juices they may be involved in the synthesis of essential amino acids. Buchner (1953), Koch (1960), Brooks (1963) and Henry (1967) give details.

In natural environments, association between the insect and its symbiotes represents a physiological entity. If the microsymbiotes are eliminated, the resulting aposymbiotic insects may show severe symptoms of malnutrition, e.g. reduced size, retarded development, deformation, reduced fecundity and enhanced larval mortality. Finally, aposymbiotic insects may die because of an acute lack of essential nutritional factors.

It is evident that a method for controlling microsymbiotes might simultaneously be a useful method for controlling their hosts too. Of all the methods that induce aposymbiosis (extirpation of mycetomes, thermo-inactivation, disinfection of eggshell, application of antibiotics) only treatment with chemicals is practical for field-application.

A very simple type of symbiosis is known from Trypetidae (Diptera) and from Coreidae, Coptosomidae and Pentatomidae (Heteroptera). Here, pseudomonads live within the intestine or its crypts. The microsymbiotes are transmitted on the egg by faecal contamination. In some trypetids (e.g. the olive fruit fly, *Dacus oleae*) a special smearing apparatus has developed during co-evolution of the symbiote and its host. Because the eggs are contaminated only externally by the symbiotic micro-organisms, aposymbiosis may be attained by surface disinfection of eggs after they have been laid, using chemicals such as mercuric chloride, sodium hypochlorite, and chloramine. An aqueous solution of crystal violet is sufficient to kill symbiotic Actinomycetes on eggs of Triatomidae (Heteroptera) resulting in aposymbiosis of the host (Harington, 1960).

Another method of obtaining aposymbiotic insects is chemotherapy, for example by oral application of sulphonamides or antibiotics. For instance Fytizas and Tzanakakis (1966) used antibiotics to eliminate pseudomonads in maggots, especially *Pseudomonas savastonoi,* the microsymbiote of *D. oleae* The bacterium is sensitive to streptomycin and experiments demonstrated that the antibiotic applied to adult flies inhibited larval development in olives. This effect lasted until aposymbiotic flies were recontaminated in the laboratory. Control of olive fruit fly with streptomycin may be promising, because under field conditions recontamination of the flies is relatively difficult. It should be mentioned that the symbiote of *D. oleae* is simultaneously a plant pathogen causing olive knot, and *D. oleae* is not essential for the existence of this disease, which may be transmitted by other means (especially in the Americas).

In many insect hosts, however, the microsymbiotes are localized in special mycetomes within the body cavity and they are transmitted to offspring by internally infected eggs. In such obligate symbiosis, disinfection of the surface of eggs does not influence the symbiotic condition of the offspring. Here, only chemotherapy may be a useful control method for symbiotes. Pilot laboratory experiments have been carried out on several storage insects. The cockroaches, *Blatta orientalis, Blattella germanica* and *Periplaneta americana* have been treated successfully with sulphathiazol, penicillin, chloromycetin, chlorotetracycline, oxytetracycline (Brooks and Richards, 1955, 1956; Frank, 1954, 1956), and the beetles, *Rhyzopertha dominica, Oryzaephilus surinamensis* and *Sitophilus oryzae* with penicillin, streptomycin, oxytetracycline, chlorotetracyline (Steinhaus and Bell, 1953; Huger, 1956; Schneider, 1956).

In similar successful experiments aposymbiosis has been obtained in plant-sucking Homoptera, especially *Pseudococcus citri,* by treatment with penicillin and chloramphenicol (Köhler and Schwartz, 1962) and *Aphis fabae,* by use of tetracycline, oxytetracycline, chlorotetracycline etc. (Ehrhardt and Schmutterer, 1966). These results, however, have no practicable value at present, because systemic application of the antibiotics would be necessary for any useful control. Unfortunately, these obligate symbiotes are also transmitted by internally infected eggs and, therefore, unlike the blood-sucking Triatomidae (Heteroptera), aposymbiosis is unattainable by disinfectants. At present no practicable way exists to control Homoptera on plants by chemically induced aposymbiosis.

More promising are experiments done by Musgrave and French (1969) with blood-sucking Heteroptera. Chloramphenicol or oxytetracycline were successfully used to eliminate *Nocardia rhodnii,* the microsymbiote of the bug *Rhodnius prolixus.* High mortality occurred after larvae (nymphs) or adults fed through an artificial membrane on defibrinated mammalian blood containing the injectable antibiotics. These results may encourage therapeutic experiments to control blood-sucking ectoparasites not only by egg-disinfection (see above) but also by systemic application of antibiotics, because systemic application to vertebrates, in contrast to plants, is a useful method.

For successful control the chemicals must eliminate all the symbiotes without selecting resistant forms. Streptomycin, but not oxytetracycline, produced aposymbiosis in *Rhyzopertha dominica* (Steinhaus and Bell, 1953). According to Huger (1956) oxytetracycline (as well as chlorotetracycline) induced resistant strains of microsymbiotes, which may recontaminate aposymbiotic cells in mycetomes, and chlorotetracycline did likewise in *Blattella germanica* (Brooks and Richards, 1955, 1966).

It should be mentioned that antibiotics may also have a direct effect on arthropods. The effect of antimicrobial agents on insects without typical microsymbiotes is different; some like the silkworm, *Bombyx mori,* grow better, others such as larvae of the codling moth, *Cydia (Carpocapsa) pomonella,* suffer intoxication. Harries (1968) studied the effect of antibiotics on the red spider mite, *Tetranychus urticae.* After some days, actinomycin D as well as nine other antibiotics produced an acaricidal effect, while sublethal doses significantly reduced the fecundity of the mites. The same author mentioned reduction of fecundity by antibiotics, such as cycloheximide, in other phytophagous mites. Boszek and Czajkowska (1968) reported similar mortality and reduction of fecundity in some stored products mites. Although no microsymbiotes are known from these mites, the pathological effect on them may be caused indirectly by a disturbance of their gut-microflora. On the other hand, it is also possible that, after absorption, the antibiotics may have interfered with the protein biosynthesis of the host organism. Thus it is possible that antibiotics may affect the host of symbiotes both indirectly by causing aposymbiosis and directly by a toxic effect.

II. Conclusions

With extracellular symbiosis, disinfection of eggs may eliminate microsymbiotes in the offspring. Application of chemotherapeutics in food, however, is a useful method of eliminating both extracellular and intracellular symbiotes. In some cases, it may be promising to treat animals and plants simultaneously against pathogens and symbiote-dependent insects. The main problem in the possible antibiotic control of symbiosis-dependent insects is the same as that in chemotherapy of insect diseases–complete elimination of the micro-organisms and the prevention of selection of resistant strains. At present, it is not clear whether or not the deleterious effect of several antimicrobial agents on certain arthropods (especially mites) without typical microsymbiotes is due to a disturbance of their gut-microflora.

References

Boczek, J. and Czajkowska, B. (1968). *Roczn. Nauk Roln.* (Warsaw) Ser. A, **93,** 597-612. (In Polish.)

Brooks, M. A. (1963). *Symp. Soc. gen. Microbiol.* **8,** 200-231.

Brooks, M. A. and Richards, A. G. (1955, 1956). *Cit. after* Brooks (1963).

Buchner, P. (1953). "Endosymbiose der Tiere mit pflanzlichen Mikroorganismen", 771 pp. Verlag Birkhäuser, Basel.

Ehrhardt, P. and Schmutterer, H. (1966). *Z. Morph. Ök. Tiere* **56,** 1-20.

Frank, W. (1954). *Cit. after* Frank (1956).

Frank, W. (1956). *Z. Morph. Ök. Tiere* **44,** 329-366.

Fytizas, E. and Tzanakakis, M. E. (1966). *Meded. Landbouwhogeschool Gent* **31,** 782-789.

Harington, J. S. (1960). *Parasitology* **50,** 279-286.

Harries, F. H. (1968). *J. econ. Ent.* **61,** 12-14.

Henry, S. M. (ed.) (1967). "Symbiosis, its Physiological and Biochemical Significance", Vol. 2, 443 pp. Academic Press, New York.

Huger, A. (1956). *Z. Morph. Ök. Tiere* **44,** 626-701.

Koch, A. (1960). *Ann. Rev. Microbiol.* **14,** 120-140.

Köhler, M. and Schwartz, W. (1962). *Zschr. allgem. Mikrobiol.* **2,** 190-208.
Musgrave, A. J. and French, E. B. (1969). *Can. Ent.* **101,** 757-759.
Schneider, H. (1956). *Z. Morph. Ök. Tiere* **44,** 555-625.
Steinhaus, E. A. and Bell, C. R. (1953). *J. econ. Ent.* **46,** 582-598.

CHAPTER 32

Co-ordination of International Effort and Industrialization

P. GRISON

Station de Recherches de Lutte Biologique et de Biocoenotique, La Minière par Versailles, France

I. Introduction

It is not my purpose to re-tell the history of the utilization of micro-organisms pathogenic to insects for the control of crop pests; the excellent work of Steinhaus (1949) and others report its various stages. These stages were marked not only by periods of disappointment and uncertainty, but also by spectacular successes like the large-scale utilization of *Bacillus popilliae* against *Popillia japonica* in the U.S.A. (e.g. Dutky, 1940). This success was the real start of "microbial control".

When Steinhaus began his work on the virus disease of *Colias eurytheme* in 1944, "everyone thought he was audacious to think it could be used to control the insect" (personal communication): he reported his first successful field trials in 1948. Later, after a previous attempt by Metalnikov and Chorine (1929a, b) he reawakened interest in the potentialities of *Bacillus thuringiensis* as an effective microbial insecticide (Steinhaus, 1951, 1960 for historical account). From this period on, national teams were set up to study insect pathology and microbial control, in place of research by individual workers.

These successes stimulated work on insect pathology in Europe. According to Franz (1961) the practical aspects of insect pathology are centred mainly in Czechoslovakia (Weiser, 1955), France (Bonnefoi and Grison, 1959; Grison and Beguin, 1954; Toumanoff and Grison, 1954), the U.S.S.R. (Evlakhova and

Shvetsova, 1953; Poltev *et al.,* 1954), and Germany (Franz, 1954). The literature is scattered through so many journals and printed in so many languages that it becomes increasingly difficult to follow new developments.

II. National and International Basis of the Developing Co-ordination

The present paper will show how rapid progress in fundamental research on different groups of pathogens laid the basis for most practical trials, and led to the organization of national teams. In contrast, the number of pathogens selected for application in microbial control has been surprisingly small. As soon as the national teams obtained their first encouraging results, personal exchange of information seemed useful and necessary to improve the co-ordination of their work. This was effected by the birth of new journals and the organization of meetings.

In 1956, the Commission Internationale de Lutte Biologique (C.I.L.B.), which later became the Organisation Internationale de Lutte Biologique (O.I.L.B.), started the journal *Entomophaga,* devoted to all aspects of biological control. In 1959, Steinhaus founded the *Journal of Insect Pathology.* Each year this journal, now called the *Journal of Invertebrate Pathology,* collects more than a hundred original papers and brief communications running to about 600 pages. Both journals also publish appropriate general news.

Beginning at Prague in 1958, a series of international meetings established personal contacts among scientific workers in this field (Table I). These meetings were held every four years and have been noteworthy as occasions when a

TABLE I

International conferences. The proceedings of these are given in Appendix 1

Conference	Venue	Countries	Participants	Organizing and participating bodies
First, 1958	Prague	17		Czechoslovak Academy of Sciences. C.I.L.B. Commonwealth Institute of Biological Control (C.I.B.C.)
Second, 1962	Paris	25	111	C.I.L.B. International Union of Biological Sciences (I.U.B.S.)
Third, 1966	Wageningen	14	94	International Agricultural Centre at Wageningen. I.U.B.S. International Commission for Biological Control (I.C.B.C.)
Fourth, 1970	Beltsville	13	177	International Minerals and Chemical Corp. I.C.B.C. I.U.B.S. Nutrilite Products Inc. U.S.D.A. Society for Invertebrate Pathology

number of regional meetings, meetings of specialists and new bodies have been arranged.

After the Prague meeting, the C.I.L.B. organized the first regional meeting; a "Colloquium on Insect Pathology and Microbial Control" in 1958 in Paris. Eleven countries were represented. At the 1962 meeting (Table I) a Scientific Committee was formed to prepare the next conference and to organize restricted working meetings. One of these meetings was held in London in 1964 with Vago as Chairman, assisted by Burges, with the joint support of the Agricultural Research Council of Great Britain (A.R.C.), the Institut National de la Recherche Agronomique of France (I.N.R.A.), and the C.I.L.B. It was a turning point in international co-ordination of the work of national teams: conditions for the practical utilization of insect viruses and *Bacillus thuringiensis* were discussed; important recommendations were made on the control of purity and non-toxicity to man and the higher animals, on the identification of strains of *B. thuringiensis* (which the C.I.L.B. had entrusted to the Pasteur Institute in Paris), on the means of standardizing bioassays, and so on.

The next full international meeting in 1966 (Table I) approved the recommendations of the working groups. It is not possible to recount here the results of a conference which led to the creation of the Society for Invertebrate Pathology, whose aims were outlined by Sparks and Steinhaus (1967). This is, perhaps, the zenith of co-ordinative efforts in the past decade and it is to be hoped that it will lead to renewed efforts in the future. A Directory, produced in 1967 (Appendix 1,G), lists 568 scientists working in this field.

The co-ordination of programmes established on a regional basis remains important in fostering closer contact between specialists. In Europe, every year, the *ad hoc* Committee of the O.I.L.B. holds a meeting on a particular subject: in 1966 on the assay of insect-pathogenic viruses and fungi; in 1967 on the action of the insect pathogens on vertebrates; in 1968 on the principles of application of microbial preparations in the field.

In the U.S.S.R., similar joint meetings are held by the various Institutes of Plant Protection (I.Z.R.). In 1964, an All-Union meeting was held in Novosibirsk on methods of biological and microbial control, at which the very interesting results obtained in the U.S.S.R. were presented, and the trends of research in the various Soviet laboratories were outlined.

In the U.S.A. in 1965, the Division of Invertebrate Pathology of the University of California invited the research workers from specialist laboratories of American universities, industry, and the U.S.D.A. to discuss the practical use of nuclear polyhedrosis for the control of *Heliothis zea* (Falcon, 1965). In 1967, a joint U.S.-Japan seminar on microbial control of insect pests was held in Fukuoka: most of the Japanese research has been concerned with disease of the silkworm, and only in recent years has Japan become more interested in microbial insecticides. Most papers were concerned with basic research. In 1966, during the 11th Pacific Scientific Congress in Tokyo, I observed excellent developments in the practical application of viruses against forest pests like *Dendrolimus spectabilis, Lymantria dispar,* etc. This work was of the same high calibre as similar work done in the U.S.S.R.

Finally, there is the important co-ordination of scientific effort by exchange of live material, in the taxonomic identification of this material, and in the field of training. Steinhaus established the first Insect Pathology course at Berkeley in 1947. It was 15 years before similar developments took place in other countries, particularly in France (Montpellier University) under the direction of Vago, and in Japan by Aizawa (Kyushu University, Fukuoka). In 1962, Laird (1965), when he was at the W.H.O., organized extensive exchange of live material for the characterization of diseases of vectors on a world-wide basis. Taxonomic identification, with the basic studies of pathogenesis which it encourages, is carried out in many countries in laboratories that keep reference collections. These, and the facilities mentioned above, are listed in detail in Appendices 4, 5 and 6 to encourage their further development.

III. Industrialization and the Future of Microbial Control

The U.S. Conference on the *Heliothis* virus is proof of the renewed industrial interest in the possibilities of the practical utilization of pathogens. We are perhaps at a decisive turning point in microbial control, although the concept is not new, *viz.* the massive multiplication of *Metarrhizium anisopliae* at Krasnodar in about 1880 (Krassilstchik, 1886) and of *Bacillus thuringiensis* in Paris in 1925-1930 ("Sporéine").

Sporéine initiated early international co-operation when some was sent to Britain before the second world war for tests against the Mediterranean flour moth (Jacobs, 1951). Industrial production of *Bacillus popilliae* was started by two firms in the U.S.A. in the late 1950's and of *B. thuringiensis* by five firms (Appendix 6, part IV). This gave great impetus to national interest, because these firms freely distributed their products for trials. Later distribution extended outside the U.S.A., and so encouraged international co-operation, particularly since the host spectrum of *B. thuringiensis* among the Lepidoptera is so wide. Industrial organizations in a number of different countries are at present keen to provide experimental quantities of microbial insecticides based on bacteria, viruses and fungi to research workers willing to test them.

Only three firms in the U.S.A. still manufacture *B. thuringiensis* for sale (Appendix 6, part IV). Home sales, while growing, are small relative to chemical insecticides. Export sales of "Thuricide" are no more than 5% of the total sales and are more or less equally divided between Europe, the Middle East and South America, although I would doubt if any one area is buying as much as $100,000 worth. In 1968-1969 sales in W. Germany were 156 gal (Schicke and Geisthardt, personal communication). In addition, there have recently been some sales of Thuricide to South East Asia. In the U.S.A., Thuricide is used mainly for looper control on lettuce and cole crops and for Lepidoptera on tobacco.

In Western Europe, there have been new industrial moves to manufacture products based on *B. thuringiensis,* notably in Germany and in France (Appendix 6). In France, a new industrial group is improving the technology of a new formula for commercial production. In Britain there is no industrial production, but Shell Research Ltd. is active in research on production for experimental use and on the toxins (Burges, personal communication). However, the problems of regulation and registration are only partly resolved in most West European countries. In this respect, much is to be gained by international exchange of views and information: once one country takes a lead in establishing regulations, others tend to follow. Many European countries import American products under licence and give them different trade names, e.g. Britain, Jugoslavia, the Netherlands and Czechoslovakia (Appendix 6). In Romania and Bulgaria manufacture is restricted by problems of industrial technology.

The best opportunities for practical utilization are to be found in the U.S.S.R. In other countries either regulations are still too strict or industrial technology has not yet advanced sufficiently. In the U.S.S.R. research successes in the V.I.Z.R. and several specialist institutes, together with the help of a fermentation industry near Moscow, led to the production of Enterobacterin 3 (Appendix 6). This amounted to 200 tons in 1968, sufficient to protect fruit and market crops on about 100,000 hectares, i.e. 247,100 acres (oral communication during a visit to the V.I.Z.R. at Leningrad, 1968; confirmed by data in Soviet literature). At the time of writing, a second product, Dendrobacillin, is about to be used against *Dendrolimus sibiricus* on the pine and larch forests of the Siberian taiga.

Following the work of Telenga (1964), and Telenga and Goral (1967), a unit was established at Krasnodar, U.S.S.R., to produce Beauverin (Appendix 6). This contains conidiospores of *Beauveria bassiana* plus amounts of chemical insecticides 4-5 times less than the normal dose. It is intended for the control of the Colorado beetle, European corn borer and codling moth. The U.S.S.R. has pioneered the use of this fungus, and also the use of mixtures of insecticides and pathogens–detailed exchanges of views with Soviet workers are desirable.

On the other hand, the principles of industrialization of insect viruses are much more advanced in the U.S.A. (Appendix 6; Ignoffo, 1965; Ignoffo and Heimpel, 1965). However, none has as yet been registered for sale, although a petition for exemption from tolerance and permanent label registration was submitted for the *Heliothis* virus on 1 January 1968 (Ignoffo, personal communication).

IV. Suggestions for the Future of International Co-operation

International co-operation should operate on two planes. The first concerns the exchange of scientific and technical information as well as fundamental and methodological discussions between scientists within the framework of conferences organized by international agencies like the O.I.L.B., the Society for Invertebrate Pathology, and the W.H.O. However, further co-ordination should also be undertaken in the field of training. On the second plane, that of industrialization and mutual benefit from technological progress, co-operation has developed between public research and industry mainly on a national basis (as in the U.S.A., U.S.S.R. and France). Except for exchanges and deliveries between various firms or production units, rapid technological co-operation on an international basis seems unlikely. This is explained partly by the uncertainties still existing on the future and profitability of microbial control, and partly on its ecological significance and status.

At the moment, the pesticide industry is too often taken to task for the problems of biosphere pollution; it must therefore act prudently in the face of governmental concern as regards the regulation and registration of microbial preparations. It is to be hoped that microbial control will rapidly adapt itself to ecological and economic conditions, to recompense the feats of imagination and perseverance by research workers all over the world and the audaciously creative expansion of industrial technology.

References

Bonnefoi, A. and Grison, P. (1959). *Phytiat. Phytophar.* **8**, 65-72.

Dutky, S. R. (1940). *J. Agric. Res.* **61**, 57-78.

Evlakhova, A. A. and Shvetsova, O. I. (1953). 80 pp. Izdatel'stvo Akademii Nauk S.S.S.R., Moscow, Leningrad, U.S.S.R.

Falcon, L. A. (1965). *Bull. ent. Soc. Am.* **11**, 84.

Franz, J. M. (1954). *Anz. f. Schädlingskunde* **5**, 27.

Franz, J. M. (1961). *Ann. Rev. Ent.* **6**, 183-200.

Grison, P. and Beguin, S. (1954). *C.r. hebd. Séanc. Acad. Agric. Fr.* **40**, 413-416.

Ignoffo, C. M. (1965). *J. Invertebrate Path.* **7**, 209-226.

Ignoffo, C. M. and Heimpel, A. M. (1965). *J. Invertebrate Path.* **7**, 329-340.

Jacobs, S. E. (1951). *Proc. Soc. appl. Bact.* **13**, 83-91.

Krassilstschik, I. M. (1886). "De insectorum morbis qui fungis parasitis efficunter", 97 pp. *Soc. Nat. Nouv. Mem. Russie,* Odessa.

Laird, M. (1965). *Proc. XIIth Int. Congr. Ent. London,* p. 730.

Metalnikov, S. and Chorine, V. (1929a). *Int. Corn Borer Investigations Sci. Rep.* **2**, 54-59.

Metalnikov, S. and Chorine, V. (1929b). *Int. Corn Borer Investigations Sci. Rep.* **2**, 60-61.

Poltev, V. I., Alexandrova, L. V. and Evlakhova, A. A. (1954). Infections and Protozoan Diseases of Insects (in Russian), Abstr. of Repts., Joint Plenary Session of the Sericulture and Apiculture, Plant Protection and Veterinary Science Sections (Vsesoyuznoi akademii Sel'skokkhozyaistvennykh Nauk imeni V.I. Lenina, Leningrad, U.S.S.R., 76 pp.)

Sparks, A. K. and Steinhaus, E. A. (1967). *J. Invertebrate Path.* **9**(2), i-iii.

Steinhaus, E. A. (1949). "Principles of Insect Pathology". McGraw-Hill, New York.
Steinhaus, E. A. (1951). *Calif. Agric.* **5**, 5.
Steinhaus, E. A. (1960). *Bact. Rev.* **24**, 365-373.
Telenga, N. A. (1964). *Entomophaga, Mém. hors Sér.* No. 2, 531 544.
Telenga, N. A. and Goral, V. M. (1967). *In* "Méth. lutte biol. contre les ravageurs forest. et agric. Conférence Samarcande", Oct. 1966, pp. 171-173.
Toumanoff, C. and Grison, P. (1954). *C.r. hebd. Séanc. Acad. Agric. Fr,* **40**, 277-280.
Weiser, J. (1955). *Acta Soc. ent. Ceskoslov.* **52**, 61-76.

CHAPTER 33

Past Achievements and Future Prospects

H. D. BURGES and N. W. HUSSEY

Pest Infestation Control Laboratory, Slough, Buckinghamshire, England
and
Glasshouse Crops Research Institute, Littlehampton, Sussex, England

I. Achievement

The contributions to this book demonstrate the value of applied microbial control as a practical weapon against some insect pests. They also reveal the extent of the active research effort, including both fundamental and practical aspects of insect pathology, that should ensure future progress. Insect pathogens that require repeated applications are termed "microbial insecticides" and those able to persist and spread among insect pests are regarded as "introductions".

A. MICROBIAL INSECTICIDES

Microbial insecticides have supplied a new lethal factor for the control of some herbivorous pests in the agricultural or forest environment (Tables I and II,

TABLE I

Some economically important Lepidoptera against which control by Bacillus thuringiensis *has been approved, or about which enough is known probably to warrant approval in addition to those registered in the U.S.A. (Table II in Chapter 3)*

Status	Scientific name	Common name
Approved in British Isles	*Hyponomeuta padellus*	small ermine moth
Approved in the Netherlands	*Malacosoma neustria*	lackey moth
Species that will probably be approved in Europe and the British Isles	*Aporia crataegi*	black-veined white butterfly
	Erannis defoliaria	mottled umber moth
	Euproctis chrysorrhoea	brown tail moth
	Hedya nubiferana	fruit tree tortrix moth
	Hyponomeuta malinellus	small ermine moth
	Lymantria dispar	gypsy moth
	Malacosoma neustria	lackey moth
	Pieris brassicae	cabbage white butterfly
	Prays citri	citrus flower moth
	Prays oleae	olive moth
	Spilonota ocellana	bud moth
	Thamnonoma wauaria	currant webworm
	Tortrix viridana	oak tortricid
Species that will probably be approved in Central America	*Ceramidia* sp.	Banana peel scarring or defoliating caterpillars
	Opsiphanes sp.	
	Platynota sp.	
Species that will probably be approved in Canada	*Acleris variana*	black headed budworm
	Thymelicus lineola	European skipper

Table II of Chapter 3). Their efficiency is unaffected by the population level of the pest. No microbial insecticides have yet been produced against insects of medical and veterinary importance, except the exotoxin of *Bacillus thuringiensis* which is active against flies and lice (not at present in commercial use).

In comparison with chemicals, microbial insecticides are few in number. However, for a limited number of uses, they are as effective as the best chemicals, though they are often more expensive. Those containing *B. thuringiensis* are registered and used commercially against some lepidopterous pests (Table I; Table II of Chapter 3). Production and formulation methods are well developed. The range of Lepidoptera known to be susceptible is wide and growing, but luckily includes very few beneficial species. The polyhedrosis and granulosis viruses are numerous (Table II), but much more specific, though collectively they have a wider host range and a similar potential for insect control to that of *B. thuringiensis.* The registration of some for practical use is being considered. The great advantage of microbial insecticides lies not only in

TABLE II

Insect viruses feasible for use as microbial insecticides[a]

Polyhedroses	Granuloses
Agrotis segetum	*Agrotis segetum*
Choristoneura fumiferana	*Argyrotaenia velutinana*
Colias philodice eurytheme	*Choristoneura fumiferana*
Dendrolimus spectabilis	*Cydia (Carpocapsa) pomonella*
Gilpinia (Diprion) hercyniae	*Eucosoma griseana*
Heliothis zea; H. virescens; H. phloxiphaga	*Hyphantria cunea*
Hemerocampa pseudotsugata	*Pieris brassicae; P. rapae*
Kotochalia junodi	*Spodoptera (Laphygma) exigua; S. (L.) frugiperda*
Lymantria dispar; L. fumida	*Trichoplusia ni*
Malacosoma fragile; M. disstria	
Mamestra (Barathra) brassicae	
Neodiprion sertifer; N. swainei; N. lecontei	
N. pratti pratti; N. pratti banksiana	
Pectinophora gossypiella	
Peridroma margaritosa	
Plusia gamma	
Prodenia eridania; P. ornithogalli; P. praefica	
Pseudaletia unipuncta	
Spodoptera (Laphygma) frugiperda; S. (L.) exigua	
Spodoptera (Prodenia) litura	
Thaumetopoea pityocampa	
Trichoplusia ni	

[a]Chapter 4; Ignoffo, 1967; Vasiljević, in press.

their safety to man and domestic animals but also in their specificity, for they appear to cause no more harm to beneficial insects than the killing of prey. However, this specificity, which is often at species level, may be a disadvantage when several pest species need to be controlled. In comparison with chemicals other disadvantages, apart from cost, are usually lack of contact action and sometimes the vulnerability of only one stage in the host's life-cycle.

Insect pathogens are relatively unaffected by chemical insecticides, although some fungicides may harm them, while some pathogens can be synergized by chemicals. In Russia, a factory is being built near Kiev to produce the fungus *Beauveria bassiana.* In 1971 and 1972, it is expected to treat 5 million acres with 250 tons of this fungus, synergized by reduced doses of chemical insecticides (Ferron, in press). This treatment should reduce chemical residues and it is possible that insecticide resistance may develop less readily.

Because the toxins of *B. thuringiensis* are stomach poisons in many insects, they could be used alone, though, at present, only spore-crystal mixtures are in commercial use because there is no good reason to remove the spores. The spores are of some importance against most insects, particularly at low dosages, and, in some insects, play a vital pathogenic role. An environment in which spores are unlikely to be desirable is the storehouse, but in preparations for use against storage pests, at least 99% of the spores could be killed by ultra-violet light, without harm to the crystals, or alternatively spore-free crystal protein of lower stability could be produced by an extraction process, though not in its original crystalline form. At present the cost of removing spores would be prohibitive. Reasonably pure exotoxin can be produced on a commercial scale, but this has not yet been justified. If exotoxin proves sufficiently safe in pure form, it may be useful against some flies, Lepidoptera and other groups.

B. MICROBIAL INTRODUCTIONS

Some insect pathogens that have proved valuable as introductions are listed in Table III, many against pests that had reached new regions. Sometimes the control achieved has been widespread and adequate, at others it has been limited either to favourable areas, favourable periods, or to times when the pest reached a high population density. Naturally-occurring pathogens also play a considerable role in curbing pest populations (Table IV), again the extent of control varying with time and region. A good illustration is the excellent ecological study of *Entomophthora floridana* on *Eutetranychus banksi* in Florida citrus groves (Muma, 1969).

About 1000 species of micro-organism pathogenic to insects and mites have been described (Ignoffo, 1967) and there are reliable methods of identification for many species and strains, but few have been purposefully introduced by man. As with introduced macrobial agents (DeBach, 1964), with which they are compared in Table V, the proportion of successes has been low. The most important features of the different groups of pathogens are compared in Table VI.

C. MICROBIAL CONTROL

We conclude that the deliberate introduction of pathogens and their use as microbial insecticides is a valuable method of control, used on a relatively small scale at present, and that pathogens are an important factor in the natural limitation of insect numbers. We further conclude that among the new methods of insect control, the achievements of applied microbial control are more modest than those due to the improved use of chemicals or applied macrobial control, but greater than those from the use of resistant varieties of plants. Similar views were expressed at a symposium in Rome in 1968 entitled: "New perspectives in the control of injurious insects" (Segre, 1969). Our achievements include expertise in using microbial control and the organizations built up to practise and extend this knowledge. We are acquiring a more thorough knowledge of ecology, a necessary adjunct because microbial control is often slower and more subtle than that of chemicals. For example, the greatest effect of an introduced

TABLE III

Examples of introductions of organisms into insect populations that resulted in lasting microbial control. Some of the introductions were made purposefully by man, others were accidental or natural

Micro-organism	Pest	Degree of success	Place	Authority[a]
VIRUS				
Polyhedrosis virus	*Gilpinia (Diprion) hercyniae*, European spruce sawfly	Control below economic and serious defoliation levels	Canada Newfoundland	Bird and Burke, 1961; Balch, 1946
Polyhedrosis virus	*Neodiprion sertifer*, European pine sawfly	Control below economic and serious defoliation levels; often replaced other methods	Canada, U.S.A., U.K.	Bird, 1953; Dowden and Girth, 1953; Bergold, 1958; Rivers, 1964a, b
Polyhedrosis virus	*Malacosoma disstria*, forest tent caterpillar	Virus spread and persisted causing heavy mortality	Canada	Stairs, 1965
Granulosis virus	*Hyphantria cunea*, fall webworm	Reduced major introduced pest to a minor level	Jugoslavia	Vasiljević, 1964, 1968, in press
BACTERIA				
Bacillus popilliae *B. lentimorbus*	*Popillia japonica* Japanese beetle	Beetle reduced from major to minor pest within three years of introduction of the bacteria	N.E. U.S.A.	Hall, 1964, Beard, 1964
FUNGI				
Entomophthora 3 species	*Therioaphis maculata*, spotted alfalfa aphid	Slow spread from centres of inoculation. Control in many areas	California	Hall and Dunn, 1957, 1958

TABLE III—*continued*

Micro-organism	Pest	Degree of success	Place	Authority[a]
FUNGI—*continued*				
Entomophthora (Empusa) erupta	*Lygus communis*, green apple bug	Lasting control after introduction into previously uninfected orchards, in others fungus can be started early	Annapolis valley	Dustan, 1924a; MacLeod, 1963; Baird, 1958 (69, 74)
Entomophthora sphaerosperma (sphaerospermia)	*Psylla mali*, European apple sucker	Near total control heavy infestations, less so light ones, marked fall of pest in Nova Scotia since fungus used.	Nova Scotia	Dustan, 1924b; MacLeod, 1963; Baird, 1958 (70, 72, 75)
Entomophthora spp.	Aphids, 4 species on potato	Of all the biological agents studied, fungi were outstanding in reducing populations	Maine	Shands *et al.*, 1958, 1963
Entomophthora aulicae	*Euproctis (Nygmia) chrysorrhoea (phaeorrhoea)* brown tail moth	Nearly freed many areas in warm moist weather, reduced damage by later invaders, over-wintered, good spring control	Maine, Massachusetts	Baird, 1958 (135, 136); Speare and Colley, 1912
Entomophthora creatonotus	*Creatonotus gangis*, tiger moth	Epizootic controlled the moth in 1960. Fungus persisted to give control in recent years	Taiwan	Yen, 1962, personal communication
Aschersonia aleyrodis	*Dialeurodes* spp. and other white-flies	Fungus effective in warm moist periods, best with shade trees, enables at least one spray to be stopped	Florida	Baird, 1958 (21-27, 29, 30, 32, 82, 83, 141, 182, 185, 245, 285, 287)
Aschersonia spp.	*Dialeurodes citri*, citrus whitefly	In 1963 $>$7000 acres treated with success. Each tree must be treated because fungus does not spread readily	Trans and N. Caucasus	Ferron, in press

Cephalosporium lecanii	Scale insect	Used frequently. Good results all over world, e.g. scales largely controlled by introduction in the Seychelles	W. Indies, U.S.S.R., Brazil, Puerto Rico, Guam, India, Ceylon	Chapter 16; Baird, 1958
Acrostalagmus aphidum	*Myzus persicae*, peach-potato aphid	Fungus sprayed in 1926 spread to control aphids. Control by fungus recurrence in 1927	Puerto Rico	Baird, 1958 (188)
Sphaerostilbe aurantiicola	*Quadraspidiotus (Aspidiotus) perniciosus*, San José scale	After distribution, this, or a native fungus, nearly exterminated the scale	S. California	Baird, 1958 (298)
Metarrhizium anisopliae	*Tomaspis saccharina*, froghopper	Fungus established. Some persistent natural control. Earlier control with extra sprays as soon as insects appear	Trinidad, Grenada	Baird, 1958 (118, 224, 225, 236, 273, 274, 293, 294)
Metarrhizium anisopliae	*Agrotis segetum*	Sprays in cold frames caused 80% mortality and reduced infestation the next year	Sweden	Baird, 1958 (189)
Spicaria prasina	*Trichoplusia ni*, cabbage looper	Larval outbreak suppressed. Fungus continued control usually below economic level	Taiwan	Yen, 1960, personal communication
PROTOZOAN				
Glugea pyraustae	*Ostrinia nubilalis*, European corn borer	Reduces population to a level that enables economic control by other means. No dramatic epizootics	Illinois	Chapter 6
NEMATODE				
Tripius sciarae	Sciarid flies	Flies in a glasshouse began to decrease after four weeks and weekly insecticide sprays could be stopped	Rothamsted, England	Poinar, 1965

[a] Numbers following Baird (1958) refer to abstracts of original papers made by Baird.

TABLE IV

Importance of naturally occurring pathogen infections in the control of insect numbers

Importance	Occurrence of natural control
Viruses: very important	Polyhedroses and granuloses very often cause population crashes of lepidopterans and sawflies during severe infestations, particularly in forests. Other viruses occasionally cause severe mortality in many insect orders. Some viruses reduce virility and fedundity of adult insects and cause important enzootic control.
Fungi: very important	Very common causes of population crashes during outbreaks of many orders of insects, particularly associated with seasonal rains, warm humid weather, cool wet spells unfavourable for rapid insect growth and hibernation quarters. Also act on low populations, when and where micro-environmental conditions favour the fungus, giving important enzootic control. Once an insect becomes infected, death tends to be rapid.
Bacteria: important	*Bacillus popilliae* group causes heavy mortality and important enzootic control of some ground beetles. *Bacillus thuringiensis* occurs only in *Lepidoptera*; outdoors, epizootics are rare and enzootic control slight; indoors, epizootics have been common in silkworm farms and in London warehouses where heavy moth infestations used to occur, still cause epizootics in grain and nut stores in Africa. Outdoors, other sporeformers and some non-sporeformers cause occasional epizootics and considerable enzootic control, particularly when weather or food plant does not favour insect growth.
Protozoans: fairly important	Common causes of low to moderate insect mortality, tending to act rather by reduction of virility and fecundity, the two factors together sometimes causing important enzootic control. Occasionally virulent protozoans kill many insects in nature. Attack most orders of insects. Importance in nature reviewed in Chapter 6.
Nematodes: fairly important	Sometimes cause epizootics and may wipe out insect populations in conditions that favour the nematode. Commonly cause variable mortality, usually in aquatic, soil- and bark-dwelling insects. May castrate insects without causing heavy mortality of reproductive stages. Natural occurrence is reviewed in Chapter 8.
Rickettsiae: some importance	Epizootics occasional. Tend to cause variable mortality and reduce fecundity, giving some enzootic control.

pathogen on a pest may be delayed for a year following treatment, as after introducing the fungus *Entomophthora* against the green apple sucker in Canada (Dustan, 1924b), and the polyhedrosis virus of the pine sawfly in Scotland (Rivers, 1964a, b, personal communications). Because a microbial insecticide might act slowly it cannot be used in certain crops. Thus the polyhedrosis virus of *Heliothis zea* shows great promise on cotton, grain sorghum and corn, where some damage can be tolerated, but not on tomato, where slight damage can reduce the value of a crop (Dulmage, 1967). Where little damage can be

TABLE V

Salient features of microbial control agents compared with those of macrobial agents

Feature	Microbial agents and nematodes	Macrobial agent
Safety	Most are safe for man and beneficial insects	Absolutely safe to man, mainly so to beneficial insects.
Effect of chemicals { insecticides	Largely unharmed	Severely harmed
Effect of chemicals { fungicides	Harmed by some	Harmed by a few
Powers of search	Lacking, except in nematodes	Good
Spread	Passive, sometimes slow	Active, by own mobility, usually rapid
Persistence in environment	Free resistant spores: spores and vegetative forms often within all stages of insect	Usually specific diapause or aestivating developmental stage
Significance of environmental conditions	Sometimes limiting	Usually limiting
Acquired resistance of host	Possible	Unlikely
Storage	Usually easy	Usually difficult
Mode of application	Apply over limited area, release infected insects, or application of microbial insecticide	Release over limited area
Cost	Introduction low: microbial insecticides moderate to high	Low, particularly if introduced only once
Predictability of control	Some introductions predictable after experience with the pathogen. Microbial insecticides predictable	Some predictable after experience with the agent—only if climate is similar to that in known satisfactory areas
Control	A few introductions give good control, others partial, many fail. Microbial insecticides give good control	A low proportion of agents tried give good control, others partial, many fail

tolerated, microbial control is possible only with a rapidly acting and reliable microbial insecticide, such as one containing *B. thuringiensis.* Similarly, the yardstick of immediate and impressive kill, as obtained with lethal chemicals, should be accepted only when this degree of kill is necessary. A less impressive immediate pest mortality that does not suppress macrobial agents is often more valuable in the long-term. For instance, the arbitrary aim of chemical control of the gypsy moth in the U.S.A. is to lower the number of egg clusters to 50/acre, whereas after treatment with *B. thuringiensis,* less damage may ensue though

TABLE VI

Salient features, in approximate order of significance, of the different groups of pathogens

Group	Features
Nematodes	Safety: for man probably absolute: for useful insects usual Some grow *in vitro* Limited powers of search Persist by free resistant stages Use: mainly trial introductions
Protozoans	Safety: for man absolute: for useful insects usual Production only *in vivo* Resistant stages moderately resistant Transmission by insect egg common Use: mainly trial introductions
Fungi	Safety: some not safe for man and useful insects Some grow *in vitro* Often limited by need of high humidity Spores remarkably persistent No transmission by eggs: aerial dispersion often good Infection commonly through the cuticle Use: mainly introductions: microbial insecticide trials variable
Bacteria (sporeforming)	Safety: most are safe for man and useful animals Many grow *in vitro* Many virulent, toxigenic Spores very resistant Transmission by eggs uncommon Use: commercial microbial insecticides, successful introductions
Viruses	Safe for man and useful animals Grow *in vivo* only Transmission by eggs common Many very virulent Inclusion bodies resistant Use: very successful introductions: trial microbial insecticides very promising
Rickettsia	Safety to man often doubtful: probably safe for useful insects Grow *in vivo* only Transmission by eggs common No highly resistant stage Many very virulent Use: introductions possible

more egg clusters occur. Where predatory or parasitic arthropods are introduced, the use of chemicals must be restricted, but microbial agents can be used instead, e.g. to control caterpillars on glasshouse chrysanthemums during the macrobial control of red spider mites and aphids.

D. SAFETY OF MICROBIAL AGENTS

As regards safety for man, the knowledge that toxins may be involved has stimulated toxicological studies in addition to the more obvious pathogenicity studies. The present mood is one of increased caution. Governments and regulating authorities have a responsibility to establish and maintain standards, but this must not be an excuse for inaction or unreasonable delay in the use of suitable pathogens. In recent years the U.S.A. has tended to lead both in the use of pathogens and in legislation governing their applications. In contrast, one of the pioneers in the trial of pathogens, France, where the first product containing *B. thuringiensis* (Sporeine) was manufactured, has lagged behind in legislation, and the use of *B. thuringiensis* was not permitted until 1970. Three aspects of safety must be considered, the health of the worker producing or applying pathogens, that of the consumer in contact with treated commodities and that of wild life. Each case must be considered individually. In general, however, most insect pathogens are harmless to both man and vertebrates and none are known to be phytotoxic or phytopathogenic. Apart from a few cases of allergy to fungal spores, the symptoms of which disappeared as soon as the agent was removed, research and application of microbial control has involved no danger or ill health. The paucity of records of vertebrates or man harmed by insect pathogens is encouraging when one realizes that insects are sought as food by vertebrates and live in and on food–man's in particular–both in the field and the store.

E. ECONOMICS

In the field of economics, some microbial agents are commercially viable; others, although desirable weapons for insect control, are not. For introduction, only one organism *(Bacillus popilliae)* has been commercially produced, but some private organizations and individuals are supplying virus for introduction into Canadian forests. As regards microbial insecticides, two commercial firms in the U.S.A. have been, and still are, prominent in the research and development of *B. thuringiensis* though other firms, some outside the U.S.A., have done limited work. Some firms are interested at the experimental level. One firm in Britain is studying *B. thuringiensis* chemically and microbiologically, as a long-term investment, without, at present, venturing into production. Currently three firms in the U.S.A. and one in France are producing *B. thuringiensis* commercially, and *Beauveria bassiana* is being produced in Russia. Several firms in the U.S.A. are developing viruses as microbial insecticides. The greatest potential for economic gain from microbial control lies in its use over wide areas so it is not surprising that government laboratories and university departments are undertaking considerably more research than industry. In one instance a government department (United States Department of Agriculture) has produced a pathogen *(B. popilliae)* in bulk and organized its introduction over wide areas of the U.S.A. Most major countries have laboratories capable of this type of programme. The World Health Organization is organizing a worldwide search for pathogens of medically important insects.

When properly conducted, control with microbial insecticides is now reliable and predictable. This is essential because the effort involved in mass-production and application is as substantial as that for chemicals. Introductions are not yet reliable and progress can, at present, be measured only in terms of the recognition of the problem.

F. TECHNICAL ACHIEVEMENTS

Finally, a number of recent technical advances rank among the most important achievements. It is sufficient here to list some of the most significant: improvements in fermentation technology, harvesting methods and formulation; standardization of products by reliable bioassays; serological and esterase typing of *B. thuringiensis*; seroassay of the crystal in unformulated *B. thuringiensis* preparations; enzymatic and other chemical studies of the crystal; purification of the exotoxin of *B. thuringiensis*; breeding of insects on artificial media and their use in producing polyhedrosis and granulosis viruses; discovery of non-occluded viruses in insects and the association of bacteria and nematodes; separation of fungal toxins.

II. Expectations

A. USES IN INTEGRATED CONTROL PROGRAMMES

The future of insect control lies, as always, in the integration of all available control methods. The use of chemicals alone is unlikely to solve pest problems permanently. Nor is any method or combination of methods likely to give perfection, the orchard of perfect trees with every apple unblemished, for instance. With biological control–both macrobial and microbial–this is because, if agents are to maintain themselves in the environment as long-term controlling forces, they need a residue of pests, which may cause some damage. Chemical insecticides kill off macrobial agents directly or affect their behaviour, allowing the pests to resurge. There is even an example of a pathogen *(Entomophthora sphaerosperma)* exterminating a pest *(Plutella maculipennis)* so effectively that macrobial agents were drastically reduced, largely by lack of food, so that eventually the pest resurged in weather conditions unfavourable to the pathogen (Ullyett and Schonken, 1940; Ullyett, 1947). A balance between the pest and all controlling forces, physical and biological, is essential. Pathogens applied as microbial insecticides can restore this balance when pests begin to increase, while pathogens applied as introductions and as supplements to enzootic organisms form part of the natural controlling complex. Chemicals inevitably have some hazards to man and useful wild life: even insect hormones may prove to be too similar to physiological regulators in mammals to be applied to food materials. We anticipate that microbial control will play a useful–and extremely safe–part in integrated control, while not replacing chemical methods against the majority of pests. However, although of early concept, applied microbial control is still in its infancy, remaining largely at the research level. As a result of their high selectivity the range of microbial insecticides, economically competitive with chemicals, should increase to fulfil specialized roles in integrated control. Their economic position will probably continue to improve as prohibitive legislation increases against the more dangerous chemicals. For instance, Allen (1968), discussing the use of polyhydrosis virus against bollworms (*Heliothis* complex) in an integrated programme on cotton, stated "the future of the virus does not depend on its fulfillment of certain criteria [of effectiveness] alone but in the eventual acceptance by the grower of a newer, more challenging approach to insect control". Reflecting an intensification of interest in non-chemical control caused by the recent refusal of West Germany and Britain to purchase tobacco containing residues of chlorinated hydrocarbons, an American corporation, formed to control agricultural insects without the use of persistent pesticides that leave residues on the tobacco, plans to use microbial insecticides in its programmes (J. W. Drawdy, personal communication).

When successful, the introduction of pathogens should be highly economic since relatively little effort is involved in making an introduction. Periodic, localized, or limited control–operating only a high population levels–may be economically worthwhile, even if only to achieve an improvement in the efficiency of other methods of control. Every likely species and improved strain of pathogen should be evaluated for the control of pests. However, judging from the experience of introducing fungi (Baird, 1958) and that of applied macrobial control, only a small proportion of attempted introductions will yield spectacular success.

B. COMPARATIVE ADVANTAGES OF DIFFERENT PATHOGEN GROUPS IN DIFFERENT GROUPS OF ARTHROPODS

The potentialities of the six major groups of pathogens are just becoming apparent (Table VI). We may expect bacteria (that form spores) and viruses (that form inclusion bodies) to be the main sources of microbial insecticides for some time to come, with some hope of candidates from among the fungi, protozoans and nematodes. Careful attention will have to be paid to the *correct* usage of bacterial and viral insecticides. They must be used against the appropriate developmental stages of susceptible species and preferably be applied late in the day to minimize the deleterious effect of the ultra-violet content of sunlight. Otherwise they are not unduly susceptible to the environment. In contrast, fungi and nematodes are much more susceptible to the environment and, as microbial insecticides, they can be successful only in regions, times, ecological niches or microenvironments with adequate free moisture or high humidity. They may be used in association with low dosages of chemical insecticides. Temperatures, particularly in summer, may affect their efficiency. Thus, these organisms may play a more specialized role than others in integrated control, being used against the aquatic stages of insects, in moist soil, during the rainy season, in geographical regions of high rainfall or even in individual orchards and plantations that are notably moist. Field tests by Dresner (1949), for instance, suggested that *Beauveria bassiana* was better for controlling the Mexican bean beetle, *Epilachna varivestis,* during frequent heavy rainfall in New York State than the insecticide rotenone. Fungi and nematodes might be used in the wet season to reduce the pest population and delay recuperation in the ensuing dry season. As microbial insecticides, except in very favourable conditions, fungi tend to be required in uneconomically high concentrations. The use of protozoans as microbial insecticides is unlikely because their spores are less virulent and tend to be more vulnerable to the environment than bacterial spores. Further they can be produced only *in vivo.*

All six groups, in this order of merit; viruses, fungi, spore-forming bacteria, nematodes, protozoans and rickettsia, hold promise for introductions, particularly in environments where moderate insect populations can be tolerated (Table VI). In these populations debilitative pathogens, and those of moderate or low pathogenicity, can persist to take a modest, but useful and sometimes critical, toll of insects. The more virulent pathogens tend to cause impressive spasmodic control. With introductions, such features as transovarial transmission that enable pathogens to act on sparse host populations are important.

As the pathogens of more and more insects are studied, a pattern is beginning to emerge. Some insect groups, e.g. Lepidoptera, sawflies, bees, Tenebrionidae and Scarabaeidae, appear to suffer greatly from disease, both in severity of attack and variety of pathogens involved: the Lepidoptera support members of almost all groups of pathogens. Some groups of pathogens, e.g. Entomophthorales, Microsporida (particularly *Nosema*), Gregarinidae and *Beauveria* are very widespread both in frequency of occurrence and in variety of insects attacked. Other insect groups, e.g. grain weevils, bean weevils, parasitic Hymenoptera, Anobiidae and Ptinidae, seem to be almost free from pathogens. Some groups of pathogens are largely restricted to a few insect groups, e.g. *Bacillus thuringiensis* and the polyhedrosis and granulosis types of virus mainly to Lepidoptera, *Coelomomyces* to mosquitoes, and the *Bacillus popilliae* group to scarabaeid beetles. Sometimes key factors can be recognized that account for these facts, e.g. the crystal of *B. thuringiensis,* the remarkable ability of *B. popilliae* spores to survive in soil and reproduction of *Coelomomyces* by zoospores.

It is almost possible to predict what pathogens should be used to attack a particular insect species and the degree of control to be expected. Against a moth pest of an apple tree, for instance, one might introduce a microsporidan and a cytoplasmic polyhedrosis virus to sap its vitality, a nuclear polyhedrosis and a granulosis virus in the hope of reducing it to sub-pest status, and an *Entomophthora* for assault in periods of humid, and otherways favourable conditions; as microbial insecticides, a *Beauveria* or a *Metarrhizium* might be sprayed on mature larvae if the species pupates in soil or litter and finally a strain of *Bacillus thuringiensis* might be sprayed on young larvae for rapid control if the pest becomes too numerous. The pest groups most susceptible to microbial control appear to be Lepidoptera to *B. thuringiensis,* polyhedrosis and granulosis virus; aphids and scale insects to fungi; scarabaeids to the *B. popilliae* group of bacteria; and sawflies to polyhedrosis virus.

All reference up to this point has been to insects. Mites are a smaller, less studied group of pests and naturally fewer pathogens have been recorded. The variety recorded has been wide, the missing pathogen groups being those mainly associated with particular groups of insects. Promising experimental control of citrus mites by virus has been obtained, but control on a commercial scale has not been attempted. Little is known about the role of naturally occurring microbial control, but we can probably expect a similar situation for mites to that already observed with insects.

The extent to which it is worth carrying the identification of pathogens depends on the circumstances. If information on the general nature and potential of a disease situation is required, identification to order, genus or species in sufficient, though it should not be overlooked that pathogenicity sometimes depends on strain. Usually, identification should be taken as far as possible by easy methods and only taken further if necessity demands, as when a pathogen is to be developed for applied microbial control. Methods for the identification of varieties, as in *B. thuringiensis,* are likely to be adequate until development is well advanced. Then, even diagnosis to variety may be insufficient, biotype being important in relation to virulence, pathogenicity in specific hosts and attenuation.

An important aspect of the development of applied microbial control is the selection of the most suitable wild biotypes or strains. Once these wild types have been exhausted, strains may be improved by genetical recombination etc., to produce artificial laboratory or industrial biotypes. These can be identified only by case histories and quantitative performances. Performance is measured by toxin production, by production of spores or equivalent bodies, or by bioassay to indicate virulence. Better strains of *B. thuringiensis* are continually being used commercially and there is scope for even further biotype improvement. Different strains of some viruses have been recorded. Particularly with viruses, improvements could be expected by seeking better strains in new natural epizootics of disease. It may be important to isolate the virus at the beginning of a disease outbreak.

Further advances, discussed in more detail in the next section, are possible from toxins. Strain selection frequently produces strains of increased toxigenicity. The identification of more toxins is certain to occur, more may be manufactured biologically and in due course some may be synthesized.

Resistance to pathogens has been detected in the laboratory, but not in practice and it is too early to speculate about its practical significance. Resistance to toxins must also be considered: flies resistant to the exotoxin of *B. thuringiensis* have been obtained in the laboratory (Harvey and Howell, 1965). It seems unlikely that resistance to existing insecticidal chemicals will influence susceptibility to pathogens or their toxins, although no evidence is available.

Improvements to *in vitro* methods of production are likely to be made in small steps though occasional jumps might occur in the more difficult of these methods. Since *in vitro* production is so much more economical than that *in vivo*, further attempts will be made to find *in vitro* methods for pathogens now grown satisfactorily only in living hosts. Alternatively, larger or more easily bred insect hosts may be found for the production of some pathogens and eventually tissue culture may be used.

Bioassay is unlikely to be superseded for the standardization of products in the near future, although quicker methods might be used as routine with periodic reference checking by bioassay. Such routine methods include counts of organisms and sero-assay. Some toxins might be measurable chemically.

III. Research

Detailed assessments of the research required in different aspects of the subject are given in each chapter. Here, our object is to discuss, with a few examples, features common to many chapters as well as important trends and principles. In general, there must be research to investigate the role that microbial control can play in integrated insect control. This includes not only trials with various crops and laboratory investigations arising from them but also fundamental work in insect pathology and ecology. A convenient starting point in this discussion is the simplest one, the use of pathogens as microbial insecticides to achieve rapid control or to restore a balance between an insect pest and its natural controlling forces.

A. *BACILLUS THURINGIENSIS*

The leading, and most studied organism in microbial insecticides—the pacemaker—is *B. thuringiensis,* the subject of several chapters. We will correlate research requirements from these chapters in some detail, because this provides a good illustration of the research potential of microbial insecticides.

During field application *B. thuringiensis* must be protected against ultra-violet radiation and weathering. It must be applied so as to give adequate cover, particularly to the under sides of leaves, because it is effective only when eaten and is most effective against the youngest larvae. Synergistic substances should be sought among harmless chemicals.

An intensive study of genetics could lead to improvements both in the yield of spores and crystals, as well as in their activities. Since different bacterial strains are active against different pests, desirable invasive properties of the spore, as well as toxic characters of the crystal, against a particular pest could be combined into one strain; or a few super-strains could be tailored against groups of host species. Strains should be sought, or fabricated, for host species at present considered not susceptible or poorly so, a hope fostered by the discovery of serotype V, a variety *(galleriae)* particularly active against *G. mellonella*, which was once regarded as only slightly susceptible to *B. thuringiensis*. Our existing knowledge of genetical tools such as bacteriophage and transformation should be extended. Except for use against storage moths, there is no point in eliminating the spore from commercial preparations; rather the crystal-synergizing and invasive properties of the spore should be improved and extended to host species at present considered susceptible mainly to crystal activity.

The most important research rewards might lie in fundamental study of the crystal, an inert protoxin. Can we release the toxic molecules from the crystal and use them more effectively? Physical data suggest that the arrangement of molecules is remarkably similar in the crystals of different bacterial varieties. Dumb-bell-shaped subunits of molecular weight in the order of 200,000 are arranged in four-fold screw symmetry. Ultra-centrifuge analyses have revealed the largest molecules, in alkaline solutions of crystals, to be about MW 200,000 (Norris, personal communication), although it is not clear whether these are re-aggregations of the smaller molecules (40,000) reported by other workers. These solutions also contain molecules of about MW 10,000, the size of individual polypeptides. These molecules, and their significance, need better definition. Most have proved toxic *per os*: more information is needed about toxicity by injection into the body cavity. These molecules need very careful comparison with antigenic molecules obtained by enzymic hydrolysis, varying in size from MW $>$ 200,000 down to peptide-sized molecules of MW 5000. Of these, molecules of MW 40,000 to MW 5000 have been toxic by injection.

There is some evidence that the same toxic antigen occurs in several varieties of *B. thuringiensis* and that some varieties acquire their toxicity mainly from unique toxic antigens. Several different toxic peptides could be located on molecules in various combinations, or possibly a single toxic peptide could be non-specifically absorbed in various amounts to different polypeptides or proteins. The isolation of the peptide(s) and polypeptide(s) and knowledge of the amino acid sequences conferring toxicity would greatly facilitate both genetical studies, investigations of mode of action and mechanisms of resistance to the crystal.

Further insight could be gained into these and other questions by unravelling the modes of release of toxic molecules from the protoxin in a number of host species of differing susceptibilities. Trypsin and chymotrypsin, as well as enzymes from *Pieris brassicae* and *Bombyx mori,* release from the crystal substances toxic to those Lepidoptera that are susceptible to the intact crystal. The moth, *Ephestia kuehniella,* is comparatively resistant to the intact crystal, yet is susceptible to crystal hydrolysates both *per os* and by injection. Are these hydrolysates stable and toxic to non-lepidopterous insects and/or to vertebrates? These are intriguing research possibilities in the search for pest-specific poisons. Because the ultimate toxic molecules may be toxic only to insects that eat them, will they be relatively safe for macrobial agents, harmless to vertebrates *per os,* yet able to limit pest complexes of diverse insect types? Will they eventually be synthesized?

It seems vital to have a better knowledge of the mode of action of the ultimate toxic molecules in the insect. Damage to the midgut epithelium of lepidopterans has often been demonstrated. Recently, products of crystal hydrolysis have been shown to block nervous conduction at synapses in the cockroach. What is the relative importance of these modes of action?

The basis for the mechanism of vertebrate resistance to the crystal needs further investigation. It is believed that the vertebrates do not possess the correct combinations of solvents and enzymes in the gut to release the toxic molecules from the protoxin and, that even if they did, stomach pepsin and acidity would destroy the crystal protein at the beginning of the alimentary tract. This needs confirmation, then extension by studying injection of enzymic-hydrolysis products of the crystal into vertebrates.

The exotoxin offers different possibilities. Its chemical nature is largely known and the details that remain to be discovered will show whether it is a single chemical or a family of extremely similar compounds. It is toxic by injection into mice, but relatively much less so orally: the exact oral LD_{50} for a number of vertebrate species should be determined. The molecular basis for its interference with insect moulting and metamorphosis should be interesting, because it is not the only poison to cause deformities. The teratogenic effects occur when exotoxin is administered *per os,* but not by injection (R. P. M. Bond, unpublished results). Extrapolation of these results with insects to the mammalian problem would be speculation but obviously the possibility of teratogenic effects of exotoxin on mammals must be investigated with care. The necessity for such an investigation is underlined by an observation which touches, albeit obliquely, on the subject. Chromomycin, an antibiotic which, like exotoxin, inhibits the RNA polymerase enzyme has been shown to bring about teratogenic effects in the sea squirt, *Ciona intestinalis* (Brahmachary, 1966).

From this synopsis of the research potential of *B. thuringiensis* as a microbial insecticide we can see the need for field trials and a concerted laboratory study to investigate the problems encountered in practical use of the bacterium, to probe ahead for new approaches and to increase fundamental information.

B. OTHER PATHOGENS

In 1950, *B. thuringiensis* was regarded only as an infectious bacterium: its toxins and their research potential were not anticipated. Research should look for similar potential in other bacteria and in other groups of pathogens that are candidate microbial insecticides, i.e. mainly viruses, fungi and nematodes. As far as practical application of these groups as microbial insecticides is concerned, priority should be given to virulence studies, strain selection, protective formulation and covering power. In addition, fungi tend to be required in heavy concentrations, so investigation of synergists is important. Fungi and nematodes are more dependant on the micro-environment than spore-forming bacteria and occluded viruses, so there should be emphasis on environmental studies.

Research is likely to be more complex with those pathogens able to persist and spread naturally. These may be used as introductions to new areas and to supplement naturally occurring enzootic pathogens. Research should examine mechanisms of transmission from insect to insect and from one generation to the next, as well as calculate the biomass of a pathogen in the environment and its distribution. Pathogens are likely to be distributed unevenly in nature, with the insect cadaver as focal unit. This may explain how insects become infected in nature and yet require very high levels of inocula in laboratory experiments. It suggests that artificial introduction of pathogens in droplets attractive to the insect would be preferable to the even distribution required for a microbial insecticide. Research on the distribution of foci of enzootic pathogens might reveal whether artificial supplementation, regulated according to the size or state of the pest population, would keep the population level tolerable and avoid outbreaks. This will obviously be related to environmental conditions. Research is required on the significance of particularly susceptible individuals for the maintenance of pathogen foci.

Of great importance is the acquisition of base-line data on the natural occurrence of pathogens before man intervenes. Equally important is a sound study of the pathogen, especially, for instance, spore viability and temperature requirements. The effective spread of pathogens is commonly thought to occur only at high host density, but often this may not be so, e.g. with the viruses of the armyworm, *Pseudaletia unipuncta* (Tanada, 1968) and the sawfly, *Gilpinia (Diprion) hercyniae* (Stairs, 1968). Diseases have usually been studied at times of spectacular outbreaks, or applied when insects are numerous, whereas studies between outbreaks are more important, the object being to prevent insects reaching numbers at which epizootics intervene. Study is needed to determine the best time to apply pathogens. This may be in seasons when insects are few or, especially with cyclic populations, during years of scarcity. When sampling populations, allowance must be made for the rapid disappearance of diseased insects and cadavers from the environment. To locate disease we may need to use novel methods, such as the serological examination of the gut contents or faeces of predators.

A variety of pathogens should be introduced for study in insect populations and their environments. An excellent example, illustrating lines of useful research, followed the first appearance of the fall webworm, *Hyphantria cunea,* in Europe in 1940. It became so numerous in orchards and forest margins that it invaded dwelling houses. A nuclear polyhedrosis was observed in 1952, and a cytoplasmic polyhedrosis in 1953, neither with dramatic effects on the population. In 1957, a granulosis appeared and subsequently reduced the moth to the status of a minor pest (Vasiljević, 1964, 1968, in press, personal communication). Recently, the pest has spread into new areas of Europe, apparently without the granulosis virus, an excellent–and probably fleeting–opportunity to gather base-line data before the virus appears, or is purposefully introduced. Also, the pest has recently increased again in old areas of infestation in Europe (Vasiljević, personal communication)–another stimulus for study. The pest occurs in the U.S.A. and a granulosis, although present, appears to be unimportant–why? Other areas of pest abundance, Japan and the U.S.S.R., offer opportunities to try granulosis. There are other pathogens that could be considered as adjuncts to virus. Vasiljević believes that *H. cunea* acquired the granulosis virus from a native European moth. If this is so, the virus acted rather like Brazilian myxomatosis in the European rabbit. Intensive study of the host ranges of many pathogens seems warranted.

Ecological studies must be backed by fundamental laboratory work. For instance, ideas that may be applicable to research on many groups of pathogens have arisen from intense efforts in the U.S.A. to sporulate *Bacillus popilliae* on artificial media. Thus, in strains of moderate virulence, the rate of sporulation in the infected larva is slow, allowing slow build up to very large numbers of spores. These spores are difficult to germinate and less than 1% germinate on media or on injection into the larval haemocoel; most spores ingested do not germinate even with repeated passage through the gut. This probably means that spores require for germination very specific or complex circumstances, maybe similar to those in the larval gut. Outside the host body, these special requirements probably prevent the germination of spores, so that a large, long-lived inoculum builds up and ensures limitation of pest populations. These observations help to explain the success of this pathogen in nature–knowledge vital to the strategy of its artificial use and encouraging to the expansion of this type of work. The failure of *B. thuringiensis* to persist outdoors contrasts sharply with the success of *B. popilliae,* probably because the *B. thuringiensis* spore germinates readily and then dies in the soil. Possibly the crystal is another way to extend the duration of pathogenicity by fixing the toxins in an inert protoxin more stable than the spore, so that the protoxin survives longer in nature than most spores and synergizes the action of those spores that survive. This offers another theory for the evolutionary development of the crystal in addition to the current idea that the crystal arose as over-production of spore protein in imbalanced cells. Can this crystal be linked with spores of other bacteria more durable in nature than those of *B. thuringiensis*? Already there is evidence that, in some lepidopteran species, the crystal damages the gut and initiates septicaemia caused more frequently by rods and cocci of other bacteria than by *B. thuringiensis.*

C. PATTERN OF FUTURE PROGRESS

Research on microbial control should not cease at a study of pathogen, pest and ecology. Man is a vital factor in the advent of pests and in their control. If he is not familiar with new methods, they will not be used. Pest control must be considered at the sociological level, affecting the whole community, not just an individual field or orchard (Smith, 1969). The combined efforts of the grower, the advisory agricultural staff, the research entomologist and insect pathologist must be harnessed to formulate and test new techniques. Over areas of dense cultivation of a single or a limited number of crops, community research projects need trial. For instance, the use of *Heliothis* virus on fields, scattered in a cotton area where chemical treatment predominates, will not reap the full benefit of the harmless nature of the virus to macrobial agents or of the possible ability of the virus to persist and spread because too many parasites and diseased pests will be killed by insecticides. In contrast, wide use of virus in a region where chemicals are banned, may so impregnate the region with virus that it may spread and persist, thus allowing macrobial agents to build up and establish an equilibrium with the pest at a low population level. Subsequently, spot treatments with virus and *B. thuringiensis* over limited areas could deal with future limited resurgences so proving less costly on an area basis, than the snowballing use of chemicals, though it might be more expensive for some individual fields. Such pest control could be financed on a regional basis, each grower paying his share of the total cost for the region. However, a single large grower restarting extensive use of chemicals could again throw the whole region into imbalance.

The experimental banning of chemicals would be difficult to initiate if left to industry because of the difficulty of organization. A further difficulty is that several pests are usually present together. Governmental organization and backing would, therefore, be required. This could also involve the production of the necessary quantities of virus or other pathogen: past experience has shown how slow progress is until large quantities of pathogen became available for study, e.g. the generous donation of *B. thuringiensis* all over the world by American firms.

International co-operation is also valuable and great hopes are pinned on the formation of the I.O.B.C. (International Organization for Biological Control), with the achievements of the European-based O.I.L.B. (Organisation International de Lutte Biologique) as its model. For instance, an intercontinental working group on the control of *H. cunea* by virus could stimulate great progress. Within the O.I.L.B., recommendations have recently been made for the formation of a working group to exploit the promising granulosis virus of the codling moth. Eventual extension of this on an intercontinental basis seems a valuable exercise against this worldwide pest of apple. There are already signs of increase in the study of the pathogens of a worldwide group of tropical pests, termites, as yet without practical results, even though the termite lives in an environment conducive to microbial control–humid, crowded, intimate. Has the termite evolved such resistance against pathogens (as far as fungal pathogens are concerned, possibly in the course of its exploitation of fungi as food) that microbial control will not be extensive, or are our methods of trial at fault? Or will the use of exotic pathogens overcome resistance? This is another case where close international co-operation is desirable both in fundamental research and at the more practical levels.

The banning of DDT in an increasing number of countries, curbs on other persistent chemicals, and an increasing awareness of the dangers of wide spectrum, highly toxic pesticides create a gap in our insect control weaponry that must be rapidly filled. In order that microbial control can play its role, there is an urgent need for more research on immediate problems with the better known microbial agents while long-term studies offer glittering prospects.

References

Allen, G. E. (1968). Proc. Joint U.S.-Japan Semin. Microbial Control Insect Pests. U.S. Committee Sci. Cooperation. Panel 8, pp. 37-41. Fukuoka, Japan.

Baird, R. B. (1958). "The Artificial Control of Insects by Means of Entomogenous Fungi: a Compilation of References with Abstracts", 300 references. Entomology Laboratory, Belleville, Ontario.

Balch, R. E. (1946). *Can. Dep. Agric. bi-m. Prog. Rep.* **2,** 1.

Beard, R. L. (1964). *Entomophaga, Mém. hors Sér.* No. 2, 47-49.

Bergold, G. H. (1958). Viruses of insects. *Handb. Virusforschung* **4,** 60-142.

Bird, F. T. (1953). *Can. Ent.* **85,** 437-446.

Bird, F. T. and Burk, J. M. (1961). *Can. Ent.* **93,** 228-238.

Brahmachary, R. L. (1966). *Acta Embryol. Morphol. Exp.* **9,** 25-30.

DeBach, P. (1964). *In* "Biological Control of Insect Pests and Weeds" (P. DeBach and E. I. Schlinger, eds), pp. 673-713. Chapman and Hall, London.

Dowden, P. B. and Girth, H. B. (1953). *J. econ. Ent.* **46,** 525-526.

Dresner, E. (1949). *Boyce Thompson Inst. Plant Res. Inc.* **15,** 319-335.

Dulmage, H. T. (1967). *In* "Insect Pathology and Microbial Control" (P. A. van der Laan, ed.), pp. 120-124. North-Holland Publ. Co., Amsterdam.

Dustan, A. G. (1924a). *Proc. Acadian ent. Soc.,* 1923, **9,** 14-36.

Dustan, A. G. (1924b). *60th Ann. Rep. Fruit Growers' Ass., Nova Scotia,* 100-104.

Ferron, P. (In press.) *Entomophaga.*

Hall, I. M. (1964). *In* "Biological Control of Insect Pests and Weeds" (P. DeBach and E. I Schlinger, eds), pp. 610-628. Chapman and Hall, London.

Hall, I. M. and Dunn, P. H. (1957). *Calif. Agric.* **11,** 5 and 14.

Hall, I. M. and Dunn, P. H. (1958). *J. econ. Ent.* **51,** 341-344.

Harvey, T. L. and Howell, D. E. (1965). *J. Invertebrate Path.* **7,** 92-100.

Ignoffo, C. M. (1967). *In* "Insect Pathology and Microbial Control" (P. A. van der Laan, ed.), pp. 91-117. North-Holland Publ. Co., Amsterdam.

MacLeod, D. M. (1963). *In* "Insect Pathology. An Advanced Treatise" (E. A. Steinhaus, ed.), Vol. 2, pp. 189-231. Academic Press, New York.

Muma, M. H. (1969). *Fla Ent.* **52,** 107-112.

Poinar, G. O. (1965). *Parasitology* **55,** 559-569.

Rivers, C. F. (1964a). *Entomophaga, Mém. hors Sér.* No. 2, 477-480.

Rivers, C. F. (1964b). *Discovery* **25,** 27-31.

Segre, B. (1969). "New Perspectives on the Control of Injurious Insects", No. 128, 276 pp. Accademia Nazionale dei Lincei, Rome.

Shands, W. A., Simpson, G. W. and Hall, I. M. (1963). *Maine Agric. Exp. Sta. Bull. T6* (Technical Series), 1-42.

Shands, W. A., Thompson, C. G., Simpson, G. W. and Wave, H. E. (1958). *J. econ. Ent.* **51,** 184-186.

Smith, R. F. (1969). *In* "New Perspectives on the Control of Injurious Insects" (B. Segre, ed.), No. 128, pp. 21-30. Accademia Nazionale dei Lincei, Rome.

Speare, A. T. and Colley, R. H. (1912). "The Artificial Use of the Brown-tail Fungus in Massachusetts, with Practical Suggestions for Private Experiment, and a Brief Note on a Fungous Disease of the Gypsy Caterpillar", 29 pp. Wright and Potter Printing Co., Boston.

Stairs, G. R. (1965). *Can. Ent.* **97,** 1059-1062.

Stairs, G. R. (1968). Proc. Joint U.S.-Japan Semin. Microbial Control Insect Pests. U.S.-Japan Committee Sci. Cooperation. Panel 8, pp. 19-23. Fukuoka, Japan.

Tanada, Y. (1968). Proc. Joint U.S.-Japan Semin. Microbial Control Insect Pests. U.S.-Japan Committee Sci. Cooperation. Panel 8, pp. 25-31. Fukuoka, Japan.

Ullyett, G. C. (1947). *Ent. Mem. Dep. Agric. Un. S. Afr.* **2,** 55-202.

Ullyett, G. C. and Schonken, D. B. (1940). *Un. S. Afr. Sci. Bull. Dep. Agr. Forestry* No. 218, 24 pp.

Vasiljević, L. (1964). *Entomophaga, Mém. hors Sér.* No. 2, 383-391.

Vasiljević, L. (1968). *Zašt. Bilja* **98,** 29-40.

Yen, D. F. (1960). *Pl. Prot. Bull.* **2,** 54-58.

Yen, D. F. (1962). *J. Insect Path.* **4,** 88-94.

APPENDIX 1

Key Publications

ALOYSIUS KRIEG

Biologische Bundesanstalt für Land- und Forstwirtschaft, Institut für biologische Schädlingsbekämpfung, Darmstadt, Germany

I. Text Books

Aoki, K. (1957). "Insect Pathology", 493 pp. Gihodo, Tokyo. (In Japanese.)

Collins, H. C. (1967). "Progress in Microbiological Techniques", 231 pp. Edition Plenum, New York.

De Bach, P. (1964). "Biological Control of Insect Pests and Weeds", 844 pp. Chapman and Hall, London.

Evlakhova, A. A., Shvetsova, O. I. and Shchepetil'nikova, V. A. (1961). "Biological Methods for Control of Harmful Insects", 96 pp. Gosudarstvennoe izdatel'stvo sel'skochozyaistvennoi literaturi, Leningrad. (In Russian.)

Franz, J. M. (1961). "Biologische Schädlingsbekämpfung". *In* "Handbuch der Pflanzenkrankheiten" (H. Richter, ed.), Vol. 6(3), 2nd edit., pp. 1-302. Verlag Parey, Berlin.

Krieg, A. (1961). "Grundlagen der Insektenpathologie. Viren-, Rickettsien- und Bakterien-Infektionen", 304 pp. Verlag Steinkopff, Darmstadt.

Lipa, J. J. (1967). "Introduction to Insect Pathology", 342 pp. Pański Wydawnictwo Rolnicze i Leśne, Warszawa. (In Polish.)

"Manual of Microbial Methods" (1957). (Soc. Am. Bacteriologists; Comm. Bacteriol. Techn. ed., 315 pp.) McGraw-Hill, New York.

Müller-Kögler, E. (1965). "Pilzkrankheiten bei Insekten. Anwendung zur biologischen Schädlingsbekämpfung und Grundlagen der Insektenmykologie", 444 pp. Verlag Parey, Berlin.

Poltev, V. I. (ed.) (1969). "Microflora of Insects", 271 pp. Izdatel'stvo Nauka, Sibirsk. Otd., Novosibirsk. (In Russian.)

Smith, K. M. (1967). "Insect Virology", 256 pp. Academic Press, New York.

Steinhaus, E. A. (1947). "Insect Microbiology", 763 pp. Comstock Publ. Co., Ithaca, New York.

Steinhaus, E. A. (1949). "Principles of Insect Pathology", 757 pp. McGraw-Hill, New York.

Steinhaus, E. A. (ed.) (1963). "Insect Pathology. An Advanced Treatise", Vol. 1, 661 pp., Vol. 2, 689 pp. Academic Press, New York.

Weiser, J. (1966). "Diseases of Insects", 554 pp. Academia Československ. Akad. VED, Prague. (In Czech.)

II. General Reviews

Cameron M. J. W. (1963). Factors affecting the use of microbial pathogens in insect control. *Ann. Rev. Ent.* 8, 265-286.

Dutky, S. R. (1959). Insect microbiology. *Adv. appl. Microbiol.* **1,** 175-200.
Franz, J. M. (1961). Biological control of pest insects in Europe. *Ann. Rev. Ent.* **6,** 183-200.
Franz, J. M. (1964). Microorganisms in the biological control of insects. *In* "Global Impacts of Applied Microbiology" (P. Starr, ed.), pp. 256-266. Almqvist and Wiksell, Stockholm.
Shvetsova, O. I., Evlakhova, A. A. and Orlovskaya, E. V. (1963). Insect diseases and their role in control of pests of the forest. *Ent. Obozr.* **42,** 5-10. (In Russian.)
Steinhaus, E. A. (1957). Microbial diseases of insects. *Ann. Rev. Microbiol.* **11,** 165-182.
Tanada, Y. (1967). Microbial pesticide. *In* "Pest Control. Biological, Physical and Selected Chemical Methods" (W. W. Kilgore and R. L. Doutt, eds), pp. 31-88. Academic Press, New York.
Telenga, N. A. and Sikura, A. I. (1968). "Combination of Biological and Chemical Preparations for Plant Protection". Vses. inst. nauchn.-techn. inform., sel'sk. choz.; Minist. sel'sk. choz. SSSR, *Obz. Lit.* (Moscow) **202,** 106. (In Russian.)

III. Reviews, Reports and Compilations of Special Topics

A. REVIEWS, REPORTS

Aizawa, K. (1967). Problems of microbial control in Japan. *Mushi, Fukuoka* **39** (Suppl.), 97-102.
Aizawa, K. and Nakasato, Y. (1963). Diagnosis of diseases in insects 1959-1962. *Mushi, Fukuoka* **37,** 155-158.
Baird, R. B. (1958). The artificial control of insects by means of entomogenous fungi. A compilation of references with abstracts (Mimeogr.), 53 pp. Ent. Lab., Belleville, Canada.
Benz, G. (1963). Arthropoden-Viren. *Vierteljahr.-schrift, Naturforsch. Ges., Zürich* **108,** 1-35.
Bergold, G. H. (1953). Insect viruses. *Adv. Virus Res.* **1,** 91-132.
Bergold, G. H. (1958). Viruses of insects. *In* "Handbuch der Virusforschung" (C. Hallauer and K. F. Meyer, eds), Vol. 4, pp. 60-142. Springer Verlag, Vienna.
Day, M. F. (1965). The use of pathogens in insect control. *Austr. J. Sci.* **28,** 241-243.
Evlakhova, A. A. and Shvetsova, O. I. (1965). "Diseases of Harmful Insects", 51 pp. Izdatel'stvo Kolos, Moscow. (In Russian.)
Franz, J. M. (1968). Zur Berechnung des Wirkungsgrades einer mikrobiologischen Bekämpfung von Schadinsekten. *Anz. Schädlingskunde* **41,** 65-71.
Heimpel, A. M. (1967). A critical review of *Bacillus thuringiensis* var. *thuringiensis* and other crystalliferous bacteria. *Ann. Rev. Ent.* **12,** 287-322.
Heimpel, A. M. and Angus, T. A. (1960). Bacterial insecticides. *Bact. Rev.* **24,** 266-288.
Krieg, A. (1961). "*Bacillus thuringiensis* Berliner. Uber seine Biologie, Pathogenie und Anwendung in der biologischen Schädlingsbekämpfung". *Mitt. biol. BundAnst. Ld–u. Forstw.* **103,** 1-79.
Kreig, A. (1967). "Neues über *Bacillus thuringiensis* und seine Anwendung". *Mitt. biol. BundAnst. Ld–u. Forstw.* **125,** 1-106.
Krieg, A. (1968). Uber die hygienische Bedeutung von insektenpathogenen Mikroorganismen zur biologischen Schädlingsbekämpfung. *Zentralbl. Bakt. Ref.* **214,** 501.
Lipa, J. J. (1963). Polish analytical bibliography of insect pathology. Part I. Diseases and microbial control of harmful insects. *Prace Nauk. Inst. Ochr. Rośl.* **5,** 3-101. (In Polish.)
Lüthy, P. (1968). "Untersuchungen an *Bacillus fribourgensis* Wille". *Zentralbl. Bakteriol.* II. **122,** 671-711.
Müller-Kögler, E. (1967). Nebenwirkungen insektenpathogener Pilze auf Mensch und Wirbeltiere: Aktuelle Fragen. *Entomophaga* **12,** 429-441.
Niklas, O. F. (1967). "Die Nematoden DD-136 (*Neoaplectana* sp.) und *Neoaplectana carpocapsae* Weiser, 1955 (Rhabditoidae als Insektenparasiten. Eine Literaturübersicht". *Mitt. biol. BundAnst. Ld–u. Forstw.* **124,** 1-40.

Rogoff, M. H. (1966). Crystal forming bacteria as insect pathogens. *In* "Advances in Applied Microbiology" (W. W. Umbreit, ed.), Vol. 8, pp. 291-313. Academic Press, New York.

Steinhaus, E. A. (1956). Microbial control–the emergence of an idea. *Hilgardia* **26,** 107-157.

Steinhaus, E. A. and Marsh, G. A. (1962). Report of diagnosis of diseased insects 1951-1961. *Hilgardia* **33,** 349-490.

Tanada, Y. (1956). An annotated list of infectious diseases of insects in Hawai. II. *Proc. Hawaiian Ent. Soc.* **16,** 149-155.

Weiser, J. (1961). "Die Mikrosporidien als Parasiten der Insekten". *Monogr. angew. Ent.* (W. Zwölfer, ed.), Vol. 17, 149 pp. Verlag Parey, Hamburg.

B. COMPILATIONS OF SPECIAL PAPERS

Gukasyan, A. B. (ed.) (1966). "Microorganisms for Control of Forest Pests", 258 pp. Izdatel'stvo Nauka, Moscow. (In Russian.)

Gukasyan, A. B. (ed.) (1967). "Crystalliferous Microorganisms and Perspectives for their Use against Forest Pests", 162 pp. Izdatel'stvo Nauka, Moscow. (In Russian.)

Maramorosch, K. (ed.) (1968). "Insect Viruses", 192 pp. Springer Verlag, Berlin.

Talalaev, E. V. (ed.) (1965). Use of microorganisms for controlling forest pests in East Siberia. *Isv. biol.-geogr. nauchn. issled. inst. Irkutsk gosudarst. univ. Irkutsk.* **19,** 1-100. (In Russian.)

Telenga, N. A., Shcherbinovskij, N. S. and Dyadechko, N. P. (eds) (1959). "Biological Method of Control of Plant Pests", 231 pp. Akad. Nauk Ukrain. SSR Kiew. (In Russian.)

Vasil'ev, V. P. *et al.* (eds) (1967). Problems of chemicobiological control of harmful insects. *Resp. Meshved. temat. nauchn. sb. Zashch. Izd. Rast. Urozhaj, Kiew.* **4,** 1-152. (In Russian.)

IV. Colloquia and Congresses

A. INTERNATIONAL CONFERENCES OF INSECT PATHOLOGY AND MICROBIAL CONTROL

Colloque international sur la pathologie des insectes et la lutte microbiologique. Paris 1962. *Entomophaga Mém. hors. Sér.* No. 2, 566 pp. (1964).

First annual meeting of *Soc. Invertebrate Path.* (with *Am. Inst. Biol. Sci.*). Columbus 1968.

International conference of biological control. *Rashch. Rast. Moscow* **11**(12), 51-53 (1966). (In Russian.)

Proc. Int. Colloq. "Insect Pathology and Microbial Control", (P. A. van der Laan, ed.), 360 pp. Wageningen 1966. North-Holland Publ. Co., Amsterdam (1967).

Proc. Joint U.S.-Japan Semin. Microbial Control of Insect Pests, 61 pp. U.S. Committee Sci. Cooperation. Panel 8. Fukuoka (1967).

Trans. "First International Conference of Insect Pathology and Biological Control", 653 pp. Prague 1958.

B. INTERNATIONAL SYMPOSIA ON STANDARDIZATION OF PREPARATIONS OF INSECT PATHOGENS

International Symposium on the identification and assay of viruses and *Bacillus thuringiensis.* London 1964. (C. Vago, H. D. Burges ref.) *J. Insect Path.* **6,** 544-547 (1964).

Symposia on the standardization of preparations of insect pathogens. Wageningen 1966. *In* "Insect Pathology and Microbial Control" (P. A. van der Laan, ed.), pp. 293-360. North-Holland Publ. Co., Amsterdam (1967).

C. SYMPOSIA OF "ORGANISATION INTERNATIONAL DE LUTTE BIOLOGIQUE" (O.I.L.B.)

Mémoires originaux présentés au "Colloque sur la pathologie des insectes". Paris 1958. *Entomophaga* **4,** 193-283 (1959).
Résolutions du Symposium sur le titrage des virus et champignons entomopathogènes. Paris 1966. *Entomophaga* **11,** 245-246 (1966).
Symposium der O.I.L.B. Uber "Prinzipielle Fragen zur Anwendung mikrobiologischer Präparate im Freiland". Darmstadt 1968. (E. Müller-Kögler ref.) *Nachrichtenbl. dtsch. Pflanzenschutzdienst* (Braunschweig) **20,** 76 (1968).
Symposium sur l'action de virus et champignons entomopathogènes sur les vertébrés. Zürich 1967. (B. Hurpin ref.) *Entomophaga* **12,** 321-323 (1967).
Symposium sur le titrage des préparations à base de *Bacillus thuringiensis.* Paris 1964. *Entomophaga* **9,** 127-129 (1964).
Symposium über Insektenpathologie in Darmstadt 1956 (J. Franz and E. Müller-Kögler, eds). *Entomophaga* **1,** 82-105 (1956).

D. SOME NATIONAL COLLOQUIA OR CONGRESSES OF INSECT PATHOLOGY AND/OR MICROBIAL CONTROL

"Biological Methods of Control in Agriculture, Forest and of Weeds". Trans. I. Int. H.S. Conf. Samarkand 1966 (M. A. Rish, ed.), 203 pp. Tashkent 1966. (In Russian.)
Conference on problems of use of microorganisms for control of insects. Moscow 1962 (V. P. Luk'yanchikov, ref.), *Mikrobiologiya* **31,** 956-957 (1962). (In Russian.)
Proc. "All-Union Conference of Agricultural Microbiology". Leningrad 1963. *Vses. nauchn.-issled. inst. sel'sk. mikrobiol. Leningrad* (1963) 247 pp. (In Russian.)
Report of second work conference on the utilization of nuclear-polyhedrosis virus for the control of *Heliothis* species. Mississippi State University 1967. (G. E. Allen, ref.) *Bull. ent. Soc. Am.* **13,** 234 (1967).
Report of work conference on the utilization of nucleopolyhedrosis virus for the control of *Heliothis zea.* Berkeley 1965 (L. A. Falcon, ref.). *Bull. ent. Soc. Am.* **11,** 84 (1965).
"Research on Methods of Biological Control of Agricultural and Forest Pests". Proc. Symp. Novosibirsk 1964 (A. I. Cherepanov, *et al.,* eds). *Akad. Nauk. SSSR, Sibirsk. Otd. Novosibirsk* (1964), Vol. 1, 224 pp. Novosibirsk (1965), Vol. 2, 157 pp. (In Russian.)
Séance sur le thème: "La lutte biologique". (Société Française de Phytiatrie et de Phytopharmacie. Versailles 1966.) *Phytiatrie-Phytopharmacie Paris* **16,** 63-123 (1967).
Symposium "Microbial Insecticides". (Ann. Meeting of *Am. Soc. Microbiol.*) Washington 1964. *Bact. Rev.* **29,** 364-405 (1965).
Techn. Rep., Conference Am. Inst. Biol. Sci. "Biological Control of Insects of Medical Importance", 144 pp. Washington (1960) (Mimeograph).

E. INTERNATIONAL CONGRESSES OF ENTOMOLOGY AND MICROBIOLOGY (WITH SPECIAL PAPERS ON INSECT PATHOLOGY AND/OR MICROBIAL CONTROL)

"XIII. Int. Congr. Ent. Abstr. Paper", 325 pp. Moscow 1968.
"IX. Int. Congr. Microbiol. Moscow 1966" (Abstr. Focal topic sessions–English edit.) (Section C4, p. 307-328). Moscow (1966).
"Proc. VII. Int. Congr. Ent. Lond. 1964" (Section 11, pp. 712-752.) London (1965).
"Proc. X. Int. Congr. Ent. Montreal 1956" (Section on Biological Control, Vol. 4, pp. 675-742). Montreal (1958).
"Recent Progress in Microbiology" (Symposia VIII. Int. Congr. Microbiol. Montreal 1962) (N. E. Gibbons, ed.) (Symposium III, pp. 131-182). Toronto (1963).
"Verh. XI. Int. Kongr. Ent. Wien 1960" (Sektion XIII, Vol. 2, pp. 669-882). Vienna (1962).

V. Special Lists of References

Bibliography on biological control (important chapters: 1. general papers, 4. fundamental research on micro-organisms as pathogens of arthropods, 5. application of microbial control of arthropods). (Documentation of O.I.L.B.[1]), J. M. Franz, ed.)

Part I: *Entomophaga* **1,** 107-112 (1956).
II: *Entomophaga* **2,** 293-311 (1957).
III: *Entomophaga* **3,** 333-364 (1958).
IV: *Entomophaga* **4,** 315-348 (1959).
V: *Entomophaga* **5,** 295-335 (1960).
VI: *Entomophaga* **6,** 277-329 (1961).
VII: *Entomophaga* **8,** 89-161 (1963).
VIII: *Entomophaga* **8,** 263-321 (1963).
IX: *Entomophaga* **9,** 311-389 (1964).
X: *Entomophaga* **11,** 11-113 (1966).
XI: *Entomophaga* **12,** 5-80 (1967).
XII: *Entomophaga* **13,** 3-87 (1968).
XIII: *Entomophaga* **14,** 5-116 (1969).

VI. Dictionaries and Directories

"Directory for Invertebrate Pathology" (Anonymous) (1970), 736 entries (Mimeogr.) Lab. Invertebrate Path. Dept. Zool. Ent. Ohio State Univ. Columbus, Ohio.

"Preliminary List for a Directory of Biological Control Workers". Simmonds, F. J. (without year), 69 pp. (Mimeogr.) Commonwealth Inst. Biol. Control Curepe, Trinidad.

Steinhaus, E. A. and Martignoni, M. E. (1967). "An Abridged Glossary of Terms Used in Invertebrate Pathology" (Mimeogr.), 22 pp. U.S.D.A. Forest Serv. Pacif. N. Forest, Range. Exp. Stn Portland, Ore.

[1] Organisation International de Lutte Biologique.

APPENDIX 2

Information Sources and Literature Searching in Biological Control

J. R. NORRIS

Shell Research Ltd., Milstead Laboratory of Chemical Enzymology, Sittingbourne, Kent, England

Biological control is a subject which attracts workers from many different disciplines. Literature sources are correspondingly diverse and the object of this appendix is to simplify the task of locating information relevant to biological control in the contemporary literature and to describe a literature search system based on computer scanning.

I. Sources of Information

Since 1956 the Journal, *Entomophaga,* has periodically published extensive classified bibliographies on biological control. The publications have been listed under a series of headings:

1. General papers on the total subject.
2. Fundamental research on the utilization of entomophagous arthropods (without taxonomy).
3. Application of biological control by means of entomophagous arthropods (including methods of checking efficiency).
4. Fundamental research on micro-organisms as pathogens of arthropods (without aiming at complete coverage of the specialized topic of diseases of honey-bees and silk-worms).
5. Application of microbial control of arthropods.
6. Work on enemies of arthropods (vertebrates, non-arthropod invertebrates, joint action of micro-organisms and metazoans).
7. Biological control of weeds.
8. Integrated control.
9. Autocidal control, including fundamental papers.

Changes in publication trends in these fields have been described by Rothman and Woodhead (1968). An analysis of a recent (1968) bibliography published in this series, reveals that 1370 papers of direct interest to workers in the biological control field were documented during a two year period in no less than 499 different publications. Of these, 332 were single papers published in minor publications of very limited circulation which cannot be regarded as major sources of information in this field. Table I gives a break-down of the distribution of papers among the journals represented. It is worth noting that 15% of all the papers appeared in three English language journals; *Academia, The Journal of Invertebrate Pathology* and the *Journal of Economic Entomology.* The inclusion of *Entomophaga* brings the total to almost 18%. Table II lists the journals which contained five or more relevant publications during the period covered.

TABLE I

The distribution of papers among source publications

No. of papers in source	No. of sources	No. of papers in source	No. of sources
1	332	9	4
2	67	10	4
3	21	11-20	9
4	23	21-30	4
5	12	31-40	4
6	9	41-50	0
7	6	51+	3
8	1		

TABLE II

Number of papers in specific journals

Journal	No. of papers
Academia, Prague	73
Journal of Invertebrate Pathology	71
Journal of Economic Entomology	66
Entomophaga	36
Dokladȳ Akademii nauk SSSR Novosibirsk	33
Proceedings of the First International Congress of Parasitology, Rome	32
Entomophaga, Mémoires hors Série	31
Canadian Entomologist	30
Annals of the Entomological Society of America	29
Zashchita rasteniĭ ot vrediteleĭ Moskva	29
Proceedings, F.A.O. Symposium on Integrated Pest Control, Rome	27
Mushi, Fukuoka Entomological Society	20
Journal of Sericultural Science, Japan	18
U.S.-Japan Committee on Science Co-operation Panel 8, Research Pesticides	18
Izvestiya Biologo-geograficheskogo nauchno-issledovatel'skogo instituta. Irkutsk	17
Izdatelstvo Nauka	15
Japanese Journal of Applied Entomology and Zoology	15
Bollettino di zoologia agraria e bachicoltura (Milano)	12
Pčelovodstvo	11
Zoolohichnyi zhurnal Ukrayiny	11
Bulletin of Apiculture	10
Dissertation Abstracts	10
Trudy Vsesoyuznogo nauchno-issledovatel'skogo instituta zashchity rasteniĭ	10
Zeitschrift für angewandte Entomologie	10
Annales de la Société entomologique de France	9
Hilgardia (America)	9
Journal of Animal Ecology	9
Nature	9
Medelingen Rijksfaculteit Landbouwwetenschappen	8

TABLE II—*continued*

Journal	No. of papers
Annales des épiphyties, Paris	7
Ekologia polska	7
Indian Journal of Entomology	7
Postepy nauki rolniczej (Warsaw)	7
Revista peruana de entomologia agricolá, Lima	7
Waldhygiene	7
Australian Journal of Science	6
Compte Rendu de l'Academie des Sciences, Paris	6
Journal of the Entomological Society of South Africa	6
Journal of Kansas Entomological Society	6
Mikrobiologiya	6
National Academy of Science, National Research Council Publication	6
Proceedings of the Hawaiian Entomological Society	6
Science	6
Technical Bulletin of the Commonwealth Institute of Biological Control	6
Agricultural Research Service, U.S. Department of Agriculture	5
Anzeiger für Schädlingskunde	5
Beiträge zur Entomologie, Berlin	5
Bollettino dell'Istituto di entomologia agraria e dell' Osservatorio di fitopathologia di Palermo	5
Bulletin of Entomological Research	5
Bulletin of the Entomological Society of America	5
Entomologicheskoe obozrenie	5
Kontyû (Tokyo) (Entomological Society of Japan)	5
Mosquito News	5
New Zealand Entomologist	5
Science Bulletin of the Faculty of Agriculture of Kyushu University	5
PANS, Pest Articles, News Summaries, Section A	5

II. Computer Techniques for Information Retrieval

With a subject in which the sources of information are so diverse the use of computer search techniques can be a most valuable asset in keeping abreast of the literature. The technique of most value for this kind of work is the selective dissemination of information method by which a computer matches a set of key words, including synonyms, associated key words, author names and key references, represented in an interest profile constructed by an individual worker for a specific purpose, with the words occurring in literature references. Three such systems, operated on a commercial basis, are particularly important to workers in the biological field. The Biosciences Information Service of Biological Abstracts, Philadelphia, cover the semi-monthly issues of Biological Abstracts and the monthly Bioresearch index. The C.B.A.C. (Chemical Biological Activities) service operated by the Chemical Abstracts Service of Columbus, Ohio, covers specifically literature dealing with the interaction of chemicals and biological systems. The A.S.C.A. (Automatic Subject Citation Alert) service provided by the Institute of Scientific Information, Philadelphia, provides complete coverage of some 1600 scientific journals including all the major ones of interest to workers in the field of biological control. Table III illustrates a profile currently in use by the author for the A.S.C.A. system. Words may be listed as full words or phrases or as word stems. Thus the term POLYHED/ will pick up "polyhedrosis", "polyhedroses", "polyhedra", "polyhedral" etc. The computer will pick out any title containing any one

TABLE III

Example of a computer search profile (A.S.C.A.)

List 1 Single terms	List 2 Double terms	List 3 Double terms
THURINGIENSIS	CRYSTAL/	VIRUS
POLYHED/	INSECT/	VIRAL
GRANULOS/	CATERPILLAR/	INSECT
POPILLIAE	LEPIDOPT/	IRIDESCENT
LENTIMORBUS	HYMENOPT/	
CEREUS	LOOPER/	
PARASPOR/	MICROB/	
BEAUVERIA	BACT/	
MILKY DISEASE	MOTH	
B. LARVAE	MOTHS	
BIOLOGICAL CONTROL	TOXIN/	
MICROBIAL CONTROL	SPOR/	
INTEGRATED CONTROL	WORM/	

term from List 1 or any combination of two or more terms from either List 2 or 3.

The object of this particular profile is to scan the literature thoroughly for references concerned with *Bacillus thuringiensis* and to pick up major publications in the related fields of insect pathology and biological control. Obviously interest profiles will reflect in detail the particular sphere of interest of an individual worker. Figure 1 shows a typical page of print-out from this profile, from which it will be seen that 8 of 11 titles detected are relevant. A certain amount of irrelevant material is inevitable but a good profile will keep this to a minimum without jeopardizing the efficiency with which relevant literature is retrieved.

The construction of an effective search profile requires some experience and it is usual for the first attempts to be modified in the light of experience. Wishing to include the terms "MOTH" and "MOTHS" I decided that they could both be covered by the abbreviated word stem "MOTH/". I discovered that a remarkable number of papers are published weekly which contain the word "mother" in their titles.

A comprehensive account of data handling and information retrieval by computer, including a detailed description of the various systems for the selective dissemination of information is given by Dammers (1971). Details of systems commercially available can be obtained from Chemical Abstracts Service (American Chemical Society) Columbus, P.O. Box 1378, Ohio, 43216, U.S.A. and from the Institute for Scientific Information, 325 Chestnut Street, Philadelphia, Pa. 19106, U.S.A. Their economic and operational merits are still under debate. This is not surprising since we know so little about the true cost of keeping up with the current literature. However, the significant increase in the use of computers for literature searching, particularly during the past two years, indicates that the number of organizations which consider this approach to be of advantage is growing rapidly. Experience at Shell Research Ltd. to date suggests that the use of computer operated services becomes economic when the effort absorbed in current awareness activities exceeds 2% of one's working time.

References

Dammers, H. (1971). *In* "Methods in Microbiology" (J. R. Norris and D. W. Ribbons, eds), Academic Press, London.

Rothman, H. and Woodhead, M. (1968). *Nature, Lond.* **220,** 1053-1054.

a s c a

AUTOMATIC SUBJECT CITATION ALERT

A SERVICE OF

isi® **INSTITUTE FOR SCIENTIFIC INFORMATION**

325 Chestnut St Philadelphia Pa 19106 USA

```
        DR. J.R. NORRIS                              Z2170 ACCT NO
        SHELL RESEARCH LTD.                            191 $ UNITS USED
        MILSTEAD LAB.                                 0000 $ UNITS UNUSED

        SITTINGBOURNE, KENT, ENGLAND                         Z2170


       REPORT FOR  18 JUL 69                  PAGE  1

     439,395 INDEXING TERMS FROM CURRENT SCIENTIFIC
             LITERATURE WERE PROCESSED FOR ASCA THIS WEEK

             FLAHERTY DL   LYNN CD       JENSEN FL      LUVISI DA
( )             CALIF AGR       23    11 69       NO R     N4       D4063
    INTEGRATED     ECOLOGY AND INTEGRATED CONTROL OF SPIDER MITES
                   IN SAN JOAQUIN VINEYARDS

             AUDETLAP.P    VAUCLAIR R
( )             B CANCER        55   457 68    R   83R     N4       D5564
    GRANULOS/      (FR) GRANULOSA CELL TUMORS . A REVIEW OF
                   LITERATURE AND REPORT OF 7 CASES

             CRAGGS RF
( )             NOT AM MATH     16   688 69    M    1R     N4       D3758
    POLYHED/       EXTENDING HOMEOMORPHISMS BETWEEN APPROXIMATING
                   POLYHEDRA

             KAWASE S      MIYAJIMA S
( )             J INVER PAT     13   330 69        12R     N3       D5348
    POLYHED/       IMMUNOFLUORESCENCE STUDIES ON MULTIPLICATION OF
                   CYTOPLASMIC-POLYHEDROSIS VIRUS OF SILKWORM
                   BOMBYX MORI

             ARNOTT HJ     SMITH KM
( )             J INVER PAT     13   345 69         7R     N3       D5348
    GRANULOS/      ULTRASTRUCTURAL OBSERVATIONS ON BRANCHED RODS
                   ASSOCIATED WITH SOME INSECT GRANULOSES

             VAIL PV       HALL IM
( )             J INVER PAT     13   358 69        13R     N3       D5348
    POLYHED/       INFLUENCE OF INFECTIONS OF NUCLEAR-POLYHEDROSIS
                   VIRUS ON ADULT CABBAGE LOOPERS AND THEIR PROGENY

             TANADA Y      HUKUHARA T    CHANG GY
( )             J INVER PAT     13   394 69        12R     N3       D5348
    POLYHED/       A STRAIN OF NUCLEAR-POLYHEDROSIS VIRUS CAUSING
                   EXTENSIVE CELLULAR HYPERTROPHY

             PENDLETO.IR
( )             J INVER PAT     13   423 69        19R     N3       D5348
    CRYSTAL/       COMPARATIVE TOXICITIES OF CRYSTAL SEROTYPES OF
                   BACILLUS THURINGIENSIS FOR LARVAE OF PHILOSAMIA
                   CYNTHIA VAR RICINI

             DOUGHERT.EM   FAUST RM
( )             J INVER PAT     13   459 69    N    4R     N3       D5348
    POLYHED/       NUCLEIC ACID IN INTACT NUCLEAR POLYHEDRAL
                   BODIES ISOLATED FROM VIRUS-INFECTED FALL
                   ARMYWORM SPODOPTERA FRUGIPERDA

             COOKSEY KE    DONNINGE.C    NORRIS JR      SHANKLAN.D
( )             J INVER PAT     13   461 69    N    5R     N3       D5348
    THURINGIEN     NERVE-BLOCKING EFFECT OF BACILLUS THURINGIENSIS
                   PROTEIN TOXIN

             DERYCKE PH    VANGREMB.G
( )             Z PARASITEN     32   128 69         6R     N2       D4436
    GRANULOS/      STUDY ON RELATION BETWEEN OSMOTIC PRESSURE AND
                   EVAGINATION OF ECHINOCOCCUS GRANULOSUS

   ACCT NO Z2170
```

Fig. 1. A typical page of print-out corresponding to the profile in Table III.

APPENDIX 3

Information Services

THE LATE EDWARD STEINHAUS

Center for Pathobiology, University of California, Irvine, California, U.S.A.

One of the main goals of the recently formed Center for Pathobiology is to collect and to preserve all books, reprints, literature, letters, film, tapes, computerized programs etc., pertaining to pathobiology. This forms the basis of its information service, which is the principal area it implemented initially. The Center is able to help insect pathologists find specific reference material from the literature and will provide Xeroxed copies of virtually any article pertaining to insect disease without charge. Of course, the request must be reasonable and for articles not ordinarily readily available to the person making the request.

In addition to the scientific literature service the Center will furnish biographical summaries of insect pathologists willing to cooperate in this part of its endeavour.

APPENDIX 4

World Teaching Facilities in Insect Pathology

L. P. S. VAN DER GEEST and P. A. VAN DER LAAN

Laboratory of Applied Entomology, University of Amsterdam, The Netherlands

The information in this appendix was obtained by circulating a questionnaire among insect pathologists throughout the world. It indicates where lecture courses in insect pathology are being offered and degrees are awarded. The field of research work is also given if this information was available.

I. Austria

ZOOLOGISCHES INSTITUT, UNIVERSITÄTSPLATZ 2, GRAZ

Course: Insect pathology, in a general course on biological control
Degrees: M.Sc. and Ph.D.
Research: Pathogenicity of fungi.

HOCHSCHULE FÜR BODENKULTUR, VIENNA AND ZOOLOGISCHES INSTITUT DER UNIVERSITÄT, INNSBRUCK

Course: General insect pathology; application of pathogens in forest pests.
Degrees: M.Sc. and Ph.D.
Research: Microbial control.

II. Canada

DEPARTMENT OF BIOLOGICAL SCIENCES, SIMON FRASER UNIVERSITY, BURNABY 2, B.C.

Course: (Graduate level). Insect pathology, in a general pathology course. Biological control.
Degrees: M.Sc. and Ph.D.

DEPARTMENT OF ZOOLOGY, UNIVERSITY OF MANITOBA, WINNIPEG, MANITOBA

Degrees: M.Sc. and Ph.D.
Research: Protozoa and Nematoda. Post-doctoral training on entomophilic nematodes.

CANADA DEPARTMENT OF AGRICULTURE, RESEARCH INSTITUTE, 228 DUNDAS STREET EAST, BELLEVILLE, ONTARIO

Research: Thesis work for advanced degree taken at Canadian Universities possible. Post-doctoral training available, work on bacterial and viral pathogens.

DEPARTMENT OF ZOOLOGY, UNIVERSITY OF GUELPH, GUELPH, ONTARIO

Degrees: M.Sc. and Ph.D.
Research: Non-microbial pathology and endosymbioses. Facilities available for post-doctoral training.

CANADA DEPARTMENT OF AGRICULTURE, RESEARCH STATION, HARROW, ONTARIO

Research: Post-doctoral training on viral pathogens.

DEPARTMENT OF MICROBIOLOGY AND IMMUNOLOGY, QUEEN'S UNIVERSITY, KINGSTON, ONTARIO

Degrees: M.Sc. and Ph.D.
Research: Immune responses in insects, mechanisms of bacterial pathogenicity and insect viruses in tissue culture. Post-doctoral training available.

INSECT PATHOLOGY RESEARCH INSTITUTE, P.O. BOX 490, SAULT STE MARIE, ONTARIO

Research: Thesis work for advanced degree taken at Canadian Universities possible. Post-doctoral training. Work in all fields of invertebrate pathology.

DEPARTEMENT DE MICROBIOLOGIE ET IMMUNOLOGIE, UNIVERSITÉ DE MONTRÉAL, MONTRÉAL, QUEBEC

Course: Invertebrate virology, incorporated in a general virology course.
Degrees: M.Sc. and Ph.D.
Research: On viruses and bacteria. Post-doctoral training.

III. Republic of China

DEPARTMENT OF PLANT PATHOLOGY AND ENTOMOLOGY, NATIONAL TAIWAN UNIVERSITY, TAPEI, TAIWAN

Course: Principles of insect pathology (with laboratory exercises)
Degrees: M.Sc.
Research: Bacterial and fungal pathogens. Microbial control.

IV. Czechoslovakia

BIOLOGICKÝ ÚSTAV ČSAV, PATHOLOGIE HMYZU, NA CVIČIŠTI 2, PRAHA 6

Degrees: M.Sc. and Ph.D.
Research: Mainly on protozoan and fungal pathogens.

V. France

STATION DE RECHERCHES DE LUTTE BIOLOGIQUE ET DE BIOCÉNOTIQUE, LA MINIÈRE, 78 VERSAILLES

Research: Preparation of dissertation for Ph.D. degree taken at a University possible. Post-doctoral training. Work on most fields of insect pathology.

FACULTÉ DES SCIENCES, UNIVERSITÉ DE MONTPELLIER, MONTPELLIER (IN CONJUNCTION WITH STATION DE RECHERCHES CYTOPATHOLOGIQUES, 30-SAINT CHRISTOL-LES ALÈS)

Course: Invertebrate pathology covering physiopathology; viruses, bacteria, rickettsiae, fungi and protozoa; immunology, transmission and practical aspects.
Degrees: M.Sc. and Ph.D.
Research: On cytopathology. Post-doctoral training.

VI. Germany

TECHNISCHE HOCHSCHULE, DARMSTADT

Course: Principles of insect pathology.

VII. Hungary

NÖVÉNYNÉDELMI KUTATÓ INTÉZET, HERMAN OTTÓ ÙT 15, BUDAPEST

Research: Work for M.Sc. and Ph.D. theses possible in conjunction with University for Agriculture and University for Horticulture.

VIII. India

DIVISION OF ENTOMOLOGY, INDIAN AGRICULTURE RESEARCH INSTITUTE, NEW-DELHI-12

Course: Insect pathology incorporated in a parasitology course.
Degrees: M.Sc. and Ph.D.

PUNJAB AGRICULTURAL UNIVERSITY, LUDHIANA, PUNJAB

Course: General insect pathology.
Degrees: No M.Sc. and Ph.D. programmes.

IX. Israel

FACULTY OF AGRICULTURE, HEBREW UNIVERSITY OF JERUSALEM, REHOVOT

Courses: Insect pathology incorporated in courses on virology, mycology and biological control.
Degrees: M.Sc. and Ph.D.
Research: Insect virology and entomogenous fungi. Post-doctoral training.

X. Italy

INSTITUTO DI MICROBIOLOGIA AGRARIA E TECNICA, UNIVERSITA DI FIRENZE, FIRENZE

Course: Insect pathology incorporated in courses on forest and industrial microbiology.

XI. Japan

INSTITUTE OF BIOLOGICAL CONTROL, KYUSHU UNIVERSITY, FUKUOKA

Course: Insect microbiology
Degrees: M.Sc. and Ph.D.
Research: Spore-forming bacteria; microbial control. Post-doctoral training.

LABORATORY OF APPLIED MICROBIOLOGY AND SILKWORM PATHOLOGY, KYOTO UNIVERSITY OF INDUSTRIAL ARTS AND TEXTILE FIBERS, GOSYO-KAIDOCHY, SAKYO-KU, KYOTO

Courses: (undergraduate): Introduction to epizootiology and silkworm pathology. Silkworm pathology.
(graduate): Applied microbiology. Insect pathology.
Degrees: M.Sc.

NAGOYA UNIVERSITY, FURO-CHO, CHIKUSA-KU, NAGOYA

Courses: (undergraduate): General insect pathology.
(graduate): Insect pathology.
Degrees: M.Sc. and Ph.D.
Research: Insect virology. Post-doctoral training.

LABORATORY OF INSECT PATHOLOGY AND BIOLOGICAL CONTROL, DEPARTMENT OF PLANT PROTECTION, TOKYO, NOKO UNIVERSITY, FUCHU, TOKYO

Courses: (undergraduate): Insect pathology I and II. Biological control.
(graduate): Biological control.
Degrees: M.Sc.
Research: Fungi, viruses, Microbial control.

XII. Netherlands

LABORATORIUM VOOR TOEGEPASTE ENTOMOLOGIE, UNIVERSITEIT VAN AMSTERDAM, AMSTERDAM

Course: Insect pathology incorporated in a course on applied entomology.
Degrees: M.Sc. and Ph.D.
Research: Viral and bacterial pathogens. Post-doctoral training.

LABORATORIUM VOOR VIROLOGIE, LANDBOUWHOGESCHOOL, WAGENINGEN

Course: Insect virology incorporated in a general virology course (with laboratory periods).
Degrees: M.Sc. and Ph.D.
Research: Insect virology. Post-doctoral training.

XIII. New Zealand

MICROBIOLOGY DEPARTMENT, UNIVERSITY OF OTAGA, DUNEDIN

Degrees: M.Sc. and Ph.D.
Research: Insect virology.

XIV. Pakistan

ZOOLOGY DEPARTMENT, PANJAB UNIVERSITY, NEW CAMPUS, LAHORE

Course: General insect pathology. (In preparation.)
Degrees: M.Sc.
Research: Effect of radiation on pathogenicity of insect pathogens.

XV. Philippines

DEPARTMENT OF ENTOMOLOGY, UNIVERSITY OF THE PHILIPPINES, COLLEGE, LAGUNA

Course: Insect pathology and microbiology including biological relationships between micro-organisms and insects.
Degrees: M.Sc.
Research: Fungal and bacterial pathogens.

XVI. Poland

INSTYTUT OCHRONY ROSLIN, UL. GRUNWALDSKA 189, POZNAN

Degrees: M.Sc. and Ph.D.
Research: On most fields of insect pathology. Post-doctoral training.

XVII. Switzerland

VETERINÄR-MEDIZINISCHE FAKULTÄT, UNIVERSITY OF BERN, BERN

Course: (undergraduate): Bee pathology.

ENTOMOLOGISCHES INSTITUT, EIDG. TECHNISCHE HOCHSCHULE, UNIVERSITÄTSSTRASSE 2, ZÜRICH

Course: Principles of insect pathology.
Degrees: M.Sc. and Ph.D.
Research: Epizootiology; viral and bacterial pathogens.

XVIII. United Kingdom

DEPARTMENT OF ZOOLOGY AND APPLIED ENTOMOLOGY, IMPERIAL COLLEGE OF SCIENCE AND TECHNOLOGY, UNIVERSITY OF LONDON (FIELD STATION, SILWOOD PARK) ASCOT, BERKS

Course: Insect nematodes and protozoa, incorporated in courses on parasitology and nematology.
Degrees: M.Sc. and Ph.D.
Research: Insect nematodes and protozoa.

BEE DEPARTMENT, ROTHAMSTED EXPERIMENTAL STATION, HARPENDEN, HERTS

Research: Work for theses of M.Sc. and Ph.D. degrees taken at London University possible. Bee diseases.

SCHOOL OF AGRICULTURAL SCIENCES, UNIVERSITY, LEEDS 2

Course: (undergraduate): Microbial control incorporated in a course on biological control.
Degrees: M.Sc. and Ph.D.
Research: Mainly on bacterial pathogens.

GLASSHOUSE CROPS RESEARCH INSTITUTE, LITTLEHAMPTON

Degrees: M.Sc. and Ph.D. in association with a University.
Research: Diseases of glasshouse and mushroom pests.

DEPARTMENT OF PARASITOLOGY, NATIONAL INSTITUTE FOR MEDICAL RESEARCH, MILL HILL, LONDON N.W.7

Research: Work for theses of M.Sc. and Ph.D. at London University possible. Insect nematodes.

INSECT PATHOLOGY UNIT, UNIVERSITY OF OXFORD, OXFORD

Course: Invertebrate virology (with laboratory periods).
Degrees: M.Sc. and Ph.D.
Research: Insect virology. Post-doctoral training facilities available (limited).

BORDEN LABORATORY, BROAD OAK ROAD, SITTINGBOURNE, KENT

Research: Work for higher degrees taken at a University possible. *Bacillus thuringiensis.*

XIX. United States of America

DIVISION OF ENTOMOLOGY, UNIVERSITY OF CALIFORNIA, BERKELEY, CALIF. 94720

Courses: (undergraduate): Principles of insect pathology and insect microbiology (infectious and non-infectious diseases, diagnoses, therapy, microbial control).
(graduate): Advanced insect pathology (as above, more advanced, symptomatology, morphopathology, physiopathology and epizootiology. Biological control).
Degrees: M.Sc. and Ph.D.
Research: All fields of invertebrate pathology. Post-doctoral training.

CENTER OF PATHOBIOLOGY, UNIVERSITY OF CALIFORNIA, IRVINE, CALIF. 92664

Courses: Regular and computerized courses on invertebrate pathology.
Degrees: M.Sc. and Ph.D.
Research: All fields of invertebrate pathology. Post-doctoral training.

DEPARTMENT OF BIOLOGICAL CONTROL, UNIVERSITY OF CALIFORNIA, RIVERSIDE, CALIF. 92502

Courses: (undergraduate): Principles of insect pathology.
(graduate): Advanced insect pathology. Details as at Berkeley.
Degrees: M.Sc. and Ph.D.
Research: Mainly on bacterial and fungal pathogens.

BIOLOGICAL SCIENCES GROUP, MICROBIOLOGY SECTION, UNIVERSITY OF CONNECTICUT, STORRS, CONNECTICUT 06268

Courses: Biological control. Pathobiology of invertebrates.
Degrees: M.Sc. and Ph.D.
Research: Mainly on crystalliferous bacteria.

DEPARTMENT OF ENTOMOLOGY AND NEMATOLOGY, UNIVERSITY OF FLORIDA, GAINESVILLE, FLORIDA

Course: Biological control of insects.
Degrees: M.Sc. and Ph.D.
Research: In conjunction with U.S.D.A. laboratory in Gainesville: pathology studies with mosquitoes.

DEPARTMENT OF BIOLOGY, BALL STATE UNIVERSITY, MUNCIE, INDIANA 47306

Degrees: M.Sc. and Ph.D.

DEPARTMENT OF ENTOMOLOGY, PURDUE UNIVERSITY, LAFAYETTE, INDIANA 47907

Course: (graduate): Principles of insect pathology (research methods and considerations of cause, symptomatology and epizootiology of insect diseases; histo- and cytopathology).
Degrees: M.Sc. and Ph.D.
Research: Fungal and viral pathogens. Post-doctoral training.

DEPARTMENT OF ENTOMOLOGY, UNIVERSITY OF MARYLAND, COLLEGE PARK, MARYLAND

Course: (graduate): General insect pathology.
Degrees: M.Sc. and Ph.D.
Research: Most fields of invertebrate pathology.

DEPARTMENT OF ENTOMOLOGY, MISSISSIPPI STATE UNIVERSITY, STATE COLLEGE, MISSISSIPPI

Course: (undergraduate): Principles of insect pathology.
(graduate): Insect pathology.
Degrees: M.Sc. and Ph.D.
Research: In conjunction with U.S.D.A. Boll Weevil Research Laboratory. Post-doctoral training.

DEPARTMENT OF ENTOMOLOGY, FISHERIES AND WILDLIFE, UNIVERSITY OF MINNESOTA, ST. PAUL, MINNESOTA 55101

Course: (graduate): Insect microbiology (includes pathology and symbiosis).
Degrees: M.Sc. and Ph.D.
Research: Emphasis on physiology and microbe-insect relationships, especially of beneficial microbes. Post-doctoral training.

ENTOMOLOGY DEPARTMENT, UNIVERSITY OF NEBRASKA, LINCOLN, NEBRASKA 68503

Degrees: M.Sc. and Ph.D.
Research: Histopathology.

DEPARTMENT OF ENTOMOLOGY AND LIMNOLOGY, CORNELL UNIVERSITY, ITHACA, N.Y. 14850

Course: General insect pathology (viruses, rickettsiae, bacteria, spirochetes, fungi, protozoa, nematodes and selected arthropods).
Degrees: M.Sc. and Ph.D.
Research: Virus diseases of muscoid flies.

BOYCE THOMPSON INSTITUTE OF PLANT RESEARCH INC., 1086 NORTH BROADWAY, YONKERS, N.Y. 10701

Research: Work for theses of M.Sc. and Ph.D. degrees taken at local Universities possible. Fungal diseases of insects. Post-doctoral training.

DEPARTMENT OF ENTOMOLOGY, NEW YORK STATE AGRICULTURAL EXPERIMENT STATION, CORNELL UNIVERSITY, GENEVA, N.Y. 14456

Degrees: M.Sc. and Ph.D.
Research: Virus diseases of insects. Milky disease bacteria.

DEPARTMENT OF ENTOMOLOGY, NORTH CAROLINA STATE UNIVERSITY, RALEIGH, N.C. 27607

Course: Principles of insect pathology.
Degrees: M.Sc. and Ph.D.
Research: Mainly on protozoan diseases of insects.

DEPARTMENT OF ZOOLOGY AND ENTOMOLOGY, OHIO STATE UNIVERSITY, COLUMBUS, OHIO, 43210

Courses: Insect microbiology and pathology. Insect pathology. Biological control of invertebrates and weeds.
Degrees: M.Sc. and Ph.D.
Research: Most fields of invertebrate pathology. Post-doctoral training.

DEPARTMENT OF ENTOMOLOGY, OREGON STATE UNIVERSITY, CORVALLIS, OREGON 97330

Course: General insect pathology.
Degrees: M.Sc. and Ph.D.
Research: Most fields of invertebrate pathology, with emphasis on diseases of forest insects.

DEPARTMENT OF ENTOMOLOGY, PENNSYLVANIA STATE UNIVERSITY, UNIVERSITY PARK, PENN. 16802

Course: Insect pathology incorporated in a course on biological control.
Degrees: M.Sc. and Ph.D.
Research: Bacterial and fungal pathogens. Post-doctoral training.

DEPARTMENT OF ENTOMOLOGY, TEXAS A & M UNIVERSITY, COLLEGE STATION, TEXAS 77843

Degrees: M.Sc. and Ph.D.
Research: Insect virology.

DEPARTMENT OF ENTOMOLOGY, 237 RUSSELL LABORATORIES, UNIVERSITY OF WISCONSIN, MADISON, WISCONSIN 53706

Course: General insect pathology (with laboratory periods).
Degrees: M.Sc. and Ph.D.
Research: Most fields of insect pathology. Post-doctoral training.

APPENDIX 5

Insect Pathogens Available for Distribution

L. P. S. VAN DER GEEST and P. A. VAN DER LAAN

Laboratory of Applied Entomology, University of Amsterdam, The Netherlands

The data listed in Appendices 5 and 6 are composed of replies to a questionnaire which was circulated among insect pathologists throughout the world. The degree of completeness largely depends on the answers received. The numbers refer to the list of laboratories where the pathogens are available. This list is given at the end of Appendix 6. Scientific names are quoted as given in the replies (out of date insect names are placed in brackets).

I. Bacteria

Aerobacter aerogenes, 66, 73
A. cloacae, 66
Alcaligenes sp., 66
A. bookeri, 66, 69
A. faecalis, 66, 73
Bacillus alvei, 61, 66, 69, 79
B. amuscatoxicus, 78
B. bombycis, 66, 69
B. brevis, 66, 69
B. cereus, 14, 21, 66, 69, 73
B. cereus, var. *mycoides*, 15, 21, 66, 93
B. circulans, 69, 73
B. ephestiae, 66, 69
B. firmus, 66, 69
B. larvae, 12, 57, 79
B. laterosporus, 66, 69, 73
B. lentimorbus, 73, 74, 79
B. maceran, 69
B. medusa, 66, 69
B. megatherium, 15, 21, 66, 69, 73
B. popilliae, 69, 74, 79, 82
B. pumilus, 66, 69
B. sphaericus, 66, 69, 73
  var. *fusiformis*, 66
B. subtilis, 66, 69, 73
  var. *aterrimus*, 66, 73
  var. *niger*, 66, 73
B. thuringiensis var. *aizawai*, 21, 78
  var. *alesti*, 14, 66, 73, 78
  var. *anagastae*, 78
  var. *darmstadiensis*, 21
B. thuringiensis var. *dendrolimus*, 14, 21, 78
  var. *entomocidus*, 13, 14, 15, 66, 73, 78
  var. *finitimus fowleri*, 69, 78
  var. *galleriae*, 21, 73, 78
  var. *pacificus*, 78
  var. *sotto*, 13, 14, 15, 29, 32, 66, 69, 73, 78
  var. *subtoxicus*, 66, 69, 78
  var. *thuringiensis*, 13, 21, 66, 78
B. thuringiensis (serotype not specified), 1, 6 (20 strains), 13, 15, 19 (196 strains), 27, 29, 35, 45, 49, 56, 58 (several strains), 63 (150 strains), 64, 66, 69 (200 strains), 73, 76, 82, 90 (100 strains), 86
Bacterium imperiale, 66
Brevibacterium imperiale, 49, 69, 73
B. incertum, 49, 73
Erwinia amylovora, 73
E. carotovora, 73
Escherichia coli, 15, 66, 73
E. communior, 73
E. freundii, 73
Flavobacterium arborescens, 79
Micrococcus aquatilis, 79
M. muscae, 15, 69
M. pyogenes var. *albus*, 66, 69
Proteus sp., 66, 69
P. mirabilis, 73
Proteus sphingidis, 79
P. vulgaris, 66, 73

II. Fungi

Nectria aurantiicola, 39
N. coccophila, 36
N. laeticolor, 39
Nocardia corralina, 73
Oospora destructor, 29, 73
Paecilomyces baarnensis, 21, 36
P. coccus, 66
P. farinosus, 18, 21 (16 strains) 29, 32, 33, 34, 36 (7 isolates), 66, 73
P. fumuso-roseus, 18, 21, 29, 32, 34, 36 (7 isolates), 66, 73
P. heliothis, 21, 36
P. javanicus, 36
Penicillium chrysogenum, 73
P. thomic, 14
Scopulariopsis insectivora, 14
Sphaerostilbe aurantiicola, 36, 79
S. coccophila, 32
S. flammea, 75
Spicaria sp., 14, 66 (for *Spicaria* see also *Paecilomyces*)
S. prasina, 15, 29, 33, 34
S. rileyi, 18, 21, 36, 75, 88
S. rubido-purpurea, 28, 29, 32, 73
S. verticillata, 36
S. violacea, 14
Sporotrichum cejpii, 36
S. paranense, 36
Streptomyces aureofaciens, 73
Syngliocladium (Sorosporella) uvella, 36, 88
Verticillium spp., 26, 66
V. album minimum, 36
V. (Cephalosporium) aphidicola, 23, 36
V. aphidum, 36
V. coccidicolum, 36
V. coccorum, 36
V. lecanii (6 isolates), 36
V. longisporum, 36

III. Protozoa

Hosts from which the protozoan pathogens have been isolated are given where these were known to the authors.

Pathogen	Host
Adelina tribolii, 67	*Tribolium confusum*
Blastocrithidia culicis, 79	*Culex pipiens*
Crithidia fasciculata, 79	*C. pipiens*
C. oncopelti, 79	*Oncopeltus fasciatus*
Eugregarinae, 64	*Tenebrio obscurus*
Eugregarinae, 64	*Tribolium castaneum*
Eugregarinae, 64	*T. confusum*
Farinocystis tribolii, 64	*T. castaneum*
Glugea fumiferanae, 13	
G. gasti, 80	*Anthonomus grandis*
Gregarina polymorpha, 64	*Tenebrio molitor*
Lankesteria sp., 60	
Lymphotropha tribolii, 52	*Tribolium castaneum*
Mattesia sp., 67	*Ephestia (Cadra) cautella*
Mattesia sp., 67	*Carpophilus* sp.
Mattesia sp., 67	*Plodia interpunctella*
M. dispora, 21	*Ephestia (Anagasta) kuehniella*
M. grandis, 80	*Anthonomus grandis*
M. trogodermae, 52, 67	*Trogoderma* sp.
Microsporida, 8	*Archips cerasivorana*
Microsporida, 8	*Choristoneura fumiferana*
Microsporida, 83	*Muscoid flies*
Microsporida, 8	*Operophtera brumata*
Microsporida, 8	*Pristiphora erichsonii*
Microsporida, 8	*P. geniculata*
Nephridiophaga blatellae, 72	*Blatella germanica*
Nosema sp., 60	

Pathogen	Host
Nosema sp., 14	*Alsophila pometaria*
Nosema sp., 14	*Anacampsis innocullela*
Nosema sp., 14	*Anathrix puta*
Nosema sp., 72	*Anopheles quadrimaculatus*
Nosema sp., 14	*Archips cerasivorana*
Nosema sp., 67	*Ephestia (Cadra) figulilella*
Nosema sp., 67	*Carpophilus freemani*
Nosema sp., 67	*C. hemipterus*
Nosema sp., 33	*Dictyoploca japonica*
Nosema sp., 14	*Hyphantria cunea*
Nosema sp., 14	*Malacosoma disstria*
Nosema sp., 21	*Phaedon cochleariae*
Nosema sp., 14	*Phigalia titea*
Nosema sp., 33	*Vespa* sp.
N. apis, 12	
N. bombycis, 13, 34	*Bombyx mori*
N. carpocapsae, 21	*Cydia (Enarmonia) pomonella*
N. heliothidis, 72, 81	*Heliothis zea*
N. heliothidis, 81	*H. virescens*
N. plodiae, 67	*Plodia interpunctella*
N. pyraustae, 13	
N. tortricis, 21	*Tortrix viridana*
N. whitei, 52, 67	*Tribolium castaneum*
Octosporea viridanae, 21	*Tortrix viridana*
Perezia pyraustae, 76	*Ostrinia (Pyrausta) nubilalis*
Plistophora sp., 14	*Archips cerasivorana*
Plistophora sp., 72	*Culiseta inornata*
Plistophora sp., 60	
P. culicis, 52, 77	*Anopheles stephensi*
Sporomyxa tenebrionis, 21	*Tenebrio molitor*
Stempellia n.sp., 72	*Culex pilosus*
S. magna, 72	*C. restuans*
Thelohania sp., 72	*Aedes taeniorhynchus*
Thelohania sp., 77	*Culex peccator*
Thelohania sp., 72	*C. salinarius*
Thelohania sp., 41	*Mosquitoes*
Thelohania sp., 67	*Plodia interpunctella*
Thelohania sp., 14	*Pristiphora erichsonii*
Thelohania sp., 14	*P. geniculata*
Thelohania sp., 72	*Psorophora confinnis*
T. legeri, 72	*Anopheles quadrimaculatus*
T. minuta, 72	*Culex erraticus*
T. obesa, 72	*Anopheles crucians*
T. opacita, 77	*Culex salinarius*
T. opacita, 72	*C. territans*
T. weiseri, 21	*Tortrix viridana*

IV. Nematoda

Agamomermis culicis, 77
Bradynema sp. ex *Megaselia halterata*, 52
Contortylenchus sp. ex *Ips sexdentatus*, 52
Corethrellonema grandispicululosum, 77
Dirofilaria immitis, 59
Dirofilaria repens, 59
Gastromermis sp., 77
Mermithids in mosquitoes, 60
Neoaplectana carpocapsae (DD 136), 7
Romanomermis sp., 77

V. Rickettsia

Unnamed rickettsia from Carabidae, 89

VI. Viruses

A. NUCLEAR POLYHEDROSIS VIRUSES *(BORRELINAVIRUSES)*: HOSTS

Adoxophyes orana (reticulana), 35, 38
Aglais urticae, 14
Anthela varia, 1
Antheraea yamamai, 33
Anticarsia gemmatilis, 66
Arctia caja, 66
Autographa sp., 66
A. biloba, 66
A. brassicae, 73
A. californica, 66, 70, 78
Blepharomastix acutangualis, 66
Bombyx mori, 2, 13, 14, 27, 30, 31, 66, 78
Catabena esula, 66
Ceramica picta, 78
Choristoneura fumiferana, 13, 14, 78
C. rosaceana, 14
Chorizagrotis auxiliaris, 66
Colias sp., 14, 66
C. lesbia, 66
C. philodice eurytheme, 66
Coloradia pandora, 66
Danaus plexippus, 13
Dasychira plagiata, 66, 78
Dendrolimus undans flaveola, 33
Dictyoploca japonica, 33
Ephestia (Cadra) cautella, 67, 78
Epiphyas postvittana, 2, 78
Errannis tiliaria, 13, 14, 78
Euproctis phaeorrhoea, 18
Galleria mellonella, 13, 14, 27, 57, 66, 78
Heliothis sp., 66, 81, 93
H. armigera, 66
H. peltigera, 26
H. phloxophaga, 73
H. virescens, 66, 73, 78, 91
H. zea, 13, 18, 66, 69, 73, 78, 91, 93
Hemerocampa sp., 66
Hemerocampa (Orgyia) antiqua, 8
H. (O.) leucostigma, 13
H. (O.) pseudotsugata, 66
H. vetusta, 66
Hemileuca tricolor, 66
Hyphantria cunea, 14, 31, 32, 33, 73
Idaea seriata, 48
Inachis io, 14
Junonia sp., 66
J. coenia, 66
Kunugia yamadai, 33
Lambdina fiscellaria, 8, 13, 66
Leucoma (Stilpnotia) salicis, 4, 8, 66
Lymantria (Porthetria) dispar, 5, 14, 18, 22, 33, 66, 71, 73, 78
L. (P.) dispar japonica, 33
Malacosoma sp., 66
M. alpicola, 48
M. americanum, 8, 14, 71, 78
M. californicum, 66
M. disstria, 8, 13, 14, 66, 71, 78
M. fragile, 66, 71
M. neustria, 18, 78
M. neustria testacea, 31
M. pluviale, 14, 66
Mamestra brassicae, 14, 21, 31, 35, 37
M. illoba, 32
M. persicaria, 14
Megalopyge sp., 66
Mythrimna (Aletia) oxygala luteopallens, 14
Neophasia menapia, 13, 14
Nymphalis antiopa, 13, 14, 66
Operophtera bruceata, 8, 14
O. brumata, 8
Orthosia hibisci, 14
Pandemis lamprosana, 14
Peridroma sp., 66, 78
P. saucia, 66, 73
Phryganidia sp., 66
P. californica, 66
Pieris brassicae, 14
Plusia gamma, 18
Prodenia ornithogalli, 69, 78
P. praefica, 66, 73
P. terricola, 66
Pseudaletia sp., 66
Pseudaletia (Leucania) unipuncta, 13, 14, 66, 73, 78
Pterolocera amplicornis, 2, 66
Pygaera anastomosis, 14
Rachiplusia ou, 75
Sabulodes caberata, 66
Selidosema suavis, 66
Sibine stimulea, 78
Sparganothis pettitana, 14
Spodoptera sp., 66
S. exempta, 78
S. exigua, 66, 69, 73, 78
S. frugiperda, 66, 73, 78

Spodoptera littoralis, 26, 78
S. mauritia, 66
Tetratopha scorpealis, 66
Tinea pellionella, 14, 27, 67
Tineola bisselliella, 66
Tortrix viridana, 21
Trichiocampus viminalis, 14
Trichoplusia ni, 13, 66, 69, 70, 73, 75, 78, 81, 82
Vanessa cardui, 66

B. NUCLEAR POLYHEDROSIS VIRUSES *(BIRDIA VIRUSES)*: HOSTS

Diprion sp., 13
Gilpinia (Diprion) hercyniae, 8, 13, 14, 78
Neodiprion abietis, 8, 13
N. banksianae, 8
N. dyari, 78
N. lecontei, 13, 14, 71
Neodiprion nannulus, 8, 13, 14
N. pratti banksianae, 13, 78
N. pratti pratti, 71, 78
N. sertifer, 8, 13, 14, 46, 71, 78
N. swainei, 13, 14, 78
N. virginiana, 13, 14

C. CYTOPLASMIC POLYHEDROSIS VIRUSES *(SMITHIA VIRUSES)*: HOSTS

Agrotis segetum, 78
Alsophila pometaria, 8
Antheraea eucalypti, 2
A. pernyi, 78
Arctia caja, 78
Bombyx mori, 27, 30, 31 (hexahedron and icosahedron polyhedra), 66, 78
Ceramica picta, 78
Choristoneura fumiferana, 8, 13
Chorizagrotis auxiliaris 89
Cingilia canisaria, 8
Colias philodice eurytheme, 66, 78
Cydia (Carpocapsa, Enarmonia) pomonella, 18, 21, 48, 78
Dendrolimus sp., 15
D. spectabilis, 18, 31, 32, 33
D. superans, 33
Erannis tiliaria, 8
Estigmene acrea, 78
Galleria mellonella, 18
Gonepteryx rhamni, 78
Heliothis zea, 73
Hemerocampa leucostigma, 8, 14
Hyalophora cecropia, 14
Hyloicus pinastri, 78
Hyphantria cunea, 8, 31
Lacanobia (Diataraxia) oleracea, 14
Lasiocampa quercus, 78
Leucoma (Stilpnotia) salícis, 18
Lymantria (Porthetria) dispar japonica, 33
Lymantria fumida, 33
Malacosoma americanum, 8
M. californicum, 66
Mamestra brassicae, 18, 31
Mania maura, 21
Nymphalis antiopa, 8, 78
Operophtera brumata, 8
Paleacrita vernata, 8
Pectinophora gossypiella, 73, 78
Phalera bucephala, 78
Phlogophora meticulosa, 78
Polia oleracea, 18
Polygonia c-album, 78
Pseudaletia unipuncta, 78
Schizura concinna, 8
Sphinx ligustri, 78
Thaumetopoea pityocampa, 18
Trichoplusia ni, 78
Vanessa cardui, 8, 13

D. GRANULOSIS VIRUSES *(BERGOLDIA VIRUSES)*: HOSTS

Agrotis segetum, 78
Amelia pallorana, 66
Argyrotaenia velutinana, 78, 82
Autographa sp., 66
A. californica, 66
Chilo suppressalis, 27
Choristoneura fumiferana, 13, 14, 78
C. murinana, 13, 14
Chorizagrotis auxiliaris, 66, 78
Erinnyis alope, 66
Estigmene sp., 66
E. acrea, 66, 73, 78
Eucosma griseana, 66
Eulype hastata, 66
Euxoa ochrogaster, 66
Gryllus sp., 66
Harrisina brillians, 66
Heliothis sp., 66
Hyphantria cunea, 31
Junonia sp., 66

Junonia coenia, 66, 78
Lamprosema (Nacoleia) diemenalis, 66
Megalopyge sp., 66
Natada nararia, 66
Nephelodes emmedonia, 66, 78
Oryctes rhinoceros, 66
Peridroma sp., 66
P. saucia, 66, 73, 78
Phthorimaea operculella, 2
Pieris brassicae, 18, 37, 48, 66, 78
P. rapae, 2, 13, 18, 66, 75, 78, 82
P. rapae crucivora, 27
Plodia interpunctella, 66, 67, 78
Prodenia androgea, 66
Pseudaletia sp., 66
P. unipuncta, 66, 78
Recurvaria milleri, 66
Sabulodes sp., 66
S. caberata, 78
Sesamia cretica, 66
Spodoptera sp., 66
S. exigua, 66
S. frugiperda, 66, 73, 78
Trichoplusia ni, 66, 70, 73, 75, 78
Zeiraphera diniana, 14, 48, 66
Z. griseana, 18

E. CYTOPLASMIC SPINDLE INCLUSION VIRUSES *(VAGOIAVIRUSES)*: HOSTS

Aphodius tasmaniae, 2
Cossus cossus (mixed with nuclear polyhedrosis virus), 5
Melolontha melolontha, 18
Othnonius batesi, 2

F. IRIDESCENT VIRUSES: HOSTS

Chilo suppressalis, 2, 27
Mosquitoes, 72 (R and T strains), 77
Sericesthis sp., 2, 21, 73
Tipula paludosa, 13, 14, 27, 51, 66, 73, 93

G. OTHER VIRUSES

Acute bee paralysis virus, 57
AV-virus *(Pseudomoratorvirus ex Antheraea eucalypti)*, 2
Chronic bee paralysis virus, 57
Dense nucleus virus of *Galleria mellonella,* 57
Flacherie virus of *Bombyx mori,* 27, 30
Non-inclusion virus of *Pseudaletia* sp., 66
Sacbrood virus of honey-bee, 57, 66

Extensive collections of pathogens, including viruses, bacteria, rickettsiae, fungi and protozoans, are also maintained in other institutes from which no detailed lists were received. Exchange, however, of pathogens with these laboratories is possible, 14, 17, 20.

APPENDIX 6

Sources of Special Materials

L. P. S. VAN DER GEEST and P. A. VAN DER LAAN

Laboratory of Applied Entomology, University of Amsterdam, The Netherlands.

I. Insects and Ticks Available for Distribution

The numbers refer to the list of laboratories at the end of this appendix. A list of species held mainly by insect toxicological laboratories is given by the "Insect Toxicologists' Information Service" (F. J. Oppenoorth and N. W. H. Houx, eds, Laboratory for Research on Insecticides, Marijkeweg 22, Wageningen, The Netherlands.)

A. THYSANURA

Lepisma saccharina, 53
Thermobia domestica, 53

B. ORTHOPTERA

Acheta domesticus, 53, 65
Locusta migratoria, 18
Schistocerca gregaria, 18, 53

C. PHASMIDA

Carausius morosus, 53

D. DICTYOPTERA

Blaberus craniifer, 53, 65
Blatella germanica, 53, 64, 65
Blatta orientalis, 64, 65
Leucophaea maderae, 53
Periplaneta americana, 53, 64, 65
P. australasiae, 64
Pycnoscelus surinamensis, 65

E. HETEROPTERA

Dysdercus fasciatus, 53
Oncopeltus fasciatus, 53
Rhodnius prolixus, 59
Triatoma infestans, 53

F. LEPIDOPTERA

Achroia grisella, 64, 65
Acrolepia assectella, 18
Adoxophyes orana (reticulana), 35, 38
Aglais urticae, 18

Agrotis ipsilon (ypsilon), 18
Agrotis (Euxoa) segetum, 18
Antherea pernyi, 18, 53
Araschnia levana, 18
Arctia caja, 18
Argyrotaenia velutinana, 82
Autographa californica, 66
Bombyx mori, 13, 15, 18, 31
Chilo suppressalis, 15
Colias philodice eurytheme, 66
Corcyra cephalonica, 65
Cossus cossus, 18
Cydia (Carpocapsa) pomonella, 18, 22, 66
Earias insulana, 18
Ephestia (Cadra) cautella, 64, 65, 67
E. elutella, 64, 65, 67
E. (Cadra) figulilella, 67
E. (Anagasta) kuehniellc, 14, 18, 64, 65, 73
Estigmene acrea, 69
Feltia exclamationis, 18
Galleria mellonella, 13, 14, 18, 31, 64, 65, 66, 67, 73
Grapholitha molesta, 82
Heliothis virescens, 73
H. zea, 15, 66, 73
Hemerocampa pseudotsugata, 87
Hibernia defoliaria, 18
H. marginaria, 18
Hyphantria cunea, 31
Hyponomeuta cognatellus, 18
H. malinellus, 18
H. padellus, 18
H. vigintipunctatus, 18
Inachis io, 18
Leucoma (Stilpnotia) salicis, 18
Lymantria (Porthetria) dispar, 18, 71
Lymantria monacha, 18
Malacosoma neustria, 18
Mamestra brassicae, 18, 34
Manduca sexta, 53
Odoptera (Ennomos) subsignarius, 85
Operophtera brumata, 18
Orgyia antiqua, 18
Orthosia gothica, 18
Ostrinia (Pyrausta) nubilalis, 15, 22, 76
Paralipsa gularis, 64, 65
Paramyelois transitella, 67
Peridroma (Lycophotia) saucia, 18, 66
Phalera bucephala, 18
Philosamia cynthia ricini, 15
Phytometra gamma, 18
Pieris brassicae, 18, 35, 53, 54
P. coerulea c/a double recessive variety, 53
P. rapae, 10, 13
Plodia interpunctella, 64, 65, 67
Plutella maculipennis, 18
Pseudaletia (Cirphis) unipuncta, 18, 66
Pygaera anastomosis, 18
Pyralis farinalis, 64
Samia (Platysamia) cynthia, 18
Saturnia pavonia, 18
S. pyri, 18
Sesamia nonagrioides, 18
Smerinthus (Sphinx) ocellata, 18
Spodoptera exigua, 66, 73
S. (Prodenia) litura, 15
Thaumetopoea pityocampa, 18
T. processionea, 18
Tinea columberiella, 64, 65
T. flavescentella, 64
T. pellionella, 65
Tineola bisselliella, 64, 65, 67, 73
Tortrix viridana, 18
Trichoplusia ni, 9, 69, 73, 82
Triphaena pronuba, 18
Zeiraphera griseana, 18

G. DIPTERA

Aedes aegypti, 59
Calliphora erythrocephala, 53, 64
Culex pipiens fatigans, 59, 73
Drosophila melanogaster, 48, 67
Microphthalma europaea, 18
Microphthalma numidica[1], 18
Musca domestica, 64, 73
M. vicina, 64
Sarcophaga argyrostoma (barbata), 53
Tipula oleraceae, 51

H. HYMENOPTERA

Athalia rosae (colibri), 18
Bracon hebetor, 64
Choristoneura fumiferana, 13
Diprion pini, 14, 18
Monomorium pharaonis, 64
Neodiprion sertifer, 71

---

[1] Undescribed species identified by L. P. Mesnil, C.I.B.C., Delemont, Switzerland.

I. COLEOPTERA

Trogoderma inclusum, 64, 65, 67
T. irroratum, 64
T. ornatum, 65, 67
T. variabile (parabile), 64, 67
T. simplex, 64, 67
Trododerma sternale, 64, 65, 67
T. sternale plagifer, 64
Typhaea stercorea, 64
Urophorus humeralis, 67
Zabrotes subfasciatus, 64

J. ACARINA (MITES AND TICKS)

Rhipicephalus appendiculatus, 55

II. Antisera Available for Distribution

For *Bacillus thuringiensis* crystal proteins, 19 (10 serotypes), 56 (12 serotypes), 63
Specific H antisera for *B. thuringiensis*, 63
For cytoplasmic polyhedrosis virus of *Bombyx mori*, strain forming hexahedron polyhedra, 30, strain forming icosahedron polyhedra, 30
For mosquito pathogens, 72
For Tipula Iridescent Virus, 62

III. Mass Cultures of Pathogens

Beauveria bassiana, 3
Metarrhizium anisopliae, 3
Isaria sp. 3

IV. Commercial Products, including Information and References

by P. Grison

Pathogen		Product	Country	Supplier	Notes
Bacillus popilliae		Doom	U.S.A.	Fairfax	a,b,c,d
		Japidemic	U.S.A.	Ditman Corp.	e.b.d
Bacillus thuringiensis serotypes	I	Biotrol	U.S.A.	Nutrilite	a,b,f
	I,III,V	Thuricide	U.S.A.	I.M.C.	a,b,g,h
	III	Dipel	U.S.A.	Abbott	a,b,i,j
	I	Bakthane	U.S.A.	Rohm and Haas	e,b
	I	Agritrol	U.S.A.	Merck	e,b,k
	I	Parasporine	U.S.A.	Grain Proc.	e,b
	I	Biospor	Germany	Hoechst	e,b,l
	?	Sporeine	France	L.I.B.E.C.	e,b,d
	I	Bactospeine	France	Roger Bellon; Péchiney Progil	e,b,d
	I	Bactospeine	France	Roger Bellon; Rhône Poulenc	a,b,d,m
	I	Plantibac	France	Procida	e,b,d
	I	Baktukal	Jugoslavia	Serum Zavod Kalinovica	a,n
	I	Bathurin	Czechoslovakia	Spolana n.p., Neratovice	a,o
	V	Entobacterin 3	U.S.S.R.	Near Moscow	a,b,g,p
	IV	Dendrobacillin	U.S.S.R.	At Novosibirsk	a,b,q,r

Pathogen	Product	Country	Supplier	Notes
Beauveria	—	U.S.A.	Nutrilite	i,b,e,f
bassiana	Beauverin	U.S.S.R.	At Krasnodar	a,b,d
Metarrhizium anisopliae		U.S.A.	Nutrilite	i,b,e,f
Nuclear polyhedrosis	*Heliothis*	U.S.A.	Nutrilite; I.M.C.; Hays-Sammons	i,b,f,h,s
viruses	*Prodenia*	U.S.A.	Nutrilite; I.M.C.	i,b,f,h
	Spodoptera	U.S.A.	Nutrilite; I.M.C.	i,b,f,h
	Trichoplusia	U.S.A.	Nutrilite; I.M.C. Biol. Control Sup.	i,b,f,h,t
	Neodiprion	U.S.A.	Indiana Farm Bur. Co-op. Assoc.	i,b,u
Neoaplectana carpocapsae	Nematode	U.S.A.	Nutrilite	i,g,f

a. On sale. b. Powder. c. Fairfax Biological Laboratory, Clinton Corners, New York. d. Information from Grison. e. Not on sale now. f. Address No. 69. g. Stabilized liquid. h. Address No. 73. i. Experimental. j. Amdal Division, Abbott Laboratories, North Chicago. k. Briggs, J. D. (1963). *Proc. North Central Br. Ent. Soc. Am.* p. 1718. l. Krieg, A. (1967). *Mitt. biol. BundAnst. Ld-u. Forstw.* No. 125, 106 pp. m. Société des Usines Chimique, Rhône Poulenc, 22, Ave Montaigne, Paris 8. n. Vasiljević (oral communication to Grison). o. Weiser (personal communication to Grison). p. Evlakhova, A. A. and Schvetsova, O. I. (1963). *Acad. Sci. U.S.S.R., Moscow,* 24-34; Leskova, A. J. (1961). *Bull. V.I.Z.R.* No. 3-4, 50-53. q Talalaev, E. V. (1965). *Novosibirsk,* Nov. 1964, 19-20. r. Gukasian, A. B. (1961). *Izvestia Akad. Nauk, U.S.S.R. Biological Series* No. 5, pp. 785-797. s. Hays-Sammons, Mission, Texas, U.S.A. t. Biological Control Supplies, Phoenix, Arizona, U.S.A. u. Indiana Farm Bureau Cooperative Association, 47 South Pennsylvania, Indianapolis 9, Indiana, U.S.A.

V. Standard Preparations of Pathogens

A. FOR *BACILLUS THURINGIENSIS*

E_{61}, international standard for spore-crystal complex, 19
Standard preparations of all known serotypes, 19
Standard preparations used in industry, 69, 73
TTB 174, standard used for thermostable exotoxin, 19
Pure thermostable exotoxin, 63

B. FOR VIRUSES

Standard preparation of nuclear polyhedrosis virus of *Heliothis zea,* 73

VI. Insects for Standardization

A. FOR SPORE-CRYSTAL COMPLEX OF *BACILLUS THURINGIENSIS*

Estigmene acrea, 69
Pieris brassicae, 18
Trichoplusia ni, 69, 73

B. FOR THERMOSTABLE EXOTOXIN OF *B. THURINGIENSIS*

Drosophila melanogaster (LC_{50} = 0.2 p.p.m.), 48

VII. Diagnostic Services

66, 78, 87

VIII. Reference Collections of Identified Material

These collections are not for supply: they can be examined at the centre holding them.

Preparations of mosquito pathogens (protozoans, viruses and fungi), 72

Microscopical and histological preparations of most diseases known to occur in invertebrates (about 5000 preparations), 20

Tumors in lower animals, 92

World Health Organisation, International Reference Center for Diagnosis of Diseased Vectors, 86

Specimens and slides of diseased arthropods and of pathogens. Xeroxed information materials, photographs etc. collected from all over the world can be supplied. This centre is eager to receive material to add to this collection, 68

IX. Laboratories Willing to Supply Items Listed in Appendices 5 and 6

1. Australia: Entomology Laboratories, Department of Primary Industries, Meirs Road, Indooroopilly, Brisbane, Queensland (4068).
2. Australia: CSIRO, Division of Entomology, P.O. Box 109, Canberra City.
3. Austria: Zoologisches Institut, Universitätsplatz 2, Graz.
4. Belgium: Centrum voor Bosbiologisch Onderzoek, Bokrijk-Genk.
5. Bulgaria: Plant Protection Institute, Kostinbrod, Sofia.
6. Canada: Forest Research Laboratory, 506 West Burnside Road, Victoria, B.C.
7. Canada: Department of Zoology, Faculty of Arts and Science, University of Manitoba, Winnipeg, Manitoba.
8. Canada: Department of Forestry and Rural Development, Forest Research Laboratories, P.O. Box 4000, Fredericton, N.B.
9. Canada: Department of Zoology, University of Guelph, Guelph, Ontario.
10. Canada: Canada Department of Agriculture, Research Station, Harrow, Ontario.
11. Canada: Department of Microbiology and Immunology, Queen's University, Kingston, Ontario.
12. Canada: Apiculture Section, Entomology Research Institute, Research Branch, Canada Department of Agriculture, Central Experimental Farm, Ottawa, Ontario.
13. Canada: Insect Pathology Research Institute, P.O. Box 490, Sault Ste. Marie, Ontario.
14. Canada: Forestry Research Laboratory, Canada Department of Forestry, P.O. Box 3800, 1080 Route du Vallon, Ste. Foy, Quebec 10.
15. China: Laboratory of Insect Pathology, Department of Plant Pathology and Entomology, National Taiwan University, Taipei, Taiwan.
16. Czechoslovakia: Hodonin, Delnicka 18.
17. Czechoslovakia: Biologický Ústav ČSAV, Pathologie Hmyzu, Praha 6, Elemingovo náměsti 2.
18. France: Station de Recherches de Lutte Biologique et de Biocoenotique, I.N.R.A., La Minière, 78 Versailles.
19. France: Laboratoire de Lutte Biologique, Centre d'Identification de *Bacillus thuringiensis,* Institut Pasteur, 25 Rue du Docteur Roux, Paris XVe.

20. France: Station de Recherches Cytopathologique, I.N.R.A., 30 Saint-Christol-Les-Alès.
21. Germany (West): Biologische Bundesanstalt für Land- und Forstwirtschaft, Institut für biologische Schädlingsbekämpfung, Kranichsteinerstrasse 81, Darmstadt.
22. Hungary: Növényvédelmi Kuatató *Intezet,* Herman Otto Ut 15, Budapest 11.
23. India: Commonwealth Institute of Biological Control, Indian Road, P.O. Box 1503, Bangalore.
24. India: Plant Pathology Section, University of Agricultural Sciences, Hebbal, Bangalore.
25. India: Research Department, Hindustan Antibiotics Ltd., Pimpri, Poona.
26. Israel: Faculty of Agriculture, Hebrew University of Jerusalem, Rehovot.
27. Japan: Institute of Biological Control, Faculty of Agriculture, Kyushu University, Fukuoka.
28. Japan: Mito Tobacco Experiment Station, Suifumura, Kujigun, Ibaragiken.
29. Japan: Laboratory of Applied Microbiology and Silkworm Pathology, Kyoto University of Industrial Arts and Textile Fibres, Gosyo-Kaidochyo, Sakyo-ku, Kyoto.
30. Japan: Sericultural Laboratory, Faculty of Agriculture, Nagoya University, Furo-Cho, Chikusa-Ku, Nagoya.
31. Japan: Laboratory of Sericulture, Faculty of Agriculture, University of Tokyo, Bunkyo-ku, Tokyo.
32. Japan: Laboratory of Insect Pathology and Biological Control, Department of Plant Protection, Tokyo Noko University, Fuchu, Tokyo.
33. Japan: Laboratory of Insect Pathology, Asakawa Forest, Government Forest Experiment Station, Nagafusacho 1833, Hachioji, Tokyo.
34. Japan: Sericultural Experiment Station, Ministry of Agriculture and Forestry, Suginami-ku, Tokyo.
35. Netherlands: Laboratorium voor Toegepaste Entomologie, Universiteit van Amsterdam, Linnaeusstraat 2 B, Amsterdam-O.
36. Netherlands: Centraal Bureau voor Schimmelcultures, Baarn.
37. Netherlands: Laboratorium voor Virologie, Landbouwhogeschool, Binnenhaven 11, Wageningen.
38. Netherlands: Proefstation voor de Fruitteelt in de volle Grond, Kerkstraat 45, Wilhelminadorp.
39. New Zealand: Plant Disease Division, D.S.I.R., Private Bag, Auckland.
40. New Zealand: D.S.I.R., Entomology Division, Private Bag, Christchurch.
41. New Zealand: Department of Microbiology, Medical School, University of Otaga, Dunedin.
42. New Zealand: Department of Botany and Zoology, Massey University, Palmerston North.
43. New Zealand: Plant Diseases Division, D.S.I.R., Palmerston North.
44. Pakistan: Zoology Department, Panjab University, New Campus, Lahore.
45. Philippines: Central Experiment Station, College of Agriculture, University of the Philippines, College, Laguna.
46. Poland: Instytut Badawczy Leśnictwa, Wery Kostrzewy 3, Warsawa.
47. Sweden: Department of Forest Entomology, Royal College of Forestry, Stockholm 50.
48. Switzerland: Entomologisches Institut, Eidg. Technische Hochschule, Universitätstrasse 2, Zürich.
49. U.K.: National Collection of Industrial Bacteria, Torry Research Station, P.O. Box 31, Aberdeen, AB9 8DG.
50. U.K.: Sirex Biological Control Unit, Silwood Park, Sunninghill, Ascot, Berks.
51. U.K.: Department of Bacteriology, West of Scotland Agricultural College, Auchincruive, Ayr.
52. U.K.: Department of Zoology and Applied Entomology Field Station, Imperial College of Science and Technology, Silwood Park, Ascot, Berks.
53. U.K.: Department of Zoology, University of Cambridge, Downing Street, Cambridge.
54. U.K.: G.C.R.I. Insect Virus Group, University Farm Road, Huntingdon Road, Cambridge CB3 0DJ.
55. U.K.: Institute for Research on Animal Diseases, Compton, Near Newbury, Berkshire.

56. U.K.: Microbiology Department, Anderson College, University of Glasgow, 56 Dumbarton Road, Glasgow, W.1.
57. U.K.: Bee Department, Rothamsted Experimental Station, Harpenden, Herts.
58. U.K.: Department of Entomology, The University, Leeds 2.
59. U.K.: School of Tropical Medicine, Pembroke Place, Liverpool 3.
60. U.K.: London School of Hygiene and Tropical Medicine, University of London, Keppel Street (Gower Street), London, W.C.1.
61. U.K.: National Collection of Type Cultures, Central Public Health Laboratory, Colindale Avenue, London, N.W.9.
62. U.K.: Insect Pathology Unit, Commonwealth Forestry Institute, University of Oxford, South Parks Road, Oxford.
63. U.K.: Milstead Laboratory of Chemical Enzymology, Broad Oak Road, Sittingbourne, Kent.
64. U.K.: Pest Infestation Control Laboratory, Ministry of Agriculture, Fisheries and Food, London Road, Slough, Bucks.
65. U.K.: Infestation Control Laboratory, Government Buildings, Block B, Tolworth, Surbiton, Surrey.
66. U.S.A.: Department of Entomology and Parasitology, Division of Entomology, University of California, Berkeley, California 94720.
67. U.S.A.: U.S.D.A., Agricultural Research Service, Market Quality Research Division, Stored Product Insects Research Laboratory, Fresno, California 93727.
68. U.S.A.: Center for Pathobiology, University of California, Irvine, California 92664.
69. U.S.A.: Nutrilite Products, Inc., P.O. Box 98, Lakeview, California 92353.
70. U.S.A.: U.S.D.A., Agricultural Research Service, Entomology Research Division, P.O. Box 112, Riverside, California 92502.
71. U.S.A.: U.S.D.A., Forest Service, Northeastern Forest Experiment Station, Forest Insect and Disease Laboratory, Hamden, Connecticut 06541.
72. U.S.A.: U.S.D.A., Agricultural Research Service, Entomology Research Division, P.O. Box 1268, Gainesville, Florida 32601.
73. U.S.A.: International Minerals and Chemical Corporation, Growth Sciences Center, Libertyville, Illinois 60048.
74. U.S.A.: Agricultural Research Service Collection, U.S.D.A., Northern Utilization Research and Development Division, Peoria, Illinois 61604.
75. U.S.A.: Department of Entomology, Purdue University, Lafayette, Indiana 47907.
76. U.S.A.: U.S.D.A., Agricultural Research Service, Corn Borer Investigations, Ankeny, Iowa 50021.
77. U.S.A.: U.S.D.A., Agricultural Research Division Temporary Building "A", Moneese State College, Lake Charles, Louisiana 70601.
78. U.S.A.: U.S.D.A., Agricultural Research Service, Entomology Research Division, Insect Pathology Pioneering Laboratory, Beltsville, Maryland 20705.
79. U.S.A.: American Type Culture Collection, 12301 Parklawn Drive, Rockville, Maryland 20852.
80. U.S.A.: U.S.D.A., Agricultural Research Service, Boll Weevil Research Laboratory, P.O. Box 5367, State College, Mississippi 39762.
81. U.S.A.: Insect Pathology Laboratory, Mississippi State University, State College, Mississippi 39762.
82. U.S.A.: Department of Entomology, New York State Agricultural Experiment Station, Geneva, New York 14456.
83. U.S.A.: Department of Entomology and Limnology, New York State College of Agriculture, Cornell University, Ithaca, New York 14850.
84. U.S.A.: Boyce Thompson Institute for Plant Research, Inc. 1086 North Broadway, Yonkers, New York 10701.
85. U.S.A.: U.S.D.A., Southeastern Forest Experiment Station, P.O. Box 12254, Research Triangle Park, N.C. 27709.
86. U.S.A.: Department of Zoology and Entomology, 1735 Neil Avenue, Ohio State University, Columbus, Ohio 43210.

87. U.S.A.: U.S.D.A., Pacific Northwest Forest and Range Experiment Station, Forestry Sciences Laboratory, 3200 Jefferson Way, Corvallis, Oregon, 97331.
88. U.S.A.: U.S.D.A., Agricultural Research Service, Entomology Research Division, P.O. Box 3187, Charleston, South Carolina 29407.
89. U.S.A.: U.S.D.A., Agricultural Research Service, Northern Grain Insects Research Laboratory, Entomology and Crops Research Division, Brookings, South Dakota, 57006.
90. U.S.A.: U.S.D.A., Agricultural Research Service, Entomology Research Division, P.O. Box 1033, Brownsville, Texas 78520.
91. U.S.A.: College of Agriculture, Texas A & M University, College Station, Texas 77843.
92. U.S.A.: Museum of Natural History, Smithsonian Institute, Washington, D.C., 20560.
93. U.S.A.: Department of Agriculture, University of Wisconsin, 237 Russell Laboratories, 1630 Linden Drive, Madison, Wisconsin, 53706.
94. Western Samoa: UN-SPC Rhinoceros Beetle Project, P.O. Box 597, Appia.

APPENDIX 7

A Bibliography on Diseases and Enemies of Medically Important Arthropods 1963-67 With Some Earlier Titles Omitted from Jenkins' 1964 List

MARSHALL LAIRD

Memorial University of Newfoundland,
St. John's, Newfoundland, Canada

This bibliography is subdivided into two sections, the first comprising references overlooked by Jenkins (1964) in his 1973-article list of the relevant literature up to 1962, and the second covering the ensuing five-year period 1963-67 inclusive (larvivorous fish, an annotated bibliography on which appeared recently–Gerberich and Laird, 1966–are not considered).

I. Titles Not Cited by Jenkins (1964), Up to the End of 1962

Abbassian-Lintzen, R. (1962). Tabanidae (Diptera) of Iran: VIII. A collection of horseflies from the Province of Fars (Southern Iran). *Bull. Soc. Path. exot.* **55**, 443-456. (Tabanids are preyed upon by certain sphecoid wasps, Oxybelidae.)

Abe, Y. (1947). On the habits of *Culex vorax* Edwards. *Seibutsukai* **1**, 22-26. (In Japanese.) (Larvae predacious on those of other mosquitoes.)

Adler, S. and Mayrink, W. (1961). A gregarine *Monocystis chagasi* n.sp. of *Phlebotomus longipalpis*. Remarks on the accessory glands of *P. longipalpis*. *Rev. Inst. Med. Trop. São Paulo* **3**, 230-238.

Akatov, V. A. (1955). On the duration of the preservation of trichomonads in the domestic fly. *Veterinariia, Moscow* **32**, 84. (In Russian.)

Akopyan, M. M. (1961). On the problem of parasitic castration of fleas. *Prirod. Ochag. Bolez. Kazakh., Alma Ata* **4**, 562-567. (In Russian.)

Alfeev, N. I. (1941). Experiments in acclimatizing the ichneumon fly *Hunterellus hookeri* in Russia as an aid to tick control. Abstr. of Report before 3rd Sovesh. Parazit. Prob. Moskva, *Vestnik Sel'sk. Nauk Vet., Mosk.* pp. 138-139. (In Russian.)

Alfeev, N. I. and Klimas, Y. V. (1938a). Experience in cultivating ichneumon flies, *Hunterellus hookeri,* obtained from the United States, which destroys ixodid ticks of the Soviet fauna. *Priroda, Mosk.* **2**, 98-101. (In Russian.)

Alfeev, N. I. and Klimas, Y. V. (1938b). On the possibility of experimental cultivation of *Hunterellus hookeri* under the climatic conditions of U.S.S.R. *Sovet. Vet., Mosk.* **15**, 55. (In Russian.)

Allen, A. A. (1962). *Ontholestes murinus* (L.) *(Col., Staphylinidae)* attacking *Lucilia sericata Meig.* (Dipt., Calliphoridae). *Ent. mon. Mag. Lond.* **98**, 87.

Altson, A. M. (1920). The life-history and habits of two parasites of blow-flies. *Proc. zool. Soc. Lond.* **15**, 195-243.

Anderson, J. R. and DeFoliart, G. R. (1962). Nematode parasitism of black fly (Diptera: Simuliidae) larvae in Wisconsin. *Ann. ent. Soc. Am.* **55**, 542-546.

Anderson, J. R. and Dicke, R. J. (1960). Ecology of the immature stages of some Wisconsin black flies (Simuliidae: Diptera). *Ann. ent. Soc. Am.* **53**, 386-404. (Reports nematode parasitism.)

Ashworth, J. H. and Rettie, T. (1912). On a gregarine: *Steinina rotunda* nov. sp., present in the mid-gut of bird-fleas of the genus *Ceratophyllus*. *Proc. R. Soc. Lond.* B **86**, No. 584, 31-38.

Axtell, R. C. (1961). Mites–enemies of house flies. *Farm Res.* **27**, 4-5.

Bal, Chandra and Rai, B. P. (1955). On the occurrence of *Stenophora* in the midgut of *Blatta orientalis*. *Proc. Ind. Sci. Cong.* **3**, 281.

Balch, H. E. (1932). Cultivation of *Nyctotherus ovalis* and *Endamoeba blattae*. *Science* **76**, 237.

Balogh, J. (1958). Macrocheliden aus Bulgarien (Acari: Mesostigmata). *Acta ent. Mus. Nat. Prague* **32**, 247-256.

Barabash-Nikiforov, I. I. (1945). Contribution to the question of the antimalaria role of bats. *Med. Parasit.* **14**, 93. (In Russian.)

Barrass, R. (1960a). The courtship behaviour of *Mormoniella vitripennis* Walk. (Hymenoptera: Pteromalidae). *Behaviour, Leiden* **15**, 185-209. (Entomophagous parasite of Muscidae.)

Barrass, R. (1960b). The effect of age on the performance of an innate behaviour pattern in *Mormoniella vitripennis* Walk. (Hymenoptera: Pteromalidae). *Behaviour, Leiden* **15**, 210-218.

Barrass, R. (1961). A quantitative study of the behaviour of the male *Mormoniella vitripennis* (Walker) (Hymenoptera: Pteromalidae) towards two constant stimulus-situations. *Behaviour, Leiden* **18**, 288-312. (Entomophagous parasite of Muscidae.)

Barthelmes, D. (1960). *Tetrahymena parasitica* (Penard, 1922) Corliss 1952 als Parasit in Larven vom *Chironomus plumosus*–Typ. *Z. f. Fischerei u. der. Hilfswiss.* **9**, N.F., 273-280.

Basir, M. A. (1940). Nematodes parasitic in Indian cockroaches. *Proc. Indian Acad. Sci.* B **12**, 8-16.

Beal, F. E. L. and McAtee, W. L. (1927). Common birds of Southeastern United States in relation to agriculture. *U.S. Dep. Agric. Farmers' Bull.* **755**, 1-44. (Avian predation on mosquitoes.)

Bedford, G. A. H. (1929). Anoplura (Siphunculata and Mallophaga) from South African hosts. *Rep. vet. Res. S. Afr.* **15**, 501-549. (Phoresy of a sucking louse on a muscoid fly.)

Bennike, S. A. B. (1943). Contributions to the ecology and biology of the Danish fresh-water leeches (Hirudinea). *Folia Limnol. Scand.* **2**, 1-109. (Leeches as predators on chironomid larvae.)

Biswas, K. (1942). Algal flora and mosquito larvae. *Sci. Cult.* **8**, 189-190.

Blagoveščenskij, D. I. (1940). Hymenopterous parasites of ticks of the family Ixodidae. 2. *Soveshch. Parazit. Prob., Moskva*, p. 23. (In Russian.)

Blickle, R. L. (1961). Parasites of the face fly, *Musca autumnalis*, in New Hampshire. *J. econ. Ent.* **54**, 802.

Borgatti, A. L. (1961). The toxicology of commercial formulations of *Bacillus thuringiensis* Berliner to Japanese quail and house fly larvae. *Diss. Abstr.* **22**, 2110-2111.

Bregatova, N. G. and Koroleva, E. V. (1960). The macrochelid mites (Gamesoidea: Macrochelidae) in the U.S.S.R. *Parazit. Sb. Zool. Inst.* **19**, 32-154. (In Russian.)

Bridges, C. H., Romane, W. M. and Emmons, C. W. (1962). Phycomycosis of horses caused by *Entomophthora coronata*. *J. Am. vet. med. Ass.* **140**, 673-677. (This fungal pathogen of muscoid flies is an important infectious agent in granulomatous lesions of horses in Texas.)

Briggs, J. D. (1960). Pathogens for the control of pests. *In* "Biological and Chemical Control of Plant and Animal Pests", pp. 137-148. AAAS, Washington, D.C.

Briscoe, M. S., Moore, R. E. and Puckett, D. E. (1961). Microbial isolations from the gut of *Blaberus craniifer* Burmeister. *J. Insect Path.* **3**, 254-258.

Bronskill, J. F. (1962). Encapsulation of rhabditoid nematodes in mosquitoes. *Can. J. Zool.* **40**, 1269-1275.

Brooke Worth, C. and Paterson, H. E. (1960). Phoresy of sucking lice (Siphunculata: Linognathidae) by a mosquito (Diptera: Culicidae). *J. ent. Soc. Sth. Africa* **23**, 228-230.

Brooks, M. A. (1954). Certain aspects of the histochemistry and metabolic significance of the intracellular bodies (bacteroids) of cockroaches (Blattariae). Ph.D. thesis, University of Minnesota.

Brooks, M. A. (1958). Nature and significance of intracellular bacteroids in cockroaches. *Proc. X Int. Congr. Ent., Montreal* 1956 **2**, 311-314.

Brooks, M. A. and Richards, A. G. (1955). Intracellular symbiosis in cockroaches. I. Production of aposymbiotic cockroaches. *Biol. Bull.* **109**, 22-39.

Brooks, M. A. and Richards, A. G. (1956). Intracellular symbiosis in cockroaches. III. Re-infection of aposymbiotic cockroaches with symbiotes. *J. exp. Zool.* **132**, 447-465.

Brumpt, E. (1945). Utilization éventuelle du batrachian *Xenopus laevis* dans la lutte contre les larves de moustiques; interactions diverse à prévoir. *C.r. hebd. Séanc. Acad. Sci. Paris* **220**, 923-925. (Use recommended for Corsica and Algeria, on basis of successful work involving *X. clivii* in Ethiopia.)

Burakova, L. V. (1931). Contribution to the biology of *Scatopse fuscipes* Meig., a possible enemy of sandflies (*Phlebotomus*). *Parazit. Sborn.* **2**, 113-118. (In Russian.)

Burtt, E. (1952). The occurrence in nature of tsetse pupae (*Glossina swynnertoni* Austen). *Acta Tropica* **9**, 304-344. (Random trampling by mammals of control significance, especially in rainy periods when pupation occurs on soil surface.)

Buyanova, O. F. (1954). The importance of ponds constructed in dry river beds from the (Ducks as predators) point of view of anophelism and malaria. *Med. Parasit.* **1**, 66-70. (In Russian.)

Bychkov, V. A. (1932). The duration of the persistence of *Bacterium prodigiosum* in flies. *Parazit. Sborn.* **3**, 149-159. (In Russian.)

Bychkov-Oreshnikov, V. A. (1934). On the microflora of the flies of some of the camps and on the role possibly played by them in the distribution of the intestinal diseases. *Trudy Voenno-Med. Akad., Leningrad* **1**, 393-400. (In Russian.)

Callot, J. (1959). Action d'un Agamomermis sur les caractères sexuels d'un cératopogonide. *Ann. Parasit. hum. comp.* **34**, 439-443.

Carpenter, G. D. H. (1920). "A Naturalist on Lake Victoria". T. Fisher Unwin, London. (Some of the Sesse Islands of Lake Victoria have large spider populations. Three of these with many webs had no tsetse and others fewer than elsewhere.)

Caullery, M. and Comas, M. (1928). Le déterminisme du sexe chez un Nématode *(Paramermis contorta)*, parasite des larves des chironomes. *C.r. hebd. Séanc. Acad. Sci., Paris* **186**, 646-648.

Chatton, E. (1912). Microsporidies considérées comme causes d'erreurs dans l'étude du cycle évolutif des trypanosomides chez les insectes. *Bull. Soc. Path. exot.* **4**, 662-664. *Correction (cited as 1911 by Jenkins, 1964).*

Chen, L. (1933). Züchtungsversuche an parasitischen Protozoen von *Periplaneta orientalis (Endamoeba blattae, Nyctotherus ovalis, Lophomonas blattarum). Z. Parasit.* **6**, 207-219.

Chernyavskya, M. A. (1957). Algological characteristics of anophelogenic reservoirs in the Irtysh River Valley. *Tr. Omst. Med. Inst.* **21**, 315-322. (In Russian.)

Chodorowski, A. (1958). Influence of the drying up of intermittent pools on the predator-prey relationship. *Ekol. Polska* B **4**, 41-44. (In Polish.)

Clarke, J. L. (1938). Mosquito control as related to marsh conservation. *Proc. N.J. Mosq. Exterm. Ass.*, 25th Ann. Mtg, 1938, pp. 139-147. (Illustrates and lists various arthropod predators, with notes on their relative efficiency, and states that a bladderwort, *Utricularia vulgaris*, destroyed all but three of 1800 small mosquito larvae in a bowl.)

Comas, M. (1927). Sur le mode de penetration de *Paramermis contorta* v. Linst. dans le larve de *Chironomus thumi* Kief. *C.r. hebd. Séanc. Soc. Biol.* **96**, 673-675.

Corbet, P. S. (1960). Recognition of nulliparous mosquitoes without dissection. *Nature, Lond.* **187,** 525-526. (Female mosquitoes in Uganda, bearing hydrachnid mites, are nearly always nulliparous.)

Corbet, P. S. and Griffiths, A. (1962). Field and laboratory observations on two species of *Toxorhynchites. E. Afr. Virus Res. Inst. Rep.* **12,** 43-44.

Corti, E. (1902). Di un nuova nematode parasita in larva di *Chironomus. R.C. reale ist. lombardo sci.,* Ser. II **35,** 105-113.

Couch, J. N. (1962). Validation of the family Coelomomycetaceae and certain species and varieties of *Coelomomyces. J. Elisha Mitchell Sci. Soc. ent.* **78,** 135-138.

Cousin, G. (1930). Le développement endoparasitaire de la larve ectoparasite de *Mormoniella vitripennis* Walk. *C.r. hebd. Séanc. Acad. Sci. Paris* **190,** 1530-1532.

Cousin, G. (1933). Etude biologique d'un chalcidien: *Mormoniella vitripennis* Walk. *Bull. biol. Fr. Belg.* **67,** 371-400.

Cowperthwaite, J., Weber, M. M., Packer, L. and Hutner, S. H. (1953). Nutrition of *Herpetomonas (Strigomonas) culicidarum. Ann. N.Y. Acad. Sci.* **56,** 972-981.

Crawley, H. (1905a). *Coelosporidium blattellae,* a new sporozoan parasite of *Blattella germanica. Proc. natn. Acad. Sci., Phila.* **57,** 158-161.

Crawley, H. (1905b). *Coelosporidium blattellae,* sp.n., a sporozoan parasite of *Blattella germanica. Science* Ser. 2. **21,** 269-270.

Daniel, M. (1962). A contribution to the problem of natural enemies of larvae of the chigger mite *Trombicula autumnalis* (Acariformes: Trombiculidae). *Věst. Čs. Spo. Zool.* **26,** 146-147. (Nymphs of the mite *Allothrombium fuliginosum* feed on chigger larvae.)

Daniel, M. and Samšiňák, K. (1955). *Phanolophus nasica* Andre (Acari: Smariidae) a new parasite of the Italian cockroach *Calliptamus italicus* L. *Zool. Zh.* **34,** 1242-1249. (In Russian.)

Das Gupta, S. K. and Ghosh, S. M. (1956). Observations on parasitisation of anopheline mosquitoes by *Culicoides anophelis. Bull Calcutta Sch. trop. Med.* **4,** 122-123.

Das Gupta, S. K. and Ghosh, S. M. (1957a). *Culicoides anophelis* Edw. as an ectoparasite of culicine mosquitoes. *Bull. Calcutta Sch. trop. Med.* **5,** 26-27.

Das Gupta, S. K. and Ghosh, S. M. (1957b). A record of *Culicoides anophelis* Edw., parasitizing *Culex fatigans* Wied. *Bull. Calcutta Sch. trop. Med.* **5,** 68-69.

Dias, E. (1937). Sobre a presenca de symbiontes em hemiptores hematophagos. *Mems Inst. Oswaldo Cruz* **32,** 164-168.

Doby, J. M. and Laurent, P. (1953). Mermithides parasites de larves de simulies en provenance de l'Avre et de la Semoy. *Annls Parasit. hum. comp.* **248,** 330-331.

Downs, A. E. and West, A. S. (1954). Progress on the use of the precipitin test in entomological studies. *Can. Ent.* **86,** 181-184. (Larval Trichoptera predacious on fourth instar mosquito larvae.)

Dubinin, V. B. (1950). Mites of the subfamily Myialgesinae parasitic on blood-sucking flies and feather lice. *Ent. Obozr. Moscow* **31,** 123-131. (In Russian.)

Duncan, J. T. (1926). On a bactericidal principle present in the alimentary canal of insects and arachnids. *Parasitology* **18,** 238-252.

Edwards, R. L. (1961). The area of discovery of two insect parasites *Nasonia vitripennis* (Walker) and *Trichogramma evanescens* Westwood, in an artificial environment. *Can. Ent.* **93,** 475-481.

Emmons, C. W. and Bridges, C. H. (1961). *Entomophthora coronata,* the etiologic agent of a phycomycosis of horses. *Mycologia* **53,** 307-312. (A coenocytic mycelium of this muscoid fly pathogen grows in mammalian tissues.)

Enigk, K. (1956). Observations of *Hunterellus hookeri* in *Ixodes ricinus. Dtsch. tiërarztl. Wscher.,* **63,** 161-162. (In German.)

Epstein, H. (1911). Beiträge zur Kenntnis von *Pleistophora periplanetae* (L. and S.). *Biol. Zent.* **31,** 676-682.

Evans, A. C. (1933). Comparative observations on the morphology and biology of some hymenopterous parasites of carrion-infesting Diptera. *Bull. ent. Res.* **24,** 385-405.

Evans, A. M. (1930). Observations on the predacious habits and prey of *Coenosia humilis* Mg. (Anthomyiidae). *Trans. R. ent. Soc. Lond.* **78,** 325-329.

Evans, G. O., Sheals, J. G. and Mcfarlane, D. (1961). "The Terrestrial Acari of the British Isles", Vol. I, 219 pp. Introduction and Biology. British Museum (Nat. Hist.). (Mentions mite infestations of Culicidae.)

Fattig, P. W. (1946). The Tabanidae or horseflies and deerflies of Georgia. *Emory Univ. Mus. Bull.* **4**, 1-26. (Random predation of adult tabanids.)

Fearnside, C. J. (1900). Parasites found on mosquitoes. *Ind. med. Gaz.* **35**, 129-130.

Feldman-Muhsam, B. and Havivi, Y. (1962). A micro-organism associated with sperm cells of *Ornithodoros. Nature, Lond.* **193**, 1095-1096.

Correction (Incorrectly cited by Jenkins, 1964).

Ferguson, M. J. and Micks, D. W. (1961). Microorganisms associated with mosquitoes: I. Bacteria isolated from the mid-gut of adult *Culex fatigans* Wiedemann. *J. Insect Path.* **3**, 112-119.

Ferrière, C. (1953). Un nouvel Encyrtidae (Hym. Chalcidoidea) de la Guinée Française. *Revue Path. vég. Ent. agric. Fr.* **32**, 116.

Filipponi, A. and Ilardi, A. (1959). Alcuni dati sulla biologia di *Macrocheles insignitus,* Berl. (Acarina: Mesostigmata). *Riv. Parassit.* **20**, 79-90.

Fitzgerald, N. W. (1952). Some new gregarines. M.Sc. Thesis, Otago University, Dunedin, New Zealand. (*Enterocystis zwetkowi* listed from "Blattidae".)

Fletcher, O. K., Jr. (1948). Ducks as mosquito predators. *J. Nat. Malar. Soc.* **7**, 186.

Floch, H. and Abonnenc, E. (1942). Ixodides de la Guyane française le "peu d'agoniti". *Publ. Inst. Pasteur, Guyane* **20**, 1-22. *(Trombidium muscae:* host, *Musca domestica.)*

Franz, D. R. and Hagmann, L. E. (1962). A microsporidian parasite of *Aedes stimulans* (Walker). *Mosquito News* **22**, 302-303.

Frohne, W. C. (1955). Ecological by-lines of an Alaskan mosquito worker. *Proc. Pap. Calif. Mosq. Contr. Ass., 23rd Ann Conf., and 11th Ann. Meet. Am. Mosq. Control Ass.* (*Rhamphomyia* spp.–Diptera, Empididae–as predators on swarming adult mosquitoes, and pupae.)

Frohne, W. C. and Frohne, R. G. (1952). Mating swarms of males of the mosquito *Aedes punctor* (Kirby), in Alaska. *Mosquito News* **12**, 248-251. (Empid predation referred to.)

Fukuda, S. (1939). Biology of *Mormoniella vitripennis* Walk., a parasite of *Sturmia sericariae* Corn. *Zool. Mag.* **51**, 185-195. (In Japanese.)

Gallagher, M. R. (1962). Vitamin synthesis by the symbionts in the fatbody of the cockroach, *Periplaneta americana* (Linnaeus). Ph.D. Thesis, Fordham Univ., New York.

Gauthier, M. (1961). Une nouvelle espèce de *Stachylina: St. minuta* n.sp., parasite des larves de chironomides tanytarsiens. *Trav. Lab. Hydrobiol. Piscicult. Univ. Grenoble* **52/53**, 4 pp. reprint.

Geigy, R., Halff, L. A. and Kocher, V. (1953). Untersuchungen uber die physiologischen Beziehungen Zwischen einem Ubertrager der Chagas-Krankheit *Triatoma infestans* und dessen Darmsymbionten. *Schwiz. Med. Wochschr.* **83**, 928-930.

Georgévitch, J. (1925). Sur la structure de la spore de *Pleistophora periplanetae. C.r. hebd. Séanc. Acad. Sci. Paris* **181**, 1191-1194.

Georgévitch, J. (1926a). Sur le cycle évolutif de *Pleistophora periplanetae. C.r. hebd. Séanc. Acad. Sci. Paris* **182**, 102-104.

Georgévitch, J. (1926b). Study of the development of *Pleistophora periplanetae* Lutz and Splend. *Glas Srpske Kral. Acad.* **122**, 1-33. (In Serbo-Croatian.)

Georgévitch, J. (1927). Recherches sur *Pleistophora periplanetae* Lutz et Splend. *Arch. Zool. exp. gen.* **66**, 1-21.

Gerhardt, R. W. (1955). Further studies during 1954 on blue-green algae–a possible anti-mosquito measure for rice fields. *Proc. Pap. Calif. Mosq. Contr. Ass., 23rd Ann. Conf., and 11th Ann. Meet. Am. Mosq. Control Ass.*, 3 pp. reprint.

Gerhardt, R. W. (1961). A resumé of studies on rice field mosquito ecology. *Calif. Vector Views* **8**, 43-47.

Gertsh, W. J. (1949). "American Spiders". Van Nostrand Co., New York.

Ghosh, S. M. and Hati, A. K. (1962). *Actinomycetes* infection in *Anopheles* and *Culex* larvae. *Bull. Calcutta Sch. trop. Med.* **10,** 171.

Gillies, M. T. (1962). Interspecific competition in mosquitoes–has it any bearing on biological control? *Verh. 11. Int. Kongr. Ent.* (Wien, 1960) **2,** 502-503.

Girault, A. A. and Sanders, G. E. (1909). The chalcidoid parasites of the common house or typhoid fly (*Musca domestica* Linnaeus) and its allies. *Psyche Camb., Mass.* **16,** 119-132.

Glaser, R. W. (1920). Biological studies on intracellular bacteria. No. 1. *Biol. Bull.* **39,** 133-145.

Glaser, R. W. (1930). On the isolation, cultivation and classification of the so-called intracellular "symbiont" or "Rickettsia" of *Periplaneta americana. J. exp. Med.* **51,** 59-82.

Glasgow, R. D. (1939). Biological control of mosquitoes; a special problem in applied ecology. *Proc. New Jers. Mosq. Exterm. Ass.*, 26th Ann. Mtg., 20-35 (including discussion).

Godoy, A. and Pinto, C. (1922). Da presenca dos symbiotes nos Ixodides. *Brasil-med.* **2,** 335.

Goodchild, A. J. P. (1955). The bacteria associated with *Triatoma infestans* and some other species of Reduviidae. *Parasitology* **45,** 441-448.

Gravely, F. H. (1911). Mosquito sucked by a midge. *Rec. Indian Mus.* **6,** 4-5.

Greathead, D. J. (1959). On *Dirhinus excavatus* Dalman (Hym., Chalcididae), and an alcocharine larva (Col., Staphylinidae), parasites of the pupae of *Stomorhina lunata* (F.) (Dipt., Calliphoridae) in Eritrea. *Ent. mon. Mag.* **95,** 105-108.

Green, E. E. (1905). On *Toxorhynchites immisericors* (Walker), the elephant mosquito. *Spolia Zeylan.* **2,** 159-164.

Greenberg, B. (1959). Persistence of bacteria in the developmental stages of the housefly. I. Survival of enteric pathogens in the normal and aseptically reared host. *Am. J. trop. Med. Hyg.* **8,** 405-411.

Greenberg, B. (1962a). Host-contaminant biology of muscoid flies. II. Bacterial survival in the stable fly, false stable fly, and the little house fly. *J. Insect Path.* **4,** 216-223.

Greenberg, B. (1962b). Host-contaminant biology of muscoid flies. III. Effect of hibernation, diapause, and larval bactericides on normal flora of blow-fly prepupae. *J. Insect Path.* **4,** 415-428.

Greenberg, B. and Carpenter, P. D. (1960). Factors in phoretic association of a mite and a fly. *Science* **132,** 738-739.

Gropengiesser, C. (1925). Untersuchungen über die Symbiose der Blattiden mit niederen pflanzlichen Organismen. *Z. Bakt. Parasit.*, Abt. II **64,** 495-511.

Groves, J. (1925). *Chara* and mosquito larvae. *J. Bot.* **63,** 56.

Gukasian, A. B. (1962). Conference on the use of microorganisms in the control of injurious insects. *Izv. Akad. Nauk. SSR, Ser. biol.* **5,** 809-812. (In Russian.)

Haas, G. E. and Dicke, R. J. (1959). Fleas collected from cottontail rabbits in Wisconsin. *Trans. Wisc. Acad. Sci. Arts Lett.* **48,** 125-133. (Pathogens mentioned.)

Halcrow, J. G. (1954). The phenomenon of metathetely, with notes on the parasites of some Mauritian mosquitoes. *Entomologist* **87,** 122-123.

Hardy, G. H. (1924). A blow-fly and some parasites. *Qd agric. J.* **2,** 22.

Hardy, G. H. (1925). The fecundity of *Mormoniella* and some problems in parthenogenesis. *Qd agric. J.* **24,** 347-348. (*Lucillia* spp. as hosts.)

Harrison, A. D. (1955). Four new species of gregarines from mountain cockroaches of the Cape Peninsula. *Ann. S. Afr. Mus.* **41,** 397-405.

Harvey, T. L. and Brethour, J. R. (1960). Feed additives for control of housefly larvae in livestock faeces. *J. econ. Ent.* **53,** 774-776.

Hati, A. K. and Ghosh, S. M. (1961). *Vorticella* infestation of mosquito larvae and its effect on their growth and longevity. *Bull. Calcutta Sch. trop. Med.* **9,** 155.

Hati, A. K. and Ghosh, S. M. (1962). Study on water scorpion *(Laccotrephes maculatus)* as a predator of mosquito larvae and pupae. *Bull. Calcutta Sch. trop. Med.* **10,** 120-121.

Haufe, W. O. (1952). Observations on the biology of mosquitoes (Diptera: Culicidae) at Goose Bay, Labrador. *Can. Ent.* **84,** 254-263. (Three species of Chaeborinae proved to prey on mosquito larvae.)

Haws, L. D. (1960). Predaceous mites for biological control of house flies. Mimeogr. docum., *Rep. Wyo. agric. Exp. Stn.*, Laramie, Wyoming.

Heimpel, A. M. (1962). General aspects of bacteriological control. *Mém. hors. Sér. Ent.* No. 2, 23-33.

Heitor, F. (1962). Parasitisme de blessure par le champignon *Mucor hiemalis* Wehmer chez les insectes. *Ann. Épiphyties* **13,** 179-203. (The cockroach *Blabera fusca* proved refractory.)

Hertig, M. (1921). Attempts to cultivate the bacteroids of the Blattidae. *Biol. Bull.* **41,** 181-187.

Hine, J. S. (1907). Second report upon the horseflies of Louisiana. *La. Bull. agric. Exp. Stn.* **93,** 59. (Reared *Telenomus tabanivorus* (Ashmead) from egg masses of *Tabanus atratus.)*

Hinman, E. H. (1932). The presence of bacteria within the eggs of mosquitoes. *Science* **76,** 106-107.

Hoare, C. A. (1921). Some observations and experiments on insect flagellates, with special reference to artificial infection of vertebrates. *Parasitology* **13,** 67.

Hocking, B. and Hocking, J. M. (1962). Entomological aspects of African onchocerciasis and observations on *Simulium* in the Sudan. *Bull. Wld Hlth Org.* **27,** 465-472. (Considers biotic control prospects and mentions various predatory insects.)

Hoffman, W. E. (1925). The life history of *Sphaerodema rusticus* Fabr. (Hemiptera: Belostomatidae). *Lingnaam Agric. Rev.* **3,** 167-179. (Fed on mosquito larvae and pupae under laboratory conditions.)

Holdaway, F. G. and Evans, A. C. (1930). Parasitism a stimulus to pupation: *Alysia manducator* in relation to the host *Lucilia sericata. Nature, Lond.* **125,** 598.

Hovasse, R. (1930). *Bacillus cuenoti* Mercier, bactéroide de *(Periplaneta orientalis),* à la morphologie d'une bactérie. *Arch. Zool. Exp.* **70,** 93-96.

Hoyte, H. M. D. (1961a). The Protozoa occurring in the hind-gut of cockroaches. I. Response to changes in environment. *Parasitology* **51,** 415-436.

Hoyte, H. M. D. (1961b). The Protozoa occurring in the hind-gut of cockroaches. II. Morphology of *Nyctotherus ovalis. Parasitology* **51,** 437-463.

Hoyte, H. M. D. (1961c). The Protozoa occurring in the hind-gut of cockroaches. III. Factors affecting the dispersion of *Nyctotherus ovalis. Parasitology* **51,** 465-495.

Huber, J. A. (1936). *Kleine plagegeister,* Dillingen. (Odonata preying on mosquito larvae.)

Hughes, T. E. (1959). "Mites or the Acari", 225 pp. Athlone Press, Univ. Lond. (Notes presence of Hydryphantidae parasitizing anopheline and culicine mosquitoes.)

Hutchison, J. A. (1962). Studies on a new *Entomophthora* attacking calyptrate flies. *Mycologia* **54,** 258-271.

Hyatt, K. H. (1956). A collection of mites from stable manure. *Ent. mon. Mag.* **92,** 36-38. (Macrochelid mite predators on muscoid fly eggs, England.)

Hynes, H. B. N. (1960). A plea for caution in the use of DDT in the control of aquatic insects in Africa. *Ann. trop. Med. Parasitol.* **54,** 331-332.

Iatsenko, F. I. (1943). Study of the mosquito microflora. *Med. Parazitol.* **12,** 59-63. (In Russian.)

Illies, J. (1955). Steinfliegen oder Plecopteren. *In* "Die Tierwelt Deutschlands" (F. Dahl, ed.), p. 43. Jena. (Larvae of *Dinocras cephalotes* Curt. and *Isoperla grammatica* Pod. prey on larval blackflies.)

Ishimura, K. (1952). On the early stage of *Megarhinus towadensis* Matsumara. *Jap. J. San. Zool.* **3,** 12-19. (In Japanese.)

Ivanič, M. (1926). Zur Kenntnis der Entwicklungsgeschichte von *Coelosporidium periplanetae* (Lutz u. Splendore). *Arch. Protistenk.* **56,** 63-89.

Iwata, K. (1938). Habits of some Japanese pemphredonids and crabronids (Hymenoptera). *Mushi* **11,** 20-41. (Sphecoid wasp, *Rhopalum nipponicum,* preying on chironomids.)

Iyengar, M. O. T. (1927). Parasitic nematodes of *Anopheles* in Bengal. *Far East Ass. trop. Med., Trans., 7th Congress British India* **3**, 128-135.

Jacobi, E. F. (1939). Über lebersweise, auffinden des Wirtes und Regulierung der Individuenzahl von *Mormoniella vitripennis* Walker. *Arch. Néerl. Zool.* **3**, 197-282.

Jafri, R. H. (1961). Synergistic action of radiation and of *Bacillus thuringiensis* toxin on protozoan diseases of insects. *Progr. Protozool., Proc. 1st Int. Conf. Protozool., Prague, August 22-31, 1961*, 510-515.

Jafri, R. H. (1964). Susceptibility of irradiated insects to *Bacillus thuringiensis* infection. *Mém. hors Sér. Ent.* No. 2, 351-354.

James, H. G. (1951). Natural control of Tabanidae (Diptera) in the region of Churchill, Manitoba, *82nd Ann. Rep. ent. Soc. Ontario*, 70-74. (Chalcidoid, *Diglochis occidentalis* (Ashm.).)

Jänner, G. (1937). *Beiträge zur Fauna Thüringens* 3, Diptera. Erfurt. (Salamanders preying on mosquito larvae.)

Javelly, E. (1914). Les corps bactéroids de la blatte *(Periplaneta orientalis)* n'ont pas encore été cultivés. *C.r. hebd. Séanc. Soc. Biol.* 77, 413-414.

Jayewickreme, S. H. and Niles, W. J. (1946). Successful feeding experiments with an adult trombiculid mite (order Acarina). *Nature, Lond.* **157**, 878. (Mite feeding on *Mansonia uniformis.*)

Jeu, M. H. (1962). The ectoparasitic mites of *Anopheles hyrcanus* var. *sinensis* Wied. and *Musca domestica vicina* Macq. and their influence on the reproduction of the hosts. *Acta ent. sin.* **11**, 135-137. (In Chinese.)

Jobbins-Pomeroy, A. W. (1916). Notes on five North American buffalo gnats of the genus *Simulium. U.S. Dep. agric. Bull. 329*, 48 pp. (Reports nematode parasitism.)

Johnson, A. A. (1955). Life history studies on *Hydromermis contorta* (Kohn), a nematode parasite of *Chironomus plumosus* (L.). Ph.D. Thesis, Univ. Illinois, Urbana.

Johnson, Phyllis T., McConnell, E. and Hertig, M. (1962). Natural and experimental infections of leptomonad flagellates in Panamanian *Phlebotomus* sandflies. *J. Parasit.* **48**, 158.

Jones, C. M. (1962). Biological control of stable flies. *Proc. 17th Ann. Meet. N. Cent. Brch, ent. Soc. Am.* **17**, 145-146.

Keilin, D. (1920). On two new gregarines. *Allantocystis dasyhelis* nov. gen. et n.sp. and *Dendrorhynchus systeni* nov. gen. et n.sp. parasitic in the alimentary canal of the dipterous larvae *Dasyhelea obscura* Winn. and *Systenus* sp. *Parasitol.* **12**, 154-158.

Keller, H. (1950). Die Kultur der intrazellularen Symbionten von *Periplaneta orientalis. Z. Naturforsch.* **56**, 269-273.

Ketchel, M. M. and Williams, C. M. (1953). Isolation of the intracellular symbiont of the roach. *Anat. Rec.* **117**, 650.

Khelevin, N. V. (1941). The hibernation shelters of *Anopheles* in the Ivanovo Region. *Med. Parasitol.* **10**, 440-444. (In Russian.) (Spider *Tegenaria derhami* Soap.—a predator of hibernating *A. maculipennis* in basements.)

Khodukin, N. I. (1927). On the intestinal protozoa of Phlebotomus. *Med. Mysl. Uzbek.*, 2(VII) Tashkent **1**, 83-87. (In Russian.)

King, P. E. (1960). The passage of sperms to the spermatheca during mating in *Nasonia vitripennis* (Walker) (Hym., Pteromalidae). *Ent. mon. Mag.* **96**, 136.

King, P. E. (1961). A possible method of sex ratio determination in the parasitic hymenopteran *Nasonia vitripennis. Nature, Lond.* **189**, 330-331. (Entomophagous parasite of Muscidae.)

King, P. E. (1962a). The structure and action of the spermatheca in *Nasonia vitripennis* (Walker) (Hymenoptera: Pteromalidae). *Proc. R. ent. Soc., Lond. (A)* **37**, 73-75.

King, P. E. (1962b). Structure of the micropyle of *Nasonia vitripennis. Nature, Lond.* **195**, 829-830.

King, P. E. (1962c). The muscular structure of the ovipositor and its mode of function in *Nasonia vitripennis* (Walker) (Hymenoptera: Pteromalidae). *Proc. R. ent. Soc., Lond. (A)* **37**, 121-128.

King, P. E. (1962d). The effect of resorbing eggs upon the sex ratio of the offspring in *Nasonia vitripennis* (Hymenoptera, Pteromalidae). *J. exp. Biol.* **39**, 161-165.

Klyushkina, E. A. (1956). An unusual case of cannibalism in ticks of the family Ixodidae. *Zool. Zh., Mosk.* **35**, 614-615. (In Russian.)

Klyushkina, E. A. (1958a). Discovery of a parasite of the ixodid tick, *Hunterellus hookeri* How., in the Crimea. *Med. Parazit. (Mosk.)* **27**, 734. (In Russian.)

Klyushkina, E. A. (1958b). *Hunterellus hookeri* How., a parasite of the ixodid tick in the Crimea. *Zool. Zh., Mosk.* **37**, 1561-1563. (In Russian.)

Kolomiyets, Y. S. (1950). *Aspergillus fumigatus* as a parasite of ticks. *Priroda, Mosk.* **39**, 64-65. (In Russian.)

Krall, E. (1959). Hairworms and mermithids–parasites of insects. *Eesti Loodus* **4**, 216-220. (In Estonian.) (Fifty per cent of an adult chironomid midge population parasitized in Estonia.)

Krantz, G. W. (1962). A review of the genera of the family Macrochelidae Vitzthum 1930 (Acarina: Mesostigmata). *Acarologia* **4**, 143-173.

Kudo, R. R. (1962). Microsporidia in southern Illinois mosquitoes. *J. Insect Path.* **4**, 353-356.

Kühlhorn, F. (1959). Beitrag zur Kenntnis der Ernährungsbiologie unserer heimischen Amphibien. *Veröff. Zool. Staatssamml. München* **5**, 145-188.

Kühlhorn, F. (1961a). Untersuchungen über die Bedentung verschiedener Vertreter der Hydrofauna und- Flora als natürliche Begrenzungsfaktoren für *Anopheles*–Larven *(Dipt., Culicidae). Z. angew. Zool.* **48**, 129-161.

Kühlhorn, F. (1961b). Uber das Verhalten sozialer Faltenwespen (Hymenoptera: Vespidae) heim Stalleinflug, innerhalb von Viehställen und beim Fliegenfang–Untersuchungen über die Insektenfauna von Räumen (5). *Z. angew. Ent.* **48**, 405-422. (Wasps and flies.)

Kühlhorn, F. (1962). Untersuchungen über die Bedentung der Vermilbung bei *Anopheles. Verhandl., XI Int. Congr. Ent.,* Wien 1960 **2**, 870-874. (Adult mosquitoes bearing a few immature water mites oviposit normally.)

Kurochkin, J. V. (1960). The nematode *Heterotylenchus pavlovskyi* sp.n., castrating flea-vectors of plague. *Dokl. Acad. Nauk. U.S.S.R.* **135**, 1281-1284. (In Russian.)

Laessle, A. M. (1961). A micro-limnological study of Jamaican bromeliads. *Ecology* **42**, 499-517. (Arthropod predators on mosquito larvae include carnivorous ceratopogonids, *Bezzia* sp., *Erythrodiplax*–Odonata–and *Diceratobasis*–Zygoptera.)

Laing, J. (1937). Host-finding by insect parasites. I. Observations on the finding of hosts by *Alysia manducator, Mormoniella vitripennis,* and *Trichogramma evanscens. J. anim. Ecol.* **6**, 298-317.

Laird, M. (1948). The occurrence of *Herpetomonas muscarum* (Leidy, 1856) in the intestine of *Calliphora quadrimaculata* (Swederus, 1787). *New Zealand Sci. Rev.* **6**, 12-13.

Laird, M. (1950). The occurrence of *Leptomonas ctenocephali* (Fantham, 1912) in the intestine and Malpighian tubules of the cat flea, *Ctenocephalides felis* (Bouché, 1835) in New Zealand. *Trans. R. Soc. N.Z.* **78**, 476-478.

Laird, M. (1959). Protozoa, including an entozoan of guinea pigs, from house flies. *Can. J. Zool.* **37**, 467-468.

Laird, M. (1962a). *Coelomomyces* fungi, an important group of mosquito parasites. W.H.O. mimeogr. docum., WHO/EBL/1, 4 pp. (Separate English and French versions.)

Laird, M. (1962b). Validation of certain species of *Coelomomyces* described from the Australian and Oriental regions. *J. Elisha Mitchell Sci. ent. Soc.* **72**, 132-133.

Laird, M. and Colless, D. H. (1962). A field experiment with a fungal pathogen of mosquitoes in the Tokelau Islands. *Proc. XI Int. Congr. Ent., Vienna,* 1960 **2**, 867-868.

Lange, R. (1962). Phasen wechselnder Jagdintensität bei Waldameisen. *Z. angew. Ent.* **50**, 56-64.

Lee, D. L. (1958a). On the morphology of the male and female and 4th stage larvae (female) of *Hammerschmidtiella diesingi* (Hammerschmidt, 1838) Chitwood, 1932, a new nematode parasitic in the cockroach. *Parasitology* **48**, 433-436.

Lee, D. L. (1958b). Digestion in *Leidynema appendiculata* (Leidy, 1850), a nematode parasitic in the cockroach. *Parasitology* **48**, 437-447.

Lee, D. L. (1959). The nervous system of *Thelastoma bulhoesi* (Magalhaes, 1900; Travassos, 1929), a nematode parasitic in cockroaches. *Parasitology* **49,** 473-476.

Lester, H. M. O. (1934). Report on the tsetse investigation. *Rep. med. Hlth Serv. Nigeria,* 1933, 74-83. (Rainy season fungal infections.)

Lewis, D. J. and Wright, C. A. (1962). A trematode parasite of *Simulium. Nature, Lond.* **193,** 1311-1312.

Linam, J. H. (1962). Hydracarinid mites parasitic on the mosquito, *Culex tarsalis* Coquillet (Acarina and Diptera: Culicidae). *Proc. ent. Soc. Wash.* **64,** 234.

Lisova, A. I. (1962). Gregarina (genus *Diplocystis*) in the body cavity of sandflies. *Zool. Zh.* **41,** 1095-1099. (In Russian.)

Lokshina, S. S. and Gorodetskii, A. S. (1956). Presence of microbes of the intestinal group in hibernating flies. *Dizenterii, Kiev, Gosmedizdat Ukr., SSR,* 242-244. (In Russian.)

Lorenc, W. (1938). Untersuchungen an Flagellaten aus dem Genus *Lophomonas*: 1. Zucht von *Lophomonas blattarum* Stein ausserhald des Wirtstieres. *Zoologica Pol.* **3,** 225-250.

Lucas, C. L. T. (1927). Two new species of amoeba found in cockroaches: with notes on the cysts of *Nyctotherus ovalis* Leidy. *Parasitology* **19,** 223-235.

Lucas, C. L. T. (1928). A study of excystation in *Nyctotherus ovalis* with notes on other intestinal protozoa of the cockroach. *J. Parasit.* **14,** 161-175.

Lyell Clarke, J. (1938). Mosquito control as related to marsh conservation. *Proc. New Jers. Mosq. Exterm. Ass., 25th Ann. Meet.* 139-147.

Lysenko, O. (1959). *Flavobacterium serpens* n.sp., an organism occurring in the microflora of flies. *Folio Microbiol.* **4,** 196-199.

McComb, C. W. and Bickley, W. E. (1959). Observations on black flies in two Maryland counties. *J. econ. Ent.* **52,** 629-632. (Reports nematode parasitism.)

McConnell, E. and Richards, A. G. (1959). The production by *Bacillus thuringiensis* Berliner of a heat stable substance toxic for insects. *Can. J. Zool.* **5,** 161-168.

MacDonald, W. A. (1957). A calliphorid host of *Thyridanthrax abruptus* (Diptera: Bombyliidae). *Bull. ent. Res.* **48,** 533.

MacDonald, W. W. (1960). On the systematics and ecology of *Armigeres* subgenus *Leicesteria* (Diptera: Culicidae). Malaysian Parasites XXXVIII. *Stud. Inst. Med. Res., Fed. Malaya, No. 29,* 110-153. (Larval cannibalism in *Leicesteria.*)

MacDonald, W. W. and Traub, R. (1960). An introduction to the ecology of the mosquitoes of the lowland dipterocarp forest of Selangor, Malaya. Malayan Parasites XXVII. *Stud. Inst. Med. Res., Fed. Malaya, No. 29,* 79-109. (Larval cannibalism in *Toxorhynchites* larvae.)

McDuffie, W. C., Gahan, J. B., Davis, A. N. and La Brecque, G. C. (1962). Highlights of recent research on mosquito control by the Entomology Research Division, U.S.D.A. *Proc. New Jers. Mosq. Exterm. Ass.* **49,** 16-27.

Makings, P. (1961). Males of *Aedes detritus* Halliday on flowers of ragwort in Cork, and notes of some predators of the mosquito. *Irish Nat. J.* **13,** 272-273.

Manier, J. F., Rioux, J. A. and Whisler, H. C. (1961). *Rubetella inopinata* n. sp. et *Carouxella scalaris* n.g., n.sp., Trichomycètes parasites de *Dasyhelea lithotelmatica* Strenzke, 1951 (Diptera: Ceratopogonidae). *Naturalia monspel. Sér. Bot.* **13,** 25-38. 25-38.

Mann, K. H. (1957). The breeding, growth and age structure of a population of the leech *Helobdella stagnalis* (L.). *J. Anim. Ecol.* **26,** 171-177. (Prey includes chironomid larvae.)

Mardzhanian, G. M. and Markosian, A. A. (1962). Bacterial insecticides and the possibilities of their use in Armenia. *Izv. Upr. Sel'khoz. Nauk. Arm. SSR.* **5,** 51-57. (In Russian.)

Martin, R. (1942). Le paludisme autochtone à Addis-Ababa. *Arch. Inst. Pasteur Algérie* **20,** 10-14. (*Xenopus* frogs as predators.)

Martini, E. (1931). Culicidae. *In* "Die Fliegen der Palaeartischen Region" (E. Lindner, ed.), pp. 1-398. E. Schweizerbart'sche (Erwin Nägler) Stuttgart. (Gives records of predation upon mosquito larvae involving *Hydra,* planarians, gammarids, various aquatic insects, salamanders, toads, tadpoles, and ducks.)

Martini, E. (1952). *Lehrbuch der Medizinischen Entomologie,* Jena. (Adult dolichopodid and ephydrid flies capture larval culicines and anophelines.)

Matikashvili, N. V. (1955). Reduviidae as the natural enemies of ticks. *Trudy Gruzinsk. Nauch.-Issled. Vet. Inst., Tbilisi* **11,** 229-230. (In Russian.)

Mel'chakeva, E. D. (1962). Cases of cannibalism in the tick *Ornithodoros papillipes* under laboratory conditions. *Trudy Inst. Zool. Akad. Nauk. Zazakh. SSR* **16,** 211-212. (In Russian.)

Mercier, L. (1906). Un organisme à forme levure parasite de la blatte (*Periplaneta orientalis* L.). Levure et *Nosema. C.r. hebd. Séanc. Soc. Biol.* **60,** 1081-1083.

Mercier, L. (1907). Recherches sur les bactéroides des Blattides. *Arch. Protistenk.* **9,** 346-358.

Merwe, J. S. van der (1943). Investigations on the biology and ecology of *Mormoniella vitripennis* Walk. *(Pteromalidae,* Hym.). *J. ent. Soc. Sth. Afr.* **6,** 49-64.

Metalnikov, S. and Chorine, V. (1929). On the infection of the gypsy moth and certain other insects with *Bacterium thuringiensis. Int. Corn Borer Invest., Sci. Rep.* **2,** 60-61. (Reference to *Anopheles maculipennis* Meig. and *Culex pipiens* L.)

Michener, C. D. (1946). The taxonomy and bionomics of some Panamanian trombidiid mites (Acarina). *Ann. ent. Soc. Am.* **39,** 349-380.

Micks, D. W. and Ferguson, J. (1961). Microorganisms associated with mosquitoes: III. Effect of reduction in the microbial flora of *Culex fatigans* Wiedemann on the susceptibility to *Plasmodium relictum* Grassi and Feletti. *J. Insect Path.* **3,** 244-248.

Mira, G. (1940). Sulla presenza di forme larvali di un acaro acquatico parassita, della famiglia degli Hydracnidae, su alcune zanzar'e del genere *Anopheles* in A.O.I. *Boll. Idrobiol. A.O.I.* **1,** 29-33. (Mites, *Atax* sp., infesting anophelines.)

Miyamoto, S. (1937). Observations on a marine water strider, *Asclepios coreanus miyamotoi* Esaki. *Mushi* **9,** 137-142. (In Japanese.) (This gerrid will take adult *Culex pipiens pallens.*)

Moggridge, J. Y. (1936). Some observations on the seasonal spread of *Glossina pallidipes* in Italian Somaliland with notes on *G. brevipalpis* and *G. austeni. Bull. ent. Res.* **27,** 449-466. (*G. brevipalpis* harbours a fungus.)

Muesebeck, C. F. W. (1961). A new Japanese *Trichopria* parasitic on the house fly (Hymenoptera: Diapriidae). *Mushi* **35,** 1-2. (*T. commoda* was being mass-produced on Kyoto for liberation in a fly control campaign.)

Mühlens, P. (1911). Zur Bekämptung der Mückenplage, Umschau, 25. (Water bugs and salamanders as mosquito larval predators.)

Mulla, M. S. (1958). Control of mites in laboratory cultures of the eye gnat, *Hippelates collusor* (Townsend). *J. econ. Ent.* **51,** 461-462.

Mulla, M. S. (1962). Recovery of a cynipoid parasite from *Hippelates* pupae. *Mosquito News* **22,** 301-302.

Muratov, E. A. and Kheisin, E. M. (1959). Discovery of *Crithidia hyalommae* O'Farrell in the ticks *Hyalomma detritum* and *H. anatolicum* in Tadzhikistan. *Dokl. Akad. Nauk. Tadzhik, SSR* (Stalinabad) **2,** 33-37. (In Russian.)

Muspratt, J. (1955). Research on South African *Culcini* (Diptera, Culicidae). *J. ent. Soc. Sth. Afr.* **18,** 149-207. (*Toxorhynchites brevipalpis.*)

Nathan, H. A. and Cowperthwaite, J. (1954). Use of the trypanosomid flagellate, *Crithidia fasciculata,* for evaluating antimalarials. *Proc. Soc. exp. Biol. Med.* **85,** 117-119.

Nowrojee, D. (1912). Life-histories of Indian insects–II. Some aquatic Rhynchota and Coleoptera. *Mem. Dep. Agric. India ent. Ser.* **2,** 165-191. *(Ranatra filiformis* Fab. readily preys on anopheline larvae.)

Ohgushi, R. I. (1959a). Effects of host upon the reproductive ability of a parasitic wasp, *Mormoniella vitripennis* (Wlk.) parasitic on fly puparia. *Jap. Zool. Mag. Zool. Soc.* **68,** 426-430. (In Japanese.)

Ohgushi, R. I. (1959b). The longevity, egg laying capacity and the number of hosts parasitized by one female of *Mormoniella vitripennis* (Walker) (Pteromalidae, Hymenoptera), reared in three species of fly puparia. *Insect Ecol., Tokyo* **8,** 46-57. (In Japanese.)

Ohgushi, R. I. (1960). Studies on the host selection by *Nasonia vitripennis* (Wlk.) parasitic on housefly pupae. *Physiol. Ecol. (Seiro-Seitai) Kyoto* **9,** 11-31. (In Japanese.)

Ohgushi, R. I. (1961). Effect of host upon the quiescence of *Nasonia vitripennis* (Wlk.), a parasitic wasp of fly pupae. *Jap. J. appl. Ent., Zool.* **5**, 154-155.

Ohgushi, R. I. and Kato, S. (1959). Ecological study on the parasitic wasp of flies. 1. Experiment on the parasitization of *Mormoniella vitripennis* against fly pupae in different media. *Jap. J. San. Zool.* **10**, 172-176. (In Japanese.)

Oliveira, S. J. de and Lent, J. (1962). Preliminary notes on chironomid (Diptera) intersexuality induced by *Agamomermis* (Nematoda). *Rev. Brasil. Biol.* **22**, 357-365.

Ostashev, S. N. (1957). Microflora of flies of pig-sties. *Sborn. Trudov, Leningrad. Nauch.-Issled. Vet. Inst., Moskva, Leningrad* **1**, 232-234. (In Russian.)

Patton, W. S. (1910). Experimental infection of the Madras bazaar fly, *Musca nebula* Fabr. with *Herpetomonas muscae domesticae* (Burnett). *Bull. Soc. path. exot.* **3**, 264-274.

Pavlov, P. (1940). Epizoozia di paralisi da zeche nelle capre in Bulgaria. *Riv. Parassit.* **4**, 227-232. (*Trombidium holosericeum* on *Musca domestica.*)

Pawlowsky, L. K. (1936). Zur Ökologie der Hirudineen-Fauna der Wigryseen. *Arch. Hydrobiol.* **10**, 1-47. (Leeches prey upon midge larvae.)

Peppler, H. J. (1944). Usefulness of microorganisms in studying dispersion of flies. *Bull. U.S. Army Med. Dep.* **75**, 121-122.

Petriščeva, P. A. (1947). Cannibalism in ticks, *Ornithodoros,* as a possible means of transmission of spirochaetes of tick relapsing fever. *Nov. Med. Mosk.* **5**, 24-26. (In Russian.)

Petriščeva, P. A. and Čagin, K. P. (1947). Some observations on *Lutzia vorax* Edwards. *Zool. Zh.* **26**, 85-86. (In Russian.)

Petrova, A. D. (1959). Interrelationships between ixodid ticks and tyroglyphid mites. *Nauch. Dokl. Vyssh. Shkoly, Biol.-Nauk., Mosk.* **1**, 17-19. (In Russian.)

Phipps, J. (1951). Some ecological aspects of anopheline breeding in the northern coastal area of Tanganyika. *E. Afr. med. J.* **28**, 341-353. (Mosquito larval predators included hemipterans dytiscid beetles, nymphs of Odonata, and the water tortoise *Pelusios sinuatus.* The numbers of anophelines and culicines consumed are contrasted.)

Pierre, L. L. (1961). Functions of symbionts in the fat body of the tropical cockroach, *Leucophaea maderae* (Fabricius). Ph.D. thesis, Fordham Univ., New York.

Pierre, L. L. (1962). Synthesis of ascorbic acid by the normal fat-body of the cockroach, *Leucophaea maderae* (F.) and by its symbionts. *Nature, Lond.* **193**, 904-905.

Pimental, D. and Cranston, F. (1960). The house cricket, *Acheta domesticus,* and the house fly, *Musca domestica,* as a model predator-prey system. *J. econ. Ent.* **53**, 171-172.

Potts, W. H. (1950a). Tsetse research, *E.A. Tsetse and Trypanosomiasis Res. Reclamation Org. Rep.,* 1949, pp. 6-13. E.A. High Commission, Nairobi.

Potts, W. H. (1950b). Tsetse research, *ibid.,* 1950, pp. 11-13. (Importance of ants of the genus *Pheidole,* especially after fires, which they survive and which change their habits so that they prey more on tsetse puparia.)

Prell, H. (1919). Anopheles und Malaria, Flugschr. *Dtsch Gesundh. f. angew Ent.,* No. 9. (Water bugs preying on mosquito larvae.)

Putman, C. D. (1959). Two aspects of the behaviour of *Aleochara bilineata* Gyll. (Coleoptera: Staphylinidae). *Anim. Behaviour* **7**, 248. (Predator on Muscidae.)

Radvan, R. (1960a). Epidemiological importance of spread and transmission of bacteria surviving during the development of flies. *Čslka. Epidem. Mikrobiol. Immunol.* **9**, 497-500. (In Czech.)

Radvan, R. (1960b). Persistence of bacteria during development in flies. I. Basic possibilities of survival. *Folia Microbiol.* **5**, 50-58.

Radvan, R. (1960c). Persistence of bacteria during development in flies. III. Localization of the bacteria and transmission after emergence of the fly. *Folia Microbiol.* **5**, 149-158.

Rašin, K. (1928). *Coelomomyces chironomi* n.sp. *Věst. VI. Sjezdu Cesk. přirodozpytců v Praze* **3**, 146.

Rašin, K. (1929). *Coelomomyces chironomi* n.sp., houba cizopasici v dutině tělni larer *Chironoma. Biol. Spis. Vys. Šk. Zvěrolék* **8**, 1-13.

Rempel, J. G. (1940). Intersexuality in Chironomidae induced by nematode parasitism. *J. exp. Zool.* **84**, 261-289.

Rempel, J. G., Naylor, J. M., Rothfels, K. and Ottonen, B. (1962). The sex chromosome constitution of chironomid intersexes parasitized by nematodes. *Can. J. Genet. Cytol.* **4**, 92-96.

Richards, A. G. and Smith, M. N. (1955). Infection of cockroaches with *Herpomyces*. I. Life history studies. *Biol. Bull.* **108**, 206-218.

Rivosecchi, L. and Bettini, S. (1958). Contributo alla conoscenza dei predatori della ova di *Latrodectus tredecimguttatus* Rossi. *Riv. Parassit.* **19**, 249-266.

Roberts, R. A. (1933). Biology of *Brachymeria fonscolombei* (Duf.), a hymenopterous parasite of blowfly larvae. *Tech. Bull. U.S. Dep. Agric.* **365**, 1-21.

Roberts, R. A. (1935). Some North American parasites of blowflies. *J. agric. Res.* **50**, 489-490.

Rodhain, J. (1913). A propos de *Leptomonas pangoniae* et *Trypanosoma denysi*. Note rectificative. *Bull. Soc. Path. exot.* **6**, 181.

Rodhain, J. (1919). Larvae de Sarcophagides probablement parasites accidentels de *Glossina palpalis* en captivité. *Bull. Soc. Path. exot.* **12**, 104.

Rodriguez, J. G. (1962). Studies on biological control of housefly eggs using macrochelid mites. (Abstract) *XI Int. Kongr. Ent.* Wien, 1960, Verhandlungen, Bd. II, 875.

Rodriguez, J. G., Wade, C. F. and Wells, C. N. (1962). Nematodes as a natural food for *Macrocheles muscaedomesticae* (Acarina: Macrochelidae), a predator of the house fly egg. *Ann. ent. Soc. Am.* **55**, 507-511.

Roshdy, M. A. (1961). Observations by electron microscopy and other methods on the intracellular Rickettsia-like microorganisms in *Argas persicus* Oken (Ixodoidea, Argasidae). *J. Insect Path.* **3**, 148-166.

Roubaud, E. (1908a). Sur un nouveau flagellé parasite de l'intestin des muscides au Congo français. *C.r. hebd. Séanc. Soc. Biol.* **64**, 1106-1108.

Roubaud, E. (1908b). *Leptomonas mesnili* n.sp. nouveau flagellé à formes trypanosomes de l'intestin de muscides non picqueurs. *C.r. hebd. Séanc. Soc. Biol.* **65**, 39-41.

Roubaud, E. (1911). *Cercoplasma* (n.g.) *caulleryi* (n.sp.) nouveau flagellé à formes trypanosomiennes de l'intestin d'*Auchmeromyia luteola* Fabr. *C.r. hebd. Séanc. Soc. Biol.* **71**, 503.

Rubtsov, I. A. (1961). The biology of *Anastatus* sp. (Eupelmidae: Hymenoptera) parasitic on the ootheca of *Supella supellectilium*. *J. zool. Soc. India* **13**, 62-69.

Sack, P. (1911). Aus dem Leben unserer Steckmücken 42. *Ber. Sencken. naturf. Ges.* **42**, 309-322. (Toad tadpoles preying on mosquito larvae.)

Sahov, S. D. (1928). On the discovery of endoparasites in the family Culicidae. *Trudy 3. Vseross. S'ezda Zool. Anat. i. Gistol, p. 163. (Leningrad, 14-20 December 1927.) (In Russian.)*

Salt, G. (1932). The natural control of the sheep blowfly, *Lucilia sericata* Meigen. *Bull. ent. Res.* **23**, 235-245.

Sandosham, A. A., Coombs, G. L. and Hassan, A. (1962). *Crithidia fasciculata* Léger, 1902 from the Malpighian tubules of *Anopheles hackeri* Edwards, 1921. *Med. J. Malaya* **17**, 95.

Sauerländer, S. and Ehrhardt, P. (1961). Reduzierung der Proteinfraktionen in der Hämolymphe bakterienkranker Blattiden. *Naturwissenschaften* **48**, 674-675.

Sauerländer, S. and Köhler, F. (1961). Erhöhung der Körpertemperatur von *Periplaneta americana* L. im Verlauf zweier Bakteriosen. *Experientia* **17**, 397.

Saunders, D. S. (1960). The "white-clubbed" form of *Syntomosphyryum* (Hym.: Eulophidae) parasitic on tsetse flies. *Bull. ent. Res.* **51**, 17-20.

Schiemenz, H. (1953). *Die Libellen unserer Heimat*, Urania Verlag, Jena. (Odonata preying on mosquito larvae.)

Schneider, F. (1950). Die Entwicklung Syrphid parasiten *Diplazon fissorius* Grav. (Hymen., Ichneum.) in uni, oligo- und polyvoltinen Wirten und sein Verhalten bei parasitärer Aktivierung der Diapauselarven durch *Diplazon pectoratorius* Grav. *Metteh. Schweiz. Ent. Gesellsch.* **23**, 155-194.

Schoof, H. F. (1962). Integration of biological and chemical control. Opportunities against medically important arthropods. *Bull. ent. Soc. Am.* **8**, 199-201.

Schuberg, A. and Kuhn, P. (1911). Die Mückenplage und ihre Bekämpfung. Über die Übertragung von Krankheiten durch einheimische stechende Insekten. Teil 1. *Arbeiten aus dem K. Gesundheitsamte, Berlin* **31**, 377-393. (Water bugs preying on mosquito larvae.)

Seguy, E. (1931). Les moustiques de la forêt Fontainebleau et de la Vallée du Loing. II. Biologie et moyens d'action contre ces insectes. *Trav. Ass. Nat. Loing famc.* **5**, 19-93 (also as *Trav. Lab. ent. Mus. nat. Hist. Nat.* **1**, 1933).

Selmair, E. (1962). Über das Verhalten von Symbionten nach dem Tode des Wirtstieres und bei gleichzeitiger Infektion mit Mikrosporidien. *Arch. Mikrobiol.* **43**, 290-293.

Sen, P. and Das Gupta, S. K. (1958). *Mermis* (Nematoda) as an internal parasite of *Culicoides alatus* (Ceratopogonidae). *Bull. Calcutta Sch. trop. Med.* **6**, 15.

Sen, P. and Das Gupta, S. K. (1959). Feeding habits of *Culicoides anophelis* (Diptera: Ceratopogonidae). *Bull. Calcutta Sch. trop. Med.* **7**, 108-109.

Shapiro, J. M., Salternik, Z. and Biferman, S. (1944). Malaria survey of the Dead Sea area during 1942, including the description of a mosquito flight test and its results. *Trans. R. Soc. trop. Med. Hyg.* **38**, 95-116. (Mites on mosquitoes.)

Shaw, F. R. and Maisey, S. A. (1961). The biology and distribution of the rockpool mosquito, *Aedes atropalpus* (Coq.). *Mosquito News* **21**, 12-16. (*A. atropalpus* larval populations were relatively low in presence of diving beetles and dragonfly naiads.)

Shiwago, P. (1909). Über Vermehrung bei *Pleistophora periplanetae* (Lutz Splendore). *Zool. Anz.* **34**, 647-654.

Shoguki, Y. (1950). Biology of *Culex vorax* Edwards. *Shin. Konchū* **3**, 282-283. (In Japanese.) (Larvae predacious on those of other mosquitoes.)

Sidorov, V. E. (1960). The body cavity of argasid ticks as a habitat for spirochaetes and brucellae. *Zh. Mikrobiol. Epidemiol. Immunobiol.* **31**, 91-96. (In Russian.)

Smith, K. G. V. (1949). Some observations on *Empis livida* Lin. (Dip., Empidae), with notes on its prey. *Ent. Rec.* **61**, 39-42. (Attacking *Culex* sp. possibly *C. pipiens* L.)

Smith, N. M. and Barrett, H. P. (1928). The cultivation of a parasitic amoeba from the cockroach. *J. Parasit.* **14**, 272-273.

Sokolov, I. I. (1952). On the discovery of fungus organisms on spermatophores of *Ornithodoros papillipes. Dokl. Akad. Nauk SSSR, Mosk.* **85**, 241-244. (In Russian.)

Sommerman, K. M. (1962). Notes on two species of *Oreogeton*, predaceous on black fly larvae (Diptera: Empididae and Simuliidae). *Proc. ent. Soc. Wash.* **64**, 123-129.

Sprague, V. (1940). Observations on *Coelosporidium periplanetae* with special reference to the development of the spore. *Trans. Am. microsc. Soc.* **59**, 460-474.

Sprague, V. (1941). Studies on *Gregarina blattarum* with particular reference to the chromosome cycle. *Illinois Biol. Monogr.* **18**, 1-57.

Sprague, V. and Ramsey, J. (1942). Further observations on *Plistophora kudoi*, a microsporidian of the cockroach. *J. Parasit.* **28**, 399-406.

Steiner, G. (1923). *Simulium* in the high Alps controlled by *Mermis* species. *J. Parasit.* **10**, 208.

Steinhaus, E. A. and Marsh, G. A. (1962). Report of diagnoses of diseased insects 1951-1961. *Hilgardia* **33**, 349-490.

Stephanides, T. (1960). On the possible influence of the Hydra in mosquito larvae control. *Praktika Hellenic Hydrobiol. Inst. Acad. Athens* **7**, 3-5.

Sternberg, S. and Tahori, A. S. (1962). Control of *Aleuroglyphus ovatus* (Troupeau) in flea cultures. *Bull. ent. Res.* **53**, 257-264.

Steve, P. C. (1959). Parasites and predators of *Fannia canicularis* (L.) and *Fannia scalaris* (F.). *J. econ. Ent.* **52**, 530-531.

Steyn, J. J. (1960). Araneophagous behaviour of *Pseudospilophorus plagosus* Boh. (Coleopt.: Cetoniidae). *J. ent. Soc. Sth. Afr.* **23**, 413-414. (This social spider destroys large numbers of houseflies.)

Strickland, C. (1912). *Agrippina bona*, n.g., n.sp., representing a new family of gregarine. *Parasitology* **5**, 97-109.

Strickland, C. (1914). The nuclear changes in *Agrippina bona* Strickland. *Parasitology* **7**, 380-382.

Suitor, E. C., Jr. and Weiss, E. (1961). Isolation of a rickettsia-like microorganism (*Wolbachia persica,* n.sp.) from *Argas persicus* (Oken). *J. inf. Dis.* **108,** 95-106.

Tanabe, J. (1931). Evaluation of *Bembix niponica* Smith as a natural enemy of horse flies. *Chûô-Jûikai Zasshi* **44,** 817-824. (In Japanese.)

Taylor, A. W. (1932). Pupal parasitism in *Glossina morsitans* and *Gl. tachinoides* at Gadau, North Nigeria. *Bull. ent. Res.* **23,** 463-467.

Theodoridès, J., Ormierès, R. and Jolivet, P. (1958). Eugrégarines parasites d'orthoptéroides. *Exploration du Parc National Albert* **2,** 1-43.

Thomson, J. G. (1935). A microsporidian *(Octosporea)* in the intestine of *Musca sorbens* Wied. *Trans. R. Soc. trop. Med. Hyg.* **29,** 6.

Treillard, M. and Lwoff, A. (1924). Sur an infusoire parasite de la cavité générale des larves de *Chironomes.* Sa sexualité. *C.r. hebd. Séanc. Acad. Sci. Paris* **178,** 1761-1764.

Trpis, M. (1960). Stechmücken der Reisfelder und Möglichkeiten ihren Bekämpfung. *Biol. prace* **6,** 1-57, (Turbellarians, trematodes, *Lymnaea,* gammarids, various aquatic insects, toad tadpoles, and ducks preying on mosquito larvae.)

Uemoto, K. (1961). Studies on the ecology of the hymenopterous parasites of flies in Japan. *J. Kyoto Pref. Univ. Med.* **70,** 1663-1712. (In Japanese.)

Umphlett, C. J. (1962a). Morphological and cytological observations on the mycelium of *Coelomomyces. Mycologia, Lancaster* **54,** 540-554.

Umphlett, C. J. (1962b). Comparative studies in the genus *Coelomomyces* Keilin. *Diss. Abstr.* **22,** 2560.

Uskakova, G. V. (1962). On the findings of *Hunterellus hookeri,* How., parasites of ixodid ticks in Kazakhstan. *Trud. Inst. Zool. Akad. Nauk Kazakh. SSR* **16,** 183-185. (In Russian.) (NAMRU 3 mimeographed document, 98–T98.)

Varley, G. C. and Butler, C. G. (1933). The acceleration of development of insects by parasitism. *Parasitology* **25,** 263-268.

Vasconcelos, A. B. (1923). The algae of the genus *Chara* and mosquito larvae. *Am. J. Publ. Hlth* **13,** 543-546.

Vercammen-Grandjean, P. H. (1955). Un genre nouveau: *Durenia,* dans la sous famille des Trombellinae (Trombidiidae: Acarina). *Revue Zool. Bot. afr.* **52,** 252-260. (Mites from culicine and aedine mosquitoes.)

Vercammen-Grandjean, P. H. (1956). Un nouveau Trombidiidae larvaire parasite de divers Culicoides originaires d'Ecosse *Evansiella culicoides* n.g., n.sp. (Acarina). *Ann. Mag. nat. Hist.* **10,** 283-286.

Veremchuk, G. V. (1962). The entomohelminth family Steinernematidae Chitwood and Chitwood, 1937. *Tezisy doklad, naučn. konf. Vses. obščč. gelmintologov, Akad. Nauk SSR, Moscow* **1,** 24-25. (In Russian.)

Wahlberg, B. (1847). Bidrag till Kännedomen om Stickmyggorna och deras fiender. Öfversigt af Kengl. *Vet.-Akad. Förhandl. Årg.* **4,** 257-259. (Records empid flies attacking mosquitoes.)

Wallace, F. G. (1961). Criteria for the differentiation of genera among the trypanosomid parasites of insects. *Prog. Protozool., Proc. 1st Int. Conf. Protozool., Prague, Aug. 22-31,* 70-74.

Walters, H. S. (1962). The morphology and life cycle of certain microsporidian parasites found in mosquitoes. Thesis, Pretoria, 126 pp.

Warren, A. (1915). A study of the food habits of Hawaiian dragonflies. *Coll. Hawaii Publ. Bull.* **3,** 1-45. (Chironomid larvae and ostracods were the commonest components of the gut contents of larval *Anax* and *Pantala anisopterans.)*

Waterston, J. (1919). Notes on the morphology of Chalcidoidea bred from *Calliphora. Parasitology* **9,** 109-198.

Watson, J. M. (1945). A new sporozoan *Gregarina rhyparobiae* n.sp. from a tropical cockroach *Rhyparobia maderae. Parasitology* **36,** 195-198.

Weidner, H. (1950). Die Malariamückenbrutplätze Nord Griechenlands und ihre Sammlung. *Z. angew. Ent.* **32,** 86-133.

Weiser, J. (1943). Zur Kenntnis der Mikrosporidien ans Chironomiden-Larven I. *Zool. Anz.* **140,** 126-128.

Weiss, E., Myers, W. F., Suitor, E. C., Jr. and Neptune, E. M., Jr. (1962). Respiration of a rickettsia-like microorganism, *Wolbachia persica*. *J. infect. Dis.* **110**, 155-164.
Welch, H. E. (1962). New species of *Gastromermis, Isomermis* and *Mesomermis* (Nematoda: Mermithidae) from blackfly larvae. *Ann. ent. Soc. Am.* **55**, 535-542.
Welch, H. E. and Bronskill, J. F. (1962). Parasitism of mosquito larvae by the nematode, DD136 (Nematoda: Neoaplectanidae). *Can. J. Zool.* **40**, 1263-1268.
Wenyon, C. M. (1912). Observations on the natural flagellates of fleas, including a confirmation of Noller's important results on the transmission of *Trypanosoma lewisi* by the dog flea. *Rep. Advis. Comm. Trop. Dis. Res. Found., Rep. Protozoologist Lond. Sch. Trop. Med.*, pp. 90-91.
Wesenberg-Lund, C. (1943). "Biologie der Süsswasserinsekten", Gyldendalske Boghandel, Copenhagen. (The leech *Erpobdella octoculata* L. is said to feed mainly on mosquito larvae.)
Weurman, C. (1946). Investigations concerning the symbiosis of bacteria in *Triatoma infestans* (Klug.) Antonie Leenuenhoek. *Ned. Tijdschri. hyg. microbiol. serologie* (Amsterdam) **11**, 129-138.
Whiting, P. W. and Bush, D. J. (1959). Maintaining stocks in *Mormoniella. Proc. Pennsylvania Acad. Sci.* **33**, 248-251. (Entomophagous parasite of Muscidae.)
Williams, J. R. and Pickering, G. (1962). An attempt to control the development of *Musca domestica* L. in poultry faeces using feed additives of *Bacillus thuringiensis* Berliner. *Brit. poultry Sci.* **3**, 195-201.
Williams, R. E., Delong, D. M. and Venard, C. (1961). Observations on *Toxorhynchites rutilus septentrionalis* (Dyar and Knab) in the field and laboratory (Diptera: Culicidae). *Ann. ent. Soc. Am.* **54**, 669-671.
Wistreich, G. A. and Chao, J. (1961). Microorganisms from the mid-gut of larval and adult *Aedes sierrensis* (Ludlow) and *Anopheles albimanus* Wiedemann. *J. Insect Path.* **3**, 274-279.
Wollman, E. (1926). Observations sur un lignée aseptique de blattes *(Blattella germanica)* datant de cinq ans. *C.r. hebd. Séanc. Soc. Biol.* **95**, 164-165.
Womersley, H. (1956). On some new Acarina-Mesostigmata from Australia, New Zealand and New Guinea. *J. Linn. Soc. Lond. Zool.* **42**, 505-599. (Ectoparasitic mite from a cockroach.)
Wülker, W. (1958). Parasitäre Intersexualität bei Chironomiden des Schluchsees. *Gew. u. Abwässer* **20**, 61-67.
Wülker, W. (1960). Neue Ergebnisse zur parasitären Intersexualität der Chironomiden (Dipt.). *Naturwissenschaften* **47**, 21-22.
Wülker, W. (1961). Untersuchungen über die Intersexualität der Chironomiden (Dipt.) nach *Paramermis*-Infektion. *Arch. Hydrobiol., Suppl.* **25**, 127-181.
Wülker, W. (1962). Parasitäre und nicht parasitäre geschlechtliche Aberrationen bei Chironomiden. *Zool. Anz. Suppl.* **25**, 132-139.
Wylie, H. G. (1962). An effect of host age on female longevity and fecundity in *Nasonia vitripennis* (Walk.) (Hymenoptera: Pteromalidae). *Can. Ent.* **94**, 990-993.
Young, M. D. (1935). Description, incidence and cultivation of *Tetratrichomastix blattidarum*, n.sp. from the cockroach *(Blattella, Periplaneta)*. *J. Parasit.* **21**, 309-310.
Zaman, V., Fernando, C. H. and Chellapah, W. T. (1962). The agar gel-diffusion technique as a means of tracing mosquito antigens in the water bug, *Anisops breddini* (Notonectidae). *Med. J. Malaya* **17**, 90.

II. List of References for 1963-1967 Inclusive

Abbassian-Lintzen, R. (1965). A male of *Tabanus* sp. was observed to be captured by a small wolf spider in Khuzestän, southwestern Iran, in the spring of 1964. (Personal commun., 22 Dec. 1965.)
Adhami, U. M. and Craig, G. B., Jr. (1965). Predation of *Bradysia coprophila* (Lint.) (Diptera: Sciaridae) on mosquito larvae. *Mosquito News* **25**, 487-488.

Amonkar, S. V. (1965). Pathogenicity of *Aspergillus flavus* Link to *Musca domestica nebulo* Fabricius. *J. Invertebrate Path.* 7, 513-514.

Anderson, J. R. (1964). The behaviour and ecology of various flies associated with poultry ranches in Northern California. *Proc. Pap. 32nd Annual Conf. Calif. Mosquito Control Ass., Inc.*, 30-34. (Pathogens and predators are mentioned, the latter including larval *Ophyra leucostoma* Wied. (Diptera) which kill maggots of, e.g. *Musca domestica, M. stabulans* and *Fannia canicularis,* apparently by injecting a toxin into the body cavity.)

Anderson, J. R. and Poorbaugh, J. H. (1964a). Biological control possibility for house flies. *California Agriculture* **18,** 2-4. (The black garbage fly, *Ophyra leucostoma,* is an efficient larval predator.)

Anderson, J. R. and Poorbaugh, J. H. (1964b). Observations on the ethology and ecology of various Diptera associated with northern Californian poultry ranches. *J. med. Ent.* **1,** 131-147. (Sticky-tape fly population sampling also caught entomophagous parasites and other natural enemies.)

Anderson, L. D., Bay, E. C. and Ingram, A. A. (1964). Studies of chironomid midge control in water-spreading basins near Montebello, California. *Calif. Vector Views* **11,** 13-20. (Mentions birds, particularly such shore birds as the least sandpiper, *Pisobia minutilla,* as midge larval predators.)

Andrade, Z. A., Paula, L. A., Sherlock, I. A. and Cheever, A. W. (1967). Nasal granuloma caused by *Entomophthora coronata. Am. J. trop. Med. Hyg.* **16,** 31-33. (First Brazilian record of human infection with this pathogen of muscoid flies.)

Anon. (1964). Research Report 1962-63, Research Institute, Belleville, Ontario. (In this and in Anon. 1967b and 1967c is much information on research concerning the natural enemies and diseases of insects of public health importance.)

Anon. (1965a). Lutte biologique contre les vecteurs des maladies. *In* "La Lutte Biologique", Chapter IX, pp. 69-72. Délégation Générale a la Recherche Sci. Tech., Rapp. Gén. Comm. d'Etudes, Suppl. *Le Progrès Scientifique,* Paris, 119 pp.

Anon. (1965b). Summary of research for 1964 and objectives for 1965. *State of California Dep. Publ. Hlth, Bur. Vector Control,* mimeographed document, 33 pp. (Microsporidan, gregarine, bacterial and viral pathogens.)

Anon. (1967a). International Advisory Committee for Biological Control, Biological Information Bulletin No. 2, 72 pp. (Secty. F. J. Simmonds, CIBC, Curepe, Trinidad). (Pp. 55-64: note several American projects in public health entomology, indicating the availability of stocks of, e.g. various entomophagous parasites of *Musca domestica, Hippelates* spp. etc.)

Anon. (1967b). Research Report 1964-65, Research Institute, Belleville, Ontario.

Anon. (1967c). Research Report 1966, Research Institute, Belleville, Ontario.

Aragâo, M. B. (1967). Equilíbrio da natureza e contróle biológico. *Malariologia e doencas tropicais* **19,** 655-695.

Artyukhovsky, A. K. and Kolycheva, R. V. (1965). On the mermitosis of mosquitoes of the genus *Aedes* in the bottomland of the Khoper River. *Zool. Zh.* **44,** 454-455. (In Russian.)

Aspöck, H. (1966). Parasitierung eines im Freiland aufgefundenen Intersexes von *Aedes (Ochlerotatus) communis* de Geer *(Insecta, Culicidae)* durch einen Pilz der Ordnung *Blastocladiales. Ztschr. Morph. Okol. Tiere* **57,** 231-243.

Axtell, R. C. (1963a). Manure-inhabiting Macrochelidae (Acarina: Mesostigmata) predaceous on the house fly. *Adv. Acarology* **1,** 55-59.

Axtell, R. C. (1963b). Effect of Macrochelidae (Acarina: Mesostigmata) on house fly production from dairy cattle manure. *J. econ. Ent.* **56,** 317-321.

Axtell, R. C. (1963c). Acarina occurring in domestic animal manure. *Ann. ent. Soc. Am.* **56,** 628-633.

Axtell, R. C. (1964). Phoretic relationship of some common manure-inhabiting Macrochelidae (Acarina: Mesostigmata) to the house fly. *Ann. ent. Soc. Am.* **57,** 584-587.

Axtell, R. C. (1966). Comparative toxicities of insecticides to house fly larvae and *Macrocheles muscaedomesticae,* a mite predator of the house fly. *J. econ. Ent.* **59,** 1128-1130.

Axtell, R. C. (1967). Macrochelidae (Acarina: Mesostigmata) as biological control agents for synanthropic flies. *Proc. 2nd Int. Congr. Acarology,* Nottingham, England, 19-25 July 1967. (40 pp. typescript.)

Azab, A. K., Tawfik, M. F. S. and Awadallah, K. T. (1964). Insect enemies of common flies in Giza Region. *Bull. Soc. ent. Egypte* **47** (1963), 277-286. (Dermestid beetle predators and various entomophaga.)

Bailey, D. L., Barnes, W. W. and Dewey, R. W. (1967a). *Stempellia magna* (Kudo) (Nosematidae: Microsporidia) in *Culex restuans* Theobald from Virginia. *Mosquito News* **27,** 111-114.

Bailey, D. L., Barnes, W. W. and Dewey, R. W. (1967b). A new Maryland record of *Thelohania* (Nosematidae: Microsporidia). *J. Invertebrate Path.* **9,** 354-356. (Host, *Aedes canadensis.*)

Balay, G. and Grenier, P. (1964). *Lispe nivalis* Wiedemann (Muscidae: Lispinae), et *Ochthera* sp. (Ephydridae), Diptères prédateurs de *Simulium damnosum* Theobald et *S. adersi* Pomeroy, en Haute-Volta. *Bull. Soc. Path. exot.* **57,** 611-619.

Batko, A. (1964a). Remarks on the genus *Entomophthora* Fresenius 1856 non Nowakowski 1883 *(Phycomycetes: Entomophthoraceae). Bull. Acad. Polon. Sci., Ser. Sci. biol.* **12,** 319-321.

Batko, A. (1964b). Remarks on the genus *Lamia* Nowakowski 1883 vs. *Culicicola* Nieuwland 1916 *(Phycomycetes: Entomophthoraceae). Bull. Acad. Polon. Sci., Sér. sci. biol.* **12,** 399-402.

Batko, A. (1964c). Some new combinations in the fungus family *Entomophthoraceae (Phycomycetes). Bull. Acad. Polon. Sci., Sér. sci. biol.* **12,** 403-406.

Batko, A. (1964d). Notes on entomophthoraceous fungi in Poland. *Entomophaga, Mém. hors. Sér.* No. 2, 129-131. (*Entomophthora calliphorae* Giard recorded from *Calliphora erythrocephala* Mg. on elm leaves.)

Batko, A. (1964e). Studies on the entomophthoraceous fungi in Poland. Ph.D. Thesis, University of Warsaw. (In Polish.)

Bay, E. C. (1964). An analysis of the "sayule" (Diptera: Chironomidae) nuisance at San Carlos, Nicaragua, and recommendations for its alleviation. *W.H.O. mimeogr. docum.,* WHO/EBL/20, 18 pp. (Potential invertebrate predators of chironomid midge larvae in this area include *Coelotanypus* larvae, leeches (*Helobdella* sp.), and other customary natural enemies including dytiscid beetles and dragonfly larvae. Communal-web spiders (*Tetragnatha* sp.) captured large numbers of adult midges. Many larvae were parasitized by mermithid nematodes.)

Bay, E. C. (1967). Potential for naturalistic control of mosquitoes. *Proc. 35th Ann. Conf. Calif. Mosq. Control Ass. Inc., and Am. Mosq. Control Ass.* pp. 34-37.

Bay, E. C. and Legner, E. F. (1963a). The prospects for the biological control of *Hippelates collusor* (Townsend) in Southern California. *Proc. 31st Ann. Conf. Calif. Mosq. Control Ass. Inc.,* pp. 76-79.

Bay, E. C. and Legner, E. F. (1963b). Quality control in the production of *Hippelates collusor* (Tsnd.) for use in the search and rearing of their natural enemies. *Proc. 50th Ann. Mtg N.J. Mosq. Exterm. Assn and 19th Ann. Meet. Am. Mosq. Control Ass.* pp. 403-410.

Bay, E. C., Legner, E. F. and Medved, R. (1964). *Hippelates collusor* (Diptera: Chloropidae) as a host for four species of parasitic Hymenoptera in Southern California. *Ann. ent. Soc. Am.* **57,** 582-584.

Beam, F. D. (1966). Mortality of *Aedes sollicitans* Walker due to a high microfilaremia of dog heartworm, *Dirofilaria immitis* Leidy. *Proc. N.J. Mosq. Exterm. Assn* **53,** pp. 117-126.

Beard, R. L. (1963). Fighting the face fly. Biological control is far from simple. *Frontiers Plant Sci.* **16,** 4.

Beard, R. L. (1964a). Pathogenic stinging of house-fly pupae by *Nasonia vitripennis* (Walker). *J. Insect Path.* **6**, 1-7.
Beard, R. L. (1964b). Parasites of muscoid flies. (Symposium on culture procedures for arthropod vectors and their biological control agents, Gainesville, Florida, 30 Sept.-4th Oct. 1963.) *Bull. Wld Hlth Org.* **31**, 491-493.
Beard, R. L. and Walton, G. S. (1965). An *Aspergillus* toxin lethal to larvae of the house fly. *J. Invertebrate Path.* 7, 522-523.
Beaucournu, J-C. and Chabaud, A-G. (1963). Infestation spontanée de puces par le spiruride *Mastophorus muris* (Gmelin). *Ann. Parasit. hum. comp.* **38**, 931-934.
Beaudoin, R. and Wills, W. (1965). A description of *Caudospora pennsylvanica* sp.n. (Caudosporidae, Microsporidia), a parasite of the larvae of the black fly, *Prosimulium magnum* Dyar and Shannon. *J. Invertebrate Path.* **7**, 152-155.
Beirne, B. P. (1964). Integrated controls for pest damage. *Agric. Inst. Rev., Nov.-Dec. 1964,* 13-15. (Joint use of mermithid nematodes and larvicides against mosquitoes.)
Beirne, B. P. (1965). Present and future role of parasites and predators for insect control. *W.H.O. mimeogr. docum.*, WHO/EBL/35.65. 12 pp.
Belizin, V. I. (1963). Cynipid parasites of synanthropic flies in Uzbekistan (Hymenoptera, Cynipoidea). *Zool. Zh.* **42,** 1652-1658. (In Russian.)
Bennett, F. D. (1966). Commonw. Inst. Biol. Control Rep., Curepe, Trinidad, pp. 1-5, mimeogr.
Bennett, F. D. (1967). Control of houseflies, stableflies and fruitflies in Mauritius (Project 9: for Mauritius) Commonw. Inst. Biol. Control, Rep. of work carried out during 1966 (p.67, in 86 pp. mimeogr. docum. 31 Jan. 1967, Curepe, Trinidad reports (introduction of *Pachycrepoides vindemiae, Spalangia cameroni* and *Muscidifurax raptor* against houseflies and stableflies.)
Bennett, F. D. and Legner, E. G. (1967). Memorandum on the possibilities of biological control of the muscoid flies by hymenopterous parasites. *W.H.O. mimeogr. docum.*, WHO/VBC/67.22. 10 pp.
Benz, G. (1963). Arthropoden-Viren. *Viert. Nat. Ges. Zurich* **108,** 1-35. (A classification.)
Bettini, S. (1965). Acquired immune response of the house fly, *Musca domestica* (Linnaeus), to injected venom of the spider *Latrodectus mactans tredecimguttatus* (Rossi). *J. Invertebrate Path.* **7**, 378-383.
Bhasker, Rao, T. (1963). On *Rhizomastix periplanetae* n.sp., from *Periplaneta americana* of Hyderabad A.P., India. *Riv. Parassit.* **24,** 159-162.
Borgatti, A. L. and Guyer, G. E. (1963). The effectiveness of commercial formulations of *Bacillus thuringiensis* Berliner on house-fly larvae. *J. Insect Path.* **5,** 377-384.
Bouček, Z. (1963). A taxomomic study in *Spalangia* Latr. (Hymenoptera, Chalcidoidea). *Acta Ent. Mus. Nat. Prague* **35,** 429-512.
Bourne, J. R. and Nielsson, R. J. (1967). *Nemobius fasciatus*—a predator on horn fly pupae. *J. econ. Ent.* **60,** 272-274. (Crickets as predators on dung-breeding flies.)
Bracken, G. K. and Barlow, J. S. (1967). Fatty acid composition of *Exeristes comstockii* (Cress) reared on different hosts. *Can. J. Zool.* **45,** 57-61.
Brady, J. (1963). Results of age-grouping dissections on four species of *Anopheles* from southern Ghana. *Bull. Wld Hlth Org.* **29,** 147-153. (*Coelomomyces* in ovaries of *Anopheles gambiae.*)
Bras, G., Gordon, C. C., Emmons, C. W., Prendegast, K. M. and Sugar, M. (1965). A case of phycomycosis observed in Jamaica; infection with *Entomophthora coronata. Am. J. trop. Med. Hyg.* **14,** 141-145. (First case of phycomycosis reported from Jamaica, and first human infection with *E. coronata.*)
Briand, L. J. and Welch, H. E. (1963). Use of rhabditoid nematode, DD136, for control of mosquitoes. (Abstract) *Proc. 99th Ann. Meet. ent. Soc. Ontario,* p. 131. (Nematodes reduced mosquito emergence in plastic pools.)
Briggs, J. D. (1964). Mass propagation of bacteria pathogenic for insects. *Bull. Wld Hlth Org.* **31,** 495-497.
Briggs, J. D. (1966). 1965 activities of the WHO International Reference Centre for diagnosis of diseases of vectors. *W.H.O. mimeogr. docum.*, WHO/EBL/66.73, 8 pp.

Briggs, J. D. (1967). 1966 activities of the WHO International Reference Centre for diagnosis of diseases of vectors. *W.H.O. mimeogr. docum.*, WHO/VBC/67.8, 8 pp.

Brooks, M. A. (1964). Symbiotes and the nutrition of medically important insects. *Bull. Wld Hlth Org.* **31**, 555-559.

Brooks, M. A. and Richards, K. (1966). On the *in vitro* culture of intracellular symbiotes of cockroaches. *J. Invertebrate Path.* **8**, 150-157.

Bucher, G. E. (1964). The regulation and control of insects by fungi. *Ann. Ent. Soc. Quebec* **9**, 30-42.

Burgerjon, A. and Galichet, P. F. (1965). The effectiveness of the heat-stable toxin of *Bacillus thuringiensis* var. *thuringiensis* Berliner on larvae of *Musca domestica* Linnaeus. *J. Invertebrate Path.* **7**, 263-264.

Burton, G. J. (1963). Feeding of *Mansonia titillans* (Wullman) on other mosquitoes. *Mosquito News* **23**, 164.

Büttiker, W. (1967). Biological notes on eye-frequenting moths from N. Thailand. *Mitt. Schweiz. Ent. Gesells.* **39**, 151-179. (Mermithid parasite.)

Cali, C. T. and Mai, W. F. (1965). Studies on the development of *Blatticola blattae* Graeffe 1860 Chitwood 1932 within its host, *Blattella germanica* L. *Proc. helminth. Soc. Wash.* **32**, 164-169.

Cantwell, G. E. and Laird, M. (1966). The World Health Organization kit for the collection and shipment of pathogens and parasites of diseased vectors. *J. Invertebrate Path.* **8**, 442-451.

Chabora, P. C. and Pimental, D. (1966). Effect of host (*Musca domestica* Linnaeus) age on the pteromalid parasite *Nasonia vitripennis* (Walker). *Can. ent.* **98**, 1226-1231.

Chao, J., Wistreich, G. A. and Moore, J. (1963). Failure to isolate microorganisms from within mosquito eggs. *Ann. ent. Soc. Am.* **56**, 559-561.

Chapman, H. C. (1964-67). Quarterly Reports, Insects Affecting Man and Animals Research Laboratory, U.S.D.A Lake Charles, Louisiana, U.S.A. (Information on candidate biological control agents, especially pathogens of mosquitoes.)

Chapman, H. C. (1967). A survey of Nauru Island for mosquitoes and their internal pathogens and parasites. *W.H.O. mimeogr. docum.*, WHO/VBC/67.28, 11 pp.

Chapman, H. C., Clarke, T. B., Woodard, D. B. and Kellen, W. R. (1966). Additional mosquito hosts for mosquito iridescent virus (MIV). *J. Invertebrate Path.* **8**, 545-546.

Chapman, H. C. and Kellen, W. R. (1967). *Plistophora caecorum* sp.n., a microsporidian of *Culiseta inornata* (Diptera: Culicidae) from Louisiana. *J. Invertebrate Path.* **9**, 500-502.

Chapman, H. C. and Woodard, D. B. (1966a). *Coelomomyces* infections in Louisiana mosquitoes. *1966 Progm, 22nd Ann. Meet. Am. Mosq. Contr. Assn. 6-9 March*, No. 10, p. 15. ENT, ARS, USDA, McNeese State College, Lake Charles, La.

Chapman, H. C. and Woodard, D. B. (1966b). *Coelomomyces* (Blastocladiales: Coelomomy*cetaceae*) infections in Louisiana mosquitoes. *Mosquito News* **26**, 121-123.

Chapman, H. C., Woodard, D. B., Kellen, W. R. and Clark, T. B. (1966). Host-parasite relationships of *Thelohania* associated with mosquitoes in Louisiana (Nosematidae: Microsporidia). *J. Invertebrate Path.* **8**, 452-456.

Chapman, H. C., Woodard, D. B. and Petersen, J. J. (1967a). Pathogens and parasites in Louisiana Culicidae and Chaoboridae. *Proc. 54th Ann. Meet. New Jers. Exterm. Assn*, pp. 55-59.

Chapman, H. C., Woodard, D. B. and Petersen, J. J. (1967b). Nematode parasites of Culicidae and Chaoboridae in Louisiana. *Mosquito News* **27**, 490-492.

Chastel, C., Rageau, J. and Abonnenc, E. (1966). Présence de *Culicoides anophelis* Edwards, 1922 (Diptera: Ceratopogonidae) au Cambodge. *Bull. Soc. Path. exot.* **59**, 151-155.

Cheng, T. H. (1963). Insect control in mainland China. *Science* **140**, 269-277. (*Pseudobagrus fulvidraco* predacious on mosquito larvae.)

Cheong, W. H. and Ganapathipillae, A. (1964). Preliminary observations on the aquatic stages of *Toxorhynchites* (Diptera: Culicidae) in Malaya. *Med. J. Malaya* **19**, 58.

Chu, Wei Shuang and Toumanoff, C. (1966). Rapport préliminaire sur la flore bactérienne accompagnant les mortalités des larves des *Culicides* dans les conditions d'élevage. *W.H.O. mimeogr. docum.*, WHO/EBL/66.74, 81 pp.

Clark, T. B. (1966). A method for the inoculation of mosquito larvae. *J. Invertebrate Path.* **8**, 425-426.

Clark, T. B. and Fukuda, T. (1967). *Stempellia magna* in the tree hole mosquito, *Aedes sierrensis. J. Invertebrate Path.* **9**, 430-431.

Clark, T. B., Kellen, W. R., Fukuda, T. and Lindegren, J. E. (1967). Experiments on the biological control of mosquitoes with the fungus *Beauveria bassiana* (Bals.) Vuill. *Proc. Calif. Mosq. Control Ass.* **35**, 99.

Clark, T. B., Kellen, W. R. and Lindegren, J. E. (1963). Axenic culture of two trichomycetes from Californian mosquitoes. *Nature, Lond.* **197**, 208-209.

Clark, T. B., Kellen, W. R., Lindegren, J. E. and Sanders, R. D. (1966). *Pythium* sp. (Phycomycetes: Pythiales) pathogenic to mosquito larvae. *J. Invertebrate Path.* **8**, 351-354.

Clark, T. B., Kellen, W. R. and Lum, T. M. (1965). A mosquito iridescent virus (MIV) from *Aedes taeniorhynchus* (Wiedemann). *J. Invertebrate Path.* **7**, 519-521.

Coelho, M. de V. and Falcão, A. L. (1964). Aspects of the life cycle of *Monocystis chagasi* Adler and Mayrink 1961, in *Phlebotomus longipalpus. Rev. Brasil Biol.* **24**, 417-421.

Cole, M. M. (1965). Biological control of ticks by the use of hymenopterous parasites. A review. *W.H.O. mimeogr. docum.*, WHO/EBL/43.65, 12 pp.

Coluzzi, M. (1963). Osservazioni sui parassiti dei Culicidi e sul loro eventuale impiego nella lotta biologica. *In* "Relazione Annuale del Lavorosvolto dalla Stazione Sperimentale di Monticelli", pp. 39-48. Frosinone, Italy. (Fungal genera *Rubetella, Saprolegnia* and *Coelomomyces.*)

Coluzzi, M. (1966). Experimental infections with *Rubetella* fungi in *Anopheles gambiae* and other mosquitoes. *Proc. 1st Int. Congr. Parasit.*, Rome, 1964, I, 592-593.

Conner, R. M. and Hansen, P. A. (1967). Effect of valine, leucine and isoleucine on the production of fly toxin by *Bacillus thuringiensis* and related organisms. *J. Invertebrate Path.* **9**, 114-125.

Corbet, P. S. (1963a). Observations on *Toxorhynchites brevipalpis conradti* Grunb. (Diptera: Culicidae) in Uganda. *Bull. ent. Res.* **54**, 9-17.

Corbet, P. S. (1963b). The reliability of parasitic water-mites (Hydracarina) as indicators of physiological age in mosquitoes (Diptera: Culicidae). *Ent. exp. appl.* **6**, 215-233.

Corbet, P. S. and Griffiths, A. (1963). Observations on the aquatic stages of two species of *Toxorhynchites* (Diptera: Culicidae) in Uganda. *Proc. R. ent. Soc. Lond.* (A) **38**, 125-135.

Cosgrove, W. B. (1966). Acriflavin-induced akinetoplasty in *Crithidia fasciculata. Acta Protozool.* **4**, 155-161.

Costa, M. (1966). Notes on macrochelids associated with manure and coprid beetles in Israel. 1. *Macrocheles robustus* (Berlese, 1904), development and biology. *Acarologia* **8**, 532-548.

Couch, J. N. (1967). Sporangial germination in *Coelomomyces punctatus* and infection of *Anopheles quadrimaculatus. Abstr. Joint U.S.-Japan Semin. Microbial Control Insect Pests,* pp. 34-35. U.S.-Japan Committee Sci. Cooperation. Panel 8. Fukuoka.

Coz, J. (1966). Contribution à l'étude du parasitisme des adultes d'*Anopheles funestus* par *Gastromermis* sp. (Mermithidae). *Bull. Soc. Path. exot.* **59**, 881-889. Also *W.H.O. mimeogr. docum.*, WHO/EBL/66.76, 11 pp.

Dabrowska-Prôt, E. (1966). Experimental studies on the reduction of the abundance of mosquitoes by spiders. II. Activity of mosquitoes in cages. *Bull. Acad. Polon. Sci.* **14**, 771-775.

Dabrowska-Prôt, E., Luczak, J. and Tarwid, K. (1966). Experimental studies on the reduction of the abundance of mosquitoes by spiders. III. Indices of prey reduction and some controlling factors. *Bull. Acad. Polon. Sci.* **14**, 777-782.

Dale, P. S. (1966). *Blatticola tuapakae* and *Protrellina gurri* n.spp., nematode parasites of the black roach. *N.Z. Jl. Sci.* **9**, 538-544.

Damodar, P., Perti, S. L. and Agarwal, P. N. (1964). The toxicity of solvent extract of the fungus, *Macrosporium* sp. to flies and mosquitoes. *Indian J. Ent.* **26**, 110-112.

Dary, M. R. and Camay, L. (1966). Preliminary note on a survey for parasites of *Anopheles* larvae in Guatemala, as a contribution to relevant biological control research. *W.H.O. mimeogr. docum.*, WHO/EBL/66.75, 6 pp.

Das Gupta, S. K. (1964a). *Culicoides (Trichecoides) anophelis* Edwards (Insecta: Diptera: Ceratopogonidae) as an ectoparasite of insect vectors. *Proc. zool. Soc., Calcutta* **17,** 1-20.

Das Gupta, S. K. (1964b). Mermithid infections in two nematoceran insects. *Curr. Sci.* **33,** 55.

Desportes, I. (1966). L'ultrastructure de la jonction entre la primite et le satellite des associations de *Gregarina blattarum* Sieb. (Eugregarines: Gregarinidae). *C.r. hebd. Séanc. Acad. Sci., Paris,* D **262,** 1869-1870.

Dinther, J. B. M. van (1965). Egg-consumption by *Bembidion ustulatum* and *B. lampros* (Fam. Carabidae) in laboratory prey-density experiments with housefly eggs. *Int. Symp. Crop Prot., 17th Symp.,* p. 103.

Dinther, J. B. M. van (1966). Laboratory experiments on the consumption capacities of some Carabidae. *Meded. Rijskfac. Landbouw. Wet Gent* **31,** 730-739. (Predators on Muscidae.)

Dinther, J. B. M. van and Mensink, F. T. (1965). Egg consumption by *Bembidion ustulatum* and *Bembidion lampros* (Fam. Carabidae) in laboratory prey density experiments with housefly eggs. *Meded. LandbHoogesch. OpzoekStns Gent* **30,** 1542-1554.

Doane, C. C. (1964). Field tests with an aerial application of *Bacillus thuringiensis. Bull. Connecticut Agric. Exp. Stn (New Haven)* **665,** 1-20.

Dodge, H. R. (1964). Larval chaetotaxy and notes on the biology of *Toxorhynchites rutilus septentrionalis* (Diptera: Culicidae). *Ann. ent. Soc. Am.* **57,** 46-53.

Drea, J. J. (1966). Studies of *Aleochara tristis* (Coleoptera: Staphylinidae), a natural enemy of the face fly. *J. econ. Ent.* **59,** 1368-1373.

Dupuis, C. (1964). Contributions a l'étude des *Phasiinae* cimicophages (Diptères Tachinaires). 30–Notes biogeographiques et taxonomiques sur quatre espèces framfaises peu connues. *Cahiers Nat. Paris* **20,** 89-98.

Dutky, S. R. (1967). An appraisal of the DD 136 nematode for the control of insect populations and some biochemical aspects of its host-parasite relationships. *In Abstr. Joint U.S.-Japan Semin. Microbial Control Insect Pests,* pp. 49-50. U.S.-Japan Committee Sci. Cooperation. Panel 8. Fukuoka. (Successful tests against houseflies in chicken houses.)

Dutky, S. R., Thompson, J. V. and Cantwell, G. E. (1964). A technique for the mass propagation of the DD-136 nematode. *J. Insect Path.* **6,** 417-422.

Efford, I. E. (1963). The parasitic ecology of some watermites. *J. anim. Ecol.* **32,** 141-156.

Emmons, C. W. (1964). Phycomycosis in man and animals. *Riv. Patol. veg, Padova* **4,** (Ser. III), 329-337. (Rhinophycomycosis caused by *Entomophthora coronata;* a new record from Nigeria is included.)

Fain, A. (1964). Observations sur la biologie de *Cordylobia ruandae* et de son hôte *Grammomys dolichurus surdanter* en Rwanda. Parasitisme des pupes de cette mouche par des chalcidoides. *Ann. Soc. Belge Méd. trop. Parasit. Mycol.* **44,** 1095-1104. (*C. ruandae* is a calliphorid.)

Farish, D. J. (1965). Some aspects of the sensory and phoretic behaviour of *Macrocheles muscaedomesticae* (Scopoli, 1772) (Acarina: Macrochelidae) with a consideration of phoresy as a phenomenon. M.S. Thesis, North Carolina State Univ., Raleigh, N.C., U.S.A. 181 pp.

Farish, D. J. and Axtell, R. C. (1966). Sensory functions of the palps and first tarsi of *Macrocheles muscaedomesticae* (Acarina: Macrochelidae), a predator of the housefly. *Ann. ent. Soc. Am.* **59,** 165-170.

Farr, D. F. and Lichtwardt, R. W. (1967). Some cultural and ultrastructural aspects of *Smittium culisetae (Trichomycetes)* from mosquito larvae. *Mycologia* **59,** 172-182.

Feigin, J. M. (1963). Exposure of the house fly to selection by *Bacillus thuringiensis. Ann. ent. Soc. Am.* **56,** 878-879.

Feldman-Muhsam, B. and Havivi, Y. (1963). On *Adlerocystis* n.gen. *(Phycomycetes)* a symbiote of *Ornithodoros* ticks. *Parasitology* **53,** 183-188.

Feldman-Muhsam, B. and Havivi, Y. (1966). Symbiotes of spermiophores of ticks of the genus *Ornithodoros. Proc. 1st Int. Congr. Parasit.,* Rome, 21-26. Sept. 1964 **2,** 1052-1055.

Fenley, W. R. (1966). Field observations of *Aedes ventrovittis* Dyar (Diptera: Culicidae) parasitized by *Panisopsis* sp. (Acarina: Thyasidae). *Mosquito News* **26,** 583-584.

Field, G., Savage, L. B. and Duplessis, R. J. (1966). Note on the cockroach mite *Pimeliaphilus cunliffei* (Acarina: Pterygosomidae) infesting oriental, German and American cockroaches. *J. econ. Ent.* **59,** 1532.

Filipponi, A. (1964). The feasibility of mass producing macrochelid mites for field trials against houseflies. *Bull. Wld Hlth Org.* **31,** 499-501.

Filipponi, A. (1967). Autoecologia e capacita' moltiplicata di *Macrocheles muscae-domesticae* (Scopoli) (Acari: Mesostigmata). *Riv. Parassit.* **28,** 129-156.

Filipponi, A. and Delupis, G. D. di (1963a). Sulla biologia e capacita' riproduttiva di *Macrocheles peniculatus* Berlese (Acari: Mesostigmata) in condizioni sperimentale di laboratorio. *Riv. Parassit.* **24,** 93-111.

Filipponi, A. and Delupis, G. D. di (1963b). Sul regime dietetico di alcuni macrochelidi (Acari: Mesostigmata) associati in natura a muscidi di interesse sanitario. *Riv. Parassit.* **24,** 277-288.

Filipponi, A. and Francaviglia, G. (1963). Oviparita' e larviparita' in *Macrocheles peniculatus* Berl. (Acari: Mesostigmata) regolate da fattori ecologici. *Riv. Parassit.* **24,** 81-104.

Filipponi, A. and Francaviglia, G. (1964). Larviparita facoltativo in alcuni Macrochelidi (Acari: Mesostigmata) associati a muscidi di interesse sanitario. *Parassitologia* **6,** 99-113.

Filshie, B. K., Grace, T. D. C., Poulson, D. F. and Rehacek, J. (1967). Virus-like particles in insect cells of three types. *J. Invertebrate Path.* **9,** 271-273. (Includes *Aedes aegypti.*)

Fischer, Z. (1964). Some observations concerning the food consumption of the dragonfly larvae of *Erythromma najas* Hans. and *Coenagrion hastulatum* Charp. *Polsk. Arch. Hydrobiol.* **12,** 253-254. (In Polish.) (*Culex* sp. among prey.)

Fisher, F. M. and Sanborn, R. C. (1964). *Nosema* as a source of juvenile hormone in parasitized insects. *Biol. Bull.* **126,** 235-252.

Fisher, T. W. (1964). Shipping techniques for entomophagous insects. *Bull. Wld Hlth Org.* **31,** 503-504.

Flanders, S. E. and Bay, E. C. (1964). Standardization of mass rearing procedures for entomophaga. *Bull. Wld Hlth Org.* **31,** 505-507.

Foster, R. (1963). Infestation of *Glossina palpalis* R.-D. 1830 (Diptera) by larval Mermithidae Braun 1883 (Nematoda) in West Africa, with some comments on the parasitization of man by the worms. *Ann. trop. Med. Parasit.* **57,** 347-358. (Reviews recorded cases of human infestation by larval mermithids, suggesting that the parasites may establish themselves in man and that infections may vary from benign–if confined to the gut–to severe, if other organs are involved.)

Fox, I. (1966). Competition and predation between mites and fleas. *Proc. 1st Int. Congr. Parasit.,* Rome, 21-26 Sept. 1964 **2,** 1022-1023. (Colonized *Xenopsylla cheopis* surviving attacks by *Laelaps nuttalli* and *Cheyletus malaccensis.*)

Fuldner, D. (1964). Geruchsorientierung einer parasitischen Käferlarve (*Aleochara curtula* Goeze) am Puparium des Writes *(Calliphora). Naturwissenschaften* **51,** 345-346.

Gad, A. M., Sadek, S. and Fateen, Y. A. (1967). The occurrence of *Coelomomyces indicus* Iyengar in Egypt, U.A.R. *Mosquito News* **27,** 201-202.

Galichet, P. F. (1966). Administration aux animaux domestiques d'une toxine thermostable sécrétée par *Bacillus thuringiensis* Berliner en vue d'empêcher la multiplication de *Musca domestica* Linnaeus dans les féces. *Ann. Zootech.* **15,** 133-145.

Geldreich, E. E., Kenner, B. A. and Kabler, P. W. (1964). Occurrence of coliforms, fecal coliforms and streptococci on vegetation and insects. *Appl. Microbiol.* **12,** 63-69. (Fecal streptococci may be transferred to growing plants by, e.g. houseflies.)

Gerberich, J. B. and Laird, M. (1966). An annotated bibliography of papers relating to the control of mosquitoes by the use of fish. (Revised and enlarged to 1965.) *W.H.O. mimeogr. docum.*, WHO/EBL/66.71, 107 pp. Also "Bibliography of Papers Relating to the Control of Mosquitoes by the Use of Fish. An Annotated Bibliography for the Years 1901-1966". *FAO Fish. Tech. Pap.* No. 75, 1968. 70 pp. FAO, Rome.

Gerling, D. (1967). The eggs of the pupal parasites of *Musca domestica* L. *Israel J. Ent.* **2,** 11-13.

Ghosh, S. M. and Hati, A. K. (1964). *Oedogonium princeps* (Chlorophycae: Oedogoniacae), a useful agent for biological control of anopheline larva. *Sci. Cult.* **30,** 461-462.

Gingrich, R. E. (1965a). *Bacillus thuringiensis* as a feed additive to control dipterous pests of cattle. *J. econ. Ent.* **58,** 363-364.

Gingrich, R. E. (1965b). *Thelohania tabani* sp.n., a microsporidian from larvae of the black horse fly, *Tabanus atratus* Fabricius. *J. Invertebrate Path.* **7,** 236-240.

Gingrich, R. E. and Eschle, J. L. (1966). Preliminary report on the larval development of the horn fly, *Haematobia irritans,* in feces from cattle given fractions of a commercial preparation of *Bacillus thuringiensis. J. Invertebrate Path.* **8,** 285-287.

Glascow, J. P. (1963). "The Distribution and Abundance of Tsetse", 241 pp. Pergamon, London. (Concludes that there is no evidence to confirm that *Trypanosoma* spp. are pathogenic to *Glossina* spp. He also refers to original observations re Sumba Island, Lake Victoria, which, in 1947, had no *Nephila* spiders and numerous *Glossina palpalis fuscipes.* Three years later *Nephila* was very abundant, and no tsetse could be found.)

Goldsmid, J. M. (1965). Hymenopterous parasites from an adult *Haemaphysalis leachii leachii* (Acarina: Ixodidae). *J. Parasit.* **51,** 259.

Goma, L. K. H. (1964a). Observations on predation of *Toxorhynchites* larvae. *E.A. Virus Res. Inst. Rep.* **13,** 59.

Goma, L. K. H. (1964b). Laboratory observations on the influence of illumination on the predatory habits of *Toxorhynchites* larvae (Diptera: Culicidae). *Ann. trop. Med. Parasitol.* **58,** 350-354.

Götz, P. (1964). Der Einfluss Unterschiedlicher Befallsbedingungen auf die Mermithogene Intersexualität von *Chironomus* (Dipt.). *Z.f. Parasitenkunde* **24,** 484-545.

Greenberg, B. (1966). Bacterial interactions in gnotobiotic flies. *Proc. IX Int. Congr. Microbiol., Moscow,* 371-380.

Greenberg, B. and Miggiano, V. (1963). Host-contaminant biology of muscoid flies. IV. Microbial competition in a blowfly. *J. infect. Dis.* **112,** 37-46.

Greenwood, E. S. (1964). *Bacillus thuringiensis* in the control of *Lucilia sericata* and *Musca domestica. N.Z. J. Sci.* **7,** 221-226.

Gregson, J. D. (1964). Problems pertaining to culture procedures for some ixodid ticks. *Bull. Wld Hlth Org.* **31,** 591-594.

Gruvel, J. and Balis, J. (1966). A note on the presence of *Thyridanthrax argentifrons* Aust. (Dipt. Bombyliidae), a parasite of the pupa of *Glossina tachinoides* West. in the region of Bas Chari, around Fort-Lamy. *Proc. 1st Int. Congr. Parasitol., Rome, 21-26 Sept. 1964,* **2,** 989.

Gugnani, H. C., Wattal, B. L. and Kalra, N. L. (1965). A note on *Coelomomyces* infection in mosquito larvae. *Bull. Ind. Soc. Mal. Other Communic. Dis.* **2,** 333-337.

Guttman, H. N. (1963). Experimental glimpses at the lower Trypanosomatidae. *Exp. Parasitol.* **13,** 129-142.

Guttman, H. N. (1966). First defined media for *Leptomonas* spp. from insects. *J. Protozool.* **13,** 390-392.

Guttman, H. N. and Eisenman, R. N. (1965). Acriflavin-induced loss of kinetoplast deoxyribonucleic acid in *Crithidia fasciculata* (*Culex pipiens* strain). *Nature, Lond.* **207,** 1280-1281.

Haeusermann, W. (1967). In 1965/1966 surveys in Tanzania revealed mermithid nematodes in adult females and larvae of *Simulium damnosum* (Mselezi Valley and Sali). *S. vorax* and *S. alcocki* also proved positive. Larval Diptera and fungi were found in adult female *S. damnosum* from Mselezi, and several species of *Simulium* larvae exhibited Microsporidia. (Personal commun., 5 February 1967.)

Hague, N. G. M. (1963). The influence of *Rhabditis (Rhabditella) axei* (Rhabditinae) on the development of *Stomoxys calcitrans. Nematologica, Leiden* **9,** 181-184.

Hair, J. A. and Turner, E. C. (1965). Attempted propagation of *Nasonia vitripennis* on the face fly. *J. econ. Ent.* **58,** 159-160.

Happold, D. C. D. (1965). Mosquito ecology in central Alberta. I. The environment, the species, and studies of the larvae. *Can. J. Zool.* **43,** 795-819. (Relationship between larvae and other aquatic animals.)

Harshbarger, J. C. and Forgash, A. J. (1964a). Effect of lindane on intestinal microorganisms of the American cockroach, *Periplaneta americana. J. econ. Ent.* **57,** 779-780.

Harshbarger, J. C. and Forgash, A. J. (1964b). Effect of lindane on the intracellular microorganisms of the American cockroach, *Periplaneta americana. J. econ. Ent.* **57,** 994-995.

Harvey, T. L. and Howell, D. E. (1965). Resistance of the house fly to *Bacillus thuringiensis* Berliner. *J. Invertebrate Path.* **7,** 92-100.

Hati, A. K. and Ghosh, S. M. (1963a). On the gregarine (*Lankesteria culicis* Ross) infection in *Aedes aegypti* mosquito in Calcutta. *Bull. Calcutta Sch. trop. Med.* **11,** 7-8.

Hati, A. K. and Ghosh, S. M. (1963b). On the life history and habits of *Sphaerodema annulatum. Bull. Calcutta Sch. trop. Med.* **11,** 58-59.

Hati, A. K. and Ghosh, S. M. (1963c). Ciliated protozoal infection in *Culex fatigans* larvae. *Bull. Calcutta Sch. trop. Med.* **11,** 109.

Hati, A. K. and Ghosh, S. M. (1965a). *Aspergillus parasiticus* infection in adult mosquitoes. *Bull. Calcutta Schl trop. Med.* **13,** 18-19.

Hati, A. K. and Ghosh, S. M. (1965b). Laboratory studies on the predaceous habits of the dragonfly nymph. *Bull. Calcutta Sch. trop. Med.* **13,** 61-62. (*Brachytron pratense* nymphs.)

Hati, A. K. and Ghosh, S. M. (1965c). Biological control of mosquitoes; effect of *Hydra. Bull. Calcutta Sch. trop. Med.* **13,** 143-144.

Hays, K. L. (1965). The frequency and magnitude of intraspecific parasitism in *Triatoma sanguisuga* (Leconte) (Hemiptera). *Ecology* **46,** 875-877.

Heimpel, A. M. (1965a). The specificity of the pathogen *Bacillus thuringiensis* var. *thuringiensis* Berliner for insects. *Proc. XII Int. Congr. Ent.,* p. 736. London 1964.

Heimpel, A. M. (1965b). Microbial control of insects. *Wld Rev. Pest Control* **4,** 150-161.

Heimpel, A. M. (1967). A critical review of *Bacillus thuringiensis* var. *thuringiensis* Berliner and other crystalliferous bacteria. *Ann. Rev. Ent.* **12,** 287-322.

Heimpel, A. M. and Harshbarger, J. C. (1965). Symposium on microbial insecticides. V. Immunity in insects. *Bact. Rev.* **29,** 397-405.

Henry, S. M. (1965). Intestinal microorganisms of the cockroach with and without intracellular symbiotes. *Proc. XII Int. Congr. Ent., London.* July 1964, p. 748.

Hilsenhoff, W. L. (1963). Predation by the leech *Helobdella stagnalis* on *Tendipes plumosus* (Diptera: Tendipedidae) larvae. *Ann. ent. Soc. Am.* **56,** 252.

Hilsenhoff, W. L. (1964). Predation by the leech *Helobdella nepheloidea* on larvae of *Tendipes plumosus* (Diptera: Tendipedidae). *Ann. ent. Soc. Am.* **57,** 139.

Hilsenhoff, W. L. (1966). The biology of *Chironomus plumosus* (Diptera: Chironomidae) in Lake Winnebago, Wisconsin. *Ann. ent. Soc. Am.* **59,** 465-473.

Hilsenhoff, W. and Lovett, O. L. (1966). Infection of *Chironomus plumosus* (Diptera: Chironomidae) by a microsporidian (*Thelohania* sp.) in Lake Winnebago, Wisconsin. *J. Invertebrate Path.* **8,** 512-519.

Hinckley, A. D. (1965). Trophic records of some insects, mites and ticks in Fiji. *Dep. Agric. Fiji Bull. No. 45,* 116 pp. (Predators and entomophaga recorded for muscoid flies. The deliberately introduced beetle *Pachylister chinensis* and the accidentally introduced ant *Pheidole megacephala* are "often quite effective" as predators on *Musca domestica* "but no substitute for sanitation in either farm or domestic situations".)

Hoare, C. A. and Wallace, F. G. (1966). Developmental stages of trypanosomatid flagellates: a new terminology. *Nature, Lond.* **212**, 1385-1386.

Hokama, Y. and Washino, R. K. (1966). Potential invertebrate predator-prey relationships in a rice field habitat (abstract). *Proc. Calif. Mosq. Control Ass.* **34**, 59.

Holling, C. S. (1965). The functional response of predators to prey density and its role in mimicry and population regulation. *Mem. ent. Soc. Can.* **45**, 1-62. (Original data on predation by mantids on adult houseflies, and on mosquito larvae by aquatic Hemiptera and Coleoptera.)

Holling, C. S. (1966). The functional response of invertebrate predators to prey density. *Mem. ent. Soc. Can.* **48**, 1-86. (Original data on predation by mantids on houseflies.)

Hooi, C. W. and Ramachandran, C. P. (1963). (Mermethid?) (sic.) from two Malayan mosquitoes. *Singapore Med. J.* **4**, 180.

Houser, E. C. and Wingo, C. W. (1967). *Aphaereta pallipes* as a parasite of the face fly in Missouri, with notes on laboratory culture and biology. *J. econ. Ent.* **60**, 731-733.

Huger, A. (1964). Eine Rickettsiose der Orientalischen Schabe, *Blatta orientalis* L., verursacht durch *Rickettsiella blattae* nov. spec. *Naturwissenshaften* **51**, 1-3.

Hutchison, J. A. (1963). The genus *Entomophthora* in the western hemisphere. *Trans. Kansas Acad. Sci.* **66**, 237-254. (Key, host list, distribution maps.)

Ignoffo, C. M. (1967). Possibilities of mass-producing insect pathogens. *In* "Insect Pathology and Microbial Control" (P. A. van der Laan, ed.), pp. 91-117. North-Holland Publ. Co., Amsterdam.

Ikeshoji, T. (1965). Predation of *Armigeres* larvae on *Culex pipiens fatigans* larvae. *W.H.O. mimeogr. docum.*, WHO/VC/134.65, 6 pp.

Ikeshoji, T. (1966). Bionomics of *Culex (Lutzia) fuscanus. Jap. J. exp. Med.* **36**, 321-334. Also: *W.H.O. mimeogr. docum.*, WHO/EBL/66.56, 21 pp. Bionomics of *Culex (Lutzia) fuscanus* in Rangoon.

Jackson, J. O. and Wilson, B. H. (1965). Observations on some predators of horse fly and deer fly (Diptera: Tabanidae) eggs in Louisiana. *Ann. ent. Soc. Am.* **58**, 934-935. (Adult coccinellid beetles, *Coeleomegilla maculata* DeGeer and *Hippodamia convergens* Guérin-Méneville.)

Jadin, J. (1966). Du rôle des bactéries dans le tube digestif des insectes vecteurs des plasmodides et des trypanosomides. *9th Int. Congr. Microbiol., Moscow,* 1966. Abstr. 325.

Jafri, R. H. (1964). Influence of pathogens on the life span of irradiated insects. *Revue Path. vég. Ent. agric. Fr.* **43**, 37-51.

Jafri, R. H. (1965a). Prospects of integrated radiation and microbial control of harmful insects. *Proc. XII Int. Congr. Ent., London,* July 1964, pp. 747-748.

Jafri, R. H. (1965b). Influence of pathogens on the life span of irradiated insects. *J. Invertebrate Path.* **7**, 66-70.

James, H. G. (1963). Larval habitats, development, and parasites of some Tabanidae (Diptera) in southern Ontario. *Can. Ent.* **95**, 1223-1232.

James, H. G. (1964). Insect and other fauna associated with the rock pool mosquito *Aedes atropalpus* (Coq.). *Mosquito News* **24**, 325-329.

James, H. G. (1965a). The role of Coleoptera in the natural control of mosquitoes in Canada. *Proc. XII Int. Congr. Ent. London,* July 1964, pp. 357-358.

James, H. G. (1965b). Predators of *Aedes atropalpus* (Coq.) (Diptera: Culicidae) and of other mosquitoes breeding in rock pools in Ontario. *Can. J. Zool.* **43**, 155-159.

James, H. G. (1966a). Location of univoltine *Aedes* eggs in woodland pool areas and experimental exposure to predators. *Mosquito News* **26**, 59-63.

James, H. G. (1966b). Insect predators of univoltine mosquitoes in woodland pools of the Pre-Cambrian Shield in Ontario. *Can. Ent.* **98**, 550-555.

James, H. G. (1967a). Bird predation on black fly larvae and pupae in Ontario. *Can. J. Zool.* **46**, 106-107.

James, H. G. (1967b). Seasonal activity of mosquito predators in woodland pools in Ontario. *Mosquito News* **27**, 454-457.

James, H. G. (1967c). Activity and sequence of mosquito predators in woodland pools in Ontario. *Proc. Calif. Mosq. Control Ass.* **35**, 95.

James, H. G. and Redner, R. L. (1965). An aquatic trap for sampling mosquito predators. *Mosquito News* **25**, 35-37.

Jarry, D. M. and Jarry, D. T. (1963). Quelques *Thelastomatidae* (Nematoda: Oxyuroidea) parasites des Blattides à l'Institut Pasteur de Tunis. *Arch. Inst. Past., Tunis* **40**, 229-234.

Jenkins, D. W. (1964). Pathogens, parasites and predators of medically important arthropods. Annotated list and bibliography. Suppl. to Vol. **30,** *Bull. Wld Hlth Org.,* 150 pp.

Johnson, A. A. (1963). *Octomyomermis itascensis* gen. et sp. nov. a parasite of *Chironomus plumosus* (L.). *Trans. Am. microsc. Soc.* **82**, 237-241.

Johnson, A. A. (1965). *Hydromermis itascensis* sp.n. (Nematoda: Mermithidae) a parasite of *Glyptotendipes lobiferus* (Say) (Diptera: Chironomidae) and the taxonomic status of *Gastromermis. J. Parasit.* **51**, 53-56.

Johnson, P. T., McConnell, E. and Hertig, M. (1963). Natural infections of leptomonad flagellates in Panamanian *Phlebotomus* sandflies. *Exp. Parasit.* **14**, 107-122.

Johnson, W. E., Jr. (1964). Parasitic Hydracarina observed on mosquitoes at the Wichita Mountains Wildlife Refuge. *Mosquito News* **24**, 336-338.

Jones, C. M. and Anthony, D. W. (1964). The Tabanidae (Diptera) of Florida. *USDA, ARS, Tech. Bull. 1295,* 85 pp. (Pp. 54-59: a review of the natural enemies of tabanids with numerous original observations.)

Jones, R. K. H. (1965). Parasitism by larvae of *Unionicola intermedia* Koenike, and another *Unionicola* sp. (Acarina: Pionae), on chironomids. *Nature, Lond.* **207**, 317-318.

Kajak, Z. and Pieczyński, E. (1966). The influence of invertebrate predators on the abundance of benthic organisms (chiefly *Chironomidae*). *Ecol. polska* **12**, 175-179. (In Polish.)

Karanukaran, L. (1966). Parasitism of *Chironomus costatus* Joh. (Diptera: Nematocera) by a mermithid. *Nematologia, Leiden* **12,** 172-174.

Kellen, W. R. (1963). Research on biological control of mosquitoes. *Proc. Pprs. 31st Ann. Conf. Calif. Mosq. Control Ass. Inc. (Jan. 28-30), 1963),* pp. 23-25.

Kellen, W. R. (1965). Microsporida as parasites of mosquitoes. *Proc. XII Int. Congr. Ent., London,* July, 1964, pp. 728-729.

Kellen, W. R., Chapman, H. C., Clark, T. B. and Lindegren, J. E. (1965). Host-parasite relationships of some *Thelohania* from mosquitoes (Nosematidae: Microsporida). *J. Invertebrate Path.* **7**, 161-166.

Kellen, W. R., Chapman, H. C., Clark, T. B. and Lindegren, J. E. (1966). Transovarian transmission of some *Thelohania* (Nosematidae: Microsporida) in mosquitoes of California and Louisiana. *J. Invertebrate Path.* **8,** 355-359.

Kellen, W. R., Clark, T. B. and Lindegren, J. E. (1963). A new host record for *Coelomomyces psorophorae* Couch in California (Blastocladiales: Coelomomycetaceae). *J. Insect Path.* **5**, 157-166.

Kellen, W. R., Clark, T. B. and Lindegren, J. E. (1966). Two previously undescribed *Nosema* from mosquitoes of California (Nosematidae: Microsporida). *J. Invertebrate Path.* **9**, 19-25.

Kellen, W. R., Clark, T. B., Lindegren, J. E., Hoe, B. C., Rogoff, M. H. and Singer, S. (1965). *Bacillus sphaericus* Neide as a pathogen of mosquitoes. *J. Invertebrate Path.* **7**, 442-448.

Kellen, W. R., Clark, T. B., Lindegren, J. E. and Sanders, R. D. (1966a). A cytoplasmic-polyhedrosis virus of *Culex tarsalis* (Diptera: Culicidae). *J. Invertebrate Path.* **8**, 390-394.

Kellen, W. R., Clark, T. B., Lindegren, J. E. and Sanders, R. D. (1966b). Development of *Thelohania californica* in two hybrid mosquitoes. *Exp. Parasit.* **18**, 251-254.

Kellen, W. R. and Myers, C. M. (1964). *Bacillus sphaericus* Neide as a pathogen of mosquitoes (summary). *Proc. Pprs. 32nd Ann. Conf. Calif. Mosq. Control Ass. Inc. (January 26-29, 1964) Calif. Mosq. Control Ass. Proc. 32, p. 37.*

Kellen, W. R. and Wills, W. (1963). Studies on the transovarial transmission of *Thelohania californica* Kellen and Lipa in *Culex tarsalis* Coquillet. *Prog. Protozool., Proc. 1. Int. Congr. Protozool. (Prague, 1961)*, pp. 490-494.

King, D. (1965). Descriptive and experimental studies on the development of the Acanthocephalan, *Moniliformis dubius* Meyer, 1933. M.Sc. Thesis, Univ. New South Wales.

King, P. E. and Hopkins, C. R. (1963). Length of life of the sexes in *Nasonia vitripennis* (Walker) *(Hymenoptera, Pteromalidae)* under conditions of starvation. *J. exp. Biol.* **40,** 751-761.

King, W. E. (1964). Studies in the behaviour of *Macrocheles muscaedomesticae,* predator of the house fly egg. M.Sc. Thesis, Univ. Kentucky.

Kinn, D. N. (1966). Predation by the mite, *Macrocheles muscaedomesticae* (Acarina: Macrochelidae), on three species of flies. *J. med. Ent.* **3,** 155-158.

Kloss, G. R. (1966). Revisao des nematóides de Blattaria do Brasil. *Pap. Avulsos Zool.* São Paulo **18,** 147-188.

Knuckles, J. L. (1967). An apparatus for rearing bacteria-free blowfly larvae and pupae. *Turtox News* **45,** 76-77.

Kovchazov, G. (1963). A parasite from Bulgarian *Anopheles maculipennis. W.H.O. mimeogr. docum.*, WHO/EBL/13, 3 pp. (Trematode ziphidocercariae.)

Kramer, J. P. (1963). A microsporidian of the genus *Octosporea,* a parasite of *Phormia regina* (Meigen) and *Callitroga macellaria* (Fabricius) (Diptera: Calliphoridae). *Prog. Protozool. Proc. 1. Int. Congr. Protozool. (Prague, 1961),* pp. 495-496.

Kramer, J. P. (1964a). The microsporidian *Octosporea muscaedomesticae* Flu, a parasite of calypterate muscoid flies in Illinois. *J. Insect Path.* **6,** 331-342.

Kramer, J. P. (1964b). *Nosema kingi* sp.n., a microsporidian from *Drosophila willistoni* Sturtevant, and its infectivity for other muscoids. *J. Invertebrate Path.* **6,** 491-499.

Kramer, J. P. (1964c). Parasites in laboratory colonies of mosquitoes. *Bull. Wld Hlth Org.* **31,** 475-478.

Kramer, J. P. (1964d). The fate of spores of *Nosema apis* Zander ingested by muscoid flies. *(Colloq. Int. Path. Insectes et la Lutte Microbiol.* Paris, Oct. 1962), *Entomophaga, Mém. hors Sér.* No. 2, 95-99.

Kramer, J. P. (1965a). The microsporidians *Octosporea muscaedomesticae* Flu and *Nosema kingi* Kramer: a comparison of their effects on muscoid flies. *In* "Progress in Protozoology". *2nd Int. Conf. on Protozool.,* London, August 1965. *Excerpta Med. Int. Congr. Ser. No. 91.* 71. (Abstract).

Kramer, J. P. (1965b). The microsporidian *Octosporea muscaedomesticae* Flu, a little-known pathogen of muscoid flies. *W.H.O. mimeogr. docum.*, WHO/EBL/53.65, 8 pp.

Kramer, J. P. (1965c). Generation time of the microsporidian *Octosporea muscaedomesticae* Flu in adult *Phormia regina* (Meigen) (Diptera: Calliphoridae. *Z. f. Parasitenkunde* **25,** 309-313.

Kramer, J. P. (1965d). Effects of an octosporeosis on the locomotor activity of adult *Phormia regina* (Meigen) (Dipt. Calliphoridae). *Entomophaga* **10,** 339-342.

Kramer, J. P. (1966). On the octosporeosis of muscoid flies caused by *Octosporea muscaedomesticae* Flu (Microsporida). *Am. midl. Nat.* **75,** 214-220.

Kramer, J. P. (1967). On microsporidian diseases of noxious invertebrates. *Abstr. Joint U.S.-Japan Semin. Microbial Control Insect Pests. U.S.-Japan Committee Sci. Cooperation, Panel 8,* p. 48. Fukuoka. (Octosporeosis of muscoid flies.)

Krieg, A. (1967). Neues über *Bacillus thuringiensis* und seine Anwendung. *Mitt aus der Biol. Bundes f. Land-u. Forst. Berlin-Dahlem* **125,** 106 pp. (Pp. 82-83 concern several dipterans of public health concern.)

Kudo, R. R. and Daniels, E. W. (1963). An electron microscope study of the spore of a microsporidian, *Thelohania californica. J. Protozool.* **10,** 112-120.

Kühlhorn, F. (1965). An investigation of the natural enemies of *Anopheles* larvae (Diptera: Culicidae) in different areas at varying altitudes in West Germany. *W.H.O. mimeogr.*

docum., WHO/EBL/37.65, 18 pp. (Reviews German-language literature and gives original observations on experimental predation on mosquito larvae by the spider *Lycosa amentata* Clerck. and the turtle *Emys orbicularis* L., the latter in Greece.)

Kuprijanova, E. S. (1966). *Entomophthora* fungus parasitizing mosquitoes of the *Culex pipiens* L. complex. *Zool. Zh.* **45,** 675-678. (In Russian.) Also: Parasitization of mosquitoes of the *Culex pipiens* L. complex by fungi of the order Entomophthorales. *W.H.O. mimeogr. docum.*, WHO/EBL/66.57, 10 pp.

Ladd, T. L., Jr. and Travis, B. V. (1965). Elimination of gregarines from the cockroach *Leucophaea maderae* (Fab.). *J. Parasit.* **51,** 569.

Laing, J. E. and Welch, H. E. (1963). A dolichopodid predacious on larvae of *Culex restuans* Theob. *Proc. ent. Soc. Ont.*, 1962 **93,** 89-90.

Laird, M. (1963a). Vector ecology and integrated control procedures. *Bull. Wld Hlth Org.* **29** (Suppl.), 147-151.

Laird, M. (1963b). Rats, coconuts, mosquitoes and filariasis. *In* "Pacific Basin Biogeography", pp. 535-542. *10th Pacific Sci. Congr.*

Laird, M. (1965a). Control of vectors of disease. *Mitt. Int. Verein. Limnol.* **13,** 63-65. (From *Symposium on Natural Populations,* Freshwat. Biol. Ass., Windermere, England, July 1964.)

Laird, M. (1965b). The role of the World Health Organization in biological control research. *In* "Progress in Protozoology". *2nd Int. Conf. Protozool.*, London, August 1965. *Excerpta Med. Int. Congr. Ser. No. 91*, p. 70.

Laird, M. (1965c). Insect pathology and vector control: an international collaborative programme of research. *Proc. XII Int. Congr. Ent., London,* July 1964, p. 730.

Laird, M. (1965d). Biotic factors in the control of the *Culex pipiens* complex. *WHO/Vector Control/125.65,* pp. 175-181. and 210-211.

Laird, M. (1966). Some protozoa from Singapore insects. *Proc. 1st Int. Congr. Parasit.*, 21-26 Sept. 1964 **1,** 595-596.

Laird, M. (1967a). A coral island experiment: a new approach to mosquito control. *Chron. Wld Hlth Org.* **21,** 18-26. (Danish and Swedish versions published as "Nye veje i myggebekaempelsen–et coralø-eksperiment". *Naturens Verden,* Sept. 1967, pp. 274-281, and "Nya metoder for myggbekämpning". *Naturens Varld* **10,** 306-313, 1967.)

Laird, M. (1967b). Biotic factors in the control of *Aedes aegypti. Bull. Wld Hlth Org.* **36,** 625-627.

Laird, M. and Briggs, J. D. (1967). Report on the World Health Organization's survey for pathogens and parasites of arthropods of public health importance. "Insect Pathology and Microbial Control" (P. A. van der Laan, ed.), pp. 4-5. North-Holland Publ. Co., Amsterdam.

Laird, M. and Wright, J. W. (1966). Integrated control and public health entomology. *Proc. FAO Symp. Integrated Pest Control,* Rome **3,** 77-79.

Lakshana, P. (1966). A new species of trombiculid mite infesting scorpions in Thailand (Acarina: Trombiculidae). *J. med. Ent.* **3,** 258-260. (Describes *Neotrombicula scorpionis* Lakshana.)

Lange, R. (1964). Der Einfluss der Nahrung von *Musca domestica* L. auf die Mortalität des Endoparasiten *Aphaereta pallipes* (Say) *(Hym., Braconidae). Z. angew. Ent.* **54,** 213-218.

Lange, R. and Bronskill, J. F. (1964). Reactions of *Musca domestica* L. (Diptera: Muscidae) to parasitism by *Aphaereta pallipes* (Say) (Hymenoptera: Braconidae), with special reference to host diet and parasitoid toxin. *Z. f. Parasitenkunde* **25,** 193-210.

Larson, L. V. (1967). Association of *Vorticella* and *Epistylis* (Protozoa: Ciliata) with mosquito larvae. *W.H.O. mimeogr. docum.*, WHO/VBC/67.20, 00 pp.

Laurence, B. R. and Samarawickrema, W. A. (1966). Predation in a mosquito community. *Bull. Wld Hlth Org.* **34,** 475-477.

Lavrentyev, P. A., Salnikov, V. G. and Anisin, S. D. (1965). The use of bacteria for mosquito control. *Veterinariya* (Mosk.) **42,** 107-108. (In Russian.)

Leão, A. E. A. and Pedroso, M. C. (1965). A new species of the genus *Coelomomyces,* parasite of the eggs of *Phlebotomus. Mycopath. Mycol. appl.,* den Haag **26,** 305-307. (In Portuguese.) (*Coelomomyces ciferri* described.)

Legner, E. F. (1966). Parasites of the house fly and other filth-breeding Diptera in Southern California. *J. econ. Ent.* **59,** 999-1001.

Legner, E. F. (1967a). The status of *Nasonia vitripennis* as a natural parasite of the house fly, *Musca domestica. Can. Ent.* **99,** 308-309.

Legner, E. F. (1967b). Behaviour changes the reproduction of *Spalangia cameroni, S. endius, Muscidifurax raptor* and *Nasonia vitripennis* (Hymenoptera: Pteromalidae) at increasing fly host densities. *Ann. ent. Soc. Am.* **60,** 819-826.

Legner, E. F. (1967c). Two exotic strains of *Spalangia drosophilae* merit consideration in biological control of *Hippelates collusor* (Diptera: Chloropidae). *Ann. ent. Soc. Am.* **60,** 458-462.

Legner, E. F. and Bay, E. C. (1964a). La primera exploración para buscar enemigos naturales de *Hippelates* en Puerto Rico *(Insecta: Chloropidae). Caribbean J. Sci.* **4,** 467-471.

Legner, E. F. and Bay, E. C. (1964b). Natural exposure of *Hippelates* eye gnats to field parasitization and the discovery of one pupal and two larval parasites. *Ann. ent. Soc. Am.* **57,** 767-769.

Legner, E. F. and Bay, E. C. (1965a). *Ooencyrtus submetallicus* Howard in an extraordinary host-relationship with *Hippelates pusio* Loew. *Can. Ent.* **97,** 556-557.

Legner, E. F. and Bay, E. C. (1965b). Predatory and parasitic agents attacking the *Hippelates pusio* complex in Puerto Rico. *J. agric. Univ. P. Rico* **49,** 368-376.

Legner, E. F. and Bay, E. C. (1965c). Culture of *Hippelates pusio* (Diptera: Chloropidae) in the West Indies for natural enemy exploration and some notes on behaviour and distribution. *Ann. ent. Soc. Am.* **58,** 436-440.

Legner, E. F., Bay, E. C., Brydon, H. W. and McCoy, C. W. (1966). Research with parasites for biological control of house flies in Southern California. *Calif. Agric.* **20,** 10-12.

Legner, E. F., Bay, E. C. and Farr, T. H. (1966). Parasitic and predacious agents affecting the *Hippelates pusio* complex in Jamaica and Trinidad. *Can. Ent.* **98,** 28-33. (Predator attack was thought significant.)

Legner, E. F., Bay, E. C. and McCoy, C. W. (1965). Parasitic natural regulatory agents attacking *Musca domestica* L. in Puerto Rico. *J. Agric. Univ. P. Rico* **49,** 368-376.

Legner, E. F., Bay, E. C. and Medved, R. A. (1966). Behaviour of three native pupal parasites of *Hippelates collusor* in controlled systems. *Ann. ent. Soc. Am.* **59,** 977-984.

Legner, E. F., Bay, E. C. and White, E. B. (1967). Activity of parasites from Diptera: *Musca domestica, Stomoxys calcitrans, Fannia canicularis* and *F. femoralis,* at sites in the Western Hemisphere. *Ann. ent. Soc. Am.* **60,** 462-468.

Legner, E. F. and Brydon, H. W. (1966). Suppression of dung-inhabiting fly populations by pupal parasites. *Ann. ent. Soc. Am.* **59,** 638-651.

Legner, E. F. and Gerling, D. (1967). Host-feeding and oviposition on *Musca domestica* (L.) by *Spalangia cameroni* Perk., *Nasonia vitripennis* Walk. and *Muscidifurax raptor* G. and S. (Hymenoptera: Pteromalidae) influences their longevity and fecundity. *Ann. ent. Soc. Am.* **60,** 678-691.

Legner, E. F. and McCoy, C. W. (1966). The house fly, *Musca domestica* Linnaeus, as an exotic species in the Western Hemisphere invites biological control studies. *Can. Ent.* **98,** 243-248.

Legner, E. F., Olton, G. A. and Eskafi, F. M. (1966). Influence of physical factors on the developmental stages of *Hippelates collusor* in relation to the activities of its natural parasites. *Ann. ent. Soc. Am.* **59,** 851-861.

Lehr, P. A. (1964). On the feeding habits and importance of Asilidae. *Trans. Ins. Sci. Studies Plant Protection* **8,** 213-244. (In Russian.)

Leong, L. and Paran, T. P. (1966). A study of the nematode parasites of cockroaches in Singapore. *Med. J. Malaya* **20,** 349.

Leskova, A. (1966). The effect of entobacteria and an entomopathogenic crystal-forming bacterium on the house fly. *In* "Biol. metod. bor'b. s vredit. sel'sk., lesn. choz. i. karant. sorn." (M. A. Ris, ed.), pp. 124-125. Izd. Fan, Tashkent. (In Russian.)

Levinson, Z. H. (1964). Some comments on Rachel Carson's "Silent Spring" and several research ideas stimulated by it. *Israel J. exptl. Med.*, 1963 **11**, 190-193.

Lewis, D. J. (1965a). Features of the *Simulium damnosum* population of the Kumba area in West Cameroon. *Ann. trop. Med. Parasit.* **59**, 365-374. (Fungal parasites were common, probably *Entomophthora* sp.)

Lewis, D. J. (1965b). Internal structural features of some Central American phlebotomine sandflies. *Ann. trop. Med. Parasit.* **59**, 375-385. (Fungal, ciliate and flagellate endoparasites and ectoparasitic mites.)

Lewis, T. (1964). What the swallows are hunting. *The Field,* April 1964. (Swifts, a nesting pair of which must each catch about 10,000 flying insects between dawn and dusk each day, destroy many midges. Sewage farms attract swifts in the early evening, when many species of midge are in flight there.)

Lichtwardt, R. W. (1964). Axenic culture of two new species of branched Trichomycetes. *Am. J. Bot.* **51**, 836-842. *(Smittium culisetae* and *S. simulii.)*

Lipa, J. J. (1964). Biological control of medically important insects. *Wiadomosci Parazytol.* **10**, 21-32. (In Polish.)

Love, J. E. and Gill, G. D. (1965). Incidence of coliforms and enterococci in field populations of *Stomoxys calcitrans* (Linnaeus). *J. Invertebrate Path.* 7, 430-436.

Luczak, J. and Dabrowska-Prôt, E. (1966). Experimental studies on the reduction of the abundance of mosquitoes by spiders. I. Intensity of spider predation on mosquitoes. *Bull. Acad. Pol. Sci. Sér. Sci. biol.* **14**, 315-320.

McConnell, E. (1963). Leptomonads of wild-caught Panamanian *Phlebotomus*: culture and animal inoculation. *Expl Parasit.* **14**, 123-128.

McConnell, E. and Correa, M. (1964). Trypanosomes and other microorganisms from Panamanian *Phlebotomus* sandflies. *J. Parasit.* **50**, 523-528.

McDuffie, W. C. and Weidhaas, D. E. (1965). The future outlook for new and improved materials and methods for mosquito control. *Mosquito News* **25**, 85-91. (Prospects for biological control employing parasites and predators in integrated control.)

McGhee, R. B., Schmittner, Stella M. and Hanson, W. L. (1965). Speciation in the genus *Crithidia. In* "Progress in Protozoology". *2nd. Int. Conf. Protozool., Lond.*, Aug 1965. *Excerpta Medica Int. Congr. Ser. No. 91,* 142, pp. 135-136. Also *W.H.O. mimeogr. docum.*, WHO/EBL/45.65, 6 pp.

Macan, T. T. (1965). Predation as a factor in the ecology of water bugs. *J. Anim. Ecol.* **34**, 691-698.

Madden, J. L. and Pimental, D. (1966). Density and spatial relationships between a wasp parasite and its housefly host. *Can. Ent.* **97**, 1031-1037.

Madelin, M. F. (1964). Laboratory studies on the infection of *Anopheles gambiae* Giles by a species of *Coelomomyces. W.H.O. mimeogr. docum.*, WHO/EBL/17, 233 pp and Corrigendum.

Madelin, M. F. (1965). Further laboratory studies on a species of *Coelomomyces* which infects *Anopheles gambiae* Giles. *W.H.O. mimeogr. docum.*, WHO/EBL/52.65, 22 pp.

Madelin, M. F. (1966). Fungal parasites of insects. *Ann. Rev. Ent.* **11**, 423-448.

Maitland, P. S. and Penney, M. M. (1967). The ecology of the Simuliidae in a Scottish river. *J. Anim. Ecol.* **36**, 179-206. (Briefly refers to parasites and predators, including leeches.)

Manier, J. F., Rioux, J. A. and Juminer, B. (1964). Presence en Tunisie de deux Trichomycètes parasites de larves de Culicides. *Arch. Inst. Pasteur Tunis* **41**, 147-152.

Marchette, N. J. and Hatié, C. (1965). Microbial isolates from the digestive tract of *Triatoma protracta* (Uhler) (Reduviidae). *J. Invertebrate Path.* **7**, 45-48.

Marr, J. D. M. and Lewis, D. J. (1964). Observations on the dry-season survival of *Simulium damnosum* Theo. in Ghana. *Bull. ent. Res.* **55**, 547-564. (Notes on parasites, including ciliate protozoans in abdomen, a nematode and a planidium.)

Martinson, F. D. and Clark, B. M. (1967). Rhinophycomycosis entomophthorae in Nigeria. *Am. J. trop. Med. Hyg.* **16**, 40-47.

Masuda, R. (1964). Studies on the parasitic enemy of flies in the rural district of Tokyo (Report 1). On the parasitic Hymenoptera of overwintering fly pupae in Ohme city and Chofu city. *Jap. J. sanit. Zool.* **15**, 145-149. (In Japanese.) (Recommends that instead of destroying fly puparia, these should be collected in a container covered with a net to retain emerging flies and allow hymenopterous parasites to escape.)

Maurand, J. and Manier, J. F. (1967). Une microsporidie nouvelle pour les larves de Simulies. (Abstract) 1 p. mimeogr. *In* "Résumé des Communications", Groupement des Protistologues de langue française, 6th Réunion Ann., Geneva, 5-7 May 1967.

Mercer, E. H. and Nicholas, W. L. (1967). The ultrastructure of the capsule of the larval stages of *Moniliformis dubius* (Acanthocephala) in the cockroach *Periplaneta americana*. *Parasitology* **57**, 169-174.

Micks, D. W. and Ferguson, M. J. (1963). Microorganisms associated with mosquitoes. IV. Bacteria isolated from the mid-gut of adult *Culex molestus* Forskal, *Aedes aegypti* (Linneaus) and *Anopheles quadrimaculatus* Say. *J. Insect Path.* **5**, 483-488.

Millar, E. S. (1965). *Bacillus thuringiensis* in the control of flies breeding in the droppings of caged hens. *N.Z. Jl agric. Res.* 8, 721-722. (Also *W.H.O. mimeogr. docum.*, WHO/EBL/40.65, 3 pp.) (*née* Greenwood, q.v.)

Min, H. S. (1965). Studies on the transport of carbohydrate in *Crithidia luciliae*. *J. cell. comp. Physiol.* **65**, 243-248.

Minár, J. (1966). Phoresis of *Damalinia (C.) meyeri* (Mallophaga) and *Lamprochernes nodosus* (Pseudoscorpionidea) on mosquitoes *Aedes sticticus* (Culicidae). *Folia Parasitol. Praha* **13**, 270-273.

Mončadskij, A. S. (1964). The role of the larvae of Chaoborinae (Diptera: Culicidae) in the destruction of the larvae of blood-sucking mosquitoes. *Zool. Zh.* **43**, 455-466. (In Russian.)

Mončadskij, A. S. and Avila, G. (1966). Las larvas de los mosquitos (Diptera: Culicidae) de Cuba, su biologia y deteminacion. *Poeyana Inst. Biol.*, Series A, No. 28, 92 pp. (Lists five mosquitoes of four genera preyed upon by larval *Psorophora howardi*.)

Morozov, V. A. (1967). Detection of a parasitic fungus, *Coelomomyces*, in *Aëdes* larvae in the Krasnodar region. *Med. Parazit. Moskva* **36**, 353. (In Russian.)

Müller-Kögler, E. (1964). Insekten-Mykologie: Streiflichter und Ausblicke. *Entomophaga, Mém. hors Sér.* No. 2, 111-124.

Müller-Kögler, E. (1965). "Pilzkrankheiten bei Insekten", XVI + 1-444. Paul Parey, Berlin.

Müller-Kögler, E. (1967). Nebenwirkungen Insektenpathogener Pilze auf Mensch und Wirbeltiere: Aktuelle Fragen. *Entomophaga* **12**, 429-441. (Warns of the hazards of using certain insect-pathogenic fungi that are also pathogenic for man and other vertebrates.)

Muspratt, J. (1963a). Destruction of the larvae of *Anopheles gambiae* Giles by a *Coelomomyces* fungus. *Bull. Wld Hlth Org.* **29**, 81-86.

Muspratt, J. (1963b). Progress Report (May 1963) on investigations concerning three mosquito pathogens at Livingstone, Northern Rhodesia. *W.H.O. mimeogr. rep.*, WHO/EBL/12, 7 pp. (*Coelomomyces, Tetrahymena,* mermithids.)

Muspratt, J. (1964). Parasitology of larval mosquitoes, especially *Culex pipiens fatigans* Wied., at Rangoon, Burma. *W.H.O. mimeogr. docum.*, WHO/EBL/18, 19 pp. (*Coelomomyces* and Entobacteriaceae.)

Muspratt, J. (1965). Technique for infecting larvae of the *Culex pipiens* complex with a mermithid nematode and for culturing the latter in the laboratory. *Bull. Wld Hlth Org.* **33**, 140-144.

Nagel, W. P. (1963). The population dynamics of an experimental parasite-host system, with *Nasonia vitripennis* (Walk.) (Pteromalidae: Hymenoptera) as the parasite and *Musca domestica* L. (Muscidae: Diptera) as the host. *Diss. Abstr.* **23**, 3563-3564.

Nagel, W. P. and Pimental, D. (1963). Some ecological attributes of a pteromalid parasite and its housefly host. *Can. Ent.* **95**, 208-213.

Nagel, W. P. and Pimental, D. (1964). The intrinsic rate of natural increase of the pteromalid parasite *Nasonia vitripennis* (Walk.) on its muscoid host, *Musca domestica* L. *Ecology* **45**, 658-660.

Nakagawa, P. Y. (1963). Status of *Toxorhynchites* in Hawaii. *Proc. Hawaiian ent. Soc. 1962* **18,** 291-294.

Nakasuji, F. (1965a). On the predacious habits of a histerid, *Saprinus speciosus* Erichson, feeding on maggots of medically important flies. *Kontyû* **33,** 131-140. (In Japanese.)

Nakasuji, F. (1965b). Difference of the activity of hymenopterous parasites with special reference to the depth of the pupation site of fly larvae. *Kontyû,* **33,** 441-445. (In Japanese.)

Newell, I. M. and Ryckman, R. E. (1966). Species of *Pimeliaphilus* (Acari: Pterygosomidae) attacking insects, with particular reference to the species parasitizing Triatominae (Hemiptera: Reduviidae). *Hilgardia* **37,** 403-436. (The Mexican mite, *P. gloriosus,* can seriously threaten laboratory colonies of the *Triatoma protracta* complex.)

Nickle, W. R. (1967). *Heterotylenchus autumnalis* sp.n. (Nematoda: Sphaerulariidae), a parasite of the face fly, *Musca autumnalis* de Geer. *J. Parasit.* **53,** 398-401.

Novak, D. (1965). Zum Auftreten der Mykosen bei Stechmücken in Mähren (Diptera: Culicidae). *Beitr. Ent.* **15,** 135-137.

Novak, D. (1967). Beobachtungen zur Verbreitung von Mykosen bei Stechmücken. *Zeits. Tropenmed. u. Parasit.* **18,** 4 pp.

Ode, P. E. and Matthysse, J. G. (1964a). Face fly control experiments. *J. econ. Ent.* **57,** 631-636.

Ode, P. E. and Matthysse, J. G. (1964b). Feed additive larviciding to control face fly. *J. econ. Ent.* **57,** 637-640.

O'Donnell, A. E. and Axtell, R. C. (1965). Predation by *Fuscuropoda vegetans* (Acarina: Uropodidae) on the house fly *(Musca domestica). Ann. ent. Soc. Am.* **58,** 403-404.

Oliver, J. N. and Krantz, F. W. (1963). *Macrocheles rodriguezi,* a new species of mite from Kansas (Acarina: Macrochelidae) with notes on its life cycle and behaviour. *Acarologia* **5,** 519-525.

Ormerod, W. E. (1965). The effect of *Trypanosoma rangeli* Tejera on the concentration of amino acids in the haemolymph of *Rhodnius prolixus* Stål. *Proc. XII Int. Congr. Ent.* London, July 1964.

Pagayon, A. U. (1963). A peculiar parasite destroying anopheline eggs. *Hlth. Dept. Bull. (Manila),* 1960-1963, pp. 32-35, 41-45. (Besides a mermithid? nematode in adult anophelines, an unidentified organism, possibly a nematode, parasitizes unlaid eggs of *Anopheles* spp. in several areas of the Philippines.)

Parenti, U. (1966). Facteurs de l'environnement dans le rapport sexes de *Paramermis contorta* parasite de *Chironomus tentans. Proc. 1st Int. Congr. Parasit.,* Rome, 1964, pp. 585-585.

Pawlik, J. (1966). Control of the nematode *Leidynema appendiculata* (Leidy) [*Nemata: Rhabditida: Thelastomatidae*] in laboratory cultures of the American cockroach. *J. econ. Ent.* **59,** 468-469.

Pérez-Reyes, R. (1966). Insect protozoa. I. *Monocercomonas* and other small flagellates of Mexican insects. *Proc. 1st. Int. Congr. Parasit.,* Rome, 21-26 Sept. 1964, **1,** 600-601. (Hosts include cockroach, *Blaberus* sp.)

Petersen, J. J., Chapman, H. C. and Woodard, D. B. (1967). Preliminary observations on the incidence and biology of a mermithid nematode of *Aedes sollicitans* (Walker) in Louisiana. *Mosquito News* **27,** 493-498. (Also *Proc. Calif. Mosq. Control Ass.,* 1967 **35,** 95.

Petrova, A. D. (1964). The part played by synanthropic flies in the spread of Macrochelidae Vitzt. (In Russian.) *Med. Parazit., Mosk.* **33,** 553-557.

Phelps, R. J. and Defoliart, G. R. (1964). Nematode parasitism of Simuliidae. *Res. Bull. agric. Exp. Stn. Univ. Wis. No. 245,* 78 pp.

Pierre, L. L. (1964). Uricase activity of isolated symbionts and the aposymbiotic fat body of a cockroach. *Nature, Lond.* **201,** 54-55.

Pierre, L. L. (1965). Guanase activity of the symbionts and fat bodies of the cockroach, *Leucophaea maderae. Nature, Lond.* **208,** 666-667.

Pimental, D. (1966). Wasp parasite *(Nasonia vitripennis)* survival on its house fly host *(Musca domestica)* reared on various foods. *Ann. ent. Soc. Am.* **59,** 1031-1038.

Pimental, D. and Al-Hafidh, R. (1965). Ecological control of a parasite population by genetic evolution in the parasite-host system. *Ann. ent. Soc. Am.* **58,** 1-6.

Poinar, G. O. (1964). A new nematode, *Orthomermis oedobranchus* gen.n., sp.n. (Mermithidae) parasitizing *Smittia* larvae (Chironomidae) in England. *Nematologica* **10,** 501-506.

Poinar, G. O. (1965a). Nematodes associated with the Psychodidae and other terrestrial nematocerous Diptera. *Proc. XII Int. Congr. Ent., Lond.* July 1964, p. 749.

Poinar, G. O. (1965b). An association between *Pelodera (Coarctadora) acarambates* n.sp. (Rhabditina: Nematoda) and macrochelid mites *Macrocheles glaber* and *M. subnotus* (Mesostigmata: Acari). *Nematologica* **10,** 507-511.

Poinar, G. O. and Ecke, D. H. (1967). Studies on a new species of *Gastromermis* (Mermithidae) parasitizing *Tanytarsus* larvae (Chironomidae) in California. *W.H.O. mimeogr. docum.*, WHO/VBC/67.27, 4 pp.

Pritchard, G. (1964). The prey of dragonfly larvae (Odonata: Anisoptera) in ponds in northern Alberta. *Can. J. Zool.* **42,** 785-800. (Dragonfly larvae are general live animal feeders, chironomid larvae being their commonest prey in nature. Culicine and anopheline larvae are commonly taken too, and some larval ceratopogonids.)

Pritchard, G. (1965). Prey capture by dragonfly larvae (Odonata: Anisoptera). *Can. J. Zool.* **43,** 271-289.

Qadri, S. S. and Bhasker Rao, T. (1963). On a new flagellate *Polymastix periplanetae* from the common cockroach *Periplaneta americana. Riv. Parassit.* **24,** 153-158.

Rageau, J. (1964). Observations biologiques sur les *Tabanidae* de l'Océanie française. *Bull. Soc. Path. exot.* **57,** 1150-1159. (Mentions an ectoparasitic mite.)

Rajapaksa, N. (1964). Survey for *Coelomomyces* infections in mosquito larvae in the south-west coastal belt of Ceylon. *Bull. Wld Hlth Org.* **30,** 149-151.

Ramalingam, S. (1966). *Coelomomyces* infections in mosquito larvae in the South Pacific. *Med. J. Malaya* **20,** 334.

Rao, T. B. (1963). On *Rhizomastix periplanetae* n.sp., from *Periplaneta americana* of Hyderabad A.P., India. *Riv. Parassit.* **24,** 159-162.

Rastagaeva, K. S. (1965). The role of the ichneumon-flies (*Telenomus* and *Trichogramma*) in the restriction of the number of horse-flies in nature. *Zool. Zh.* **44,** 1870-1871. (In Russian.)

Rees, D. M., Smith, D. A. and Low, J. B. (1963). Report of the Utah mosquito control–fish and wildlife management coordination committee. *Proc. 16th Ann. Meet. Utah Mosq. Abatement Ass.* pp. 33-35.

Restrepo, A., Greer, D. L., Robledo, M., Diaz, C., Lopez, R. and Bravo, C. (1967). Subcutaneous phycomycosis: report of the first case observed in Colombia, South America. *Am. J. trop. Med. Hyg.* **16,** 34-39. *(Entomophthora coronata.)*

Reynolds, D. G. (1966). Infection of *Culex fatigans* with a microsporidian. *Nature, Lond.* **210,** 967. (Successful laboratory infections using *Plistophora culicis* derived from anophelines.)

Richards, J. G. and King, P. E. (1967). Chorion and vitelline membranes and their role in resorbing eggs of the *Hymenoptera. Nature, Lond.* **214,** 601-602. (Entomophagous parasites of Muscidae.)

Roberts, D. R., Smith, L. W., Jr. and Enns, W. R. (1967). Laboratory observations on predation activities of *Laccophilus* beetles on the immature stages of some dipterous pests found in Missouri oxidation lagoons. *Ann. ent. Soc. Am.* **60,** 908-910.

Roberts, D. W. (1967). Some effects of *Metarrhizium anisopliae* and its toxins on mosquito larvae. *In* "Insect Pathology and Microbial Control" (P.A. van der Laan, ed.) pp. 243-246. North-Holland Publ. Co. Amsterdam. (Müller-Kögler, 1967, recommends that this fungal species should be screened to assess its possible hazard to warm-blooded animals.)

Roberts, L. W. and Wilson, B. H. (1967). Predation on horse flies by two bembicine wasp species in certain areas of southern Louisiana. *J. econ. Ent.* **60,** 412-415.

Roshdy, M. A. (1963). Feulgen-Schiff's technique for examination of the distribution of intracellular *Rickettsia*-like micro-organisms in whole mounts of ticks, or their tissues. *Nature, Lond.* **199,** 827.

Rubtsov, I. A. (1963). On mermithids parasitizing simuliids. *Zool. Zh.* **42,** 1768-1784. (In Russian.) Also: Observations on mermithid nematodes parasitizing blackflies. *W.H.O. mimeogr. docum.,* WHO/EBL/19. (Average of 17% parasitism, ranging up to 99% in rivers of Leningrad area.)

Rubtsov, I. A. (1966a). Nematodes of the family Tetradonematidae, parasitizing members of the family Simuliidae (Diptera). *Helminthologia* **7,** 165-198.

Rubtsov, I. A. (1966b). Mermithids (Mermithidae) parasitizing black flies (Simuliidae). New species of the genus *Mesomermis* Dad. *In* "Novye Vidy fauny Sibiri i prilegajusich Regionov" (A. I. Cerepanov, ed.), pp. 109-147. *Izd. Nauka, Sib. Otd.,* Novosibirsk. (In Russian.)

Rubtsov, I. A. (1967a). Mermithidae (Nematoda), endoparasites of blackflies (Diptera: Simuliidae). II. New species of genus *Gastromermis* Micoletzky, 1923. *Acad. Nauk. U.S.S.R., Trudi Zool. Inst.* **43,** 59-92.

Rubtsov, I. A. (1967b). Natural enemies and methods of biological control of insects of medical importance. *Medicina, Moscow,* 120 pp. (In Russian.)

Santis, L. De (1965). Himenópteros parásitos de ootecas de cucarachas domesticas en la República Argentina. *Fitosanitarias* **4,** 8-10.

Sanders, D. P. and Dobson, R. C. (1966). The insect complex associated with bovine manure in Indiana. *Ann. ent. Soc. Am.* **59,** 955-959. (Biotic control of Muscidae.)

Sandner, H. (1966). Remarks on the possibility of biological control of sanitary pests in the temperate zone. *Mimeogr. docum.,* 8 pp., *1st Symp. Med. Vet. Acaroentomol.,* Gdomsk, Poland, Oct. 1966. (Polish Parasitological Society.)

Sasa, M., Kurihara, T., Dhamvanij, O. and Harinasuta, C. (1964). Observations on a mosquito-eating fish *(Lebistes reticulatus)* breeding in polluted waters in Bangkok. *W.H.O. mimeogr. docum.,* WHO/EBL/26.64, 22 pp. (Integrated control possibilities considered.)

Saunders, D. S. (1964). Rearing tsetse fly parasites in blowfly puparia. *Bull. Wld Hlth Org.* **31,** 509-510.

Schober, H. (1967). Observations on *Culex pipiens* larvae infested with *Vorticella* sp. *Mosquito News* **27,** 523-524.

Service, M. W. (1965a). Predators of the immature stages of *Aedes (Stegomyia) vittatus* (Bigot) (Diptera: Culicidae) in water-filled rock-pools in Northern Nigeria. *W.H.O. mimeogr. docum.,* WHO/EBL/33.65, 19 pp.

Service, M. W. (1965b). *Tachydromia* spp. (Diptera: Empidae) as predators of adult anopheline mosquitoes. *W.H.O. mimeogr. docum.,* WHO/EBL/34.65, 4 pp.

Shafti, R., Siddiqui, M. A. and Ahmed, Z. (1966). Studies on the bacterial isolates of the common mosquitoes of Pakistan. *Zentralbl. Bakt. Abt. I, Orig.* **199,** 514-521.

Shaikh, M. U. and Morrison, F. O. (1966). Susceptibility of nine insect species to infection by *Bacillus thuringiensis* var. *thuringiensis. J. Invertebrate Path.* **8,** 347-350.

Shamsuddin, M. (1966). A *Bathymermis* species (Mermithidae: Nematoda) parasitic on larval tabanids. *Quaestiones ent.* **2,** 253-256. (Parasite of larval *Chrysops* in Alberta.)

Shida, T. (1963). Prey list of *Vespula lewisi* Cameron in the suburbs of Tokyo. *Kontyû* **31,** 198-199. (In Japanese.) (Prey includes muscoid flies, tabanids and *Culex tritaeniorhynchus.*)

Shipitsina, N. K. (1963). Infection of blackflies (Simuliidae: Diptera) with parasites and its effect on the function of ovaries. *Zool. Zh.* **42,** 291-294. (In Russian.)

Shoemaker, W. E. (1964). A biological control for *Aedes sollicitans* and the resulting effect upon wildlife. *New Jers. Mosq. Exterm. Ass. Proc.* **51,** 93-97.

Simmonds, F. J. (1964). Mass production of insect parasites and predators. *Bull. Wld Hlth Org.* **31,** 511-512.

Singer, S., Goodman, N. S. and Rogoff, M. H. (1966). Defined media for the study of bacilli pathogenic to insects. *Ann. N.Y. Acad. Sci.* **139,** 16-23. (Culture of *Bacillus sphaericus* Neide, derived from a moribund larva of *Culiseta incidens.*)

Singh, P., King, W. E. and Rodriguez, J. G. (1966a). Biological control of muscids as influenced by host preference of *Macrocheles muscaedomesticae* (Acarina: Macrochelidae). *J. med. Ent.* **3,** 78-81.

Singh, P., King, W. E. and Rodriguez, J. G. (1966b). Biological control of muscids with *Macrocheles muscaedomesticae* (Macrochelidae: Acarina). *Proc. ent. Soc. Am., N. Cent. Brch* **20,** 79.

Smith, K. M. (1967). "Insect Virology", 256 pp. Academic Press, New York. (Material concerning mosquitoes included.)

Smith, W. W. (1966). Mermithid-induced intersexuality in *Culicoides stellifer* (Coquillett). *Mosquito News* **26,** 442-443.

Smith, W. W. and Perry, V. G. (1967). Intersexes in *Culicoides* spp. caused by mermithid parasitism in Florida. *J. econ. Ent.* **60,** 1025-1027.

Sol, R. (1963). Neuere Erkenntnisse über Eiablage und biotische Begrenzungsfaktoren bei der Brachfliege (*Phorbia coarctata* Fall.). *Mitt Biol. Bundesanst.* **108,** 163-166.

Sonleitner, F. J. (1964). The stress factor in insect colonies. *Bull. Wld Hlth Org.* **31,** 545-549.

Spiller, D. (1963). A difficulty in rearing *Rhodnius prolixus. N.Z. Ent.* **3,** 28-31.

Spiller, D. (1964). Bacterial status of a housefly rearing medium. *N.Z. Ent.* **3,** 33-38.

Srinivasun, M. C., Narasimhan, M. J. and Thirumalachar, M. J. (1964). Artificial culture of *Entomophthora muscae* and morphological aspects for differentiation of the genera *Entomophthora* and *Conidiobolus. Mycologia* **56,** 683-691.

Stejskal, M. (1965). Eine neue Gregarine, *Fusiona geusi* n.sp., n.gen., n.fam., n.superfam., aus der Südamerikanischen Schabe *Pycnoscelus surinamensis* L. 1758. *Z. f. Parasitenkunde* **26,** 215-220. (This South American cockroach is parasitized in Venezuela.)

Stephanides, T. (1964). Some further notes on the possible influence of the Hydra in mosquito larvae control. *Praktika Hellenic Hydrobiol. Inst. Acad. Athens* **9,** 3-7.

Stoffolano, J. G., Jr. and Nickle, W. R. (1966). Nematode parasite (*Heterotylenchus* sp.) of face fly in New York State. *J. econ. Ent.* **59,** 221-222.

Strawinski, K. (1964). Zoophagism of terrestrial *Hemiptera-Heteroptera* occurring in Poland. *Ekologia Polska,* Seria A **12,** 429-452. (Diet of *Empicoris culiciformis* (Deg.) includes adult mosquitoes.)

Suitor, E. C., Jr. (1964). The relationship of *Wolbachia persica* Suitor and Weiss to its host. *J. Insect Path.* **6,** 111-124.

Sychevskaya, V. I. (1963). Some Chalcidoidea reared from puparia of synanthropic flies in Uzbekistan. *Zool. Zh.* **42,** 858-864. (In Russian.)

Sychevskaya, V. I. (1964a). Hymenopterous parasites of synanthropic flies in Central Asia. *Ent. Obozr.* **43,** 391-404. (In Russian.)

Sychevskaya, V. I. (1964b). Mites found on synanthropic flies in Uzbekistan. *Med. Parazitol.* **33,** 557-560. (In Russian.)

Sychevskaya, V. I. (1966). The biology of *Brachymeria minuta* (L.) (Hymenoptera, Chalcidoidea), a parasitoid of synanthropic flies of the family Sarcophagidae (Diptera). *Ent. Obozr.* **45,** 752-762. (In Russian.) Also *W.H.O. mimeogr. docum.,* WHO/EBL/66.60, 3 pp.

Takahashi, F. and Pimental, D. (1967). Wasp preference for black-, brown-, and hybrid-type pupae of the house fly. *Ann. ent. Soc. Am.* **60,** 623-625.

Tamashiro, M. (1964). Observations on the larval ecology of *Aedes (Stegomyia) polynesiensis* Marks on Aitutaki, Southern Cook Islands. *W.H.O. mimeogr. docum.,* WHO/EBL/22, 29 pp. (No pathogens were found. The only potential larval predators, besides introduced fish, were dytiscid beetles and Odonata.)

Tavares, I. I. (1966). Structure and development of *Herpomyces stylopygae* (Laboulbeniales). *Am. J. Bot.* **53,** 311-318. (Cockroach parasite.)

Teernstra-Eeken, M. H. and Engel, A. (1967). Notes on entomophthorous fungi on Heleomyzidae and Culicidae (Diptera). *J. Invertebrate Path.* **9,** 431-432.

Thomas, V. (1966). A note on an egg parasite of *Megynenum subpurpurascens* West. (Pentatomidae: Rhynchota). *Med. J. Malaya* **20,** 335.

Turnbull, A. L. (1965). Effects of prey abundance on the development of the spider *Agelenopsis potteri* (Blackwall) (Araneae: Agelenidae). *Can. Ent.* **97,** 142-147. (*Aedes aegypti* as sole prey in laboratory feeding experiments.)

Turnbull, A. L. (1966). A population of spiders and their potential prey in an overgrazed pasture in eastern Ontario. *Can. J. Zool.* **44,** 557-583. (Prey includes muscoid flies, reduviid bugs, ceratopogonid midges, blackflies, horse flies and mosquitoes.)

Tuzet, O. and Ormières, R. (1964). *Stylocystis riouxi* n.sp. Grégarine parasite de *Dasyhelea lithotelmatica* Strenzke 1951 (Diptera: Ceratopogonidae). *Bull. Soc. Zool.* **89,** 163-166.

Tuzet, O. and Rioux, J. A. (1965). Les grégarines des Culicidae, Ceratopogonidae, Simuliidae et Psychodidae. *In* "Progress in Protozoology". *2nd Int. Conf. on Protozool.,* Lond. Aug. 1965. *Excerpta Medica International Congress Series No. 91,* 164, p. 150 (Abstract). Also full text as *W.H.O. mimeogr. docum.,* WHO/EBL/66.50, 18 pp.

Tuzet, O., Rioux, J. A. and Manier, J. F. (1964). La parasitisme fongique chez quelques nématocères vulnerants. *W.H.O. mimeogr. docum.,* WHO/EBL/25, 6 pp. Also *Proc. 1st Int. Congr. Parasit.,* Rome, 1964 **I,** 590-591.

Vago, C. (1964). Emploi des virus contre les insectes nuisibles et possibilités d'adaptation de cette méthode à la lutte contre les vecteurs de maladies. *Bull. Wld Hlth Org.* **31,** 513-517.

Vago, C. (1965). Viroses d'insectes à importance medicale. *Proc. XII. Int. Congr. Ent., Lond.,* July 1964, pp. 732-734.

Vago, C. (1966). Les problèmes de la lutte microbiologique contre les vecteurs de maladies vus à travès l'expérience agricole. *Proc. 1st Int. Congr. Parasit., Rome,* 21-26 Sept. 1964 **1,** 594-595.

Vávra, J. (1965). Recent contributions to the morphology and development of some Microsporidia. *In* "Progress in Protozoology", *2nd Int. Congr. Protozool.,* Lond., Aug. 1965. *Excerpta Med. Int. Congr. Ser., No. 91,* 59, pp. 66-67. (Cytological studies of microsporidians from larval chaoborines and blackflies, with clarification of the taxonomic status of *Caudospora simulii.)*

Velasquez, C. C. (1964). Observations on the life history of *Plagiorchis dilimanensis* sp.n. (Trematoda: Digenea). *J. Parasit.* **50,** 557-563.

Velthuis, H. H. W., Velthuis-Kluppell, F. M. and Bossink, G. A. H. (1965). Some aspects of the biology and population dynamics of *Nasonia vitripennis* Walker (Hymenoptera: Pteromalidae). *Ent. exp. appl.* **8,** 205-227.

Walker, I. (1967). Effect of population density on the viability and fecundity in *Nasonia vitripennis* Walker (Hymenoptera: Pteromalidae). *Ecology* **48,** 294-301.

Walker, I. and Pimental, D. (1966). Correlation between maternal longevity and incidence of diapause in *Nasonia vitripennis* Walker (Hymenoptera: Pteromalidae). *Gerontologia* **12,** 89-98.

Wallace, F. G. and Todd, S. R. (1964). *Leptomonas mirabilis* Roubaud 1908 in a Central American blowfly. *J. Protozool.* **11,** 502-505.

Wallwork, J. H. and Rodriguez, J. G. (1963). The effect of ammonia on the predation rate of *Macrocheles muscaedomesticae* (Acarina: Macrochelidae) on house fly eggs. *Adv. Acarology* **1,** 60-69.

Warhurst, D. C. (1963). The biology of *Endolimax blattae* Lucas, an endocommensal of cockroaches. *J. Protozool.* **10,** 28.

Warhurst, D. C. (1964). Appendix 2. A list of protozoa described from the hindgut of *Periplaneta americana, Blatta orientalis* and *Blattella germanica.* Ph.D. Thesis, Univ. Leicester, pp. 238-246.

Warhurst, D. C. (1966). A note on *Polymastix* Bütschli, 1884, from the colon of *Periplaneta americana* (Insecta: Dictyoptera). *Parasitology* **56,** 21-23.

Warhurst, D. C. (1967). Cultivation *in vitro* of *Endolimax blattae* Lucas, 1927 from the cockroach hind gut. *Parasitology* **57,** 181-186.

Weiser, J. (1963a). Diseases of insects of medical importance in Europe. *Bull. Wld Hlth Org.* **28,** 121-127.

Weiser, J. (1963b). Zur Kenntnis der Mikrosporidien aus Chironomiden-Larven III. *Zool. Anz.* **170,** 226-230.

Weiser, J. (1964a). Protozoonosen und Nematodenbefall bei Insekten. *Entomophaga, Mém. hors Sér.* No. 2, pp. 67-75.

Weiser, J. (1964b). Problèmes de controle biologique des insectes vecteurs. *Annls Parasit. hum. comp.* **39,** 211-219.

Weiser, J. (1964c). Parasitology of blackflies. *Bull. Wld Hlth Org.* **31,** 483-485.

Weiser, J. (1965a). Influence of environmental factors on protozoan diseases of insects. *XII Int. Congr. Ent., Lond.,* July 1964, p. 726.

Weiser, J. (1965b). A new virus infection of mosquito larvae. *Bull. Wld Hlth Org.* **33,** 586-588.

Weiser, J. (1966a). *Nemoci Hymzu.* Academia, CAV, Prague 1966, 554 pp.

Weiser, J. (1966b). Microbial pathogens of invertebrates. *Proc. 1st Int. Congr. Parasit.* Rome, 21-26 Sept. 1964 **1,** 589-590.

Weiser, J. and Batko, A. (1966). A new parasite of *Culex pipiens* L., *Entomophthora destruens* sp. nov. *(Phycomycetes, Entomophthoraceae). Folia Parasit.* **13,** 144-149.

Weiser, J. and Coluzzi, M. (1964). *Plistophora culisetae* n.sp., a new microsporidian (Protozoa Cnidosporidia) in the mosquito *Culiseta longiareolata* (Macquart, 1838). *Riv. Malariol.* **43,** 51-55.

Weiser, J. and Coluzzi, M. (1966). *Plistophora culisetae* in the mosquito *Culiseta longiareolata* Macqu.–further remarks. *Proc. 1st Int. Congr. Parasit.,* Rome, 21-26. Sept. 1964 **1,** 596-597.

Weiser, J. and Novak, D. (1963). Auftreten vom Mykosen bei Stechmücken. *Entomophaga, Mém. hors Sér.* No. 2, 149-150.

Welch, H. E. (1963). A survey of mermithid nematodes of blackflies. (Abstract). *Proc. 99th Ann. Mtg. Ent. Soc. Ontario,* p. 131.

Welch, H. E. (1964a). Mermithid parasites of blackflies. *Bull. Wld Hlth Org.* **31,** 857-863.

Welch, H. E. (1964b). *Romanomermis iyengari,* species nov. (Nematoda: Mermithidae, Braun, 1883). *Pilot Register of Zoology Card No. 4.*

Welch, H. E. (1965). Entomophilic nematodes. *Ann. Rev. Ent.* **10,** 275-302.

Welch, H. E. and Poinar, G. O. Jr. (1965). The role and use of nematodes in the regulation and control of insects of medical importance. *Proc. XII Int. Congr. Ent., Lond.,* July 1964, p. 732.

Welch, H. E. and Rubtsov, I. A. (1965). Mermithids (Nematoda: Mermithidae) parasitic in blackflies (Insecta: Simuliidae). I. Taxonomy and bionomics of *Gastromermis boophthorae* sp. nov. *Can. Ent.* **97,** 581-596.

White, E. B. and Legner, E. F. (1966). Notes on the life history of *Aleochara taeniata,* a staphylinid parasite of the housefly, *Musca domestica. Ann. ent. Soc. Am.* **59,** 573-577.

Whiting, A. R. (1967). The biology of the parasitic wasp *Mormoniella vitripennis =Nasonia brevicornis* (Walker). *Quart. Rev. Biol.* **42,** 333-406. (An exhaustive review, with a 7-page bibliography including much pertinent material not given herein.)

Whitsel, R. H. (1965). A new distribution record and an incidence of mermithid nematode parasitism for *Leptoconops kerteszi* Kieffer (Diptera: Ceratopogonidae). *Mosquito News* **25,** 66-67.

Whitsel, R. H. and Schoeppner, R. F. (1967). Parasitic trombidiid mites on *Dasyhelea mutabilis* (Coquillet) (Diptera: Ceratopogonidae). *Proc. ent. Soc. Wash.* **69,** 284-286.

Williams, P., Lewis, D. J. and Garnham, P. C. C. (1965). On dermal leishmaniasis in British Honduras. *Trans. R. Soc. trop. Med. Hyg.* **59,** 64-71. (Mites were occasionally present on sandflies and blackflies.)

Willis, R. R. and Axtell, R. C. (1967). Evaluation of *Fuscuropoda vegetans* (Acarina: Uropodidae) as a predator of the immature stages of the housefly. *J. Elisha Mitchell Sci. Soc.* **83,** 165.

Wills, W. and Beaudoin, R. (1965). Microsporidia in Pennsylvania mosquitoes. *J. Invertebrate Path.* **7,** 10-14.

Wilson, F. (1965). Biological control and the genetics of colonizing species. *In* "The

Genetics of Colonizing Species" (H. G. Baker and G. L. Stebbins, eds), pp. 307-329. Academic Press, New York. (Includes a section on *Gambusia affinis.*)

Wistreich, G. A. and Chao, J. (1963). Microorganisms from the midgut of larval and adult *Aedes aegypti* (Linnaeus). *J. Insect Path.* **5**, 56-60.

Woolever, P. S. (1966a). Life history and electron microscopy of a haplosporidian, *Nephridiophaga blattellae* (Crawley) (new combination) in the Malpighian tubules of the German cockroach, *Blattella germanica* (L.). *Diss. Abst.* **26**, 7514.

Woolever, P. S. (1966b). Life history and electron microscopy of a haplosporidian, *Nephridiophaga blattellae* (Crawley) (n. comb.), in the Malpighian tubules of the German cockroach, *Blattella germanica* (L.) *J. Protozool.* **13**, 622-642.

Wülker, W. (1963a). Parasitologische und biochemische Verwandtschaft in der Gattung *Chironomus* (Dipt.). *Naturwissenschaften* **50**, 49-50.

Wülker, W. (1963b). Prospects for biological control of pest Chironomidae in the Sudan. *W.H.O. mimeogr. docum.*, WHO/EBL/11, 23 pp.

Wülker, W. (1964). Parasite-induced changes of internal and external sex characters in insects. *Exp. Parasit.* **15**, 561-597.

Wülker, W. (1965). Der Mechanismus des Eindringens parasitärer mermithiden (Nematoda) in *Chironomus*-larven (Dipt., Chironomidae). *Z.f. Parasitenkunde* **26**, 29-49.

Wülker, W. (1966). Lähmung des Wirtes durch endoparasitäre Nematoden. *Umschau* **66**, 775. (Parasitization of chironomids.)

Wylie, H. G. (1963). Some effects of host age on parasitism by *Nasonia vitripennis* (Walk.) (Hymenoptera: Pteromalidae). *Can. Ent.* **95**, 881-886.

Wylie, H. G. (1965a). Discrimination between parasitized and unparasitized house fly pupae by females of *Nasonia vitripennis* (Walk.) (Hymenoptera: Pteromalidae). *Can. Ent.* **97**, 279-286.

Wylie, H. G. (1965b). Effects of superparasitism on *Nasonia vitripennis* (Walk.) (Hymenoptera: Pteromalidae). *Can. Ent.* **97**, 326-331.

Wylie, H. G. (1965c). Some factors that reduce the reproductive rate of *Nasonia vitripennis* (Walk.) at high adult population densities. *Can. Ent.* **97**, 970-977.

Wylie, H. G. (1966a). Some effects of female parasite size on reproduction of *Nasonia vitripennis* (Walk.) (Hymenoptera: Pteromalidae). *Can. Ent.* **98**, 196-198.

Wylie, H. G. (1966b). Survival and reproduction of *Nasonia vitripennis* (Walk.) at different host population densities. *Can. Ent.* **98**, 275-281.

Wylie, H. G. (1966c). Some mechanisms that affect the sex ratio of *Nasonia vitripennis* (Walk.) (Hymenoptera: Pteromalidae) reared from superparasitized housefly pupae. *Can. Ent.* **98**, 645-653.

Yasumatsu, K. and Watanabe, C. (Compilers) (1964-1965). "A Tentative Catalogue of Insect Natural Enemies of Injurious Insects in Japan. Parts 1-3", pp. vii + 1-166, vii + 1-116, and iv + 1-64. Ent. Lab. Fac. Agric., Kyushu Univ.

Yasuno, M. (1965). Ecological studies of *Culex (Lutzia) vorax,* with special reference to the dispersion pattern and the predatory behaviour. *Jap. J. Sanit. Zool.* **16**, 274-281. (In Japanese.)

Yendol, W. G. and Miller, E. M. (1967). Susceptibility of the face fly to commercial preparations of *Bacillus thuringiensis. J. econ. Ent.* **60**, 860-864.

Zaka-ur-Rab, M. (1963). Arachnoid parasites and predators of Insecta: a bibliography of literature. *Beitr. Ent.* **13**, 873-889.

Zaman, V., Fernando, C. H. and Chellappah, W. T. (1963). The agar gel-diffusion technique as a method of tracing mosquito antigens in the water bug *Anisops breddini* (Notonectidae). *Experientia* **19**, 106.

Zilton, A., Paula, L. A., Sherlock, I. and Cheever, A. (1967). Nasal granuloma caused by *Entomophthora coronata. Am. J. trop. Med. Hyg.* **16**, 31-33.

Acknowledgements

My thanks are due to numerous friends in many countries who brought to my attention earlier papers not cited by Jenkins (1964); to Miss Janet Marshall, Student Assistant, Memorial University of Newfoundland, and Miss Carolyn Farrow, formerly of WHO Headquarters, Geneva, for assistance in the preparation of the first draft; to Dr. Helen Sollers-Riedel, Assistant Editor, *Mosquito News,* for her kindness in checking the manuscript and advising me of omissions therein; and to the WHO, in the service of which I assembled much of the material now presented.

Author Index

Asterisks indicate pages at the end of chapters where References are listed

C

D

E

F

G

H

K

L

Q

R

X

Y

Subject Index

B

D

F

G

H

I

M

N

S